Aneurysmal Subarachnoid Hemorrhage

Aneurysmal Subarachnoid Hemorrhage

Report of the Cooperative Study

Edited by

Adolph L. Sahs
Donald W. Nibbelink
James C. Torner

Associate Editors

Harold P. Adams, Jr.
Pasquale A. Cancilla
Carl J. Graf
William G. Henderson
George E. Perret
John C. VanGilder

Urban & Schwarzenberg • Baltimore-Munich 1981

Urban & Schwarzenberg, Inc.
7 E. Redwood Street
Baltimore, Maryland 21202
USA

Urban & Schwarzenberg
Pettenkoferstrasse 18
D-8000 München 2
Germany

Printed in the United States of America

Library of Congress Cataloging in Publication Data

Aneurysmal subarachnoid hemorrhage.

  Continues: Intracranial aneurysms and subarachnoid
hemorrhage.
  Includes index.
  1. Intracranial aneurysms.
  2. Subarachnoid hemorrhage.
I. Sahs, Adolph L. [DNLM: 1. Cerebral aneurysms.
2. Subarachnoid hemorrhage. WL 200 A579]
RC693.A53   616.8'1   81–2354
ISBN 0–8067–1861–7   AACR2

ISBN 0-8067-1861-7 Baltimore

ISBN 3-541-71861-7 Munich

Contents

Authors

Harold P. Adams, Jr., M.D.
Department of Neurology
University of Iowa
Iowa City, Iowa

Pasquale A. Cancilla, M.D.
Department of Pathology
University of Iowa
Iowa City, Iowa

Carl J. Graf, M.D.
Division of Neurosurgery
Department of Surgery
University of Iowa
Iowa City, Iowa

William G. Henderson, M.P.H., Ph.D.
Biostatistics Division
Veterans Administration Hospital
Hines, Illinois

Donald W. Nibbelink, M.D., Ph.D.
Clinical Research Laboratories
Merck, Sharp & Dohme
West Point, Pennsylvania

George E. Perret, M.D., Ph.D.
Division of Neurosurgery
Department of Surgery
University of Iowa
Iowa City, Iowa

Adolph L. Sahs, M.D.
Department of Neurology
University of Iowa
Iowa City, Iowa

James C. Torner, M.S.
Department of Neurology
University of Iowa
Iowa City, Iowa

John C. VanGilder, M.D.
Division of Neurosurgery
Department of Surgery
University of Iowa
Iowa City, Iowa

Acknowledgments

The authors and participants in this study gratefully acknowledge the generous support and encouragement of the National Institute of Neurological Diseases and Blindness (now National Institute of Neurological and Communicative Disorders and Stroke). Without such assistance this cooperative institutional clinical study would not have been possible.

They are particularly indebted to the following for continuing interest, support and advice:

Murray Goldstein, D.O., M.P.H.
Deputy Director
National Institute of Neurological and Communicative Disorders and Stroke
Bethesda, Maryland

Elsa O. Keiles, Sc.D.
Chief, Special Programs, Extramural Programs
National Institute of Neurological and Communicative Disorders and Stroke
Bethesda, Maryland

Jean Benedict, M.S.
Stroke Program Coordinator, Stroke and Trauma Program
National Institute of Neurological and Communicative Disorders and Stroke
Bethesda, Maryland

The Central Registry also acknowledges the contributions of the following statistical consultants: David D. Rutstein, M.D., and Lloyd A. Knowler, Ph.D.

Data managers who assisted in the program at various intervals were: Reginald Yoder, Robert Ford, John Ashenbrenner, John Brumbach and Rick Pearson.

Four medical students who provided valuable assistance were: Donna Drees, Earl Kemp, Evan Reinders and Brian Vonk.

The following secretaries have contributed generously of their time and effort: Mrs. Hattie Jones, Mrs. Mildred Beem, Mrs. Louise Gustaffson, Mrs. Jean Radtke, Mrs. Donna Daniels, Miss Judy Davis, Miss Mary Sahs, Miss Marian Smith, Mrs. Victoria Barthelow, Miss Beatrice Martin, Mrs. Margaret Hayes, Miss Karalee White and Ms. Patricia Piper.

The authors and publisher gratefully acknowledge permission to republish material which has appeared through the following sources:

Chapter 2. This appeared as: Sahs, Adolph L.: Cooperative Study of Intracranial Aneurysms and Subarachnoid Hemorrhage. Report of a Randomized Treatment Study. I. Introduction. *Stroke* 5:550–551, 1974. Republished by permission of American Heart Association, Inc.

Chapter 3. Appeared as: Nibbelink, D.W., and Knowler, L.A.: Cooperative Study of Intracranial Aneurysms and Subarachnoid Hemorrhage. Report on a Randomized Treatment Study. II. Objectives and Design of Randomized Aneurysm Study. *Stroke* 5:552–556, 1974. Republished by permission of American Heart Association, Inc.

Chapter 4. Appeared as: Nibbelink, D.W., Torner, J.C., and Henderson, W.G.: Cooperative Study of Intracranial Aneurysms and Subarachnoid Hemorrhage—Report on a Randomized Treatment Study. IV–A. Regulated Bed Rest. *Stroke* 8:202–218, 1977.

Republished by permission of American Heart Association, Inc.

Chapter 5. Published as: Henderson, W.G., Torner, J.C., and Nibbelink, D.W.: Intracranial Aneurysms and Subarachnoid Hemorrhage—Report on a Randomized Treatment Study. IV–B. Regulated Bed Rest—Statistical Evaluation. *Stroke* 8:579–589, 1977. Republished by permission of American Heart Association, Inc.

Chapter 9. Published as: Graf, C.J., and Nibbelink, D.W.: Cooperative Study of Intracranial Aneurysms and Subarachnoid Hemorrhage. Report on a Randomized Treatment Study. III. Intracranial Surgery. *Stroke* 5:557–601, 1974. Republished by permission of American Heart Association, Inc.

Chapter 13. Appeared as: Nibbelink, D.W.: Considerations in the Treatment of Stroke. Cooperative Aneurysm Study: Antihypertensive and Antifibrinolytic Therapy Following Subarachnoid Hemorrhage from Ruptured Intracranial Aneurysm. In: Whisnant, J.P., and Sandok, B.A.: Cerebral Vascular Diseases. New York, Grune & Stratton, Inc., 1975, pp 155–165. Republished by permission of American Heart Association, Inc.

Chapter 14. Published as: Nibbelink, D.W., Torner, J.S., and Henderson, W.G.: Intracranial Aneurysms and Subarachnoid Hemorrhage. A Cooperative Study. Antifibrinolytic Therapy in Recent Onset Subarachnoid Hemorrhage. *Stroke* 6:622–629, 1975. Republished by permission of American Heart Association, Inc.

Chapter 16. This appeared as: Adams, H.P. Jr., Nibbelink, D.W., Torner, J.C., and Sahs, A.L.: Antifibrinolytic Therapy in Patients with Aneurysmal Subarachnoid Hemorrhage. A Report of the Cooperative Aneurysm Study. *Archives of Neurology* 38:25–29, 1981. Republished by permission of American Medical Association, copyright 1981.

Table of Organization

Central Registry

Members Who Have Participated

Harold P. Adams, Jr., M.D.*
Leon F. Burmeister, Ph.D.
Pasquale Cancilla, M.D.*
Carl J. Graf, M.D.*
William G. Henderson, M.P.H., Ph.D.
Neal Kassell, M.D.*
Andres Keichian, M.D.
Lloyd A. Knowler, Ph.D.
Paul Leaverton, Ph.D.
Herbert Locksley, M.D.

William F. McCormick, M.D.
Russell Meyers, M.D.
Donald W. Nibbelink, M.D., Ph.D.
Hiro Nishioka, M.D.
George Perret, M.D.*
Adolph L. Sahs, M.D.*
James Torner, M.S.*
M. W. Van Allen, M.D.*
John VanGilder, M.D.*

*Present Members

Advisory Committee and Special Consultants to the Central Registry

Richard G. Cornell, Ph.D.
Charles Drake, M.D.
William Fields, M.D.
Anthony P. Fletcher, M.D.
Ray Gifford, M.D.

Albert Heyman, M.D.
Walter M. Kirkendall, M.D.
Sean Mullan, M.D.
M. Dean Nefzger**

**Deceased 1974

Participating Investigators and Centers

Randomized Treatment Study

NIH Grant Number	Investigators	Centers
NB 04347	Mark L. Dyken, M.D. Robert L. Campbell, M.D.	Indiana University Medical Center, Indianapolis, Indiana
	Milton Ettinger, M.D.*	Minneapolis General Hospital, Minneapolis, Minnesota
NB 04373	Adolph L. Sahs, M.D. George E. Perret, M.D. Carl J. Graf, M.D. Herbert B. Locksley, M.D. Donald W. Nibbelink, M.D. Hiro Nishioka, M.D.* Lloyd A. Knowler, Ph.D.	University of Iowa, Iowa City, Iowa
	Mr. Wylie McKissock Mr. Lawrence Walsh Mr. Alan Richardson	Atkinson Morley's Hospital, London, England
	Paul Slosberg, M.D.*	Mt. Sinai Hospital of New York, New York, New York
NB 04345	Marshall B. Allen, Jr., M.D.	Medical College of Georgia, Augusta, Georgia
NB 04937	Albert Cook, M.D. Reza Khatib, M.D.	State University of New York, Downstate Medical Center, Brooklyn, New York
NB 04708	Hubert L. Rosomoff, M.D. Labe Scheinberg, M.D.	Albert Einstein College of Medicine, Bronx, New York
	Lars Leksell, M.D. R. Galera, M.D. Ladislau Steiner, M.D.	Karolinska Institute, Stockholm, Sweden
	Mr. Keith Bradley Mr. W. L. Elrick	University of Melbourne, Melbourne, Australia
NB 04343	Joseph Ransohoff, M.D. Clark Randt, M.D. Albert Goodgold, M.D.	New York University, New York, New York
	Erik Kågström, M.D. Nils Lundberg, M.D.	University of Lund, Lund, Sweden

NIH Grant Number	Investigators	Centers
NB 02413	Edwin B. Boldrey, M.D.	University of California Medical Center, San Francisco, California
NB 07135	Robert McLaurin, M.D. James Salmon, M.D.	University of Cincinnati, Cincinnati, Ohio
NB 07113	Orlando Andy, M.D. Robert R. Smith, M.D.	University of Mississippi Jackson, Mississippi

* Ceased participation during the study.

Antifibrinolytic and Later Studies

NIH Grant Number	Investigators	Centers
NS-09435-02	Guy O. Odom, M.D. Wesley A. Cook, Jr., M.D. Robert H. Wilkins, M.D.	Duke University Medical Center, Durham, North Carolina
NS-09437	Mark L. Dyken, M.D. Robert Campbell, M.D.	Indiana University Medical Center, Indianapolis, Indiana
NS-09431, NS-12456	Donald W. Nibbelink, M.D. Adolph L. Sahs, M.D. George E. Perret, M.D. Carl J. Graf, M.D. Andres Keichian, M.D. Harold Adams, M.D. Maurice Van Allen, M.D. John VanGilder, M.D. Neal Kassell, M.D. Pasquale Cancilla, M.D. Lloyd A. Knowler, Ph.D. Paul Leaverton, Ph.D. William G. Henderson, Ph.D. Leon F. Burmeister, Ph.D. James C. Torner, M.S. William F. McCormick, M.D.	University of Iowa Hospitals, Iowa City, Iowa
	Wylie McKissock, FRCS Lawrence S. Walsh, FRCS Alan E. Richardson, FRCS, MRCS David Uttley, FRCS, MBChB	Atkinson Morley's Hospital, London, England

NIH Grant Number	Investigators	Centers
NS-09432-02	Marshall B. Allen, Jr., M.D.	Medical College of Georgia, Augusta, Georgia
	Albert Cook, M.D. Reza Khatib, M.D.	State University of New York, Downstate Medical Center, Brooklyn, New York
NS-09439-01	Hubert L. Rosomoff, M.D. Labe Scheinberg, M.D. Kenneth Shulman, M.D.	Albert Einstein College of Medicine, Bronx, New York
	Lars Leksell, M.D. Rafael Galera, M.D. Ladislau Steiner, M.D.	Karolinska Institute, Stockholm, Sweden
	Keith Bradley, FRACS W. L. Elrick, FRCS	University of Melbourne, Alfred Hospital, Prahran, Victoria, Australia
NS-09433	Edwin B. Boldrey, M.D.	University of California Medical Center, San Francisco, California
NS-09438	Orlando Andy, M.D. Robert R. Smith, M.D.	University of Mississippi, Jackson, Mississippi
	John Riishede, M.D. Aage Harmsen, M.D.	University Hospital, Copenhagen, Denmark
	S. Peerless, M.D., FRCS	University of British Columbia, Vancouver, B.C., Canada University Hospital, London, Ontario, Canada
	Henry Troupp, M.D. Gunnar Af Björkesten, M.D.*	Neurosurgical Clinic, Helsinki, Finland
	J.W.F. Beks, M.D.	University Hospital, Groningen, Holland

*Deceased 1974

Foreword

The first monograph of the study on Intracranial Aneurysms and Subarachnoid Hemorrhage from the Central Registry at the University of Iowa is now known to all neurosurgeons as the Cooperative Study and has become a constant source of reference, particularly as to the natural history of these disorders. It was the first such in-depth study supported by the National Institutes of Health (NIH) of a major human disorder "seen too infrequently to permit individual or small groups of investigators to gain sufficient experience for statistically valid conclusions as to pathologic biology and the preferred therapy of the morbid condition of its variables." While recording the rather dismal results of surgical repair in that period, its most significant contribution was to focus attention on the importance and timing of disastrous rebleeding from cerebral aneurysm, as well as the additional calamity of progressive neurologic decline and high morbidity from major cerebral ischemia associated with arterial spasm.

The present volume continues this tradition of exploration, by randomized study for the most part, of the natural history of aneurysms and the results of conservative methods of preventing rebleeding. In addition, more detail is provided on the early results of carotid ligation and intracranial surgery. Most notably revealed is that antifibrinolysins, on current evidence, reduce the incidence of rebleeding by about 50%, which must be considered a real achievement in the alteration of the history of such a critical human disorder.

Although the results of treatment in the 1960's left much to be desired, through steady, continuing progress in neurosurgical technique, involving great effort and cost, it is becoming apparent that most aneurysms now can be obliterated safely regardless of site, size or complexity. Even so, this ability has had little impact on the whole aneurysm story. The reasons for this are multiple, but chiefly entail the failure to recognize the initial hemorrhage (about one third are missed initially and many more go unrecognized), a persistent rate of rebleeding around 10% in spite of antifibrinolytic therapy and blood pressure control, the cerebral ischemic syndrome associated with vasospasm, and other continuing medical complications with a much lower surgical morbidity.

This volume should point the way to the 1980's, providing a program of education for the public and physicians to recognize the initial onset of the disorder and a relentless attack on rebleeding and vasospasm.

The first issue to be addressed will be the timing of surgery in a multicentered study which has now been funded by the NIH as the first study of the Central Registry in Iowa in the 1980's. Although early surgery in the 1950's and 60's proved to have too high a morbidity, it must be looked at again in the light of modern neuroanaesthesia and microneurosurgery. Although sure to prevent most rebleeding, its new safety must be shown, as well as its effect on the ischemic syndrome, salutary or otherwise, perhaps based on the CT scan.

Unquestionably, other avenues will appear for exploration, and with NIH support, the Iowa group should remain in the forefront of a scientific approach to answers, utilizing randomized control studies from multiple centers.

October, 1980

CHARLES G. DRAKE, M.D.

Preface

In the United States the yearly incidence of all types of stroke has been recorded as approximately 500,000 and the death rate about 200,000. Statistics on the incidence of subarachnoid hemorrhage vary considerably. For example, Kurtzke[1] indicated at one time that subarachnoid hemorrhage comprised some 12% of cerebrovascular disease cases. This would have placed the annual figure at approximately 60,000 cases. In a later report, Kurtzke[2] wrote that the weighted averages would indicate that some 8% of the incident strokes are subarachnoid hemorrhage. Thus, if the incidence of stroke is 200, then for subarachnoid hemorrhage the incidence should be near 16 per 100,000 population per year. This is higher than the figures cited by Garraway et al.[3] in the Rochester study indicating approximately 11 per 100,000. One should note that although other types of stroke appear to be declining, subarachnoid hemorrhage apparently is not following that pattern.

The members of the Central Registry have used a figure of 80% to apply to those cases of nontraumatic hemorrhage caused by ruptured aneurysms. The remaining cases are due to ruptured arteriovenous malformations, bleeding diatheses, tumors and "cause undetermined." The figure of 26,000 has been used by us as the yearly incidence of aneurysmal subarachnoid hemorrhage in the United States. This number is higher than the 20,000 figure cited by Sypert,[4] who also indicated that in the United States there are an estimated 400,000 adults who are harboring unruptured cerebral aneurysms, and every year 5% of these people will undergo a major neurologic catastrophe.

Careful postmortem studies showed aneurysms in 8.0% of the specimens from an autopsied population one year of age and older. Ruptures had occurred in 40% of this series. One fourth of these people had more than one aneurysm.[5]

The bright part of this picture relates to: (1) the remarkable progress made in the diagnosis of these lesions, in that cerebral angiography and computed axial tomography have provided clinical diagnostic accuracy unheard of one generation ago, and (2) the spectacular progress which has been made in surgical treatment. Numerous publications call attention to the advances made possible by microscopy, superior anesthesia, controlled hypotension and improved general care, including monitoring. Yet, satisfaction with advances in the treatment of aneurysmal subarachnoid hemorrhage can be realized only when improved survival rates can be shown in *all* cases of aneurysm, regardless of the therapy employed. Statistics on intracranial aneurysms often emanate from tertiary referral centers where the processes of attrition and careful selection have eliminated a large number of poor-risk and desperately ill patients. Thus, of the 26,000 cases of aneurysmal subarachnoid hemorrhage yearly, approximately one third can expect to reach the status of "good-result" surgery. The others die acutely at home or at work, while others deteriorate and die in a local hospital. Still others survive long enough to reach a referral center, only to expire there. A certain number are too ill for surgery, have complicating diseases, or refuse operation. The profession cannot disregard this large group. Many of the interests and activities of the Central Registry and participating centers have been directed toward the medical aspects of care of the patient with subarachnoid hemorrhage.

On the gloomy side, one encounters such items as: failure to identify the warning aneurysmal leak,[6] rapid deterioration of some patients so that surgery is impossible and development of vascular spasm and other complications which delay or prevent surgery.

The members of the Central Registry and others hope that the information contained in the following reports will serve as a baseline with which to compare the progress that is certain to take place in this field during the decade of the 80's.

February, 1981

ADOLPH L. SAHS, M.D.

References

1. Kurtzke, J.F.: Epidemiology of Cerebrovascular Disease. Springer-Verlag, New York, 1969, p 117.
2. Kurtzke, J.F.: Epidemiology of Cerebrovascular Disease. Joint Council C.V.D. Survey Report, Whiting Press, Inc., Rochester, Minn., 1980, p. 157.
3. Garraway, W.M., Whisnant, J.P., Furlan, A.J. et al.: The declining incidence of stroke. N Eng J Med 300: 449–452, 1979.
4. Sypert, G.W.: Intracranial aneurysms: Natural history and surgical management. Compr Ther 4: 64–73, (May) 1978.
5. McCormick, W.F.: The natural history of intracranial saccular aneurysms. Weekly Update, Neurology and Neurosurgery 1: No. 3, 1–8, 1978.
6. Adams, H.P. Jr, Jergenson, D.D., Kassell, N.F., Sahs, A.L.: Pitfalls in the recognition of subarachnoid hemorrhage. JAMA 244: 794–796, 1980.

Section I

Historical Background

Chapter 1

History of the Cooperative Aneurysm Study and Central Registry

Adolph L. Sahs, M.D.

Introduction

In 1951, Dr. Lester Mount[1] assembled a group of 752 cases of subarachnoid hemorrhage from the literature and from the cases at the Neurological Institute of New York. In this group of conservatively treated patients, the mortality rate was 48%. In the series of 469 cases treated surgically, there was a mortality of 14%. It was obvious to Dr. Mount that the two series were not matching, and that a cooperative study would be useful to provide statistically valid conclusions. A protocol was constructed and all board-certified neurosurgeons were contacted at that time. However, the project was not implemented, mainly because of lack of funds.

In 1956, Dr. A. E. Walker requested that the National Institute of Neurological Diseases and Blindness (NINDB), as it was designated at that time, call a meeting of physicians interested in subarachnoid hemorrhage. The writer attended the meeting in Bethesda, Maryland, and expressed interest in pursuing the matter further. Following negotiations which were carried out between the Department of Neurology of the University of Iowa College of Medicine and Drs. Pearce Bailey and Gordon Seger,

the Cooperative Aneurysm Study evolved. By May 1957, a Central Registry was established at the University of Iowa. Dr. R. A. Utterback devoted much time and effort toward the development of the Central Registry. After many months of planning and negotiations with various centers, together with the unstinting support of the NINDB, 19 participating centers were enrolled and began to forward completed protocols. The group included 18 institutions from the United States and one from Europe (Dr. McKissock's service at Atkinson Morley's Hospital in London).[2]

Phase I: Nonrandomized Project

This initial phase was essentially a data-collecting effort. A total of 6,368 protocols was received in the ensuing eight years. Intracranial aneurysms numbered 3,265 in this series, arteriovenous malformations 507, and 56 had both conditions. The available statistics on July 28, 1965, at the conclusion of the study, indicated that the gross survival

3

rate was 54% (death rate 46%). All patients were hospitalized at major medical centers with neurologic and neurosurgical expertise. At that time, we also processed a series of 2,540 cases of intracerebral hemorrhage and miscellaneous nontraumatic conditions.

A series of publications emanated from the Central Registry, beginning with a short report by Locksley[3] in 1961, which was published in *Neurology*. In 1965, Sahs[4] contributed a chapter to the monograph on *Intracranial Aneurysms and Subarachnoid Hemorrhage,* edited by Fields and Sahs. In the next year, the group at the Central Registry published a series of reports[5-18] in the *Journal of Neurosurgery*. This series was collected into monograph form, *Intracranial Aneurysms and Subarachnoid Hemorrhage*[2] (published in 1969), and has been quoted widely as representing the "natural history" of the disease as it appears in referral centers. For example, Stehbens[19] has made numerous references to the Cooperative Study in his book entitled *Pathology of the Cerebral Blood Vessels,* published in 1972.

A capsule account of Phase I can be found in Nibbelink's[20] report of the Cooperative Study under the heading of "A. Nonrandomized Project."

Comments on Phase I:

Many lessons were learned during this data-collection period:

1. This study gave all participants considerable experience in conducting a cooperative study. This information comprised the background for a presidential address before the American Neurological Association in 1968.[21] A critique on the advantages and pitfalls of cooperative studies was discussed at that time.
2. An objection was raised that since London was such a heavy contributor, we were biasing the study by including such a large number of patients from Atkinson Morley's Hospital.
3. The risk of rebleeding at the end of the first week was illustrated graphically.
4. The need for randomization of selected treatments became more evident, particularly when it was pointed out that surgical therapy was accumulating a morbidity figure of 53% and a mortality rate of 46%.
5. The participants became convinced that the clinical condition of the patient, especially his state of consciousness, was the important prognostic factor.
6. The selection process of good-risk patients was all important in the surgical management of this condition, but what should be done with the seriously ill, poor-risk patients?
7. A good working relationship was established among the neurologists and neurosurgeons in the group. The free exchange of ideas proved mutually beneficial.

Phase II: Randomized Treatment Study

Plans were developed over a period of several years and interested participants were enrolled. This study was designated Phase II, and there was temporal overlap with Phase I. In essence, the Central Registry was collecting data from two programs concurrently for a period of time (Table 1–1). A group of 10 centers proceeded with the proposed format and began to submit protocols to the Central Registry on June 15, 1963. This program continued until February 1, 1970, but follow-up evaluations in some patients were maintained over a 9.5-year period. The four treatment types were: regulated bed rest, drug-induced hypotension with regulated bed rest, carotid ligation and intracranial surgery. A total of 1,665 protocols was available, from which 660 were excluded for a variety of reasons. The remaining 1,005 cases were allocated randomly among the four treatment categories. An additional 33 cases were disqualified after allocation of treatment, leaving a total of 972 for detailed analysis of comparative treatments.

Category	Designation	Years	No. of Protocols Received	References
Phase I	Nonrandomized Data Collection Study	1957–1965	6,368	Sahs, Perret, Locksley, et al[2]
Phase II	Randomized Treatment Study	1963–1970	1,665	Sahs;[22] Nibbelink, Knowler;[23] Graf, Nibbelink;[24] Nibbelink, Torner, Henderson[29] Nibbelink, Torner, Henderson (Chapter 6); Perret, Nibbelink (Chapter 8)
Phase III	Drug-Induced Hypotension and Antifibrinolytic Therapy	1970–1972	242	Nibbelink, Sahs;[33] Nibbelink[34] Nibbelink (Chapter 13)
Phase IV	Antifibrinolytic Therapy	1972–1974	502	Nibbelink, Torner, Henderson[48] Nibbelink, Torner, Henderson (Chapter 14)
Phase V	Antifibrinolytic Therapy Plus Modest Fluid Restriction	1974–1977	601	Nibbelink, Torner, Burmeister (Chapter 15)
Phase VI	Seriously Ill Patients: Treatment by Reduction of Intracranial Pressure. Pilot Study	1977–1979	63	VanGilder, Torner, (Chapter 18)
Phase VII	Timing of Surgery	1980–		Kassell, et al (In Preparation)

One of the controversial sections in this study involved the allocation of patients to the surgical category. The mere fact that a patient was allocated randomly to a treatment did not necessarily mean that such treatment was *actually* carried out on that particular patient. For example, a patient assigned to intracranial surgery might not have had an operation because the surgeon deemed the lesion inoperable.

The first reports on Phase II began to appear in print in 1974: an introduction,[22] design of the program[23] and the results of intracranial surgery.[24] We were dealing with a pool of 972 cases, as indicated previously, and eventually received the majority of our cases from 14 centers, 10 of which were in the United States and 4 were elsewhere. The largest contributor, again, was Atkinson Morley's Hospital in London. Two hundred sixty-eight patients with a single aneurysm located on the anterior portion of the circle of Willis were allocated randomly to intracranial surgery. Thirty died before surgery could be accomplished and 10 were considered unsuitable for intracranial operation. Among 40 in whom treatment was not accomplished (surgery not performed), but who were allocated to surgery, 32 (80%) died. Intracranial operative treatment was accomplished in 228 patients. The technical approach of the operation remained entirely with the individual surgeon. The average overall mortality was 36.8% over a 9.5-year period, distributed as follows: anterior communicating, 34.2%; middle cerebral, 35.3%; internal carotid, 46.7%. The overall mortality in patients operated upon within 14 days from the last bleed was 44.5%; for those operated upon beyond the 14-day interval, it was 23.2%. Thus, there was a conspicuous drop in mortality from operations performed at the end of the 14-day period. In patients whose medical condition was appraised on the day of surgery, 31.1% died who were in good condition, 40.8% in fair condition and 64.7% in poor condition. In this group of 228 operations, there were 19 examples (8.3%) of proved or suspected rebleeding episodes following surgery (5 days to 4 years), with 16 deaths.

Release of this information on surgical therapy created consternation and disbelief. One should remember that we were covering the period from 1963 to 1970, and that some patients were actually not operated upon, but were charged to surgery because of the randomization techniques employed. However, these figures are not too far removed from the statistics presented by Klafta and Hamby,[25] and by Paul and Arnold.[26] One should note, however, that the figures just cited do not approach the lower figures reported by Pool[27] (7% for all grades of risk among 56 anterior communicating artery patients) and Krayenbühl et al.[28] (5%) in 1972.

In our Phase II (Randomized) Study,[29] bed rest continued to fare badly. A group of 124 patients was assigned randomly to treatment within 7 days of the bleed, 49 between 8 and 21 days, and 14 between 22 and 92 days. During the mean follow-up interval of 6.5 years, the mortality was 55.1%. A total of 47.1% died of causes attributed directly to the cerebral effects of the ruptured aneurysm.

The results of two other treatments are being reported in this monograph. Chapters 6 and 7 contain information on drug-induced hypotension. Of the 309 patients allocated to drug-induced hypotension, 143 (46.3%) died during a mean period of 6.5 years following three weeks of antihypertensive treatment.

The results from carotid ligation are reported in Chapter 8. In the entire group of 187 patients assigned to this form of therapy, there was a death rate of 39.6%. One should note, however, that 62 patients could not undergo carotid ligation for various reasons.

The long-term follow-up evaluation is reported in Chapter 10. The cumulative mortality rates showed that over a five-year period carotid ligation patients fared best, while patients treated by bed rest did very poorly.

A preliminary report of the results of Phase II can be found in Nibbelink's[20] report under "B. Randomized Treatment Study (Phase II)."

Phase III: Randomized Treatment Study With Drug-induced Hypotension and Antifibrinolytic Treatment

The rationale for this and most of the subsequent aspects of our program was succinctly recorded by Drake[30] independently in 1968: "It is probably true that if we could learn how to keep a patient safe from rebleeding for a week, or longer, in obtunded patients with cerebral symptoms, the problem of surgery of ruptured intracranial aneurysms would nearly be solved." The present state of the art is summarized, again by Drake,[31] as follows: "There can be no question now in experienced hands utilizing modern resources, most aneurysms can be dealt with safely (mortality and disabling morbidity less than 5%) provided the patient reaches the good operative risk period in good condition. This is now true, as well, for aneurysms on the basilar vertebral circulation."

The participants in the Cooperative Study became interested in the possible use of antifibrinolytic agents after noting the encouraging report by Mullan and Dawley.[32] The Cooperative Aneurysm Group agreed to study the effect of antifibrinolytic therapy during the period immediately following a subarachnoid hemorrhage from ruptured intracranial aneurysm. As a result, Phase III was inaugurated.[33] Among 242 patients randomized between three treatment programs, 28.9% of patients allocated to drug-induced hypotension died within 14 days following the hemorrhage; 5.8% of those allocated to antifibrinolytic therapy died during this period; and 23.8% of those who received the combined program of drug-induced hypotension *and* antifibrinolytic therapy expired.

Controversy surrounded, and still surrounds, the use of this drug for the prevention of rebleeding during the period immediately following rupture of a saccular aneurysm. One of the most spirited discussions took place at the Princeton Conference in 1974, following Dr. Nibbelink's presentation.[34] At that time, Girvin[35] made the statement that in his experience the advantages claimed for epsilon-aminocaproic acid (EACA) could not be substantiated. In the summary of the Ninth Princeton Conference, Dr. C. H. Millikan[36] indicated skepticism that the mortality from subarachnoid hemorrhage could be reduced to 5% by the use of epsilon-aminocaproic acid.

It was shown later by us that the 5.8% death rate listed in the preliminary report was indeed low, and with the initiation of Phase IV and a more extensive input of cases, the mortality figure in the first two weeks became 11.6%, where it tended to remain. The best available figures which we can use for comparison are those from regulated bed rest statistics from our Phase II study showing a 21.1% mortality in a two-week period (27 of 128 patients). The data indicated a reduction in mortality of approximately 50% through the use of an antifibrinolytic agent during this critical period.

The following questions then arise: (1) Is the reduction in mortality the result of antifibrinolytic therapy, better patient care, or possibly the antihypertensive/dehydrating effect of the drug? (2) What are the possible toxic reactions of antifibrinolytic drugs? (3) Can the drug be used with equal effectiveness by all physicians? If not, why do the negative reports continue to appear?

Rationale of Antifibrinolytic Therapy

Aminocaproic acid is similar to lysine, except that it lacks an alpha-amino group. As early as 1959, Alkjaersig et al.[37] showed that aminocaproic acid acts mainly as a competitive inhibitor of plasminogen activity. In higher concentrations this substance is said to be a noncompetitive inhibitor of plasmin and other enzymes such as trypsin and pepsin. Aminocaproic acid does not appear to have anticoagulant action when used in therapeutic concentrations.[38]

Aminocaproic acid is rapidly absorbed from the gastrointestinal tract, and peak levels are found two hours after a single dose.[39] The absorption, distribution and excretion of epsilon aminocaproic acid following its oral or intravenous administration to man was studied. Clearance is mainly through the kidney, and a large portion of a single dose is excreted within 12 hours. For this reason, the continuous intravenous infusion route is preferable.

Tovi and colleagues[40-44] published a series of basic and clinical observations on this subject. Most authors are now agreed that the antifibrinolytic drug enters the subarachnoid space after a subarachnoid hemorrhage, and that fibrinolysis is thereby inhibited.

Supportive Publications

Reports which support the use of antifibrinolytic therapy for subarachnoid hemorrhage are numerous. The publications emanating from the Cooperative Aneurysm Study are as follows: Nibbelink and Sahs;[33] Nibbelink;[34,45] Nibbelink and Jacobsen;[46] Nibbelink, Sahs and Knowler;[47] Nibbelink, Torner and Henderson.[48] Section III of this book contains additional information generated by the Cooperative Aneurysm Study on the use of antifibrinolytic agents. As indicated previously, the stimulus for this study arose from the report of Mullan and Dawley.[32] In that series of 35 patients treated with EACA, 3 died of progressive deterioration, 1 died of rebleeding on the 25th day, and 1 rebled but did not die on the 7th day. In the second report by Mullan,[49] encompassing 117 patients, there were 31 deaths under drug management, which included a combination of antifibrinolytic and antihypertensive treatment. Our Phase III study[33,34] indicated that 23.8% of patients who received a combined antifibrinolytic-antihypertensive program died.

It is difficult to analyze many of the reports because of selection factors, dosages of medication and length of therapy, but some of the recent reports appear important. Ransohoff et al.[50] treated 50 nonconsecutive patients in preliminary fashion with EACA and antihypertensive measures, with 12 instances of rebleeding (24%); in a subsequent series of 50 patients there were 6 instances of rebleeding, 5 of them fatal.

Smith and Upchurch[51] treated 21 patients with ruptured intracranial aneurysms. One rebled during the acute treatment period. They suggested frequent measurement of the fibrinolytic activity in patients receiving antifibrinolytic drugs. Sengupta et al.[52] reported on the use of EACA in 66 patients. There was no recurrent hemorrhage in the EACA-treated group, while 17 in the control group rebled. Tovi[53] treated 32 patients with tranexamic acid. No rebleeding occurred during the first week. Hemorrhage occurred in 2 patients during the second week of treatment. Corkhill[54] reported that of 20 consecutive cases arriving at one center from all parts of Tasmania, there were no recurrent hemorrhages within a period of six weeks or more after the presenting hemorrhage. All had surgery. Two patients died, the first from pulmonary embolism three weeks after operation, and the second patient died three weeks after operation following rupture of his middle cerebral aneurysm during release of the clip applicator. Chowdhary et al.[55] had excellent results from the use of epsilon-aminocaproic acid.

Negative Reports

The report by Girvin[35] has been mentioned above. Another negative report by Girvin is available.[56] Others have emerged, including those by Gibbs and O'Gorman,[57] and Profeta et al.[58]

Wintzen and Van Rossum[59] challenged the publication by Chowdhary et al., and pointed to their previous report[60] on the failure of tranexamic acid to favorably affect the outcome. Similarly, Kaste and Ramsay[61] issued a negative report on the value of tranexamic acid. In a recent review by Ramirez-Lassepas he questioned the efficacy of antifibrinolytic therapy (see Reference 21a, Chapter 16).

Concerns

Most of the concerns about the use of antifibrinolytic drugs after subarachnoid hemorrhage are directed toward: (1) drug toxicity; (2) intracranial vascular spasm; (3) intracerebral thrombosis, venous thrombosis and pulmonary embolism; and (4) hydrocephalus caused by adhesive arachnoiditis.

Drug Toxicity

The potential dangers of this drug have been recognized since the utilization of epsilon-aminocaproic acid in hemorrhagic states.[62-67] Rhabdomyolysis during treatment with epsilon-aminocaproic acid has been reported.[68-70] On the other hand, Nilsson et al.[71] had extensive experience with the use of the drug and reported a minimal number of complications. After five years' experience with EACA in over 700 cases of various hemorrhagic disorders, the authors concluded that EACA could not be regarded as a significant thrombotic agent.

Intracranial Vascular Spasm

This is a very controversial subject because the parameters used to define vascular spasm after subarachnoid hemorrhage are still poorly defined. The report by Nibbelink et al.[47] indicated that of the 242 patients studied, 36% had vasospasm. There were no unusual trends in respect to cerebrovascular spasm so far as the antifibrinolytic-treated group was concerned.

Arteriopathic Complications: Intracranial Thrombosis, Venous Thrombosis, Pulmonary Embolism

A cautiously negative report originated from Kagström and Palma.[72] Sonntag and Stein[73] reported on 3 patients out of 7 receiving antifibrinolytic therapy who developed arteriopathic complications. Hood[74] questioned these observations, and attributed the changes to spasm.

Norlen and Thulin[75] reported 1 death in 14 patients receiving EACA therapy. The cause of death was bilateral thrombosis of the anterior cerebral arteries 10 days after surgery. Herring[76,77] cited Smith as indicating that in the series of 92 patients receiving EACA, pulmonary emboli occurred at a frequency of two to three times the expected rate. Mortality occurred in 4 of the 6 patients who developed emboli. Six patients developed uremia; 2 of these required renal dialysis. Major peripheral arterial occlusion occurred in 2 patients. There were no myocardial infarctions. Myocardial infarction plus pulmonary embolism was reported by Farina et al.[78]

Hydrocephalus

Hydrocephalus was not a significant factor in the report submitted by Herring,[76] citing Smith. However, Park[79] has recently raised the question of the role of EACA in the production of communicating hydrocephalus.

Phase IV: Analysis of Additional Patients Treated With Antifibrinolytic Medication (Nonrandomized)

In this cooperative study among 13 institutions, 502 patients were treated with epsilon-aminocaproic acid or tranexamic acid.[48] Thirty-one protocols were disqualified, leaving 471 eligible cases. The mortality at the end of 14 days was 11.6%, and the proved rebleed rate was 12.7%. Comparison of the mortality and rebleed rates between this group and the group of patients allocated to regulated bed rest within 7 days[29] reveals the rates to be decreased by one-half among patients treated with antifibrinolytic therapy.

An effort was made to record all the complications of this medication. The most frequent drug-related complication was diarrhea in 24.3% of the patients, but in only 2.4% was this severe. Hemiparesis was reported in 17% and hemiplegia in 11.2%. Particular attention was directed to certain hematologic factors such as clotting derangements, bleeding time abnormalities, evaluation of certain coagulation disorders and the occurrence of pulmonary embolism. So-called clotting derangements were reported in 3 patients; one had an elevated partial thromboplastin time of 88 sec (with a control of 37), another had a prothrombin time of 8 sec (with a control of 12) and in the third patient no information was specified. Coagulation factor abnormalities were classified as minor in 2 patients. These were manifested in one patient as a mild gastrointestinal hemorrhage; the other had marked increase in serum fibrinogen and platelet count without clinical manifestations. Two patients developed pulmonary emboli. One was subclinical, i.e., the pathological report described multiple small lung emboli, and in the other patient cardiorespiratory difficulties alerted the attending physician to this diagnosis. The condition was confirmed by a radioactive lung scan. Both of these patients were poorly responsive as a result of the intracranial event, and one was excessively obese as well.

The 16.8% incidence of ischemic neurologic deficit, the 17% occurrence of hemiparesis and the 11% incidence of hemiplegia warranted careful attention. A perusal of the literature of the 1960's indicates an exceedingly high incidence of intracranial infarction in those patients dying of ruptured aneurysms. This unusually high occurrence has been documented by Schneck (55% of 105 cases),[80] Schneck and Kricheff[81] and Crompton (75% of 159 cases).[82]

A short review of Phase IV can be found in Nibbelink's[20] section of the 1976 edition of the Cerebrovascular Survey Report.

Phase V: Antifibrinolytic Therapy Plus Modest Fluid Restriction (Randomized Study)

Between 1974 and 1977, the protocols of 601 patients were received as in accordance with a modification of the treatment pattern. These patients were randomized into three treatment categories: (1) antifibrinolytic therapy with fluid restriction, (2) antifibrinolytic therapy without fluid restriction and (3) glycerol with fluid restriction. Seventy-five patients did not satisfy eligibility criteria. The glycerol-with-fluid-restriction group suffered a higher than expected rebleed rate, and patient entry was suspended after 16 months. Fourteen-day mortality for the 245 patients in the non-fluid-restricted group was 10.6% and 9.4% for the 266 in the fluid-restricted group. Rebleeding during the same period was 8.2% and 9.4%, respectively. A significant change in neurologic status was demonstrated in patients in the fluid-restricted category. The results suggested that lowering the fluid input resulted in a slightly lower death rate but increased the risk of recurrent hemorrhage.

A detailed report by Nibbelink, Torner and Burmeister can be found in Chapter 15 of this book.

Phase VI: Seriously Ill Patients— Treatment by Reduction of Increased Intracranial Pressure

Introduction

Increased knowledge of cerebral physiology, medical therapy and improved surgical technique for the management of subarachnoid hemorrhage secondary to ruptured intracranial aneurysms have improved the prognosis of this entity. However, there remains a population of patients with significant neurologic deficits and decreased levels of consciousness following ruptured intracranial aneurysm who have a poor prognosis. The purpose of the pilot study was to investigate the significance of increased intracranial pressure in patients with poor neurologic condition and to evaluate the effectiveness of treatment.

Background and Rationale

Poor neurologic condition is one of the major risk factors which determines survival. The patient at risk is dependent partially on the elapsed time after subarachnoid hemorrhage. One day following the initial ictus, 44.7% of patients with subarachnoid hemorrhage attributed to ruptured intracranial aneurysms are seriously ill or moribund.[2] At the time of first angiography, 22.1% are responsive only to noxious stimuli or are unresponsive. The natural history of this population at one year is a predicted survival rate of 25 to 29%.[2] Similarly, surgical intervention in this population has been unrewarding. The mortality in patients with disturbance of consciousness but responding, unresponsive or moribund on the day of intracranial surgery for the treatment of aneurysms is 55.1%.[18] Delay of surgical intracranial intervention significantly decreases the operative mortality and morbidity when patients are allowed to achieve a good neurologic condition.[18,24,83]

The use of antifibrinolytic medication has significantly reduced the incidence of rebleeding during the initial two weeks following rupture of an intracranial aneurysm.

Several studies have suggested that the majority of patients with significant neurologic deficit and altered levels of consciousness have associated increased intracranial pressure.[25,84–88] Increased intracranial pressure is a result of either cerebral edema, hydrocephalus, intracerebral and intraventricular hemorrhage, infarction, increased intracerebral blood volume and/or a combination of these factors. The subsequent neurologic status and intracranial pressure measurements are determined by volume and site of extravasated blood, the vasomotor reaction and intracranial compensatory pressure buffering capacity. Cerebral blood flow, cerebral perfusion pressure, cerebral edema, cerebral metabolic rate of oxygen utilization and amount of PCO_2 accumulation are the prime factors requiring control for optimum neurologic function.

Objectives of the Study

1. To determine if increased intracranial pressure is a common denominator in patients with poor neurologic condition following a ruptured intracranial aneurysm.
2. To determine if reduction of increased intracranial pressure will lower the morbidity and mortality in patients in poor neurologic condition following subarachnoid hemorrhage from a ruptured aneurysm when compared to present levels using epsilon-aminocaproic acid and dexamethasone as a standard.

Results

Patient Population Characteristics

From May 1977 to October 1978, 63 patients entered the study from 10 participating institutions. The majority had aneurysms located on the internal carotid or anterior cerebral-anterior communicating arteries. Forty-three patients (68% of 63) were female and 37 patients (59% of 63) were less than 50 years of age. Vasospasm present on cerebral angiography was reported in 30 patients (48% of 63). Of these, 18 had localized vasospasm (segmental or involving individual vessels) and 12 had diffuse vasospasm (narrowed main ipsilateral vessels or all major vessels). Neurologic status at time of entry into the study was Condition C in 49 patients and Condition D in 14 patients. Patients in Condition C had the following characteristics: impaired state of alertness but capable of protective or other adaptive responses to noxious stimuli; or, poorly responsive but with stable vital signs. Patients in Condition D had the following characteristics: no response to address or shaking, nonadaptive response to noxious stimuli and instability of vital signs.

Intracranial pressure measurements were reported in 62 patients. The first measurement was made during the first 3 days in 33 patients, during days 4 through 7 in 18 patients, during days 8 through 11 in 10 patients, and during day 14 in 1 patient.

Measurement techniques for evaluating intracranial pressure were determined by the participating institution and investigator. Intraventricular recording was done in 25 patients (40% of 63) and epidural pressure transducer was done in 18 (29% of 63). Other techniques utilized were subarachnoid screw (6 patients), translumbar catheter (2), subdural pressure transducer (7) and epidural fiberoptic sensor (4).

Proportion with Elevated Intracranial Pressure

The average intracranial pressure (ICP) level for the first two days of measurement was equal to or greater than 20 mm Hg in 48 patients (77% of 62). A test of the hypothesis that the percentage of Conditions C and D is equal to 50% demonstrated a statistically significant level of $P < 0.0001$. Hence, a poor-condition patient is more likely to have elevated ICP than not.

Treatment Program

Therapies utilized for the reduction of elevated ICP consisted of the use of mannitol in 75% of the patients, controlled respiration in 50%, fluid restriction in 48%, cerebrospinal fluid drainage in 38%, surgical decompression in 3% and other therapies (glycerol, furosemide, low-molecular-weight dextran, phentobarbital) in 8%. Eight of the 14 patients with normal ICP also received one of the therapies considered for reducing ICP.

Adjunctive therapies utilized were antifibrinolytic therapy (epsilon-aminocaproic acid or tranexamic acid), dexamethasone and antihypertensive agent when necessary.

Mortality

Mortality was assessed at two weeks and four weeks post-subarachnoid hemorrhage. A comparison of mortality rates between normal ICP and elevated ICP patients revealed a lower mortality for Condition C patients at the two-week and four-week intervals in the elevated-ICP group. A comparison of the mortality rates of the ICP study patients (normal and elevated ICP) with the mortality rates of the antifibrinolytic studies (Phases III, IV, V) of the Cooperative Aneurysm Study demonstrated a lower mortality for Condition C patients (statistically nonsignificant) and very little difference for Condition D patients and for the overall group.

A comparison of the reported cause of death in the ICP study and the antifibrinolytic studies indicated possible changes in the cause of mortality, but the number of deaths was too small for valid statistical comparison. The results of this study are reported in Chapter 18 of this book.

Phase VII: Timing of Surgery

In September 1980, a grant was obtained from the National Institute of Neurological and Communicative Disorders and Stroke to study the timing of cerebral aneurysm surgery.

Each year in the United States 26,000 individuals have subarachnoid hemorrhage from a ruptured aneurysm. Many are young, healthy people at the peak of productivity in their lives. Approximately 11,000 will die or be permanently disabled as a result of the initial insult of the hemorrhage, leaving approximately 15,000 potential functional survivors available for treatment. Most of these have good neurologic function post-hemorrhage, with the potential for returning to a vigorous and productive life. However, us-

ing contemporary medical and surgical therapy with operation planned no sooner than one to two weeks after the hemorrhage, many will develop devastating neurologic deficits or perish from rebleeding or vasospasm. Ultimately, more than 50% of those who reach a hospital (8,000 per year) will have a favorable outcome. Recent reports challenging the time-honored principle of delayed surgery suggest that an overall favorable outcome among patients available for treatment can be improved to 75% if surgery is performed in the first several days after the hemorrhage. If these results are reproducible and generally applicable, the impact of timing of surgery represents approximately 4,000 lives salvaged per year.

Sporadic recent reports have indicated interest in early operation.[89] Hunt and Miller[90] reported in 1976 that, "Early intervention is justified in a small percentage of cases with aneurysmal hemorrhage." Samson and colleagues[91] retrospectively reviewed 106 consecutive patients in good clinical condition, comparing early operation with late operation and finding no significant difference in the operative mortality in each group (early surgery 5%, late surgery 4%). A much more aggressive surgical approach has been suggested, particularly by the Japanese neurosurgeons.[92]

The purpose of this study is to define the relationship between the interval of surgery following aneurysm rupture and the overall outcome in terms of survival and disability. Specifically, the investigators hope to identify those intervals when surgery produces optimal results as well as those intervals when the results are likely to be adverse. The secondary objective of the study is to document the contemporary results of modern medical and surgical therapy.

In order to accomplish these objectives, a prospective, multicenter, international survey will be performed. Randomized controlled clinical trials are generally accepted to be the most efficient mechanism for determining the appropriateness of new therapeutic modalities. However, early in the planning stages of this study it became apparent that this technique could not be applied to the timing of surgery problem, for several reasons. First, from a purely theoretical point of view, there is insufficient supportive evidence that the timing of surgery affects outcome to warrant a randomized study. Furthermore, randomization would have to be made to at least four different intervals, thus producing great difficulties in obtaining a sufficient number of cases. But more importantly, there are two additional practical considerations precluding a randomized study at this time. The neurosurgical community was approached regarding the possibility of randomizing patients to different intervals of surgery. Very little interest could be elicited in such a study. Also, it was felt that extreme difficulties would be encountered in obtaining the cooperation of patients and their families during the randomized process and still fully comply with the present requirements for informed consent.

Accordingly, it was decided to perform a prospective survey of the influence of timing of surgery on outcome. In this study, patients will be managed according to the individual surgeons' practices as modified by the patients' condition. Data will be collected prospectively in a predetermined format on patients with ruptured aneurysms admitted within three days of their first subarachnoid hemorrhage. At the time of initial evaluation, surgeons will specify at which interval they anticipate performing surgery, but of course they will be free to modify this as conditions dictate. Patients' status will be evaluated on admission, immediately pre- and postoperatively, and at 14 days and 6 months following the hemorrhage. The 6-month evaluation will be performed by an independent observer not involved with the patient's management who is blind to the time of surgery.

Approximately 3,000 cases will be required in order to detect differences of 10% in outcome between surgery performed in different intervals. To perform the study in a reasonable time frame, an international cooperative effort utilizing data from approximately 30 North American and 30 foreign centers will be performed.

This project was in the planning and development stage for 36 months. Approximately 6 months has been allocated for project initiation (including final recruitment and training of centers), 36 months for data collection and 12 months for data analysis and dissemination of results. Accordingly, the results of the study should be available in the spring or summer of 1985.

References

1. Mount, L.A.: Treatment of spontaneous subarachnoid hemorrhage. JAMA 146:693–698, 1951.
2. Sahs, A.L., Perret, G.E., Locksley, H.B., et al.: Intracranial Aneurysms and Subarachnoid Hemorrhage. A Cooperative Study. J.B. Lippincott Co., Philadelphia, 1969.
3. Locksley, H.: Cooperative clinical study of intracranial aneurysms and subarachnoid hemorrhage. Neurology 11:162–164, (April) 1961.
4. Sahs, A.L.: Preliminary report of National Institutes of Health Cooperative Study of Intracranial Aneurysms and Subarachnoid Hemorrhage. In: Fields, W.S., Sahs, A.L.: Intracranial Aneurysms and Subarachnoid Hemorrhage. Charles C Thomas Publisher, Springfield, Ill, 1965, pp 486–501.
5. Sahs, A.L., Perret, G., Locksley, H.B., Nishioka, H., Skultety, F.M.: Section I. Preliminary remarks on subarachnoid hemorrhage. J Neurosurg 24:782–788, 1966.
6. Knowler, L.A.: Section I. Some statistical aspects of a cooperative study. J Neurosurg 24:789–791, 1966.
7. Sahs, A.L.: Section I. Observations on the pathology of saccular aneurysms. J Neurosurg 24:792–806, 1966.
8. McCormick, W.F.: Section I. The pathology of vascular ("arteriovenous") malformations. J Neurosurg 24:804–816, 1966.
9. Locksley, H.B., Sahs, A.L., Knowler, L.: Section II. General survey of cases in the Central Registry and characteristics of the sample population. J Neurosurg 24:922–932, 1966.
10. Locksley, H.B., Sahs, A.L., Sandler, R.: Section III. Subarachnoid hemorrhage unrelated to intracranial aneurysm and A-V malformation. A study of associated diseases and prognosis. J Neurosurg 24:1034–1056, 1966.
11. Perret, G., Nishioka, H.: Section IV. Cerebral an-

giography. An analysis of the diagnostic value and complications of carotid and vertebral angiography in 5,484 patients. J Neurosurg 25:98–114, 1966.

12. Locksley, H.B.: Section V, Part 1. Natural history of subarachnoid hemorrhage, intracranial aneurysms, and arteriovenous malformations. J Neurosurg 25:219–239, 1966.

13. Locksley, H.B.: Natural history of subarachnoid hemorrhage, intracranial aneurysms and arteriovenous malformations. Based on 6,368 cases in the Cooperative Study. J Neurosurg 25:321–368, 1966.

14. Perret, G., Nishioka, H.: Section VI. Arteriovenous malformations. An analysis of 545 cases of cranio-cerebral arteriovenous malformations and fistulae reported to the Cooperative Study. J Neurosurg 25:467–490, 1966.

15. Nishioka, H.: Section VII, Part 1. Evaluation of the conservative management of ruptured intracranial aneurysms. J Neurosurg 25:574–592, 1966.

16. Sahs, A.L.: Section VII, Part 2. Hypotension and hypothermia in the treatment of intracranial aneurysms. J Neurosurg 25:593–600, 1966.

17. Nishioka, H.: Section VIII, Part 1. Results of the treatment of intracranial aneurysms by occlusion of the carotid artery in the neck. J Neurosurg 25:660–682, 1966.

18. Skultety, F.M., Nishioka, H.: Section VIII, Part 2. The results of intracranial surgery in the treatment of aneurysms. J Neurosurg 25:683–704, 1966.

19. Stehbens, W.E.: Pathology of the cerebral blood vessels. C.V. Mosby Co, St. Louis, 1972.

20. Nibbelink, D.F.: Intracranial Hemorrhage. In: Siekert, R.G.: Cerebrovascular Survey Report (Revised) 1976. Whiting Press, Inc, Rochester, Minnesota, pp 179–180.

21. Sahs, A.L.: Presidential address: Observations on cooperative studies. Trans Am Neurol Assoc 93:1–15, 1968.

22. Sahs, A.L.: Cooperative study of intracranial aneurysms and subarachnoid hemorrhage. Report on a randomized treatment study. I. Introduction. Stroke 5:550–551, 1974.

23. Nibbelink, D.W., and Knowler, L.A.: Cooperative study of intracranial aneurysms and subarachnoid hemorrhage. Report on a randomized treatment study. II. Objectives and design of randomized aneurysm study. Stroke 5:552–556, 1974.

24. Graf, C.J., Nibbelink, D.W.: Cooperative study of intracranial aneurysms and subarachnoid hemorrhage. III. Intracranial surgery. Stroke 5:557–601, 1974.

25. Klafta, L.A., Jr., Hamby, W.B.: Significance of cerebrospinal fluid pressure in determining time for repair of intracranial aneurysms. J Neurosurg 31:217–219, 1969.

26. Paul, R.L., Arnold, J.G., Jr.: Operative factors influencing mortality in intracranial aneurysm surgery: analysis of 186 consecutive cases. J Neurosurg 32:289–294, 1970.

27. Pool, J.L.: Bifrontal craniotomy for anterior communicating artery aneurysms. J Neurosurg 30:212–220, 1972.

28. Krayenbühl, H.A., Yasargil, M.G., Flamm, E.S., et al.: Microsurgical treatment of intracranial saccular aneurysms. J Neurosurg 37:678–686, 1972.

29. Nibbelink, D.W., Torner, J.C., Henderson, W.G.: Intracranial aneurysms and subarachnoid hemor-

rhage. Report on a randomized treatment study. VI-A. Regulated bed rest. Stroke 8:202–218, 1977.

30. Drake, C.G.: Discussion of Hunt, W.E., Hess, R.M.: Risk related to time of surgery in intracranial aneurysms. J Neurosurg 28:19–20, 1968.

31. Drake, C.G.: Intracranial aneurysms. In: Tower, D.B.: The Nervous System. Vol 2, The Clinical Neurosciences. Raven Press, New York, 1975, pp 287–295.

32. Mullan, S., Dawley, J.: Antifibrinolytic therapy for intracranial aneurysms. J Neurosurg 28:21–23, 1968.

33. Nibbelink, D.W., Sahs, A.L.: Antifibrinolytic therapy and drug-induced hypotension in treatment of ruptured intracranial aneurysms. Trans Am Neurol Assoc 97:145–151, 1972.

34. Nibbelink, D.W.: Cooperative Aneurysm Study: Antihypertensive and antifibrinolytic therapy following subarachnoid hemorrhage from ruptured intracranial aneurysm. In: Whisnant, J.P., Sandok, B.A.: Cerebral Vascular Diseases. Grune & Stratton, Inc., New York, 1975, pp 155–165.

35. Girvin, J.: Formal discussion—Cooperative Aneurysm Study. In: Whisnant, J.P., Sandok, B.A.: Cerebral Vascular Diseases. Grune & Stratton, Inc., New York, 1975, pp 165–167.

36. Millikan, C.H.: Summary of the Ninth Princeton Conference on Cerebral Vascular Diseases, January 9–11, 1974. Stroke 5:429–438, 1974.

37. Alkjaersig, N., Fletcher, A.P., Sherry, S.: E-aminocaproic acid: An inhibitor of plasminogen activation. J Biol Chem 234:832–837, 1959.

38. Egeblad, K.: Effects of epsilon-aminocaproic acid on fibrin clot lysis. Thromb Diath Haem 15:173–191, 1966.

39. McNicol, G.P., Fletcher, A.P., Alkjaersig, N., et al.: The absorption, distribution and excretion of e-aminocaproic acid following oral or intravenous administration to man. J Lab Clin Med 59:15–24, 1962.

40. Tovi, D., Nilsson, I.M.: Increased fibrinolytic activity and fibrin degradation products after experimental intracerebral haemorrhage. Acta Neurol Scand 48:403–415, 1972.

41. Tovi, D., Nilsson, I.M., Thulin, C–A.: Fibrinolysis and subarachnoid haemorrhage. Inhibitory effect of tranexamic acid. A clinical study. Acta Neurol Scand 48:393–402, 1972.

42. Tovi, D., Nilsson, I.M., Thulin, C–A.: Fibrinolytic activity of the cerebrospinal fluid after subarachnoid haemorrhage. Acta Neurol Scand 49:1–9, 1973.

43. Tovi, D.: Fibrinolytic activity of human brain. A histochemical study. Acta Neurol Scand 49:152–162, 1973.

44. Nilsson, I.M.: Local fibrinolysis as a mechanism for haemorrhage. Thromb Diath Haem 34:623–633, 1975.

45. Nibbelink, D.W.: Antifibrinolytic activity during administration of epsilon-aminocaproic acid Stroke 2:555–558, 1971.

46. Nibbelink, D.W., Jacobsen, C.D.: Plasminogen depletion during administration of epsilon-aminocaproic acid. Thromb Diath Haem 29:598–602, 1973.

47. Nibbelink, D.W., Sahs, A.L., Knowler, L.A.: Antihypertensive and antifibrinolytic medications in subarachnoid hemorrhage and their relation to ce-

rebral vasospasm. A report of the Cooperative Aneurysm Study. In: Smith, R.R., Robertson, J.T.: Subarachnoid Hemorrhage and Cerebrovascular Spasm. Charles C Thomas, Springfield, Ill, 1975, pp 177–205.

48. Nibbelink, D.W., Torner, J.C., Henderson, W.G.: Intracranial aneurysms and subarachnoid hemorrhage. A cooperative study. Antifibrinolytic therapy in recent onset subarachnoid hemorrhage. Stroke 6:622–629, 1975.

49. Mullan, S.: Conservative management of the recently ruptured aneurysm. Surg Neurol 3:27–32, 1975.

50. Ransohoff, J., Goodgold, A., Benjamin, M.V.: Preoperative management of patients with ruptured intracranial aneurysms. J Neurosurg 36:525–530, 1972.

51. Smith, R.R., Upchurch, J.J.: Monitoring antifibrinolytic therapy in subarachnoid hemorrhage. J Neurosurg 38:339–344, 1973.

52. Sengupta, R.P., So, S.C., Villarejo-Ortega, F.J.: Use of epsilon aminocaproic acid (EACA) in the preoperative management of ruptured intracranial aneurysms. J Neurosurg 44:497–484, 1976.

53. Tovi, D.: The use of antifibrinolytic drugs to prevent early recurrent aneurysmal subarachnoid haemorrhage. Acta Neurol Scand 49:163–175, 1973.

54. Corkill, G.: Earlier operation and antifibrinolytic therapy in the management of aneurysmal subarachnoid haemorrhage. Med J Aust 1:468–470, 1974.

55. Chowdhary, U.M., Cary, P.C., Hussein, M.M.: Prevention of early recurrence of spontaneous subarachnoid haemorrhage by e-aminocaproic acid. Lancet 1:741–743, 1979.

56. Girvin, J.P.: The use of antifibrinolytic agents in the preoperative treatment of ruptured intracranial aneurysms. Trans Am Neurol Assoc 98:150–152, 1973.

57. Gibbs, J.R., O'Gorman, P.: Fibrinolysis in subarachnoid hemorrhage. Postgrad Med J 43:779–784, 1967.

58. Profeta, G., Castellano, G., Guarnieri, L., et al.: Antifibrinolytic therapy in the treatment of subarachnoid haemorrhage caused by arterial aneurysms. J Neurosurg Sci 19:77–78, 1975.

59. Wintzen, A.R., Van Rossum, J.: E-Aminocaproic acid in prevention of subarachnoid haemorrhage. Lancet 1:1084, 1979.

60. Van Rossum, J., Wintzen, A.R., Endtz, L.J., Schoen, J.H.R., de Jonge, H.: Effect of tranexamic acid of rebleeding after subarachnoid hemorrhage: A double-blind controlled clinical trial. Ann Neurol 2:242–245, 1977.

61. Kaste, M., Ramsay, M.: Tranexamic acid in subarachnoid hemorrhage. A double-blind study. Stroke 10:519–522, 1979.

62. McNicol, G., Fletcher, A., Alkjaersig, N., et al.: The use of epsilon-aminocaproic acid, a potent inhibitor of fibrinolytic activity in the management of postoperative hematuria. J Urol 86:829–837, 1961.

63. Naeye, R.L.: Thrombotic state after a haemorrhagic diathesis, a possible complication of therapy with epsilon-aminocaproic acid. Blood 19:694–701, 1962.

64. Bergin, J.J.: The complications of therapy with epsilon-aminocaproic acid. Med Clin North Am 50:1669–1678, 1966.

65. Charyton, C., Purtilo, D.: Glomerular capillary thrombosis and acute renal failure after epsilon aminocaproic therapy. N Engl J Med 280:1102–1104, 1969.

66. Ratnoff, O.: Epsilon aminocaproic acid: A dangerous weapon. N Engl J Med 280:1125–1126, 1969.

67. Gralnick, H.R., Greipp, P.: Thrombosis with epsilon aminocaproic acid therapy. Am J Clin Pathol 56:151–154, 1971.

68. Britt, C.W., Jr., Light, R.R., Peters, B.H., Schochet, S.S., Jr.: Rhabdomyolysis during treatment with epsilon-aminocaproic acid. Arch Neurol 37:187–188, 1980.

69. Biswas, C.K., Milligan, D.A.R., Agte, S.D., Kenward, D.H.: Acute renal failure and myopathy after treatment with aminocaproic acid. Brit M J 281:115–116, 1980.

70. Swash, M.: Aminocaproic acid myopathy. Brit M J 281:454, 1980.

71. Nilsson, I.M., Anderson, L., Bjorkman, S.E.: Epsilon-aminocaproic acid (EACA) as a therapeutic agent based on 5 years' clinical experience. Acta Med Scand (Suppl) 448:5–46, 1966.

72. Kagström, E., Palma, L.: Influence of antifibrinolytic treatment on the morbidity in patients with subarachnoid hemorrhage. Acta Neurol Scand 48:257–258, 1972.

73. Sonntag, V.K.H., Stein, B.M.: Arteriopathic complications during treatment of subarachnoid hemorrhage with epsilon-aminocaproic acid. J Neurosurg 40:480–485, 1974.

74. Hood, R.S.: Arteritis due to EACA therapy. Letter to the Editor. J Neurosurg 42:117, 1975.

75. Norlen, G., Thulin, C–A.: The use of antifibrinolytic substances in ruptured intracranial aneurysms. Neurochirugia 12:100–102, 1969.

76. Herring, M.: Withdrawal of EACA favored in intracranial aneurysms. Hospital Tribune, Feb. 2, 1976, p 24.

77. Herring, M.: Withdrawal of EACA favored in intracranial aneurysms. Medical Tribune, Jan 7, 1976, p. 12.

78. Farina, M.L., Levati, A., Piano, R.: Myocardial infarction during antifibrinolytic treatment. Thromb Haemost 42:1347–1348, 1979.

79. Park, B.E.: Spontaneous subarachnoid hemorrhage complicated by communicating hydrocephalus: Epsilon-aminocaproic acid as a possible predisposing factor. Surg Neurol 11:73–80, 1979.

80. Schneck, S.A.: On the relationship between ruptured intracranial aneurysm and cerebral infarction. Neurology 14:691–702, 1964.

81. Schneck, S.A., Kricheff, I.I.: Intracranial aneurysm rupture, vasospasm, and infarction. Arch Neurol 11:668–680, 1964.

82. Crompton, M.R.: Cerebral infarction following rupture of cerebral berry aneurysms. Brain 87:263–280, 1964.

83. Hunt, W.E., Hess, R.M.: Surgical risk as related to time of intervention in the repair of intracranial aneurysms. J Neurosurg 28:14–20, 1968.

84. Botterell, E.H., Loughheed, W.M., Scott, J.W., et al.: Hypothermia and interruption of carotid, or carotid and vertebral circulation, in the surgical

management of intracranial aneurysms. J Neurosurg 13:1–42, 1956.

85. Nornes, H., Magnaes, B.: Intracranial pressure in patients with ruptured saccular aneurysms. J Neurosurg 36:537–547, 1972.

86. Nornes, H.: The role of intracranial pressure in the arrest of hemorrhage in patients with ruptured intracranial aneurysms. J Neurosurg 39:221–234, 1973.

87. Stornelli, S.A., French, J.D.: Subarachnoid hemorrhage—Factors in prognosis and management. J Neurosurg 21:769–780, 1964.

88. Kaufmann, G.E., Clark, K.: Continuous simultaneous monitoring of intraventricular and cervical subarachnoid cerebrospinal fluid pressure to indicate development of cerebral or tonsillar herniation. J Neurosurg 33:145–150, 1970.

89. Suzuki, J., Yoshimoto, T.: Early operation for the ruptured intracranial aneurysm. Jpn J Surg 3:149–156, 1973.

90. Hunt, W.E., Miller, C.A.: The results of early operation for aneurysm. Clin Neurosurg 24:208–215, 1976.

91. Samson, D.S., Hodosh, R.M., Reid, W.R., Beyer, C.W., Clark, W.K.: Risk of intracranial aneurysm surgery in the good grade patient: Early versus late operation. Neurosurg 5:422–426, 1979.

92. Suzuki, J., Yoshimoto, T.: Early operation for the ruptured intracranial aneurysm. In: Suzuki, J.: Cerebral Aneurysms. Neuron Publishing Co., Tokyo, 1979, pp 224–230.

Section II

Report of Randomized
Treatment Study

Chapter 2

Randomized Treatment Study. Introduction

Adolph L. Sahs, M.D.

Abstract

Fifteen institutions participated in a cooperative study for treatment of single ruptured intracranial aneurysms. Between June 1963 and February 1970, 1,005 protocols were submitted to the Central Registry. All patients had a single ruptured aneurysm on the internal carotid, middle cerebral, anterior cerebral-anterior communicating or vertebral-basilar arteries. The four treatments allocated randomly were regulated bed rest, drug-induced hypotension, carotid ligation and intracranial surgery. This study was an attempt to determine the relative merits of these several modes of therapy.

Introduction

Phase I was the report on a data-collection study which covered a series of observations of patients with cerebral aneurysms and other disorders producing spontaneous subarachnoid hemorrhage extending over a period of 8 years. During that interval, 6,368 cases were reported to the Central Registry. From these, 3,265 aneurysm cases were identified. A group of 2,951 patients bled from a ruptured aneurysm, and in 314 patients the aneurysm had not bled. This group incorporated seriously ill and poor-risk patients. The report was entitled *Intracranial Aneurysms and Subarachnoid Hemorrhage*, by Drs. Sahs, Perret, Locksley and Nishioka, and was published in monograph form in 1969. The gross mortality of patients managed conservatively ranged from 36% in the middle cerebral to 42% in the anterior cerebral-anterior communicating group.

Of those patients subjected to intracranial surgery, the following mortality rates occurred: years 1956 to 1957, 33%; 1958, 30%; 1959, 36%; 1960, 34%; 1961 to 1964, 26%.

These statistics were questioned because of the possible variety of skills which were applied at various centers for both good-risk and poor-risk patients. It became evident after the project was underway that a randomized treatment study was indicated to provide more information concerning the relative merits of various modes of therapy.

Treatment of saccular aneurysms is a complex problem which involves variables such as age and sex, specific aneurysm site, elapsed time since hemorrhage and clinical condition of the patient. These, and probably other factors, influence the natural outcome of a ruptured aneurysm and have considerable impact on the prognosis of medical and surgical treatment. At the commencement of the original study, many of the group anticipated this problem and recognized the greater efficiency and scientific validity of a treatment study which, by proper design, would attempt to obviate factors of individual selection and also carefully define each mode of treatment according to standards most commonly employed. At that time, however, there existed such strongly conflicting and impressionistic opinions regarding treatment that the compromises and cooperation needed for a well-designed study of treatment were not immediately forthcoming. However, over a period of four or five years of individual and collective study, there evolved a more widespread awareness of the necessity for such a study and conviction as to its feasibility.

By December 1961, an ad hoc committee devised a plan for a controlled comparative study of medical and surgical treatments of bleeding intracranial aneurysms. This was designated Phase II. Six months later, the detailed program was accepted in principle. A nucleus of 10 centers proceeded with the proposed format, and began to submit protocols on June 15, 1963. The program was continued until February 1, 1970.

Table 2–1.   Case Registrations Excluded.

	No.
Died before randomization	101
Multiple aneurysms	300
Arteriovenous anomaly in addition to aneurysm	13
Intracranial mass lesion requiring immediate surgery	49
Inability to obtain comprehensive treatment permit	147
Unrelated disease sufficiently compromising to hypotensive or surgical treatments	25
Previous aneurysm treatment other than bed rest	7
Aneurysm of posterior circle	13
Patient set aside according to prearranged schedule	4
Unknown	1
Total	660

Patients meeting the criteria for admission to the study were allocated randomly to one of four treatment categories. These included regulated bed rest, drug-induced hypotension with regulated bed rest, carotid ligation and intracranial surgery.

The sites chosen for study were single aneurysms located on the internal carotid, middle cerebral and anterior cerebral-anterior communicating arteries, plus aneurysms of the posterior portion of the circle of Willis. Intervals from last bleed to allocated treatment were subdivided into three time periods as follows: (1) within 7 days following the last bleed, (2) 8 to 21 days after the hemorrhage and (3) 22 to 92 days. An original estimate of 1,000 cases was indicated to answer the question regarding which treatment would be most favorable. A statistical method utilizing sequential analysis was considered by our statistician to be most efficient in terms of number of cases, time and effort. These determinations were monitored closely in order to assess any factors responsible for any statistically significant undesirable outcome.

Case registrations were forwarded to the Central Registry from 1963 through the first six weeks of 1970. During this period, a total of 1,665 cases was available, from which 660 were excluded (Table 2–1). The remaining 1,005 cases were randomly allocated among the four treatment categories. In this group, 33 cases were disqualified after allocation of treatment, leaving a total of 972 for detailed analysis of comparative treatments.

The mere fact that a patient was allocated randomly to a treatment category did not necessarily mean that such treatment was actually carried out on that particular patient. For example, a patient assigned to intracranial surgery might not have received such definitive treatment for a number of reasons. This problem will be discussed in detail in the sections that follow, but the reader should be aware at the onset that the "allocated treatment" could not be followed according to protocol in all instances.

Chapter 3

Randomized Treatment Study. Objectives and Design of Randomized Aneurysm Study

Donald W. Nibbelink, M.D. Ph.D. and Lloyd A. Knowler, Ph.D.

Abstract

Four selected treatments—regulated bed rest, drug-induced hypotension, carotid ligation, and intracranial surgery—were randomly allocated with respect to location of the aneurysm and interval following last bleed. The objective of the study was to answer the question, "What mode of treatment offers a patient with a single ruptured intracranial aneurysm during the previous three months the highest probability of optimal results with respect to survival, residual neurologic deficit, capacity for self-care and gainful employment?" Various treatments were suspended at specific intervals when a particular mode of therapy became inferior to the others.

A group of 33 patients was disqualified after treatment was randomly allocated. The numbers of protocols remaining for analysis within each treatment category were 202 for regulated bed rest, 309 for drug-induced hypotension, 187 for carotid ligation, and 274 for intracranial surgery.

Introduction

Evaluation of surgical and nonsurgical treatment of ruptured intracranial aneurysms has been the primary objective of the Cooperative Aneurysm Study since 1958. Uncontrolled clinical variables have always made the development of a properly designed treatment study very difficult. For nonsurgically treated patients with a single aneurysm, a mortality of 38% was observed in the previous Cooperative Study[1] within 14 days following the last bleed, and 68% at the end of 8 years; whereas mortality following intracranial operation was 30% during the interval from surgery to time of discharge. However, it was emphasized that "selective withdrawal of cases favorable for surgery is likely to affect the data and probability calculations based thereon, in the direction of making them more pessimistic than would be obtained from a completely undistorted sample." Because of theoretical and practical limitations of "case matching" on a statistical basis, the present study was established so that selected treatments were randomly allocated with respect to location of the aneurysm and interval from last bleed.

Table 3–1.   Definition of Aneurysm Site.

1. Internal carotid—a single aneurysm located on the internal carotid artery distal to its emergence from the cavernous sinus to its terminal bifurcation, and including those aneurysms at the junction of the posterior communicating artery with the internal carotid artery. Infundibular dilatations 2 mm in diameter or less were not included.
2. Middle cerebral—a single aneurysm on the middle cerebral artery and its branches.
3. Anterior cerebral-anterior communicating—a single aneurysm on the anterior cerebral artery and its branches, the anterior communicating artery, and its junction with the anterior cerebral artery.
4. Vertebral-basilar—a single aneurysm on the vertebral, basilar, posterior communicating-posterior cerebral artery junction; posterior cerebral artery, and all its branches.

Objective

The principal objective of the study was to provide an answer to the question, "What designated mode of treatment offers a patient with a single ruptured intracranial aneurysm during the previous three months the highest probability of optimal results with respect to survival, residual neurologic deficit and capacity for self-care and gainful employment?" The four modes of treatment recommended for random allocation were: (1) regulated bed rest, (2) drug-induced hypotension with regulated bed rest, (3) ipsilateral common carotid artery occlusion with bed rest and (4) intracranial surgery. Definition of each treatment category will be provided in the forthcoming reports.

The relative value of each treatment was expected to remain usefully represented so that the effects of various factors not directly related to a ruptured aneurysm or its treatment would tend to cancel out. In that sense, the study was designated a "randomized study." To minimize the effects of any dissimilarities among participating centers, such variables as professional skill, hospital facilities, biologic differences among racial groups and economic class were balanced to assure that each individual center constituted, of itself, a small "randomized study."

Design of Randomization

The aneurysm sites chosen for this investigation were located on the internal carotid, middle cerebral and anterior cerebral arteries, plus single aneurysms on the posterior portion of the circle of Willis (see Table 3–1 for definition of each site). Intervals from last bleed to allocation of treatment were designated as follows: 0 to 7 days, 8 to 21 days and 22 to 92 days (Table 3–2). A statistical method utilizing sequential analysis[2] was engaged to compare one treatment with another with respect to mortality at 30, 90 and 180 days following the last bleed. Additional analyses were performed on a yearly basis until five years following the bleed. The sequential plan was used in order to terminate the study as soon as feasible after a sufficient number of cases had been accumulated. Each treatment at each site and at each time interval was compared to each and every other treatment with respect to the principal objective of the study. Any evidence of inferiority comparing one treatment with another at a statistically signifi-

Table 3–2 Stratification of Design for Randomization.

Site:	1	Internal carotid
	2	Middle cerebral
	3	Anterior cerebral-anterior communicating
	4	Posterior circle
Interval:*	1	0–7 days
	2	8–21 days
	3	22–92 days
Treatment:	1	Regulated bed rest
	2	Drug-induced hypotension with regulated bed rest
	3	Ipsilateral common carotid artery occlusion with regulated bed rest
	4	Intracranial surgery

* From day of last bleed to date admitted to treatment study.

Table 3–3.   Designated Treatments for Each
Aneurysm Site and Interval from Last Bleed.

Site	Interval (days)	Treatment*
Internal carotid	0–7	1 2 3 4
	8–21	1 2 3 4
	22–92	1 2 3 4
Middle cerebral	0–7	1 2 3 4
	8–21	1 2 3 4
	22–92	1 2 3 4
Anterior cerebral-anterior communicating	0–7	1 2 3 4
	8–21	1 2 3 4
	22–92	1 2 3 4
Posterior circle	0–7	1 4
	8–21	1 4
	22–92	1 4

cant level ($P = 0.05$) was immediately called
to the attention of the participants. Mortality
and morbidity were continuously monitored
in order to assess those factors potentially
deleterious in executing the treatment programs.

Within each interval following the last
bleed, patients with a single aneurysm on
the anterior portion of the circle of Willis
were randomly allocated to one of four treatment categories (Table 3–3). For those with

an aneurysm on the posterior portion of the
circle, only two alternatives were recommended: (1) regulated bed rest, and (2) intracranial surgery (Table 3–3).

Each patient with subarachnoid hemorrhage underwent a prescribed protocol of
clinical and laboratory evaluations. These
included lumbar puncture with findings consistent with grossly bloody cerebrospinal
fluid and xanthochromic supernatant, followed by angiographic visualization of the
anterior and posterior cerebral circulations.
Following visualization of a single aneurysm
by cerebral angiography, and provided each
patient was a candidate for any of the four
treatment programs, the allocation of treatment was determined randomly, and the
course of therapy instituted. Between June
15, 1963, and February 1, 1970, 1,005 protocols were presented to the Central Registry for analysis. A preliminary statistical
analysis was reported in 1972.[3]

During the study, treatments were suspended in specific categories for various reasons. In the column designated "treatment
suspensions" in Table 3–4, ipsilateral common carotid ligation was discontinued in the
group with an anterior cerebral-anterior
communicating aneurysm on December 1,

Table 3–4.   Intervals Various Treatments Were Suspended.

Aneurysm Site	Interval from Last Bleed to Randomization (days)	Treatment* (Beginning 6–15–63*)	Treatment Suspension†	Treatment 1–1–69 to 2–15–72
Internal carotid	0–7	1 2 3 4	B 2 3 B	2 3 X
	8–21	1 2 3 4	C 2 3 4	2 3 4
	22–92	1 2 3 4	C 2 3 4	2 3 4
Middle cerebral	0–7	1 2 3 4	D 2 3 4	2 3 4
	8–21	1 2 3 4	D 2 3 4	2 3 4
	22–92	1 2 3 4	D 2 3 4	2 3 4
Anterior cerebral	0–7	1 2 3 4	D 2 A 4	2 X 4
	8–21	1 2 3 4	D 2 A 4	2 X 4
	22–92	1 2 3 4	D 2 A 4	2 X 4
Posterior circle	0–7	1 4	C C	
	8–21	1 4	C C	
	22–92	1 4	C C	
Total		42		23

* Treatment designation:
  1 = regulated bed rest   3 = carotid ligation
  2 = drug-induced hypotension 4 = intracranial surgery

† Suspended treatments:
  A   12–1–66   C   6–19–67
  B   3–19–67   D   1–1–69

1966 (A). This action followed a decision by the participants, and was *not* on the basis that carotid ligation was an inferior treatment. The rationale for the majority of participants at that time was the premise that ipsilateral common carotid ligation was ineffective in prevention of rebleeding in anterior communicating aneurysms. On March 19, 1967 (B, Table 3–4), regulated bed rest and intracranial surgery were suspended for the internal carotid group because both treatment modes were significantly inferior to drug-induced hypotension (Treatment 2) and carotid ligation (Treatment 3). Regulated bed rest in the 8 to 21-day interval and 22 to 92-day intervals was suspended later in the internal carotid group (June 19, 1967) following a statistically significant difference in mortality. Collection of single aneurysms on the posterior portion of the circle of Willis was also suspended on June 19, 1967. The number of cases was too few to have any statistical meaning. Later, on January 1, 1969, regulated bed rest was discontinued for all intervals in patients with an aneurysm located on the middle cerebral distribution and the anterior cerebral complex. For these reasons the number of cases for each site were not similar, especially with regard to the regulated bed rest and carotid ligation treatment categories.

Participating Institutions and Distribution of Cases

Fifteen institutions (see Participating Investigators and Centers, p. xii) began to submit protocols when the study was initiated. One institution (Center 14) ceased participation after contributing 1 protocol (Table 3–5), and a second institution (Center 22) submitted no more protocols after contributing 12 cases with the Central Registry. Centers 31, 32 and 33 began to contribute protocols after the study was in progress.

Overseas participants collectively contributed 587 protocols (58.4% of 1,005). Without their high-quality material, this study could not have been completed. The remaining 418 protocols were from 10 institutions in the United States. As noted in

Table 3–5.   Distribution of Cases With Respect to Aneurysm Site for Each Participating Center.

| Center | Aneurysm Site | | | | |
	Internal Carotid	Middle Cerebral	Anterior Cerebral	Vertebral Basilar	Total
12	21	10	20	0	51
14	0	0	0	1	1
19	30	18	25	2	75
20*	0	0	314	0	314
22	4	2	6	0	12
24	19	9	20	1	49
25	38	4	20	2	64
26	36	13	25	0	74
27*	27	22	37	5	91
28*	51	30	57	4	142
29	13	5	12	1	31
30*	8	10	22	0	40
31	5	1	13	0	19
32	7	0	7	0	14
33	9	4	15	0	28
Total	268	128	593	16	1,005

* Overseas participants.

Table 3–6.   Distribution of Allocated Treatments for each participating Center.

| | Treatment Allocation | | | | |
Center	Regulated Bed Rest	Drug-Induced Hypotension	Carotid Ligation	Intracranial Surgery	Total
12	10	17	8	16	51
14	0	0	0	1	1
19	15	23	18	19	75
20	77	97	46	94	314
22	6	4	1	1	12
24	9	13	10	17	49
25	11	21	16	16	64
26	14	21	19	16	70
27	20	29	13	29	91
28	27	49	32	34	142
29	8	6	9	8	31
30	10	11	7	12	40
31	3	5	3	8	19
32	1	5	4	4	14
33	3	14	5	6	28
Total	214	315	191	281	1,001
Allocated to special study					4
					1,005

Table 3–5, the variation in numbers of protocols from various centers was considerable. Center 20 submitted anterior cerebral-anterior communicating aneurysms only per arrangement at the outset of the study.

By random allocation, patients at each center were assigned to one of four treatment programs. The allocated treatment distribution for each center (Table 3–6) reveals similar proportions. Total accumulations for each treatment were 214 for regulated bed rest, 315 for drug-induced hypotension, 191 for carotid ligation and 281 for intracranial surgery.

Within this group of 1,005 patients, 33 were disqualified (Table 3–7). Disqualification signifies that following allocation of treatment, certain conditions or events arose which precluded the continuation of allocated therapy. These items (Table 3–7) were similarly distributed among the four treatment categories. Subtracting these 33 pa-

Table 3–7.   Tabulation of Disqualified Cases.

8	Surgery required
7	Previous hypotensive treatment
4	Refused treatment
4	Incorrect allocation of treatment
4	Special study
3	Multiple aneurysms found
1	Extracranial aneurysm
1	Refused hospitalization
1	Uremia
33	Total disqualified

tients leaves a total of 972 for analysis. The distribution for each aneurysm site and treatment allocation is represented in Table 3–8.

The following reports will include a detailed analysis of all patients included in each treatment category. Each presentation will discuss factors primarily concerned with medical parameters, followed later by the details of statistical analysis.

Table 3–8.   Distribution of Patients Allocated to Specified Therapy Program for Each Aneurysm Site.

Aneurysm Site	Treatment Allocation				Total
	Regulated Bed Rest	Drug-Induced Hypotension	Carotid Ligation	Intracranial Surgery	
Internal carotid	37	82	88	50	257
Middle cerebral	23	35	27	38	123
Anterior cerebral-anterior communicating	135	192	72	180	579
Vertebral basilar	7	0	0	6	13
Total	202	309	187	274	972

References

1. Sahs, A.L., Perret, G.E., Locksley, H.B., et al: Intracranial Aneurysms and Subarachnoid Hemorrhage. A Cooperative Study. Lippincott Co, Philadelphia, 1969.
2. Wald, A.: Sequential Analysis. Wiley and Sons, New York, 1947.
3. Sahs, A.L., Nibbelink, D.W., Knowler, L.A.: Cooperative aneurysm project: Introductory report of a randomized treatment study. In McDowell, F.H. Brennan, R.W.: Cerebral Vascular Diseases. Transactions of the Eighth Princeton Conference. Grune & Stratton, New York, 1972, pp 33–41..

Chapter 4

Randomized Treatment Study. Regulated Bed Rest

Donald W. Nibbelink, M.D., Ph.D., James C. Torner, M.S. and William G. Henderson, Ph.D.

Abstract

Three weeks of regulated bed rest was one of four treatments evaluated in the Cooperative Aneurysm Study.

A total of 187 patients with a recently ruptured intracranial aneurysm had subarachnoid hemorrhage confirmed by lumbar puncture. A group of 124 patients was assigned to treatment within 7 days after the bleed, 49 between 8 and 21 days and 14 between 22 days and 92 days.

During the mean follow-up interval of 6.5 years, mortality was 55.1%. A proved rebleed was the cause of death in 34.2%, progressive deterioration from aneurysm rupture in 8.0% and a suspected rebleed in 4.8%. A total of 47.1% died of causes attributed directly to the cerebral effects of the ruptured aneurysm.

of four selected treatments to be evaluated in patients with a recently ruptured intracranial aneurysm. A specific format of therapy was followed during the 21-day period of bed rest. The remaining three treatment categories included drug-induced hypotension with bed rest, ipsilateral common carotid ligation and bed rest, and intracranial surgery. The results from patients allocated to each treatment category are discussed in separate sections in a series of reports. Chapter 2 of this volume presents a general outline of rationale and purpose of the study.[3] Chapter 3 includes the design and objectives of this aneurysm study.[4] Chapter 9 deals with the results of those patients who were allocated to intracranial surgery.[5] The present section includes the medical evaluation of patients allocated to regulated bed rest. The next chapter will include the statistical analysis.

Introduction

McKissock and collaborators[1,2] were the first investigators to stress the importance of controlled clinical trials for evaluation of certain treatments in patients with a ruptured intracranial aneurysm. In the present study, regulated bed rest was recommended as one

Clinical Material

Between June 15, 1963, and February 15, 1970, data forms from 202 patients who received bed rest treatment were submitted to the Central Registry for analysis. All but 8

27

Table 4–1. Distribution of Aneurysm Site.

Site	No.	%
IC	35	18.1
MC	22	11.3
AC	130	67.0
VB	7	3.6
Total	194	100.0

IC = internal carotid; MC = middle cerebral; AC = anterior cerebral; VB = vertebral-basilar.

patients were allowed to complete their designated course of treatment. Among these 8 patients, 2 experienced repetitive seizure activity, 1 was discharged 9 days after randomization, 2 were restless and uncooperative and 3 failed to be admitted to the reporting hospital within 5 weeks after the last bleed. The distribution of the major aneurysm locations is shown in Table 4–1. Further details on specific aneurysm locations appear in Table 4–2.

As of June 19, 1967, the allocation of patients with a vertebrobasilar aneurysm was suspended because an insufficient number of patient data forms were submitted to the Central Registry for statistical purposes. The 7 patients allocated before the suspension date were in good neurologic condition (Grade 2, see Table 4–3 for definition). One was in poor medical condition with severe

Table 4–2. Distribution of Patients with Specific Intracranial Aneurysm Location.

Specific Site	Major Distribution			Total
	Right	Center	Left	
INTERNAL CAROTID				
Subclinoid	1	—	1	2
Supraclinoid, ophthalmic region	1	—	0	1
Supraclinoid, posterior communicating junction	16	—	11	27
Supraclinoid, at bifurcation	2	—	2	4
Posterior communicating (distinct from internal carotid junction)	0	—	1	1
Subtotal	20		15	35
MIDDLE CEREBRAL				
Proximal to first main branching	1	—	0	1
At main branching	12	—	8	20
Distal to main branching	0	—	1	1
Subtotal	13		9	22
ANTERIOR CEREBRAL-ANTERIOR COMMUNICATING				
Proximal to anterior communicating	1	—	3	4
At anterior communicating junction	29	—	34	63
Distal to anterior communicating	4	—	6	10
At anterior communicating	0	53	0	53
Subtotal	34	53	43	130
VERTEBRAL - BASILAR				
Basilar artery termination	0	2	0	2
Posterior inferior cerebellar artery	2	—	1	3
Basilar, trunk	0	1	0	1
Vetebral	0	—	1	1
Subtotal	2	3	2	7
Total	69	56	69	194

Table 4–3.   Definition of Neurologic Condition.

Grade	Definition
1	Symptom-free
2	Minor symptoms (headache, meningeal irritation, diplopia)
3	Major neurologic deficit but fully responsive
4	Impaired state of alertness but capable of protective or other adaptive responses to noxious stimuli
5	Poorly responsive but with stable vital signs
6*	No response to address or shaking, nonadaptive response to noxious stimuli and progressive instability of vital signs

* Grade 6 patients excluded because they were expiring.

pneumonia, but the remaining 6 were in good or fair condition (defined in section on "Age and Medical Condition"). Five were women, and 2 were men. Three died following a proved rebleed at 1 day, 36 days and 150 days, respectively, after the day of allocation to treatment. These 7 patients with a vertebrobasilar aneurysm will be eliminated from further analyses. The remaining 187 patients were included for detailed evaluation.

The distribution of the interval from the last bleed to randomization is shown in Table 4–4.

Neurologic Condition and Interval Between Last Bleed and Allocation to Treatment

The distribution of patients in each neurologic condition was analyzed with respect to various intervals from last bleed to day of randomization. For patients randomized

within 7 days after the hemorrhage, 69.3% (86 of 124) were in good condition (Grades 1 and 2, Table 4–5). For those patients randomized during the 8 through 21-day interval, 73.5% were in good condition, and in the group allocated to treatment during the 22 through 92-day interval, 42.8% were in such condition. Only 14 patients were included in the latter interval. The average distribution of patients in good neurologic condition for the entire group was 68.4% (128 of 187).

Definition of Regulated Bed Rest

The following criteria were included in the regulated bed rest treatment program: (1) hospitalization for three weeks; (2) subdued lighting for three weeks; (3) head of bed elevated no more than 30°; (4) patient allowed to turn but not to sit up or feed himself; (5) proper regulation of bowel movements with commonly used stool softeners; (6) after the first week, the patient could be

Table 4–4.   Distribution of Interval from Last Bleed to Randomization.

Days*	No.	%
0–7	124	66.3
8–21	49	26.2
22–92	14	7.5
Total	187	100.0

* From last bleed to randomization.

Table 4–5.   Distribution of Patients in Various Neurologic Conditions for Each Interval from Last Bleed to Randomization.

Days*	Neurologic Condition†					Total
	1	2	3	4	5	
0–7	4	82	22	10	6	124
8–21	6	30	9	3	1	49
22–93	1	5	5	3	0	14
Total	11	117	36	16	7	187

* From last bleed to randomization.
† See Table 4–3 for definition.

Table 4–6.   Mortality Distribution for Each Aneurysm Site and Interval to Randomization.

Days*	Site			Total	% Deaths
	IC	MC	AC		
0–7	25(14)†	12(8)	87(56)	124(78)	62.9
8–21	6(1)	7(4)	36(15)	49(20)	40.8
22–92	4(3)	3(1)	7(1)	14(5)	35.7
Total	35(18)	22(13)	130(72)	187(103)	
% of Deaths	51.4	59.1	55.4	55.1	

IC = internal carotid; MC = middle cerebral; AC = anterior cerebral.
* From last bleed to randomization.
† Number in parentheses denotes deaths.

helped to a bedside commode; (7) maintenance of adequate airway and oxygenation as necessary; (8) prophylaxis of seizures by administration of phenytoin, 100 mg tid, for at least four weeks; (9) maintenance of 1,800 to 2,000 ml of fluids per 24 hr by mouth, nasogastric tube or intravenously; (10) maintenance of 1,000 calories of nutrition per day, either by oral diet or tube feeding formula; (11) if sedation was required for restlessness, paraldehyde, phenobarbital or chloral hydrate was administered in usual dosage; (12) condom drainage for men and catheter drainage for women was ordered for patients with incontinence; (13) proper analgesia was maintained by administration of acetylsalicylic acid, codeine or meperidine hydrochloride; (14) every effort was made by each contributing center to provide a sustained high standard of nursing care encompassing frequent checking of vital signs, level of responsiveness, neurologic assessment of verbal requests, pupil size, reactivity to light, ability to move extremities and relative strength of grip; and (15) no agents such as osmotic diuretics, corticosteroids, or similar medications were permitted.

tients allocated to treatment within 7 days after the last bleed (Table 4–6). Mortality among patients who were allocated to treatment during the 8 to 21-day interval and 22 to 92-day interval was considerably less (40.8 and 35.7%, respectively). Mortality among patients with an internal carotid aneurysm was 51.4%; for those with a middle cerebral aneurysm it was 59.1%, and in the group with an aneurysm on the anterior cerebral complex it was 55.4% (Table 4–6). These figures are not significantly different. Among the group of patients who were hospitalized and who had their diagnostic workup completed within one week after onset of symptoms, mortality was appreciably higher.

Several clinical parameters were analyzed with respect to potential influence on mortality: age, sex, aneurysm site, neurologic and medical conditions, systolic and mean blood pressures, interval between last bleed and randomization, cerebral vasospasm, size of aneurysm, cause of death and associated medical disorders. In the discussion to follow, each parameter is analyzed with respect to mortality and rebleed rate.

Age, sex distribution and aneurysm site are displayed in Tables 4–7 and 4–8.

Results

Mortality was 55.1% among the 187 patients treated with regulated bed rest during a mean follow-up interval of 6.5 years. The highest mortality (62.9%) occurred in pa-

Age and Neurologic Condition

The severity of each neurologic condition was correlated with respect to age. The age group 50 to 59 had the highest number of patients in each neurologic condition (Table

Table 4–7. Age and Sex Distribution with Number of Deaths Among All Sites Combined.

Age	Men	Women	Total	% Deaths
9–19	4(1)*	2(0)	6(1)	16.7
20–29	10(6)	5(1)	15(7)	46.7
30–39	5(2)	12(6)	17(8)	47.1
40–49	17(9)	26(11)	43(20)	46.5
50–59	34(21)	30(18)	64(39)	60.9
60–69	10(9)	22(12)	32(21)	65.6
70–79	2(2)	7(4)	9(6)	66.7
Total	82(50)	104(52)	186(102)	
Unknown	1(1)		1(1)	
	83(51)		187(103)	
% Deaths	61.4	50.0	55.1	

* Number in parentheses denotes deaths.

4–9). As expected, mortality was lowest in Grade 1 patients (36.4%) and highest in Grade 5 (100%). With each increase in severity of neurologic deficit, a proportionate rise in mortality was noted (Table 4–9). For the group with relatively minor symptoms (Grades 1 and 2), 61 died (47.7% of 128), while of those in poor condition (Grades 3, 4, and 5), 41 died (70.7% of 58). This difference was highly significant ($P<0.01$). For patients 50 years of age or over who were in poor neurologic condition, the chance of survival was less than 30%.

For all aneurysm sites combined, a proved rebleed was the cause of death in 34.2% (64 of 187) of all patients, or 62.1% of the 103 deaths. Progressive decline in clinical condition following the direct cerebral effects of the original bleed was reported in 8.0% (15 of 187) or 14.6% of 103 deaths. Death

following a suspected rebleed was reported in 9 patients. Therefore, 47.1% (88 of 187) of deaths were directly related to the cerebral effects of the ruptured aneurysm.

Age and Medical Condition

Some medical conditions were present prior to the onset of symptoms of subarachnoid hemorrhage, while other conditions appeared during the initial phases of the illness. As the specific medical condition was recognized, it was regarded as an associated condition necessary for consideration as the course of treatment was followed.

At the time of treatment allocation, each patient was appraised as to the degree of risk for a major surgical procedure, using the rating scale of *good, fair, poor* and *prohib-*

Table 4–8. Sex Distribution by Site of Aneurysm.

Sex	Aneurysm Site			Total
	IC	MC	AC	
Males	8(2)*	11(7)	64(42)	83(51)
	25.0%	63.6%	65.6%	61.4%
Females	27(16)	11(6)	66(30)	104(52)
	59.3%	54.5%	45.5%	50.0%
Total	35(18)	22(13)	130(72)	187(103)
% Deaths	51.4	59.1	55.4	55.1

IC = internal carotid; MC = middle cerebral; AC = anterior cerebral.
* Number in parentheses denotes deaths.

Table 4–9. Deaths by Age and Severity of Neurologic Condition with All Aneurysm Sites Combined.

Age	Neurologic Condition* 1	2	3	4	5	Total
9–19	1 (0)†	4 (1)	1 (0)	0	0	6 (1)
20–29	2 (2)	12 (5)	0	1 (0)	0	15 (7)
30–39	1 (0)	10 (3)	4 (3)	1 (1)	1 (1)	17 (8)
40–49	2 (0)	31 (16)	6 (1)	3 (2)	1 (1)	43 (20)
50–59	5 (2)	40 (22)	12 (10)	4 (2)	3 (3)	64 (39)
60–69	0	17 (8)	10 (9)	4 (3)	1 (1)	32 (21)
70–79	0	3 (2)	3 (1)	2 (2)	1 (1)	9 (6)
Total	11 (4)	117 (57)	36 (24)	15 (10)	7 (7)	186 (102)
Unknown						1 (1)
						187 (103)
% Deaths	36.4	48.7	66.7	66.7	100	55.1

* Defined in Table 4–3.
† Number in parentheses denotes deaths.

Table 4–10. Distribution by Age and Medical Condition with All Aneurysm Sites Combined.

Age	Medical Condition* Good	Fair	Poor	Prohibitive	Total
9–19	6 (1)†	0	0	0	6 (1)
20–29	11 (6)	3 (1)	1 (0)	0	15 (7)
30–39	12 (4)	4 (3)	1 (1)	0	17 (8)
40–49	28 (12)	12 (6)	3 (2)	0	43 (20)
50–59	30 (16)	23 (13)	10 (9)	1 (1)	64 (39)
60–69	15 (6)	11 (10)	5 (4)	1 (1)	32 (21)
70–79	0	2 (0)	6 (5)	1 (1)	9 (6)
Total	102 (45)	55 (33)	26 (21)	3 (3)	186 (102)
Unknown		1 (1)			1 (1)
		56 (34)			187 (103)
% Deaths	44.1	60.7	80.8	100	55.1

* See text for definition.
† Number in parentheses denotes deaths.

Table 4–11. Distribution of Cause of Death by Severity of Medical Condition.

Cause of Death	Medical Condition* Good	Fair	Poor	Prohibitive	Total
Proved rebleed	36	20	6	2	64
Progressive decline	2	4	9	0	15
Suspected rebleed	4	3	2	0	9
Unrelated cause	1	4	2	1	8
Unknown	2	3	2	0	7
Total	45	34	21	3	103
Total patients each condition	102	56	26	3	187

* See text for definition.

itive. This classification was unrelated to the aneurysm per se. A *good*-condition patient was alert and normotensive. He had no more than a degree of fever and was considered to be in good health prior to his subarachnoid hemorrhage. In general, patients in *fair* condition had a single underlying medical problem such as hypertension, cirrhosis of the liver, mild to moderate anemia, poor nutrition, generalized atherosclerosis or chronic pulmonary disease. A patient with more than one adverse medical factor or a single condition which was moderately severe (e.g., recent myocardial infarction, electrolyte abnormalities, malignant hypertension, advanced atherosclerotic disease) was regarded as being in *poor* condition. Patients in the *prohibitive* category had a complicated and serious illness with one or more medical disorders.

Among 187 patients, 102 (54.5%) were in good condition, 56 (30.0%) in fair condition and 26 (13.9%) in poor condition; in 3 patients (1.6%) the medical condition was categorized as prohibitive (Table 4–10). With an overall mortality of 55.1%, good-condition patients alone had a mortality of 44.1%, whereas in fair-condition patients it was 60.7%. For patients in poor condition, mortality was 80.8%. All patients with a prohibitive medical status died. Clearly, medical disorders associated with subarachnoid hemorrhage had considerable influence on mortality. This pattern was consistent for all age groups. The number of deaths below age 50 as compared with those age 50 or above revealed the death rate to be significantly higher in the older group. Age was not a significant factor after analyzing the number of deaths above (22 of 45, or 48.9%) or below (23 of 57, or 40.4%) age 50 in good-medical condition patients alone. However, for patients in the fair, poor and prohibitive-medical conditions combined, 54.2% (13 of 24) died in the group below age 50, whereas 73.3% (44 of 60) died in the group age 50 or above ($P = 0.109$).

Patients in good and fair medical conditions had a higher proportion of deaths after a rebleed (70.9%, or 56 of 79, Table 4–11)

as compared with patients in poor and prohibitive conditions (33.3%, or 8 of 24). Comparison of the distribution of deaths which followed a proved rebleed among various medical conditions shows no significant difference among all patients in good, fair or poor medical condition.

Cause of Death

The major cause of death for patients with an aneurysm at various sites was a proved rebleed. Table 4–12 shows the distribution of the cause of death for each aneurysm site.

Evaluation of the interval to death following allocation to formal bed rest therapy revealed that the major proportion of patients died during the three-week period of bedrest. During the first 14 days after randomization, 27 died (26.2% of 103) following a proved rebleed; 40 died (38.8% of 103) within 29 days (Table 4–13). From day 30 and after, there were 24 more deaths which followed a recurrent hemorrhage (23.3% of 103). Analysis of the remaining causes of death reveals that among the 9 patients who died following a suspected rebleed, 4 succumbed within 14 days after randomization and the remaining 5 after the 44-day interval. Among 15 patients who died following progressive deterioration in clinical condition, 11 deaths were reported within 19 days, and the remaining 4 died after the 44-day interval. Two of these developed hydrocephalus (one required a ventriculopleural shunt), and 2 remained poorly responsive following the last prerandomized bleed. Eight patients died from unrelated causes. Five of these occurred after the one-year interval following randomization.

Mortality and Blood Pressure on Day of Randomization

The level of blood pressure as measured within 7 days after the last bleed was another variable which was related to differences in mortality. The average value of four systolic

Table 4-12.   Distribution of Cause of Death for Each Aneurysm Site.

Aneurysm Site	Cause of Death					
	Proved Rebleed	Suspected Rebleed	Progressive Decline	Unrelated Cause	Unknown	Total
Internal carotid (35)*	7 (20.0%)	2 (5.7%)	5 (14.3%)	2 (5.7%)	2 (5.7%)	18 (51.4%)
Middle cerebral (22)	9 (40.9%)	1 (4.5%)	2 (9.1%)	1 (4.5%)	0 (0%)	13 (59.1%)
Anterior cerebral (130)	48 (36.9%)	6 (4.6%)	8 (6.2%)	5 (3.8%)	5 (3.8%)	72 (55.4%)
Total (187)	64 (34.2%)	9 (4.8%)	15 (8.0%)	8 (4.3%)	7 (3.7%)	103 (55.1%)

* Total patients allocated to bed rest for each aneurysm site.

Table 4-13.   Interval to Death Following Randomization for Each Cause of Death with All Sites Combined.

Days from Randomization to Death	Proved Rebleed	Suspected Rebleed	Progressive Decline	Unrelated Cause	Unknown	Total
0–4	5	3	5	0	0	13
5–9	12	0	3	0	0	15
10–14	10	1	2	0	0	13
15–19	2	0	1	1	0	4
20–24	5	0	0	0	0	5
25–29	6	0	0	0	0	6
30–34	8	0	0	0	0	8
45–59	2	2	1	0	2	7
60–120	2	1	0	2	0	5
121–365	2	0	2	0	2	6
1–3 yr	6	0	0	4	2	12
Over 3 yr	4	2	1	1	1	9
Total	64	9	15	8	7	103

Table 4–14. Distribution of Death Rates Tabulated with Respect to Interval After Last Bleed, Neurologic Condition and Blood Pressure.

Systolic Blood Pressure (mm Hg)	Allocation to Treatment After Last Bleed						Total
	0–7 Days			8–92 Days			
	Neurologic Condition*			Neurologic Condition*			
	Good	Poor	Subtotal	Good	Poor	Subtotal	
140 or below	18/40 (45.0%)	6/12 (50.0%)	24/52 (46.1%)	9/26 (34.6%)	7/12 (58.3%)	16/38 (42.1%)	40/90 (44.4%)
Over 140	29/46 (63.0%)	25/26 (96.2%)	54/72 (75.0%)	5/16 (31.2%)	4/9 (44.0%)	9/25 (36.0%)	63/97 (64.9%)
Total	47/86 (54.6%)	31/38 (81.6%)	78/124 (62.9%)	14/42 (33.3%)	11/21 (52.4%)	25/63 (39.7%)	103/187 (55.1%)

* See text for definition.

blood pressures taken at intervals of 4 hours or more was calculated at the Central Registry. For this analysis patients were subdivided into two groups. One group had average systolic blood pressures of 140 mm Hg or below, and the other had average values above that level. Table 4–14 shows that the mortality was 44.4% in patients with average systolic values of 140 mm Hg or below, while in the group with levels above 140 mm Hg it was 64.9%. This difference was highly significant ($P<0.01$).

Rebleed Rate, Neurologic Condition and Blood Pressure

The highest percentage of patients who rebled were those allocated to treatment within 7 days and whose average systolic blood pressures were over 140 mm Hg (Table 4–15). However, these percentages were not statistically different from the group whose blood pressure was 140 mm Hg or below. By comparison with the mortality table (Table 4–14), a proved rebleed as a cause of death remained the nearest association for patients who were in good neurologic condition, no matter what the interval following randomization. If systolic blood pressure alone had more direct influence on rebleeding, one would have expected a more direct relationship between mortality and rebleeding.

Recurrent Hemorrhage Following Randomization

The frequency distribution of recurrent hemorrhages as associated with mortality was presented in the previous discussion (p. 33). Whenever deterioration in mental status and/or neurologic condition was noted, a lumbar puncture was performed as conditions permitted. When significant increase in red cell count was noted in the cerebrospinal fluid or recent gross hemorrhage was observed at postmortem examination, these findings were designated as a proved re-

Table 4-15. Distribution of Rebleed Rates Tabulated with Respect to Interval After Last Bleed, Neurologic Condition and Blood Pressure.

Systolic Blood Pressure (mm Hg)	Allocation to Treatment After Last Bleed								Total
	0–7 Days				8–92 Days				
	Neurologic Condition*				Neurologic Condition*				
	Good	Poor	Subtotal		Good	Poor	Subtotal		
140 or below	18/40 (45.0%)	3/12 (25.0%)	21/52 (40.4%)		9/26 (34.6%)	3/12 (25%)	12/38 (31.6%)		33/90 (36.7%)
Over 140	25/46 (54.3%)	14/26 (53.8%)	39/72 (54.2%)		3/16 (18.8%)	1/9 (11.1%)	4/25 (16.0%)		43/97 (44.3%)
Total	43/86 (50.0%)	17/38 (44.7%)	60/124 (48.4%)		12/42 (28.6%)	4/21 (19.0%)	16/63 (25.4%)		76/187 (40.6%)

* See text for definition.

Table 4-16. Distribution of Patients with a Proved Rebleed for Each Neurologic Condition and Aneurysm Site with Respect to Interval After Last Prerandomized Bleed.

Days After Last Bleed	Internal Carotid Neurologic Condition*					Middle Cerebral Neurologic Condition					Anterior Cerebral Neurologic Condition					Total
	1	2	3	4	5	1	2	3	4	5	1	2	3	4	5	
0–4	0	0	0	0	0	0	1	0	0	0	1	0	1	0	0	2
5–9	0	3	0	0	0	0	1	1	0	0	1	5	3	3	1	18
10–14	0	2	0	0	0	0	1	0	0	0	0	5	1	1	0	10
15–29	0	1	1	0	0	0	4	0	0	0	2	12	0	1	0	20
30–59	0	2	0	0	0	0	0	0	0	0	0	3	5	0	0	11
60–265	0	0	0	0	0	0	0	0	0	0	0	3	1	0	0	5
1–3 yr	0	0	0	0	0	0	0	0	0	0	0	5	0	0	1	6
Over 3 yr	0	0	0	0	0	0	1	0	0	1	1	2	0	0	0	4
Total	0	8	1	0	0	0	8	1	0	1	4	35	11	5	2	76

* See Table 4-3 for definition.

bleed. Whenever deterioration in clinical condition was not followed by a lumbar puncture or postmortem examination, a suspected rebleed was reported. The foregoing discussion is an analysis of proved rebleeds which followed the *last prerandomized bleed* responsible for hospitalization. Neurologic condition, aneurysm site and interval following last bleed were the most important parameters related to recurrent hemorrhage.

Inspection of Table 4–16 reveals that the number of rebleeds for all aneurysm sites was 40.6% (76 of 187). The highest frequency occurred during the 5 through 9-day interval when 18 (23.7% of 76) patients rebled during this period alone. The frequency distribution gradually diminished in the subsequent intervals. The majority (65.8%, or 50 of 76) occurred within 29 days after the last bleed.

The percentage of patients who rebled was 25.7% for the internal carotid group, 45.4% for the middle cerebral group and 43.8% for the anterior cerebral complex. Rebleed rate in Grade 2 patients was 34.8% for the internal carotid group, 72.7% for the middle cerebral group and 42.2% for the anterior cerebral complex. The higher percentage in the middle cerebral group may be influenced by the smaller number of patients for this site. The overall rebleed rate for good-condition patients (Grades 1 and 2) was 43.0% (55 of 128). Comparison of rebleed rate among poor-condition patients (Grades 3, 4, and 5) reveals that 8.3% (1 of 12) rebled among the internal carotid group, 25.0% (2 of 8) in the middle cerebral group and 46.1% (18 of 39) among patients with an anterior cerebral-anterior communicating aneurysm, for an overall rate of 35.6% (21 of 59). Therefore, no significant difference in rebleed rate occurred among good and poor-neurologic condition patients (43.0% vs 35.6%).

Mortality after recurrent hemorrhage was high for all aneurysm sites. Seven of 9 patients died from the cerebral effects of the rebleed in the internal carotid group, 9 of 10 patients in the middle cerebral group and 49 among 57 patients in the anterior cerebral

group, for a mortality of 85.5% (65 of 76 rebleeds). These 65 deaths followed a proved rebleed, with an additional 9 deaths which followed a suspected rebleed, for an overall mortality of 39.6% (74 of 187). For comparison with the gross mortality of 55.1% among patients in the entire bed rest treatment category, the difference of 15.5% includes such causes as progressive deterioration from the direct cerebral effects of the prerandomized bleed and from unrelated and unknown factors.

Interval to Randomization and Recurrent Hemorrhages

Rebleeding was the major cause of morbidity and mortality during the bed rest treatment period. For all aneurysm sites, the group of patients allocated to bed rest within 7 days after bleed had the highest mortality and rebleed rate in the follow-up period. Figure 4–1 presents schematically the rebleed rate for each aneurysm site among patients allocated to treatment within 7 days. The group of 87 patients with an aneurysm on the anterior cerebral complex had the slowest rise during the 5 through 29-day interval following the last bleed. The curves in Figure 4–1 represent the data in Table 4–17 for patients randomized within 7 days. This table contains the percentages in proved rebleed rate during the 62 days after the last prerandomized bleed for patients randomized within each interval. Among patients randomized within 7 days in the internal carotid group, 36% rebled; 20% rebled by day 11. No rebleeds were noted among the 6 patients allocated to treatment during the 8 to 21-day interval or in the 4 patients allocated during the 22 to 92-day interval. Therefore, those percentages are not included in Table 4–17. Although the number of patients with a middle cerebral aneurysm was small, a relatively high proportion rebled. Of the 12 patients randomized within the 7-day interval, 5 rebled, with 1 additional patient who rebled at 75 days (not shown in Table 4–17). Three of 7 patients rebled who were randomized within the 8 to 21-day in-

Table 4-17. Cumulative Rebleeds After Allocation to Bed Rest Treatment.

Days After Last Bleed	Internal Carotid (25)* 0-7†		Middle Cerebral (12) 0-7		Middle Cerebral (7) 8-21		Anterior Cerebral (87) 0-7		Anterior Cerebral (36) 8-21		Total (187)	
	No.	%	No.	%	No.	%	No.	%	No.	%	No.	%
0-2	0	0	0	0	0	0	0	0	0	0	0	0
3-5	2	8.0	1	8.3	0	0	3	3.4	0	0	6	3.2
6-8	2	8.0	2	16.7	0	0	11	12.6	0	0	15	8.0
9-11	5	20.0	3	25.0	0	0	16	18.4	0	0	24	12.8
12-14	5	20.0	3	25.0	1	14.2	19	21.8	2	5.6	30	16.0
15-17	5	20.0	4	33.3	1	14.2	20	23.0	3	8.3	33	17.6
18-20	6	24.0	5	41.6	2	28.6	24	27.6	3	8.3	40	21.4
21-23	6	24.0	5	41.6	3	42.8	25	28.7	3	8.3	42	22.5
24-26	6	24.0	5	41.6	3	42.8	28	32.2	4	11.1	46	24.6
27-29	6	24.0	5	41.6	3	42.8	31	35.6	5	13.9	50	26.7
30-32	8	32.0	5	41.6	3	42.8	32	36.8	5	13.9	53	28.3
33-35	8	32.0	5	41.6	3	42.8	32	36.8	5	13.9	53	28.3
36-38	9	36.0	5	41.6	3	42.8	32	36.8	6	16.7	55	29.4
39-41	9	36.0	5	41.6	3	42.8	34	39.1	7	19.4	58	31.0
42-44	9	36.0	5	41.6	3	42.8	34	39.1	7	19.4	58	31.0
45-47	9	36.0	5	41.6	3	42.8	34	39.1	7	19.4	58	31.0
48-50	9	36.0	5	41.6	3	42.8	35	40.2	7	19.4	59	31.5
51-53	9	36.0	5	41.6	3	42.8	36	41.4	7	19.4	60	32.1
54-56	9	36.0	5	41.6	3	42.8	36	41.4	7	19.4	60	32.1
57-59	9	36.0	5	41.6	3	42.8	36	41.4	8	22.2	61	32.6
60-62	9	36.0	5	41.6	3	42.8	36	41.4	8	22.2	61	32.6

* Total patients allocated to specific interval to randomization.
† Days to randomization after last bleed.

terval. Of the 3 patients allocated to treatment during the 22 to 92-day interval, 1 rebled 4 years later. Therefore, a total of 45.5% (10 of 22) rebled in the middle cerebral group.

Patients with an aneurysm on the anterior cerebral complex who were randomized within 7 days had a high rebleed rate. Forty-one percent rebled during the 53-day interval following the prerandomized bleed (Table 4–17). Over 20% rebled within 14 days. Patients allocated to bed rest during the 8 to 21-day interval had a lower rebleed rate. Only 22% rebled by the 59th day following last bleed. None of the 7 patients rebled who were allocated to bed rest during the 22 to 92-day interval. Therefore, this interval was not included in Table 4–17.

For all sites combined, for patients randomized following the 21st day (when all patients randomized within this interval were allocated to treatment), 10% rebled between days 21 and 59 (Table 4–17). Following the initial two-month interval, more patients with an aneurysm on the anterior cerebral-anterior communicating complex rebled than those with an aneurysm at the remaining two major sites. From the 3rd

Table 4–18. Frequency Distribution of Proved Rebleeds for Patients Randomized at Specified Intervals—Anterior Cerebral Aneurysms Only.

Months After Last Bleed	Interval to Randomization After Last Bleed (days)		
	0–7	8–21	Total
1–2	36	8	44
3–4	1	1	2
5–6	0	0	0
7–12	2	0	2
13–18	1	0	1
19–24	3	1	4
25–36	0	1	1
37–48	2	1	3
Total	45	12	57

through 48th month following last bleed, 9 patients rebled who were allocated to treatment within 7 days, and 4 patients rebled in the group originally allocated to treatment during the 8 to 21-day interval (Table 4–18). No late rebleeds were reported among patients allocated to treatment within the 22 to 92-day interval. As mentioned previously for the middle cerebral group, 1 patient rebled on the 75th day, and 1 rebled 4 years later. No other late rebleeds occurred.

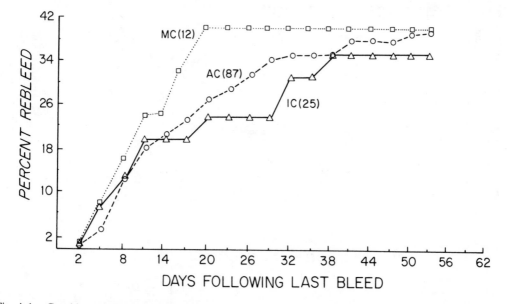

Fig. 4–1. Graphic comparison of rebleed rates at specific intervals following last bleed for each aneurysm site in patients randomized within seven days after last bleed. MC = middle cerebral, AC = anterior cerebral-anterior communicating, IC = internal carotid.

Table 4-19. Cumulative Deaths After Allocation to Bed Rest Treatment.

Days After Last Bleed	Internal Carotid (25)* 0–7‡		Middle Cerebral (12)* 0–7‡		Middle Cerebral (7)* 8–12‡		Anterior Cerebral (87)* 0–7‡		Anterior Cerebral (56)* 8–21‡		Total (187)†	
	No.	%	No.	%	No.	%	No.	%	No.	%	No.	%
0–2	0	0	0	0	0	0	0	0	0	0	0	0
3–5	0	0	0	0	0	0	1	1.1	0	0	1	0.1
6–8	3	12.0	2	16.7	0	0	7	8.0	0	0	12	6.4
9–11	8	32.0	2	16.7	0	0	11	12.6	0	0	21	11.2
12–14	9	36.0	3	25.0	0	0	15	17.2	0	0	27	14.4
15–17	9	36.0	5	41.7	1	14.3	17	19.5	0	0	32	17.1
18–20	10	40.0	6	50.0	2	28.6	19	21.8	2	5.6	39	20.9
21–23	10	40.0	6	50.0	3	42.9	23	26.4	2	5.6	44	23.5
24–26	10	40.0	6	50.0	3	42.9	23	26.4	3	8.3	45	24.1
27–29	10	40.0	6	50.0	3	42.9	27	31.0	4	11.1	50	26.7
30–32	10	40.0	6	50.0	3	42.9	30	34.5	4	11.1	53	28.3
33–35	11	44.0	6	50.0	3	42.9	31	35.6	4	11.1	55	29.4
36–38	11	44.0	6	50.0	3	42.9	31	35.6	5	13.9	56	29.9
39–41	12	48.0	6	50.0	3	42.9	32	36.8	6	16.7	59	31.5
42–44	12	48.0	6	50.0	3	42.9	33	37.9	6	16.7	60	32.0
45–47	12	48.0	6	50.0	3	42.9	33	37.9	7	19.4	61	32.6
48–50	12	48.0	6	50.0	3	42.9	34	39.1	7	19.4	62	33.1
51–53	12	48.0	6	50.0	3	42.9	36	41.4	7	19.4	64	34.2
54–56	12	48.0	6	50.0	3	42.9	37	42.5	7	19.4	65	34.7
57–59	12	48.0	6	50.0	3	42.9	38	43.7	8	22.2	67	35.8
60–62	12	48.0	6	50.0	3	42.9	38	43.7	8	22.2	67	35.8

* Number of patients allocated to interval of randomization.
† Total patients for all aneurysm sites and treatment intervals.
‡ Interval to randomization after last bleed.

Interval to Randomization and Subsequent Mortality

The mortality distribution was variable for specific intervals following last bleed at each aneurysm site. Twenty-five percent of patients with a middle cerebral aneurysm allocated to bed rest within 7 days actually died within 14 days; 17.2% died in the anterior cerebral group (Table 4–19). Thirty-six percent of patients with an internal carotid aneurysm died during that interval. By the 20th day following last bleed, 21.8% of patients died in the anterior cerebral group. Among those with an internal carotid and middle cerebral aneurysm, the mortality was 40.0 and 50.0%, respectively (Table 4–19). After the 20th day, mortality continued to rise gradually among the anterior cerebral group, whereas mortality among patients with an internal carotid and middle cerebral aneurysm remained similar through the 62nd day. Figure 4–2 represents schematically the death rate for patients randomized within 7 days (Table 4–19). Mortality between the 5th and 20th day was most frequent among patients with an internal carotid and middle cerebral aneurysm. However, patients with an anterior cerebral aneurysm had a more gradual rise which did not reach its maximum until the 62nd day.

Table 4–20 includes a summary distribution of deaths at monthly intervals for all patients with an aneurysm at each location and interval following last bleed. The group of 20 patients who were randomized in the 8 to 21-day and 22 to 92-day intervals with an internal carotid or middle cerebral aneurysm was too small for secondary statistical analysis. However, 20% (4 of 20) died within 2 months and 35% within 4 months. A lower rebleed rate was the reason for the lower mortality 2 months following last bleed in the group of 36 patients with an anterior cerebral aneurysm allocated to treatment during the 8 to 21-day interval. After the 62nd day, mortality stabilized for all groups, with the exception of patients

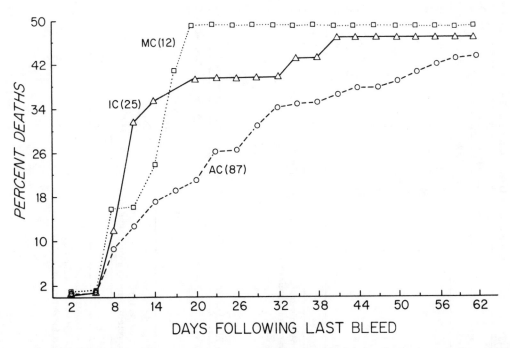

Fig. 4–2. Distribution of deaths at specific intervals following last bleed for each aneurysm site in patients randomized within seven days after last bleed. MC = middle cerebral, IC = internal carotid, AC = anterior cerebal-anterior communicating.

Table 4-20.   Frequency Distribution of Deaths After Last Bleed for Patients Randomized During Specific Intervals.

Months After Last Bleed	Internal Carotid			Middle Cerebral			Anterior Cerebral			Total (187)
	(25)* 0–7†	(6) 8–21	(4) 22–92	(12) 0–7	(7) 8–21	(3) 22–92	(87) 0–7	(36) 8–21	(7) 22–92	
1–2	12	0	1	6	3	0	38	8	0	68
3–4	1	1	1	1	1	0	2	1	0	8
5–6	0	0	0	0	0	0	1	1	0	2
7–12	0	0	0	0	0	0	3	0	0	3
13–18	1	0	0	1	0	0	0	1	1	3
19–24	0	0	0	0	0	0	6	0	0	7
25–36	0	0	0	0	0	0	1	2	0	3
37–48	0	0	0	0	0	0	4	1	0	5
49–60	0	0	0	0	0	1	1	1	0	3
Over 60	0	0	1	0	0	0	0	0	0	1
Total	14	1	3	8	4	1	56	15	1	103

* Total patients analyzed during each interval to randomization.
† Interval to randomization.

Table 4-21.   Distribution of Clinical Characteristics in Patients with Pre-existing Hypertension.

	Average Age (yr)	Neurologic Condition		Medical Condition‡			Average Blood Pressure		Total Deaths
		Good*	Poor†	Good	Fair	Poor	Systolic (mm Hg)	Diastolic (mm Hg)	
Internal carotid (9)	57.1	4	5	1	4	4	181	104	8
Middle cerebral (3)	49.0	2	1	1	1	1	145	94	2
Anterior cerebral-anterior communicating (24)	55.0	16	8	11	8	5	167	96	12
Total (36)		22	14	13	13	10			22

* Good = Grades 1 and 2.
† Poor = Grades 3, 4, and 5 (see Table 4-3 for definition).
‡ See text for definition.

allocated to treatment within 7 days with an anterior cerebral-anterior communicating aneurysm. For patients with this aneurysm site, 49 survived the initial 62 days. Between the 3rd and 60th month, 18 additional patients (36.7%) died following a rebleed. These data suggest that during the initial 8-week period, patients with an anterior cerebral-anterior communicating aneurysm had a slower rebleed rate than those with an internal carotid or middle cerebral aneurysm. After this 8-week interval, patients with an aneurysm on the anterior cerebral complex had comparatively more recurrent hemorrhages than those with aneurysms at the remaining two sites.

Overall Medical Condition of Patients with Ruptured Intracranial Aneurysm

Each medical disorder was reported which existed prior to treatment or which was acquired during treatment. In an earlier section, the relationship of mortality to overall medical condition was analyzed. The foregoing analysis includes data on various medical conditions as they relate to age, neurologic condition, recurrent hemorrhage and cause of death. Those conditions recognized prior to or at the time of randomization will be discussed separately from those which developed during the bed rest treatment program.

Medical Disorders at Randomization

Pre-existing hypertension was the most frequently reported medical condition prior to allocation to treatment. No information was supplied with respect to duration or type of antihypertensive medication prescribed.

Internal Carotid Aneurysm

In these 35 patients, 9 (25.7%) had known pre-existing hypertension, and in 23 a definite history of hypertension was negative. No information was available in 3. Among the 9 patients with pre-existing hypertension, 2 had systolic levels in the range of 160 to 180 mm Hg, 2 in the range of 180 to 200 mm Hg, and 2 over 200 mm Hg. In 3 patients this information was incomplete. Average age in these 9 patients was 57.1 years (range 40 to 79). There were 2 males and 7 females. Four patients were in Grade 2 neurological condition, 2 in Grade 3, and 3 in Grade 4. One patient was in good medical condition, 4 were in fair condition and 4 in poor condition. Average systolic pressure prior to randomization was 181 mm Hg systolic (range 127 to 215) and 104 mm Hg diastolic (range 78 to 158). Average mean blood pressure was 129 mm Hg. All 9 patients had one bleed prior to hospitalization. Eight of the 9 patients died: 2 following a proved rebleed at 11 and 20 days after the last bleed, respectively; 1 following a suspected rebleed; 2 following progressive deterioration in clinical condition; and 1 each died with pneumonia, pulmonary edema and from unknown cause.

Middle Cerebral Aneurysm

Three of 22 patients (13.6%) had pre-existing hypertension; in 16 patients there was no history of hypertension. No information was available in 3. Among the 3 patients with pre-existing hypertension, 1 had known systolic levels in the range of 160 to 180 mm Hg, 1 in the range of 180 to 200 mm Hg, and in the other the range was unknown. Average age was 49 years (range 42 to 55), and all were females. Two were in Grade 2 neurologic condition, and 1 was in Grade 5. One patient was in good medical condition, 1 in fair condition and 1 in poor condition.

Average systolic blood pressure at randomization was 145 mm Hg (range 120 to 175), and average diastolic blood pressure was 94 mm Hg (range 79 to 109). Average mean blood pressure was 111 mm Hg. Two patients had had one previous bleed, and 1 patient had two bleeds. Two patients died following proved rebleed 18 and 75 days after their last prerandomized bleed. One patient remained alive.

Anterior Cerebral Aneurysm

Among 130 patients, 24 (18.5%) had known pre-existing hypertension. Eighty-eight patients had no history of hypertension. No information was reported in 18. Among the 24 patients with pre-existing hypertension, 5 had systolic levels between 160 and 180 mm Hg, 1 between 160 and 180 mm Hg and 1 between 180 and 200 mm Hg. In 7 patients systolic levels were over 200 mm Hg. In 10 patients the levels were unknown. Average age was 55.1 years (range 42 to 72). Nineteen were females; 5 were males. One patient was in Grade 1 neurologic condition, 15 in Grade 2, 2 in Grade 3, 5 in Grade 4, and 1 in Grade 5. Eleven patients were in good medical condition, 8 in fair condition, 4 in poor condition and 1 was in prohibitive condition. Average systolic pressure at randomization was 167 mm Hg (range 130 to 204), and average diastolic pressure was 96 mm Hg (range 55 to 116). Average mean blood pressure was 120 mm Hg. Three patients had two previous bleeds, and 21 had one bleed. Ten of the 24 had a rebleed following randomization; 2 rebled 5 days after last bleed, 1 at 9 days, 1 at 10 days, 2 at 18 days, and 1 each at 39 days, 40 days, 594 days and 752 days. Seven of the 10 patients died following their proved rebleed. In addition, 2 died following progressive clinical deterioration, 1 following a suspected rebleed and 2 from unknown cause, for a total of 12 deaths (50% of the 24 patients with pre-existing hypertension).

Summary

This analysis reveals that among a total of 36 patients with known pre-existing hypertension (Table 4–21), 22 (61.1%) were in good neurologic condition at the time of initial evaluation, and most patients (23 of 36, or 63.8%) were in fair or poor medical condition. There were 22 deaths. This number

of deaths (61.1% of 36) was not significantly greater than the 55.1% for the entire treatment group. Therefore, pre-existing hypertension prior to treatment did not significantly influence mortality over the mean 6.5-year interval.

Medical Disorders Acquired During Bed Rest Treatment

For all aneurysm locations, 37.4% (70 of 187) acquired various medical disorders during the bed rest treatment program. A genitourinary tract infection was reported in 37 patients, pulmonary infection in 19 and a lower frequency of several other conditions for each aneurysm site. An acquired infectious disorder was the usual medical condition which complicated this course of treatment.

Cerebral Angiography

The technique of cerebral angiography was not specified according to protocol. Some institutions pursued the angiographic study within several hours of admission to the hospital, while others followed routine scheduling. In spite of these variables, several important factors relating to these procedures were analyzed. These analyses include number of procedures, complications, associated abnormalities (whether or not related to the aneurysm), vasospasm, interval after last bleed to first angiographic procedure, interval after last bleed to randomization, neurologic condition, systolic and mean blood pressures and size of the aneurysm. These analyses are based on the sample of 195 patients. This number includes the 194 patients who completed their course of treatment, plus 1 patient who was discharged 9 days after randomization. Occasionally, a result will be based on a total of 193 patients because insufficient angiographic information was reported on 2 patients.

Multiple angiographic procedures (more than one) were performed on 57 of 193 patients (29.5%) allocated to bed rest for a number of reasons. These procedures were distributed in similar proportions among the three aneurysm sites. In some institutions, each carotid system was studied at separate intervals. Some patients were re-evaluated for deterioration in neurologic condition associated with a rebleed or ischemic neurologic deficit. Other patients had their vertebral-basilar system visualized angiographically during later procedures. Although the protocol suggested complete cerebral angiographic surveys, vertebral-basilar visualization was completed in only 66 of 193 patients (34.2%). Therefore, the presence of a single aneurysm was certain in these patients only. As each aneurysm was discovered, a complete angiographic survey was not always pursued when the clinical presentation was consistent with the angiographic findings.

The number of multiple angiographic procedures (29.5%) may have been one factor responsible for delay in formal allocation to treatment. Another possible reason for delay was poor neurologic and/or medical condition prior to transfer from the local hospital to the participating institution. The distribution was similar in patients allocated to drug-induced hypotension, carotid ligation and intracranial surgery. The interval from the first angiographic procedure to the day of randomization (the formal beginning of bed rest) was no more than two days in 69.2%, five days in 85.6% and eight days in 92.8%. Assuming that the first angiographic procedure was pursued in the uniform manner at each participating institution, the delay in randomization of more than five days in 14.4% was not unusual. The reasons for delay in those instances were not clarified.

Post-treatment Angiography

Among 76 patients who had post-treatment angiographic surveys for determination of the volumetric size of the aneurysm, the fundus portion of the aneurysm enlarged in 20 (26.3%), the dimensions remained unchanged in 16 (21.1%) and the aneurysm was smaller in 36 (47.3%). Information on the patient data form was insufficient for three patients. Although patients who died prior to post-treatment angiography did not have follow-up studies, among the survivors 26.3% (20 patients) had angiographic evidence of increased volume in the fundus portion of the aneurysm.

Morbidity Associated with Angiography

Unexpected deterioration in neurologic condition was regarded as a complication when it occurred during or within 24 hours after the angiographic procedure. Among 195 patients subjected to 268 procedures, 21 (10.8% of 195) had unexpected complications (Table 4–22). Among patients with an internal carotid aneurysm, 2 acquired hemiplegia and aphasia. In 1 patient the condition cleared eventually, and in the other it remained permanent and the patient died. One additional patient had transient hemiparesis which cleared in three hours. No patient rebled or had recognized hypotensive episodes. In the middle cerebral group, 1 patient had temporary hemiplegia and aphasia which cleared in 3 hours, 1 acquired permanent hemiparesis, 1 became poorly responsive without focal manifestations and died and 1 had a proved rebleed 18 hours after cerebral angiography. In the anterior cerebral group, 4 patients developed hemiparesis alone; in 2 the hemiparesis remained permanent, and in 2 it cleared within 3 hours. Three patients acquired temporary dysphasia which cleared in 3 to 6 hours. One patient acquired permanent hemiparesis and asphasia, 1 was lethargic following a left pneumothorax and died 4 days later, and 1 had temporary diplopia and increased headache. Three patients rebled, 1 fatally, and the other 2 became poorly responsive. One of these 2 patients died 5 days later, and the other died

Table 4–22.   Distribution of Patients with Complications Which Occurred During or Within 24 Hours After Angiographic Procedure.

Complicating Event	Internal Carotid	Middle Cerebral	Anterior Cerebral	Total
		Aneurysm Site		
Hemiplegia and aphasia	2	1	0	3
Hemiparesis alone	1	1	4	6
Hemiparesis and aphasia	0	0	1	1
Dysphasia alone	0	0	3	3
Rebleed (remained alive)	0	1	2	3
Rebleed (fatal)	0	0	1	1
Convulsions	0	0	1	1
Poorly responsive	0	1	0	1
Left pneumothorax and poorly responsive	0	0	1	1
Diplopia and headache	0	0	1	1
Total	3	4	14	21

5 months later. One additional patient developed convulsions during the procedure.

In summary, 5 patients (2.6%) died after their rebleed or ischemic deficit. Morbidity was 10.8%. It must be emphasized that the mortality and morbidity were associated with multiple angiographic procedures in acutely ill patients with a hemorrhagic cerebral vascular disorder. Many patients with subarachnoid hemorrhage are also at greater risk than those with an ischemic vascular disorder or with normal intracranial pressure.

Angiographic Abnormalities Associated with the Aneurysm

Abnormalities associated with single ruptured intracranial aneurysms were noted in 52 patients. A total of 54 lesions were reported among all aneurysm sites (Table 4–23). Intracerebral mass lesions were noted in 12.3% (24 of 195). Most lesions were consistent with a hematoma and/or localized area of cerebral swelling. Sixteen patients (8.2%) had increased sweep of the anterior cerebral vessels; 11 (5.6%) had evidence of an extracerebral mass lesion. Only 2 patients had an irregular intima consistent with intracranial atherosclerosis, and 1 had an infundibular dilatation.

For each aneurysm location, the most frequent abnormality was an intracerebral mass lesion as determined by angiographic examination. Correlation of intracerebral mass lesions (24), extracerebral mass lesions (11) and stretching of the anterior cerebral vessels (16) revealed that these lesions occurred 51 times in 54 patients. Such lesions are commonly associated with poor neurologic condition. Therefore, one would expect increased mortality with progressive clinical deterioration from direct cerebral effects of the bleed. Among 8 patients with an internal carotid aneurysm, 6 died: 4 after progressive deterioration in neurologic condition and 1 each from unrelated and unknown causes. Among 6 patients with a middle cerebral aneurysm, 5 died: 3 after a proved rebleed and 1 each after a suspected rebleed and unrelated cause. Among 31 patients with an anterior cerebral aneurysm, 19 died: 13 after a proved rebleed, 3 after a suspected rebleed, 2 from unrelated causes and 1 after progressive clinical deterioration. In summary, 30 deaths (66.7% of 45 patients) were associated with these angiographic findings. Sixteen of these deaths followed a proved rebleed, 5 followed progressive deterioration, 4 followed a suspected rebleed, and 4 were from unrelated and 1 from unknown causes. Comparison of the overall mortality of 55.1% in the bed rest treatment group with the 66.7% figure cannot be regarded as a statistically significant increase. Most deaths (16 of 30) followed a proved rebleed.

Cerebral Vasospasm

The angiographic demonstration of decreased intra-arterial size is usually regarded as cerebral vasospasm. Although the primary objective of this study was not the evaluation of vasospasm, the degree of arterial narrowing as interpreted on the cerebral angiogram was reported to the Central Registry. We are cognizant of the pitfalls in the analysis of the data submitted due to variation in the interpretation between one observer and another as to what actually constitutes vasospasm. Cerebral vasospasm was categorized on each angiogram as one of three degrees of severity: no vasospasm; localized vasospasm (narrowing of intra-arterial diameter over 1 to 3-cm distances on the proximal portions of the intracranial portion of the internal carotid artery, middle cerebral, anterior cerebral and vertebral-basilar artery); and diffuse vasospasm (narrowed diameter of the intracranial internal carotid artery and all the main ipsilateral branches). Various degrees of vasospasm were correlated with age, sex, neurologic condition, systolic and mean blood pressures, interval from last bleed to angiography, size of the aneurysm (mm^3) and mortality.

Age

The frequency of vasospasm among all aneurysm sites and age groups was 42.5% (82 of 193). The proportion of patients with vasospasm increased proportionately with age. A low figure of 16.7% was observed in the age group 10 to 19, with the highest incidence of 57.1% in the age group 60 to 69 (Table 4–24). Among the 7 patients in the age group 70 to 79, only 2 had localized involvement. Analysis of the entire group be-

Table 4-23.   Distribution of Associated Lesions in Addition to a Single Aneurysm at Angiographic Survey for Each Site.

Site	Angiographic Abnormality					
	Extracerebral Mass	Intracerebral Mass	Stretching of Anterior Cerebral	Irregular Intima (atherosclerosis)	Infundibular Dilatation	Total
Internal carotid (37)*	0	4	3	1	0	8
Middle cerebral (23)	0	4	2	0	0	6
Anterior cerebral (135)	11	16	11	1	1	40†
Total (195)	11	24	16	2	1	54‡

* Number of patients allocated to each site.
† Nine patients had more than one angiographic abnormality.
‡ Additional patients with miscellaneous findings included 4 with nonfilling of one anterior cerebral artery, 1 with displacement of midline vessels, 1 an occluded right internal carotid artery in the neck and 1 a superficial temporal artery aneurysm.

Table 4–24.   Age Distribution with Respect to Each Category of Vasospasm.

Age	Cerebral Vasospasm None	Localized*	Diffuse*	Total	% with Vasospasm
10–19	5	0	1	6	16.7
20–29	10	4	1	15	33.3
30–39	13	3	4	20	35.0
40–49	24	10	7	41	41.5
50–59	39	23	7	69	43.5
60–69	15	12	8	35	57.1
70–79	5	2	0	7	28.6
No data	—	—	—	2	—
Total	111	54	28	195	

* See text for definition. (p. 47).

low age 50 reveals 36.6% (30 of 82) had some degree of vasospasm, whereas in those patients who were 50 years of age or over, 46.8% had this condition. This difference was not statistically significant. However, vasospasm was present in all age groups, with a higher frequency among the older groups, especially among females (see Summary, p. 53).

Sex Distribution

Evaluation of sex distribution with each aneurysm site revealed that patients with an internal carotid aneurysm included 9 males and 28 females. In contrast, the proportion of males and females in the middle cerebral and anterior cerebral groups was very similar (Table 4–25). The distribution of patients with various degrees of vasospasm was proportional among each aneurysm location with the exception of females in the middle cerebral group, where 4 patients had no vasospasm, 3 had localized vasospasm and 4 had diffuse vasospasm. For all aneurysm sites combined, 37% (32 of 87) of men had variable degrees of vasospasm in comparison with 46.7% (50 of 107) of women.

Localized spasm must be clarified, particularly in relation to the A_1 segment of the anterior cerebral arteries. Differentiation between congenital narrowing of this segment and localized vasospasm was difficult in some instances. Analysis of the patient

Table 4–25.   Sex Distribution for Aneurysm Site and Degree of Vasospasm.

Aneurysm Site	Cerebral Vasospasm None	Localized	Diffuse	Total*
		MALES		
Internal carotid	7	2	0	9
Middle cerebral	8	3	1	12
Anterior cerebral	40	19	7	87
Total	55	24	8	87
		FEMALES		
Internal carotid	15	9	4	28
Middle cerebral	4	3	4	11
Anterior cerebral	38	18	12	68
Total	57	30	20	107

* There was insufficient information on 1 patient, making a total of 195.

Table 4–26.   Distribution of Patients with Respect to Interval from Last Bleed to First Angiographic Procedure Tabulated for Various Degrees of Vasospasm Among All Aneurysm Sites.

Interval*	Cerebral Vasospasm			Total	% Initial Angiogram Completed
	None	Localized	Diffuse		
0	4	3	0	7	
1	19	8	3	30	19.1
2	26	8	4	38	
3	15	4	3	22	50.0
4	7	8	2	17	
5	9	3	5	17	67.5
6	5	3	0	8	
7	9	0	1	10	76.8
8	2	1	0	3	
9	1	1	2	4	80.4
10	4	3	1	8	
11	1	1	1	3	86.1
12	1	2	2	5	
13	0	1	0	1	89.2
14	1	1	1	3	
Over 14	8	7	3	18	100.0
Total	112	54	28	194†	
%	57.7	27.8	14.4		

* Days from last bleed to first cerebral angiogram.
† No information was available on 1 patient, making a total of 195.

report forms reveals that unilateral narrowing of the A_1 segment proximal to the anterior communicating artery was observed in 8 of 37 patients with an aneurysm on the anterior cerebral complex. In 2 additional instances localized spasm was bilateral, and in 1 patient with an internal carotid aneurysm it was also bilateral. No instances of selected A_1 narrowing were reported in the middle cerebral group. Therefore, a total of 11 patients with "localized vasospasm" conceivably had congenital narrowing of the A_1 segment. This would reduce the total number of patients with localized and diffuse vasospasm to 71 (36.8% of 193) instead of 82 (42.5%), a difference which is not significant. Therefore, this observation can be disregarded in various correlative analyses.

Interval from Last Bleed to Initial Angiography

Analysis of the number of patients with and without vasospasm at specific intervals following last bleed revealed that 50% had their initial angiographic procedure within 3 days after the bleed. During this interval, 64 patients (66.0% of 97) had no vasospasm, 23 (23.7%) had localized vasospasm and 10 (10.3%) had diffuse involvement (Table 4–26). By comparison, among the 50% who had their initial angiographic procedure after the 3-day interval, 48 (49.5% of 97) had no vasospasm, 31 (32.0%) had localized spasm and 18 (18.6%) had diffuse vasospasm. Thus, a total of 49 patients (50.5%) had localized or diffuse vasospasm when the initial angiogram was performed 4 or more days after the last bleed. For all sites combined, this percentage was a 16.5% increase. Particularly during the 8 to 14-day interval (Fig. 4–3), the percentage of patients with vasospasm increased appreciably. The appearance of intraarterial narrowing, as demonstrated by cerebral angiography, had its peak incidence during that interval.

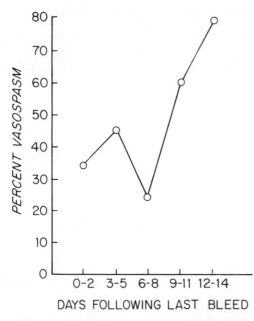

Fig. 4–3.   Percent of patients with localized and diffuse vasospasm at specific intervals after last bleed. Percentages plotted in the figure were calculated from the data in Table 4–26. For intervals greater than 6 days, small numbers represented.

Neurologic Condition

Correlation of neurologic deficit with specific degree of vasospasm reveals that patients in poor neurologic condition (Grades 3, 4 and 5) had a greater frequency of localized and diffuse arterial narrowing. Among various neurologic conditions, 30.6% of patients in Grade 2 had localized or severe vasospasm, 65.7% in Grade 3 and 58.8% in Grade 4 (Table 4–27). Comparison of good-condition patients (Grades 1 and 2) with those in poor condition (Grades 3, 4 and 5) reveals that in the former group 32.1% (43 of 134) had vasospasm (mostly localized), whereas 65.0% (39 of 60) of those in the latter group had localized or diffuse vasospasm in similar proportions (Table 4–27). The frequency and severity of arterial narrowing were significantly increased ($P < 0.001$) in poor-condition patients.

Systolic Blood Pressure

Four representative blood pressures, taken at more than 4-hour intervals between hospital admission and randomization, were recorded by the usual manometric technique. These four readings were averaged at the Central Registry. Average systolic values at various increments were tabulated with various degrees of cerebral vasospasm for all sites combined. Most patients (117 of 194, or 60.3%) had systolic values between 121 and 160 mm Hg (Table 4–28). Ninety-four patients (48.5% of 194) had systolic values of 140 mm Hg or below, 83 (42.8%) between 141 and 180 mm Hg and 17 (8.8%) had systolic values over 180 mm Hg. Therefore, nearly one-half of all patients had systolic values of 140 mm Hg or below. The percentage of patients with vasospasm at various increments varied between 31.3 and

Table 4–27.   Distribution of Neurologic Condition with Respect to Degree of Vasospasm for All Aneurysm Sites.

Neurologic Grade*	Cerebral Vasospasm			Total	% with Vasospasm
	None	Localized	Diffuse		
1	7	5	1	13	46.2
2	84	28	9	121	30.6
3	12	13	10	35	65.7
4	7	5	5	17	58.8
5	2	3	3	8	75.0
Total	112	54	28	194†	

* See Table 4–3 for definition.
† There was no information on 1 patient, making a total of 195.

Table 4–28. Distribution of Patients with Various Degrees of Vasospasm Tabulated with Respect to Designated Levels of Systolic Blood Pressure for All Aneurysm Sites.

Systolic Blood Pressure (mm Hg)	Cerebral Vasospasm			Total	% with Vasospasm
	None	Localized	Diffuse		
101–120	22	7	3	32	31.3
121–140	33	17	12	62	46.8
141–160	35	13	7	55	36.4
161–180	13	11	4	28	53.6
Over 180	9	6	2	17	47.1
Total	112	54	28	194*	42.3

* No information on 1, making a total of 195.

53.6% (Table 4–28). No association could be established whereby elevated systolic blood pressure suggested increased incidence of vasospasm.

Mean Blood Pressure

Mean blood pressures were calculated, using the data compiled for systolic and diastolic determinations. In order to determine the relationship of vasospasm to systolic and diastolic values, mean blood pressure distribution was compared with various degrees of vasospasm.

Forty-nine patients (25.3% of 194) had mean blood pressures varying from 95 to 104 mm Hg (Table 4–29). Most patients (81.4% or 158 of 194) had mean pressures between 85 and 124 mm Hg. In this group, 42.4% (67 of 158) had localized or diffuse vasospasm. The ratio of patients with vasospasm versus those without vasospasm varied among various values of mean blood pressure. No evidence of an association was observed between elevated mean pressure and severity of vasospasm.

Size of Aneurysm

Measurements of the intraluminal diameter of the aneurysm on the cerebral angiogram were recorded at each participating institution. We are cognizant of variations in measurements taken from one institution to an-

Table 4–29. Distribution of Mean Blood Pressure Tabulated with Respect to Various Degrees of Vasospasm for All Aneurysm Sites.

Mean Blood Pressure	Cerebral Vasospasm			Total	% with Vasospasm
	None	Localized	Diffuse		
65–74	2	0	0	2	0.0
75–84	6	2	2	10	40.0
85–94	25	12	4	41	39.0
95–104	24	14	11	49	51.0
105–114	26	8	4	38	31.6
115–124	16	11	3	30	46.7
125–134	12	3	2	17	29.4
135–144	1	2	2	5	80.0
Over 144	0	2	0	2	100.0
Total	112	54	28	194*	

* No information on 1, making a total of 195.

Table 4–30. Distribution of Aneurysm Size Tabulated with Respect to Degree of Vasospasm for All Sites Combined.

Size (mm³)*	Cerebral Vasospasm			
	None	Localized	Diffuse	Total
1–100	29	18	6	53
101–200	26	11	5	42
201–300	21	5	8	34
301–400	9	4	2	15
401–600	9	3	3	15
601–900	5	3	1	9
901–1400	5	3	1	9
1401–2200	3	5	1	9
Over 2200	5	2	1	8
Total	112	54	28	194†

* See text for method of calculation. (p. 51)
† Insufficient information on 1, making a total of 195.

other. Each dimension was reported to the nearest fraction of a millimeter. All volumetric determinations were calculated at the Central Registry. The median volumetric size was 200 mm³. The group with an aneurysmal volume below 200 mm³ had a 42.1% incidence of vasospasm (Table 4–30). The group of patients with volumetric measurements above 200 mm³ had a similar frequency of vasospasm (42.4% or 42 of 99). Therefore, aneurysm size was unrelated to the incidence of vasospasm.

Mortality

Increased mortality and degree of vasospasm were related to poor neurologic condition. The relationship of mortality to various degrees of vasospasm was also analyzed.

In patients with no vasospasm, 52.3% died among all aneurysm sites combined. This figure compares with 57.4% and 61.5% among those patients with localized and diffuse vasospasm, respectively (Table 4–31). Therefore, vasospasm alone was unrelated to mortality on a statistical basis.

Summary of Vasospasm Data

The role of vasospasm in the production of neurologic dysfunction in patients with subarachnoid hemorrhage has not been fully investigated in this study, and only some general statements can be made. Neither does this analysis fully contribute to a clear understanding of the problem. However, these data suggest that poor neurologic condition

Table 4–31. Distribution of Degree of Vasospasm with Respect to Each Aneurysm Site.

Aneurysm Site	Cerebral Vasospasm			
	None	Localized	Diffuse	Total
Internal carotid	21 (6)*	11 (9)	3 (3)	35 (18)
Middle cerebral	11 (9)	6 (2)	5 (2)	22 (13)
Anterior cerebral	75 (41)	37 (20)	18 (11)	130 (72)
Total	107 (56)	54 (31)	26 (16)	187† (103)
%	52.3	57.4	61.5	55.1

* Number in parentheses denotes deaths.
† Total patients with treatment followed according to protocol.

has a close relationship to vasospasm in comparison with other variables under consideration. The severity of neurologic deficit correlated highly with the presence of some degree of vasospasm. Analysis of sex distribution shows that females with an internal carotid aneurysm had a higher incidence of vasospasm than males. Too few patients with a middle cerebral aneurysm were collected for making a definite conclusion. There was no correlation between males and females with a ruptured aneurysm on the anterior cerebral complex. The parameter of age and the severity of vasospasm revealed no statistical relationship, but the average percentage of patients with vasospasm was 10% higher in those above 50 years of age versus those in the 5th decade or below. No relationship to vasospasm was observed for variables such as average systolic or mean blood pressures, aneurysm size or mortality.

Discussion

Patients allocated to regulated bed rest provided a baseline and control for comparison of effectiveness of the other treatment modalities. Every effort was made by each participating institution to conduct this therapeutic program in as uniform a manner as possible. The adequacy of randomization was evaluated with respect to age, sex, aneurysm site, neurologic and medical conditions and vasospasm. These parameters were all found to be in proper distribution for all aneurysm sites.

Patient distribution in the bed rest treatment group was 9.1% for those in the age group 30 to 39, 23.1% in the age group 40 to 49, 34.4% in the age group 50 to 59 and 17.2% in the age group 60 to 69. This distribution was similar to that reported by Pakarinen[6] (14.0, 29.8, 30.9 and 12.1%, respectively), and it also concurs with his review of several published reports.

Comparison of the results of this study with nonrandomized published reports is somewhat hazardous because conservatively treated patients usually form a highly selected portion of the representative sample undergoing analysis. Therefore, the results for morbidity and mortality tend to be inordinately high in such groups. Patients in Logue's series[7] who were treated conservatively and followed 17 months to 9 years had a 59% (20 of 34) recurrent bleed rate, with a mortality of 41% from such recurrences. In a series of 115 patients[8] treated conservatively and followed an average of 5 years (varying from 1.5 to 23 years), 55% (63 of 115) had a recurrent bleed. Forty-eight of these (42%) were fatal. In Parkarinen's series,[6] the 116 patients treated conservatively (i.e., 1 month of bed rest) included a very selected group. Sixty-four deaths occurred before angiographic demonstration of the aneurysm. Furthermore, 66 patients were more than 50 years of age. Among the 68 deaths, 60 occurred during the 1st week after onset of symptoms. Recurrent bleeding episodes for the total series were at 51.7%, with an incidence of 40.1% at 8 weeks. Cumulative mortality 2 weeks after last bleed was 21.6%, at the 4th week 39.7%, and at the 6th week 47.4%. These figures did not include the preoperative patients. By comparison, the cumulative mortality in the present study was 14.4% at the end of the 2nd week, 27.7% at the 4th week and 32.3% at the 6th week. However, comparison of all conservatively treated patients in Pakarinen's series (including all those prior to operation) reveals that 13.2% died within 2 weeks, 26.6% within 4 weeks and 36.7% within 6 weeks after the last bleed. These percentages, interestingly, show a striking similarity to those of the present study. The values presented in this study probably represent a mortality which is nearest to the actual natural course following subarachnoid hemorrhage from a ruptured intracranial aneurysm in patients admitted to referral centers. After this 6-week interval mortality rises slowly.

In a randomized trial[2] stratified with respect to age, hypertension, clinical condition and interval following last bleed to the beginning of treatment, 42 patients with an aneurysm at the junction of the internal carotid and posterior communicating artery were treated with 6 weeks of bed rest. Six months after the bleed, 35.7% had died. In the present study, 48.6% (18 of 37) died during the 6-month interval following last bleed. With regard to patients with a middle cerebral aneurysm,[9] 36.9% died within 6 months after the last bleed. In this study, 50.0% (11 of 22) died during that interval. Mortality in patients with an anterior cerebral-anterior communicating aneurysm in the randomized trial of McKissock et al.[10] was 39.8% (61 of 153) at 6 months (28.7% died following a rebleed within 28 days after the last bleed). In this study, aneurysms on the anterior cerebral-anterior communicating complex had a cumulative mortality of 23.1% at 4 weeks, 30.0% at the end of 6 weeks and 39.2% (51 of 130) at 6 months. These figures compare favorably with the series from London for each aneurysm site.

Recurrent hemorrhage within 2 months after the bleed has been the major cause of death in many published reports of unoperated patients. In undifferentiated subarachnoid hemorrhage reviewed by Pakarinen,[6] an average of 32.3% rebled within 8 weeks after their initial bleed, the major proportion occurring in the 2nd and 3rd weeks (10.1% and 8.0%, respectively). In Pakarinen's series of patients who had proved aneurysm (107), including preoperative recurrences in patients eventually treated operatively, 83 patients (77.5%) had a recurrent bleed within 8 weeks. Fourteen (13.1%) occurred during the 1st week, 19 (17.8%) during the 2nd, 14 (13.1%) during the 3rd and 21 (19.6%) during the 4th. Therefore, a total of 63.5% rebled within 4 weeks, with an additional 14.0% in the following 2 weeks. This high rebled rate shows the importance of differentiating subarachnoid hemorrhage due to ruptured aneurysm alone, rather than including all cases in an undifferentiated series. In addition, the influence of patient selection (nonsurgical patients) was also apparent. Furthermore, aneurysm location can be influential. In the random-

ized series[2] of 42 conservatively treated patients with an internal carotid aneurysm, 21 (50%) rebled within 6 weeks, and 15 of these died (71.4%, 15 of 21). Most of them (12) occurred during the 4 to 6-week interval. In the present study, 5 patients (14.3%) with an internal carotid aneurysm rebled within 2 weeks, 6 (17.1%) in 4 weeks and 9 (25.7%)in 6 weeks, with no further rebleeds to the end of the 8-week interval. Essentially, these percentages relate the number of rebleeds which occurred during treatment with bed rest. Twenty-six patients began their official period of bed rest within 7 days after last bleed. However, when consideration was given to the number of rebleeds which occurred during the interval prior to hospitalization, 8 patients had clinical neurologic symptoms or signs of an initial bleed during a 60-day interval preceding the bleed prompting admission to the reporting hospital. Among all 37 patients with an internal carotid aneurysm, 8 had two bleeds prior to official commencement of bed rest. Nine additional patients rebled within 6 weeks after entry into the study. Therefore, a total of 17 patients (48.6%) with recurrent hemorrhage was reported over a period of 14 weeks.

Analysis of those patients from the study who started their bed rest program within 7 days after the last bleed showed that 5 of 26 patients (20.0%) rebled in 14 days, 6 (24.0%) rebled within 4 weeks, and a total of 9 (36.0%) in 8 weeks. The rebleed rate among patients with an internal carotid aneurysm in the Cooperative Study[11] (nonrandomized) was 19.6% (70 of 358) at 14 days and 24.3% (87 of 358) at the end of 28 days (4 weeks). The rebleed rate at 6-week interval was not reported.

In the randomized trial of McKissock et al.,[9] 18 of 55 (32.7%) conservatively treated patients with a middle cerebral aneurysm rebled during the initial 2-week interval, 40.0% (22 of 55) during the 3-week interval and 41.8% (23 of 55) during the 4-week interval, with no recurrent hemorrhages to the end of 6 weeks. In the present study, 13.6% (3 of 22) rebled during the initial 14-day period, 36.4% (8 of 22) at 30 days, with no further rebleeds to the end of 6 weeks. In the Cooperative Study series[11] (nonrandomized), 13.8% (49 of 355) rebled during the 14-day interval, and 16.9% (60 of 355) by the end of 4 weeks. The data at 6 weeks were not reported.

The randomized series[10] of anterior communicating aneurysms treated conservatively had a rebleed rate of 24.2% (37 of 153) during the first 14 days, with 34.6% (53 of 153) having a rebleed during the 4-week interval following the bleed prior to hospitalization. In the present study, 16.2% (21 of 130) rebled during the first 2 weeks following last bleed and a total of 27.7% (36 of 130) within 30 days. In the previous Cooperative Study,[11] 24.5% (130 of 530) rebled within 14 days and 27.0% (143 of 530) within 4 weeks. No statistical differences were observed among the three studies at these intervals following the bleed.

Mortality among patients following recurrent hemorrhages in the previous Cooperative Study[11] was 46% for internal carotid aneurysms, 41% for middle cerebral aneurysms and 42% for anterior cerebral-anterior communicating aneurysms. In the present study, death due to rebleeding at 30 days was 14.3% (5 of 35) for patients with an internal carotid aneurysm, 31.8% (7 of 22) for those with a middle cerebral aneurysm and 19.2% (25 of 130) for patients with an anterior cerebral-anterior communicating aneurysm. In Pakarinen's series,[6] 77.5% died following recurrent hemorrhage. Mortality during the 6-week interval in the conservatively treated patients in the randomized trial[2,9,10] among those who had a second bleed was 50.0% (21 of 42, Category B) for patients with an internal carotid aneurysm, 32.7% (18 of 55) for those with a middle cerebral aneurysm and 34.0% (52 of 153) for the anterior cerebral-anterior communicating group. In general, mortality of nonsurgically treated patients is lower in studies conducted with a design of randomization in comparison with the number of deaths reported from a nonrandomized selection.

The wide spectrum of clinical manifestations of subarachnoid hemorrhage following ruptured intracranial aneurysm was confirmed in this investigation. Most patients were in good neurologic condition after their initial bleed. Sixty-seven percent were in Grades 1 and 2, 19.5% (38 of 195) were in Grade 3 and 13.3% (26 of 195) were lethargic with varying degrees of neurologic deficit (Grades 4 and 5). The number of patients with severe central nervous system deficits from the initial rupture was small. More patients experience minimal symptoms frequently, which is consistent with minor bleeding episodes. A timely report[12] suggests that such symptoms occur in 21.4% (24 of 112) as a warning sign. In the present study, 14.8% (30 of 202) had a recent history of symptoms characterized by headache or neck or back pain as manifestations of meningeal irritation. In at least one fourth of patients with initial rupture of an intracranial aneurysm, symptoms and signs are relatively minor. By far, the most typical presentation was that complex of symptoms shown by patients in Grade 2, namely, severe headache, meningeal signs and varying degrees of nausea and vomiting, with a transient episode of amnesia in some instances.

Sex distribution has been of particular interest among patients with an internal carotid-posterior communicating aneurysm. For this treatment category, 8 were males and 27 were females. This distribution was similar among all four treatment categories. Sex distribution among patients with a middle cerebral and anterior cerebral-anterior communicating aneurysm was nearly equal. The reason for this peculiar distribution of more females among patients with rupture of an internal carotid aneurysm remains unexplained.

Among 76 patients who rebled, 65 died. Twenty-eight patients (36.8%, Table 4–16) rebled during the interval from the 5th through the 14th day following last bleed. The most crucial interval was this period. A unique feature was the distribution of rebleeds among patients with an anterior cerebral-anterior communicating aneurysm. These patients continued to have the most prolonged interval to recurrent hemorrhage, an observation which remains unexplained.

This study appraises and confirms the variation in intervals to recurrent hemorrhages among aneurysm sites. At one end of this spectrum were the so-called "minor bleeds" which may herald a warning sign an average of two weeks prior to the more severe ictus.[12] At the opposite end were those who had one severe hemorrhagic catastrophe with devastating effects to the central system at the initial rupture. Between these two extremes was the large group of patients with symptoms characterized by headache, nausea, vomiting and usually transient loss of consciousness which prompted medical attention. This group comprised nearly 70% of the entire patient population.

Particular attention must be focused on those patients who had their work-up completed and were allocated to therapy within 7 days following subarachnoid hemorrhage. This group probably provides the most important information with respect to the number of concrete observations that are associated with subarachnoid hemorrhage following a ruptured intracranial aneurysm. In the group with minor symptoms, too many factors may not appear clinically distinct from other common disorders. In the severe catastrophic lesions, the central nervous system was too extensively and too rapidly damaged to make a definite course of therapy of any value. Patients allocated to treatment within 7 days after last bleed had the highest death rate during the 5th through 20th day (Fig. 4–2). During this interval, rebleeding was the most frequent cause of death for all aneurysm sites. Patients allocated to treatment after the 7-day interval were distributed similarly among the various neurologic conditions as compared with those patients allocated to treatment within 7 days. With 66% of all patients allocated to treatment during the 7-day interval, the risk of rebleeding was most substantial among patients with an internal carotid aneurysm, followed by those with a middle cerebral

aneurysm. Patients with an anterior cerebral-anterior communicating aneurysm had the lowest rate of recurrent hemorrhage.

Various medical conditions which were present prior to rupture were relatively infrequent. The most frequent condition prior to rupture was pre-existing hypertension. Only 18% had known hypertension, a frequency which would not lead one to designate hypertension as an underlying cause for an aneurysm to rupture. Mortality in this group was 61.1%, a percentage not significantly different from the gross mortality of 55.1%

Conclusions

1. During the interval from June 15, 1963, through February 15, 1970, 202 patients with a single intracranial aneurysm were randomly allocated to regulated bed rest. After the last bleed, 124 were allocated to treatment within 7 days, 49 during the 8 to 21-day interval and 14 during the 22 to 92-day interval.
2. Thirty-seven patients had a single aneurysm on the intracranial portion of the internal carotid system, 23 had an aneurysm on the middle cerebral distribution, 135 on the anterior cerebral-anterior communicating complex and 7 on the vertebral-basilar system. There were 90 men and 112 women.
3. Eight patients failed to receive their designated treatment. Subtracting these 8 patients, in addition to the 7 with a vertebral-basilar aneurysm, allowed a remainder of 187 for correlative analysis.
4. During the mean follow-up interval of 6.5 years, mortality was 55.1%. Cumulative mortality was 62.9% for those patients randomized within 7 days, 40.8% for those randomized during the 8 to 21-day interval and 35.7% for those allocated to treatment during the 22 through 92-day interval.
5. Eleven patients in Grade 1 neurologic condition had a 36.4% mortality. Among

117 patients in Grade 2, 48.7% died; among 36 patients in Grade 3 and 15 patients in Grade 4, 66.7% died; and among 7 patients in Grade 5, all died.

6. For all aneurysm sites, a proved rebleed was the cause of death in 34.2%, progressive deterioration from aneurysm rupture in 8.0% and a suspected rebleed in 4.8%. A total of 47.1% died from causes related directly to the cerebral effects of the ruptured aneurysm.

7. Mortality in good-medical-condition patients was not significantly different in the groups below or above age 50. Among patients in fair and poor medical conditions, mortality above age 50 was significantly higher than for those below that age.

8. For all aneurysm sites, patients allocated to bed rest within 7 days after last bleed had the highest mortality and rebleed rate.

9. In 37.4% of patients, several medical disorders needed medical attention during the treatment period. The most frequent conditions were pulmonary or genitourinary tract infections.

10. Unexpected deterioration in neurologic condition occurred during or within 24 hours after angiography in 10.8%. Mortality associated with this procedure was 2.6%.

11. The incidence of vasospasm as demonstrated by cerebral angiography was 42.5%. In patients below age 50, 36.6% had definite evidence of vasospasm; for those age 50 or above, 46.8% had this condition.

12. For patients in good neurologic condition (Grades 1 and 2), 32.1% had vasospasm, whereas in poor-condition patients (Grades 3, 4, 5), 65.0% had some degree of vasospasm.

13. Systolic and mean blood pressures were statistically unrelated to the frequency or severity of vasospasm.

14. Aneurysm size was unrelated statistically to the incidence of vasospasm.

15. Mortality among patients with no vasospasm was 52.3%. In the group of patients with localized vasospasm, 57.4% died. In patients with diffuse vasospasm, the mortality was 61.5%

References

1. McKissock, W., Paine, K., Wash, L.: Further observations on subarachnoid haemorrhage. J Neurol Neurosurg Psychiat 21:239–248, 1958.
2. McKissock, W., Richardson, A., Wash, L.: "Posterior-communicating" aneurysms: Controlled trial of the conservative and surgical treatment of ruptured aneurysms of the internal carotid artery at or near the point of origin of the posterior communicating artery. Lancet 1:1203–1206, 1960.
3. Sahs, A.L.: Cooperative study of intracranial aneurysms and subarachnoid hemorrhage: Report on a randomized treatment study: I. Introduction. Stroke 5:550–551, 1974.
4. Nibbelink, D.W., Knowler, L.A.: Cooperative study of intracranial aneurysms and subarachnoid hemorrhage: Report on a randomized treatment study: II. Objectives and design of randomized aneurysm study. Stroke 5:552–556, 1974.
5. Graf, C.J., Nibbelink, D.W.: Cooperative study of intracranial aneurysms and subarachnoid hemorrhage: Report on a randomized treatment study: III. Intracranial surgery. Stroke 5:557–601, 1974.
6. Pakarinen, S.: Incidence, aetiology, and prognosis of primary subarachnoid haemorrhage. Acta Neurol Scand Suppl 29, pp 1–128, 1967.
7. Logue, V.: Surgery in spontaneous subarachnoid haemorrhage: Operative treatment of aneurysms on the anterior cerebral and anterior communicating artery. Brit Med J 1:473–479, 1956.
8. Tappura, M.: Prognosis of subarachnoid haemorrhage: Study of 120 patients with unoperated intracranial arterial aneurysms and 267 patients without vascular lesions demonstrable in bilateral carotid angiograms. Acta Med Scand Suppl 392, pp 1–75, 1962.
9. McKissock, W., Richardson, A., Walsh, L.: "Middle cerebral" aneurysms: Further results in the controlled trial of conservative and surgical treatment of ruptured intracranial aneurysms. Lancet 2:417–421, 1962.
10. McKissock, W., Richardson, A., Walsh, L.: "Anterior communicating" aneurysms: Trial of conservative and surgical treatment. Lancet 1:873–876, 1965.

11. Sahs, A.L., Perret, G.E., Locksley, H.B. et al.: Intracranial Aneurysms and Subarachnoid Hemorrhage. A Cooperative Study. J.B. Lippincott Co, Philadelphia, 1969.

12. Okawara, S.: Warning signs prior to rupture of an intracranial aneurysm. J Neurosurg 38:575–580, 1973.

Chapter 5

Randomized Treatment Study. Regulated Bed Rest: Statistical Evaluation

William G. Henderson, M.P.H., Ph.D., James C. Torner, M.S. and Donald W. Nibbelink, M.D., Ph.D.

Abstract

Regulated bed rest was one of four treatment modalities evaluated in a randomized clinical trial for patients with a ruptured intracranial aneurysm conducted between 1963 and 1970. A life table method of statistical analysis was used to determine cumulative mortality and rebleeding rate during a 5-year follow-up period for 187 patients in this treatment program and for subgroups of this patient sample. Linear discriminant function analysis was used to develop equations of clinical variables to predict mortality and rebleeding during the 90-day period following the bleed.

The clinical variables found to be most indicative of mortality included a poor initial neurologic and medical state and sex (male). Other variables somewhat indicative of high mortality but not reaching statistical significance included a short interval from last bleeding to treatment, high mean blood pressure and a large aneurysm. Aneurysm site, age, number of bleeds, pre-existing hypertension and evidence of vasospasm were not indicative of higher mortality.

The clinical variables found to be most related to rebleeding included a short interval from the last bleed to treatment and sex (male). Other variables less related to rebleeding but not reaching statistical significance included a high mean blood pressure and the number of bleeds in the medical history. Aneurysm site, initial neurologic and medical state, age, aneurysm size, pre-existing hypertension and evidence of vasospasm did not appear to be related to rebleeding.

The discriminant functions derived were used to reclassify the subjects into dead and alive, and rebleeding and no rebleeding, 90 days after initial hemorrhage. The misclassification percentages were substantial, making doubtful the prediction of mortality and rebleeding.

Introduction

Regulated bed rest was one of four treatment modalities studied in a randomized clinical trial conducted between 1963 and 1970 in patients with a ruptured intracranial aneurysm. The other three treatment programs were: (1) drug-induced hypotension with regulated bed rest, (2) ipsilateral common carotid artery occlusion with bed rest and (3) intracranial surgery. An introduction to the study,[1] the objectives and design of the study,[2] a comparison of the treatment groups,[3] a detailed analysis of intracranial surgery[4] and a medical analysis of bed rest[5] can be found in appropriate chapters. The purpose of this report is to provide a statistical analysis of the clinical factors associated with mortality and rebleeding in those treated with bed rest. Although bed rest therapy alone is outmoded as an early treatment of recently ruptured intracranial aneurysms, the results of this analysis are considered to be of importance, because the outcome of patients treated with regulated bed rest most closely approximates the natural history of the disease.

Methods

Between June 15, 1963, and February 15, 1970, 202 patients were assigned randomly to the regulated bed rest treatment category. All patients except 8 completed their designated period of bed rest. Among the remaining 194 patients, 35 had an internal carotid artery aneurysm, 22 had a middle cerebral artery aneurysm, 130 had an anterior cerebral-anterior communicating artery aneurysm and 7 had an aneurysm on the vertebral-basilar arterial system (Table 5–1). On June 19, 1967, collection of protocols from patients with a vertebral-basilar aneurysm was suspended, and this group was

eliminated from all statistical analyses because the sample size was too small.

Patients allocated to the bed rest treatment program remained at regulated bed rest for 21 days following formal initiation of this therapeutic program. Details of the treatment were described in a previous report.[5] Characteristics of the patient sample, including specific aneurysm location, interval from last bleed to treatment, initial neurologic condition, initial medical condition (Table 5–2), age, sex, blood pressure, size of aneurysm, number of previous bleeds, pre-existing hypertension and evidence of vasospasm, were also presented.[5]

The individual effects of selected clinical variables on mortality and rebleeding were analyzed statistically using a method adapted from the transient survivorship analysis of Mantel and Byar.[6] The mortality and rebleeding rates were calculated on the basis of the interval from the day of the last bleed prior to randomization to the day of death or rebleeding. A patient was only considered at risk after the day of randomization. Statistical testing of differences in 5-year mortality and rebleed rates was done using a method reported by Koch, Johnson, and Tolley.[7] The reported probability level (P-value) was interpreted as a suggestion of a trend in mortality or rebleeding rate and was not considered a test for a hypothesis of no difference in mortality or rebleeding among variables. Adequate sample sizes for testing hypotheses of clinical variables within treatment categories were not specified in the original protocol, since the primary purpose of the study was to compare the number of

Table 5–1. Distribution of Patients Allocated to Bed Rest Therapy by Site and Interval from Last Bleed to Randomization.

Days to Randomization	Aneurysm Site			
	Internal Carotid No. (%)	Middle Cerebral No. (%)	Anterior Cerebral No. (%)	Total No. (%)
0–7	25 (71.4)	12 (54.6)	87 (66.9)	124 (66.3)
8–21	6 (17.1)	7 (31.8)	36 (27.7)	49 (26.2)
22–92	4 (11.5)	3 (13.6)	7 (5.4)	14 (7.5)
Total	35 (100.0)	22 (100.0)	130 (100.0)	187 (100.0)

deaths and rebleedings among four treatment modalities.

Linear discriminant function analysis was used to develop equations of the clinical variables to predict early mortality and rebleeding. The program used was a modification of the subroutine of La Motte and Hocking[8] which was originally developed for regression analysis. The adaptation was done by Ramberg and Enochson.[9] Misclassification rates for the discriminant analysis were calculated using a procedure reported by Lachenbruch.[10]

Results

Mortality

The cumulative mortality, computed from deaths directly related to the ruptured aneurysm, was analyzed during a 5-year period following the bleed. Incremental mortality was greatest (29%) during the 1st month following the initial bleed (Table 5–3). Between the 1st and 3rd months, the incremental mortality was 9%. Following the initial 3-month interval, mortality was 3% between 3 and 6 months, 1% between 6 months and 1 year and 1 to 3% for each yearly interval thereafter up to 5 years. At the end of the 5th year, cumulative mortality was 50%.

Rebleeding

Rebleeding during the follow-up interval followed a trend similar to that of mortality (Table 5–6). Thirty percent of the patients rebled during the 1st month. The increment to cumulative rebleeds was 7% between the 1st and 3rd months, and 1% between the 3rd and 6th months. The increment also remained at 1% between 6 months and 1 year. The incidence of rebleeding varied from 1 to 3% for each yearly interval thereafter up

Table 5–2. Definitions.

Rebleed (Proved):
First recurrent hemorrhage following the last prerandomization bleed diagnosed by lumbar puncture or postmortem examination

Aneurysm-Related Death:
Primary cause of death noted to be from a proved rebleed, an episode highly suggestive of rebleeding, or progressive clinical deterioration from complications of the prerandomization bleed

Neurologic Condition on day of randomization:
Grade
1 = symptom-free
2 = minor symptoms (headache, meningeal irritation, diplopia)
3 = major neurologic deficit but fully responsive
4 = impaired state of alertness but capable of protective or other adaptive responses to noxious stimuli
5 = poorly responsive but with stable vital signs
6 = no response to address or shaking, non-adaptive response to noxious stimuli *and* progressive instability of vital signs

Medical Condition:
Good—patients who were alert, normotensive, with no more than a degree of fever, and in good health prior to subarachnoid hemorrhage
Fair—patients with a single underlying medical problem such as hypertension, cirrhosis of the liver, advanced age, anemia, poor nutrition, generalized atherosclerosis or chronic pulmonary disease
Poor—patients with more than one adverse factor or one medical condition which was particularly severe
Prohibitive—patients with a complicated illness with one or more undesirable conditions

to 5 years. At the end of the 5th year, cumulative rebleeding was 47%.

Effect of Selected Clinical Variables Upon Mortality

Variables with a potential relationship to mortality and rebleeding included the aneurysm site, the interval from last bleeding to treatment, the initial neurologic condition, initial medical condition, age, sex, mean blood pressure, size of aneurysm, number of proved and suspected bleedings, pre-existing hypertension and vasospasm. The influence of these variables was analyzed individually with respect to mortality and rebleeding. The combined influence of these variables upon mortality and rebleeding, using the statistical technique of discriminant function analysis, will be described below.

Aneurysm Site

In Table 5–3, cumulative mortality is presented for the aneurysm site. Mortality for patients with a middle cerebral artery aneurysm (47% at the end of 1 month to 63% at the end of 5 years) was highest during all follow-up periods. Mortality during the 1st month for patients with an anterior cerebral-anterior communicating artery aneurysm was less than for patients with an internal carotid aneurysm (26 vs 32%). However, at the end of 6 months the mortality among patients with an anterior cerebral-anterior communicating aneurysm was similar to that of patients with an internal carotid aneurysm. The percentage of deaths was higher for those with anterior cerebral-anterior communicating artery aneurysm during the 1-year to 5-year follow-up period. The chi-square test comparing the three mortality curves was not statistically significant ($P = 0.596$).

Interval from Last Bleeding to Treatment

The interval from last bleeding to treatment (Table 5–3) appeared to be related to mortality. Except for the first time period ($1/12$ year) when mortality for patients allocated to treatment during the 8 to 21-day and 22 to 92-day interval was reversed, mortality declined as the interval from last bleeding to treatment increased. One explanation may be that patients who were more severely ill may have sought treatment sooner than those in better condition. Also, patients with a longer interval following last bleeding survived the critical early period immediately following a bleeding episode, and may thus have had a better prognosis. The latter hypothesis is more likely, because the percentage of patients in poor neurologic condition allocated to treatment within the 8 to 21-day interval was not significantly different from the percentage of patients with the

Table 5–3. Aneurysm-Related Cumulative Mortality Rates (%) for Variables Specific to the Aneurysm and Interval to Treatment.

Variable	Initial Sample Size	Follow-up Period (Years)								Significance Level
		$1/12$	$1/4$	$1/2$	1	2	3	4	5	
Aneurysm site										
Internal carotid	35	32	38	38	38	38	38	38	38	$\chi^2 = 1.035$
Middle cerebral	22	47	56	56	56	56	56	56	63	$P = 0.596^*$
Anterior cerebral-anterior communicating	130	26	36	39	40	44	46	49	51	
Size of aneurysm										
$\leqq 200$ mm^3	75	30	36	36	36	38	39	41	45	$\chi^2 = 2.357$
> 200 mm^3	94	34	44	49	50	54	55	58	58	$P = 0.125$
Number of proved and suspected bleeds in history										
1	160	29	37	39	40	43	45	47	49	$\chi^2 = 1.030$
2 or 3	27	31	47	50	50	50	50	56	56	$P = 0.310$
Interval from last bleed to treatment										
0–7 days	124	36	45	47	49	53	53	55	56	$\chi^2 = 3.877$
8–21 days	49	14	27	29	29	29	34	37	39	$P = 0.144$
22–92 days	14	20	20	20	20	20	20	20	31	
Overall	187	29	38	41	42	44	45	48	50	

* Statistical test of the difference in 5-year mortality rates based on the mortality rates at each specified interval adjusted for lost-to-follow-up and deaths of unrelated causes.

Table 5-4.   Aneurysm-Related Cumulative Mortality Rates (%) for Clinical Variables Related to the Patient's Condition.

Variable	Initial Sample Size	Follow-up Period (Years)								Significance Level
		1/12	1/4	1/2	1	2	3	4	5	
Initial neurologic condition (Grade)*										
1, 2	128	24	32	33	35	38	39	42	45	$\chi^2 = 4.011$
3, 4, 5	59	40	52	58	58	58	61	61	61	$P = 0.045$
Initial medical condition*										
Good	102	20	30	31	33	37	38	40	45	$\chi^2 = 5.229$
Fair	56	36	43	45	45	47	47	50	50	$P = 0.073$
Poor or prohibitive	29	51	58	66	66	66	75	75	75	
Evidence of vasospasm										
None	106	29	33	35	37	42	43	46	49	$\chi^2 = 0.528$
Local	54	30	45	49	49	49	49	49	49	$P = 0.768$
Diffuse	26	32	48	48	48	48	53	53	59	
Mean blood pressure										
≤110 mm Hg	127	26	37	40	40	41	42	44	47	$\chi^2 = 2.000$
>110 mm Hg	60	36	41	43	45	51	54	57	60	$P = 0.157$
Overall	187	29	38	41	42	44	45	48	50	

* See Table 5-2.

same condition allocated within 7 days following last bleed. The overall chi-square test was close to being statistically significant at the 5% level.

Neurologic Condition

Patients in good neurologic condition (Grades 1 and 2, Table 5-4) had a 24% mortality at the end of 1 month following last bleeding. Those with more severe initial neurologic deficits had a 40% mortality at the end of 1 month. The cumulative mortality increased in both groups with time. The initial difference in mortality was maintained throughout the 5-year period. The overall chi-square test was statistically significant at the 5% level.

Medical Condition

Initial medical condition on day of randomization was classified as good, fair, poor and prohibitive (see Table 5-2 for definition). The last two categories were combined because the patient sample was small in each group. A pronounced effect of medical condition upon mortality was observed. One month following last bleeding, mortality among the three groups (good, fair, poor/ prohibitive medical conditions) was 20, 36 and 51%, respectively (Table 5-4). These differences remained unchanged throughout the 5-year period, although the cumulative mortalities for patients in good and fair medical conditions tended to converge by the end of the 5th year (45 and 50%, respectively). Seventy-five percent of patients in the poor/prohibitive group died during the 5-year interval. The overall chi-square test was close to significance at the 5% level ($P = 0.073$), while the tests for groups taken two at a time were significant at the 5% level.

Age

Patients were divided into four groups by age for purposes of this analysis. These groups included patients whose age was less than 20, 20 to 39, 40 to 59 and 60 or over

Table 5-5. Aneurysm-Related Cumulative Mortality Rates (%) for Variables Related to the Patient's Characteristics.

Variable	Initial Sample Size	Follow-up Period (Years)								Significance Level
		1/12	1/4	1/2	1	2	3	4	5	
Sex of patient										
Male	83	32	40	45	46	50	52	57	59	$\chi^2 = 3.410$ $P = 0.065$
Female	104	27	37	37	38	39	40	40	43	
Age of patient										
<20 yr	6	20	20	20	20	20	20	20	20	$\chi^2 = 1.378$ $P = 0.711$
20–39	32	29	38	38	38	38	38	38	38	
40–59	107	28	39	41	42	45	47	51	53	
≥60	41	33	41	46	49	52	52	52	57	
Pre-existing hypertension										
Absent	127	28	36	39	40	42	43	46	48	$\chi^2 = 0.376$ $P = 0.540$
Present	36	26	37	37	40	44	48	48	53	
Overall	187	29	38	41	42	44	45	48	50	

Table 5-6. Cumulative Rebleeding Rates (%) for Variables Specific to the Aneurysm and Interval from Last Bleed to Treatment.

Variable	Initial Sample Size	Follow-up Period (Years)								Significance Level
		1/12	1/4	1/2	1	2	3	4	5	
Site of aneurysm										
Internal carotid	35	19	30	30	30	30	30	30	30	$\chi^2 = 2.615$ $P = 0.270^*$
Middle cerebral	22	44	49	49	49	49	49	49	58	
Anterior cerebral-anterior communicating	130	30	37	38	40	44	46	49	49	
Size of aneurysm										
≤200 mm³	75	35	39	39	39	41	43	45	45	$\chi^2 = 0.582$ $P = 0.445$
>200 mm³	94	31	39	41	42	47	49	52	52	
Number of proven or suspected bleeds in history										
1	160	29	35	36	37	41	42	44	45	$\chi^2 = 1.948$ $P = 0.163$
2 or 3	27	37	50	50	50	50	50	57	57	
Interval from last bleed to treatment										
0–7 days	124	37	45	46	48	52	52	55	55	$\chi^2 = 6.174$ $P = 0.045$
8–21 days	49	16	25	25	25	25	30	33	33	
22–92 days	14	0	0	0	0	0	0	0	13	
Overall	187	30	37	38	39	42	43	46	47	

* Statistical test of difference in 5-year rebleeding rates based on rebleeding rates at each specified interval adjusted for lost-to-follow-up and deaths of all causes.

(Table 5–5). With few exceptions, cumulative mortality increased with age and at each follow-up interval. However, the differences did not reach statistical significance.

Sex

Cumulative mortality with respect to sex is presented in Table 5–5. Males had higher cumulative mortality than females at all follow-up intervals. The differences were small in the early periods, but they increased at later follow-up intervals. The chi-square test was close to significance at the 5% level ($P = 0.065$).

Mean Blood Pressure

Mean blood pressure is a weighted average of the pretreatment diastolic and systolic pressures, with the systolic having a weight of one and a diastolic having a weight of two. This variable was subdivided into two groups: (1) less than or equal to 110 mm Hg, and (2) greater than 110 mm Hg. Cumulative mortality was greater for patients with higher mean blood pressures at all follow-up intervals (Table 5–4). The difference in mortality was 10% at 1 month, 3% at 6 months, and then the difference increased gradually to 13% at 5 years. The chi-square test was close to significance ($P = 0.157$).

Size of Aneurysm

Aneurysm size was measured in cubic millimeters (volumetric calculation of intraluminal diameters determined from cerebral angiograms), and the group was subdivided into those with aneurysms which were less than or equal to 200 mm³, and those over 200 mm³. Cumulative mortality was greater for patients with large aneurysms at all follow-up intervals (Table 5–3). The differences in mortality between the two groups increased from 4% at 1 month to 13% at the 5-year follow-up interval. The chi-square test was close to significance ($P = 0.125$).

Proved and Suspected Bleedings

Patients with proved and suspected bleedings were subdivided into those with one bleed, and those with two or three bleeds. No patients had more than three proved or suspected bleedings. Cumulative mortality was greater at all follow-up intervals for the group of patients with two or three bleedings than for those with only one bleed (Table 5–3). However, the differences did not reach statistical significance.

Pre-Existing Hypertension*

In Table 5–5, the cumulative mortality is classified by the presence or absence of pre-existing hypertension. Up to 1 year after the initial bleed, little or no difference in mortality was found between the two groups. In long-term follow-up (5 years), the hypertensive patients had a slightly higher mortality (53 vs 48%) than the group of nonhypertensive patients. These differences were not statistically significant.

Vasospasm†

Cumulative mortality among patients with no cerebral vasospasm and those with localized and diffuse cerebral vasospasm was 29, 30 and 32%, respectively, at the end of 1 month (Table 5–4). During the interval from 3 months to 1 year, patients with no vasospasm had a lower mortality than those with localized or diffuse vasospasm. There was little difference in mortality between the groups of patients with localized and diffuse vasospasm. At the end of the 5-year follow-

* Pre-existing hypertension: existence in patient's history of hypertension ($\geq$ 160 mm Hg systolic) either treated or untreated.
† Vasospasm was determined on angiograms by the demonstration of decreased intra-arterial size and was categorized as *no vasospasm, local vasospasm* (narrowing of intra-arterial diameter over one to three-centimeters on the proximal segments of the intracranial portion of the internal carotid, middle cerebral, anterior cerebral or vertebral-basilar arteries) and *diffuse vasospasm* (narrowed diameter of the intracranial internal carotid artery and all the main ipsilateral branches).[5]

up interval, mortality among patients with no vasospasm (49%), and the patients with diffuse vasospasm exhibited the highest mortality (59%). None of the observed differences was statistically significant.

Summary of Effect of Clinical Variables on Mortality

These data show the mortality in patients with recent subarachnoid hemorrhage following treatment with a 3-week program of regulated bed rest was, over a 5-year interval, related to specific clinical variables. The patients with least good prognosis might be characterized as those with:

1. Middle cerebral artery aneurysm
2. Early presentation for treatment
3. Poor initial neurologic condition
4. Poor initial medical condition
5. Advanced age
6. Male sex
7. High mean blood pressure
8. Large aneurysm size
9. Multiple proven or suspected bleedings in history
10. Evidence of diffuse vasospasm

Only initial neurologic and medical conditions and sex were significantly related to mortality on a statistical basis. The remaining seven variables showed trends related to higher mortality. Little or no difference in mortality was found among patients with or without pre-existing hypertension.

Effect of Selected Clinical Variables Upon Rebleeding

Following entry into the study, the patients with recurrent hemorrhage died in the greatest numbers. A statistical analysis was made using selected clinical parameters and relating them to rebleeding. In this analysis, recurrent hemorrhage was proved during hospitalization by lumbar puncture, or in some instances was suspected clinically. In situ-

ations where a suspected rebleeding was reported as a cause of death, a precipitous clinical deterioration prior to death was believed to be sufficient evidence for the reporting investigator to regard the cause of death as recurrent hemorrhage, even if lumbar puncture or postmortem examination could not be performed.

Aneurysm Site

The cumulative rebleeding rate by aneurysm site was highest among patients with middle cerebral artery aneurysms throughout all follow-up periods (Table 5–6). The rate for anterior cerebral-anterior communicating artery aneurysms was intermediate, and the rate for internal carotid artery aneurysms was lowest. The differences remained uniform throughout the 5-year follow-up. Interestingly, the rebleeding rate remained the same during the 3-month to 4-year interval for patients with an internal carotid (30%) and middle cerebral artery aneurysm (49%). During that same interval, the rebleeding rate for patients with an anterior cerebral-anterior communicating artery aneurysm increased from 37 to 49%. The overall chi-square test was not statistically significant ($P = 0.270$).

Interval from Last Bleed to Treatment

The interval from last bleed to treatment had a profound effect upon rebleeding rate. Of the 14 patients allocated to regulated bed rest during the 22 to 92-day interval following the initial bleeding, no patients rebled until the 5th year of follow-up (Table 5–6). Patients allocated to treatment during the 8 to 21-day interval had an intermediate rebleeding rate throughout the 5-year interval (range 16 to 33%). In contrast, patients allocated to treatment within 7 days after an initial bleed had the highest rebleeding rate throughout the follow-up period (range 37 to 55%). The chi-square test was significant at the 5% level ($P = 0.045$).

Neurologic Condition

Cumulative rebleeding rates were analyzed for patients whose neurologic condition was recorded initially on the day of randomization. Some patients were reported to be in good neurologic condition (Grades 1 and 2, Table 5–7) and the others in poor condition (Grades 3 to 6). Patients with various minor neurologic symptoms had a higher rebleeding rate (32%) in the 1st month than those with a more severe initial neurologic condition (25%). This trend was reversed at the 3rd month and continued through the 5th year of follow-up. The differences in rebleeding rates between the two groups were never more than 8%, and the chi-square test was not significant ($P = 0.429$). These results were in marked contrast to the corresponding results for mortality.

Medical Condition

General medical condition (as defined in Table 5–2) was designated for each patient on the day of randomization. When the medical condition was analyzed with respect to rebleeding rate, no consistent differences in recurrent subarachnoid hemorrhage were found throughout the 5-year interval between the respective medical conditions (Table 5–7). Prior to the 3rd year, patients in fair medical condition had the highest rebleeding rate. Patients in good or poor/prohibitive condition had similar rebleeding rates during that interval which were lower than the rates among patients in fair condition. After the 3rd year of follow-up, the poor/prohibitive patients had the highest rebleeding rate; patients in fair condition had an intermediate rate, and patients in good condition had the lowest rate. The overall chi-square test was not significant ($P = 0.432$). These results were also in marked contrast to the corresponding results for mortality.

Age

Selected age groups were compared with respect to rebleeding rates throughout the 5-

year interval. Neglecting the constant 40% rebleeding rate for the age group under 20 because of the small sample size (n = 6), there was a trend toward an increased rebleeding rate with advanced age (Table 5–8). The age group 20 to 39 consistently had the lowest rebleeding rate, while the age groups 40 to 59 and 60 and above had the highest rates. However, the differences were not statistically significant.

Sex

Men consistently had a higher rebleeding rate than women (Table 5–8). The differences were small within the 1st year of follow-up, but they increased appreciably during the 2nd through 5th year of the follow-up (from 5% at year 1 to 17% at year 5). The difference in mortality curves was close to statistical significance ($P = 0.059$).

Mean Blood Pressure

Patients with mean blood pressure greater than 110 mm Hg at randomization had a higher rebleed rate than those with a mean pressure of less than 110 mm Hg. The difference was large in the 1st month (36 vs 27%, respectively, Table 5–7). However, this proportion diminished to a difference of one percentage point at the end of the 1st year (40 vs 39%, respectively), but increased again by the end of the 5th year (54 vs 44%, respectively). The chi-square test was not significant ($P = 0.216$).

Size of Aneurysm

During the 1st month following bleeding, patients with an aneurysm size of less than 200 mm^3 had a rebleeding rate of 35% compared to 31% for patients with aneurysms greater than 200 mm^3 (Table 5–6). At the end of the 3rd month, rebleeding rates were 39% in both groups. After the 3rd month, the rebleeding rate was higher in the group with large aneurysms, reaching a difference

Table 5–7.   Cumulative Rebleeding Rate (%) for Variables Related to the Patient's Condition.

Variable	Initial Sample Size	Follow-up Period (Years)								Significance Level
		$\frac{1}{12}$	$\frac{1}{4}$	$\frac{1}{2}$	1	2	3	4	5	
Initial neurologic condition*										
1, 2	128	32	36	37	37	41	42	45	46	$\chi^2 = 0.625$ $P = 0.429$
3, 4, 5	59	25	42	42	45	45	49	49	49	
Initial medical condition*										
Good	102	26	33	34	36	40	41	44	45	$\chi^2 = 1.677$ $P = 0.432$
Fair	56	37	45	45	45	47	47	50	50	
Poor or Prohibitive	29	30	37	37	37	37	53	53	53	
Vasospasm										
None	106	35	38	38	40	44	46	50	51	$\chi^2 = 1.433$ $P = 0.488$
Local	54	25	36	38	38	38	38	38	38	
Diffuse	26	22	41	41	41	41	48	48	48	
Mean Blood Pressure										
≦110 mm.	127	27	36	37	39	40	41	43	44	$\chi^2 = 1.533$ $P = 0.216$
>110 mm.	60	36	40	40	40	48	51	54	54	
Overall	187	30	37	38	39	42	43	46	47	

* See Table 5–2.

Table 5–8.   Cumulative Rebleeding Rates (%) for Variables Related to the Patient's Characteristics.

Variable	Initial Sample Size	Follow-up Period (Years)								Significance Level
		$\frac{1}{12}$	$\frac{1}{4}$	$\frac{1}{2}$	1	2	3	4	5	
Sex of patient										
Male	83	32	39	40	42	47	48	55	57	$\chi^2 = 3.567$ $P = 0.059$
Female	104	28	36	36	37	38	40	40	40	
Age of Patient										
<20 yr	6	40	40	40	40	40	40	40	40	$\chi^2 = 2.654$ $P = 0.448$
20–39	32	24	28	28	32	32	32	32	32	
40–59	107	31	38	38	40	43	45	49	51	
≦60	41	29	41	44	44	48	48	48	48	
Pre-existing hypertension										
Absent	127	29	34	35	37	40	41	43	44	$\chi^2 = 0.459$ $P = 0.498$
Present	36	29	39	39	39	42	47	47	47	
Overall	187	30	37	38	39	42	43	46	47	

of seven percentage points by the 5th year. The difference in mortality curves was not statistically significant ($P = 0.445$).

Number of Proved or Suspected Bleeds in History

Patients having multiple bleeds had consistently higher rebleeding rates throughout the 5-year follow-up period as compared to those having rebleeds in their history (Table 5–6). The difference in mortality curves was close to statistical significance ($P = 0.163$).

Pre-existing Hypertension

The rebleeding rate was 29% for those patients with or without pre-existing hypertension at the end of the 1st month (Table 5–8). From the 3rd month through the 5th year of follow-up, patients with pre-existing hypertension had a higher rebleeding rate, the difference varying between two and six percentage points. Statistical significance was not reached ($P = 0.498$).

Vasospasm

No consistent differences in rebleeding rates were observed among patients with variable degrees of vasospasm (Table 5–7). The rate was occasionally higher among patients without vasospasm than for those with vasospasm.

Summary of Effect of Selected Clinical Variables upon Rebleeding

Well-defined relationships between patient characteristics and rebleeding rates were fewer than between these same patient characteristics and mortality. Patients treated with regulated bed rest had the poorest prognosis in terms of the following characteristics:

1. Middle cerebral artery aneurysms
2. Early presentation for treatment
3. Advanced age
4. Male sex
5. High mean blood pressure

6. Multiple proved or suspected bleeds
7. Pre-existing hypertension.

Only the interval from last bleed to treatment and sex distribution reached statistical significance. The variables below showed no consistent relationship to the rebleeding rate, initial neurologic condition, initial medical condition, aneurysm size and degree of vasospasm.

Prediction of Mortality and Rebleeding

We sought to derive a linear function of the 11 factors considered in the previous sections which would predict the prognosis of a patient with a ruptured intracranial aneurysm treated with bed rest. Outcome is determined by mortality and rebleeding within 90 days after initiation of treatment. The statistical methodology used has been previously described. Since aneurysm site is a three-category, nominal variable, it is included as two separate variables for the purpose of these analyses.

The variables and their corresponding abbreviations and codings are given below as used for Tables 5–9 to 5–11:

Variable Name	Abbreviation	Coding
Outcome variables:		
Dead at 90 days	D90	1 = dead, 0 = alive
Rebleed at 90 days	RB90	1 = rebleed, 0 = no rebleed
Predictor variables:		
Internal carotid artery aneurysm	IC	1 = IC, 0 = MC, 0 = AC-AC
Middle cerebral artery aneurysm	MC	1 = MC, 0 = IC, 0 = AC-AC
Interval last bleed to randomization	LBRD	0–92 days
Neurologic condition	NEURC	1 = I, 2 = II, 3 = III, 4 = IV, 5 = V
Medical condition	MEDC	1 = good, 2 = fair, 3 = poor, 4 = prohibitive
Age	AGE	In years

Table 5–9. Correlation Coefficients of Outcome and Predictor Variables (n = 187).

	Predictor Variables										Outcome Variables			
	IC	MC	LBRD	NEURC	MEDC	AGE	SEX	MBP	VOL	PB	HYPER	SPASM	D90	RB90
IC	1.00										-.07	-.06	.00	-.08
MC	-.18**	1.00									.06	.08	.10	.06
LBRD	-.03	.18**	1.00								.02	.13*	-.25***	-.26***
NEURC	.05	.02	-.06	1.00							-.22**	.30***	.17**	.02
MEDC	.04	.07	.00	.61***	1.00						-.26***	.23***	.20**	.02
AGE	-.05	-.15*	-.01	.24***	.38***	1.00					-.29***	.13*	.07	.06
SEX	.21**	-.04	-.04	.08	.05	.15*	1.00				-.26***	.13*	-.03	.02
MBP	.09	-.04	-.09	.16**	.27***	.31***	.10	1.00			-.53***	.07	.13*	.08
VOL	-.04	.17*	.03	.13*	-.00	.02	-.09	-.04	1.00		.03	.09	-.07	.12
PB	.03	.01	-.09	.05	-.00	-.14*	-.02	-.03	-.04	1.00	.08	-.07	.06	.06
HYPER											1.00	-.02	-.02	-.05
SPASM												1.00	.12*	-.01

Asterisks indicate that the correlation is significantly different from zero. *0.01 < P ≤ 0.05; **0.001 < P ≤ 0.01; ***P ≤ 0.001.

Table 5–10. Discriminant Equation Coefficients for the Prediction of 90-Day Mortality (n = 145).

Number of Variables in Equation	Discriminant Predictor Variables												CONSTANT
	IC	MC	LBRD	NEURC	MEDC	AGE	SEX	MBP	VOL	PB	HYPER	SPASM	
1			-.0646		.4009								.5003
2			-.0673		.3592								-.1258
3			-.0707		.3830								-.3856
4			-.0671		.3681			.0156			.5304		-2.679
5		.4959	-.0701		.3325			.0161			.4998	.2283	-2.692
6		.4780	-.0728		.3268			.0155			.4685	.1932	-2.790
7		.5619	-.0733		.3178			.0150			.4601	.2162	-2.690
8	.3487	.6439	-.0752		.3194			.0142	-.0001		.4663	.2277	-2.690
9	.4028	.6642	-.0750		.3182		-.2250	.0138	-.0001		.3874	.2462	-2.194
10	.3870	.6598	-.0744		.3194		-.2223	.0137	-.0001	.1895	.3613	.2510	-2.382
11	.3906	.6484	-.0745	-.0346	.3390		-.2183	.0136	-.0001	.1945	.3596	.2599	-2.343
12	.3855	.6382	-.0745	-.0351	.3463	-.0014	-.2129	.0138	-.0001	.1902	.3553	.2605	-2.304

Variable Name	Abbreviation	Coding
Sex	SEX	1 = male, 2 = female
Mean blood pressure	MBP	In mm. Hg $\frac{(SYST + 2 \times DIAST)}{3}$
Aneurysm size	VOL	mm^3
Number of previous bleeds	PB	1 to 3
Pre-existing hypertension	HYPER	1 = yes, 2 = no
Vasospasm	SPASM	1 = none, 2 = local, 3 = diffuse

Table 5–9 presents the intercorrelations of the outcome and predictor variables. Several relationships are of interest, both among the predictor variables and between the predictor and outcome variables. Initial neurologic condition and initial medical condition are highly associated (0.61), almost to the extent that they are measuring the same characteristic. A poor initial neurologic status is significantly related to advanced age (0.24), high mean blood pressure (0.16), large aneurysm size (0.13) and the presence of hypertension (0.22) and vasospasm (0.30). A poor initial medical condition is also significantly related to all of these variables except aneurysm size. Advanced age is significantly related to high mean blood pressure (0.31), the presence of hypertension (0.29) and vasospasm (0.13). Curiously, the greater the age, the fewer the number of previous bleeds in the medical history (0.14). Being female is related to the presence of hypertension (0.26) and vasospasm (0.13). When the outcome variables are related to the predictor variables, death at 90 days is associated significantly with a short interval between the last bleeding before randomization (0.25), a poor initial neurologic status (0.17), a poor medical condition (0.20), a high mean blood pressure (0.13) and the presence of vasospasm (0.12). A rebleeding within 90 days is associated significantly only with a short interval between last bleeding to randomization (0.26).

The results of the discriminant analyses for the prediction of 90-day mortality are presented in Table 5–10. Only those cases with complete information on all variables were used (n = 145). A discriminant analysis was done for each number of variables from one to 12; at each step, the analysis chose the combination of variables which best discriminates between the patients who died versus those who survived. Table 5–10 gives the coefficients for the variables chosen and the constant term in the linear equation.

An example for the use of these results is as follows: Suppose one wishes to use the best six variables to predict a patient's survival status at 90 days. These variables are aneurysm site, interval from last bleeding to randomization, initial medical condition, mean arterial blood pressure, presence or absence of pre-existing hypertension, and vasospasm (six variables, Table 5–10). Suppose, further, that a patient had the following scores on these six variables: middle cerebral artery aneurysm = 1, interval from last bleeding to randomization = 5 days, poor medical condition = 3, mean arterial blood pressure = 108 mm Hg, presence of hypertension = 1, and no vasospasm = 1. The patient's discriminant score is computed as follows:

$$D = (.4780) \times \text{(aneurysm site score)}$$
$$+ (-.0728) \times \text{(interval last bleed to randomization)}$$
$$+ (.3325) \times \text{(medical condition)}$$
$$+ (.0155) \times \text{(mean blood pressure)}$$
$$+ (.4685) \times \text{(hypertension score)}$$
$$+ (.1932) \times \text{(vasospasm score)}$$
$$+ \text{constant}$$
$$= (.4780)(1) + (-.0728)(5)$$
$$+ (.3325)(3) + (.0155)(108)$$
$$+ (.4685)(1) + (.1932)(1) + (-2.790)$$
$$= + .6572$$

If a prior distribution of death (D) and survival is assumed to be 50–50, the decision rule for prediction is as follows: *When a patient's discriminant score is greater than zero, death within 90 days is predicted; when the score is negative, survival is predicted. Since the patient's score is + 0.6572, his death within the first 90 days is more likely than his survival, and some particular means of treatment might be indicated.*

Discriminant scores were computed for the 145 patients, and these patients (for whom the survival status at 90 days was already known) were classified into deceased and survivors. The overall percent misclassification ranged between 37.9 and 44.1% for the 12 discriminant analyses. Misclassification of the patients who were deceased at 90 days ranged from 19.9 to 47.2%, and misclassification of the patients who were alive at 90 days ranged from 41.3 to 57.6%.

Order of entry of the variables in the 12 discriminant analyses gives some indication about the relative importance of the variables in predicting mortality. The interval from last bleeding to randomization, medical condition, vasospasm, mean arterial blood pressure, pre-existing hypertension and middle cerebral artery aneurysm seem to be the best predictors. Internal carotid artery aneurysm, age, sex, aneurysm size, number of previous bleeds and neurologic condition entered at later stages. Neurologic condition probably entered artifically at a very late stage, because the information contained in this variable was largely accounted for by medical condition which entered at an early stage.

The results of the discriminant analyses for the prediction of 90-day rebleeding are presented in Table 5–11. The interval from last bleed to randomization again appears to be the most significant predictor of outcome. Other variables which contribute most to prediction of rebleeding include vasospasm, aneurysm size, middle cerebral artery aneurysm and mean arterial blood pressure. However, the direction of the relationship between rebleeding and the former two factors is contrary to intuition (i.e., rebleeding is more likely with a smaller aneurysm size and no vasospasm). When the 145 patients are classified by the discriminant equations, the overall percent misclassification ranges from 37.9 to 46.2%. Misclassification of the patients who rebled during the 90-day period ranged from 16.3 to 40.8%, and misclassification of the patients who did not rebleed ranged from 46.9 to 57.3%.

Table 5–11. Discriminant Equation Coefficients for the Prediction of 90-Day Rebleeding (n = 145).

Number of Variables in Equation	Discriminant Predictor Variables												
	IC	MC	LBRD	NEURC	MEDC	AGE	SEX	MBP	VOL	PB	HYPER	SPASM	CONSTANT
1			-.0726										.5463
2		.6095	-.0682									-.4019	1.1146
3		.6448	-.0685						-.0002			-.3734	1.168
4		.5618	-.0720						-.0002			-.3874	1.160
5		.5512	-.0715					.0094	-.0002			-.4093	.1925
6	-.3813	.5961	-.0708					.0106	-.0002			-.4205	.1621
7	-.4114	.6187	-.0697					.0111	-.0002	.3472		-.4163	-.3243
8	-.3970	.6070	-.0700			.0071		.0093	-.0002	.3731		-.4276	-.4921
9	-.3422	.5867	-.0704			.0085	-.2133	.0096	-.0002	.3684		-.4159	-.2726
10	-.3483	.6070	-.0704		.0420	.0078	-.2126	.0093	-.0002	.3660		-.4240	-.2595
11	-.3426	.5867	-.0707	-.0595	.0782	.0077	-.2051	.0092	-.0002	.3743	-.0180	-.4089	-.2019
12	-.3422	.5879	-.0707	-.0598	.0776	.0077	-.2082	.0090	-.0002	.3756		-.4078	-.1425

Discussion

Mortality and rebleeding rates during a 5-year period were analyzed by a life table method of statistical analysis following a 3-week period of bed rest in patients with a recently ruptured aneurysm. Linear discriminant function analysis was used to develop equations of clinical variables which could be utilized to predict mortality and rebleeding.

Five years following subarachnoid hemorrhage, 50% of all patients were dead from causes directly related to aneurysm rupture. A total of 47% rebled. The incidence of death or rebleeding varied from 1 to 3% for each yearly interval between 6 months and 5 years.

The mortality and rebleeding rates among patients with internal carotid artery aneurysms remained unchanged (38 and 30%, respectively) during the period between 3 months and 5 years following the initial bleeding. In contrast, mortality and rebleeding rates among patients with an anterior cerebral-anterior communicating artery aneurysm increased progressively during the 5-year interval. The results of mortality and rebleeding rates among patients with a middle cerebral artery aneurysm were the poorest among the three aneurysm sites. However, the number of patients included with aneurysm at this site (22) was less than the number of patients at the remaining two sites.

The interval from last bleed to treatment had a highly significant relationship to death and rebleeding. This fact is related to the known observation that recurrent hemorrhages and deaths from the original bleeding occur at a peak incidence between 5 and 10 days following the original bleeding.

Cumulative mortality and recurrent hemorrhage increased during the 5-year follow-up period in patients with both good and poor neurologic condition. Patients with poor neurologic condition had a higher mortality than those in good condition. The patient's medical condition had a similar relation between mortality and rebleeding patterns and good, fair and poor/prohibitive medical condition as observed for patients with different neurologic conditions. The unexpected finding was that patients in fair condition (patients with a single underlying medical problem) had higher mortality and rebleeding rates throughout the 5-year period than patients in good condition.

With few exceptions, cumulative mortality and rebleeding rates increased with age. Throughout the 5-year period, men had a higher mortality and rebleeding rate than women. Furthermore, higher mean blood pressure at randomization carried a worse prognosis for both mortality and rebleeding.

Cumulative mortality was greater in patients with large aneurysms than small aneurysms (< 200 mm^3) at all follow-up intervals. The differences in mortality were greater than those observed for cumulative rebleeding rate. Patients with multiple bleedings prior to hospitalization had consistently higher mortality and rebleeding rates than the group of patients with one bleeding.

The presence of pre-existing hypertension was not strongly associated with a higher mortality and rebleeding rate during the 5-year period. The percentage of deaths and rebleedings was only slightly higher in the hypertensive group. Patients with diffuse vasospasm tended to have higher mortality than those with no vasospasm or local vasospasm. However, no consistent differences in rebleeding rates were observed among patients with various degrees of vasospasm during the 5-year period.

The relationships among selected clinical characteristics, mortality and rebleeding rate had a high degree of association. The order of importance of the clinical variables was similar for cumulative mortality and rebleeding rate. The major exceptions were neurologic and medical conditions, which were more significant in the prognosis associated with cumulative mortality than with cumulative rebleeding rate.

These data were derived from patients who were randomly allocated to regulated bed rest in the Cooperative Aneurysm Study conducted between June 1963 and February 1970. Comparison of these results with others should be done with caution, since most other patient samples reported in the literature result from a selected series rather than from randomization. However, a randomized study design comparable to that described in this paper was reported by Winn, et al.[11] Their data indicated that deaths from rebleeding occurred on an average of 3 to 4% per year. Furthermore, elevated systolic blood pressure had a higher association with recurrent hemorrhage than that demonstrated in patients from the Cooperative Study. Our study demonstrated mortality from recurrent hemorrhage to vary from 1 to 3% per year after the first 6-month period following the bleeding, and that the interval from last bleeding to treatment, initial neurologic and medical conditions, and sex distribution had a higher association with mortality than blood pressure. Our calculations of mean blood pressure included those at the time of the original bleed.

Discriminant function analysis has also been applied to data from patients with recently ruptured cerebral aneurysm by Richardson et al.[12, 13] However, their method of analysis and the prognostic factors used in their study differed from those used in this report. Because recently ruptured middle cerebral artery aneurysms were not evaluated in their studies, detailed comparison of aneurysm site must be deferred. Notwithstanding, prognosis in our patients with an anterior cerebral-anterior communicating artery aneurysm was worse during the 3-month to 5-year interval (Tables 5–3 and 5–6) when compared to the group with internal carotid artery aneurysm. Our patients with an internal carotid artery aneurysm had a better prognosis than those reported by Richardson et al.[12] The neurologic and medical conditions had a high degree of influence on mortality in the Cooperative Study, but the level of consciousness in Richardson's study appeared to have less importance.

Review and analysis of these data suggest that multiple clinical variables can be useful when an attending physician must discuss and evaluate specific treatment programs for patients with recent subarachnoid hemorrhage. The interval following last bleed, initial neurologic and medical conditions, sex and mean blood pressure possess the highest value in assessment of long-term prognosis for patients with recently ruptured aneurysm, according to our study.

Linear discriminant function analysis was used to develop equations which would best predict mortality and rebleeding. The misclassification rates were substantial, indicating that the practicality of these equations may be doubtful for making specific clinical judgments at the bedside.

Conclusions

The purpose of this report was to describe the effect of various factors on the outcome of 187 patients having a ruptured intracranial artery aneurysm and treated with regulated bed rest, and to develop linear equations of these factors which could best predict outcome. These factors included aneurysm site, interval from last bleed to treatment, initial neurologic condition, initial medical condition, age, sex, mean blood pressure, aneurysm size, number of previous bleedings, pre-existing hypertension and evidence of vasospasm. Outcome was determined by survival status and rebleeding.

The variables which were found to be most indicative of mortality included: a short interval from last bleed to treatment, poor initial neurologic and medical conditions, high mean blood pressure, sex (male) and large aneurysm size. Interval from last bleed to treatment, sex, mean blood pressure and number of bleedings in medical history were most indicative of rebleeding.

Linear equations for any number of variables (1 to 12) were developed which best predicted mortality and rebleeding. The original patients used to develop these equations were reclassified using the equations as a test of the usefulness of the equations.

The misclassification rates were substantial, indicating that the practicality of these equations is doubtful for use as a basis for making clinical judgments. These results underscore further the complexity of the problem of determining accurately the prognosis of patients with ruptured intracranial aneurysms on a statistical basis.

References

1. Sahs, A.L.: Cooperative study of intracranial aneurysms and subarachnoid hemorrhage. Report on a randomized treatment study. I. Introduction. Stroke 5: 550–551, 1974.
2. Nibbelink, D.W., Knowler, L.A.: Cooperative study of intracranial aneurysms and subarachnoid hemorrhage. Report on a randomized treatment study. II. Objectives and design of randomized aneurysm study. Stroke 5: 552–556, 1974.
3. Sahs, A.L., Nibbelink, D.W., Knowler, L.A.: Cooperative Aneurysm Project: Introductory report of a randomized treatment study. In: Cerebral Vascular Disease (Eighth Princeton Conference), January 5–7, 1972, pp 33–41.
4. Graf, C., Nibbelink, D.W.: Cooperative study of intracranial aneurysms and subarachnoid hemorrhage. Report on a randomized treatment study. III. Intracranial surgery. Stroke 5: 559–601, 1974.
5. Nibbelink, D.W., Torner, J.C., Henderson, W.G.: Cooperative study of intracranial aneurysms and subarachnoid hemorrhage. Report on a randomized treatment study. IV–A. Regulated bed rest. Stroke 8: 202–218, 1977.
6. Mantel, N., Byar, D.: Evaluation of response-time data involving transient states: An illustration using heart transplant data. J Am Stat Assoc 69: 81–86, March 1974.
7. Koch, G.G., Johnson, W.D., Tolley, H.D.: A linear models approach to the analysis of survival and extent of disease in multidimensional contigency tables. J Am Stat Assoc 67: 783–796, December 1972.
8. La Motte, L.R., Hocking, R.R.: Computational efficiency in the selection of regression coefficients. Technometrics 12: 83–94, 1970.
9. Enochson, G.H.B.: A two population discriminant analysis subset selection program. Unpublished master's thesis, Department of Industrial and Management Engineering, University of Iowa, 1971.
10. Lachenbruch, P.A.: An almost unbiased method of obtaining confidence intervals for the probability of misclassification in discriminant analysis. Biometrics 23: 639–645, December 1967.
11. Winn, H.R., Richardson, A.E., Jane, J.A.: Late morbidity and mortality in cerebral aneurysms: A ten-year follow-up of 364 conservatively treated patients with a single cerebral aneurysm. Trans Am Neurol Assoc 98: 148–150, 1973.
12. Richardson, A.E., Jane, J.A., Yashon, D.: Prognostic factors in the untreated course of posterior communicating aneurysms. Arch Neurol 14: 172–176, 1966.
13. Richardson, A.E., Jane, J.A., Payne, P.M.: Assessment of the natural history of anterior communicating aneurysms. J Neurosurg 21: 266–274, 1964.

Chapter 6

Randomized Treatment Study. Drug-induced Hypotension

Donald W. Nibbelink, M.D., Ph.D., James C. Torner, M.S. and William G. Henderson, Ph.D.

Abstract

From 1963 through 1970, 309 patients with subarachnoid hemorrhage were allocated randomly to treatment with drug-induced hypotension. Eighty-two patients had a recently ruptured intracranial internal carotid artery aneurysm, 35 had a middle cerebral aneurysm and 192 had an aneurysm on the anterior cerebral-anterior communicating complex. Antihypertensive medications included chlorothiazide, reserpine, methyldopa and/or hydralazine given alone or in combination.

Thirty-three percent of patients had their blood pressure reduced according to protocol, while 56% did not achieve the specified reduction in systolic blood pressure. The remaining 11% did not meet the requirements for subgroup analysis, but were included in the overall results.

For the entire group, mortality was 46.3% during a mean period of 6.5 years following 3 weeks of antihypertensive treatment. Death caused by a proved or clinically suspected rebleed occurred in 29.8%. Deaths following a proved rebleed were reported with greatest frequency between the 6th and 30th day following the initial bleed.

Patients with an aneurysm on the anterior cerebral-anterior communicating artery complex had a greater number of deaths and/or rebleeds after the initial 30-day interval following the bleed than those with an internal carotid or middle cerebral artery aneurysm. The highest proportion of patients with proved rebleeding was reported in the subgroup whose blood pressure changed no more than 20% during treatment in comparison with control values. The lowest proportion of patients who rebled (14.7%) was reported among those without vasospasm who were in poor neurologic condition. In patients with vasospasm, 32.7% rebled.

Introduction

Recurrent hemorrhage has been the major cause of morbidity and mortality in patients with recently ruptured intracranial artery aneurysm.[1,2] Antihypertensive medication has been used to decrease the rebleed rate in such patients. In this study, we have called

Table 6–1. Aneurysm Site Distribution with Respect to Interval from Last Bleed to Randomization.

Days Last Bleed to Randomization	Aneurysm Site			Total
	Internal Carotid	Middle Cerebral	Anterior Cerebral	
0–7	56	16	118	190 (61.5%)
8–21	18	13	57	88 (28.5%)
22–92	8	6	17	31 (10.0%)
Total	82 (26.5%)	35 (11.3%)	192 (62.1%)	309

administration of antihypertensive medication "drug-induced hypotension." In reality, a better designation would be *drug-induced blood pressure reduction*, because arterial hypotension in the clinical sense was not carried out.

This report discusses the results of several clinical factors responsible for the outcome of patients treated with antihypertensive medication for a period of at least three weeks following a ruptured intracranial artery aneurysm. Various dosages of antihypertensive medication were administered by the participants so that the welfare of the patient was always of highest priority. The objective of this therapy was to decrease systolic blood pressure a specified percentage, based upon the average systolic level prior to treatment.

The need for a detailed report on this study is twofold. It is necessary to know, first, the effects of drug-induced blood pressure reduction upon mortality and rebleed rate following a recently ruptured intracranial aneurysm, and second, how such patients compare with a comparable group treated with bed rest alone, or with surgical treatment (carotid ligation or intracranial surgery). The medical and statistical analyses of patients treated with bed rest alone have been published.[2,5] The report on patients treated with intracranial surgery has also been completed.[6] The participants who made this Cooperative Study possible have been published previously.[7]

Table 6–2. Interval from Last Bleed to Randomization with Each Neurologic Condition for All Sites Combined.

Days to Randomization	Neurologic Condition*					Total
	1	2	3	4	5	
0–7	2	129	31	19	9	190
8–21	7	60	15	1	5	88
22–92	13	9	4	4	1	31
Total	22	198	50	24	15	309
%	7.1	64.1	16.2	7.8	4.8	

* Definition of Neurologic Condition:

1 = symptom-free.
2 = minor syptoms (headache, meningeal irritation, diplopia).
3 = major neurologic deficit but fully responsive.

4 = impaired state of alertness but capable of protective or other adaptive responses to noxious stimuli.
5 = poorly responsive but with stable vital signs.

Table 6–3. Distribution of Medical Condition for Each Aneurysm Site.

Medical Condition*	Aneurysm Site			Total
	Internal Carotid	Middle Cerebral	Anterior Cerebral	
Good	35 (43%)	16 (46%)	120 (63%)	171
Fair	39 (47%)	15 (43%)	54 (28%)	108
Poor	8 (10%)	4 (11%)	10 (5%)	22
Prohibitive	0	0	8 (4%)	8
Total	82	35	192	309

* Definition of medical condition: *good*—alert, normotensive, and good health prior to subarachnoid hemorrhage; *fair*—patients with single underlying medical disorder such as hypertension, cirrhosis, anemia, atherosclerosis or pulmonary disease; *poor*—patients with more than one adverse factor or one serious disorder; *prohibitive*—patients with one or more complicating illness which pre-existed the onset of subarachnoid hemorrhage.

Patient Selection

From June 1963 through February 1970, 309 patients were allocated to treatment by drug-induced hypotension. The details on the design and objectives of randomization in this study have been reported.[7,8] Eighty-two patients had a recently ruptured intracranial internal carotid artery aneurysm, 35 had a middle cerebral aneurysm and 192 had an aneurysm on the anterior cerebral-anterior communicating distribution (Table 6–1). Most patients (61.5%) were allocated to treatment within 7 days following last bleed, while 28.5% were randomized within the 8 through 21-day interval. Ten percent were allocated to treatment during the 22 through 92-day period.

The neurologic condition was determined for each patient on the day of treatment allocation. Most patients (64.1%) were in Grade 2 (Table 6–2). Comparison of general medical condition and aneurysm site reveals that a lower proportion of patients with an internal carotid or middle cerebral artery aneurysm were in good medical condition as compared to the number of patients with an aneurysm on the anterior cerebral complex (Table 6–3).

Definition of Drug-induced Hypotension

Four representative blood pressures were taken at more than 4-hour intervals by the usual manometric method during the interval between hospital admission and day of randomization. A 20% reduction was required for patients with average systolic values of 140 mm Hg or below, a 25% reduction for those with average systolic values between 141 and 180 mm Hg and a 30% reduction for systolic values over 180 mm Hg. Antihypertensive medications were used alone and in combination. Chlorothiazide, reserpine, methyldopa and/or hydralazine were used in dosages appropriate to achieve the desired reduction in systolic blood pressure and patient response. Antihypertensive treatment was continued for a minimum of 3 weeks.

Results

After a mean interval of 6.5 years, mortality among 309 patients allocated to drug-induced hypotension was 46.3% (Table 6–4).

Poor-neurologic-condition patients (Grades 4 and 5) had the highest mortality (69.2%, Table 6–5), while in mentally alert patients (Grades 1, 2 and 3) mortality was 43.0%.

Table 6–4.   Distribution of Patients in Each Aneurysm Site by Interval Following Last Bleed.

Days Last Bleed to Randomization	Aneurysm Site			Total	% Deaths
	Internal Carotid	Middle Cerebral	Anterior Cerebral		
0–7	56 (24)*	16 (7)	118 (65)	190 (96)	50.5
8–21	18 (9)	13 (8)	57 (24)	88 (41)	46.6
22–92	8 (2)	6 (2)	17 (2)	31 (6)	19.4
Total	82 (35)	35 (17)	192 (91)	309 (143)	
% Deaths	42.7	48.6	47.4	46.3	

* Number in parentheses denotes deaths.

This difference was highly significant ($P = 0.003$). Patients without impairment of mentation had significantly better survival as compared to patients with various degrees of lethargy and stupor. Mortality was not significantly different between aneurysm sites in each neurologic condition (Table 6–6).

Death caused by a proved or clinically suspected rebleed was reported in 29.8% of patients (92 of 309). Rebleeding in 70 deaths was proved by lumbar puncture or by postmortem examination; rebleeding was suspected clinically as a cause of death (without documentary evidence of lumbar puncture or postmortem examination) in 22. Twenty-two had progressive decline in clinical status without evidence of a rebleed, and 21 died of causes unrelated to bleeding (Table 6–6). In 8 patients the cause of death was unknown. Drug-induced blood pressure reduction did *not* increase the number of deaths in the category of progressive decline in neurologic condition (7.1%) when compared to a similar group of patients treated with regulated bed rest (8.5%).[2]

The distribution of patients was analyzed with respect to the interval to death for each cause. As shown in Table 6–7, the major proportion of deaths following progressive decline occurred during the 9th through 14th day following the last bleed; deaths following a proved rebleed were reported with greatest frequency between the 9th and 30th day. Deaths from a suspected rebleed, unrelated or unknown cause were scattered throughout the 6-year period.

A total of 190 patients were allocated to treatment within 7 days following last bleed. Within 14 days after the bleeding episode,

Table 6–5.   Distribution of Patients in Each Neurologic Condition and Aneurysm Site.

Aneurysm Site	Neurologic Condition*					Total
	1	2	3	4	5	
Internal Carotid	5 (0)†	51 (22)	14 (5)	5 (4)	7 (4)	82 (35)
Middle Cerebral	3 (2)	17 (9)	12 (5)	3 (1)	0	35 (17)
Anterior Cerebral	14 (0)	130 (59)	24 (14)	16 (12)	8 (6)	192 (91)
Total	22 (2)	198 (90)	50 (24)	24 (17)	15 (10)	309 (143)
% Deaths	9.1	45.5	48.0	70.8	66.7	46.3
		43.0			69.2	

* See Table 6–2 for definition of neurologic condition.
† Number in parentheses denotes deaths.

Table 6–6.   Distribution of Cause of Death for Each Aneurysm Site.

Aneurysm Site	Cause of Death					Total
	Proved Rebleed	Suspected Rebleed	Progressive Decline	Unrelated Cause	Unknown	
Internal Carotid (82)	19	4	3	8	1	35
Middle Cerebral (35)	8	3	3	2	1	17
Anterior Cerebral (192)	43	15	16	11	6	91
Total	70	22	22	21	8	143
% of 309	22.7	7.1	7.1	6.8	2.6	46.3

10 of 56 patients with an internal carotid artery aneurysm died, 4 of 16 with a middle cerebral aneurysm died and 29 of 118 who had an aneurysm on the anterior cerebral complex died. Fewer deaths occurred from all causes during the 15 through 30-day interval as compared to the initial 14-day period.

A summary analysis for each aneurysm site and interval following last bleed is represented in Figure 6–1. Patients with an anterior cerebral-anterior communicating artery aneurysm who were randomized within 7 days had the highest mortality through the first year following the last bleed. Patients with an internal carotid or middle cerebral artery aneurysm and randomized within 7 days had a similar mortality within the first year following the last bleed as compared to those with an anterior cerebral-anterior

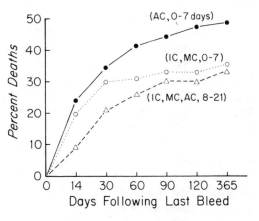

Fig. 6–1.   Cumulative percent of deaths at specified intervals following last bleed for patients randomized within 7 days and those randomized during the 8 to 22-day interval.

AC = anterior cerebral-anterior communicating aneurysm;
MC = middle cerebral aneurysm;
IC = internal carotid aneurysm.

Table 6–7.   Distribution of Cause of Death for Specified Intervals Following Last Bleed.

Days Following Last Bleed	Cause of Death					Total
	Proved Rebleed	Suspected Rebleed	Progressive Decline	Unrelated Cause	Unknown	
0–8	7	1	5	0	2	15
9–14	19	3	10	3	0	35
15–20	13	2	3	0	1	19
21–30	11	1	0	1	0	13
31–90	9	7	1	3	2	22
91–365	4	2	2	4	2	14
366+	7	6	1	10	1	25
Total	70	22	22	21	8	143

communicating aneurysm randomized during the 8 through 21-day interval.

Mortality and Blood Pressure

Mortality was determined for all patients with specified changes in blood pressure following administration of antihypertensive medication. The average of four prerandomized blood pressure recordings was calculated at the Central Registry. On the day the average systolic values were maintained at reduced levels, the difference with the pretreatment values was calculated and the percent change determined. Patients were subdivided into categories of: (1) equal to or less than ($\leq$) 20% change in systolic blood pressure after control levels were determined, (2) a decrease of more than 20% to less than 25%, (3) over 25% to less than 30% and (4) over 30% (Table 6–8). In the group with $\leq$ 20% change, survival was lowest (45.0%) at all intervals during the mean 6.5-year period of follow-up. Those with more than 20% decrease had an average survival of 61.8% (range 51.5 to 67.2%). The difference in survival between patients with 20% or more decrease in systolic blood pressure as compared to those with less than 20% was statistically significant ($P <0.01$). This difference may not be as clinically significant as it appears, since some patients either rebled or suffered a progressive clinical decline before antihypertensive medication was given or before there was opportunity for such medication to produce the specified reduction in blood pressure.

Mortality and Clinical Characteristics

Age and Sex

The sex distribution for patients treated with drug-induced hypotension was similar for men and women (Table 6–9). The greatest number of males and females was in the 50

Table 6–8.   Frequency Distribution of Deaths Following Last Bleed for Specified Percent Change in Systolic Blood Pressure.

Percent Change in Systolic Blood Pressure	Total Patients	Alive	Interval from Last Bleed to Death															Total Deaths
			0–2	3–5	6–8	9–11	12–14	15–17	18–20	21–23	24–26	27–29	30–60	61–90	91–180	181–365	>365	
$\leq$20% decrease	151	68 (45.0%)	2	2	6	13	16	6	3	5	1	2	5	4	2	4	12	83
>20 to 25% decrease	66	41 (62.1%)	0	1	1	0	1	2	4	1	1	1	2	2	1	3	5	25
>25 to 30% decrease	58	39 (67.2%)	0	0	1	2	1	0	2	0	1	0	6	0	0	2	4	19
>30% decrease	33	17 (51.5%)	0	0	2	2	0	0	2	1	0	0	2	1	2	0	4	16
Total	308*	165	2	3	10	17	18	8	11	7	3	3	15	7	5	9	25	143
Total patients at risk for each interval following last bleed			50	149	208	250	263	270	277	281	288	290	304	309				

* One patient had no blood pressure information.

Table 6–9. Age and Sex Distribution (with the Number of Deaths) for All Sites Combined.

| Age | Sex Distribution | | |
	Males	Females	Total
10 — 19	3 (2)*	2 (0)	5 (2)
20 — 29	10 (2)	9 (2)	19 (4)
30 — 39	33 (14)	22 (8)	55 (22)
40 — 49	35 (18)	37 (17)	72 (35)
50 — 59	49 (22)	59 (31)	108 (53)
60 — 69	18 (7)	23 (14)	41 (21)
70 — 79	4 (2)	5 (4)	9 (6)
Total	152 (67)	157 (76)	309 (143)
% Deaths	44.1	48.4	46.3

* Number in parentheses denotes deaths.

to 59-year age group. As expected, average mortality was slightly higher in the older age groups. Comparison of the number of deaths among patients above and below age 50 revealed no statistically significant difference. Women age 50 or above had the highest mortality (56.3%, or 49 of 87). The mortality was 38.6% in women below age 50. This difference was statistically significant (P =

0.04). The proportion of deaths among men below and above age 50 was 44.4 and 43.7%, respectively. Age appeared related to mortality more among women than men.

Sex and Aneurysm Site

The group of patients with an internal carotid artery aneurysm contained more than twice as many women (59) as men (23). There was an approximately equal number of men and women with a middle cerebral artery aneurysm, and slightly more men (109) than women (83) had an anterior cerebral artery aneurysm. This distribution was similar to the groups of patients allocated to treatment with regulated bed rest, carotid ligation and intracranial surgery.

Neurologic Condition

The distribution of deaths for each grade of neurologic condition shows that patients with a moderate to severe neurologic deficit

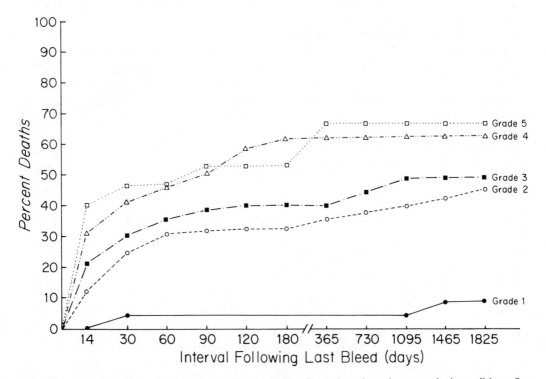

Fig. 6–2. Schematic representation of mortality distribution for patients in various neurologic conditions. See Table 6–2 for definition of each grade.

Table 6–10.   Distribution of Deaths for Patients of Various Medical Conditions and Blood Pressure Levels.

Medical Condition*	Systolic Blood Pressure at Randomization (mm Hg)					Total	%
	101–120	121–140	141–160	161–180	>180		
Good	20 (7)†	54 (18)	57 (19)	25 (11)	14 (6)	170 (61)	35.9
Fair	6 (1)	30 (13)	38 (21)	22 (16)	12 (9)	108 (60)	55.6
Poor	0	7 (6)	10 (6)	2 (2)	3 (2)	22 (16)	72.7
Prohibitive	0	0	3 (1)	2 (2)	3 (3)	8 (6)	75.0
Total	26 (8)	91 (37)	108 (47)	51 (31)	32 (20)	308 (143)	
%	30.7	40.7	43.5	60.8	62.5		

* See Table 6–3 for definition.
† Number in parentheses denotes deaths.

had a higher mortality than those with no neurologic deficit. There was a rapid rise in mortality among all grades of neurologic deficit within the first 14-day interval, followed by a distinctly slower rise from the 14 through 30-day interval (Fig. 6–2). A gradual sustained increase in mortality was observed following day 30 for patients with all grades of neurologic conditions.

Medical Condition and Blood Pressure

Mortality was significantly different among various medical conditions (defined in Table 6–3). A nearly 20% increase in deaths was observed between patients with good and fair medical condition, as well as between patients in fair and poor medical condition ($P < 0.005$, Table 6–10). Mortality was also increased for each increment in the level of systolic blood pressure prior to treatment, particularly in patients whose systolic levels

were below 180 mm Hg. Mortality in the group with blood pressure *above* 180 mm Hg was 62.5%. A difference in mortality in patients with blood pressures above as compared to those below 160 mm Hg was statistically significant ($P = 0.002$). The data suggest that among patients with elevated blood pressure (> 160 mm Hg systolic), mortality may have an important relationship with elevated systolic blood pressure in the first few days of the illness.

Systolic Blood Pressure and Vasospasm

Patients with localized and diffuse vasospasm had a 54.5% mortality (Table 6–11), whereas in those without vasospasm mortality was 40.2%. The interrelationship of vasospasm and mortality was significant ($P = 0.018$). A comparison of mortality rates for patients with and without vasospasm was

Table 6–11.   Distribution of Deaths for Patients With and Without Vasospasm at Specified Levels of Systolic Blood Pressure.

Vasospasm	Systolic Blood Pressure at Randomization					Total	%
	101–120	121–140	141–160	161–180	Over 180		
Present	8 (5)*	43 (19)	44 (22)	22 (15)	17 (12)	134 (73)	54.5
Absent	18 (3)	48 (18)	64 (25)	29 (16)	15 (8)	174 (70)	40.2
Total	26 (8)	91 (37)	108 (47)	51 (31)	32 (20)	308 (143)	
%	117 (45) 38.5			191 (98) 51.3			

* Number in parentheses denotes deaths.

Table 6–12.   Distribution of Deaths for Patients With and Without Vasospasm in Each Neurologic Condition.

Vasospasm	Neurologic Condition*					Total
	1	2	3	4	5	
Present	6 (2)†	74 (37)	32 (16)	13 (11)	10 (7)	135 (73)
Absent	16 (0)	124 (53)	18 (8)	11 (6)	5 (3)	174 (70)
Total	22 (2)	198 (90)	50 (24)	24 (17)	15 (10)	309 (143)

* See Table 6–2 for definition.
† Number in parentheses denotes deaths.

plotted for specified amounts of systolic blood pressures at the time of allocation to treatment. Patients with vasospasm had significantly higher mortality over the entire range of systolic blood pressures as compared to those without spasm (Fig. 6–3).

Vasospasm and Neurologic Condition

The percentage of patients with vasospasm in poor neurologic condition (Grades 3, 4 and 5) was 40.7% (55 of 135, Table 6–12), whereas for those without vasospasm only 19.5% (34 of 174) were in poor neurologic condition. For patients in good neurologic condition, 36.4% had vasospasm (80 of 220); but among patients in poor neurologic condition, 61.8% (55 of 89) had vasospasm ($P < 0.005$). A statistically significant interrelationship exists between vasospasm and increased neurologic deficit. Blood pressure reduction in the presence of vasospasm with a neurologic deficit does not appear to produce improved survival for these patients. Figure 6–4 illustrates that the greatest number of deaths occurred among patients in poor neurologic condition (Grades 4 and 5) who had localized and diffuse vasospasm.

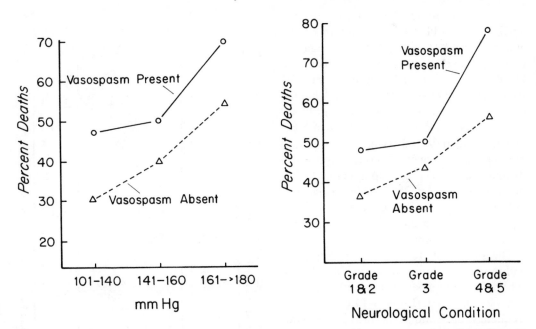

Fig. 6–3. Schematic representation of mortality rates for patients at various initial systolic blood pressure levels with regard to the presence or absence of vasospasm.

Fig. 6–4. Schematic representation of mortality comparing patients in various neurologic conditions with and without vasospasm. See Table 6–2 for definition.

Recurrent Subarachnoid Hemorrhage

Recurrent Hemorrhage During Antihypertensive Treatment

A comparison of the frequency of proved rebleeds for patients with a decrease in systolic blood pressure of 20% or less was compared with those who had more than 20% decrease during the treatment period. The overall rebleed rate was not significantly different among the four groups (Table 6–13) with designated changes in systolic blood pressure during treatment. However, an analysis of rebleed rate at certain intervals for selected subgroups did show considerable variation. For example, in the group whose blood pressure fluctuated $\leq 20\%$ from average control values, 26 of 151 (17.2%) rebled within 14 days (Table 6–13); a slightly less frequent rebleed rate (15.2%, 5 of 33) was reported in patients with reduction in systolic values more than 30% in the same 14-day period. Rebleeding in patients whose blood pressure decreased from 20 to 25% was 7.6%, and for those with a 25 to 30% decrease, the rebleed rate was 8.6%. One could question whether or not administration of antihypertensive medication had any alleviating effect on recurrent bleeds during this 14-day period, because the mean interval between the last bleed and the day of maintained reduction of systolic blood pressure was 13 days. The rebleed rate between day 15 and day 29 (when drug-induced blood pressure reduction should have shown its maximum effect) was appreciably higher in patients with a 25% decrease or less (10.6% rebleed rate) as compared to those with more than a 25% decrease in blood pressure (5.5% rebleed rate).

The number of proved rebleeds in patients within specified limits of systolic blood pressure before antihypertensive medication began was analyzed. Table 6–14 contains the frequency distribution of proved rebleeds for patients with average systolic values below 140 mm Hg, 140 to 180 mm Hg, and more than 180 mm Hg prior to treatment.

Table 6-13. Frequency Distribution of Patients with a *Proved Rebleed* at Specific Intervals Following the Prerandomization Bleed for Each Designated Change in Systolic Blood Pressure During Treatment.

Percent Change in Systolic Blood Pressure	Total Patients	No. of Rebleeds	Days Following Prerandomization Bleed														
			0–2	3–5	6–8	9–11	12–14	15–17	18–20	21–23	24–26	27–29	30–60	61–90	91–180	181–365	>365
≤20% decrease	151	50 (33.1%)	1	3	6	10	6	6	2	3	2	2	3	1	0	1	4
>20 to 25% decrease	66	22 (33.3%)	0	0	3	1	1	1	3	2	1	1	2	2	1	2	2
>25 to 30% decrease	58	14 (24.1%)	0	1	0	3	1	0	2	0	2	0	3	0	0	1	1
>30% decrease	33	11 (33.3%)	0	3	1	1	0	0	1	0	0	0	1	1	0	0	3
Total	308*	97 (31.5%)	1	7	10	15	7	7	8	5	5	3	9	4	2	4	10
Cumulative rebleeds			1	8	18	33	40	47	55	60	65	68	77	81	83	87	97

* One patient had no blood pressure information.

Table 6–14.   Frequency Distribution of Proved Rebleeds in Patients with Percent Change in Average Systolic Blood Pressure During the Treatment Period for Each Designated Range of Average Systolic Pressure Before Treatment.

Percent Decrease in Systolic Blood Pressure	Average Systolic Blood Pressure Before Treatment			Total Patients
	<140 mm Hg (99)*	140–180 mm Hg (174)	>180 mm Hg (35)	
≤20% decrease	17 (17.2%)†	30 (17.2%)	3 (8.6%)	50 (51.5%)
>20 to 25% decrease	4 (4.0%)	17 (9.8%)	1 (2.9%)	22 (22.6%)
>25 to 30% decrease	2 (2.0%)	9 (5.2%)	3 (8.6%)	14 (14.4%)
>30% decrease	1 (1.0%)	10 (5.7%)	0 (0%)	11 (11.3%)
Total	24 (24.2%)	66 (37.9%)	7 (20.0%)	97

* Number of patients with average level of designated systolic blood pressure.
† Percent of patients who rebled for each category of average systolic blood pressure before treatment.

The highest percentage of proved rebleeds was reported in patients whose blood pressure did not change more than 20% in comparison to control values. The highest percentage of rebleeds occurred in patients with average systolic values between 140 and 180 mm Hg (37.9%, or 66 of 174, Table 6–14).

Vasospasm and Systolic Blood Pressure

A comparison of rebleed rates among patients with and without cerebral vasospasm at specific levels of systolic blood pressure revealed that the number of rebleeds in patients with vasospasm was 34.3% as compared to 29.3% in those with no vasospasm (Table 6–15). Among patients with an average systolic blood pressure of 101 to 140 mm Hg, 29.4% (15 of 51) rebled in the group with vasospasm and 25.8% (17 of 66) rebled

among those without spasm. This difference was not statistically significant. In the group with an average systolic level between 140 and 180 mm Hg, those with spasm had a 42.4% rebleed rate (28 of 66); in patients without spasm 30.1% (28 of 93) rebled. Neither was this difference statistically significant ($P = 0.152$). The rebleed rate was appreciably higher than average among patients with more elevated levels of systolic blood pressure in the presence of vasospasm (141 to 160 and 161 to 180 mm Hg, but not in the group over 180 mm Hg).

Neurologic Condition and Vasospasm

Patients in good neurologic condition (Grade 2) had the highest rebleed rate (36.4%, or 72 of 198, Table 6–16). Rebleed rates were similar among patients with and without

Table 6–15.   Distribution of patients With and Without Vasospasm with the Number of Patients Who Rebled for Each Level of Average Systolic Blood Pressure at Randomization.

Vasospasm	Systolic Blood Pressure (mm Hg) at Randomization					Total	% Rebleeds
	101–110	121–140	141–160	161–180	Over 180		
Present	8 (3)*	43 (12)	44 (17)	22 (11)	17 (3)	134 (46)	34.3
Absent	18 (4)	48 (13)	64 (17)	29 (11)	15 (6)	174 (51)	29.3
Total	26 (7)	91 (25)	108 (34)	51 (22)	32 (9)	308 (97)	

* Number in parentheses denotes patients who rebled.

Table 6–16.   Distribution of the Number of Rebleeds for Patients With and Without Vasospasm in Each Neurologic Condition.

Vasospasm	Neurologic Condition*					Total
	1	2	3	4	5	
Present	6 (1)†	74 (27)	32 (10)	13 (6)	10 (2)	135 (46) 34.1%
Absent	16 (1)	124 (45)	18 (5)	11 (0)	5 (0)	174 (51) 29.3%
Total	22 (2)	198 (72)	50 (15)	24 (6)	15 (2)	309 (97) 31.4%

* See Table 6–2 for definition
† Number in parentheses denotes rebleeds.

vasospasm (34.1 vs 29.3%, respectively). The lowest number of rebleeds was reported among patients in poor neurologic condition (Grades 3, 4 and 5) without vasospasm. Only 14.7% (5 of 34) rebled in this category, whereas in the group with vasospasm 32.7% (18 of 55) rebled. Although patients in poor neurologic condition with vasospasm had a higher rebleed rate as compared to those without vasospasm, the difference was not statistically significant ($P > 0.10$).

Medical Condition and Blood Pressure

A comparison of rebleed rates in patients with various grades of medical condition at specified levels of systolic blood pressure revealed no significant interrelationships. Even among patients with an average sys-tolic blood pressure between 140 and 180 mm Hg, no differences were observed among patients in good, fair and poor medical condition. As expected, the greatest proportion of patients in fair and poor condition tended to have higher levels of systolic blood pressure than those in good condition.

Aneurysm Site and Rebleeding

For all aneurysm sites, the frequency of re-current aneurysm rupture following the last bleed before randomization diminished gradually following the 9 to 11-day interval (Table 6–13). Since these rates appear to differ among patients randomized within 7 days compared to those randomized during the 8 through 21-day interval, separate com-putations were carried out to correlate re-

Table 6–17.   Interval to Rebleed for Patients Randomized Within 7 Days Following Last Bleed for Each Aneurysm Site.

Interval Last Bleed to Rebleed (Days)	Aneurysm Site			Total (190)
	Internal Carotid (56)*	Middle Cerebral (16)	Anterior Cerebral (118)	
0–14	10	2	21	33 (17.4%)
15–30	7	1	9	17 (8.9%)
31–60	0	0	4	4 (2.1%)
61–90	1	0	2	3 (1.6%)
91–180	0	0	1	1 (0.5%)
181–365	1	0	1	2 (1.1%)
Total	19	3	38	60
%	33.9	18.7	32.2	31.6

*Total patients randomized at each site.

Table 6–18.   Interval to Rebleed for Patients Randomized During the 8 to 21-Day Interval Following Last Prerandomized Bleed for Each Aneurysm Site.

Interval Last Bleed to Rebleed (Days)	Aneurysm Site			
	Internal Carotid (18)	Middle Cerebral (13)	Anterior Cerebral (57)	Total (88)
8–14	0	3	5	8 (17.0%)*
15–30	2	4	5	11 (12.5%)
31–60	2	0	3	5 (5.7%)
61–90	0	0	1	1 (1.1%)
91–180	0	0	0	0 (0%)
181–365	0	0	2	2 (2.3%)
Total	4	7	16	27
%	22.2	53.8	28.1	30.7

* Percentage calculated on basis of 47 patients randomized during the 8 to 14-day interval.

bleed rate at specific periods for each aneurysm site and interval to randomization. Table 6–17 contains a frequency distribution of proved rebleeds at each aneurysm site for patients randomized within 7 days. The middle cerebral artery aneurysm group was comparatively small; therefore, the interpretation of results at that site remains inconclusive. The results of the groups with internal carotid and anterior cerebral artery aneurysms show very similar patterns, with no appreciable difference in rebleed rates at the end of one year (33.9 vs 32.2%, respectively). Table 6–18 shows a similar distribution for each aneurysm site in patients randomized during the 8 through 21-day interval. These data illustrate primarily that recurrent hemorrhage remained the highest within 14 days following the hemorrhage before randomization for aneurysms at all sites.

Table 6–19.   Distribution of Neurologic Deficits Observed in 22 Patients During Antihypertensive Therapy.

Signs	No.
Cerebral Infarction	8
Confusion	5
Coma	3
Hemiparesis	3
Dysphasia	3
Hemiplegia	3
Aphasia	1
Decerebration	1
Homonymous Hemianopsia	1
Total	28

Clinical Complications Acquired During Antihypertensive Treatment

Although antihypertensive medication was administered cautiously, a number of patients developed neurologic deficits during therapy. Eight patients became less responsive and their level of consciousness deteriorated to varying levels of stupor. The most frequent impression as to the etiology in the decline of mental status in these patients was cerebral infarction (Table 6–19). The nine signs listed in this table were observed among 22 patients. In 14 the deficit remained at least through hospitalization, in 6 the deficit was less than 24-hours' duration, and in 2 patients the condition was longer than 24 hours but cleared by the time of discharge. To attribute these neurologic deficits to the result of administration of antihypertensive medication might be unwarranted, since other factors such as cerebral vasospasm, cerebral edema or mass effect from a localized hematoma could produce similar clinical results without reduction in blood pressure.

During the course of treatment, cerebral edema sufficiently severe to produce tentorial herniation was reported in 27 patients. Five patients had seizures concomitant with or following a rebleed and 9 additional patients developed seizures associated with a rebleed between hospital admission and the day of randomization. Other miscellaneous conditions reported in one instance each were delirium tremens, diabetes insipidus, urinary retention, perforation of a duodenal ulcer, parotitis, viral infection, tuberculosis, polycystic kidneys, amyotrophy of the shoulder and vitreous hemorrhage. Seventeen patients required tracheostomy for respiratory care. Two patients had a shunt procedure for hydrocephalus, and 1 patient each had a ventricular tap, suprapubic cystotomy, and evacuation of a subdural hematoma.

Miscellaneous Clinical Conditions Acquired During Treatment

During the administration of antihypertensive therapy, a diminished state of alertness in the form of lethargy was observed in 28 patients (Table 6–20). Depression of mood was noted in 9 instances; syncope was reported in 9 additional patients. Low systolic blood pressure was associated with syncope in 9 patients, but in 6 additional subjects hypotension requiring corrective measures was reported without syncope. Electrocardiographic evidence of myocardial ischemia

was observed in 4 patients. None of these patients was proved to have a myocardial infarction. Patients in this study were not followed with cardiac monitoring devices; therefore, the true frequency of electrocardiographic abnormalities remains unknown. All conditions in Table 6–20 occurred among 66 patients (21.4% of 309). To state categorically that all of these conditions were drug-induced is unjustified. Patients with acute subarachnoid hemorrhage frequently have such clinical conditions without treatment with antihypertensive medication.[2]

Other medical conditions as diagnosed and treated in patients during antihypertensive therapy (and requiring corrective measures) were as follows: pulmonary infections in 19 patients, genitourinary tract infections in 41, electrolyte imbalance in 14, gastrointestinal hemorrhage in 5 and peripheral venous thrombosis in 5. Only 1 patient had a pulmonary embolus.

Table 6–20. Medical Symptoms or Signs Observed During Treatment with Antihypertensive Medication Among 309 Patients.

Symptom/Sign	No.
Lethargy	28
Mood depression	9
Syncope	9
Hypotension	6
Myocardial ischemia (EEG evidence)	4
Stuffiness of nose	4
Nightmares	3
Behavior changes	2
Cardiac arrhythmia	2
Epigastric distress	2
Vertigo	2
Appetite change	1
Gout	1
Palpitations	1
Rigidity and dyskinesia	1
Diarrhea	1
Dermatitis	1
Anuria	1
Hiccoughs	1
Anemia	1
Azoturia	1
Total	81

Subgroup Analysis in Drug-induced Hypotension

Introduction

In the preceding discussion, mortality and rebleeding were analyzed for all patients allocated to treatment with drug-induced antihypertensive medication. Antihypertensive medications were administered in various combinations in the dosages considered appropriate for the individual patient. A total of 70.7% received a chlorothiazide preparation, 53.3% received oral methyldopa, 22.9% were given intramuscular reserpine and 21.9% oral reserpine. No particular combination of these agents was more effective than another. With this therapeutic approach toward blood pressure reduction, success in decreasing systolic blood pressure to the level specified according to protocol was not achieved in all patients. For example, following 8 days of antihypertensive therapy, only 53.4% had their systolic blood pressure levels stabilized (Table 6–21). During this 8-day interval of antihypertensive therapy, only 113 patients had 20% or more decrease in systolic blood pressure (calculated from Table 6–21). The 69 patients in Table 6–21 with no maintenance blood pressure never achieved a specified reduction.

Among the 309 patients, 22 received no antihypertensive medication. Fourteen did not receive the designated period of bed rest (Fig. 6–5). These 36 patients were excluded from further analyses. Both of these subgroups are analyzed briefly in the following discussion.

Patients Who Received No Antihypertensive Medication

No antihypertensive medication was given in 22 patients. Eight of these died within 24 hours of allocation to treatment and prior to administration of antihypertensive medication; 8 additional patients were considered unsuitable for the treatment program. Insufficient information about treatment was received in 6 patients. Among the entire group of 22 patients, 3 had a rebleed within 14 days following the last prerandomized bleed and 6 rebled during the 15 to 30-day interval. Eight died during the initial 14-day interval, 7 during the 15 to 30-day interval and 1 at 564 days. Several clinical parameters

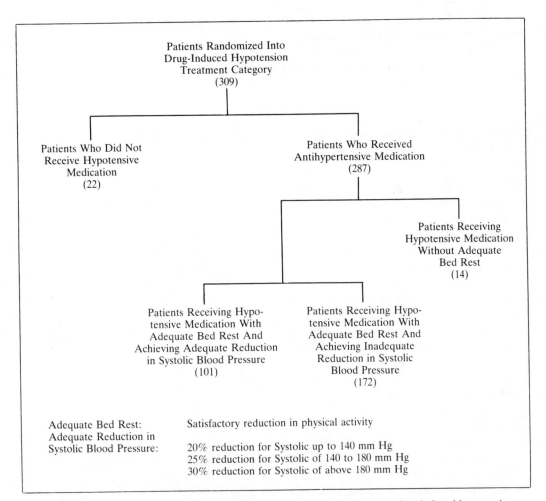

Fig. 6–5. Schematic representation of design for analysis of patients allocated to drug-induced hypotension.

were reviewed within this group, but none was found responsible for causing a disproportion of deaths or rebleeds.

Patients Who Received Antihypertensive Medication but in Whom Bed Rest was Not Accomplished

In 14 patients, bed rest therapy was not carried out satisfactorily as part of drug-induced antihypertensive treatment. Nine were too restless or uncooperative because of disorientation, agitation or hallucinations; 2 patients had recurrent seizures; and 3 were not admitted within 5 weeks following the last bleed. Four of the 14 had a proved rebleed within 34 days following the prerandomized bleed. Six of the 14 died, 2 each following a proved rebleed, a suspected rebleed, and progressive decline in clinical condition. Four deaths occurred within 34 days following the bleed, and 1 each during the 10th and 14th month, respectively.

Patients With Adequate Reduction in Systolic Blood Pressure and Proper Bed Rest

Adequate reduction in blood pressure as specified according to protocol was achieved in 101 patients (32.7%). Adequate reduction was defined as discussed on page 79. The following analysis presents a summary of clinical parameters as they relate to mortality and rebleeding in this group of patients.

A total of 69.3% had an aneurysm on the anterior cerebral artery complex, 26.7% on the intracranial portion of the internal carotid and 4.0% had a middle cerebral artery aneurysm. Seventy-eight patients (77.2%) were in good neurologic condition (Grades 1 and 2); 23 (22.8%) were in poor condition (Grades 3, 4 and 5). At the time of randomization, 27.7% had an average systolic blood pressure below 140 mm Hg, 61.4% had average systolic values between 140 and 180 mm Hg, and 10.9% had average values over 180 mm Hg. Fifty-two of the patients were men; 49 were women. The age distribution

Table 6–21. Frequency Distribution of Patients with Each Range in Percent Change in Blood Pressure from Day Antihypertensive Medication Started to Day Blood Pressure Was Maintained.

Percent Change in Systolic Blood Pressure	Interval From Day Antihypertensive Medication Started to Day Blood Pressure Maintained											
	0–2	3–5	6–8	9–11	12–14	15–17	18–20	21–23	24–26	27–29	30–60	Total
+20% to >−20%	18	17	17	8	3	5	3	3	0	0	2	76
−20% to >−25%	24	17	5	3	3	4	1	4	2	1	2	66
−25% to >−30%	14	23	5	5	5	4	1	0	1	0	0	58
≤−30%	12	10	3	0	0	2	2	1	1	1	1	33
Total	68	67	30	16	11	15	7	8	4	2	5	233
% of 309	22.0		53.4		62.1		69.3		73.1		75.4	

No maintenance blood pressure recorded	69
Insufficient information	7
Total	309

Table 6–22.   Distribution of Cause of Death for Specific Intervals Following Last Bleed in the Adequately Controlled Group.

Days Following Last Bleed	Cause of Death					Total
	Proved Rebleed	Suspected Rebleed	Progressive Decline	Unrelated Event	Unknown	
0–14	5	1	2	0	0	8
15–28	3	0	1	1	1	6
29–44	4	2	0	0	0	6
45–90	2	2	1	0	0	5
91–180	0	0	0	0	2	2
>180	2	2	1	3	1	9
Total	16	7	5	4	4	36

revealed that 5.9% were between 20 and 29 years, 15.8% between 30 and 39, 26.7% between 40 and 49, 33.7% between 50 and 59, 16.8% between 60 and 69 and 1.0% between 70 and 79. The general medical condition on the day of randomization (defined in Table 6–3) was categorized as good in 59.4%, fair in 33.7%, poor in 5.9% and prohibitive in 1.0% of patients. Pre-existing hypertension was noted in 19.8%, and 68.3% had no history of hypertension. In 11.9%, knowledge of pre-existing hypertension was unknown. No angiographic evidence of cerebral vasospasm was noted in 57.4% of patients. Spasm was localized in 23.8% and diffuse in 18.8%.

Mortality during the 6.5-year interval was 35.6% (36 of 101, Table 6–22). Most deaths (44.4%) followed recurrent hemorrhage. A total of 13.9% (14 of 101) died within 28 days following the last bleed; 24.8% died within 90 days. The combined total of suspected and proved rebleeds as the cause of

death was 22.8% (23 of 101). This figure compares with 30.1% (93 of 309) for all patients allocated to treatment with drug-induced antihypertensive medication. The distribution of deaths with proved rebleeds remained very similar for patients allocated to therapy within 7 days (Table 6–23). Thirty-one patients were allocated to drug-induced hypotension during the 8 through 21-day interval. The distribution of deaths and rebleeds was also closely related in this small group of patients (Table 6–24).

Neurologic Condition, Death and Rebleeding.

Deaths among patients in good neurologic condition (Grades 1 and 2) were compared with those in poor condition (Grades 3, 4 and 5). Mortality was 47.8% (11 of 23) among patients in poor condition; among those in good condition 32.0% died ($P = 0.25$).

Table 6–23.   Distribtuion of Deaths and Proved Rebleeds for the 63 Patients Allocated to Treatment Within 7 Days Following Last Bleed in the Adequately Controlled Group.

Days Following Last Bleed	Deaths	Proved Rebleed
0–8	3	5
9–14	5	3
15–30	5	5
31–90	8	3
91–365	3	0
366+	3	2
Total	27	18

Table 6–24.   Distribution of Deaths and Proved Rebleeds for the 31 Patients Allocated to Treatment During the 8 to 21-Day Interval Following Last Bleed in the Adequately Controlled Group.

Days Following Last Bleed	Deaths	Proved Rebleed
15–30	1	0
31–90	3	3
91–365	0	0
366+	5	3
Total	9	6

The major cause of death among patients in good neurologic condition was rebleeding. Progressive decline in neurologic status and/or infectious disease was more frequent as a cause of death in the poor-condition group.

Mortality and Rebleeding Related to Individual Patient Characteristics.

The following discussion relates mortality and proved rebleed rate during the *90-day interval* following last bleed in adequately controlled patients.

Mortality in patients below age 50 was 28.6% (14 of 49), and for those age 50 or above it was 21.2% (11 of 52). Rebleed rate in the lower age group was 26.5% (13 of 49), whereas in the older group it was 11.5% (6 of 52). Mortality was 25.0% (13 of 52) among men and 24.5% among women. Rebleed rate was 17.3% (9 of 52) for men and 20.4% for women. Sex distribution was unrelated to rebleed rate or mortality.

The average systolic blood pressure at randomization was unrelated to subsequent rebleed rate. Among patients with average systolic pressures below 140 mm Hg, 21.4% (6 of 28) rebled; for those with average systolic pressures between 140 and 180 mm Hg systolic, 21.0% (13 of 62) rebled. No patient in the group of 11 with systolic blood pressure above 180 mm Hg rebled. Mortality in the group of patients with a systolic blood pressure below 140 mm Hg was 17.9% at 90 days following the initial bleed (5 of 28), whereas in the group with pressures between 140 and 180 mm Hg mortality was 30.6% (19 of 62). Only 1 death (9.1%) occurred among 11 patients who had systolic pressures over 180 mm Hg. None of these results was significantly different statistically.

Rebleed rate was not significantly different among aneurysm sites. In the combined internal carotid and middle cerebral artery aneurysm groups, 16.1% (5 of 31) rebled within 90 days following the last bleed. In the anterior cerebral group, 20.0% (14 of 70) rebled. Mortality was higher in patients with an anterior cerebral artery aneurysm (30%, or 21 of 70) in comparison to the combined internal carotid and middle cerebral groups (12.9%, or 4 of 31). This difference was not statistically significant ($P = 0.113$).

Rebleed rate was not appreciably different among patients with various medical conditions. The rate was 18.3% (11 of 60) for patients in good condition, 20.6% (7 of 34) for those in fair condition, and 14.3% (1 of 7) in the combined poor and prohibitive groups. In contrast, mortality was 15.0% (9 of 60) in the good-condition group, 38.2% (13 of 34) in the fair-condition group, and 42.9% (3 of 7) in the combined poor and prohibitive group. More deaths in the fair and poor-medical condition groups were associated with other medical disorders superimposed upon or associated with the original bleed.

Rebleed rate in patients without angiographic evidence of cerebral vasospasm was 20.7% (12 of 58). In patients with spasm, rebleed rate was 16.3% (7 of 43). Mortality in patients without spasm was 17.2% (10 of 58), whereas in those with spasm it was 34.9% (15 of 43, $P = 0.07$). Thus, the difference in mortality was appreciable, but statistically the difference was only marginally significant.

Prior to the day antihypertensive medication was started, most patients in this treatment category (56.3% of 309 patients) had average systolic pressures in the range of 140 to 180 mm Hg. Among the 101 patients who had blood pressure reduced according to protocol, a similar proportion (61.4%) had average systolic pressures in the same range prior to treatment. An analysis of deaths and rebleeds in these 101 patients reveals that mortality and rebleed rate were not significantly different between specific increments in systolic blood pressure (Table 6–25). A comparative analysis of percentages in mortality in this table reveals no more than a 6.3% difference among average levels of systolic blood pressure, and for proved rebleeds no more than a 5.2% difference.

Rebleed rate was also unrelated to the diastolic pressure at randomization. In 63

Table 6–25.   Distribution of Deaths and Proved Rebleeds Within 90 Days Following Last Bleed in Patients with Average Systolic Blood Pressure at Randomization in Adequately Controlled Group.

Average Systolic Blood Pressure (mm Hg)	Total No. Patients	Deaths	Proved Rebleeds
101–140	36	8 (22.2%)	7 (19.4%)
141–160	37	9 (24.3%)	6 (16.2%)
Over 160	28	8 (28.6%)	6 (21.4%)
Total	101	25 (24.8%)	19 (18.8%)

patients with average diastolic pressures of 90 mm Hg or below, 17.4% rebled; in those with pressures above 90 mm Hg, 21.6% rebled (8 of 37). Similarly, mortality was 23.8% (15 of 63) in the group with average diastolic pressures below 90 mm Hg, whereas in the group above 90 mm Hg it was 27.0% (10 of 38).

Analysis relating proved rebleeds and mortality to various levels of mean blood pressure also shows no statistically significant difference (Table 6–26). The greatest difference in rebleed rate between any two increments in mean blood pressure was 7.8%; for mortality, 4.2%. Therefore, the various blood pressure levels *prior to treatment* were unrelated to subsequent mortality and rebleed rate within 90 days following last bleed. The question arises as to how much effect decreased systolic blood pressure had upon prevention of rebleeding or

death. Discussion of that subject will follow after presentation of the data among patients who achieved inadequate control of blood pressure during antihypertensive treatment.

Patients With Proper Bed Rest But Inadequate Reduction in Systolic Blood Pressure

Patients with inadequate reduction in blood pressure (defined in Fig. 6–5) did not achieve the designated decrease in systolic blood pressure during the three-week treatment period. A group of 172 patients form the basis for this analysis relating clinical characteristics to mortality and proved rebleeds. Forty-five patients had an internal carotid artery aneurysm, 28 had an aneurysm on the middle cerebral distribution and 99 on the anterior cerebral complex. Neurologic condition was classified as good in 119 patients

Table 6–26.   Distribution of Proved Rebleeds and Deaths Within 90 Days Following Last Bleed for Specified Levels of Mean Blood Pressure at Randomization in Adequately Controlled Group.

Mean Blood Pressure at Randomization	Total No. Patients	Proved Rebleed	Deaths
71–90	10	0	0
91–110	50	9 (18.0%)	14 (28.0%)
111–130	31	8 (25.8%)	8 (25.8%)
>130	10	2 (20.0%)	3 (30.0%)
Total	101	19 (18.8%)	25 (24.7%)

Table 6–27.   Distribution of Cause of Death at Specific Intervals Following Last Bleed for Patients with Inadequate Blood Pressure Reduction.

Days Following Last Bleed	Cause of Death					
	Proved Rebleed	Suspected Rebleed	Progressive Decline	Unrelated Cause	Unknown	Total
0–7	3	0	3	0	1	7
8–14	15	2	6	2	0	25
15–28	14	2	2	0	0	18
29–44	2	0	0	2	0	4
45–90	1	2	0	1	2	6
91–180	0	0	1	2	0	3
>180	9	5	0	8	0	22
Total	44	11	12	15	3	85

(69.2% of 172, Grades 1 and 2) and poor in 53 (30.8%, Grades 3, 4 and 5). General medical condition (defined in Table 6–3) on the day of allocation to treatment was classified as good in 53.5%, fair in 34.9%, poor in 8.1% and prohibitive in 3.5%. Analysis of age distribution reveals 8.7% were in the 2nd and 3rd decades of life, 20.3% in the 4th, 21.5% in the 5th, 35.5% in the 6th and 14.0% in the 7th and 8th decades. Eighty-two patients were men; 90 were women. A positive history for pre-existing hypertension was reported in 24.4%, whereas 61.6% had no such history. In 14.0% no information about pre-existing hypertension was available. Cerebral vasospasm was reported as being absent in 57.0% of patients on the initial cerebral angiogram, whereas in 26.2% spasm was present and localized and in 16.9% it was diffuse. The average systolic blood pressure at randomization was in the range of 141 to 160 mm Hg in 36.6% of patients; 37.8% were below this range and 25.6% were above. Mean blood pressure distribution was highest among patients between 91 and 110 mm Hg (43.0%). All clinical parameters were distributed in similar proportions to the number of patients with adequate blood pressure reduction. No specific parameter could be found responsible for failure of adequate reduction in systolic blood pressure during the three-week treatment period.

Mortality during the mean 6.5-year interval was 49.4% (85 of 172) among patients with inadequate reduction in systolic blood pressure. Most deaths were caused by a proved rebleed (51.8%, or 44 of 85, Table 6–27). The majority of deaths from rebleeding occurred between the 8th and 28th day (65.9%, or 29 of 44) following the prerandomized bleed. The remaining deaths occurred at irregular intervals.

For patients randomized within 7 days following last bleed, the majority had a proved rebleed between the 9th and 30th day (Table 6–28). Following day 30, the number of deaths due to a proved rebleed diminished.

For patients randomized during the 8 through 21-day interval, 17 of 43 patients (39.5%) rebled during the mean 6.5-year follow-up period and 23 patients died (53.5%, Table 6–29). Deaths and rebleeds in patients with inadequate reduction of blood pressure were appreciably higher beginning at the 9

Table 6–28.   Distribution of Deaths and Proved Rebleeds for the 110 Patients Allocated to Treatment Within 7 Days Following Last Bleed.

Days Following Last Bleed	Deaths	Proved Rebleed
0–8	9	11
9–14	19	13
15–30	11	9
31–90	6	3
91–365	5	3
366+	7	3
Total	57	42

Table 6–29.   Distribution of Deaths and Proved Rebleeds for the 43 Patients Allocated to Treatment Between the 8th and 21st Day Following Last Bleed.

Days Following Last Bleed	Deaths	Proved Rebleed
9–14	4	5
15–30	8	7
31–90	3	1
91–365	3	2
>365	5	2
Total	23	17

through 14-day interval following the pre-randomization bleed in the 0 through 7-day group than in the 8 through 21-day interval when the major increase occurred at the 15 through 30-day period (Table 6–29). These were the only major differences observed between the adequately and inadequately treated patients.

For the 19 patients randomized during the 22 through 92-day interval, no recurrent hemorrhages were reported but 5 deaths occurred. Two patients died between the 91st and 180th day following last bleed; 1 died during the 3rd year, and 2 died during the 5th year following the bleed.

Neurologic Condition, Death and Rebleeding.

Mortality among patients in good neurologic condition (Grades 1 and 2) was 46.2% (55 of 119), and for those in poor condition (Grades 3, 4 and 5) mortality was 56.6% (30 of 53). These results show a slightly lower mortality among those with adequate reduction in blood pressure (32.0% for good-condition patients vs 47.8% for those in poor condition). Statistical differences between these values were not significant. The frequency distribution of deaths for each neurologic condition differed somewhat in comparison to those who received adequate reduction. Within 20 days following last bleed, deaths occurred in 63.3% (19 of 30) of the poor-condition patients and 45.5% (25 of 55) of those in good condition.

For patients who attained adequate reduction in blood pressure, 45.4% (5 of 11) of poor-condition patients died and only 28% (7 of 25) of good-condition subjects expired.

The percentage of patients with a proved rebleed for those in good and poor neurologic condition during the 6.5-year interval did not differ significantly (37.0% for patients in good condition, 28.3% for those in poor condition). More rebleeds occurred within 20 days in the poor-condition group (93.3%, or 14 of 15), and only 54.5% (24 of 44) rebled in the good-condition group. For patients with adequate blood pressure control, the proportion of proved rebleeds within 20 days in good-condition patients was 38.1%. Therefore, an important difference between the adequately and inadequately controlled groups was the number of rebleeds which occurred within 20 days following last bleed. The primary reason for increased mortality among patients inadequately controlled was the higher rebleed rate among patients in poor neurologic condition within three weeks following the last bleed. In addition, patients in good neurologic condition with adequate blood pressure control had a reduced rebleed rate during this interval.

Mortality and Rebleeding Related to Individual Patient Characteristics.

With 70.6% of deaths and 83.1% of proved rebleeds observed within 90 days following last bleed, several secondary analyses of specific clinical parameters were related to mortality and rebleed rate. For all aneurysm sites, the mortality was 34.9% and the rebleed rate was 28.5%. Patients in good medical condition had a 19.6% (18 of 92) proved rebleed rate; those in fair condition, 43.3% (26 of 60); and those in poor and prohibitive condition, 25% (5 of 20). Mortality was 23.9% (22 of 92) for patients in good medical condition, 41.7% (25 of 60) for those in fair condition and 65.0% (13 of 20) for patients in poor and prohibitive condition. The proved rebleed rate below age 50 was 28.7% (25 of 87), and for those age 50 or above it was

28.2% (24 of 85). Mortality in patients below age 50 was 32.2% (28 of 87), whereas for those age 50 or above it was 37.6% (32 of 85). Rebleed rate was 29.3% (24 of 82) among men and 27.8% (25 of 90) for women. Mortality was 32.9% (27 of 82) for men and 36.7% (33 of 90) for women.

A higher percentage of proved rebleeds was observed among patients with higher ranges of average systolic blood pressure. For patients with average systolic blood pressure below 140 mm Hg, 21.5% (14 of 65) had a proved rebleed and 26.2% died. In patients with an average systolic blood pressure between 141 and 180 mm Hg, 33.7% (30 of 89) had a proved rebleed and 39.3% died. The differences between proved rebleed rate and mortality in these two groups were not statistically significant ($P = 0.14$ for rebleed rate and $P = 0.12$ for deaths).

An analysis of diastolic blood pressure related to rebleed rate did not show as much difference as the results with systolic pressure. Although the trend toward an increased number of rebleeds was seen with diastolic levels up to 105 mm Hg, there were fewer rebleeds in the group with diastolic levels above 105 mm Hg. Patients with diastolic blood pressure of 90 mm Hg or below had a 24.2% (24 of 99) rebleed rate and a mortality of 29.3% (29 of 99). Patients with diastolic blood pressure between 91 and 120 mm Hg had a 34.8% (24 of 69) rebleed rate and 43.5% died (30 of 69). These differences were not statistically significant.

Mean blood pressure below 110 mm Hg was associated with a proved rebleed rate of 23.2% (22 of 95), but in patients with mean blood pressure between 111 and 150 mm Hg, 35.6% (26 of 73) rebled. Mortality for patients with mean pressures of 110 mm Hg or below was 28.4% (27 of 95); for those with mean pressures between 111 and 150 mm Hg, 42.5% (31 of 73) died. The differences for rebleed rate and for mortality were not statistically significant.

Cerebral vasospasm was related statistically to mortality, but not for rebleeding. Mortality was 45.9% for patients with vaso-

spasm and 26.5% ($P = 0.01$) for those without spasm. Rebleed rate for those with vasospasm was 35.1%; for those without spasm it was 23.5% ($P = 0.13$).

Mortality and Rebleeding Among Centers

Comparison of proved rebleeds and deaths among participating centers reveals no statistically significant differences. Eleven centers (less than 20 patients each) had a total of 84 patients with 21 (25.0%) who rebled within 90 days following the last bleed. Of the three other centers which had more than 20 patients, there was one with a rebleed rate of 25.6% (10 of 39), one with 34.8% (8 of 23) and another with 38.5% (10 of 26). Mortality among the group of 84 patients from 11 centers was 35.7%. One center with 39 patients had a 33.3% mortality, another with 26 patients had a 38.5% rate and one with 23 patients had a mortality of 30.4%.

Cerebral Angiography

Of 414 angiographic studies performed on 309 patients, 23 (7.4%) had complications during or within 24 hours following the procedure. These complications were as follows: 5 patients acquired hemiparesis alone or hemiplega and aphasia (in 2 the deficits cleared within 3 hours, but in 3 they were permanent); transient aphasia was observed in 2 patients, but in both instances it cleared prior to discharge; 4 patients had severe hypotension requiring vasopressor medication; 4 rebled but remained alive; 2 had transient confusion; 1 developed permanent brain stem ischemia and frontal lobe infarction; 1 developed temporary right homonymous hemianopsia; 1 had transient apnea; 1 had unspecified complications. Among these 21 patients, morbidity was permanent in 6 and transient in 15 (duration no more than 24 hours) or cleared prior to discharge. Two patients died during angiography (0.6%).

In addition to the demonstration of a single intracranial aneurysm, displacement of the cerebral arteries was reported in 55 of 309 patients (17.8%). In 7, vessel displacement was consistent with an extracerebral mass. Thirty-seven reported the abnormality consistent with an intracerebral mass, and 11 had a widened sweep of the anterior cerebral arteries. The extracerebral mass lesions were interpreted as hematoma formation outside of the cerebral hemispheres, and the intracerebral mass lesions were believed to be regional cerebral edema, hematoma formation or a combination of both. An increase in ventricular size evidenced by increased sweep of the anterior cerebral arteries was noted in 11 patients (3.5%).

Cerebral angiography was performed more than once in 88 of 309 patients (28.5%). The reasons for multiple procedures included the performance of one carotid system at a time at some institutions. Some patients were reevaluated after deterioration in neurologic condition associated with a rebleed or ischemic deficit, and others had their vertebral-basilar system visualized at later intervals. These were not unusual circumstances given the years (1963 to 1970) when these angiographic studies were performed.

Vertebral-basilar visualization was performed in 37.2% of patients (115 of 309). Therefore, the presence of a single aneurysm was certain in these patients only.

Thirty-nine percent (120 of 309) had selected post-treatment cerebral angiograms at a mean interval of 3 months following the first angiogram. In this group of 120 patients, 41 had more than 20% enlargement in the size of the aneurysm; in 40 patients the aneurysm size remained the same (± 20%); and in 25 patients the size was at least 20% less compared to the determination on the initial study. In 14 patients, no information was available on aneurysm size. The mean interval between initial angiography and the follow-up study was 109.4 days. These data illustrate that aneurysm size following a rupture may not remain the same, but may enlarge (38.6%) or diminish (23.6%).

Cerebral Vasospasm

Intra-arterial narrowing (interpreted as vasospasm by the attending physician at each investigating institution) was reported on the patient data forms. There are a number of pitfalls in presentation and interpretation of data such as these, with potential discrepancies due to variation in techniques for taking angiographic measurements of vessels, size of radiographs and location of measurements on the vessel.

The angiograms were classified into one of three categories: (1) no vasospasm, (2) localized vasospasm (narrowing of intra-arterial diameter over 1 to 3 cm on the proximal portion of the intracranial internal carotid artery, middle cerebral, anterior cerebral-anterior communicating or vertebral-basilar artery), and (3) diffuse vasospasm (narrowed diameter of the internal carotid artery and all main ipsilateral branches). The frequency of localized vasospasm was 24.9% for all aneurysm sites combined, and the proportion of patients with diffuse spasm was 17.9%. The largest proportion of patients had localized spasm during the 6 through 8-day interval (39.1%, Table 6–30), and for diffuse spasm the highest number occurred during the 9 through 14-day interval (31.8%). For the entire group, the highest number of patients with spasm had their initial angiograms during the 6 through 14-day interval.

The incidence of vasospasm was correlated with age. The frequency distribution of vasospasm for patients below and above age 50 was 41.1 and 46.2%, respectively. Women had a slightly higher percentage than men (48.4 vs 38.8%). No significant differences in the frequency of spasm were observed between one aneurysm site and another. The incidence of vasospasm was 42.7% among patients with an internal carotid artery aneurysm, 40.0% among patients with a middle cerebral artery aneurysm and 44.8% among patients with an aneurysm on the anterior cerebral complex. Patients in fair or poor medical condition

Table 6–30.   Distribution of Patients with Localized or Diffuse Vasospasm at Specific Intervals Following Last Bleed.

Type of Vasospasm	Days Following Last Bleed						Total
	0–2	3–5	6–8	9–14	15–30	31–60	
Localized	20	25	18	6	5	1	75
Diffuse	19	12	11	7	5	0	54
Total	39	37	29	13	10	1	129
Total patients each interval	105	96	46	22	24	8	301
% with spasm	37.1	38.5	63.0	59.1	41.7	12.5	42.9

had an increased frequency of vasospasm as compared to those in good condition. The frequency of vasospasm in patients who were symptom-free or had minor neurologic symptoms (headache, stiff neck, photophobia) was 36.4% (80 of 220); 61.8% of patients in poor neurologic condition (major neurologic deficit, poorly responsive, or seriously ill) had spasm.

Systolic Blood Pressure and Vasospasm

The incidence of vasospasm was not appreciably higher among patients with elevated systolic blood pressure. The percentages of patients with spasm at systolic pressures above 140 mm Hg varied from 40.7 to 53.1%; for patients with average systolic pressures of 140 mm Hg or below, the range was 30.8 to 47.2%.

Analysis of vasospasm in patients whose blood pressure was controlled (as specified in the protocol) showed that localized and diffuse spasm occurred most frequently between the 6th and 14th day following the last bleed. A similar distribution was observed in patients with blood pressure controlled inadequately.

Some variation in the distribution of spasm among patients who achieved adequate or inadequate blood pressure reduction was observed between aneurysm sites; however, the differences were not statistically significant. Comparison of patients with an internal carotid artery aneurysm and the group with an anterior cerebral-anterior communicating artery aneurysm revealed that the percentage of patients with vasospasm was 33.3% for the former group and 47.1% for the latter. For the inadequately controlled group, 53.3% of patients with an internal carotid artery aneurysm had spasm vs 38.4% of those with an anterior cerebral-anterior communicating artery aneurysm.

Mean Blood Pressure and Vasospasm

Except for patients with mean blood pressures below 90 mm Hg, no appreciable differences were observed at various levels from 90 to over 150 mm Hg (Table 6–31). For the number of patients at each specified range of mean blood pressure, no significant differences in the distribution of vasospasm were noted between those with adequately and inadequately controlled blood pressure.

Angiographic Size of Aneurysm and Vasospasm

Measurements of aneurysm size on radiographs from the lateral and anterior-posterior projections were recorded on the patient data forms in their dimensions (mm). The volume (mm^3) was calculated at the Central Registry and analyzed with the various clinical parameters. Comparison of the incidence of vasospasm and aneurysm size at specific size ranges revealed no significant differences in the frequency of vasospasm.

Table 6–31.   Distribution of Vasospasm as Related to Mean Blood Pressure in the Entire Treatment Group.

Mean Blood Pressure (mm Hg)	Total No. Patients	Patients with Vasospasm
71–90	36	8
91–110	140	67
111–130	103	47
121–150	24	10
>150	5	2
Total	308*	134

* Insufficient information in 1 patient

Summary

Multiple angiographic procedures (more than one) were performed in 28.5% of patients prior to randomization. Selected post-treatment angiograms revealed that the size of the aneurysm increased in 34.2% of patients within 3 months following last bleed and decreased in 20.8%. Complicating events during or within 24 hours of the angiogram occurred in 7.4%. Mortality associated with the study was 0.6%.

Cerebral vasospasm of the localized variety was observed more frequently (24.9%) than the diffuse form (17.9%). Vasospasm was observed most frequently when the initial angiographic study was performed during the 6 through 14-day period following the last bleed. A higher than average frequency of cerebral vasospasm was observed among patients in fair and poor medical condition, and in subjects with poor neurologic condition. No statistically significant differences in frequency of vasospasm were observed among aneurysm sites, age and sex distribution, specific increments of systolic or mean blood pressure, or various aneurysm sizes.

Discussion

Drug-induced reduction in systolic blood pressure has been used frequently as part of a medical regimen in the treatment of patients with recently ruptured intracranial aneurysm. The frequency of recurrent hemorrhage has been reported to be significantly diminished with this treatment, particularly for patients not amenable to surgical therapy.

Among 109 patients reported in the previous Cooperative Study,[9] 52 died (48%). Mortality varied from 13% among Grade 2 patients to 78% for those in Grade 5. The same combinations of antihypertensive medication were used as in the present study, with the addition of methyldopa and hydralazine. In the earlier study, 47% had treatment initiated within 4 days following the last bleed and 70.6% within 10 days. Seventy-seven percent of survivors had no disability, or were able to perform previous work with modification.

Mortality during the mean 6.5-year follow-up period was 55.1% (103 of 187) in the bed rest group and 44.3% (121 of 273) for patients with drug-induced hypotension. This difference was statistically significant ($P = 0.03$). This reduction in mortality among patients who received antihypertensive medication with adequate blood pressure reduction was believed to be the reason for this difference. The primary reason for improved survival was the decrease in rebleed rate in adequately controlled patients when compared to the rate observed in those inadequately controlled.

Rebleeding and Mortality

Among 101 patients who achieved adequate blood pressure control in the present study,

16 died following a rebleed. A total of 24 had a proved rebleed; the mortality was 66.7% (16 of 24). Among the 172 patients with inadequately controlled blood pressure, 44 deaths (25.6%) followed a proved rebleed. For all patients allocated to drug-induced hypotensive treatment, 97 rebled (Table 6–13), and 70 of these (72.2%) died (Table 6–6). Therefore, not only was recurrent hemorrhage the major morbidity factor, but death following rebleeding was of major consequence among the entire treatment group. This compares with an 83.8% mortality (62 of 74) following recurrent hemorrhage among patients allocated to regulated bed rest.[2] Thus, drug-induced blood pressure reduction as an overall treatment program had no significant effect upon survival *following recurrent hemorrhage.*

Medical Condition and Rebleed Rate

Rebleed rate was not significantly different among various patients with different medical conditions in the adequately controlled patients. However, among inadequately controlled patients in good medical condition, the proved rebleed rate was 19.6%; for patients in fair condition, it was 43.3%. The reason for the high mortality of 65.0% (13 of 20) in patients with poor and prohibitive medical condition was the increased number of patients who were in poor neurologic condition. Death due to rebleeding occurred in 5 of 20 patients.

Vasospasm, Rebleed Rate and Mortality

Comparison of proved rebleeds and mortality among patients with vasospasm reveals a lower than average rebleed rate in the adequately controlled group (16.3%), but mortality was 34.9%. This suggests that drug-induced blood pressure reduction in the presence of cerebral vasospasm may have been detrimental in this group of patients.

Pre-existing Hypertension, Rebleed Rate and Mortality

As a predisposing medical factor, there was no evidence that pre-existing hypertension had any influence on rebleeding. However, mortality was increased by 13.3% in patients with pre-existing hypertension in the group adequately controlled and by 9.8% in the inadequately controlled group. Statistically, these differences were not significant, but the trend toward higher mortality was apparent.

Antihypertensive Medication Used

The antihypertensive medications used during the treatment period and for variable intervals following discharge were reserpine, chlorothiazide, methyldopa and hydralazine, alone and in combination. Dosages of these medications were monitored as clinically indicated by the attending physician for proper blood pressure control. The wide variation of response to various antihypertensive agents did not permit use of restricted dosage schedules for each medication. The most frequently used preparations were chlorothiazide and methyldopa. These medications, alone or in combination, were the most effective in reducing blood pressure in the adequately controlled group. A more detailed analysis of the distribution of specific combinations revealed no evidence that one combination was more effective than another. In the adequately controlled group, chlorothiazide was used in 84.2% of patients and methyldopa in 67.3%. A similar proportion of patients was treated with these agents in the inadequately controlled group. There was no difference in the frequency of treatment with reserpine between the adequately and inadequately controlled groups, or between the oral and intramuscular preparations of this drug.

The interval between the last bleed and the beginning of antihypertensive medication was 11 days or less in 80% of patients for each medication in both the adequately and inadequately controlled groups. The combination of a chlorothiazide and methyldopa was also the most frequent combination used in both groups.

The usual approach for administration of these medications was a cautious decrease in systolic blood pressure without causing further neurologic deficit. In the inadequately controlled group, antihypertensive medication was abandoned in only 8 patients because of an increase in neurologic deficit. Eight others were regarded as unsuitable for treatment because their systolic pressure was already below 120 mm Hg. Death occurred in 5 patients following the first few doses of antihypertensive medication, but the cause of death was not attributed to the medication.

Among 309 patients allocated randomly to drug-induced hypotension, 22 had inadequate bed rest, 14 received no antihypertensive medication and 172 had inadequate reduction in systolic blood pressure, leaving 101 patients with systolic blood pressure reduction as specified according to protocol. Within the latter group, mortality was significantly decreased. The major reason was a significantly lower rebleed rate within the 3-week interval following last bleed.

The question of whether the differences reported in this study are truly the result of effective lowering of blood pressure remains unanswered. The data show the importance of several clinical variables which are necessary to consider when evaluating patients with subarachnoid hemorrhage following a ruptured intracranial aneurysm. These include medical and neurologic condition of the patient, aneurysm location, vasospasm, age, sex and the interval following last bleed. Any one of these may have selective influence upon outcome at various intervals following the rupture of an intracranial aneurysm.

Conclusions

I. Patients allocated to drug-induced hypotension in this Cooperative Study had the following characteristics:

1. Among 309 patients, 82 had a recently ruptured internal carotid artery aneurysm, 35 had a middle cerebral artery aneurysm and 192 had an aneurysm on the anterior cerebral-anterior communicating artery complex.

2. Sixty-one percent of the patients were allocated to treatment within 7 days following the last bleed, 29% between the 8th and 21st day and 10% during the 22nd and 92nd day.

3. At entry into the study, 71% were in good neurologic condition (minor symptoms such as headache, meningeal irritation or diplopia); 29% were in poor condition.

4. Fifty-five percent were in good medical condition at entry into the study; 35% were in fair condition and 10% were in poor and prohibitive condition.

5. Localized or diffuse vasospasm was present in 43.6% of patients.

6. Among patients in good neurologic condition, 36.4% had vasospasm; whereas in subjects in poor neurologic condition, 61.8% had vasospasm.

7. An analysis of sex distribution revealed that 49.2% of patients were men and 50.8% were women.

8. The average systolic blood pressure at entry into the study was as follows: 140 mm Hg or below in 38% of patients, 141 through 160 mm Hg in 35%, 161 through 180 mm Hg in 16.6%, and, over 180 mm Hg in 10.4%.

II. Among 309 patients, overall mortality during a mean period of 6.5 years was 46.3%.

1. Mortality was 42.7% among patients with an internal carotid artery aneurysm, 48.6% among those with a middle cerebral artery aneurysm, and 47.4% among patients with an aneurysm on the anterior cerebral-anterior communicating artery complex.

2. Mortality was 50.5% among patients randomized within 7 days, 46.6% in patients randomized between 8 and 21 days, and 19.4% for those allocated to treatment during the 22 to 92-day period.

3. Mortality was 43.0% in mentally alert patients (Grades 1, 2 and 3), but 69.2% in poor-condition patients (Grades 4 and 5).

4. Death caused by a proved or clinically suspected rebleed was reported in 29.8% (22.7% proved and 7.1% suspected clinically).

5. Deaths following a proved rebleed were reported with greatest frequency between the 6th and 23rd day following the initial bleed.

6. Among the 189 patients allocated to treatment within 7 days following the initial bleed, 50% of deaths in patients with an internal carotid artery aneurysm, 66.7% in patients with a middle cerebral artery aneurysm and 50% of those with an aneurysm on the anterior cerebral artery complex occurred within 14 days.

7. Patients with an aneurysm on the anterior cerebral-anterior communicating artery had a greater number of deaths and/or rebleeds after the initial 30-day interval following the prerandomized bleed than those with an internal carotid or middle cerebral artery aneurysm.

8. Survival among patients with a 20% decrease or more in systolic blood pressure was significantly superior to those with a less than 20% decrease in blood pressure.

9. Mortality among patients with systolic blood pressure of 140 mm Hg or below at entry into the study was 38.5%. For patients with an average systolic pressure over 140 through 160 mm Hg, mortality was 43.5%; for patients with an average systolic pressure between 160 and 180 mm Hg, mortality was 60.8%. In patients with average systolic pressure over 180 mm Hg, mortality was 62.5%.

10. Mortality in patients with localized and diffuse vasospasm was 54.4%; in those without spasm, mortality was 40.2%.

11. Average mortality was slightly higher in the older age groups. Comparison of the number of deaths among patients above and below age 50 revealed no statistically significant difference.

12. The number of proved rebleeds in patients with vasospasm was 34.3%, compared to 29.3% among those with no vasospasm.

13. The proportion of rebleeds among patients in Grades 1 and 2 neurologic condition was 33.6%; for those in Grades 3 through 5, the average percentage was 25.8%.

14. The lowest proportion of rebleeds (14.7%) was reported among patients without vasospasm in poor neurologic condition; in those with vasospasm, 32.7% rebled.

15. During the 60-day interval following the bleed, 28.4% of patients rebled in the group randomized within 7 days; 27.3% rebled in the group randomized in the 8 to 21-day interval.

16. No statistically significant differences in rebleed rate were found among patients in good, fair or poor medical condition.

17. During a mean interval of 6.5 years, 31.4% of patients rebled. Within 14 days following the prerandomized bleed, 12.9% of pa-

tients rebled; within 23 days, a total of 19.4% rebled.

18. The proved rebleed rate among patients with systolic blood pressure of 140 mm Hg or below at entry into the study was 27.4%. For patients with an average systolic pressure over 140 and below 160 mm Hg, the rebleed rate was 31.5%; for patients with systolic pressure between 160 and 180 mm Hg, the rebleed rate was 43.1%. In patients with an average systolic pressure above 180 mm Hg, the rebleed rate was 28.1%.

19. Neurologic deficits acquired during drug-induced antihypertensive therapy were observed in 7.1% of patients.

III. Analysis of the 101 patients who received drug-induced blood pressure reduction as specified according to protocol revealed the following:

1. Mortality during the mean 6.5-year interval was 35.6%. Forty-four percent of these deaths followed a recurrent hemorrhage.

2. Proved rebleeds occurred in 24 patients (23.7%) during the mean period of 6.5 years.

3. During the 90-day period following the bleed, mortality was 21.8% among patients in good neurologic condition and 34.8% among those in poor neurologic condition; the rebleed rate was 20.5 and 13.0%, respectively. Mortality was 25.0% among men and 24.5% among women, with a rebleed rate of 17.3% among men and 20.4% among women. Mortality was 15.0% among patients in good medical condition, 38.2% for patients in fair medical condition and 42.9% for those in poor and prohibitive medical condition. The rebleed rate was not significantly different between various medical conditions. A comparative analysis of patients with average blood pressure levels prior to treatment (140 mm Hg systolic or below, > 140 to 180 mm Hg, and over 180 mm Hg) revealed no significant difference in mortality or rebleed rate. The mortality among patients with known pre-existing hypertension was 35.0%, compared to 21.7% among those without pre-existing hypertension. The rebleed rate was 20.0% in the former group and 20.3% in the latter.

IV. Analysis of the 172 patients who did not receive drug-induced blood pressure reduction revealed the following:

1. Mortality during the mean 6.5-year interval was 49.4%. Fifty-two percent of these deaths followed a recurrent hemorrhage.

2. Proved rebleeds occurred in 59 patients (34.3%) during the mean follow-up period of 6.5 years.

3. During the 90-day period following the bleed, mortality was 30.3% among patients in good neurologic condition and 45.3% among those in poor neurologic condition; the rebleed rate was 28.6 and 28.3%, respectively. Mortality was 32.9% among men and 36.7% among women with a rebleed rate of 29.3% among men and 27.8% among women. Mortality was 23.9% among patients in good medical condition, 41.7% for patients in fair medical condition and 65.0% for those in poor and prohibitive medical condition. The rebleed rate was 19.6% among patients in good medical condition, 43.3% for those in fair medical condition and 25.0% among patients in poor and prohibitive medical condition. Of patients with an average systolic blood pressure below 140 mm Hg prior to entry into the study, 26.2% died and 21.5%

had a proved rebleed. In the group with an average systolic pressure above 140 to 180 mm Hg, 39.3% died and 33.7% had a proved rebleed. For patients with an average systolic pressure over 180 mm Hg, 44.4% died and 27.8% had a proved rebleed. Mortality among patients with known pre-existing hypertension was 38.1%, compared to a mortality of 28.3% for those without pre-existing hypertension. The rebleed rate was 26.2% in the former group and 25.5% in the latter.

V. Mortality during a mean 6.5-year follow-up period for all patients randomized to drug-induced hypotensive therapy (309) was 46.3%. Mortality for those randomized to regulated bed rest (202) was 55.0%. This difference was close to statistical significance ($P = 0.07$). Mortality among all patients who received antihypertensive medication (273) was 44.3%. Mortality among patients who received regulated bed rest[2] (187) was 55.1%. This difference was statistically significant ($P = 0.03$).

VI. Recurrent hemorrhage for the overall group of patients randomized to drug-induced hypotension was 31.4% (97 of 309). Of those patients randomized to regulated bed rest, 38.1% rebled (77 of 202). This difference was not statistically significant ($P = 0.14$). Of the 273 patients who received antihypertensive medication, 30.4% had a recurrent hemorrhage; 40.6% in the group treated with regulated bed rest rebled ($P = 0.03$). Therefore, overall rebleed rate was significantly reduced in patients given drug-induced hypotension.

VII. It is reasonable to assume that with the recently developed agents for blood pressure reduction, the number of patients who did not achieve satisfactory control in this study could be reduced appreciably.

References

1. Sahs, A.L., Perret G., Locksley, H.B., Nishioka, H.: Intracranial Aneurysms and Subarachnoid Hemorrhage. A Cooperative Study. J. B. Lippincott Co., Philadelphia, 1969.
2. Nibbelink, D.W., Henderson, W.G., Torner, J.C.: Cooperative study of intracranial aneurysms and subarachnoid hemorrhage. Report on a randomized treatment study. IV–A Regulated bed rest-medical evaluation. Stroke 8:202–218, 1977.
3. Slosberg, P.S.: Treatment of ruptured intracranial aneurysms by induced hypotension. Mount Sinai J Med. N.Y. 40:82–90, 1973.
4. Nibbelink, D.W., Knowler, L.A.: Cooperative aneurysm project: Introductory report of a randomized treatment study. Cerebral Vascular Diseases (Eighth Princeton Conference), January 5–7, 1972, pp. 33–41.
5. Henderson, W.G., Torner, J.C., Nibbelink, D.W.: Cooperative study of intracranial aneurysms and subarachnoid hemorrhage. Report on a randomized treatment study. IV–B Regulated bed rest-statistical evaluation. Stroke 8:579–589, 1977.
6. Graf, C.J., Nibbelink, D.W.: Cooperative study of intracranial aneurysms and subarachnoid hemorrhage. Report on randomized treatment study. III. Intracranial surgery. Stroke 5:557–601, 1974.
7. Nibbelink, D.W., Knowler L.A.: Cooperative Study of intracranial aneurysms and subarachnoid hemorrhage. Report on a randomized treatment study. II. Objectives and design of randomized aneurysm study. Stroke 5:552–556, 1974.
8. Nibbelink, D.W.: Cooperative Aneurysm Study. Antihypertensive and antifibrinolytic therapy following subarachnoid hemorrhage from ruptured intracranial aneurysm. In: Whisnant, J.P., Sandok, B.A.: Cerebral Vascular Diseases, Grune & Stratton, Inc., New York, 1975, pp 155–165.
9. Sahs, A.L.: Hypotension and hypothermia in the treatment of intracranial aneurysms. In: Sahs, A.L., Perret, G., Locksley, H., Nishioka, H.: Intracranial Aneurysms and Subarachnoid Hemorrhage. J. B. Lippincott Co., Philadelphia 1969, pp 143–149.

Chapter 7

Randomized Treatment Study. Drug-induced Hypotension: Statistical Evaluation

James C. Torner, M.S., William G. Henderson, M.P.H., Ph.D. and Donald W. Nibbelink, M.D., Ph.D.

Abstract

Mortality and proved rebleed rate were analyzed statistically in relation to several clinical variables in patients with recently ruptured intracranial aneurysms. A total of 309 patients were treated with antihypertensive therapy for a 3-week period. The outcomes of the clinical variables were analyzed statistically by a life table method.

Medical condition prior to treatment, cerebral vasospasm and large aneurysm size (> 200 mm^3) were the most significant parameters causing increased mortality during long-term follow-up. Elevated mean blood pressure (> 110 mm Hg) and large aneurysm size (> 200 mm^3) prior to treatment were the most significant factors responsible for a high rebleed rate. When systemic blood pressure could not be maintained within the 30-day interval following the bleed, mortality and rebleed rate were significantly higher at 1 month as compared to patients with blood pressure controlled according to protocol.

Introduction

The medical treatment of recently ruptured intracranial aneurysms with antihypertensive drugs has been one of the usual therapeutic measures used in the early prevention of recurrent hemorrhage and death. This therapy was one of four treatment modalities studied in a randomized clinical trial conducted by the Cooperative Aneurysm Project from 1963 to 1970.[1] The design of the study,[2] preliminary results,[3] detailed analyses of intracranial surgery,[4] regulated bed rest,[5,6] and an overall discussion of drug-induced hypotension (Chapter 6) have been reported. This paper describes the statistical results of a 5-year follow-up period after 3 weeks of antihypertensive therapy.

Treatment Definition

Patients with proved subarachnoid hemorrhage from a single ruptured intracranial aneurysm were allocated to antihypertensive therapy in a randomized treatment program (Chapter 6). Drug-induced hypotension was defined as achieved when systolic blood pressure was decreased a minimum of 20% for patients with an average systolic blood pressure less than 140 mm Hg, a minimum of 25% for patients with an average systolic level of 140 to 180 mm Hg, and a minimum of 30% for patients with average systolic levels greater than 180 mm Hg. The baseline blood pressure value was determined by calculating the average of four blood pressures taken at more than 4-hour intervals by the usual manometric method prior to treatment. Completion of the regulated bed rest program was also a necessary requirement for this analysis. The detailed criteria of regulated bed rest are contained in a previous report.[5] Patients with an inadequate reduction in blood pressure were those who had a maintenance blood pressure reduction less than that specified above.

The antihypertensive medications used in this study were reserpine, chlorothiazide, methyldopa and/or hydralazine. These medications were given in dosages appropriate for each patient considering his/her condition and response to treatment.

Statistical Methodology

The data were obtained through computer-based programs which provided frequency information and statistical analyses. The outcome of clinical variables was analyzed statistically by a clinical life table method similar to that of Cutler and Ederer.[7] The method adopts an ideology of Mantel and Byar[8] which recognizes that each patient is not at risk until treatment has begun. Statistical testing of differences in recurrent hemorrhage or death at the specified intervals was accomplished by the LINCAT program described by Grizzle, Starmer, and Koch,[9] and Koch, Johnson, and Tolley.[10] The statistically significant differences represent trends in mortality or recurrent hem-

orrhage. The primary purpose of this Cooperative Study was the comparison of results of treatments with respect to incidence of recurrent hemorrhage and death, and not a test of hypotheses of clinical factors relating to rebleeding and death.

Patient Selection

Of the 1,005 patients eligible for treatment, 315 were allocated randomly to drug-induced antihypertensive therapy. Six of these patients were disqualified. Of the remaining 309 patients, 82 had an internal carotid aneurysm, 35 had a middle cerebral aneurysm and 192 had an anterior cerebral-anterior communicating aneurysm. One hundred and ninety patients were randomized within 7 days from their last prerandomization bleed, 88 were randomized within the 2nd and 3rd week and 31 were randomized between the 4th and 12th week. The percentage distribution of these randomization variables and those variables considered to be significantly at risk are presented in Table 7–1. In summary, 28.8% of the patients randomized to drug-induced hypotension were in poor neurologic condition (Grades 3 to 5), 44.7% had a complicating medical condition, 23.9% had a history of previously documented hypertension, 43.7% had localized or diffuse vasospasm at angiography and 62.1% had a prerandomization systolic blood pressure of greater than 140 mm Hg. Patient groups were subdivided on the basis of accomplished treatment according to protocol (Fig. 7–1). Detailed explanation of these patient groups is included in the clinical discussion (Chapter 6).

Results

Mortality and rebleed rate were analyzed separately in relation to several clinical variables.

Mortality

Cause of Death

Of the 273 patients who received antihypertensive treatment with adequate bed rest (Fig. 7–1), 115 died during a 5-year follow-up period (Table 7–2). Sixty-six percent of those deaths were due to recurrent hemorrhage, either proved or suspected. Fifteen percent of all deaths in 5 years were due to progressive decline in clinical condition after the prerandomization bleed.

During the first 30 days after the bleed, 56.5% of the 5-year deaths occurred. Within the 30-day interval, 63.1% of all deaths were due to a proved rebleed, 7.7% were due to a suspected rebleed and 21.5% were due to progressive clinical deterioration following the bleed.

Aneurysm-Related Deaths

Deaths related directly to aneurysm rupture (Table 7–3) were due primarily to the pathologic changes resulting from the pretreatment bleed. In 273 patients, a mortality of 23% occurred within 30 days after the bleed. At the end of 5 years, 37% died (Table 7–4).

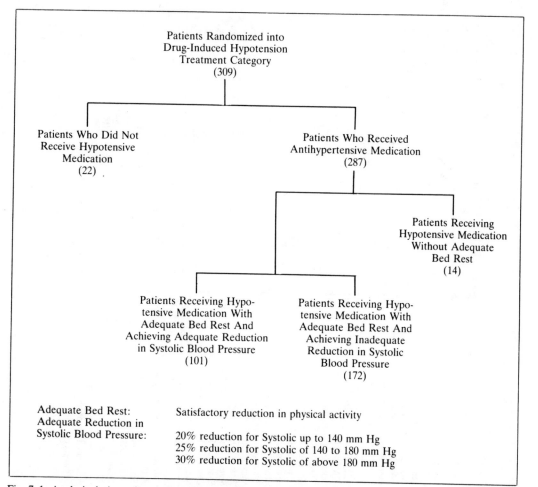

Fig. 7–1. Analysis design—drug-induced hypotension.

Table 7-1.   Characteristics at Randomization of Patients Allocated to Drug-Induced Hypotension by Study Subgroups.*

Category	Overall Group % of n=309	No Hypotensive Therapy % of n=22	No Bed Rest with Hypotensive Therapy % of n=14	Adequate Reduction with Hypotensive Therapy % of n=101	Inadequate Reduction with Hypotensive Therapy % of n=172	P Value‡
Randomization Variables						
Site						
Internal carotid	26.5	22.7	35.7	26.7	26.2	.008
Middle cerebral	11.3	13.6	0.0	4.0	16.3	
Anterior cerebral	62.2	63.6	64.3	69.3	57.6	
Interval to randomization (Days)						
0-7	61.5	59.1	28.6	62.4	64.0	.383
8-21	28.5	36.4	42.8	30.7	25.0	
22-92	10.0	4.5	28.6	6.9	11.0	
Risk Variables						
Neurologic condition— Grades 3-5	28.8	45.4	21.4	22.8	30.8	.197
Medical condition—fair, poor, prohibitive†	44.7	50.0	42.9	40.6	46.5	.410
Sex—males	49.2	45.5	57.1	51.5	47.7	.629
Bleeds in history (2-4)	17.5	4.5	14.3	18.8	18.6	.906
Pre-existing hypertension	23.9	36.4	28.6	19.8	24.4	.396
Vasospasm	43.7	45.5	57.1	42.6	43.0	.957
Age ≥ 50 yrs	51.1	50.0	71.4	51.5	49.4	.838
Size of aneurysm > 200 mm³	49.8	45.5	64.3	47.5	50.6	.632
Systolic blood pressure > 140 mm	62.1	54.5	50.0	64.4	62.2	.822
Diastolic blood pressure > 90 mm	40.1	36.4	35.7	37.6	42.4	.513
Mean blood pressure > 110 mm	42.7	40.9	35.7	40.6	44.8	.585
	$\bar{x}$ / $\tilde{x}$	$\bar{x}$ / $\tilde{x}$	$\bar{x}$ / $\tilde{x}$	$\bar{x}$ / $\tilde{x}$	$\bar{x}$ / $\tilde{x}$	
Interval to randomization	9.41 / 5.71	7.86 / 6.00	18.43 / 11.50	7.82 / 5.55	9.80 / 5.57	.184
Age	47.65 / 49.73	47.27 / 49.00	53.43 / 55.00	48.14 / 49.80	46.94 / 49.00	.438
Size of aneurysm	545 / 211	684 / 165	409 / 318	488 / 198	573 / 234	.640
Systolic blood pressure	149.2 / 145.6	151.8 / 148.25	145.9 / 142.5	149.5 / 145.4	149.0 / 146.0	.843
Diastolic blood pressure	89.5 / 88.3	87.2 / 84.00	86.2 / 88.0	89.0 / 87.6	90.1 / 89.2	.504
Mean blood pressure	109.1 / 107.3	108.5 / 106.25	107.7 / 107.0	109.4 / 105.7	108.9 / 108.1	.785

$\bar{x}$ = mean $\tilde{x}$ = median
* See figure 7-1.

† For definition, see Table 7-3.
‡ Adequate vs inadequate.

Table 7-2. Cause of Death and Time to Death for Patients Who Had Bedrest and Hypotensive Therapy According to Protocol.

Days from Last Bleed to Death	Cause of Death										
	Proved Rebleed		Suspected Rebleed		Progressive Decline		Unrelated Cause*		Unknown		Total	% of Five-year Deaths
	No.	%	No.	%	No.	%	No.	%	No.	%	No.	
0–30	41	(63.1)	5	(7.7)	14	(21.5)	3	(4.6)	2	(3.1)	65	56.5
31–90	8	(40.0)	6	(30.0)	1	(5.0)	3	(15.0)	2	(10.0)	20	17.4
91–180	0		0		1	(20.0)	2	(40.0)	2	(40.0)	5	4.4
181–365	4	(50.0)	1	(12.5)	1	(12.5)	2	(25.0)	0		8	6.9
366–730	3	(75.0)	0		0		1	(25.0)	0		4	3.5
731–1095	1	(16.7)	1	(16.7)	0		3	(50.0)	1	(16.7)	4	5.2
1096–1460	2	(33.3)	3	(50.0)	0		1	(16.7)	0		6	5.2
1461–1825	1	(100.0)	0		0		0		0		1	0.9
Total	60	(52.2)	16	(13.9)	17	(14.8)	15	(13.0)	7	(6.1)	115	(100)

* Unrelated causes listed in order (earliest death first): gastrointestinal bleeding; bilateral pulmonary embolism; myocardial infarction (two patients); pneumonia; ventricular fibrillation during anesthesia; pneumonia; acute cardiac insufficiency; suicide; inanition; renal failure; acute pyelonephritis; multiple myeloma; lung cancer; bronchitis-emphysema-heart failure.

Table 7–3.   Definitions of Clinical Variables.

Rebleed (Proved):
First recurrent hemorrhage following the last prerandomization bleed diagnosed by lumbar puncture or postmortem examination

Aneurysm-related Death:
Primary cause of death noted to be from a proved rebleed, an episode highly suggestive of rebleeding, or progressive clinical deterioration from complications of the prerandomization bleed

Neurologic Condition on Day of Randomization:
Grade
1 = symptom-free
2 = minor symptoms (headache, meningeal irritation, diplopia)
3 = major neurologic deficit but fully responsive
4 = impaired state of alertness but capable of protective or other adaptive responses to noxious stimuli
5 = poorly responsive but with stable vital signs

Medical Condition:
Good—patients who were alert, normotensive, with no more than a degree of fever, and in good health prior to subarachnoid hemorrhage
Fair—patients with a single underlying medical problem such as hypertension, cirrhosis of the liver, advanced age, anemia, poor nutrition, generalized atherosclerosis or chronic pulmonary disease
Poor—patients with more than one adverse factor or one medical condition which was particularly severe
Prohibitive—patients with a complicated illness with one or more undesirable conditions

Clinical Variables

Clinical variables included age, sex, aneurysm site, interval from last bleed to treatment, initial neurologic condition, initial medical condition, mean blood pressure, size of aneurysm, number of proved and suspected bleeds in history, pre-existing hypertension, presence of vasospasm at angiography and percent change in blood pressure during treatment. These factors were analyzed as dependent variables potentially affecting mortality.

Age, Sex and Pre-Existing Hypertension

Patients 60 years of age or more had a higher risk of death at all intervals than those below 60. These differences were not statistically

Table 7–4.   Cumulative Aneurysm-Related Mortality Rate (%) For Variables Related to Characteristics Prior to the Bleed.

Variable	Sample Size*	Follow-up Period (years)							
		$1/12$	$1/4$	$1/2$	1	2	3	4	5
Age (years)									
≤ 39	72	20	26	26	26	27	27	29	31
40–59	159	24	30	30	33	34	36	39	39
≥ 60	42	27	31	34	40	40	40	40	40
Sex									
Male	134	20	26	27	28	29	29	32	33
Female	139	27	32	32	36	37	39	41	41
Pre-Existing hypertension									
Present	62	28	31	31	33	33	33	37	37
Absent	175	20	25	26	29	30	32	34	35
Total	273	23	29	29	32	33	34	36	37

* Sample size of those with data recorded; may not total 273.

significant at any interval (Table 7–4). Females also demonstrated a higher risk, but the difference between males and females was not statistically significant. Pre-existing hypertension presented as a higher risk than no pre-existing hypertension, but as time from the bleed progressed, the difference was smaller. At all intervals the differences were not statistically significant.

Neurologic Condition

Patients in good neurologic condition at randomization (Grades 1 and 2) had a 21% mortality 1 month following the bleed (Table 7–5). Patients with poor neurologic condition (Grades 3 to 5) had a 30% mortality during the same period. A maximum difference of 11% was found at 3 months; how-

Table 7–5.   Cumulative Aneurysm-Related Mortality Rates (%) For Variables Related to the Patient's Condition at Randomization.

Variable	Sample Size	Follow-up Period (years)							
		$1/12$	$1/4$	$1/2$	1	2	3	4	5
Neurologic condition*†									
Grades 1, 2	197	21	26	27	30	31	32	35	36
Grades 3–5	76	30	37	37	37	37	39	39	39
Medical condition†									
Good	152	16	19	19	22	23	24	27	28
Fair	94	34	40	41	44	45	46	48	48
Poor, Prohibitive	27	38	46	46	46	46	46	46	46
		***	***	***	***	***	***	***	***
Mean blood pressure									
≤ 110 mm Hg	155	19	25	26	29	29	31	33	34
> 110 mm Hg	118	29	34	34	36	38	38	41	41
Vasospasm									
None	156	17	21	22	24	25	26	30	31
Local	69	30	33	33	35	35	36	38	38
Diffuse	48	32	48	48	53	56	56	56	56
		*	**	**	**	**	**	*	*
Total	273	23	29	29	32	33	34	36	37

Level of statistical significance between rates: * $P < 0.05$ ** $P < 0.01$ *** $P < 0.005$
† See Table 7–3 for definition.

Table 7–6.   Cumulative Aneurysm-Related Mortality Rates (%) For Variables Specific to the Aneurysm.

Variable	Sample Size	Follow-up Period (years)							
		$\frac{1}{12}$	$\frac{1}{4}$	$\frac{1}{2}$	1	2	3	4	5
Aneurysm site									
Internal carotid	72	21	23	23	24	27	31	33	33
Middle cerebral	32	35	35	35	35	35	35	39	39
Anterior cerebral-									
anterior communicating	169	22	31	31	35	35	35	38	39
No. of proved or suspected bleeds in history									
1	222	24	30	30	32	34	35	37	38
2–4	51	18	25	25	30	30	30	32	32
Size of aneurysm									
≤ 200 mm³	125	18	23	24	27	27	27	29	29
> 200 mm³	135	28	35*	35	36	39*	41*	44*	44*
Total	273	23	29	29	32	33	34	36	37

* $P < 0.05$

ever, the difference was 7% at 1 year and 3% at 5 years (36 vs 39%). These differences were not statistically significant at any period.

Medical Condition

Patients in good medical condition suffered a 16% mortality at 1 month (Table 7–5), while fair-condition patients had a 34% mortality, and those with a poor or prohibitive condition demonstrated a mortality of 38%. At 3 months, the good-condition patients had a 3% increase, fair-condition patients had a 6% increase and poor/prohibitive-condition patients had an 8% increase. Beyond the 3-month interval, the good and fair-condition patients showed an average 2% yearly increase through the 5-year follow-up. However, the poor/prohibitive patients had no increase in mortality, which suggests they were at high risk early in their post-treatment phase and at low risk after 3 months post-bleed.

Mean Blood Pressure

Baseline mean blood pressure was calculated from the prerandomization blood pressures (⅓ × systolic + ⅔ × diastolic). Patients with a mean blood pressure over 110 mm Hg had a 29% mortality at 1 month (Table 7–5). This figure was 10% higher than

in patients with mean blood pressure less than or equal to 110 mm Hg. This difference had a P-value of 0.09, and as time progressed the difference between the two groups decreased to 7% at 5 years, with a P-value of 0.24.

Cerebral Vasospasm

The presence of vasospasm had a significant influence on death at all periods (Table 7–5). Patients with localized and diffuse vasospasm had a 30 and 32% mortality, respectively, after 1 month. In contrast, a 17% mortality was shown for those with no vasospasm reported. At 3 months, patients with no vasospasm had a 4% increase, while those with localized and diffuse vasospasm had a 3 and 16% increase, respectively. Increases of 3, 2 and 5%, respectively, were shown over the next 9 months.

Aneurysm Site

No statistical difference in aneurysm-related mortality occurred among the three aneurysm sites (Table 7–6). Middle cerebral aneurysms showed a higher initial risk, but no increase occurred after the initial 30-day period. This result should be examined with caution, since only 32 patients with a middle cerebral aneurysm were included.

Number of Bleeds

No statistically significant differences were observed between patients with one bleed as compared to those with more than one bleed prior to treatment (Table 7–6).

Aneurysm Size

The size (volume) of the aneurysm as measured at angiography appeared to influence subsequent survival. Dividing the patient sample with aneurysm sizes at 200 mm³, those with a larger aneurysm had a 10% greater chance of death at 1 month (28%) compared to those with sizes less than 200 mm³ (18%, Table 7–6). By the end of 5 years, the risk had increased to a 15% difference (44 vs 29%).

Treatment-Related Variables

One of the variables for which patients were randomized was the number of days between last bleed and day of treatment allocation. A substantial relationship of time to risk of

death was noted (Table 7–7). However, the relatively small number of patients entering the study after the 1st week places limitations on the meaning of statistical significance. Of note is the difference between those who entered the study during the 1st week compared to patients who entered during the 2nd and 3rd weeks, when a difference of 15% at 1 year diminished to 8% at 5 years. These differences were not statistically significant.

Pretreatment Systolic Blood Pressure

When patients were subdivided according to pretreatment systolic blood pressure (i.e., patients with average systolic pressure of less than 140 mm Hg, 140 to 180 mm Hg, and over 180 mm Hg) and the percent reduction calculated, the cumulative aneurysm-related mortality shows no statistically significant difference at any interval among groups with *more* or *less than* 20% reduction (Table 7–7). The sample size in the 180 mm Hg group

Table 7–7. Cumulative Aneurysm-Related Mortality Rates (%) For Variables Specific to Treatment.

Variable	Sample Size	Follow-up Period (years)							
		$\frac{1}{12}$	$\frac{1}{4}$	$\frac{1}{2}$	1	2	3	4	5
Interval from bleed to treatment allocation (days)									
0–7	173	28	35	36	39	39	40	42	42
8–21	74	16	21	21	24	27	29	32	34
22–92	26	0	0	0	0	0	0	0	0
		*	*						
% decrease in SBP and initial SBP									
< 140 mm Hg									
< 20% decrease	39	5	8	8	11	14	18	18	22
≥ 20% decrease	28	3	18	18	18	18	18	22	22
No maintenance level	16	31	37	37	37	37	37	37	37
140–180 mm Hg									
< 25% decrease	73	24	26	28	32	31	34	37	37
≥ 25% decrease	62	18	28	28	30	31	31	34	34
No maintenance level	25	83	83	83	83	83	83	83	83
		**	**	**	**	**	**	**	**
> 180 mm Hg									
< 30% decrease	13	15	15	15	23	31	31	41	41
≥ 30% decrease	11	0	10	10	10	10	10	10	10
No maintenance level	6	83	83	83	83	83	83	83	83
Total	273	23	29	29	32	33	34	36	37

* $P < 0.05$ ** $P < 0.01$

Table 7–8. Cumulative Rebleed Rates (%) for Variables Specific to the Patient's Characteristics.

Variable	Sample Size	Follow-up Period (years)							
		$1/12$	$1/4$	$1/2$	1	2	3	4	5
Age (years)									
≤ 39	72	24	27	27	27	29	29	29	32
40–59	159	25	30	31	33	34	37	38	39
≥ 60	42	14	14	14	21	21	21	25	25
			*	*					
Sex									
Male	134	23	27	28	28	29	30	30	31
Female	139	24	28	28	31	33	35	37	39
Pre-existing hypertension									
Present	62	25	27	29	31	31	31	34	34
Absent	175	21	26	26	27	29	30	31	33
Total	273	23	27	28	30	31	33	34	35

* $P < 0.05$

was too small to establish any conclusions on the effect of a 30% decrease. Of note is the percent mortality for patients not reporting a maintenance blood pressure in each of the categories. Clearly, mortality occurring prior to attainment of reduced blood pressure was of major importance in this analysis. The sample size in the 180 mm Hg group was too small in any of the three blood pressure categories to draw definite conclusions.

Recurrent Hemorrhage

Fifty-two percent of all deaths and 64.5% of all aneurysm-related deaths at 5 years were caused by a proved rebleed. Twenty-three percent of patients at risk at 1 month had a rebleed (Table 7–8). Between 1 and 3 months, 4% of those at risk rebled; between 3 months and 5 years, an additional 8% rebled (average of 1.8% per year).

Age, Sex and Pre-Existing Hypertension

The variables of age, sex and pre-existing hypertension showed no overall statistical difference in recurrent hemorrhage over the follow-up period (Table 7–8). Although patients 60 years of age or more exhibited a lower initial rebleed rate as compared to the lower age groups, their pattern of rebleeding was not statistically different at 1 year

through 5 years following the prerandomization bleed.

Neurologic and Medical Condition

Neurologic and medical conditions at randomization had no statistically significant influence on recurrence of hemorrhage at 1 month (Table 7–9). However, statistical differences in rebleed rate did occur between 3 months and 3 years after the bleed among patients in good, fair or poor medical condition at the time of the initial bleed. At 3 months, patients in fair medical condition showed an increased risk of rebleeding, and this difference (as compared with the good and poor-condition patients) continued through the 3-year interval. These results suggest that fair and poor-medical condition patients suffered the highest rate of rebleeding during the first 3 months. Patients in poor condition showed no further risk of rebleeding after 1 month. However, patients in fair condition had a rebleed rate of less than 1% per year, whereas those in good condition had an approximate rebleed rate of 2% per year.

Mean Blood Pressure

Patients with a mean blood pressure over 110 mm Hg had a 30% rebleed rate at 1 month (Table 7–9). This figure was 12% higher than in patients with average mean

Table 7-9.　Cumulative Rebleed Rates (%) for Variables Specific to the Patient's Condition at Randomization.

Variable	Sample Size	Follow-up Period (years)							
		$^1/_{12}$	$^1/_4$	$^1/_2$	1	2	3	4	5
Neurologic condition†									
Grades 1, 2	197	23	28	28	30	32	34	36	37
Grades 3–5	76	25	27	27	27	27	27	27	27
Medical condition†									
Good	152	18	20	21	23	25	26	28	30
Fair	94	32	39	39	41	42	44	44	44
Poor, Prohibitive	27	27	27	27	27	27	27	27	27
			*		*	*	*	*	
Mean blood pressure									
≤ 110 mm Hg	155	18	22	22	24	25	27	29	31
> 110 mm Hg	118	30	35	36	37	39	40	40	40
		*	*	*	*	*	*		
Vasospasm									
None	156	22	25	25	27	28	29	29	30
Local	69	25	27	27	29	29	32	37	39
Diffuse	48	25	39	39	42	46	46	46	46
Total	273	23	27	28	30	31	33	34	35

* $P < 0.05$
† See Table 7–3 for definition.

blood pressure equal to or less than 110 mm Hg. The difference in rebleed rate between these two groups remained significantly different ($P < 0.05$) through the 3-year interval. During the 4th and 5th years no statistical differences were observed (Table 7–9).

Cerebral Vasospasm

Although the presence or absence of vasospasm showed a significant influence on mortality (Table 7–5), no such influence was observed with regard to recurrent hemorrhage. Patients with diffuse vasospasm showed a 14% increase between 1 and 3 months as opposed to a 3% increase for those with no vasospasm (Table 7–9). Only a 2% increase was noted for those with localized spasm during the same interval. Following the 3-month period, patients with no vasospasm had a 5% increase in recurrent hemorrhage

Table 7-10.　Cumulative Rebleed Rates (%) for Variables Specific to the Aneurysm.

Variable	Sample Size	Follow-up Period (years)							
		$^1/_{12}$	$^1/_4$	$^1/_2$	1	2	3	4	5
Aneurysm site									
Internal carotid	72	26	29	29	31	34	36	36	36
Middle cerebral	32	30	30	30	30	30	30	30	30
Anterior cerebral-									
anterior communicating	169	21	26	27	30	30	32	34	36
No. of proved or suspected bleeds in history									
1	222	24	28	28	30	32	33	35	37
2–4	51	21	26	26	28	28	28	28	28
Size of aneurysm									
≤200 mm³	125	17	20	20	22	22	23	24	24
>200 mm³	135	29	34	34	36	39	41	42	43
		*	*	**	**	***	***	***	***
Total	273	23	27	28	30	31	33	34	35

* $P < 0.05$　　** $P < 0.01$　　*** $P < 0.005$

as compared to a 12% increase in those with localized spasm. Among patients with diffuse vasospasm, a 7% increase in rebleeding was observed between 3 months and 5 years.

Aneurysm Site

No statistical differences in the percentage of rebleeding occurred with regard to aneurysm site. However, aneurysms of the anterior cerebral complex showed a slower rate of rebleeding up to 1 year following the pre-study hemorrhage, at which time their rate equaled those aneurysms in patients on the internal carotid and middle cerebral distribution (Table 7–10).

Number of Bleeds

No statistically significant differences in rebleed rate were observed between patients with one bleed compared to those with more than one bleed prior to treatment (Table 7–10). Between 1 and 5 years, patients with only one bleed (that bleed qualifying the patient for this study) showed a 1.75% rebleed rate per year, while those with more than one bleed had no recurrent hemorrhages.

Aneurysm Size

The size (volume) of the aneurysm (smaller vs larger than 200 mm^3) showed a significant difference of 12% at 1 month (Table 7–10). The risk of rebleeding for aneurysms greater than 200 mm^3 at initial rupture becomes proportionately larger during follow-up, with a calculated difference of 19% at 5 years.

Treatment-Related Variables

No recurrent hemorrhage was reported in the 26 patients who entered the study during the 22 to 92-day period after the bleed (Table 7–11). This group may represent a select group of patients by means of their survival and rebleed status. Due to the small sample size, no statistically significant differences were demonstrated, despite the increased risk among patients who entered the study during the first 3 weeks.

Pretreatment Systolic Blood Pressure

When analysis of initial systolic blood pressure and percent change was calculated in accordance with protocol guidelines, a sim-

Table 7–11.   Cumulative Rebleed Rates (%) for Variables Specific to Treatment.

Variable	Sample Size	Follow-up Period (years)							
		$1/12$	$1/4$	$1/2$	1	2	3	4	5
Interval from last bleed to treatment allocation (days)									
0–7	173	28	32	33	35	35	37	38	39
8–21	74	17	23	23	26	29	31	33	35
22–92	26	0	0	0	0	0	0	0	0
% decrease SBP and initial SBP									
<140 mm Hg									
<20% decrease	39	6	8	8	12	15	15	15	25
≥25% decrease	28	12	22	22	22	22	22	27	27
No maintenance level	16	32	32	32	32	32	32	32	32
140–180 mm Hg									
<25% decrease	73	24	28	30	34	34	35	35	35
≥25% decrease	62	17	22	22	22	24	28	31	31
No maintenance level	25	83	83	83	83	83	83	83	83
		**	**	**	**	**	**	**	**
>180 mm Hg									
<30% decrease	13	24	24	24	32	41	41	41	41
≥30% decrease	11	0	0	0	0	0	0	0	0
No maintenance level	6	25	25	25	25	25	25	25	25
Total	273	23	27	28	30	31	33	34	35

** $P < 0.01$

ilar result appeared as with mortality. Only patients in the 140 to 180 mm Hg group had an adequate sample size to determine a statistically significant difference among subgroups (Table 7–11). During the 5-year follow-up, the percentage difference in rebleed rate varied from 4 to 12% between patients with less as compared to more than 25% decrease in blood pressure during the treatment period. Those not achieving a maintenance level had an 83% rebleed rate.

Discussion

Prevention of recurrent hemorrhage and death were the primary objectives of treatment in patients with recently ruptured int acranial aneurysm. The data reported in this study define statistically the more important medical variables responsible for the outcome of such patients.

Age, sex, pre-existing hypertension and neurologic condition had no statistically significant effect on recurrent hemorrhage or death during the five-year follow-up period. However, medical condition did have a significant effect. Patients in fair, poor and prohibitive medical condition had a significantly higher mortality throughout the 5-year period when compared to the group in good medical condition prior to treatment. Recurrent hemorrhage and progressive decline in clinical condition were the primary factors responsible as the cause of death. Cerebral complications from vasospasm also had a significant effect on mortality, whereas this had no statistically significant influence on rebleed rate. There was a trend for mortality (without rebleeding) to be higher in poor-neurologic condition patients, and for rebleeding to be higher in good-neurologic condition patients.

Elevated mean blood pressure (>110 mm Hg) had a marginal effect on mortality but a statistically significant effect on rebleed rate. This suggests that increased blood pressure after the bleed would have a predictive influence upon patient outcome in the long-term follow-up period. Most patients were not treated with antihypertensive medication on a long-term basis.

Aneurysm site and number of bleeds in the patient's history had no significant effect on mortality or rebleed rate. However, aneurysm size (>200 mm^3) did have a significant effect on rebleed rate throughout the 5-year period. This is an expected result, in that larger aneurysms tend to rebleed more often than smaller aneurysms (≤200 mm^3).

Statistically significant differences in aneurysm-related mortality and rebleed rate were observed during the 5-year period for patients achieving a maintenance systolic blood pressure during the 3-week treatment period when compared to those not achieving a maintenance level.

Mortality and rebleed rate for patients with decrease in systolic pressure according to protocol during the treatment period were not significantly different statistically from those with less than the designated decrease in systolic blood pressure 1 month following the bleed. This was true for patients with average systolic blood pressures prior to treatment being less than 140 mm Hg, 140 to 180 mm Hg, and over 180 mm Hg. Therefore, the level of pretreatment systolic blood pressure and amount of decrease in blood pressure had no significant effect on mortality and rebleed rate after the 1-month follow-up period.

The statistical analyses in this report address the results of the long-term follow-up period (5 years) in patients with a ruptured intracranial aneurysm followed by 3 weeks of antihypertensive therapy. Comparison of results with the statistical report of patients treated with regulated bed rest[6] shows no significant differences at the 1-month follow-up, but significant differences are present in mortality and rebleeding rate at the 3-month follow-up and at subsequent intervals. These results indicate that a greater risk of rebleeding and subsequent related mortality occurs for a longer period with bed rest alone as compared to drug-induced hypotension therapy.

Winn et al.[11] recently reported that 6 months after the bleed, a 3.5% yearly rebleed rate was observed in patients with anterior communicating and posterior communicating artery aneurysms. Some of the patients presented in their analysis are part of the randomized trial. Given that certain patients are counted in both studies, the bed rest report showed an annual rate of 2.4% for anterior communicating aneurysms and the drug-induced hypotension data reported a 2% rate in this study. The discrepancy between investigations may be due to the inclusion of patients with definite proof of rebleeding and not those with suspected rebleeding episodes.

From the results of mortality and rebleed rate after 3 weeks of antihypertensive therapy, the outcome at specific intervals during a 5-year period suggests the following conclusions:

1. Fair, poor or prohibitive medical condition prior to treatment; diffuse vasospasm; or large aneurysm size (>200 mm^3) were the most significant factors causing high mortality in long-term follow-up.

2. Elevated mean blood pressure (>110 mm Hg) and large aneurysm size (>200 mm^3) prior to treatment were the most significant factors responsible for a high rebleed rate during long-term follow-up.

3. When systemic blood pressure could not to be maintained within the 30-day interval following the bleed, mortality and rebleed rate were significantly greater at 1 month in this group of patients when compared to patients with blood pressure more adequately controlled.

References

1. Sahs, A.L.: Cooperative study of intracranial aneurysms and subarachnoid hemorrhage. Report on a randomized treatment study. I. Introduction. Stroke 5:550–551, 1974.
2. Nibbelink, D.W., Knowler, L.A.: Cooperative study of intracranial aneurysms and subarachnoid hemorrhage. Report on a randomized treatment study. II. Objectives and design of randomized aneurysm study. Stroke 5:552–556, 1974.
3. Sahs, A.L., Nibbelink, D.W., Knowler, L.A.: Cooperative aneurysm project: Introductory report of a randomized treatment study. In: McDowell, F.H., Brennan, R.W. (eds): Cerebral Vascular Diseases. Eighth Conference. Grune & Stratton, New York, 1973, pp 33–41.
4. Graf, C., Nibbelink, D.W.: Cooperative study of intracranial aneurysms and subarachnoid hemorrhage. Report on a randomized treatment study. III. Intracranial surgery. Stroke 5:557–601, 1974.
5. Nibbelink, D.W., Torner, J.C., Henderson, W.G.: Cooperative study of intracranial aneurysms and subarachnoid hemorrhage. Report on a randomized treatment study. IV-A. Regulated bed rest. Stroke 8: 202–218, 1977.
6. Henderson, W.G., Torner, J.C., Nibbelink, D.W.: Cooperative study of intracranial aneurysms and subarachnoid hemorrhage. Report on a randomized treatment study. IV-B. Regulated bed rest—Statistical evaluation. Stroke 8:579–589, 1977.
7. Cutler, S.J., Ederer, F.: Maximum utilization of the life table method in analyzing survival. J. Chron Dis 8:699–710, (December) 1958.
8. Mantel, N., Byar, D.: Evaluation of response-time data involving transient states: An illustration using heart transplant data. J Am Statist Ass 69:81–86, (March) 1974.
9. Grizzle, J.E., Starmer, C.F., Koch, G.G.: Analysis of categorical data by linear models. Biometrics 25:489–503, 1969.
10. Koch, G.G., Johnson, W.D., Tolley, H.D.: A linear models approach to the analysis of survival and extent of disease in multidimensional contingency tables. J Am Statist Ass 67:783–796, (December) 1972.
11. Winn, H.R., Richardson, A.E., Jane, J.A.: The long-term prognosis in untreated cerebral aneurysms: I. The incidence of late hemorrhage in cerebral aneurysm: A 10-year evaluation of 364 patients. Ann Neurol 1:358–370, 1977.

Chapter 8

Randomized Treatment Study.
Carotid Ligation

George E. Perret, M.D., Ph.D., and Donald W. Nibbelink, M.D., Ph.D.

Abstract

A series of 187 patients with a single ruptured intracranial aneurysm on the anterior portion of the Circle of Willis was allocated randomly to be treated by carotid artery ligation. Included among the 62 patients who did not have carotid ligation were 15 found unsuitable and 21 who could not tolerate attempted carotid occlusion. Tolerance to carotid ligation could not be predicted. Ischemic cerebral complications related to attempted and completed treatment occurred in 36.3% of patients with a mortality rate of 6.4%. These complications were permanent in two thirds of the cases. Recurrent rupture of the aneurysm after carotid occlusion took place in 10.4% of 125 patients with a mortality rate of 7.2%. Of these, 11 bled within 32 days of carotid ligation; one rebled on day 356 and one on day 3,195 after ligation.

ities resulting from rebleeding, ischemic cerebral infarctions or complications resulting from pulmonary and cardiac abnormalities. A number of patients were unable to tolerate carotid occlusion and the procedure was abandoned. Many patients were left disabled after permanent carotid occlusion and were not able to return to gainful employment. Postoperative angiographic studies performed in 166 of 385 successfully treated patients revealed that 28 of 41 internal carotid aneurysms decreased in size after carotid occlusion; in 12 patients the size of the aneurysm was unchanged, and in 1 patient it was larger. Ischemic neurologic complications were found to be: (1) higher in elderly patients, (2) more common in those patients whose arteries were occluded in the first few days after the subarachnoid hemorrhage, (3) higher when the occlusion was carried out abruptly than when the artery was occluded gradually and (4) significantly higher with internal carotid than with common carotid occlusions. The chances of recovering from an ischemic neurologic deficit were significantly better if the occlusion was released than if the artery was left occluded. Nishioka reported an incidence of 7.8% recurrent subarachnoid hemorrhage following common carotid artery occlusion. Rebleeding was significantly higher for middle ce-

Introduction

Ligation of the common carotid artery in the neck has been reported as an effective method of treatment of recently ruptured intracranial aneurysms.[1-8] In 1966 Nishioka[5] reported the results of 814 patients treated with carotid ligation. He showed that the treatment was successful in 56% and failed in 36%. The majority of failures were fatal-

rebral and anterior cerebral-anterior communicating aneurysms than it was for internal carotid aneurysms.

The treatment of each patient suffering from a ruptured intracranial aneurysm depends on many factors, such as age, condition, potential complications and preference of the surgeon. However, in order to overcome the bias inherent to the preselection of patients with recent subarachnoid hemorrhage and to obtain a more objective evaluation of various methods of treatment, a randomized study was instituted in which patients were allocated randomly to regulated bed rest,[9] drug-induced hypotension (Chapters 6, 7), carotid ligation and intracranial surgery.[10] Each patient had only one aneurysm which had ruptured on the anterior cerebral circulation.

Of the 972 patients collected in this study, 187 were randomly allocated to treatment by common carotid ligation. This report presents analysis of the outcome, complications and rebleed rate for the 187 patients allocated to common carotid ligation between June 1963 and February 1970 in the Cooperative Aneurysm Study.

Clinical Material

A total of 95 female and 92 male patients entered the study. Eighty-eight had an internal carotid aneurysm, 27 a middle cerebral aneurysm and 72 an aneurysm on the anterior cerebral-anterior communicating arteries (Table 8–1). The 45 patients provided by the Atkinson Morley's Hospital were all anterior cerebral-anterior communicating aneurysms, while the majority of aneurysms provided by the other centers were on the internal carotid artery.

The specific site of the aneurysm on the internal carotid artery, the middle cerebral artery and the anterior cerebral-anterior communicating arteries is presented in Table 8–2. As expected, the majority (71 out of 88) of internal carotid aneurysms were in the region of the branching of the posterior communicating artery. Forty-eight of the 72 anterior cerebral-anterior communicating aneurysms were at the junction of one of the anterior cerebral arteries with the anterior communicating artery. Internal carotid aneurysms were more common in women (53) and anterior cerebral-anterior communicating aneurysms more common in men (44). The middle cerebral aneurysms were

Table 8–1.   Aneurysm Site and Contribution by Investigating Center.

	ICA*	MCA*	ACA*	Total
Indiana University Medical Center	6	1	1	8
University of Iowa Hospitals	11	4	3	18
Atkinson Morley's Hospital	0	0	45	45
Mount Sinai Hospital, N.Y.	0	0	1	1
Medical College of Georgia	5	2	3	10
State University, New York (Downstate)	12	0	4	16
Albert Einstein University	11	3	4	18
Karolinska Institute	5	3	3	11
University of Melbourne	18	7	7	32
New York University	6	2	1	9
University of Lund	3	4	0	7
University of California (S.F.)	3	0	0	3
University of Cincinnati	4	0	0	4
University of Mississippi	4	1	0	5
Total	88	27	72	187
%	47.1	14.4	38.5	

* ICA = internal carotid aneurysm; MCA = middle cerebral aneurysm; ACA = anterior cerebral-anterior communicating aneurysm

Table 8–2.   Aneurysm Site.

	Right	Left	Midline	Total
Internal carotid artery (88)				
Ophthalmic	1	3		4
Posterior communicating	37	34		71
Bifurcation	5	8		13
Middle cerebral artery (27)				
Proximal to main branching	1	2		3
At main branching	15	9		24
Anterior cerebral-anterior communicating (72)				
Proximal to anterior communicating	1	0		1
Anterior communicating junction	19	29		48
Anterior communicating artery			19	19
Distal to anterior communicating	4	0		4
Total	83	85	19	187

equally distributed among men (14) and women (13).

The age distribution of the patients varied between 13 and 77 years. One hundred three of the 187 aneurysms (55%) bled in patients between the ages of 40 and 60. As seen in Table 8–3, 50 of the 88 internal carotid aneurysms (57%) ruptured in patients 30 to 49 years old. Fourteen of 27 patients with a middle cerebral aneurysm and 27 of 72 patients with an anterior cerebral-anterior communicating aneurysm were in this age group.

Pretreatment Studies

A number of determinations were made on each patient before allocation to specific treatment: recording of the exact date of the subarachnoid hemorrhage for which the patient was hospitalized; report of lumbar puncture and studies of the cerebrospinal fluid; three or four-vessel angiography to rule out multiplicity of aneurysms, the presence of arteriovenous malformation, intracranial hematoma, vasospasm and sclerotic stenosis. Furthermore, the integrity of cross-circulation had to be determined between right and left internal carotid systems to evaluate anomalies in the circle of Willis. An estimate of operability by common carotid ligation had to be made. Matas test was recommended to determine clinical tolerance or intolerance to unilateral digital carotid compression. Neurologic complications occurring during or within 24 hours of angiography were assessed. Determinations of blood pressures (4 readings taken at least 4 hours apart), the medical condition, the presence of complicating medical conditions and the neurologic status of the patient were recorded on the day of evaluation for admission to the treatment study.

Table 8–3.   Distribution of Aneurysm Site by Age.

	Age							
Site*	10–19	20–29	30–39	40–49	50–59	60–69	70–79	Total
ICA	5	7	24	26	15	9	2	88
MCA	0	3	3	11	6	4	0	27
ACA	2	3	10	17	27	11	2	72
Total	7	13	37	54	48	24	4	187

* See Table 8–1.

Medical Condition

Medical condition was subdivided into four groups: A—good (alert, normotensive, good health prior to subarachnoid hemorrhage), B—fair (single underlying medical problem such as hypertension, anemia, generalized atherosclerosis, chronic pulmonary disease), C—poor (more than one adverse factor or one severe medical condition) and D—prohibitive (complicated illness with one or more undesirable condition). Of the 187 patients, 112 were in good and 49 in fair condition, while only 23 were in poor and 3 in prohibitive condition. Aneurysm site had no relation to medical condition. However, the percentage of patients in poor condition was greater above the age of 60 (25%) than between the ages of 10 and 59 (11.9%).

Neurologic Condition

Table 8–4 shows that 130 of the 187 patients were in good neurologic condition (Grades 1 and 2). The mortality increased with age and in patients with altered state of consciousness. Major neurologic deficit (Grade 3) was most common in patients with middle cerebral aneurysms (25.9%) and impaired or poor responsiveness in patients with anterior cerebral-anterior communicating aneurysms (16.7%).

In the entire group of 63 patients who died, 23 (26.1%) bled from an internal carotid aneurysm, 10 from a middle cerebral aneurysm (37.0%) and 30 from anterior cerebral-anterior communicating aneurysm (41.7%). There seems to be no doubt that the neurologic condition, the site of the aneurysm and the age of the patient were related to survival.

Matas Test

The Matas test consisted of digital compression of the common carotid artery on the side of the ruptured aneurysm, and was used as an indicator of tolerance to carotid occlusion. It was performed in 27 patients with an internal carotid aneurysm, 9 patients with middle cerebral aneurysm and 53 patients with anterior cerebral-anterior communicating aneurysm. In 61 patients with internal carotid aneurysm, 18 patients with middle cerebral aneurysm and 19 patients with

Table 8–4. Neurologic Condition and Age.

Age	Neurologic Condition*						Total	% Deaths
	1	2	3	4	5	6		
10–19	1	5	1	0	0	0	7 (0)†	0.0
20–29	0	10 (1)	2 (1)	1 (1)	0	0	13 (3)	23.1
30–39	1	24 (4)	3 (1)	7 (4)	2 (1)	0	37 (10)	27.0
40–49	2 (1)	36 (6)	10 (5)	4 (4)	2 (2)	0	54 (18)	33.3
50–59	3 (1)	31 (8)	8 (5)	3 (2)	3 (2)	0	48 (18)	37.5
60–69	1	14 (4)	7 (5)	0	2 (2)	0	24 (11)	45.8
70–79	0	2 (1)	0	1 (1)	0	1 (1)	4 (3)	75.0
Total	8 (2)	122 (24)	31 (17)	16 (12)	9 (7)	1 (1)	187 (63)	
Death Rate	25.0%	19.7%	54.8%	75.0%	77.8%	100.0%	33.7%	
				76.9%				

* Definition of neurologic condition:
1 = symptom-free.
2 = minor symptoms (headache, meningeal irritation, diplopia).
3 = major neurological deficit but fully responsive.
4 = impaired state of alertness but capable of protective or other adaptive responses to noxious stimuli.

5 = poorly responsive but with stable vital signs.
6 = no response to address or shaking, nonadaptive response to noxious stimuli and progressive instability of vital signs.
† Number in parentheses denotes deaths.

Table 8–5.   Age and Systolic Blood Pressure.

Age	Systolic Blood Pressure (mm Hg)					Total	Hypertension
	<120	121–140	141–160	161–180	>180		
10–19	4	2				6	
20–29	4	7	3			14	
30–39	8	17	8	2	2	37	4
40–49	9	14	15	13	5	56	18
50–59	7	14	9	9	7	46	16
60–69	2	10	5	1	6	24	7
70–79	1	1	0	2	0	4	2
Total	35	65	40	27	20	187	47 (25.1%)
	100 (53.5%)		67 (35.8%)		20 (10.7%)		
			87 (46.5%)				

anterior cerebral-anterior communicating aneurysm, a Matas test was not performed. In the 89 patients who had the test carried out, it was well tolerated for a period of over 5 minutes in 76 patients and could not be tolerated more than 1 minute in 5, from 1 to 3 minutes in 4, and from 3 to 5 minutes in 4. The diagnostic value of the Matas test in preventing ischemic neurologic deficit associated with common carotid occlusion will be reported later in conjunction with ischemic neurologic deficits (p. 136).

Blood Pressure

On the day of randomization, 4 blood pressure determinations were made at 4-hour intervals.

Tabulation of the systolic blood pressure (Table 8–5) shows that 53.5% of the patients had a low or normal blood pressure. Elevation of systolic blood pressure between 141 and 180 mm Hg occurred in 35.8% of patients, and 10.7% had a high blood pressure above 180 mm Hg. Thus, hypertension was present in 46.5% of patients between last bleed and allocation to treatment. Thirty-nine percent of the patients with internal carotid aneurysm, 63% of patients with middle cerebral aneurysm and 48.5% of patients with anterior cerebral-anterior communicating aneurysm had a systolic blood pressure above 140 mm Hg. Sixty-four percent of patients above the age of 40 had systolic pressures above 140 mm Hg after aneurysm rupture. No data are available on blood pressures prior to the subarachnoid hemorrhage. Thus, the rate of hypertensive patients before the bleed is unknown.

The mean blood pressure was determined by dividing by 3 the sum of the systolic blood pressure and twice the diastolic pressure. A mean blood pressure below 100 mm Hg was found in 44.4% of patients. Mild elevation of the mean blood pressure between 101 and 120 mm Hg was found in 33.2% of patients, and elevated mean blood pressure above 121 mm Hg was found in 22.5%. Age of the patient remains a related variable in arterial hypertension. Increased mean blood pressure was found in 62.3% of 130 patients above the age of 40.

The influence of blood pressure on neurologic complications of carotid occlusion and on recurrent subarachnoid hemorrhage will be discussed later.

Vasospasm

The diagnosis of intracranial aneurysm was made by cerebral angiography. The degree of arterial narrowing produced by vasospasm was also reported. Thus, one could determine whether or not the patient had spasm, whether the spasm was localized or segmental in one or more vessels, or whether the spasm was diffuse, involving the internal carotid and the main ipsilateral arteries.

Localized spasm was seen in the angiograms of 49 patients (26.2%) and diffuse generalized spasm in 27 patients (14.4%). There was no reported spasm in 111 patients. Vasospasm was most common in patients with a middle cerebral aneurysm (48.1%). It was reported in 42% of patients with internal carotid aneurysm and in 36.1% of patients with an anterior cerebral-anterior communicating aneurysm (Table 8–6).

Table 8–7 correlates the presence of localized and generalized vasospasm with neurologic condition. It appears that localized and generalized vasospasm is more frequent in the patient with an impaired state of responsiveness, i.e., Grades 4, 5 and 6, than in patients who are symptom-free or have only minor symptoms (Grades 1 and 2).

The relation of spasm and ischemic complications will be studied later (p. 136).

Complications of Angiography

Angiographic complications were reported in 15 patients (8%): 5 with an internal carotid aneurysm, 3 with a middle cerebral aneurysm and 7 with an anterior cerebral-anterior communicating aneurysm. The same incidence was reported in 1966.[11] They occurred in patients 36 to 63 years of age, 1 to 25 days after the subarachnoid hemorrhage. There were 6 lasting neurologic complications (2 hemiparesis, 3 hemiparesis with dys-

Table 8–6. Vasospasm.

Vasospasm	Aneurysm Site*				
	ICA	MCA	ACA	Total	%
Localized	20	8	21	49	26.2
Generalized	17	5	5	27	14.4
Total No. of aneurysms	37/88	13/27	26/72	76/187	
%	42.0	48.1	36.1	40.6	

* See Table 8–1.

phasia and 1 hemiplegia with aphasia) and 4 temporary complications (3 hemiparesis with dysphasia and 1 deterioration from stupor to coma). The 5 other complications were convulsions in 1, temporary anoxia in 1, subintimal injection in 1, generalized erythema in 1 and a recurrent subarachnoid hemorrhage during angiography in 1. In this group of patients, 4 died shortly after the angiographic studies.

Intravascular Pressure Measurements

Intravascular pressure measurements within the internal carotid artery were made using a low-displacement strain gauge at the time of placement of the clamp on the exposed common carotid artery. The measurements were made with the common carotid artery open and when fully occluded. A systolic and diastolic pressure was obtained and reported in mm Hg. Concomitant blood pressure cuff measurements were taken on the arm on the side of the exposed carotid. Such

Table 8–7. Vasospasm and Neurologic Condition.

Vasospasm	Neurologic Condition*						Total
	1	2	3	4	5	6	
Localized	2	28	10	4	5	0	49
Generalized	1	15	6	3	1	1	27
Total/No. of aneurysms	3/8	43/122	16/31	7/16	6/9	1/1	76/187

* See Table 8–4.

measurements were obtained in 39 of the 88 internal carotid aneurysms, 13 of the 27 middle cerebral aneurysms and 35 of the 72 anterior cerebral-anterior communicating aneurysms. Thus, the pressure within the internal carotid artery was obtained in 46.5% of the patients.

The mean intravascular pressures fluctuated in the internal carotid aneurysm group between 63 and 128 mm Hg. The average was 93.1 mm Hg. The mean pressures fluctuated between 93 and 130 mm Hg in the middle cerebral aneurysm group, with an average of 107 mm Hg. In the anterior communicating aneurysm group the mean intravascular pressure fluctuated between 60 and 190 mm Hg, with an average pressure of 121.6 mm Hg. The percent change in intravascular measurement between the open and occluded carotid arteries fluctuated between 23.0 and 81.7 in the group of internal carotid aneurysms, between 10.7 and 54.3 in the middle cerebral aneurysms and between 20.5 and 58.3 in the anterior cerebral-anterior communicating aneurysms. In 2 patients with internal carotid aneurysms, the percent of change increased 5.3% and 14.3%, respectively, meaning that the pressure within the internal carotid was higher when the common carotid was occluded than when it was open. In all the other instances there was a drop in pressure.

In most instances the intravascular pressure coincided with the cuff blood pressure obtained on the arm on the same side as the carotid artery measurement. In 7 instances the mean intracarotid pressure was 20 mm Hg or more higher than the mean external (arm) blood pressure, and in 4 instances it was 20 mm Hg or more lower than the cuff pressure. In 65% of the patients the mean blood pressure taken by cuff on the arm was approximately the same or slightly lower at the time of carotid exposure than at the time of randomization. However, in 31 patients the mean external blood pressure was 10 or more mm Hg higher at the time of operation than at the time of randomization.

Ophthalmodynamometry

In 18.2% of patients, retinal blood pressures were obtained by ophthalmodynamometry at the same time intracarotid pressures were measured. Two measurements were obtained: the minimum pressure required to collapse the retinal arteries completely, and the minimum pressure required to produce physical pulsation of arterial flow, both with the common carotid artery open and occluded. These studies were done in 19 of the 88 internal carotid aneurysms, in 8 of the 27 middle cerebral aneurysms and in 7 of the 72 anterior cerebral-anterior communicating aneurysms. The difference in mean ophthalmodynamometric measurements between open and occluded carotid artery varied between 9 and 59 g. In only 1 patient was there no difference, and in 2 patients the difference was less than 10 g. This suggests that the retinal artery pressure drops with common carotid occlusion in the majority of cases.

Randomization

After completion of all preliminary tests, including three- or four-vessel angiography and evaluation of the angiographically demonstrable patent anterior communicating artery, randomization was carried out. One hundred eighty-seven patients were randomly allocated to be treated by common carotid ligation. Randomization was done within 6 days of the last hemorrhage in 59.9% of patients, 15 days in 84.5% and 21 days in 91.4% of patients (Table 8–8).

Randomization was delayed 22 to 70 days in 16 patients (8.6%). The delay arose from late admission of the patient to the Cooperative Study or from delay in performing the diagnostic angiographic studies because of the poor or precarious condition of the patient.

Table 8–8.   Interval from Last Bleed to Randomization.

Days	Aneurysm Site*			Total	%	Cumulative %
	ICA	MCA	ACA			
0–3	31	7	23	61	32.6	
4–6	26	3	22	51	27.3	59.9
7–9	6	8	10	24	12.8	
10–12	9	0	2	11	5.9	
13–15	5	4	2	11	5.9	84.5
16–18	3	2	4	9	4.8	
19–21	1	1	2	4	2.1	91.4
22–70	7	2	7	16	8.6	100.0
Total	88	27	72	187	100.0	

* See Table 8–1.

Untreated Patients

Of the 187 patients allocated by randomization to be treated by carotid occlusion, 62 could not undergo treatment for the following reasons: 21 patients died before carotid ligation was scheduled or attempted; 15 patients were found not to be suitable for carotid ligation; 21 patients had carotid occlusion attempted, but it was not tolerated; 4 patients died during the course of carotid artery occlusion and 1 patient died after carotid occlusion, following a recurrent hemorrhage which occurred before treatment was started.

Of the 62 patients, 21 had an internal carotid aneurysm, 11 a middle cerebral aneurysm and 30 an anterior cerebral-anterior communicating aneurysm. There were 32 patients in Neurologic Conditions 1 and 2, 14 in Condition 3 and 16 (25.8%) in Conditions 4, 5 and 6. There were 43 patients in good or fair medical condition and 19 (30.6%) in poor medical condition. The number of patients in poor condition (both neurologic and medical) was significantly higher than it was in the overall group of 187 patients, where Neurologic Conditions 4, 5 and 6 represented 13.9% and Medical Conditions C and D were also reported at 13.9%.

The age of the patients who died before carotid occlusion was scheduled varied between 24 and 74 years. Six had an internal carotid aneurysm, 5 a middle cerebral aneurysm and 10 an aneurysm of the anterior cerebral-anterior communicating complex. Eleven died within a week from the original subarachnoid hemorrhage, and another 6 within the 2nd week of the hemorrhage. Sixteen died during the 1st week after randomization.

Fifteen of 62 patients died of recurrent hemorrhage: 3 from an internal carotid aneurysm, 2 from a middle cerebral aneurysm and 10 from an anterior cerebral-anterior communicating aneurysm. The cause of death in 5 patients was a gradual downhill course following the initial subarachnoid hemorrhage. One other patient died of pulmonary emboli. In these 21 patients, 10 were in Neurologic Condition 2, 4 were in Neurologic Condition 3 and the other 7 were in Neurologic Conditions 4, 5 and 6. Thirteen were in Medical Conditions A and B, and the other 8 in Medical Conditions C and D. Recurrent hemorrhage occurred in 12 of the 15 patients within 10 days after the original hemorrhage.

Of the 15 patients who were considered unsuitable for carotid occlusion, 3 had an internal carotid aneurysm, 2 a middle cerebral aneurysm and 10 an anterior cerebral-anterior communicating aneurysm. The reasons for unsuitability for carotid occlusion were the following: poor neurologic and medical conditions in 4, intolerance of digital compression in 6, absence of cross-circulation between right and left carotid systems in 4 and convulsive seizure in 1 patient. Eight of these patients eventually died, 3 within the first 2 weeks after the original subarachnoid hemorrhage. Three patients died later than 3 months after the original hemorrhage: 1 of urinary and electrolyte problems, 1 of respiratory and urinary tract infections and 1 of unknown cause. There were 4 recurrent hemorrhages in this group, 4, 6, 8 and 24 days after the original bleed. Of these 15 patients, 6 were over the age of 60 and 4 were between 50 and 60. These findings are summarized in Table 8–9.

In 21 patients, carotid occlusion was attempted but was not tolerated (Table 8–10). Their ages ranged from 16 to 66 years. Only 3 patients were in Neurologic Condition 4; the majority were in good neurologic condition. Eighteen were in good or fair medical condition.

Fifteen of these patients were randomized within the 1st week after subarachnoid hemorrhage. Carotid occlusion was attempted within 5 days of randomization. The complications of attempted occlusion were the following: hemiplegia or hemiparesis with aphasia or dysphasia in 6 (lasting in 5), hemiplegia or hemiparesis in 5 (lasting in 4), temporary loss of consciousness in 4, decerebration in 3, temporary confusion in 2. Carotid thrombosis was found in 2 patients. When the abrupt occlusion could not be tolerated, gradual carotid occlusion was tried but was also not tolerated, and the clamp was left open in 18 patients. The clamp was partially closed in 3 patients. The carotid artery was found thrombosed in 2 patients, and an internal carotid endarterectomy was successfully carried out in 1. In another 3 patients, the carotid bifurcation was re-exposed and vessels found patent.

In this group of 21 patients, there were 8 recurrent hemorrhages: 4 in the presence of an internal carotid aneurysm, 2 of a middle cerebral aneurysm and 2 of an anterior communicating aneurysm. Three of the recurrent hemorrhages occurred on the 5th and 6th days after the original hemorrhage.

Ten of the 21 patients died while in the hospital: 4 of recurrent hemorrhage, 4 of a gradual downhill course following a complication of the original hemorrhage or of the carotid ligation attempt and 2 of other causes (perforated duodenal ulcer and cardiopulmonary disease). One other patient died 7 years, 8.5 months later of cardiac problems.

These last two groups of patients show the limitation of the treatment of intracranial aneurysm by carotid occlusion; thus, 21.7% of 166 living patients could not undergo the prescribed treatment and should be considered as failures of treatment. These patients should be excluded from those who underwent complete carotid ligation in the evaluation of the effectiveness of carotid ligation in the treatment of intracranial aneurysm.

There are two other small categories of patients which should also be excluded from this evaluation. One is a group of patients who died of a subarachnoid hemorrhage during the course of gradual occlusion of the carotid artery, and in which the carotid artery clamp was either left partly closed or reopened. In this group of 5 patients, 2 had an internal carotid aneurysm and 3 an anterior cerebral-anterior communicating aneurysm. Their ages ranged from 25 to 74 years. Two patients were in Neurologic Condition 2, 2 in Condition 3, and 1 in Condition 4. Two were in Medical Condition A, 2 in Condition B, and 1 in Condition C. One rebled the day the clamp was applied on the carotid, 2 rebled the day after the clamp was applied, 1 rebled 3 days after application of the clamp, and another 6 days after application of the clamp but before complete occlusion.

The other category consisted of 1 patient with internal carotid aneurysm who rebled before the treatment was started. The clamp was applied to the carotid artery on the day of the recurrent hemorrhage, but the patient died 1 day later after the clamp had been completely closed. He died of the effect of the recurrent hemorrhage before treatment was started. His medical condition was considered to be fair when the clamp was applied, although his original condition at the

Table 8-9.   Patients Considered Unsuitable for Carotid Ligation.

Age	Sex	Neurologic Condition*	Medical Condition+	Days			Reason for Unsuitability
				SAH to Randomization	SAH to Rebleed	SAH to Death	
Internal carotid Aneurysm							
46	M	4	C	1	6	6	Poor condition; no cross-circulation
37	M	2	A	2			Seizures on Matas Test; no cross-circulation
58	M	3	B	18			Digital compression not tolerated
Middle cerebral aneurysm							
64	F	2	B	3			Digital compression not tolerated
64	M	2	C	13	24	24	Digital compression not tolerated; no cross-circulation
Anterior cerebral aneurysm							
46	F	5	C	1		6	Poor condition; poor cross-circulation
56	M	3	B	3	4	14	No cross-circulation
60	M	2	A	7			Digital compression not tolerated
66	F	2	C	8		161[1]	Digital compression not tolerated
69	F	5	D	8		210[2]	No cross-circulation
64	M	2	B	16			Digital compression not tolerated; severe general vasospasm
54	F	5	D	16		23	Poor condition; generalized vasospasm
59	M	2	B	22			No cross-circulation
43	F	2	A	47			No cross-circulation
38	M	5	C	49	8	100[3]	Poor condition

Cause of death: 1 = unknown; 2 = respiratory and urinary infections; 3 = urinary and electrolyte problems.
* Defined in Table 8-4.
+ Defined on p. 124.

Table 8–10.   Occlusion Attempted But Not Tolerated (Carotid Left Open).

Age	Sex	Neurologic Condition*	Medical Condition†	Days				Complications of Attempted Occlusion
				SAH to Random.	Random. to Attempt	SAH to Rebleed	SAH to Death	
Internal carotid aneurysm								
44	F	2	B	2	2	5		Carotid thrombosis, hemiparesis, aphasia
57	M	4	C	2	3		7[1]	Hemiplegia
38	M	2	A	3	0			Hemiplegia, aphasia
43	M	2	A	4	1			Hemiplegia, aphasia
56	M	2	B	5	1	5		Temporary coma
48	F	3	B	6	0		14[2]	Coma, decerebration
39	F	4	C	5	2		12[3]	Coma, decerebration
61	F	3	B	12	1	0	7[3]	Stupor, decerebration
38	F	1	A	22	1		17[1]	Hemiplegia
25	M	3	A	7	3	13	13[2]	Carotid thrombosis, endarterectomy
Middle cerebral aneurysm								
49	F	2	B	2	1	26	27[2]	Hemiplegia
37	M	2	A	8	5			Temporary confusion
48	F	2	A	16	1			Hemiparesis
66	M	3	B	1	5	6	6[2]	Confusion
Anterior cerebral aneurysm								
16	F	2	A	1	2			Hemiparesis
57	F	3	B	1	4		8[1]	Hemiplegia, aphasia
47	M	2	B	2	2			Not tolerated
59	F	2	B	4	1		10[1]	Hemiparesis, dysphasia
36	M	4	C	11	5		2813[3]	Temporary coma
62	M	1	B	23	1	48		Hemiparesis, dysphasia
33	M	2	A	6	3	14	20[2]	Not tolerated

Cause of death: 1 = downhill course; 2 = rebleed; 3 = others: cardiopulmonary problems, perforated duodenal ulcer.
* Defined in Table 8–4.
† Defined on page 124.

time of randomization was considered good.

It is difficult to assess the judgment of the surgeon in his decision to treat a patient who is on a downhill course following a second subarachnoid hemorrhage before surgical treatment. It is not believed that these last 6 cases reflect a failure of treatment or help to evaluate the value of carotid ligation.

Intracarotid pressure measurements were obtained in 19 of the 63 patients in whom carotid occlusion was not accomplished. The mean blood pressure at the time the clamp was tried was 10 or more mm Hg higher than at randomization in 7 of these 19 patients, and the mean intracarotid pressure fluctuated between 72 and 160 mm Hg (average of 116.3 mm Hg). The percentage drop of mean intracarotid pressure between open and occluded carotid artery fluctuated also between 20.4 and 80.0 mm Hg. The patient with the lowest drop in pressure between open and occluded artery developed temporary neurologic complications on carotid occlusion. Eleven patients had an over 50% drop in intracarotid pressure when the carotid was occluded, and 6 of them developed neurologic complications; 5 patients had neurologic complications with a pressure

drop of 20.4 to 41.4%. Complications of carotid occlusion could not be assessed ahead of time by evaluating the difference between the intravascular pressure of the open or occluded carotid artery.

Ophthalmodynamometry was carried out in 7 of these patients; 6 showed a drop in retinal artery pressures varying between 28.6 and 49.2%, and there was no change in 1. No conclusions can be drawn from this small number of patients.

Treatment Accomplished

Carotid occlusion was accomplished in 125 patients (60 males and 65 females). Seventy-eight were below and 47 were above age 50. Aneurysm location was on the intracranial portion of the internal carotid artery in 67 patients, the middle cerebral artery in 16 and the anterior cerebral-anterior communicating complex in 42. The majority (99) of these patients were in good neurologic condition (Grades 1 and 2). Only 26 were in Conditions 3, 4 and 5. Medical condition was reported as being good in 92 and fair and poor

Table 8–11.   Treatment Accomplished Distribution of 125 Patients.

		Abrupt Occlusion	Gradual Occlusion	Total
No. of patients		42	83	125
Age	Below 50	28	50	78
	Above 50	14	33	47
Sex	Males	29	31	60
	Females	12	53	65
Aneurysm site	Internal carotid artery	17	50	67
	Middle cerebral artery	8	8	16
	Anterior cerebral artery	17	25	42
Neurologic Condition*	1 and 2	33	66	99
	3, 4, 5 and 6	9	17	26
Medical Condition	Good	29	63	92
	Fair and poor	13	20	33
Vasospasm	None	30	49	79
	Local	7	22	29
	Generalized	5	12	17

* Defined in Table 8–4.

Table 8–12. Neurologic and Medical Condition in Relation to Age.

Age	Neurologic Condition*						Medical Condition†				Type of Occlusion		Total
	1	2	3	4	5	6	A	B	C	D	Abrupt	Gradual	
Internal carotid aneurysm													
10–19	1	3	1				4	1			3	2	5
20–29		4	1				5				2	3	5
30–39		13	4	2	1		13	3	4		6	14	20
40–49	1	15	4	1			14	7			3	18	21
50–59	1	8		1			6	4			1	9	10
60–69		3	1		1			4	1		2	3	5
70–79		1						1				1	1
Total	3	47	11	4	2	0	42	20	5	0	17	50	67
Middle cerebral aneurysm													
10–19													0
20–29		2		1			2		1		2	1	3
30–39													0
40–49	1	4	2				6	1			3	4	7
50–59		4	1				4	1			2	3	5
60–69			1				1				1		1
70–79													0
Total	1	10	4	1	0	0	13	2	1	0	8	8	16
Anterior cerebral aneurysm													
10–19		1					1				1		1
20–29		3					3				2	1	3
30–39		4		1			5				3	2	5
40–49		8					6	2			3	5	8
50–59	2	13	4	1			17	2	1		8	12	20
60–69		4	1				5				0	5	5
70–79													0
Total	2	33	5	2	0	0	37	4	1	0	17	25	42

* Defined in Table 8–4.
† Defined on page 124.

in 33. No vasospasm was seen in the initial cerebral angiograms of 79 patients. Localized spasm was reported in 29 and diffuse spasm in 17 (Table 8–11). Initial total abrupt occlusion of the common carotid artery was carried out in 42 patients, while gradual occlusion with a clamp applied to the common carotid artery was carried out in 83. Some of the contributing centers performed gradual occlusions predominantly, while others preferred immediate total occlusion. Abrupt occlusion of the common carotid artery was reported in 17 of 67 patients with internal carotid aneurysm, 8 of 16 patients with middle cerebral aneurysm and 17 of 42 patients with anterior cerebral-anterior communicating aneurysm.

The age of these patients in relation to their neurologic and medical conditions is presented in Table 8–12. For the internal carotid aneurysms, the age of the majority of patients (41) was between 30 and 49 and the majority (41) were in Neurologic Conditions 1 and 2 and Medical Condition A. Five patients were below age 20, and 6 were above age 60. Gradual occlusion was carried out in 50 patients and initial abrupt occlusion in 17. There were only 16 patients with a middle cerebral aneurysm; 8 had gradual and 8 abrupt occlusion. In the anterior cerebral-anterior communicating aneurysm group, gradual occlusion was reported in 25 and abrupt occlusion in 17. The majority of patients (28) were between the ages of 40 and 59 and belonged to Neurologic Conditions 1 and 2 and Medical Condition A.

Seventy-eight of the 125 patients were randomized within 7 days after the initial subarachnoid hemorrhage, and 28 during the 2nd week after hemorrhage. The interval between randomization and application of the clamp on the common carotid artery for gradual occlusion of the vessel was 1 to 3 days in 68 patients and 4 to 6 days in 10. In 4 patients the application of the clamp was delayed beyond 10 days, possibly because of their clinical condition. The interval between application of the clamp and total occlusion was more variable. The interval was 1 to 3 days in 38 patients, 4 to 6 days in 24, 7 to 9 days in 13 and 10 to 25 days in 8. The interval between randomization and total occlusion for the total group of 125 patients was 0 to 7 days for 91, 8 to 14 days for 23 and 15 to 35 days for 11; thus, treatment was accomplished within 7 days of randomization in 73% of patients and within 14 days of randomization in 91%.

The interval between the subarachnoid hemorrhage for which the patient was hospitalized and treatment accomplished was 0 to 7 days in 30% and 0 to 15 days in 61% of patients. A fairly large number of patients were not randomized before the 16th day after hemorrhage.

The method of carotid occlusion varied from center to center. The surgeon's preference, condition of the patient, tolerance of carotid ligation, drop in intracarotid pressure over 50% between no occlusion and total occlusion, and the complication that occurred in the patient during the course of occlusion were factors relating to the method of common carotid occlusion. This can best be summarized as follows:

1. Initial total occlusion tolerated with no subsequent neurologic complications in 41 patients.

2. Initial total occlusion tolerated with late neurologic complications (178 days after occlusion) in 1 patient.

3. Initial total occlusion was not tolerated, but gradual occlusion was tolerated in 6 patients.

4. Initial total occlusion was not tried due to the surgeon's preference and the gradual occlusion was tolerated in 50 patients.

5. Initial total occlusion was not tried due to intracarotid pressure drop greater than 50% and gradual occlusion was tolerated in 9 patients.

6. Initial total occlusion was tolerated, but a delayed neurologic deficit was produced:

   A The clamp was reopened;
      a) Deficit cleared; gradual re-occlusion was tolerated in 1 patient with anterior communicating artery aneurysm.
      b) The deficit did not clear; the artery was re-occluded to protect the aneurysm in 5 patients with internal carotid aneurysms.

   B The internal carotid artery was exposed and found to be patent; the clamp was reopened;
      The deficit did not clear; the artery was re-occluded to protect the aneurysm in 2 patients with anterior communicating aneurysms.

   C The internal carotid was exposed and found to be thrombosed;
      a) Thromboendarterectomy was done; the deficit did not clear; the artery was re-occluded to protect the aneurysm in 2 patients with anterior communicating aneurysms.
      b) Thromboendarterectomy was not done; the artery was re-occluded in 2 patients with anterior communicating aneurysms, 1 with middle cerebral aneurysm and 1 with internal carotid aneurysm.

7. Initial gradual occlusion was not tolerated, the patient developed delayed neurologic deficit, the artery was slowly re-occluded to protect the aneurysm in 4 patients with internal carotid aneurysm.

Total occlusion of the common carotid artery was tolerated in 106 patients. In 41 patients this was accomplished by abrupt closure of the vessel, whereas in 65 the occlusion was gradual.

Complications of Treatment

Thirty-one ischemic complications were reported in the 83 patients undergoing gradual common carotid occlusion (Table 8–13). This represents a complication rate of 37.3%. Twenty-one of these 31 complications persisted while the patient was in the hospital; 10 were temporary.

One persisting neurologic complication following initial abrupt occlusion of the common carotid artery occurred in a patient who had an anterior cerebral-anterior communicating aneurysm. This represents a 2.4% complication rate for the 42 patients who underwent this type of carotid occlusion. One must remember that this group of patients was able to tolerate initial total occlusion.

Thus, the complication rate of carotid ligation for the 67 patients with an internal carotid aneurysm was 23.9%; for the 16 patients with a middle cerebral aneurysm it was 6.3%, and for the 42 patients with an anterior cerebral-anterior communicating aneurysm it was 35.7%. The total complication rate was 25.6%. The persistent neurologic complication rate was 17.6%. Although this complication rate is high, it was certainly not as high as the neurologic complication rate of direct surgical treatment of the aneurysm intracranially (47.8%).[10]

The main neurologic complications were: hemiplegia in 6 patients; hemiplegia with aphasia in 6 (2 temporary); hemiparesis in 6 (3 temporary); hemiparesis with dysphasia in 8 (2 temporary); temporary dysphasia alone in 1 patient; hemianopsia alone in 1 patient; convulsions alone in 2 patients; and temporary confusion alone in 2 patients. One patient with hemiplegia also became comatose. Another patient with hemiparesis developed convulsions and confusion, and 1 of the patients with convulsions also had temporary confusion. Persistent hemiplegia occurred mostly in patients with anterior cerebral-anterior communicating aneurysms.

Six of these patients died of their complications, 3 with an internal carotid aneurysm and 3 with an anterior cerebral-anterior communicating aneurysm. Thus, the mortality rate secondary to neurologic complication of treatment was 4.8%.

If one considers all the neurologic complications which arose in patients with completed as well as attempted treatment, the rate increases from 25.6 to 33.8%, as 17 of the 20 patients in whom carotid occlusion was attempted had developed neurologic complications; 13 of them persisted and 4 were temporary. Thus, the persistent neurologic complication rate for completed and attempted carotid occlusion was 24% and the temporary complication rate 9.6%.

Table 8–13.   Complications of Accomplished Treatment.

Site*	Abrupt Occlusion		Gradual Occlusion		Total	%
	Complication		Complication			
ICA	17	0	50	16	67	16	23.9
MCA	8	0	8	1	16	1	6.3
ACA	17	1	25	14	42	15	35.7
Total	42	1 (2.4)	83	31 (37.3)	125	32	25.6

	Temporary	Persisting
ICA	7	9
MCA	0	1
ACA	3	12
Total	10	22
%	8.0	17.6

* See Table 8–1.

Vasospasm may have been related to the neurologic complications following completed carotid occlusion. However, 24 of the 32 patients had no vasospasm in the original diagnostic cerebral angiogram. Localized spasm was recorded in 6 and generalized spasm in 2. One of the patients with generalized spasm developed a persisting hemiparesis and dysphasia, while the other had only a temporary dysphasia. The relation of vasospasm to complications according to the site of aneurysm is shown in Table 8–14. It appears that the complication rate is greatest in patients who had no vasospasm.

Preocclusion Matas test was performed in 27 patients with internal carotid aneurysm, and 9 developed post-occlusion ischemic complications. These complications were persistent and severe in 6 and temporary in 3 patients. In 7 of them digital carotid compression was tolerated over 5 minutes; in 1 it was tolerated 3 to 5 minutes, and in 1 less than 1 minute. Thus, it was significant in only one or two instances. A hemiparesis developed in the case which could not tolerate the test over 1 minute.

Among the 9 patients with a middle cerebral aneurysm in which the test was performed, 1 severe complication was reported in a patient who could tolerate the digital compression more than 5 minutes.

In the 42 patients with anterior cerebral-anterior communicating aneurysms, 10 had severe and persistent ischemic complications and 5 had temporary complications. Two of the persisting complications occurred in patients who tolerated digital compression less than 1 minute, and in 1 who tolerated it 3 to 5 minutes. This high incidence of complications may be related to the caliber of the anterior communicating artery or the predominant blood flow in that vessel.

The Matas test appeared to be of diagnostic value in 5 of 89 patients. One must also bear in mind that it is difficult to keep the common carotid artery completely occluded for 5 minutes by percutaneous digital compression. It seems that the Matas test or angiographic cross-flow had little value in predicting tolerance to carotid ligation.[8,12,13]

Blood pressure had no apparent influence on ischemic complications of carotid occlusion. Blood pressure in patients with complications varied from 95/70 to 210/104 mm Hg. Mean blood pressure varied from 79 to 149 mm Hg. There were 17 patients with systolic blood pressures above and 15 below 140 mm Hg, and 17 with a mean blood pressure above and 15 below 100 mm Hg. Permanent complications occurred in 12 patients with a blood pressure above 140 mm Hg systolic or above 100 mm Hg mean blood pressure. Temporary complications occurred in 15 patients with a blood pressure below 140 mm Hg systolic or a mean pressure below 100 mm Hg. Only 1 patient (aged 52) with a blood pressure below 100 mm Hg systolic (mean blood pressure below 80 mm Hg) developed permanent complications.

Other complications of treatment occurred in 69 instances. Most of them were temporary. There were 4 immediate oper-

Table 8–14.   Vasospasm and Complications in Completed Occlusion.

Site*		None	Local	General	Total	%
			Vasospasm			
ICA	Complications	14	1	1	16	23.9
	No complications	26	14	11	51	
MCA	Complications	1	0	0	1	6.3
	No complications	10	3	2	15	
ACA	Complications	9	5	1	15	35.7
	No complications	19	6	2	27	
Total		79	29	17	125	

* See Table 8–1.

ative complications: 1 cardiac arrhythmia, 1 agitation, 1 local hemorrhage and 1 hypotension. Other postoperative complications were wound infection in 12, wound hematoma in 5 (1 of which is included in wound infection) and arterial bleeding around the clamp in 1. One patient had a postoperative thrombosis of the internal carotid artery, 1 a thrombosis of the middle cerebral artery, 1 embolization of the middle cerebral artery from an internal carotid artery thrombosis. One patient who had a wound infection developed an aneurysm on the common carotid artery with an eventual rupture of that aneurysm. In 1 patient the stem of the common carotid clamp was pulled off by the patient.

Other complications during the postoperative period which may not have been related directly to the carotid occlusion were disorientation in 1, psychosis in 1, pulmonary infections in 14, urinary tract infections in 8, septicemia in 2, electrolyte imbalance in 1, transient hypotension in 1, gastrointestinal tract hemorrhage in 3, peripheral venous thrombosis in 1, deep venous thrombosis with pulmonary emboli in 3 and a posterior neck abscess in 1.

Treatment of the complications of the subarachnoid hemorrhage or the carotid occlusion required surgical procedures in 20 instances. Sixteen patients needed tracheostomy; 12 of these had an internal carotid aneurysm, 3 an anterior cerebral-anterior communicating aneurysm and 1 a middle cerebral aneurysm. One patient developed hydrocephalus which required shunting. One patient had a pre-occlusion trephination and aspiration of an intracranial hematoma. The clamp had to be replaced in 1 patient. One patient who had developed a common carotid aneurysm needed ligation of the common carotid artery. The common carotid was injured in 1 patient at the site of the clamp and the artery had to be ligated. Thromboendarterectomy of the common carotid artery had to be done in 1 patient, and thromboendarterectomy of the internal carotid artery in 2 patients. In another 5 patients, the internal carotid artery was exposed after the vessel had been occluded in order to rule out a thrombosis of the vessel.

Recurrent Hemorrhage

Carotid occlusion may occasionally fail to protect the patient from a rerupture of the aneurysm. Nishioka,[5] in his previous analysis of the cases of the Cooperative Study treated by carotid ligation, found post-occlusion subarachnoid hemorrhage in 41 of 526 patients with common carotid occlusion, representing a rebleed rate of 7.8%, and in 5 of 51 patients (9.8%) with internal carotid occlusion. Thus, the total rebleeding rate follow-

Table 8–15. Total Rebleeds in Relation to Treatment and Site.

Rebleed	ICA*	Deaths	MCA*	Deaths	ACA*	Deaths	Total	Deaths
Before treatment scheduled	4	4	3	3	11	11	18	18
Before occlusion started	3	2	1	0	3	0	7	2
Occlusion not tolerated	1	0	2	2	2	1	5	3
During occlusion	3	2	0	0	4	3	7	5
Subtotal	11/88	8	6/27	5	20/72	15	37/187	28
After occlusion (within 30 days)	4	3	2	2	4	3	10	8
After occlusion (later than 30 days)	2	1	1	0	0	0	3	1
Subtotal	6/67	4	3/16	2	4/42	3	13/125	9
Total	17/88	12	9/27	7	24/72	18	50/187	37

* See Table 8–1.

ing carotid occlusion was 8%. However, in 7 instances of rebleeding, the hemorrhage occurred from another aneurysm than the one for which the occlusion was performed. Post-ligation hemorrhages have been reported by numerous investigators.[1,4,6-8,14,15]

The overall rebleed rate was 19.8% before complete occlusion was accomplished. Rebleeding was reported in 11 of 88 internal carotid aneurysms (12.5%), in 6 of 27 middle cerebral aneurysms (22.2%) and in 20 of 72 anterior cerebral-anterior communicating aneurysms (27.8%). Table 8–15 summarizes all the cases of recurrent hemorrhage in relation to treatment and to aneurysm site. It does not seem pertinent to analyze recurrent hemorrhages in patients following carotid ligation together with patients in whom the ligation was never accomplished, as the former were protected from recurrent hemorrhage while the latter were not.

Recurrent Hemorrhage in Non-treated Patients

Eight of the 88 internal carotid aneurysms (9.1%), 6 of the 27 middle cerebral aneurysms (22.2%) and 16 of the 72 anterior cerebral-anterior communicating aneurysms reruptured (22.2%), resulting in 23 deaths. Thus, it appears that middle cerebral and anterior cerebral-anterior communicating aneurysms have a greater tendency to rerupture than the internal carotid aneurysms.

Twelve females and 18 males were in this group. Seventeen of the 30 aneurysms reruptured within 6 days of the initial subarachnoid hemorrhage or 21 within the first 10 days. Seventeen of these patients were in Neurologic Condition 1 or 2, and 21 were in good or fair medical condition. Eleven of these patients had a systolic blood pressure above 161 mm Hg (Table 8–16). The mean blood pressure of this group of patients suggests that half the patients were hypertensive (above 111 mm Hg), and 8 had a mild increase in blood pressure.

Recurrent Hemorrhage During Treatment

Rebleeding during gradual occlusion of the common carotid artery occurred in 7 patients, 3 with internal carotid aneurysms and 4 with anterior cerebral-anterior communicating aneurysms. There were 5 deaths in this group. Rebleeding occurred at any age. These recurrent hemorrhages occurred 2 to 19 days after the initial subarachnoid hemorrhage. The majority of these patients were in Neurologic Conditions 2 and 3 and in good medical condition. Four of the 7 patients had a systolic blood pressure above 141 mm Hg. In evaluating their mean blood pressure, 2 were hypertensive and 3 had a mild increase in blood pressure.

Table 8–16.   Rebleed, Systolic Blood Pressure and Age Before Treatment.

| Age | Systolic Blood Pressure (mm Hg) | | | | | |
	120 or less	121–140	141–160	161–180	181 +	Total
20–29		1				1
30–39	2	2	1		1	6
40–49	1	3	4	2	1	11
50–59			1	1	3	5
60–69	1	2			3	6
70–79		1				1
Total	4	9	6	3	8	30

Table 8–17. Rebleed After Total Occlusion.

Days After Occlusion	Site*						Total	Deaths
	ICA	Deaths	MCA	Deaths	ACA	Deaths		
1–3	2	1					2	1
4–6	1	1					1	1
7–9			1	1	2	1	3	2
10–12							0	0
13–19	1	1					1	1
20–26			1	1	2	2	3	3
27–42	1						1	0
42 +	1 +	1	1‡				2	1
Total	6	4	3	2	4	3	13	9
No Cases	67		16		42		125	
%	9.0		18.8		9.5		10.4	

* See Table 8–1.
+ Suspected rebleed after 356 days.
‡ Rebleed after 3,195 days.

Recurrent Hemorrhage After Treatment

Thirteen of the 125 patients rebled after completed occlusion of the common carotid artery. This represents a rebleed rate of 10.4%. Nine of these patients died of the recurrent hemorrhage. Recurrent hemorrhage occurred in 6 (9%) of the 67 patients with internal carotid aneurysms, in 3 of 16 patients with middle cerebral aneurysms (18.8%) and in 4 of 42 anterior cerebral-anterior communicating aneurysm patients (9.5%). The age of these patients varied between 20 and 59 years. Six rebleeds occurred within 9 days of total occlusion of the carotid artery. One patient with an internal carotid aneurysm died of a suspected rebleed 356 days after carotid ligation, and another patient with a middle cerebral aneurysm suffered a nonfatal hemorrhage 3,195 days (8 years, 9 months) after carotid ligation. Nine of the 13 patients died (Table 8–17). Nine of these patients were in Neurologic Conditions 1 and 2, and 10 were in good medical condition at time of randomization. The systolic blood pressure was mildly elevated in 6 and above 161 mm Hg in 3. Evaluation of the mean blood pressure suggested that hypertension was present in 4 of the 13 patients and mild elevation in blood pressure in another 4. Five were reported to have normal blood pressure at the time of randomization.

It was thought that the degree of reduction of intracarotid pressure could play a role in post-occlusion recurrent hemorrhage. Six of 9 patients in whom the intracarotid pressure was measured at the time the clamp was applied had a reduction of intracarotid pressure of 41 to 60% after common carotid occlusion. One patient had a reduction of 10 to 20%, while 2 others had a reduction of 21 to 30%.

Carotid occlusion greatly reduces the rate of recurrent aneurysm rupture (10.4%) when compared to the pre-occlusion rate of 19.8%. It is also obvious that carotid occlusion does not prevent recurring rupture and subarachnoid hemorrhage. If one adds the recurrent bleeding which occurred during gradual occlusion of the carotid artery to the post-occlusion ruptures, rebleeding represents a total treatment failure rate of 15.4% (20 of 130). It is not possible to assess the number of recurrent hemorrhages which could have occurred in the same group of patients if they had not been treated by carotid ligation. Henderson et al.,[16] reporting on regulated bed rest, found a cumulative rebleeding incidence of 47% at the end of 5 years. The rebleed rate was 30% during the 1st month after randomization.

Mortality

Of the original 187 patients allocated randomly to carotid ligation, 74 died (39.6%). Thirty died before treatment, 14 after treatment was attempted or during the course of gradual carotid occlusion and 30 after completed carotid occlusion (Table 8–18).

Blood pressure was elevated in approximately half of the patients who died (38 of 74 patients). There were 36 women and 38 men, and their ages were between 22 and 74 years.

Thirty deaths among 125 treated patients represents an incidence of 24.0%. However, the mortality directly caused by the treatment (9 patients) was 6.0% (9 of 151 patients). Four of these deaths occurred in patients with internal carotid aneurysms and 5 in patients with anterior cerebral-anterior communicating aneurysms. Seven patients died of recurrent aneurysm rupture and 2 of suspected rupture (7.2%) after completed ligation. Two patients died of complications of a recurrent pretreatment hemorrhage after completed occlusion. Ten patients died of unrelated causes and 1 of unknown cause.

Death from recurrent subarachnoid hemorrhage occurred within 60 days of the original hemorrhage. Rerupture of the aneurysm took place 2, 4, 7, 14, 18, 22 and 22 days after completed carotid occlusion. Death from rebleed was more common in middle

Table 8–18. Cause of Death in Relation to Treatment and Aneurysm Site.

Cause of Death	Aneurysm Site*			Total	%Deaths
	ICA	MCA	ACA		
I. Untreated					
Proved rebleed	3	2	8	13	
Suspected rebleed	1	1	3	5	
Complication of SAH	1	3	4	8	
Unrelated cause	2		2	4	
Unknown				0	
Total	7/9†	6/7	17/20	30/36	83.3
II. Attempted or incomplete treatment					
Proved rebleed	2	1	4	7	
Suspected rebleed		1		1	
Complication of SAH	2		2	4	
Complication of treatment	1			1	
Unrelated cause			1	1	
Unknown				0	
Total	5/12	2/4	7/10	14/26	53.8
III. Fully treated					
Proved Rebleed	5	2	2	9	
Suspected rebleed	1		1	2	
Complication of SAH				0	
Complication of treatment	3		5	8	
Unrelated cause	3	4	3	10	
Unknown	1			1	
Total	13/67	6/16	11/42	30/125	24.0
TOTAL	25/88	14/27	35/72	74/187	39.6
%	28.4	51.9	48.6		

* See Table 8–1.

$$\dagger \quad \frac{\text{no. of deaths}}{\text{total no. of patients}}$$

Table 8–19. Cause of Late Deaths.

	Days SAH to Death	Age	Sex	Cause	Site of Aneurysm*
Not treated	3,355	68	M	Myocardial infarction	ACA
	2,813	44	M	Myocardial infarction	ACA
	210	69	F	Complication of SAH	ACA
Treated	3,003	59	M	Myocardial infarction	ACA
	2,219	64	M	Myocardial infarction	MCA
	1,840	63	F	Bronchopneumonia	ICA
	1,566	68	F	Unknown	ICA
	1,123	61	M	Myocardial infarction	MCA
	1,040	62	M	Myocardial infarction	ACA
	361	43	F	Suspected rebleed	ICA
	335	60	M	Suicide	MCA
	268	62	M	Myocardial infarction	MCA

* See Table 8–1.

cerebral and anterior cerebral-anterior communicating aneurysms than in internal carotid aneurysms. The causes of the late deaths are listed in Table 8–19; 1 rebleed was suspected.

Follow-up

Follow-up information was obtained on 107 patients allocated to treatment with carotid ligation (treated or not treated). As of February 1, 1977, 95 patients were followed 1 to 10 years; 53 had an internal carotid aneurysm, 10 a middle cerebral aneurysm and 32 an anterior cerebral-anterior communicating

Table 8–20. Treated Patients Follow-Up (to February 1977).

	Aneurysm Site*			
Years	ICA	MCA	ACA	Total
1	6			6
2	1			1
3	5			5
4	7	3	1	11
5	4	1	24	29
6	13	2	1	16
7	2			2
8	8		3	11
9	2	1	1	4
10	5	3	2	10
Total	53	10	32	95

* See Table 8–1.

aneurysm. The average length of follow-up was 5.75 years (Table 8–20). Twelve untreated patients were followed 1 to 10 years; an average of 5.6 years. Six of them had an anterior cerebral-anterior communicating aneurysm, 3 a middle cerebral and 3 an internal carotid aneurysm. The employment capability of these patients is reported in Table 8–21. Fifty-two percent of all treated patients are reported as working full time at a similar occupation as before their subarachnoid hemorrhage (65 of 125), representing 68.4% of surviving patients (65 of 95). Five of 95 patients (5.3%) are unfit for gainful employment. Two of 12 surviving nontreated patients are unable to work, while 5 are fully employed at a similar occupation as before the hemorrhage.

In summary, 56.7% (38 of 67) of all treated patients with internal carotid aneurysm are fully employed, representing 71.7% of surviving patients, and 9.4% are unable to work. Of all treated patients with middle cerebral aneurysm 31.3% are fully employed (5 of 16), representing 50% of surviving patients.

Fifty-two percent of all treated patients with anterior cerebral-anterior communicating aneurysm are fully employed (64.3%, if one counts houseworking women), representing 84.4% of surviving patients. Three patients with treated middle cerebral aneurysm had 9-month pregnancies with normal deliveries.

Table 8–21.   Treated and Untreated Patient Employment Capabilities (to February 1977).

	Aneurysm Site*			
	ICA	MCA	ACA	Total
1 Working full time at same or equivalent occupation as before bleed	38	5(2)†	22(3)	65(5)
2 Working part time at same or equivalent occupation as before bleed	2[1]	2	2[1](2)	6(2)
3 Unable to perform previous work, but working at physically less strenuous job	3[2]	1		4
4 Unable to perform previous work, but working steadily at special job consistent with neurologic deficit		1[5]		1
5 Not gainfully employed, but capable of working	5[3](1)	1[6](1)	7[7](1)	13(3)
6 Unfit for gainful employment	5[4](2)		1[8]	6(2)
Total	53(3)	10(3)	32(6)	95(12)

* See Table 8–1.
† Data for untreated patients' employment in parentheses.
[1] 4 mild hemiparesis
[2] 1 convulsive disorder, 1 disc operation
[3] 1 unemployed, 1 diplopia, 1 convulsive disorder
[4] 2 hemipareses, 1 memory loss, 1 leg pain, 1 convulsions
[5] Memory loss
[6] Hemiparesis following recurrent bleed
[7] 5 houseworking, 1 hemiparesis
[8] Hemiplegia

Summary and Conclusions

1. During the 7-year period from 1963 to 1970, 187 patients with single ruptured intracranial aneurysms were allocated randomly to treatment with common carotid artery ligation. Eighty-eight patients had a recently ruptured aneurysm on the internal carotid artery, 27 on the middle cerebral artery and 72 on the anterior cerebral-anterior communicating complex. Twenty-one patients died (11.2%) before receiving any treatment for their initial subarachnoid hemorrhage. Fifty-five percent of the aneurysms ruptured in patients aged 40 to 60. The site of the aneurysm, the neurologic condition and the age of the patient were directly related to survival.

2. Sixty-two patients did not have common carotid ligation: 21 died, 15 were found unsuitable for this type of treatment because of anatomic anomalies impairing right and left carotid cross-circulation, 21 could not tolerate carotid occlusion when it was attempted and 5 died during the course of the carotid occlusion. Angiographic visualization of cross-circulation, digital carotid compression, drop in intracarotid pressure and ophthalmodynamometry did not test the efficiency of collateral circulation or predict tolerance to carotid ligation.

3. The complications caused by cerebral ischemia after common carotid ligation occurred in 25.6% of patients, with a mortality of 6.4%, and the persisting neurologic complication rate was 17.6%. Vasospasm and blood pressure did not seem to influence the condition of the patient after operation.

4. Carotid ligation did not prevent recurrent aneurysm rupture or intracranial hemorrhages. After completed common carotid artery occlusion, the rebleed rate was 10.4%, with a mortality of 7.2%. The anterior cerebral-anterior communicating and middle cerebral aneurysms have a greater tendency to rerupture than the internal carotid aneurysms.

5. Of the 95 treated patients followed 1 to 10 years after ligation (average follow-up of 5.75 years), 65 (68.4%) were working full time at a similar occupation as before the original subarachnoid hemorrhage and 6 (6.3%) were unfit for gainful employment.

6. Although direct surgical approach is today's preferred method of definitive aneurysm treatment, common carotid ligation remains an effective procedure for the treatment of intracranial aneurysms in selected individuals, especially those patients with an aneurysm on the internal carotid artery.

References

1. Gurdjian, E.S., Lindner, D.W., Thomas, L.M.: Experiences with ligation of common carotid artery for treatment of aneurysms of the internal carotid artery. J Neurosurg 23:311–318, 1965.
2. German, W.J., Black, S.P.W.: Cervical ligation for internal carotid aneurysms. An extended follow-up. J Neurosurg 23:572–577, 1965.
3. Somach, F.M., Shenkin, H.A.: Angiographic end-results of carotid ligation in the treatment of carotid aneurysms. J Neurosurg 24:966–974, 1966.
4. Tindall, G.T., Goree, J.A., Lee, J.F., Odom, G.L.: Effect of common carotid ligation on size of internal carotid aneurysms and distal intracarotid and retinal artery pressures. J Neurosurg 24:503–511, 1966.
5. Nishioka, H.: Report on the cooperative study of intracranial aneurysms and subarachnoid hemorrhage. Section VIII, Part 1. Results of treatment of intracranial aneurysms by occlusion of the carotid artery in the neck. J Neurosurg 25:660–682, 1966.
6. Love, J.G., Dart, L.H.: Results of carotid ligation with particular reference to intracranial aneurysms. J Neurosurg 27:89–93, 1967.
7. Tytus, J.S., Reifel, E., Spencer, M.P., Burnett, L.L., Hungerford, L.N.: Common carotid ligation for intracranial aneurysms. J Neurosurg 32:63–73, 1970.
8. Kak, V.K., Taylor, A.R., Gordon, D.S.: Proximal carotid ligation for internal carotid aneurysms. J Neurosurg 39:503–513, 1975.
9. Nibbelink, D.W., Torner, J.C., Henderson, W.G.: Intracranial aneurysms and subarachnoid hemorrhage. Report on a randomized treatment study. IV-A. Regulated bed rest. Stroke 8:202–218, 1977.
10. Graf, C.J., Nibbelink, D.W.: Cooperative study of intracranial aneurysms and subarachnoid hemorrhage. III. Intracranial surgery. Stroke 5:557–601, 1974.
11. Perret, G.E., Nishioka, H.: Section IV. Cerebral angiography. An analysis of the diagnostic value and complications of carotid and vertebral angiography in 5,484 patients. J Neurosurg 25:94–114, 1966.
12. Dandy, W.E.: Results following ligation of the internal carotid artery. Arch Surg 45:521–533, 1942.
13. Beatty, R.A., Richardson, A.E.: Predicting intolerance to common carotid artery ligation by carotid angiography. J Neurosurg 28:9–13, 1968.
14. McKissock, W., Richardson, A., Walsh, L.: Anterior communicating aneurysms. A trial of conservative and surgical treatment. Lancet 1:873–876, 1965.
15. Winn, H.R., Richardson, A.E., Jane, J.A.: Late morbidity and mortality of common carotid ligation for posterior communicating aneurysms. J Neurosurg 47:727–736, 1977.
16. Henderson, W.G., Torner, J.C., Nibbelink, D.W.: Intracranial aneurysms and subarachnoid hemorrhage. Report on a randomized treatment study. IV-B. Regulated bed rest. Statistical evaluation. Stroke 8:579–589, 1977.

Chapter 9

Randomized Treatment Study. Intracranial Surgery

Carl J. Graf, M.D. and Donald W. Nibbelink, M.D., Ph.D.

Abstract

A group of 274 patients with a single intra-cranial aneurysm was randomly allocated to intracranial surgery. Forty patients had no surgical procedure. Only 6 had a vertebral-basilar aneurysm. The remaining 228 patients had an aneurysm on the anterior portion of the circle of Willis. Mortality during the 6.5-year interval was 36.8%. When the operation was performed within 14 days following the last bleed, mortality was 44.5%; for those operated upon after the 14-day interval, mortality was 23.2%. Postoperative complications occurred in 47.8%.

Introduction

The evaluation of a disease process may be difficult even under ideal conditions. The natural history of the disease should be known, and a treatment should be designed and employed only if it can improve the prognosis of the natural course of the disorder. If more than one treatment is available, determining which is better may compound an already complex problem. Furthermore, a specific treatment can be evaluated and compared to another only if the criteria for each are the same.

A critical evaluation of the treatment of cerebral aneurysms by intracranial operation is attempted here through a careful analysis of a large number of patients treated by a number of neurosurgeons from different areas of this country and abroad, as part of a Cooperative Treatment Study.

Following Dandy's[1] monograph in 1944, sporadic reports of surgically treated aneurysms by the direct intracranial approach appeared in the early 1950's. In the main, these reports indicated principally that intracranial operation for aneurysm was feasible. They indicated that in experienced hands an operative approach could be executed successfully by removing the aneurysm from the circulation, thereby preventing recurrent hemorrhage and at the same time preserving the parent vessel which also supplied the brain. Under certain circumstances, the patient with an aneurysm, particularly one that had ruptured, could then be given assurance that he would have no further difficulty from that aneurysm.

It is difficult to know if any other message was conveyed by these reports, except to suggest that this lesion might one day be "routinely" treated by the direct approach. During the ensuing three decades, it became evident that this was not easily accomplished. Mortality rates remained high, and questions continued to be raised concerning the wisdom of treating aneurysms in this manner. Mortality rates following intracranial operation covered a wide range, and it was apparent that many factors were responsible for a successful outcome. The information given by various writers was so heterogeneous that no conclusions could be drawn. For example, some authors discussed only operative mortality; others reported overall mortality. The specific site of the aneurysm was defined clearly in some series; in others it was not. Operative procedures were not always described precisely, so that interpretation of what the surgeon had actually done was difficult. In some instances, extracranial carotid ligation was performed as well as intracranial operation, or only a hematoma may have been evacuated and the aneurysm left untreated. Immediate and late complications following operation were not indicated or fully described. Reports of treatment frequently did not take into account the condition of the patient at the time of operation, or how soon after a bleeding insult the operation was carried out. Proper comparisons could not be made because the criteria were not the same.

In 1955, Graf[2] raised questions regarding the validity of such statistics. There was concern that as greater enthusiasm to attack aneurysms by the "direct approach" developed among neurosurgeons, ideas and impressions conveyed by these reports might be misleading. Because of the unlimited number of variables involved and the painfully slow accumulation of a significantly representative number of aneurysms at various sites on the circle of Willis necessary to provide meaningful data, the evaluation of this form of treatment presented an almost insurmountable task for any one neurosurgeon during his lifetime. Some suggestions were proposed as to how more significant evaluations of this form of treatment might be accomplished. The ponderous nature of the problem was evident. It was recognized that extraordinarily rigid criteria and absolute objectivity were necessary to bring about reliable conclusions. As greater experience with intracranial surgery accumulated, the problems became more imposing. It was apparent even then that the most important factors governing the success or failure of surgical treatment were: (1) the patient's condition, especially the neurological deficit, after the subarachnoid hemorrhage and particularly at the time of operation; (2) the presence of intracerebral hematoma; (3) "vasospasm"; (4) the time elapsed between subarachnoid hemorrhage and operation; (5) the age of the patient and the state of his cerebral blood vessels; (6) the intracranial pressure at the time of operation; and (7) the site of the aneurysm. To this list was added: (8) whether or not the aneurysm had ruptured. Although these conditions were considered most important, others could have been added. Thus, the great number of variables makes comparisons of results of treatment extremely difficult to interpret. It was further evident that a much wider experience in the management of large numbers of patients under comparable conditions was needed to obtain the information necessary to determine the efficacy of this particular treatment. The Cooperative Study of Subarachnoid Hemorrhage and Intracranial Aneurysms[3] was established and designed to find answers to questions of this nature.

Although a great deal of statistical information was gathered, it became apparent that answers to many questions were unsatisfactory because: (1) opinions and bias frequently entered into the results as described; (2) the nature of the questions was such that they could not be answered without qualification; (3) interpretation of the questions varied; and (4) questions were simply left unanswered because of lack of information, or a positive answer was not considered possible or available. Perhaps this was due to improper design of the study. In the Cooperative Study of Subarachnoid Hemorrhage and Intracranial Aneurysms,[3] 697 patients with single aneurysms at three major sites had intracranial operation. The mortality for 180 patients in the year 1956 to 1957 was 33%. In 1958 (128 patients), it was 30%; in 1959 (132 patients), 36%; and in 1960 (128 patients), 34%. In the interval between the years 1961 and 1964 (129 patients), the mortality remained rather constant at about 26%. The decreasing mortality appeared encouraging, as it represented gross mortality rates which included deaths occurring during the follow-up period after discharge from the hospital. However, the lower mortality rate in the 1961 to 1964 period was probably due to fewer follow-up reports, and those reports that were available covered a shorter period of time in general than those in the years prior to 1961.

These figures, which represented the results for intracranial operation, were justifiably criticized. Critical examination revealed that the statistics were invalid and misleading. Since intracranial surgery for aneurysms at various sites was done by surgeons with different techniques and experience under conditions comprising a host of variables, and accurate appraisal of its value represented only what was accomplished in isolated groups of patients under "uncontrolled" circumstances. Concepts concerning the type of patient subjected to intracranial operation changed during the study period. For example, a subject who was younger and in good condition was more readily acceptable than one who was older, in poor general condition, or who had severe neurologic disability. Surgeons' attitudes and decisions toward operation became more cautious and critical. Concern with "optimal" timing for operation after subarachnoid hemorrhage, the characteristics of the aneurysm and other angiographic findings (vasospasm, atherosclerosis, and so forth) became prominent in patient assessment.

The Cooperative Study[3] revealed that although the nonsurgically treated population was "adversely distorted by a tendency to select more favorable cases for operation, this selection was mitigated to some degree by the fact that nearly one half of the surgical cases were from a clinical trial designed to avoid selection." It appeared that although a high percentage of patients considered suitable for operation were relegated to a nonsurgical treatment category, their inclusion did not make the *whole group entirely unselected*. This favorably influenced the prognosis of the total nonsurgical group of patients because they were patients in better condition. Furthermore, patients reported by McKissock et al.,[4-6] who were considered likely to die from the immediate effects of the hemorrhage or were unable to tolerate digital carotid occlusion, were excluded from randomization and assigned to a conservative treatment category. This indicates to the authors that selection phenomena favorably influenced the prognosis of the surgical group and that the differences in survival were directly related to such selection. It is our opinion that the exclusion of such a selective group of patients, whose fate is predictable, is biased and invalidates making a comparative evaluation of surgical versus nonsurgical treatment because it was carried out under different conditions. A more significant study was made by Troupp and af Björkesten,[7] in which they reported the results of a controlled trial of late surgical versus conservative treatment of intracranial aneurysms. Only about one third of the patients with subarachnoid hemorrhage seen by them were acceptable for the trial, and all were good-condition patients. The decision for surgical or conservative treatment was made on the average of 51 and 50 days, respectively, following subarachnoid hemorrhage. They adhered to a specific technical surgical regimen. Comparing intracranial operation to conservative treatment (bed rest) in good-condition patients who survived at least 15 days (with intervals to 127 days for the surgical and 171 days for the nonsurgical group, when a decision of a specific treatment was made), it was their opinion that neither treatment was superior to the other. In their conservatively treated group of 92 patients, 9 died of recurrent hemorrhage—5 during the 2nd month after the initial bleed, 3 in the 3rd and 4th months and another 17 months after the first bleed. In 86 surgically treated patients, there were 5 deaths: 1 occurring in the hospital, and 4 between 1 month and 4 years after what was considered to be an unsuccessful aneurysm stalk ligature. These figures may be more significant because the authors approached the problem by defining rigidly the conditions for selection of patients and relegating patients to a specific type of surgical treatment.

In the present study, an attempt was made to appraise meticulously a mode of treatment of intracranial aneurysms under the confining rules of a protocol intended to be scrupulously objective. It is evident that an endless number of variables makes an absolute comparison unlikely. Objections to the method of evaluation will undoubtedly be raised because of defects inherent in any study of this type.

It must be remembered that intracranial surgery was a treatment program placed in the design of the study; however, all patients allocated to intracranial surgery did not have such treatment accomplished. Experience has shown that early (1 to 7 days) surgical treatment is more hazardous than when applied later. Under circumstances such as this, can one justifiably include a predictable biological fact in a statistical mathematical formula? The design of a protocol may call for precise answers to questions, but dependent information necessary for an answer may not be available. A question may be asked in such a way, for example, that an unqualified answer cannot be given. However, if each treatment category is considered in the same way, each failure theoretically cancels the other. Although this may be the case when numbers are the same at a particular point in time, can this be applied to a complex comparative analysis? For example, if intracranial surgery was not accomplished, can this be the same as treating the patient by bed rest, or is it noted as a failure of surgical treatment whether the patient survives or not? In the present study, 40 patients failed to receive intracranial sur-

Table 9–1.   Case Registrations Excluded.

101	Died before randomization
300	Multiple aneurysms
13	Arteriovenous anomaly in addition to aneurysm
49	Intracranial mass lesion requiring immediate surgery
147	Inability to obtain comprehensive treatment permit
25	Unrelated disease sufficiently compromising to hypotensive or surgical treatments
7	Previous aneurysm treatment other than bed rest
13	Aneurysm of posterior circle
4	Patient set aside according to prearranged schedule
1	Unknown
660	Total

gery for one reason or another. This does not mean, however, that intracranial operation was of no value, but only that one or many factors precluded surgical management.

Clinical Material

From June 15, 1963, through February 15, 1970, 1,665 case registrations of patients with single ruptured intracranial aneurysms were submitted to the Central Registry. Six hundred and sixty (Table 9–1) were excluded for the reasons listed. Of the remaining 1,005 cases, 33 were disqualified (Table 9–2), leaving 972 (Table 9–3), from which 274 were randomly assigned to treatment by intracranial surgery. Subarachnoid hemorrhage was

Table 9–2.   Tabulation of Disqualified Cases.

8	Surgery required
7	Previous hypotensive treatment
4	Refused treatment
4	Incorrect allocation of treatment
4	Special study
3	Multiple aneurysms
1	Extracranial aneurysm
1	Refused hospitalization
1	Uremia
33	Total disqualified

Table 9–3.   Case Registrations Randomized.

Center	Retained	Disqualified	Total
12	50	1	51
14	1	0	1
19	72	3	75
20*	308	6	314
22	12	0	12
24	47	2	49
25	61	3	64
26	70	5	75
27*	87	5	92
28*	139	3	142
29	30	0	30
30*	39	1	40
31	16	2	18
32	13	1	14
33	27	1	28
Total	972	33	1,005

* Centers outside of USA.

proved by lumbar puncture prior to demonstration of a single aneurysm by angiography of three or four vessels. Specific aneurysm locations were grouped into one of four major sites: internal carotid, middle cerebral, anterior cerebral-anterior communicating and vertebral-basilar arteries. Analysis of aneurysm location (Tables 9–4 to 9–7) reveals the origin of most defects to be at major arterial bifurcations in the majority of instances. Overall distribution by sex shows slightly more females (Table 9–8). The internal carotid group alone had 64% females.

Several factors were considered in the comparative evaluation. These included age, sex, blood pressure, neurologic and medical conditions, state of the patient's blood vessels as noted by physical examination and

Table 9–4.   Distribution of Specific Location of Each Aneurysm on the Intracranial Portion of the Internal Carotid Artery.

Right	Left	Location
0	2	Subclinoid
1	3	Supraclinoid, ophthalmic region
20	16	Supraclinoid, posterior communicating region
1	7	Supraclinoid at bifurcation
22	28	Total = 50

Table 9–5.   Distribution of Specific Location of Each Aneurysm on the Middle Cerebral Artery.

Right	Left	Location
4	1	Proximal to first main branching
19	13	At main branching
1	0	Distal to main branching
24	14	Total = 38

Table 9–6.   Distribution of Specific Location of Each Aneurysm on the Anterior Cerebral-Anterior Communicating Artery.

Right		Left	Location
1		1	Proximal to anterior communicating
47		51	At anterior communicating junction
6		7	Distal to anterior communicating
	67		At anterior communicating
54	67	59	Total = 180

Table 9–7.   Posterior Circle: Distribution of Specific Location of Each Aneurysm on the Vertebral-Basilar System.

Total	Location
4	Basilar artery termination
1	Right posterior cerebral artery
1	Left vertebral-basilar artery junction
6	

angiography and presence of "spasm" of the cerebral vessels. Included also was the interval between subarachnoid hemorrhage and randomization; interval between subarachnoid hemorrhage and operation; technical aspects of the operative procedure; complications before, during and after operation; surgical morbidity; and mortality.

Table 9–8.   Distribution of Patients by Sex and Aneurysm Site.

	Male	Female	Total
Internal carotid	18	32	50
Middle cerebral	17	21	38
Anterior cerebral	95	85	180
Vertebral-basilar	2	4	6
	132	142	274

Site of Aneurysm, Interval from SAH to Randomization

Table 9–9 compares the number of patients for each aneurysm site with interval to randomization from last bleed. There were 152 patients (55.5%) allocated to intracranial surgery within 7 days, 90 patients (32.8%) in the 8 to 21-day interval and 32 patients (11.7%) in the 22 to 92-day interval. Fifty (18.2%) had an aneurysm on the internal carotid distribution, 38 (13.9%) on the middle cerebral, 180 (65.7%) on the anterior cerebral-anterior communicating complex and 6 (2.2%) on the vertebral-basilar-posterior cerebral circulation, for a total of 274. Due to the paucity of cases collected with a single aneurysm located on the posterior portion of the circle of Willis, analysis of patients at this site was discontinued (June 19, 1967). Four of the 6 patients died subsequent to intracranial operation, 1 remained alive and 1 had no operation due to anticipated difficulty in access to the aneurysm.

The foregoing analysis includes the 268 patients with a single aneurysm located on the anterior portion of the circle of Willis. The overall mortality was 43.3% (116 of 268) in January 1973. Included in this figure are 40 patients who never had the surgical procedure to which they were allocated. Thirty-one patients had an aneurysm on the anterior cerebral complex, 5 on the internal carotid system and 4 on the middle cerebral distribution. Treatment was not accomplished in 24 patients because they died after randomization and before surgery could be undertaken (Table 9–10). The remaining 16 were considered unsuitable for intracranial operation. The mortality in those patients in whom treatment was not accomplished was 80% (32 of 40). Of the 24 patients who died before surgery could be undertaken, 6 succumbed to "progressive deterioration" from the direct cerebral effects of the original bleeding episode between the 2nd and 7th day following the initial bleed. Thirteen deaths were associated with proved rebleeding occurring in 4 instances within 2 to 7 days, in 7 instances between the 10th and the 16th day, and 1 each on the 22nd and 92nd day after the initial insult. Three patients died from a suspected recurrent hemorrhage 3, 10 and 16 days, respectively, from the initial bleed, and 1 each died with a pulmonary embolism and with cardiorespiratory arrest. Of the 24, 8 initially had minimal symptoms and signs, whereas 16 had conditions which varied from a major neurologic deficit to 1 in which the patient was unlikely to survive. The medical condition was classified as good in 7, fair in 5, poor in 5 and prohibitive in 7. Fifty percent (12 of 24) of the patients were considered in poor and prohibitive medical condition and 54% (13 of 24) were in poor neurologic condition. Their age distribution was in the latter 5th, 6th, and 7th decades. Therefore, one can say with reasonable certainty that surgical treatment would have been associated with a high mortality in this group.

Analyzing the 16 patients considered unsuitable for intracranial operation, there were 8 deaths (50%). Three died from the direct cerebral effects of the original bleeding episode in an interval ranging from 17

Table 9–9. Distribution of Patients by Aneurysm Site With Respect to Interval from Last Bleed to Randomization.

Days to Randomization	Internal Carotid	Middle Cerebral	Ant. Cerebral-Ant. Comm.	Posterior Circulation	Total
0–7	23	13	113	3	152
8–21	20	15	53	2	90
22–92	7	10	14	1	32
Total	50	38	180	6	274

Table 9–10.   Distribution of Patients Who Had No Operation After Allocation to Intracranial Surgery.

Internal Carotid	Middle Cerebral	Ant. Cerebral- Ant. Comm.	Reason Surgery Not Performed	Total
2	2	20	Patient died before surgery could be performed	24
3	2	11	Patient considered unsuitable for intracranial surgery	16
5	4	31	Total	40

days in 2 instances to 9 months in 1. Three subjects in good medical and neurologic condition rebled and died, 2 on the 27th day after the initial SAH and another 3 years later. Two died of severe pneumonia. The specific reasons for exclusion from operation include 9 in whom surgery was prohibitive because of profound neurologic deterioration, 3 who refused surgery, and in 1 instance each one of the following: aneurysm at the take-off of anterior choroidal artery, myocardial infarction, chronic lung disease and pulmonary infarction, and anterior spinal artery occlusion syndrome at angiography. Eight patients remained alive.

Within the 3-week interval following randomization, 19 subjects with an anterior communicating artery aneurysm and 2 each with an aneurysm on the internal carotid and middle cerebral artery died. Nine deaths occurred after the 3-week period, 4 following recurrent hemorrhage from an anterior communicating artery aneurysm and 1 from an aneurysm on the internal carotid. Death in 9 of the 40 patients was due to progressive deterioration. Four deaths were attributed to severe medical causes, all in patients with anterior cerebral complex aneurysms—1 before and 3 after the 3rd week following their last SAH. In this small group of patients, it appears that the anterior cerebral complex aneurysm is the most lethal when left untreated. Death occurred from progressive deterioration or from rebleeding in 62.5% (25 of 40) of patients who did not have a definitive surgical procedure.

Thirty-one (17.2%) of 180 patients with anterior cerebral complex aneurysms were not operated upon for the reasons stated (Table 9–10). For example, 11 were in such poor neurologic or medical condition that operation was considered fruitless. Twenty rebled and died after randomization and before operation was carried out. Statistically, these are considered failures of operation when the entire treatment group is considered. A progressive downhill course in 8 instances and prolonged coma in 1 precluded operation. Pulmonary embolism caused the death of 1 patient, and 1 had a cardiopulmonary arrest. Twenty-seven of 31 unoperated patients died (87.1%), 13 of the 27 (48.1%) from recurrent SAH.

In summary, deaths in this group of 40 patients total 32. Twenty-six were considered to be in poor neurologic condition after SAH and therefore not considered good surgical candidates. Sixteen of the 32 (50%) died after recurrent hemorrhage. If these 32 deaths are excluded from the total of 116 in the intracranial surgical treatment category, the mortality falls to 36.8% (84 of 228).

We believe there is a valid objection to including in the comparative evaluation of a particular treatment patients who never *had* allocated treatment. In defense of including in the total mortality those patients who died before surgery could be performed, it has been argued that they *could* have been operated upon earlier in the course of the disease once a proper diagnosis was made. This reasoning might be questioned. This might mean that immediately after the diagnosis of aneurysm was secure, an intracranial operation should have been executed regardless of the patient's condition. In this comparative study, it appears that patients allocated to intracranial surgery were for the most part in good (130) or fair (84) medical condition. An uncomfortable bias begins to appear. The knowledge that the fate of patients in poor medical and neurologic condition with or without operation is highly predictable makes their inclusion in the total mortality questionable.

Treatment Followed According to Protocol

Intracranial operative treatment was accomplished in 228 patients. A definitive operation was performed, but the specific method of approach was left entirely to the judgment of the surgeon. A planned procedure, e.g., obliteration of the neck of an aneurysm, may have been changed because of the risk of hemorrhage or of compromising the circulation, and another tactic ("trapping" or "coating") substituted. A definitive procedure was done in an effort to prevent rebleeding from the aneurysm, but it may have been considered inadequate. A specific surgical procedure was performed in 45 patients

with an aneurysm on the internal carotid artery, 34 patients with an aneurysm on the middle cerebral artery and 149 patients with an aneurysm on the anterior cerebral complex. Therefore, intracranial surgery was employed four times more frequently for anterior cerebral complex aneurysms than for those of the middle cerebral, and three times more frequently than for internal carotid aneurysms, indicating the relatively large number of anterior cerebral aneurysms in this series.

The interval between SAH and definitive treatment has been a crucial factor in evaluation of various modes of therapy, especially in relationship to surgical treatment. In this study, it was the surgeon's obligation to pursue definitive treatment as soon as possible subsequent to treatment allocation. The interval from randomization to surgery (Table 9–11) was 7 days or less in 86.0% (196 of 228). Reasons for delay beyond 7 days are as follows: in 5 patients with an internal carotid aneurysm, operation was delayed in 1 instance each for a scalp infection, a rebleed after randomization, cerebral

Table 9–11. Distribution of Patients by Aneurysm Site With Regard to Interval (Days) from Randomization to Surgery.

Days	Internal Carotid	Middle Cerebral	Ant. Cerebral-Ant. Comm.	Total
0–1	13	7	45	65
2–3	17	14	39	70
4–5	4	7	22	33
6–7	6	1	21	28
8–9	0	1	5	6
10–11	0	0	3	3
12–13	2	1	6	9
14–15	0	0	4	4
16–17	1	0	1	2
18–19	0	1	1	2
20–21	0	1	0	1
22–23	0	0	0	0
24–25	1	0	0	1
26–27	1	0	0	1
28–29	0	1	0	1
30 or more	0	0	2	2
Subtotal	45	34	149	228
No surgery	5	4	31	40
Total	50	38	180	268

Table 9–12.   All Aneurysm Locations: Distribution of Cause of Death With Respect to Interval from Surgery.

Days from Surgery to Death	Progressive Deterioration	Proved Rebleed	Suspected Rebleed	Unrelated Cause	Unknown	Total
0–2	9	0	0	1	0	10
3–5	13	0	0	0	0	13
6–8	7	2	0	1	0	10
9–11	5	1	0	0	0	6
12–14	2	1	0	1	0	4
15–17	2	0	0	0	0	2
18–20	0	1	0	0	0	1
21–23	0	0	0	0	0	0
24–26	1	0	0	0	0	1
27–29	0	0	0	0	0	0
30–32	0	0	0	0	0	0
33–35	0	0	0	0	0	0
36–38	0	0	0	0	0	0
39–41	1	0	0	0	0	1
42–44	0	0	0	0	0	0
45–47	0	1	0	0	0	1
48–50	0	0	0	0	0	0
Over 50	8	5	5	15	2	35
Total	48	11	5	18	2	84

vasospasm, preoperative treatment with epsilon-aminocaproic acid and poor neurologic condition; in 5 with middle cerebral aneurysms, operation was delayed due to poor neurologic condition in 2 patients, a death in the family in 1 and no reason was given in 2 instances; in the 22 patients with anterior cerebral complex aneurysms, 5 were in poor neurologic condition, 4 had severe vasospasm, 3 rebled soon after randomization and 1 each had an ileus, fever of unknown origin, poorly controlled diabetes mellitus and lower gastrointestinal bleeding. In 6 instances, no reason was given in spite of each patient being in good neurologic condition at the time of randomization.

Eighty-four patients (36.8%) had died as of January 1973. Forty-eight deaths (57.1% of 84) followed progressive neurologic deterioration after surgery (Table 9–12). Thirty-eight of this group (79.2%) died within 17 days following the surgical procedure. The remaining 10 remained in poor neurologic condition and died at various intervals; 5 deaths occurred between 18 days and 3 months after surgery, 4 occurred during the 3 to 5-month interval and 1 occurred 2 years

after surgery. Eleven deaths were preceded by a proved rebleeding episode (Table 9–12): 5 within 20 days from the surgical procedure, 2 during the 21 to 62-day interval, 2 during the 6th month after surgery and 1 each at the 28th and 45th month after surgery. Five deaths followed suspected rebleeding; 4 occurred between the 2nd and 13th month after surgery and another 47 months later. Eighteen patients died from unrelated causes; 3 died within 14 days following surgery and the remaining 15 died 70 days to 62 months later. The 3 deaths within the 14-day period were due in 1 instance each to pneumonia, pontine hemorrhage and myocardial infarction. The remaining 15 deaths were caused by myocardial infarction in 6, pneumonia in 3, pulmonary embolism in 2, carcinoma of lung in 2 and 1 each from carcinoma of ovary and cerebral embolism. If the unrelated and unknown causes are excluded, a forbidding mortality figure of 76.2% (64 of 84) was produced by progressive deterioration, recurrent or suspected rebleeding. The *overall* mortality from these causes was 28.1% (64 of 228), and clearly reflects a failure of certain operations.

Table 9–13. All Sites Combined: Distribution of Patients With Respect to Neurologic Condition and Age.

Age	Neurological Condition*					Total	%
	1	2	3	4	5		
10–19	2 (0)†	5 (1)	0	0	0	7 (1)	14.3
20–29	5 (1)	14 (0)	5 (1)	0	0	24 (2)	8.3
30–39	1 (0)	23 (7)	6 (1)	4 (0)	0	34 (8)	23.5
40–49	5 (0)	33 (12)	15 (6)	3 (2)	0	56 (20)	35.7
50–59	3 (1)	47 (23)	15 (8)	2 (1)	1 (1)	68 (34)	50.0
60–69	3 (0)	24 (12)	5 (1)	2 (1)	1 (1)	35 (15)	42.8
70–79	0	3 (3)	0	0	1 (1)	4 (4)	100.0
Total	19 (2)	149 (58)	46 (17)	11 (4)	3 (3)	228 (84)	36.8

* Definition of neurological condition:
1 = Symptom-free.
2 = minor symptoms (headache, meningeal irritation, diplopia).
3 = major neurologic deficit but fully responsive.
4 = impaired state of alertness but capable of protective or other adaptive responses to noxious stimuli.
5 = poorly responsive but with stable vital signs.
† Number in parentheses denotes deaths.

Age and Neurologic Condition Related to Mortality

We wish to emphasize that when one speaks of the "condition of the patient" before operation, this refers to his neurologic condition at the time of randomization, *not* to his condition on the day the operation was performed. In some cases condition between the day of randomization and the day of operation may have changed—in some better and in others worse. The data in the protocols do not give precise information in this regard, a fact which must be considered an omission. Since treatment allocation was determined after the angiographic diagnosis of a single aneurysm, the interval between SAH and operation was obviously greater than that between randomization and operation.

The mortality was 36.8% under all neurologic conditions in 228 patients with an aneurysm at one of three major sites, and in whom an intracranial operation was performed. There were 73.7% (168 to 228) in Neurologic Conditions 1 and 2 (Table 9–13). Only 14 were in a variable state of responsiveness with a neurologic deficit (Grades 4 and 5). The mortality in this group was 50% (7 of 14), while the age distribution for this same group extended from the 4th through 8th decades (Table 9–13). Although the younger age group had a tendency to be in better neurologic condition than the older group, this tendency was not as great as expected.

At all sites, aneurysms were found most frequently in patients 40 to 59 years of age, with about equal frequency in the 4th and 7th decades. After the 3rd decade, there was a progressive rise in mortality. Despite the high incidence of aneurysms in the latter decades (6th and 7th), it was evident that age became as important as the neurologic condition at the time of operation (Fig. 9–1).

Internal Carotid Aneurysm

In the internal carotid group, the gross mortality for intracranial operation was 46.7% (21 of 45, Table 9–14). In the 2nd through 4th decades, 2 of 11 patients with internal carotid artery aneurysm died following progressive deterioration after the surgical procedure. Three of these had preoperative major neurologic deficits; 1 died. Among 25

Table 9–14. Internal Carotid: Distribution of Patients With Respect to Neurologic Condition by Age in Decades.

Age	Neurologic Condition					
	1	2	3	4	5	Total
10–19	1 (0)*	1 (1)	0	0	0	2 (1)
20–29	1 (0)	2 (0)	1 (1)	0	0	4 (1)
30–39	1 (0)	2 (0)	2 (0)	0	5 (0)	5 (0)
40–49	0	6 (1)	3 (2)	2 (2)	0	11 (5)
50–59	0	9 (5)	4 (2)	0	1 (1)	14 (8)
60–69	0	4 (4)	2 (0)	1 (0)	0	7 (4)
70–79	0	1 (1)	0	0	1 (1)	2 (2)
Total	3 (0)	25 (12)	12 (5)	3 (2)	2 (2)	45 (21)

* Number in parentheses denotes deaths.

patients in the 5th and 6th decades, there were 13 deaths. Ten subjects had major preoperative deficits (Grades 3, 4 and 5). One of these was poorly responsive. Three of 7 who deteriorated progressively were seriously ill from the very outset (Grades 4 and 5).

Four fatalities occurred in the 60 to 69-year age group. All died following progressive deterioration within 17 days after surgery. Both patients in the 70 to 79-year-old group died within 11 days of the surgical procedure following progressive deterioration. The mortality among those in all age groups in poor neurologic condition (Grades 3, 4 and 5) was 52.9% (9 of 17). Seven of the 9 deaths occurred in the 40 to 59-year age interval.

Thirty-eight percent (17 of 45) of patients with internal carotid artery aneurysm were in poor neurologic condition at the time of operation, an indication that selection or bias did not enter into the problem of aneurysms in this location.

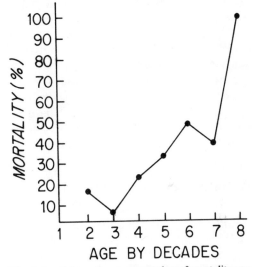

Fig. 9–1. Schematic representation of mortality presented in Table 9–13.

Middle Cerebral Aneurysm

Operative repair of aneurysms on the middle cerebral distribution was associated with a gross mortality of 35.3% (12 of 34, Table 9-15). Six deaths occurred among 17 patients who were in good condition (Grades 1 and 2). Among the 16 patients in poor condition (Grades 3 to 5) before operation, there were 6 deaths. Therefore, the proportion of deaths in the two groups was approximately the same for this relatively small group.

Twenty-one aneurysms were found in patients in the 5th and 6th decades combined, 9 in the 3rd and 4th decades combined and 4 in the 7th decade. In the 3rd and 4th decades, there was 1 death among the 9 patients, and that death was due to a proved rebleed 8 days after surgery. In the 5th and 6th decades, 9 fatalities among 21 patients

Table 9–15.   Middle Cerebral: Distribution of Patients With Respect to Neurologic Condition by Age in Decades.

| Age | Neurologic Condition | | | | | Total |
	1	2	3	4	5	
10–19	0	0	0	0	0	0
20–29	0	3 (0)*	2 (0)	0	0	5 (0)
30–39	0	2 (1)	1 (0)	1 (0)	0	4 (1)
40–49	1 (0)	5 (2)	4 (1)	0	0	10 (3)
50–59	0	7 (3)	3 (2)	1 (1)	0	11 (6)
60–69	0	0	3 (1)	1 (1)	0	4 (2)
70–79	0	0	0	0	0	0
Total	1 (0)	17 (6)	13 (4)	3 (2)	0	34 (12)

* Number in parentheses denotes deaths.

(42.9%) were observed, 6 associated with a progressive deteriorating state, 2 from unrelated causes and 1 following recurrent SAH. The 2 deaths occurring in the 7th decade were attributed 1 each to progressive deterioration and unrelated cause. Age differences in the 4th through 7th decades again appeared to influence mortality. The prognosis was better in patients who were younger than 40 years of age than in the older group.

Anterior Cerebral Aneurysm

Among this group, the gross mortality was 34.2% for all ages (51 of 149, Table 9-16). The frequency of anterior cerebral complex aneurysms was slightly greater in the 6th than in the 5th decade of life (43 and 35 cases, respectively). In the 2nd, 3rd and 4th decades combined, the mortality was 17.8% (8 of 45); in the 5th and 6th decades combined, it was 41.0% (32 of 78). In making the calculation for each decade, one notes a progressive rise in mortality. In the 2nd decade, for example, there were no deaths. However, the number of patients was small (5). In the 3rd decade, mortality was 6.7% (1 of 15); in the 4th, 28.0% (7 of 25); in the 5th, 34.3% (12 of 35); in the 6th, 46.5% (20 of 43); in the 7th, 37.5% (9 of 24); and in the 8th, 100%, with death in both subjects.

In contrast to the middle cerebral and internal carotid groups, of whom 52.9% and 62.2%, respectively, were considered in good condition at the time of operation, 81.9% (122 of 149) were so considered in the anterior cerebral category (Table 9-16).

Table 9–16.   Anterior Cerebral-Anterior Communicating: Distribution of Patients With Respect to Neurologic Condition by Age in Decades.

| Age | Neurologic Condition | | | | | Total |
	1	2	3	4	5	
10–19	1 (0)*	4 (0)	0	0	0	5 (0)
20–29	4 (1)	9 (0)	2 (0)	0	0	15 (1)
30–39	0	19 (6)	3 (1)	3 (0)	0	25 (7)
40–49	4 (0)	22 (9)	8 (3)	1 (0)	0	35 (12)
50–59	3 (1)	31 (15)	8 (4)	1 (0)	0	43 (20)
60–69	3 (0)	20 (8)	0	0	1 (1)	24 (9)
70–79	0	2 (2)	0	0	0	2 (2)
Total	15 (2)	107 (40)	21 (8)	5 (0)	1 (1)	149 (51)

* Number in parentheses denotes deaths.

The number of patients considered in good neurologic condition (122) was 4.5 times those in poor condition (27). The mortality among those with no or minimal symptoms was 34.4% (42 of 122), and 33.3% in those with a major deficit (9 of 27). One patient who was poorly responsive at the time of operation died from progressive deterioration 11 days after surgery.

The 8 deaths which occurred in the 3rd and 4th decades were all due to progressive deterioration postoperatively, with 1 exception. That patient died from a proved rebleed 18 days after surgery. Among the 32 patients who died in the 5th and 6th decades, 14 died following progressive deterioration, 9 from unrelated causes (with all but 3 occurring more than 50 days following the surgical procedure), 7 from a proved rebleed and 2 from a suspected rebleed. In the 60 to 69-year-old group, there were 9 deaths; 6 followed progressive deterioration and 1 each after a proved rebleed, suspected rebleed and an unrelated cause. Both patients in the 8th decade died, 1 each from progressive deterioration and a suspected rebleed.

The much greater number of patients in good condition in the anterior cerebral complex category would suggest that a ruptured aneurysm on the anterior cerebral artery may be a less lethal lesion than that of the internal carotid or middle cerebral artery.

However, the analysis of good-condition patients with respect to age reveals there is an important difference in the age group above or below 50. A mortality of 25.4% was observed in good condition patients below the age of 50, while those who were 50 years of age or more had a mortality of 44.1% (Table 9-17). This same difference in mortality was noted in the poor-condition group. A mortality of 23.5% was observed in poor-condition patients below the age of 50, and 50% in those age 50 or above. A similar observation was seen in the middle cerebral group (Table 9-17). However, those patients with an internal carotid aneurysm did poorly in all categories except in the group below 50 years of age in good condition. The mortality in that group was 14.3%, whereas in the remaining three categories the range was 44.4 to 71.4%. It is clear that age was a factor as important in prognosis as was neurologic condition, so that poor condition and older age influence the prognosis more adversely than either alone.

Age and Medical Condition Related to Mortality

The introductory remarks made with regard to neurologic condition (page 154) also apply

Table 9–17. Mortality With Respect to Age, Site and Neurologic Condition.

Site	Age Below 50			Age 50 or Above		
	Patients	No. Dead	%	Patients	No. Dead	%
	Good Condition (Grades 1 and 2)					
Internal carotid	14	2	14.3	14	10	71.4
Middle cerebral	11	3	27.3	7	3	42.9
Anterior cerebral	63	16	25.4	59	26	44.1
Subtotal	88	21	23.9	80	39	48.7
	Poor Condition (Grade 3, 4 and 5)					
Internal carotid	8	5	62.5	9	4	44.4
Middle cerebral	8	1	12.5	8	5	62.5
Anterior cerebral	17	4	23.5	10	5	50.0
Subtotal	33	10	30.3	27	14	51.8
Total	121	31	25.6	107	53	49.5

Table 9–18.   All Sites Combined: Distribution of Patients With Respect to Medical Condition and Age.

Age	Medical Condition				Total
	Good	Fair	Poor	Prohibitive	
10–19	7 (1)*	0	0	0	7 (1)
20–29	17 (2)	7	0	0	24 (2)
30–39	21 (4)	11 (4)	2	0	34 (8)
40–49	30 (10)	25 (9)	1 (1)	0	56 (20)
50–59	36 (16)	26 (15)	5 (3)	1	68 (34)
60–69	18 (4)	13 (7)	4 (4)	0	35 (15)
70–79	1 (1)	2 (2)	1 (1)	0	4 (4)
Total	130 (38)	84 (37)	13 (9)	1	228 (84)
	(29.2%)	(44%)	(69.2%)		(36.8%)

* Number in parentheses denotes deaths.

to the overall medical status of the patient. A major difference is that most medical conditions are less likely to fluctuate to the same degree. In general, once a medical condition is recognized, it must be taken into consideration with other factors as a course of therapy is outlined.

At the time of treatment allocation, each patient was appraised as to the degree of risk for a major surgical procedure using the rating scale of "good," "fair," "poor" and "prohibitive." This classification had nothing to do with the aneurysm per se. A good-condition patient was alert and normotensive. He had no more than a degree of fever and was considered to be in good health prior to his subarachnoid hemorrhage. In general, patients in fair condition had a de-

gree of underlying medical disease such as hypertension, cirrhosis of the liver, advanced age, mild to moderate anemia, poor nutrition, generalized atherosclerosis or chronic pulmonary disease. A patient with more than one adverse factor or the presence of one heavily weighted factor (e.g., recent myocardial infarction, electrolyte abnormalities, malignant hypertension, advanced atherosclerotic disease) was regarded as being in poor condition. Patients in a prohibitive category had a complicated illness with one or more undesirable factors which were pre-existing or which developed during the interval prior to allocation of treatment and subsequent to hospital admission.

The presence of various medical factors had a clear influence upon mortality (Table

Table 9–19.   Internal Carotid: Distribution of Patients With Respect to Medical Condition by Age in Decades.

Age	Medical Condition				Total
	Good	Fair	Poor	Prohibitive	
10–19	2 (1)*	0	0	0	2 (1)
20–29	3 (1)	1	0	0	4 (1)
30–39	4	1	0	0	5 (0)
40–49	5 (2)	5 (2)	1 (1)	0	11 (5)
50–59	6 (3)	5 (3)	3 (2)	0	14 (8)
60–69	3 (1)	4 (3)	0	0	7 (4)
70–79	0	1 (1)	1 (1)	0	2 (2)
Total	23 (8)	17 (9)	5 (4)	0	45 (21)
	(34.8%)	(52.9%)	(80%)		(46.7%)

* Number in parentheses denotes deaths.

Table 9–20.   Middle Cerebral: Distribution of Patients With Respect to Medical Condition by Age in Decades.

| Age | Medical Condition | | | | Total |
	Good	Fair	Poor	Prohibitive	
10–19	0	0	0	0	0
20–29	4	1	0	0	5 (0)*
30–39	3 (1)	1	0	0	4 (1)
40–49	3 (1)	7 (2)	0	0	10 (3)
50–59	5 (2)	5 (3)	1 (1)	0	11 (6)
60–69	2	0	2 (2)	0	4 (2)
70–79	0	0	0	0	0
Total	17 (4) (23.5%)	14 (5) (35.7%)	3 (3) (100%)	0	34 (12) (35.3%)

* Number in parentheses denotes deaths

9-18). For all sites, patients in good condition had a mortality of 29.2% (38 of 130); those in fair condition, 44.0% (37 of 84); and those in poor condition, 69.2% (9 of 13). Of considerable interest is the number of patients in fair and poor conditions. Within the total 228 patients, 97 (42.5%) were in these two conditions, and 130 (57.0%) were in good medical condition (Table 9-18). Compared with good-condition patients, those in fair medical condition had a higher mortality in each site category (Tables 9-19 to 9-21). For each site, mortality was 50% or more in those 50 years of age and older. Therefore, for medical as well as neurologic condition, mortality is greatly influenced by age.

Further analysis was made statistically after grouping all cases into good neurologic condition (Grades 1 and 2) and poor neurologic condition (Grades 3, 4 and 5). These were tabulated with respect to two age groups: below 50 years, and age 50 or above. Medical condition was also subdivided into two subgroups for purposes of this analysis. Good-medical condition patients were placed in Group 1, and those listed as fair and poor medical conditions were designated as Group 2. The data used for this analysis are listed in Table 9–22. By means of various chi-square contingency tables, there was a significant increase ($P < 0.05$) in mortality in those age 50 or above who were in good neurologic condition. Mortality in Group 2 medical condition was also significantly increased in the older age group. Analysis of

Table 9–21.   Anterior Cerebral-Anterior Communicating: Distribution of Patients With Respect to Medical Condition by Age in Decades.

| Age | Medical Condition | | | | Total |
	Good	Fair	Poor	Prohibitive	
10–19	5	0	0	0	5 (0)*
20–29	10 (1)	5	0	0	15 (1)
30–39	14 (3)	9 (4)	2	0	25 (7)
40–49	22 (6)	13 (5)	0	0	35 (11)
50–59	25 (12)	16 (9)	1	1 (0)	43 (21)
60–69	13 (3)	9 (4)	2 (2)	0	24 (9)
70–79	1 (1)	1 (1)	0	0	2 (2)
Total	90 (26) (28.9%)	53 (23) (43.4%)	5 (2) (40%)	1 (0)	149 (51) (34.2%)

* Number in parentheses denotes deaths.

mortality with respect to age and medical and neurologic condition revealed that age over 50 years and Group 2 medical condition had greater adverse effect upon survival than neurologic condition.

The number of deaths for each medical condition was proportional to the total number of patients in each site (Table 9–23). Progressive deterioration or complications of treatment other than rebleeding was the major cause of death at each site category (48 of 84, 57.1%, Table 9–23). Eighteen (21.4%) died from unrelated causes, 11 (13.1%) followed a proved rebleed and 5 (6.0%) followed suspected rebleed.

In addition to medical condition *at the time of randomization,* a general question was asked of the surgeon *at the time of operation* concerning his impression of the patient as a candidate for major surgery, *disregarding the technical operability of the aneurysm.* One of three general medical conditions was designated: good, fair or poor. By referring to Table 9–18, the mortality in patients with good, fair or poor medical conditions *at the time of allocation of treatment* was 29.2, 44.0 and 69.2%, respectively. Table 9–24 reveals that in patients whose medical conditions were appraised on the day of surgery, 31.1%

died who were in good condition, 40.8% in fair condition and 64.7% in poor condition. Perusal of all patients in each medical condition reveals no important differences developed between the day of allocation of treatment and the day of surgery (see Tables 9–18 and 9–24). Analysis of deaths in patients who had surgery performed at specific

Table 9–22. Mortality Among Subgroups of Neurologic and Medical Condition: Patients Above and Below Age 50.

	Below Age 50 Medical Condition	
Neurologic Condition	1	2
Good	64 (15)* 23.4%	26 (8) 30.8%
Poor	12 (4) 33.3%	22 (6) 27.3%

	Age 50 or Above Medical Condition	
Neurologic Condition	1	2
Good	44 (15) 34.1%	33 (21) 63.6%
Poor	9 (4) 44.4%	18 (11) 61.1%

* Number in parentheses denotes deaths.

Table 9–23. Cause of Death With Respect to Aneurysm Location in Each of Four Medical Conditions.

	Progressive Deterioration	Proved Rebleed	Suspected Rebleed	Unrelated Cause	Unknown	Total Deaths	Total Patients Each Site	% Deaths
Good								
IC*	7	0	0	1	0	8	23	29
MC	3	1	0	0	0	4	17	
AC	15	6	0	5	0	26	90	
Fair								
IC	6	0	1	1	1	9	17	44
MC	2	1	0	2	0	5	14	
AC	10	3	4	6	0	23	53	
Poor								
IC	1	0	0	2	1	4	5	69
MC	2	0	0	1	0	3	3	
AC	2	0	0	0	0	2	5	
Prohibitive								
IC	0	0	0	0	0	0	0	0
MC	0	0	0	0	0	0	0	
AC	0	0	0	0	0	0	1	
Total	48	11	5	18	2	84	228	36

* IC = internal carotid; MC = middle cerebral; AC = anterior cerebral-anterior communicating.

Table 9–24.   Distribution of Patients in Various Medical Conditions on Day of Surgery

| Site | Medical Condition | | | |
	Good	Fair	Poor	Total
Internal carotid	21 (7)*	21 (11)	3 (3)	45 (21)
Middle cerebral	18 (4)	11 (3)	5 (5)	34 (12)
Anterior cerebral-anterior comm.	96 (31)	44 (17)	9 (3)	149 (51)
Total	135 (42)	76 (31)	17 (11)	228 (84)
	(31.1%)	(40.8%)	(64.7%)	

* Number of deaths for each subgroup in parentheses.

intervals following the last bleed was also significant. For all patients operated upon within 14 days from their last bleed, 44.5% died (65 of 146), and for all patients operated on beyond the 14-day interval, 23.2% (19 of 82) died (Table 9–25). Therefore, regardless of site or condition, more deaths occurred in patients operated on within the 14-day period than in those who had their operations subsequent to this interval, particularly in those who were regarded to be in fair or poor medical condition.

The medical disorder associated with or present at the time of acute hemorrhage was designated on the registration fascicle. The most frequently noted condition was pre-existing hypertension. In many instances the magnitude and duration of hypertension were unknown. Table 9–26 shows the distribution of pre-existing hypertension among the total group with respect to aneurysm site and medical condition. There were 13.8% good-condition patients with pre-existing hypertension, 27.4% in fair condition and 46.1% in poor condition. The 1 patient in prohibitive condition later improved and was operated on 87 days after his last bleed. The significance of these figures remains to be fully explained. Yet, there appears to be a clear correlation between overall medical condition and the existence of some degree of previously observed elevated blood pressure.

Further details on specific medical disorders which were known previously or discovered at the time of subarachnoid hemorrhage are tabulated in Table 9–27. The

category with pre-existing hypertension had a 55.3% mortality (26 of 47). The next most frequent condition was heart disease and arteriosclerosis. Although these groups had a high mortality, their incidence was low. The frequency of various disorders was considerable in the fair-condition and poor-condition groups. In the good-condition category, 25.4% (33 of 130) had various medical disorders; in the fair-condition group, 46.4% (39 of 84); and in the poor-condition group, 61.5% (8 of 13). There were 27 patients with miscellaneous conditions in the group designated "other." Included were patients with diabetes mellitus, alcoholism and psychiatric disorders. Other isolated conditions noted were obesity, hernia, emphysema, dermatitis, arthritis, gout and pregnancy.

Mortality With Respect to Neurological Condition and Interval from Last Bleed to Surgery

Internal Carotid Aneurysm

Fifty patients with an internal carotid aneurysm were allocated to intracranial operation. In 5, treatment was not accomplished for reasons previously noted (Table 9–10), leaving 45 for analysis. The mortality in January 1973 was 46.7% (21 of 45, Table 9–28). Eleven were operated on within 5 days of

Table 9-25. Medical Condition on Day of Surgery Irrespective of Operability of the Aneurysm.

Interval SAH to surgery	Internal carotid			Middle cerebral			Anterior cerebral			Total
	Good	Fair	Poor	Good	Fair	Poor	Good	Fair	Poor	
0-2	0	2 (2)*	1 (1)	0	0	0	5 (1)	1 (1)	0	9 (5)
3-5	7 (2)	1 (1)	0	3 (0)	0	0	20 (9)	4 (2)	3 (2)	38 (16)
6-8	2 (0)	1 (1)	0	1 (0)	5 (2)	1 (1)	16 (6)	6 (3)	1 (1)	33 (14)
9-11	1 (1)	8 (6)	0	0	1 (1)	1 (1)	17 (6)	10 (4)	2 (0)	40 (19)
12-14	2 (1)	1 (0)	0	3 (1)	2 (0)	0	10 (5)	7 (4)	1 (0)	26 (11)
15-17	1 (1)	3 (0)	0	2 (1)	1 (0)	0	9 (1)	5 (1)	0	21 (4)
18-20	3 (0)	2 (1)	0	2 (0)	0	0	4 (0)	3 (0)	0	14 (1)
21-23	0	0	0	1 (0)	0	0	5 (1)	0	2 (0)	8 (1)
24-26	2 (1)	0	0	0	0	1 (1)	2 (0)	3 (2)	0	9 (4)
27-29	1 (1)	1 (0)	1 (1)	0	0	1 (1)	3 (1)	1 (0)	0	8 (4)
30-32	0	0	0	0	1 (0)	0	2 (0)	1 (0)	0	4 (0)
33-35	0	1 (0)	0	0	0	0	0	0	0	1 (0)
36-38	0	0	0	0	0	0	0	0	0	0 (0)
39-41	0	1 (0)	0	0	0	0	1 (0)	0	0	2 (0)
42 and over	2 (0)	0	1 (1)	5 (2)	1 (0)	1 (1)	2 (1)	3 (0)	0	15 (5)
Subtotal Percent deaths	21(7) (33.3)	21 (11) (52.4)	3 (3) (100)	18 (4) (22.2)	11 (3) (27.2)	5 (5) (100)	96 (31) (32.3)	44 (17) (38.6)	9(3) (33.3)	228 (84)
Total	45 (21) (46.7%)			34 (12) (35.3%)			149 (51) (34.2%)			

* Number in parentheses denotes deaths.

Table 9–26.   Distribution of Patients With Pre-Existing Hypertension for Each Site.

| Site | Medical Condition | | | | |
	Good	Fair	Poor	Prohibitive	Total
Internal carotid	23 (4)*	17 (8)	5 (3)	0	45 (15)
Middle cerebral	17 (2)	14 (5)	3 (1)	0	34 (8)
Anterior cerebral- anterior comm.	90 (12)	53 (10)	5 (2)	1 (1)	149 (25)
	130 (18) (13.8%)	84 (23) (27.4%)	13 (6) (46.2%)	1 (1)	228 (48) (21.1%)

* Number of patients with pre-existing hypertension in each subgroup in parentheses.

the last SAH and of these 6 died (54.5%). There were 8 deaths among 12 patients who had surgery during the 6 to 11-day interval. Two patients died among the 6 operated on 12 to 17 days from the last SAH. There were 16 patients who had their operation after 17 days; 5 died.

Table 9–28 also shows the distribution of patients with respect to neurologic condition at the time of randomization. Mortality was high for patients in any condition if the operation was performed within 14 days from the last bleed. A surprising number of patients died who were in good condition (10 of 15, Grade 2). The average time between SAH and angiography was 6.4 days (range

0 to 35); between first angiographic procedure and surgery, 10.2 days (range 0 to 64); and between SAH and operation, 16.6 days (range 0 to 72).

Middle Cerebral Aneurysm

Of 38 subjects with a middle cerebral artery aneurysm, 2 died before surgery could be performed and 2 were considered unsuitable due to poor neurologic condition (Table 9–10), leaving 34 patients for detailed analysis. The mortality was 35.3% (12 of 34, Table 9–29). No deaths occurred in the 3 patients

Table 9–27.   All Sites Combined: Distribution of Patients in Each Medical Condition With Known Pre-existing Medical Disease (Some Patients Had Multiple Conditions).

| Medical Disorder | Medical Condition | | | | |
	Good (130)*	Fair (84)	Poor (13)	Prohibitive (1)	Total
Pre-existing hypertension	18 (10)†	22 (10)	6 (6)	1 (0)	47 (26)
Upper respiratory infection	2 (1)	0	0	0	2 (1)
Pulmonary infection	2 (2)	4 (2)	0	0	6 (4)
Heart disease	1 (1)	6 (4)	4 (4)	0	11 (9)
Renal disease	2 (0)	1 (0)	1 (1)	0	4 (1)
Hepatic disease	0	2 (0)	0	0	2 (0)
Gastrointestinal bleeding	1 (1)	0	0	0	1 (1)
Malignant neoplasm	1 (1)	0	0	0	1 (1)
Arteriosclerosis	2 (1)	3 (3)	3 (3)	0	8 (7)
Other	11 (5)	14 (9)	2 (1)	0	27 (15)
Total conditions	40	52	16	1	109
Number of patients	33 (14)‡	39 (18)	8 (7)	1 (0)	

* Total patients in each condition.
† Number in parentheses denotes deaths in each subgroup.
‡ Actual mortality in patients with one or more medical conditions.

Table 9–28. Internal Carotid: Distribution of Patients With Respect to Neurological Condition and Interval Between Last Bleed to Surgery.

Days from Last bleed to Surgery	Neurologic Condition*					Total
	1	2	3	4	5	
0–2	0	0	3 (2)†	0	1 (1)	4 (3)
3–5	0	5 (2)	0	1 (0)	1 (1)	7 (3)
6–8	0	3 (1)	0	0	0	3 (1)
9–11	0	6 (6)	2	1 (1)	0	9 (7)
12–14	0	1 (1)	1	0	0	2 (1)
15–17	0	2	2 (1)	0	0	4 (1)
18–20	1 (0)	2 (1)	1	0	0	4 (1)
21–23	0	0	0	0	0	0
24–26	0	2	1 (1)	0	0	3 (1)
27–29	0	1	1 (1)	1 (1)	0	3 (2)
30–32	0	0	0	0	0	0
33–35	0	1	0	0	0	1 (0)
36–38	0	0	0	0	0	0
39–41	0	1	0	0	0	1 (0)
42 and over	1 (0)	2 (1)	1	0	0	4 (1)
Total	2 (0)	26 (12)	12 (5)	3 (2)	2 (2)	45 (21)

* See Table 9–13 for definition.
† Number in parentheses denotes deaths

who had an operation within 5 days of last bleed. However, there were 6 deaths among 14 patients who had their operation between 6 and 14 days following their last bleed. Mortality in the 17 patients operated on 15 days or more following the last bleed was 35.3% (6 of 17).

Six deaths occurred in 18 patients in good condition (Grades 1 and 2); in 13 patients who had a major neurologic deficit (Grade 3), there were 4 deaths; in 3 patients in Grade 4, there were 2 deaths.

Intracerebral hematoma, the result of a ruptured middle cerebral aneurysm, was

Table 9–29. Middle Cerebral: Distribution of Patients With Respect to Neurologic Condition and Interval Between Last Bleed to Surgery.

Days from Last bleed to Surgery	Neurologic Condition					Total
	1	2	3	4	5	
0–2	0	0	0	0	0	0
3–5	0	3 (0)	0	0	0	3 (0)*
6–8	0	5 (2)	0	2 (1)	0	7 (3)
9–11	0	1 (1)	0	1 (1)	0	2 (2)
12–14	0	2 (1)	3 (0)	0	0	5 (1)
15–17	0	2 (1)	1 (0)	0	0	3 (1)
18–20	0	0	1 (0)	0	0	1 (0)
21–23	0	0	1 (0)	0	0	1 (0)
24–26	0	0	2 (1)	0	0	2 (1)
27–29	0	1 (1)	0	0	0	1 (1)
30–32	0	1 (0)	0	0	0	1 (0)
33–35	0	0	0	0	0	0
36–38	0	0	0	0	0	0
39–41	0	0	0	0	0	0
42 and over	1 (0)	2 (0)	5 (3)	0	0	8 (3)
Total	1 (0)	17 (6)	13 (4)	3 (2)	0	34 (12)

* Number in parentheses denotes deaths.

found in 10 of the 34 patients (29.4%). In 1, the hematoma was not recognized at angiography. Although the presence of an intracerebral hematoma indicates a destructive lesion, the expected hemispheric defects did not appreciably influence mortality. Four of the 10 patients died after surgery: 2 from a progressive downhill course, 1 due to a proved rebleed 8 days after surgery and 1 from a cerebral embolism 8 months later.

Seven of the 12 deaths in this middle cerebral group were associated with progressive deterioration; 2 had proved rebleeding episodes, and the remaining 3 died of unrelated causes (1 each due to cerebral embolism, myocardial infarction and pulmonary embolism). Since the smallest collection of aneurysms occurred at this site, specific conclusions from detailed analysis are limited. However, nearly one half (16 of 34) of the patients at the time of operation had major defects or were poorly responsive. The average time between SAH and angiography was 7.5 days (range 0 to 47); between first angiographic procedure and surgery, 16.3 days (range 0 to 113); and between hemorrhage and operation, 23.8 days (range 0 to 113).

Anterior Cerebral Aneurysm

One of the greatest neurosurgical challenges resides in the surgical repair of an aneurysm at the anterior cerebral-anterior communicating region. The mortality in 149 patients treated by direct intracranial attack was 34.2% (51 of 149). This figure reflects the mortality in those who had their surgical procedure accomplished and died prior to January 1, 1973. Thirty-eight percent (56 of 149) were operated on within 8 days from their last bleed, 69.1% (103 of 149) were operated on within 14 days and 82.5% (123 of 149) were operated on within 20 days (Table 9–30). Eighty-two percent (122 of 149, including 15 who were symptom-free, Grades 1 and 2, Table 9–30) were in good neurologic condition. The mortality in this group was 34.4% (42 of 122, Table 9–30). This compares with a mortality of 33% (6 of 18) for the same group of patients with a middle cerebral aneurysm in similar neurologic condition (Table 9–29), and a mortality of 42.9% (12 of 28) for the internal carotid group (Table 9–28). By far, most patients (111) were operated on during the 14-day interval from 3 to 17 days following

Table 9–30.   Anterior Cerebral-Anterior Communicating: Distribution of Patients With Respect to Neurological Condition and Interval Between Last Bleed to Surgery.

Days from Last Bleed to Surgery	Neurologic Condition					
	1	2	3	4	5	Total
0–2	0	6 (2)*	0	0	0	6 (2)
3–5	2 (1)	18 (9)	5 (2)	1 (0)	1 (1)	27 (13)
6–8	2 (0)	19 (9)	2 (1)	0	0	23 (10)
9–11	1 (0)	23 (8)	3 (2)	1 (0)	0	28 (10)
12–14	1 (0)	15 (8)	3 (1)	0	0	19 (9)
15–17	0	10 (1)	2 (1)	2 (0)	0	14 (2)
18–20	1 (0)	4 (0)	1 (0)	0	0	6 (0)
21–23	2 (0)	4 (1)	1 (0)	0	0	7 (1)
24–26	0	5 (2)	0	0	0	5 (2)
27–29	1 (0)	1 (0)	2 (1)	0	0	4 (1)
30–32	1 (0)	1 (0)	1 (0)	0	0	3 (0)
33–35	0	0	0	0	0	0
36–38	0	0	0	0	0	0
39–41	1 (0)	0	0	0	0	1 (0)
42 and over	3 (1)	1 (0)	1 (0)	1 (0)	0	6 (1)
Total	15 (2)	107 (40)	21 (8)	5 (0)	1 (1)	149 (51)

* Number in parentheses denotes deaths.

their last SAH. Of this group, 6 were symptom-free (Grade 1) with 1 death, 85 had minor symptoms (Grade 2) with 35 deaths (41.2%), 15 had a major neurologic deficit but were fully responsive (Grade 3) with 7 deaths (46.7%), 4 had impaired mental status and were in a lethargic state (Grade 4) but there were no deaths, and 1 was poorly responsive and died 11 days after surgery. In the group of patients operated on after 17 days from their last SAH (32 patients), there were 5 deaths (15.6%): 3 due to a progressive downhill course after surgery and 2 from a suspected rebleed.

The average time between SAH and angiography was 5.1 days (range 0 to 42); between angiography and surgery, 8.7 days (range 0 to 86); and between SAH and operation, 13.2 days (range 0 to 87). On the average, the anterior cerebral group of patients had the diagnosis of aneurysm made earlier and had definitive treatment sooner than did those patients with an internal carotid or middle cerebral artery aneurysm. The reason for this is not entirely clear, particularly since the number of patients in the treated anterior cerebral group was, respectively, about three and four times greater than the internal carotid and middle cerebral groups. This might be explained by the fact that one large contributor submitted only anterior cerebral-anterior communicating cases.

Early (1st week) surgical treatment of intracranial aneurysms has been considered to be more hazardous than when applied later, that is, 2 or 3 weeks after SAH. Following the 2-week or 3-week interval, patients are generally in better condition. Many who in the early days following SAH would not be good candidates for operation improve to a point more favorable for intracranial surgery. Many who early might have been operated on in poor condition go on to die during the first days following the initial bleed. Those patients initially relegated to conservative treatment because of poor condition may therefore be considered surgical candidates because they have improved after the 2nd or 3rd week. Such uncontrolled trials have distorted figures favorably or unfavorably for surgery, depending upon the approach in making comparative evaluations.

Rebleeding Prior to Surgery

The number of proved bleeds in the patient's history was requested specifically on each protocol. The interval between bleeds (where at least two occurred) was noted with respect to the episode which brought the patient to the reporting hospital. This information was analyzed in order to determine what influence multiple episodes of prior bleeds may have on postoperative mortality.

Internal Carotid Aneurysm

Eight patients had an initial subarachnoid hemorrhage an average of 19.7 days (range 3 to 46 days) prior to the episode which prompted admission to the reporting hospital. Three additional patients had their initial bleed 2 to 3 years previously. These 11 patients (24.4% of 45) were distributed among the following neurologic conditions at the time of randomization: 1 in Grade 1, 6 in Grade 2, 2 in Grade 3, 1 in Grade 4 and 1 in Grade 5. Therefore, previous bleeds in the recent history had no influence on neurologic condition or mortality. The 24.4% with more than one bleeding episode prior to hospitalization, obviously characterized by minor symptoms only, should make one aware that multiple ruptures of single aneurysms may occur without association of severe neurologic deficit. Three deaths occurred in this group during the postoperative period: 2 due to progressive deterioration and 1 from a suspected rebleed.

Middle Cerebral Aneurysm

Analysis of total bleeding episodes in the past history in this group reveals that 8 patients (23.5% of 34) had two or more bleeding episodes within 21 days of the bleed that prompted hospital care. The average interval between the two bleeds was 9.8 days (range 2 to 21 days). One additional patient bled 4.5 years previously. Another patient rebled between randomization and surgery, but there were no reports of rebleeding between hospital admission and randomization. Two patients in this group had three episodes (dates unknown). Four patients were in Grade 2 and 5 were in Grade 3 at the time of entry into the study. There were 3 postoperative deaths: 2 from progressive deterioration and 1 due to cerebral embolism.

Anterior Cerebral Aneurysm

Among the surgical group (149), 26 patients (17.4%) had two or more bleeding episodes prior to admission. Following admission, 3 patients rebled between hospital admission and the angiographic procedure, 5 others rebled between the first angiographic procedure and randomization (4 occurred at the time of angiography) and 9 patients (6%) rebled during the interval between allocation of treatment and surgery. Therefore, 34 patients (22.8% of 149) had two or more bleeds prior to or during angiography, with an additional 9 (total of 43, or 28.9% of 149) who had two or more bleeds prior to operation. The distribution of neurologic conditions in the operated group was as follows: 4 patients in Grade 1, 12 in Grade 2, 8 in Grade 3 and 2 in Grade 4. There were 11 deaths (32.4% of 34), a proportion similar to the internal carotid (3 of 11) and middle

cerebral group (3 of 9). Seven died from progressive deterioration postoperatively, 2 had a proved rebleed and 1 each died of pneumonia and carcinoma of the ovary.

Cerebral Angiography

All patients with subarachnoid hemorrhage had a cerebral angiographic survey for determination of the location and size of the single aneurysm. No standard format was used in the technical approach to these studies among the various centers. Variations in technique, such as local versus general anesthetic, bilateral common carotid and direct vertebral angiography versus three-vessel retrograde femoral studies, duration of angiographic procedure, amount of contrast medium used and number of procedures to visualize the entire cerebral circulation, varied among centers. Some centers pursued angiography within hours of admission to the hospital; others allowed routine scheduling of the procedure. Because of these variables, an analysis was made with respect to several important factors which were related to subsequent management of the patient. These included number of procedures performed, complications, associated abnormalities (whether or not related to the aneurysm), vasospasm, interval from last bleed to first angiographic procedure, interval from last bleed to randomization, systolic and mean blood pressure and size of the aneurysm.

Multiple angiographic procedures were performed on 109 of the 268 patients (40.7%)

Table 9–31.   Distribution of Angiographic Surveys for Each Site.

Site	No. of Pretreatment Angiographic Procedures				Patients with Vertebral-Basilar Angiogram	Patients with Post-Treatment Angiogram
	1	2	3	4		
Internal carotid (50)	29	8	12	1	31	25
Middle cerebral (38)	21	12	3	2	20	23
Anterior cerebral-anterior comm. (180)	109	57	9	5	79	103
Total (268)	159	77	24	8	130	151

allocated to intracranial surgery (Table 9–31). These were distributed proportionately among the three aneurysm sites: 42.0% (21 of 50) for the internal carotid group, 44.7% (17 of 38) for the middle cerebral group and 39.4% (71 of 180) for the anterior cerebral group. Although the protocol stipulated complete cerebral angiographic surveys, vertebral-basilar visualization was completed in only 130 of 268 (48.5%, Table 9–31). Therefore, the presence of a single aneurysm was assured only in these patients. Evidently, when an aneurysm was discovered, if the clinical presentation was consistent with the angiographic findings, complete cerebral angiography was not always pursued. In 56.3% (151 of 268), a post-treatment angiogram was done.

Multiple pretreatment angiographic surveys were made for various reasons. Some centers did one carotid system at a time, some patients were restudied after a deteriorating neurologic condition associated with a rebleed or ischemic deficit (including changes in mental status) and in a few instances a repeat procedure followed the failure of an initial attempt. With the passage of time, these procedures were completed sooner with improved equipment and the more frequent use of the retrograde femoral technique for complete surveys.

The high number of multiple angiographic procedures inherently caused a delay in allocation of treatment. The interval was 3 days or less in the majority of instances, but in some it was considerably longer. Table 9–32 shows the details of the distribution for each aneurysm site. Fifty percent were allocated to surgery within 1 day of the first angiographic procedure, 69.4% in 3 days, 78.4% in 5 days and 88.8% in 10 days. Therefore, 30 patients (11.2% of 268) had a delay in allocation of treatment beyond the 10-day interval. This is a relatively small number when considering the multiple factors responsible for causing such delays.

Table 9–32.   Distribution of Patients by Aneurysm Site and Interval Between First Angiographic Procedure and Date of Randomization.

Interval (Days) First Angiogram to Date of Randomization	Aneurysm Site				
	Internal Carotid	Middle Cerebral	Anterior Cerebral	Total	Percent of Total
0	14	5	43	62	
1	10	10	52	72	50.0
2	3	2	26	31	
3	2	3	16	21	69.4
4	2	2	9	13	
5	5	4	2	11	78.4
6	2	2	8	12	
7	2	1	8	11	
8	2	0	0	2	
9	0	0	1	1	
10	1	1	0	2	88.8
12	2	0	0	2	
14	0	0	3	3	
16	1	1	1	3	
18	1	1	3	5	
20	0	0	0	0	
Over 20	3	6	8	17	
Total	50	38	180	268	

Table 9–33. Distribution of Complications Occurring During or Within 24 Hours After the Angiographic Procedure.

Internal Carotid	Middle Cerebral	Anterior Cerebral	Total	Complicating Event
1	0	4	5	Rebleed with no neurologic deficit
2	0	1	3	Rebleed with permanent hemiplegia and aphasia
0	0	2	2	Fatal rebleed
2	0	1	3	Transient hemiparesis only
1	1	0	2	Permanent hemiparesis
1	0	1	2	Temporary hemiplegia (one with amaurosis three hours)
1	1	0	2	Confusion for few hours which cleared in four days
0	0	1	1	Permanent tetraplegia
0	0	1	1	Transient drowsiness, cleared in 12 hours
0	0	1	1	Transient unresponsiveness
0	0	1	1	Rebled with convulsions
0	1	0	1	Temporary dysphasia
8	3	13	24	Totals

Complications

Among the 268 patients who were subjected to a total of 417 procedures, there were 24 patients (9.0% of 268) who experienced temporary or permanent undesirable events. Eleven patients rebled during or within 24 hours following the procedure, 5 of whom had no neurologic sequelae; 3 had permanent hemiplegia and aphasia, 1 had convulsive activity and 2 died (Table 9–33). Six others had temporary hemiparesis, hemiplegia or dysphasia which subsequently cleared. Two additional patients had permanent hemiparesis and 1 had tetraplegia at the time of vertebral-basilar angiography. Therefore, within the entire group, 6 patients had permanent neurologic sequelae and 2 died. This is a remarkably low mortality (2 of 268) and permanent (6 of 268) morbidity rate.

Associated Lesions

On each protocol for the angiographic survey, provision was made to note associated vessel shifts or other lesions which might influence the result of treatment.

Thirty-eight (14.2% of 268) had associated lesions interpreted as an intracerebral or extracerebral mass lesion, stretching of anterior cerebral arteries in 11 (4.1%), irregular intima (atherosclerosis) of cavernous or supraclinoid portion of the internal carotid artery in 5 (1.9%), and 7 patients had infundibular dilatations (less than 3 mm in diameter) at the anterior choroidal or posterior communicating arteries which were not regarded as aneurysms in this study (Table 9–34). Most of the mass lesions were interpreted as hematomas; many actually represented localized brain swelling. Hematomas documented at operation are discussed under morbidity.

The highest frequency of extracerebral and intracerebral mass lesions as interpreted angiographically occurred in the middle cerebral group (23.7%, or 9 of 38). The frequency with the anterior cerebral group was 13.9% (25 of 180). Stretching of the anterior cerebral vessels in 9 patients was important because rupture of an anterior cerebral-anterior communicating aneurysm not infrequently presents with a deep frontal lobe hematoma with rupture into a frontal horn of the lateral ventricle. Most of these patients were in poor neurologic condition and several died prior to surgery.

Table 9–34.   Distribution of Associated Lesions in Addition to a Single Aneurysm at the Angiographic Survey.

Site	Extra-cerebral Mass	Intra-cerebral Mass	Stretching of Anterior Cerebral	Irregular Intima (Atherosclerosis)	Infundibular Dilation	Total
Internal carotid (50)*	2	2	1	3	5	13
Middle cerebral (38)	0	9	1	1	2	13
Anterior cerebral-anterior comm. (180)	8	17	9	1	0	35†
Total (268)	10	28	11	5	7	61‡

* Total patients allocated to intracranial surgery.
† Other items in additional patients included absent right or left anterior cerebral artery in 3, multiple (3) anterior cerebral arteries in 1, absent right posterior cerebral in 1, occluded right middle cerebral artery in 1 and right hemisphere atrophy in 1.
‡ 14 patients had duplicate findings.

Cerebral Vasospasm

Introduction

Decrease in intra-arterial diameter over limited or extensive regions of the cerebral vasculature in patients with subarachnoid hemorrhage has usually been defined as "spasm" when other causes have been eliminated. We are cognizant of the pitfalls in presentation of data such as these, due to variation in interpretation of a cerebral angiographic survey from one observer to another, yet the importance of vasospasm in subarachnoid hemorrhage almost demands that such analyses be done. Cerebral vasospasm was defined as one of three categories: no vasospasm, localized vasospasm (narrowing of intra-arterial diameter over 1-cm to 3-cm distance on the proximal portions of the intracranial internal carotid artery, middle cerebral, anterior cerebral or vertebral-basilar artery) and diffuse vasospasm (narrowed diameter of the internal carotid and all the main branches). Various degrees of vasospasm were correlated with age, sex, neurologic condition, systolic and mean blood pressures, interval from last bleed to angiography, size (mm³) of the aneurysm and mortality.

Results

The incidence of vasospasm among males (39.2%, or 51 of 130) was virtually identical to that in females (39.4%, or 54 of 137, Table 9–35). Interestingly, in the internal carotid group, 64% (32 of 50) were females, with 53.1% (17 of 32) manifesting some degree of vasospasm. Although there were only 18 males in the internal carotid group, the trend toward the presence of increased incidence of vasospasm also existed (44.4%, or 8 of 18). In summary, 50% (25 of 50) of the internal carotid group had localized or diffuse vasospasm in similar proportions between the two sexes, 44.7% (17 of 38) of the middle cerebral group and 35.2% (63 of 179) of the anterior cerebral complex. This last group must be clarified with respect to localized vasospasm. Differentiation between congenital narrowing of the A_1 segment of the anterior cerebral arteries and localized vasospasm is difficult in many instances. Perusal of these protocols reveals that unilateral narrowing of the A_1 segment proximal to the anterior communicating aneurysm occurred in 7 of 48 patients in the anterior cerebral group, and in 2 instances it was bilateral. The possibility exists that in these 9 instances, congenital narrowing could have been the "cause" of "localized" vasospasm. In only 1 internal carotid aneurysm was lo-

Table 9–35. Aneurysm Site Distribution With Respect to Vasospasm in Males and Females.

Site	Cerebral Vasospasm			Total
	None	Localized	Diffuse	
	Males			
Internal carotid	10	4	4	18
Middle cerebral	7	5	5	17
Anterior cerebral-anterior comm.	62	26	7	95
Subtotal	79	35	16	130
	Females			
Internal carotid	15	7	10	32
Middle cerebral	14	2	5	21
Anterior cerebral-anterior comm.	54	22	8	84
Subtotal	83	31	23	137
Total	162	66	39	267
Insufficient Information				1
				268

calized vasospasm so interpreted to involve the proximal segment of the anterior cerebral artery alone. There was none listed in the middle cerebral group. Elimination of the 9 patients in the anterior cerebral group would diminish the total percentage with localized and diffuse vasospasm from 35.2 to 30.2% (54 of 179). Considering the internal carotid group where 60% (27 of 45) of patients had undesirable postoperative events from 3 to 72 hours after operation, one must regard vasospasm as highly suspicious in causing these conditions. However, as discussed in the section on morbidity, localized and diffuse vasospasm was noted in 5 instances each, for a total of 10 of the 27 with complicating postoperative events. The remaining 17 had no vasospasm at the time of their angiographic survey. Therefore, it is unlikely that vasospasm per se was a primary cause for precipitating these events.

Mortality and Vasospasm

For all aneurysm sites combined, mortality in the group operated upon with no vasospasm was 38.7%; 37.0% in the group where vasospasm was localized, and 29.0% where it was diffuse. Therefore, vasospasm apparently had no influence upon mortality. This may be an unexpected finding, since the presence of severe arterial narrowing demonstrated angiographically has been the reason for delay of operation by most surgeons. It is important to recognize, however, that the same degree of vasospasm at angiography may not have been the same as at operation, due to the interval between angiography and surgery in this study. In our opinion, there is no way to determine the exact condition of the intracerebral vessels, especially as to how they will respond to mechanical manipulation at operation.

Age and Cerebral Vasospasm

The age distribution (Table 9–36) with respect to the various categories of vasospasm shows good correlation with presence of vasospasm in each decade. Each aneurysm site was analyzed in this regard, and similar proportions within each site were noted. Therefore, a summary of all sites combined is presented. Within each decade, the percentages of patients with localized or diffuse vasospasm were distributed between 14.3 and 52.5% (average 39.3%). The higher ratios were present in the 4th, 5th and 6th decades (range 40.9 to 52.5%). After subdividing the entire group into those below 50 years of age and those 50 and over, 41.3%

Table 9–36. Distribution of Patients by Age Interval With Respect to Each Category of Vasospasm—All Aneurysm Sites Included.

Age	Cerebral Vasospasm			Total	Percent with Vasospasm
	None	Localized	Diffuse		
10–19	6	1	0	7	14.3
20–29	17	3	5	25	32.0
30–39	19	13	8	40	52.5
40–49	39	14	13	66	40.9
50–59	43	22	8	73	41.1
60–69	35	13	4	52	32.7
70–79	3	0	1	4	25.0
Total	162	66	39	267	39.3
Insufficient information				1	
				268	

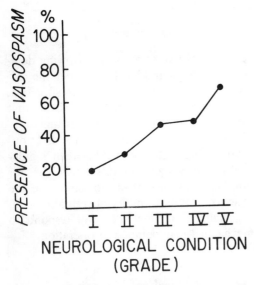

Fig. 9–2. Presence of vasospasm with respect to clinical grade.

(57 of 138) had localized or diffuse vasospasm in the younger group, and 37.2% (48 of 129) had vasospasm in the older (Table 9–36). Therefore, it is doubtful that age has any influence on appearance of vasospasm.

Neurologic Condition and Cerebral Vasospasm

Cerebral vasospasm as defined previously was present in increasing proportions with increase in neurologic deficit. The proportion of patients with and without vasospasm was similar when comparison was made between each aneurysm site. By combining all sites, it was observed with each grade of deteriorated neurologic condition that the presence of vasospasm increased. The ratio

Table 9–37. Distribution of Patients by Neurologic Condition With Respect to Each Category of Vasospasm.

Neurological Condition	Cerebral Vasospasm			Total	Percent with Vasospasm
	None	Localized	Diffuse		
Grade 1	14	3	1	18	22.2
Grade 2	110	40	14	164	32.9
Grade 3	25	14	13	52	51.9
Grade 4	8	3	6	17	52.9
Grade 5	4	6	5	15	73.3
Total	161	66	39	266	39.5
Grade 6				1	
Insufficient information				1	
				268	

of patients with, versus those without vaso-spasm progressively increases from the lowest value of 22.2% (Table 9–37) to the highest level of 73.3%. For convenience, these percentages are plotted in Figure 9–2 for each clinical grade. Although cerebral vasospasm has been suspected to play a role in the production of neurologic deficits, many severe deficits may be present without vasospasm, or vice versa.

Interval from Last Bleed to Initial Angiography

The average interval from last bleed to the first angiographic procedure was 5.8 days (range 0 to 47 days). Forty-seven percent had their initial angiogram in 3 days, 77.2% in 7 days, 86.9% in 10 days and 93.6% in 14 days (Table 9–38). Inspection of this table reveals that a higher proportion of patients have no evidence of vasospasm within 6 days of their last bleed in comparison with the group having their angiographic procedure after this interval. Analysis of these two groups reveals 66.1% (127 of 192) had no evidence of vasospasm when angiography

was performed within 6 days of the last bleed, but in the group whose angiography was done after the 6-day interval, 46.7% (35 of 75) had no vasospasm. Especially in the group whose studies were done in the interval from day 7 through 14, only 37.9% (22 of 58) had no evidence of vasospasm. Therefore, the interval between 7 and 14 days appeared to show the highest percentage (62.1%) of vasospasm in the localized and diffuse category. No differences in proportions were noted when each aneurysm site was evaluated. Therefore, the data for all aneurysm sites are presented.

Systolic Blood Pressure and Vasospasm

Four representative blood pressures at 4-hour intervals or more were recorded by the usual manometric method during the interval between admission and randomization. These four readings were transposed to the protocol at the participating center and the average calculated at the Central Registry. Average systolic values at specific increments were correlated with various cate-

Table 9–38. Distribution of Patients With Respect to Interval From Last Bleed to First Angiographic Procedure Tabulated Against Degree of Vasospasm—All Sites Combined.

Days Last Bleed to Angiography	Cerebral Vasospasm			Total	% of 267
	None	Localized	Diffuse		
0	14	1	5	20	
1	34	8	3	45	
2	20	11	0	31	
3	22	7	1	30	47.2
4	14	7	7	28	
5	9	5	4	18	
6	14	3	3	20	
7	5	5	4	14	77.2
8	3	4	3	10	
9	2	3	2	7	
10	6	2	1	9	86.9
11	1	2	3	6	
12	2	2	0	4	
13	2	1	0	3	
14	1	2	2	5	93.6
Over 14	13	3	1	17	
Total	162	66	39	267	100.0
Insufficient information				1	
				268	

Table 9–39.   Distribution of Patients' Categories of Vasospasm Tabulated With Respect to Various Levels of Systolic Blood Pressure.

Systolic BP (mm Hg)	Cerebral Vasospasm			
	None	Localized	Diffuse	Total
Below 100	0	2	0	2
101–120	20	7	8	35
121–140	67	29	14	110
141–160	41	12	11	64
161–180	23	11	5	39
Over 180	11	5	1	17
Total	162	66	39	267
Insufficient information				1
				268

gories of cerebral vasospasm for all sites combined.

A group of 54.9% (147 of 268) had average systolic blood pressure of 140 mm Hg or below prior to allocation of treatment, 103 (38.4% of 268) had average systolic pressures between 141 and 180 mm Hg, and only 17 (6.3% of 268) had over 180 mm Hg systolic (Table 9–39). Therefore, the majority of this group did not have significantly elevated systolic pressures. A total of 60 patients (40.8% of 147) had localized or diffuse vasospasm in the group with average systolic blood pressure of 140 mm Hg or below, and 45 patients (37.5% of 120) had vasospasm to some degree in the group with average

Table 9–40.   Distribution of Mean Blood Pressure Tabulated With Respect to Various Degrees of Vasospasm.

Mean BP	Cerebral Vasospasm			
	None	Localized	Diffuse	Total
65–74	0	1	0	1
75–84	8	4	1	13
85–94	34	12	8	54
95–104	44	21	11	76
105–114	34	12	10	56
115–124	23	9	6	38
125–134	14	5	2	21
135–144	4	0	1	5
Over 144	1	2	0	3
Total	162	66	39	267
Insufficient information				1
				268

systolic levels above 140 mm Hg. This difference is not significant.

Mean Blood Pressure

The analysis of the relationship between mean blood pressure and vasospasm was based on the same average blood pressures from which the systolic values were determined. Cross-tabulation of mean blood pressures among all aneurysm sites reveals similar proportions of patients with vasospasm (Table 9–40). No direct relationship between increment in mean blood pressure and vasospasm appeared. The peak incidence of mean blood pressures was in the range of 95 to 104 mm Hg. Twenty-eight percent (76 of 267) were in this range alone. The distribution began at a low value of 66 mm Hg to a high of 171 mm Hg. One hundred eighty-six patients (69.7% of 267) had mean blood pressures between 85 and 114 mm Hg. Inspection of the ratios between each degree of vasospasm reveals that in the 85 to 114 mm Hg range (Table 9–40), 60.2% (112 of 186) were without vasospasm, 24.2% (45 of 186) had localized vasospasm and 15.6% (29 of 186) had diffuse vasospasm. For patients with mean blood pressure above 114 mm Hg, 62.6% had no vasospasm, 23.8% had localized vasospasm and 13.4% had diffuse vasospasm. Therefore, a high degree of vasospasm does not signify a greater tendency toward increased blood pressure.

Size of Aneurysm and Vasospasm

The average size of the aneurysm by angiographic determination was 250 mm³. The angiographic dimensions of the intraluminal diameter were recorded by each participating center. The volumetric analysis of each aneurysm was calculated at the Central Registry. As inspection of Table 9–41 reveals, no correlation can be made with regard to aneurysm size and various degrees of vasospasm. The ratio of patients with vasospasm versus those without remains proportional

Table 9–41. Distribution of Patients in Each Category of Vasospasm Tabulated Against the Size (mm³) of Each Aneurysm.

Size (mm³) of aneurysm	Cerebral Vasospasm			
	None	Localized	Diffuse	Total
0–100	29	11	10	50
101–200	31	13	12	56
201–300	23	17	4	44
301–400	18	3	5	26
401–500	14	4	2	20
501–600	7	2	1	10
601–700	7	5	0	12
701–800	3	2	0	5
801–900	1	0	0	1
901–1000	8	0	1	9
1,001–1200	5	0	1	6
1,201–1,400	2	0	1	3
1,401–1,600	1	1	0	2
1,601–1,800	0	0	0	0
1,801–2,000	1	2	0	3
2,001–2,200	0	1	1	2
2,201–2,400	0	0	0	0
2,401–2,600	1	0	0	1
2,601–2,800	1	0	0	1
2,801–3,000	2	2	0	4
Over 3,000	3	2	0	5
Subtotal	157	65	38	260
Insufficient information				8
Total				268

among increments in aneurysm size. It appears, therefore, that intraluminal volume as determined angiographically has no effect upon appearance of cerebral vasospasm.

Surgical Techniques

General Remarks

By its nature, intracranial surgery is perhaps the least well-controlled method of treating an intracranial aneurysm. Ideal treatment consists of removing the aneurysm from the circulation without compromising the blood supply to the brain. The exigencies that may attend intracranial operation frequently preclude "standardization" of a surgical technique. A well-laid plan for a specific attack upon an aneurysm may have to be abandoned under certain circumstances and an-

other, less satisfactory one applied. A "tight, swollen and angry" brain may preclude satisfactory exposure of the aneurysm and require the execution of a less desirable or effective procedure. In some instances resection of a part of the brain may be necessary, adding a risk of permanent neurologic damage.

There is little question that the interval from last bleed to operation is vital. Early operation (3 to 7 days after SAH) may be hazardous when vasospasm is often present and associated with cerebral swelling. Although manipulation of vessels about an aneurysm may at any time induce or aggravate vasospasm, there is considerable difference when this occurs in patients who are operated upon in the early days after SAH than in those who have their operation 2 or 3 weeks later. Nor would it appear that such vasospasm is influenced favorably at the time of early operation by any adjunct to the surgical procedure. The question of operation early after SAH in the presence of raised intracranial pressure (which has not been considered in this study) is another matter. From the technical standpoint alone, such increased tension may prevent satisfactory exposure of the aneurysm. Certainly the skill and experience of the surgeon must be considered. In this Cooperative Study, the operations were performed by surgeons with considerable experience in the intracranial management of these lesions. It is evident, therefore, that in a study such as this, adherence to rigid control of variable conditions is most desirable. Yet, that which was least well controlled (intracranial surgery) signifies more difficulty in evaluation.

It is noteworthy that in this group of patients, in only two instances was a definitive operation not completed. This attests to the technical ability of the various surgeons engaged in this study and would suggest that with a "technically good" operation, a good result should have been anticipated in patients who were in good condition at the time of operation. As expected, when there were difficulties at operation, particularly in situations where major vessels were temporarily or permanently interrupted, patients were often left with serious neurologic deficits. However, in a respectable number in whom operation appeared uncomplicated, problems ensued within a few days after the procedure. It was not always clear why these developed. Because of the time factor, it was difficult to invoke the matter of vessel manipulation with attendant mechanical vasospasm. On this basis, it would have been expected that such problems would occur early after operation. Unanswered questions are raised relative to vasospasm due to the combined effects of the initial SAH, bleeding with operative exposure and mechanical vessel manipulation. It is not known how "spasm" from operative manipulation of vessels is affected by further bleeding, or vice versa.

It was considered important to know whether a particular technique or the employment of ancillary surgical procedures influenced the results of intracranial operation. It was expected that operative techniques would be varied because of the anatomical location of the aneurysm as well as the experience and approach of the individual surgeon. Table 9–42 presents the type and number of accessory procedures performed at the time of operation.

Brain Resection

This particular feature of operative technique stands out in the anterior cerebral group, i.e., in almost one half (69 of 149 or 46.3%), various degrees of resection of the brain (frontal lobe) were carried out in order to accomplish the procedure (Table 9–42). In the case of middle cerebral aneurysms, temporal (or frontal) resection was made in 17.6% (6 of 34), and in only 4.4% (2 of 45) of the internal carotid group. What lesser or greater morbidity accrued from such deliberate resection of the brain compromising anatomical or functional integrity is difficult to determine. Be this as it may, the surgeon deemed it necessary to sacrifice a portion of the brain in order to expose the aneurysm properly. By comparison, destructive lesions of the brain produced by hematoma were another matter. Patients with such complication of aneurysmal rupture fared poorly despite the removal of the clot. The incidence of hematoma was greatest among middle cerebral (6 of 34) and anterior cerebral aneurysm (21 of 149) patients (18 and 14%, respectively) who had a preoperative hemispheric deficit.

Vessel Occlusion

Temporary intracranial and/or extracranial carotid occlusion made presumably as protection against aneurysmal rupture (less commonly after rupture) was performed in 54 patients (Table 9–42). It is difficult to assess the effect of vessel occlusion and its possible relationship to postoperative complications. There is no definite information

Table 9–42.   Number of Accessory Procedures Associated With Primary Operation.

Aneurysm Site				
Internal Carotid	Middle Cerebral	Anterior Cerebral	Total	Accessory Procedure
7	1	5	13	Temporary occlusion of extracranial carotid or vertebral artery
10	8	23	41	Temporary occlusion of intracranial vessels
2	6	69	77	Resection of temporal lobe or frontal pole
4	2	5	11	Removal of bone flap at closure
1	6	21	28	Evacuation of preoperative hematoma
0	0	0	0	Ligation cervical carotid as part of "trap" procedure
24	23	123	170	

Table 9–43. Type of Surgical Procedure Accomplished at Each Aneurysm Site.

Internal Carotid	Middle Cerebral	Anterior Cerebral	Definitive Procedure
	Aneurysm Site		
0	1	22	Proximal ligation in continuity of parent vessel
3	1	6	Proximal and distal ligation of parent vessel ("trap" procedure)
33	13	50	Ligation of the neck of aneurysm
3	2	10	Clip occlusion of fundus of the sac
0	4	35	Investment of the sac with muscle, gauze, fascia, etc.
0	2	0	Investment of sac with plastics
6	9	26	Multiple
45	32	149	
	2*		
	34		

* In 1 patient the aneurysm ruptured and the patient died; in 1 the aneurysm was not found.

to indicate that such occlusion (with potential vessel injury) increased morbidity on the basis of infarction or anoxemia. Temporary extracranial carotid occlusion was employed 13 times: in 7 instances in the management of internal carotid aneurysm, 5 for anterior cerebral and 1 for middle cerebral artery aneurysms. This was done undoubtedly to control hemorrhage during exposure of an aneurysm rather than as a prophylactic measure in most instances.

Removal of Bone Flap

The bone flap was not replaced in 11 patients among 228 operations, presumably because of uncontrolled cerebral swelling.

Type of Surgical Procedure

Seven types of surgical procedures were utilized in which a single, definitive method of management was employed. One category was designated as "multiple," in which a combination of two or more of the other six was used (Table 9–43). The procedure most commonly employed at the three major sites was ligation of the neck of the aneurysm. It is presumed that this was usually

accomplished by clip occlusion, and in a few instances by means of a thread ligature.

Internal Carotid Aneurysm

In the case of internal carotid artery aneurysms (45 patients), 33 (73.3%, Table 9–43) were treated by aneurysm neck ligation, at the same time preserving the major arterial supply to the brain. In only 3 instances was the aneurysm trapped intracranially so that the carotid artery was sacrificed. In no instance was intracranial and extracranial trapping of the aneurysm accomplished. In those cases where the aneurysm was trapped, it is clear that this procedure was made of necessity in an attempt, for example, to control hemorrhage that occurred when the neck of the aneurysm was torn at its origin from the carotid rather than as a deliberate tactic to exclude carotid inflow to an unruptured aneurysm. One of these 3 patients died, and 1 remained hemiplegic and aphasic. The infrequent use of this operation is interesting since the "trapping" procedure in the earlier days of intracranial surgery for carotid aneurysm was commonly and successfully applied as a deliberate measure. The lower occurrence of trapping in this series reflects most probably the bolder, positive approach by the more experienced surgeon. In 3 instances, the fundus of the aneurysm was clipped. It is assumed that this was done to control hemorrhage from rupture during exposure of the lesion and that the neck for one reason or another could not be safely occluded by clip or ligature.

In 6 instances, more than one procedure was performed. Five patients had a ligation procedure (clipping) of the neck of the aneurysm and in addition had an investment with plastics in 1 instance, a trapping procedure in 2, clip occlusion of the fundus of the sac, and investment with muscle, gauze or fascia in 2. One patient had investment of the aneurysm with muscle and clipping of the anterior cerebral artery distally due to the anatomical relationship of the aneurysm to surrounding vessels.

Middle Cerebral Aneurysm

Thirty-four patients with a middle cerebral aneurysm had an intracranial operation; in 2 a definitive attack on the aneurysm was not performed (see Table 9–43).

Among the remaining 32 patients, ligation or clipping of the neck of the aneurysm alone was the operation of choice in 13 instances. Other procedures, such as plastic investment (2), investment with gauze, muscle or fascia (4), and clip occlusion of the fundus of the sac (2) were accomplished less frequently. Proximal ligation of the vessel from which the aneurysm arose and trapping by proximal and distal ligation of the parent vessel were made only once each. The investment technique was evidently, in the opinion of the surgeon, the most expedient that he could employ in a situation where: (1) the sac or its neck could not be safely dissected because of important blood vessels adherent to its walls, or (2) the sac could not be isolated well enough to apply a ligature without compromising the blood supply to the brain. In all instances where an investment procedure was made, the aneurysm was at the main branching of the middle cerebral artery. The "trapping" and proximal ligation operations were probably made in cases of aneurysms associated with relatively "minor" and distal arterial trunks where occlusion would leave a lesser deficit, rather than in cases where occlusion of vessels close to the first bifurcation of the middle cerebral artery would be necessary.

Nine patients had more than one procedure on the aneurysm per se (Table 9–43). Four had investment of the sac with muscle, gauze or fascia in addition to ligation or clip occlusion of the neck, 2 had clip occlusion of the fundus with clipping of the neck and 2 had clip occlusion of the fundus of the aneurysm with investment. One additional patient had investment of the aneurysm with plastics and gauze.

Intraoperative difficulties evidently were not considered major surgical problems. In 6 cases, the aneurysm ruptured at the time of exposure, but hemorrhage was readily controlled. All 6 aneurysms were located at the branchings of the main trunk. Four of these 6 patients did not survive. It should be noted, however, that whereas 2 were poorly responsive at the time of operation, 2 had only minimal symptoms. Of the 2 survivors, 1 had a major neurologic deficit and the other had minor symptoms when operated on. Three of the 4 deaths occurred in patients who had an associated intracerebral hematoma documented at surgery; 2 of the 3 were poorly responsive at the time of surgery.

Anterior Cerebral Complex Aneurysm

In this group, as in the case of internal carotid and middle cerebral artery aneurysms, clipping (ligation) of the neck alone was most commonly employed (33.6%, 50 of 149). This relatively low figure might imply difficulty in the execution of the clipping procedure and that the surgeon considered it too risky, fearing a complication resulting from occlusion of the anterior cerebral vessels. Investment of the aneurysmal sac was made in 23.5% (35 of 149). This figure is influenced by one center using primarily the investment technique. Ligation of the proximal anterior cerebral artery was carried out in 22 cases (14.8%). It is assumed that this was done: (1) as a deliberate definitive procedure for an anterior communicating artery aneurysm filling from one side only but with a contralateral anterior cerebral artery present, or (2) after inspection of the aneurysm disclosed that its relationship to both anterior cerebral arteries prevented obliteration of the aneurysm only. It was evidently considered a safer yet not entirely satisfactory operation because the aneurysm was yet within the circulation. The surgeon, however, considered it best in that particular situation. The fundus of the sac was clipped in 10 instances, indicating most probably that rupture had occurred and bleeding could be controlled only in this way, or that the neck could not be fully exposed. It is further likely that the surgeon considered this adequate protection against rebleeding and that clipping of the neck was neither necessary nor feasible. Only 6 cases in this group of 149 (4%) anterior complex aneurysms were trapped. It is not clear how this was done, except in cases where the aneurysm was distal to the anterior communicating artery or that it may have been possible in the rare situation to place a clip in the small space on either side of an aneurysm at the anterior communicating artery.

In 26 patients, more than one (multiple) operative procedure was performed in order to prevent rebleeding of the aneurysm. Twenty-four had investment of the sac with muscle, gauze or fascia; in addition, 4 patients had proximal ligation of the parent vessel, 10 had ligation of the neck of the aneurysm and 10 had clip occlusion of the fundus of the sac. Two additional patients had a clip occlusion of the neck of the aneurysm with proximal ligation of the parent vessel, indicating that the clip occlusion alone was not successful.

From these data, it appears that by and large the procedure most commonly utilized was that of aneurysm neck clipping (ligation) in 42.5% (96 of 226). This was considered the best treatment to apply in the case of aneurysms at the three major sites. Forty-one (18.1%) had multiple procedures.

Multiple Operations

Additional surgical procedures directly and indirectly related to the original operation were necessary in 46 patients. Sixteen patients (35.6% of 45) with an internal carotid aneurysm had two or more procedures, 20.6% (7 of 34) with a middle cerebral aneurysm and 15.4% (23 of 149) with an aneurysm on the anterior cerebral complex.

Internal Carotid Aneurysm

In the 45 patients where the internal carotid artery was the site of origin of the aneurysm, two operations were made in 11 instances. The second was that of tracheostomy in 8 patients, 5 of whom died. Three of the latter were in good condition at the time of operation, indicating that operation made the patient worse and was the immediate factor contributing to his death. The other 2, 1 of whom expired, were poorly responsive at the time of surgery. Although tracheostomy was necessary to support them, it is not clear how much the operative procedure influenced their deterioration to require respiratory assistance. In 1 of the 3 remaining patients in this group, the second operation was a definitive one to occlude the neck of the aneurysm; the first step was to evacuate a temporal lobe hematoma. In the 2nd patient, the bone flap was replaced. Both patients survived. The 3rd patient had a craniotomy and ligation of the aneurysm with removal of the bone flap 3 days after the last bleed. The second operation, 5 days later, was a re-exploration with resection of the frontal and temporal lobes for decompression.

Three operations were made on 4 patients in the internal carotid group, 3 of whom had a tracheostomy following operation. One of these had bilateral common carotid artery exposure at the time of operation, 1 had removal of the bone flap postoperatively and 1 had a shunt procedure for hydrocephalus. The remaining patient in this series had a right frontal resection one day after operation for clipping of the aneurysm, and a repeat resection 8 days later. Three patients died and 1 survived.

Four operations were made in 1 patient who was in Grade 3 preoperatively. Tracheostomy was performed at the time of craniotomy on the day after the bleed. On the following day, the bone flap was removed and the dura opened, presumably as a decompressive measure for cerebral swelling. The flap was replaced 34 days later.

Middle Cerebral Aneurysm

Five patients with an aneurysm on the middle cerebral artery had two operative procedures. In 4, the second procedure was a tracheostomy; 2 were in Grade 2 preoperatively and 2 in Grade 4. In 1 patient, the second procedure was evacuation of a postoperative hematoma.

Three operations were perfomed in 2 patients who had middle cerebral artery aneurysms. In 1, the first was that of subtemporal decompression for cerebral edema 7 days after hemorrhage. Fifty-two days later, the aneurysm was invested with "plastic." Seventy-one days after the bleed, another craniotomy was made to remove a "hematoma from the frontal lobes." The aneurysm in the 2nd patient was partially occluded by clips and invested with gauze 4 days after SAH. Eight and 10 days later, respectively, an intracerebral clot was removed and right temporal lobe resection was accomplished. Both patients survived.

Anterior Cerebral Aneurysm

A second operation was required in 19 patients, all noted to be in good preoperative condition except 2 who were in Grade 3. Thirteen died (68.4%). In 11 patients, a tracheostomy was performed as a second operation; in 3, a postoperative hematoma was removed; in 2, the bone flap was replaced; and in 1 instance each, a ventriculopleural shunt was placed, a chest drain was

inserted for pneumothorax and a surgical wound was re-explored.

In 3 patients, three operative procedures were required. Preoperatively, 2 were in Grade 2 and 1 in Grade 5; all 3 died. Each had a tracheostomy as a second procedure. The third procedure consisted of biparietal burr holes with evacuation of a subdural hematoma 4 days after operation, and 2 had removal of the bone flap as a decompressive procedure.

One patient in good condition had four operative procedures; the inital one included aneurysm clipping 24 days after SAH. Three, 6 and 9 days later, re-operation was necessary, the first time because of an epidural hematoma and cerebral swelling, the second to remove a subdural hematoma and the third to treat a sterile epidural abscess and remove the bone flap. This patient did not survive.

Summary

Mortality among the 46 patients requiring two or more procedures was 67.4% (31 of 46). In 30 (65.2%), the neurologic condition at the time of the first operation was good (Grades 1 and 2). Multiple procedures were made comparatively less frequently in the case of anterior cerebral complex aneurysms than for those at the internal carotid site: 23 of 149 (15.4%) and 16 of 45 (35.6%), respectively. This suggests (1) that complications at the anterior cerebral site occurred less frequently, or (2) that patients with internal carotid aneurysms were more ill and that a greater effort was expended in an attempt to salvage them. Indeed, relatively more patients with internal carotid artery aneurysms were in poor condition than were those with anterior cerebral complex aneurysms. Among the 149 anterior cerebral complex aneurysms, 18.1% (27 of 149) were described as having major neurologic deficits or as being poorly responsive and seriously ill, whereas this state existed in 37.8% (17 of 45) of those with internal carotid artery aneurysms. The conclusion might also be drawn that the internal carotid artery aneurysm was technically a greater challenge to successful surgical management than was one at the other two major sites.

Surgical Adjuncts

Agents to Reduce Intracranial Pressure

Introduction

A number of factors may prevent exclusion of an aneurysm from the circulation, such as adherence to major arteries, atherosclerotic plaques and in some instances aneurysm size. Yet, the optimum therapeutic maneuver upon an aneurysm requires its isolation from surrounding structures. Increased intracranial pressure from hydrocephalus or a swollen brain may interfere with adequate dissection of the aneurysm and prevent optimal placement of a ligature or investment of an aneurysm. Techniques to reduce intracranial pressure were utilized in 171 (75%)

of the 228 operations performed in this study. These techniques included the use of hyperosmotic agents (urea, mannitol, glycerol), steroids (dexamethasone, methylprednisolone sodium succinate, hydrocortisone), hyperventilation and spinal drainage. Fifty-seven operations were accomplished without these ancillary agents. Among the 171 operations in which they were employed, hypertonic urea alone or in combination was used in 68, mannitol alone or in combination in 64 and hyperventilation alone or in combination in 70. Dexamethasone, the most commonly used steroid, was used in combination with other agents in all but three of 31 operations. Methylprednisolone sodium succinate, hydrocortisone, cortisone and glycerol were each used once.

It is difficult to assess fully the effects of surgical adjunctive therapy. However, in analyzing deaths within the 14-day interval after surgery, it was discovered that differences existed as various adjuncts to reduce intracranial pressure were compared. The following section discusses these adjuncts with respect to mortality in the 14-day postoperative interval, neurologic condition and cause of death.

Table 9–44. Distribution of Deaths Within 14 Days Following Surgery in Patients Subjected to Various Adjuncts to Reduce Intracranial Pressure.

Days from Surgery to Death	No Adjuncts Used	Urea	Mannitol	Hyperventilation
0	1	1	1	1
1	0	1	0	1
2	1	1	2	1
3	0	2	1	0
4	0	6	1	2
5	2	3	1	1
6	1	1	0	0
7	0	1	0	1
8	2	2	1	0
9	0	0	0	0
10	0	1	1	1
11	0	2	1	0
12	0	1	0	0
13	0	0	0	0
14	1	1	0	0
Subtotal	8 (14%)	23 (33.8%)	9 (14.1%)	8 (11.4%)
Total cases in category	57	68	64	70

None Utilized

In 57 patients, measures aimed at reducing intracranial pressure were not utilized at the time of operation. Evidently, in the judgment of the surgeon, such adjuncts were not necessary. Adequate and satisfactory access to the aneurysm was accomplished without them. Within the 14-day interval after surgery, there were 8 deaths (14%, Table 9–44). In 6 of the 8, death followed postoperative deterioration. One died following recurrent SAH 8 days after surgery, and 1 expired from pneumonia and gastrointestinal bleeding. Forty-two had aneurysms of the anterior cerebral complex, 5 of whom died—an operative mortality of 11.9%. Of note is the fact that 37 were in good condition (Grades 1 and 2), while 4 had a major neurologic deficit but were fully alert (Grade 3), and 1 was poorly responsive (Grade 4) at the time of surgery. In the 7 patients with a middle cerebral artery aneurysm, 1 died on the day of surgery from uncontrollable bleeding from the aneurysm. Among 8 patients with internal carotid artery aneurysm, there were 2 fatalities, 1 of whom had a major preoperative deficit, the other being described as "seriously ill" (Grade 5). Both died within 6 days of surgery from postoperative cerebral effects.

Frequently the surgeon employed measures to reduce intracranial pressure in order to gain easier and better exposure of the lesion. A total of 171 patients were included in this category, and the following discussion pertains to those in whom anti-edema agents were utilized.

Hyperventilation

The technique of hyperventilation was not described, but indication of its use was noted in 70 operations, in 26 of which no other adjuncts were utilized. Mortality within 14 days after operation was 11.4% (8 of 70, Table 9–44). All died from progressive deterioration following the surgical procedure, except 1 who died from a pontine hemorrhage. One of these was seriously ill (Grade 5) prior to operation, but the remainder were in good condition. In the entire group (26 had hyperventilation alone and 44 had the combination of hyperventilation and other adjuncts), 54 were in good neurologic condition (Grades 1 and 2), 12 had a major neurologic deficit but were fully responsive (Grade 3), 3 were lethargic in association with a hemiparesis or hemiplegia (Grade 4) and 1 was in Grade 5 (seriously ill). There were 3 deaths among 26 patients who had hyperventilation alone (11.5%), and 5 deaths in 44 who had hyperventilation in combination with multiple adjuncts. In 3, hyperventilation was used in conjunction with urea, and one each with steroids and mannitol.

Mannitol

The amount of mannitol or duration of treatment with this hyperosmotic solution was not indicated, but its use alone (26 patients) or in combination with other adjuncts (38 patients) was the choice of the surgeon in 64 instances. Mortality within the 14-day postoperative period was 14.1% (9 of 64, Table 9–44). One died following a proved rebleed 8 days after surgery (middle cerebral aneurysm), and the remaining 8 patients died from complications of treatment. One of those who died was seriously ill and 1 had a major neurologic deficit prior to surgery, but the remaining 7 were in good condition (Grades 1 and 2). In the entire group, 49 were in good condition (Grades 1 and 2), 12 had a major neurologic deficit but were fully alert (Grade 3), 2 were lethargic in addition to a hemiparesis or hemiplegia (Grade 4) and 1 was seriously ill (Grade 5). There were 5 deaths in 26 patients (19.2%) who had mannitol alone, and 4 deaths in 38 patients (10.5%) who had mannitol in combination with other agents. Two patients in the latter group of 4 deaths had mannitol and urea, and 1 each with hyperventilation and hydrocortisone.

Urea

Urea is a relatively short-acting hyperosmolar agent which was used alone as a surgeon's choice in 51 operations, and in combination with other agents in 17, for a total of 68. The mortality in the former group was 33.3% (17 of 51) and in the latter 35.3% (6 of 17), for a combined mortality of 33.8% (23 of 68, Table 9–44). Twenty patients died in the 14-day postoperative period following a progressive downhill course (complications of treatment other than a rebleed), 2 patients had a proved rebleed 11 and 12 days after surgery, respectively, and 1 died following a myocardial infarction 8 days after surgery, although no postmortem examination was allowed for confirmation. The neurologic condition prior to surgery was good (Grades 1 and 2) in 15 patients; 5 had a major neurologic deficit (Grade 3) and in 3 patients a significant impairment of consciousness (2 cases) or seriously ill condition (1 case) existed. The percentage of deaths in patients in whom urea was used alone and in combination was similar.

Dexamethasone (Decadron) Alone and in Combination

Dexamethasone was used during operation in 31 cases. In 6 it was employed alone; in 25 in combination with urea, mannitol and hyperventilation. The dosage and route of administration of dexamethasone are unknown. Where employed alone, there were no deaths (6 cases). There were too few instances of its use with other adjuncts to warrant detailed discussion. However, 3 of 5 patients who died had the combination of urea and dexamethasone. Two of these 3 were Grade 1 and 2 patients and the other was moribund; all expired in a progressively deteriorating pattern following surgery.

Spinal Drainage

Spinal or ventricular drainage was not frequently used as a means to reduce intracranial pressure or aid in surgical exposure. Some surgeons utilize this adjunct as an effective means to reduce brain volume. In this series, spinal drainage was used only 9 times, 7 in combination with hypothermia, 2 times

with dexamethasone. Four cases involved the internal carotid artery. In 2, the patients were in good condition; the others were in poor condition. One of the latter succumbed, being poorly responsive at the time of operation. A Grade 3 patient with middle cerebral artery aneurysm and 2 with an anterior cerebral complex aneurysm (Grades 2 and 3) survived. There was not one recorded instance of ventricular puncture and drainage alone.

Discussion

There is little question that these agents have been helpful to the surgeon in combating a "tight" swollen brain that hinders exposure of the aneurysm. The overall mortality was 14% when none was employed. When urea was used, a distinctly higher mortality (33.8%) was noted. Fifteen of the 23 deaths in patients who received urea were in good-condition patients. In those patients who received mannitol, 9 deaths (14.1%) occurred among 64 patients, 49 of whom were in Grades 1 and 2. Seven of the 9 fatalities were graded similarly. Of particular interest was the group of patients who received mannitol and hyperventilation. These two agents were employed in 20 cases; 1 death occurred. These facts suggest that the use of urea, although effective for the surgeon when he attempts to expose an aneurysm, may be more hazardous than formerly believed. Although urea has been used rather "routinely" for many years, perhaps the secondary phenomena related to electrolyte shifts and rebound swelling require reevaluation. Furthermore, it is possible that there are poorly understood deleterious or physiological disturbances related to the use of urea in the function of the blood-brain barrier and cell membranes. Condemnation of the drug on the basis of the above may be premature. It is possible that if the surgeon has been able to better expose an aneurysm with the use of urea, he may also become bolder in attempting to exclude it from the circulation. This may lead to difficulty. In such attempts, he may run a greater risk of producing vessel injury or interfering with cerebral circulation, particularly the fine perforating vessels supplying the basal structures and the brain stem. A secondary small or large vessel constriction with hypovolemia could produce inadequate regional perfusion.

Hypothermia

Hypothermia was employed in 94 (41.2%) of 228 operations. It was used with equal frequency during the latter half as compared with the first half of the study. In 91, hypothermia for the operative procedure was induced to the 27° to 32° C level, and in 3 operations, deep hypothermia (less than 23° C) was employed. The mortality in the 14-day postoperative interval in the 91 patients who received moderate hypothermia was 26.4% (24 of 91). There were no deaths in the 3 patients who received deep hypothermia. Twenty-one of the 24 deaths were noted as "complications of treatment other than rebleed," 2 patients died of a proved rebleed and 1 died of bronchial pneumonia and gastrointestinal bleeding. Sixteen of the 24 deaths occurred in patients who were in good neurologic condition (Grades 1 and 2) prior to operation; 4 had a major neurologic deficit, 2 were lethargic with an associated hemiparesis, and although 2 were regarded as seriously ill, their condition was stable. The distribution of deaths for each aneurysm site was 34.6% (9 of 26) for the internal carotid group, 20.0% (4 of 20) for the middle cerebral group and 24.4% (11 of 45) for patients who received moderate hypothermia in the anterior cerebral-anterior communicating group. The mortality within 14 days

following operation for patients who received no hypothermia was as follows: 21.1% (4 of 19) for patients with an internal carotid aneurysm, 21.4% (3 of 14) for middle cerebral aneurysm and 11.9% (12 of 101) for anterior cerebral-anterior communicating aneurysm, for an overall mortality of 14.2% (19 of 134).

Antishivering drugs were given only during the operation in 25 cases; in 9 additional patients, such agents were used during and after the operation. In 4, such drugs alone were used without other methods to produce a hypothermic state. To what degree the temperature was lowered is unknown. It is not clear why antishivering drugs only were employed in the intraoperative period in these 4 instances, as these agents alone would ordinarily be insufficient to depress body-brain temperature to the degree which would be considered protective.

Aside from what may be the general protective effect of hypothermia to a compromised brain, its maximal advantage is anticipated in protecting an area of the brain during temporary vessel occlusion while the aneurysm is being dissected or obliterated. Referring to Table 9–45, temporary occlusion of vessels was made 44 times. In 36, this involved the intracranial vessels in the immediate proximity of or in continuity with the aneurysm; in 8, it involved the extracranial carotid artery. Hypothermia was apparently employed for reasons other than temporary vessel occlusion in 47 of 91 (51.6%) patients. It can be assumed that this was hoped-for protection of the brain and perhaps an aid in the technical aspects of the operation by reducing intracranial tension and producing a brain with diminished vol-

Table 9–45. Distribution of Patients Who Received Hypothermia During Temporary Occlusion of Extracranial Carotid (A) or Intracranial Carotid (B) for Each Aneurysm Site.

Aneurysm Site	Total Patients With Hypothermia	(A)	(B)
Internal carotid	26	4	8
Middle cerebral	20	1	8
Anterior cerebral-anterior comm.	45	3	20
Total	91	8	36

Table 9–46.   Distribution of Patients Who Received Hypothermia With Cerebral Edema Reducing Agents.

Site	Patients With Anti-edema Agents	Patients Without Anti-edema Agents
Internal carotid	37(21)*	8 (5)
Middle cerebral	27(16)	7 (5)
Anterior cerebral	107(37)	42(11)
Total	171(74)	57(21)

* Number in parentheses denotes those who received hypothermia.

ume. These aspects were not the only reasons for its use, since hypothermia was employed in combination with other "brain volume reducing" agents, as indicated in Table 9–46. Such agents were used in 74 patients (43.3%). Among the 21 patients of the internal carotid group in Table 9–46, there were 9 deaths within 14 days after surgery; among 16 patients of the middle cerebral group, there were 4 deaths; and among 37 patients of the anterior cerebral group, there were 9 deaths. Therefore, among the 74 patients who had the combination of hypothermia and anti-edema agents, there were 22 deaths (29.7%). Among the 21 patients who had no anti-edema agents but did undergo hypothermia (Table 9–46), there was 1 death in the anterior cerebral group due to pneumonia and gastrointestinal bleeding 14 days after surgery. From this relatively small and obviously select group of patients, no specific conclusions can be made.

Hypothermia was carried below 23°C in 1 Grade 1 patient with an anterior cerebral complex aneurysm, and in 2 others with an aneurysm at the same site in Grades 1 and 4, respectively; the degree of hypothermia was not recorded. All survived.

Other Adjuncts

Hypotension

In 47 patients, intraoperative reduction of blood pressure was accomplished. The gan-glionic blocking agent most commonly utilized was trimethaphan camsylate in 27 instances. Additional drugs included d-tubocurarine twice; a combination of d-tubocurarine and succinylcholine chloride once, succinylcholine chloride alone three times; and prostigmine and atropine once each. Hypotension was induced by increasing the depth of anesthesia using fluothane and halothane once each. In 10 cases in which hypotension was utilized, the nature of its induction and the drug employed were not specifically indicated.

Hypotensive measures were not used in 180 of the 228 patients. In 1 instance, there was no indication whether or not hypotensive measures were used. It is interesting to note that in such a high percentage (78.9%) hypotensive measures were not included as an adjunct to the operation. Some surgeons who use hypotension are convinced of its value in protection against premature rupture of the aneurysm, and that it facilitates manipulation of the aneurysm more freely during dissection. Therefore, why hypotension was not employed more often in this series is not clear. Furthermore, information was not provided in the protocols to indicate how long and to what depth hypotension was carried out during the operative procedures. The metabolic effects of prolonged hypotension as related to impaired perfusion raises questions with respect to its safety, although it appears that the degree and duration of hypotension were not of a magnitude known to produce such effects in the experimental animal. Experience with the method in the hands of those who employ it widely without gross or apparent neurologic difficulties has made it widely accepted.

Deaths among the 47 patients who received hypotension during operation were distributed by aneurysm site as follows: 2 among 8 patients with internal carotid aneurysm, none of 2 patients with middle cerebral aneurysm and 9 of 37 patients with anterior cerebral-anterior communicating aneurysm (Table 9–47). Of considerable interest is the distribution of deaths during the postoperative period in the group with and without hypotension. When combining all sites, the mortality in the group who did not receive hypotension (17.8%) is not significantly different from those who did receive ganglionic blocking agents during surgery (23.4%). Distribution of deaths within each category of neurologic condition reveals that hypotensive techniques during operation neither favorably nor adversely influenced the surgical mortality (Table 9–48).

Table 9–48. Distribution of Deaths Within the 14-Day Postoperative Interval for All Sites Combined.

Days After Surgery	Number of Deaths	
	No Hypotension	Received Hypotension
0	3	0
1	2	0
2	4	1
3	2	1
4	5	1
5	5	1
6	0	1
7	2	1
8	3	2
9	0	0
10	2	1
11	1	2
12	1	0
13	0	0
14	2	0
Subtotal	32	11
Total cases	180 (17.8%)	47 (23.4%)

Morbidity

Introduction

Major postoperative neurologic deficits included hemiparesis, hemiplegia, dysphasia and aphasia of varying degrees and duration. Other effects sometimes as devastating were characterized by varying states of stupor, coma, behavioral disorder, confusion and convulsive activity. The incidence of surgical complications produced a remarkable state of affairs. Such neurologic difficulties occurred in 109 patients (47.8% of 228 operations). Patients who had a major deficit prior to surgery and continued to have the same deficit after surgery were *not* included in this analysis. A number of less frequent complications, such as anosmia (3), meningitis (2), visual loss (1), third cranial nerve palsy (3), pneumonia (3), pneumothorax (1), diabetes insipidus (1), myocardial infarction (1) and postoperative hematoma (3), also were reported.

The following discussion presents a detailed analysis of the more frequent and major findings associated primarily with neurologic dysfunction immediately or soon after (within 72 hrs) intracranial operation.

Table 9–47. Comparison of Patients With and Without Hypotension.

	Internal Carotid	Middle Cerebral	Anterior Cerebral Complex	Total
No hypotension	37 (11)* 29.7%	32 (7) 21.9%	111 (14) 12.6%	180 (32) 17.8%
Received hypotension	8 (2) 25%	2 (0) 0%	37 (9) 24.3%	47 (11) 23.4%

* Number in parentheses denotes deaths within 14 days after surgery; insufficient information was noted in 1 protocol.

Coma

Postoperative coma of more than 24 hours' duration occurred in 45 patients (19.7% of 228 operations). Only 7 of these were alive as of January 1973. In the remaining 38 patients who died, 31 had a progressive downhill course and 7 died from other causes; 2 died from a proved rebleed, and 1 each from a suspected rebleed, pontine hemorrhage, pneumonia, pulmonary embolus and respiratory arrest.

Internal Carotid Aneurysm

The frequency of this complication among patients with an internal carotid aneurysm was 26.7% (12 of 45). Seven patients had only minimal neurologic findings (Grade 2), 4 were in Grade 3 and 1 was seriously ill (Grade 5) but his clinical condition was stable. Seven were in good medical condition, and 5 were in fair condition. None had a preoperative hematoma. Age range was 13 to 62 years, with a mean of 45.1 years. The average interval from last bleed to surgery was 9.7 days (range 2 to 29 days). Ten of the 12 patients with postoperative coma died, 9 from a progressive downhill course within 16 days following operation and 1 with pneumonia 161 days following surgery. Eight of the 10 deaths had no vasospasm at initial angiography, and 2 had localized vasospasm. In the 2 survivors, 1 had no vasospasm and 1 had diffuse (bilateral) vasospasm.

Middle Cerebral Aneurysm

In this group of 34 patients, 3 (8.8%) had postoperative coma. Two deaths occurred within 4 days; 1 died from a pulmonary embolus 79 days following operation. The interval from last bleed to surgery was 6, 10 and 26 days respectively. One patient had a preoperative hemiparesis, and the other 2 were poorly responsive but had good adaptive responses. All 3 were in poor medical condition, with known pre-existing renal disease, atherosclerosis and/or heart disease. Their average age was 63 years (range 59 to 66). Two patients had no cerebral vasospasm at initial angiography, and 1 had diffuse vasospasm.

Anterior Cerebral Aneurysm

Among the 149 patients with an anterior cerebral-anterior communicating aneurysm, 30 (20.1%) were in comatose condition immediately following or within 72 hours after operation. There were 25 deaths, 20 due to progressive deterioration, 2 due to a proved rebleed 8 and 11 days after operation, and 1 each from a pontine hemorrhage (1 day after operation), respiratory arrest and pneumonia (14 days after operation) and a suspected rebleed (146 days after operation). Twenty-four of the 25 deaths occurred within 54 days following operation. One suspected rebleed occurred 146 days later. The average interval from operation to death was 10.9 days (range 1 to 54 days). Average age distribution was 49.4 years (range 21 to 76 years). Most patients were in good neurologic status initially. Twenty-six (86.7% of 30) were in Grades 1 and 2 prior to surgery, 2 had a major neurologic deficit (Grade 3) and 2 were poorly responsive (Grades 4 and 5). One of the latter remains alive. Eighteen (60% of 30) were in good medical condition, 9 (30%) were fair and 3 were in poor medical condition. The average interval from last bleed to surgery was 10.8 days (range 2 to 51 days). Sixteen (53.3% of 30) had no vasospasm, 12 (40.0%) had localized vasospasm and 2 had diffuse vasospasm. In 13 patients (43.3%) the comatose condition was immediately postoperative; in 17 it developed within a few hours to 72 hours following surgery.

Discussion

Postoperative coma can be caused by several factors. It is assumed that in this study, problems with cerebral swelling, difficulty in lobe retraction with cerebral infarction and/or tearing of perforating arteries to the hypothalamus were not overcome satisfactorily. A hematoma can be a possibility. However, in only 9 patients was a hematoma found at operation.

The factor of age is always important in surgical mortality, yet the average ages among the group with internal carotid aneurysms (45.1 years), middle cerebral aneurysms (56.1 years) and anterior cerebral aneurysms (49.4 years) were not significantly different.

The group of patients with a middle cerebral aneurysm was unusual in that only 3 of the 34 (8.8%) had coma postoperatively. All 3 were in poor neurologic and medical condition, and their average age was 63. Such outcome can be expected. Surprisingly, despite the presence of a hematoma of varying size found at operation in 6 patients, postoperative coma developed in only 1.

Hemiplegia

Serious neurologic deficit such as hemiplegia can be expected to occur for reasons similar to those responsible for production of a comatose condition. A total of 11.4% (26 of 228) developed a hemiplegic state immediately (18 cases) or within 6 to 72 hours (8 cases) following operation. In only 3 patients did the hemiplegia clear prior to discharge from the hospital. In the remaining 23 it was permanent (throughout the hospitalization period). Thirteen deaths (50%) occurred within 14 days after surgery, all following progressive deterioration in this postoperative period. Seven of the 26 patients with hemiplegia were also comatose after operation; 1 was stuporous.

Internal Carotid Aneurysm

Among the 45 patients in this group, postoperative hemiplegia developed in 10 (22%).

Seven were in good neurologic condition preoperatively (Grades 1 and 2), 1 had a major neurologic deficit in the form of a mild hemiparesis (Grade 3) and 2 were poorly responsive. Five were in good medical condition, 4 were in fair condition and 1 was in poor condition with heart disease and atherosclerosis. The average interval from last bleed to surgery was 17 days (range 3 to 42 days). In 3 patients the hemiplegic condition was associated with stupor, and in 3 with aphasia. All patients remained hemiplegic until death or throughout their hospitalization. Six died within 14 days after surgery. Average age of the entire group was 47.7 years (range 13 to 69). Six patients had no vasospasm at the time of initial angiography, 1 had localized vasospasm, and in 3 it was diffuse. In the 10 patients with postoperative hemiplegia, 2 had temporary occlusion of the intracranial portion of the internal carotid artery during operation. One died 2 days after operation. Five patients had ligation of the neck of the aneurysm only, 3 were subjected to a "trapping" procedure and 2 had ligation of the neck and fundus clipping or investment. One patient had an intracerebral hematoma.

Middle Cerebral Aneurysm

Postoperative hemiplegia among the 34 patients with middle cerebral aneurysm occurred in 3 instances (8.8%). One patient in good neurologic condition (Grade 2) died 10 days after surgery following progressive deterioration; the 2 others had a preoperative hemiparesis (Grade 3). One patient was in good medical condition, 1 in fair condition; the one in poor condition died from pulmonary embolism 79 days after surgery. In 1 patient the hemiplegia cleared prior to discharge from the hospital, but in the 2 others it remained permanent. The average age was 60.3 years (range 52 to 65). One patient had no vasospasm and 2 had localized vasospasm at initial angiography. At operation, none of these patients had an intracerebral hematoma. The average interval from last bleed to surgery was 17.3 days (range 8 to 26). The one who died from a pulmonary embolus also had prolonged postoperative coma.

Anterior Cerebral Complex

Postoperative hemiplegia occurred in 13 (8.7%) of the 149 patients who had an operation for an aneurysm on the anterior cerebral complex. Nine patients were in good neurologic condition (Grades 1 and 2), 3 had a major deficit (hemiparesis, Grade 3) and 1 was seriously ill (Grade 5). The medical condition was good in 6 patients, fair in 6 and poor in 1. The average interval from last bleed to surgery was 8 days (range 1 to 27). All patients remained hemiplegic throughout hospitalization, except 1 in whom it cleared. Six died within 11 days after operation, following a progressive downhill course. The average age was 46.8 years (range 17 to 67). Nine patients had no vasospasm at initial angiography, 3 had localized vasospasm and in 1 it was diffuse. In no instance was a hematoma found at operation. However, 2 patients in poor neurologic condition and 1 in good condition had a hemiplegic state associated with coma. In 7 patients the hemiplegic state was discovered immediately after operation; in 6 instances it developed between 3 and 72 hours.

Discussion

Among the three major aneurysm sites, the internal carotid group had the highest rate of postoperative hemiplegia (22%), followed by the middle cerebral and anterior cerebral group, with 8.8 and 8.7%, respectively. No single factor such as age, neurologic or medical condition, interval from last bleed to operation or cerebral vasospasm alone influenced the development of this postoperative complication. In 5 of 10 patients with internal carotid aneurysm, the aneurysm ruptured during the operation. In each of the following instances, temporary

intracranial carotid occlusion was made; a clip was misplaced on the intracranial portion of the internal carotid artery as shown by postoperative angiography, and 1 had occlusion of the middle cerebral artery distal to the location of the aneurysm. One additional patient developed occlusion of the internal carotid artery at its bifurcation in the neck, and in 1 case no factors could be determined after detailed analysis of the entire protocol and operative report. Although these were the outstanding features likely to cause the hemiplegic state in the internal carotid aneurysm patients, they were not the explanations at the other two aneurysm sites. The most likely events responsible for the middle cerebral cases were age as well as medical and neurologic condition. However, little can be stated with regard to three cases in this group, a surprisingly small number for aneurysms located at this site. Patients with anterior cerebral aneurysm who developed a hemiplegic state postoperatively were generally in good neurologic and medical condition, with no or localized vasospasm. The interval between last bleed and operation did not influence the development of the hemiplegic state. Aneurysm rupture during operation was not reported in the group with hemiplegia, and neither was the presence of a preoperative hematoma an influential factor. In essence, no preoperative factors could be found responsible. One can hypothesize that remote effects of operation, cerebral edema and/or vasospasm worked alone or in combination to produce the hemiplegic deficit.

Hemiparesis

Although the presence of unilateral limb weakness is indicative of major neurologic dysfunction, it generally denotes a reversible process and is considered to be less severe than the previously discussed complications, coma and hemiplegia.

Postoperative hemiparesis occurred in 14.9% (34 of 228). This observation was noted immediately after surgery in 29 patients, and several hours later in 5. There were 9 deaths within 16 days following surgery among the three aneurysm sites; 8 followed progressive deterioration and 1 a proved rebleed 8 days after operation. In 21 patients the hemiparesis persisted throughout the postoperative period of hospitalization, and in 13 it cleared by the time of discharge.

Internal Carotid Aneurysm

Among the 12 patients with postoperative hemiparesis in the internal carotid group (45 cases, 26.7%), 4 were associated with a comatose condition. Seven patients were in good neurologic condition (Grades 1 and 2), and 5 were in Grade 3 (major neurological deficit). It must be emphasized that in these latter cases the hemiparesis was definitely worse postoperatively. Six were in good medical condition, 5 were in fair condition and 1 was in poor condition. The average interval from last bleed to surgery was 16.6 days (range 2 to 29 days). There were 5 deaths in this group following progressive decline in cerebral function within 16 days after operation. In 2 patients the hemiparesis cleared by the time of discharge; in 10 it was permanent. The average age was 53.2 years (range 26 to 71). Eight patients had no vasospasm at initial angiography, 2 had localized vasospasm and in 2 it was diffuse. As in the group of patients with postoperative hemiplegia, there were 5 whose aneurysm ruptured at the time of surgery. Whether or not there is a direct relationship, each patient had immediate postoperative hemiparesis.

Middle Cerebral Aneurysm

In only 3 patients (8.8%) in the group of 34 with a middle cerebral aneurysm did postoperative hemiparesis arise as a complica-

tion. In 2 instances a less severe hemiparesis existed prior to surgery; in 1 no deficits were noted except for signs of meningeal irritation (Grade 2). Two patients were in good medical condition and 1 was in fair condition. The average interval to surgery was 15 days (range 4 to 24). In 2 cases the hemiparesis remained throughout hospitalization; in 1 it cleared. Average age was 48 years (range 44 to 51). Two patients had localized vasospasm and 1 had diffuse vasospasm.

Anterior Cerebral Complex

Among the 149 patients with anterior cerebral aneurysm, 19 (12.7%) had postoperative hemiparesis. In 13 it was noted immediately after the operation; in 6 it appeared during the 48 hours following the operative procedure. There were 4 deaths within 14 days following the operation: 3 following progressive postoperative decline, and 1 from a proved rebleed.

All patients in this group of 19 were in good neurologic condition preoperatively (Grades 1 and 2). Nine were in comatose condition after operation. Twelve were in good medical condition; 7 were in fair condition. Average interval from last bleed to surgery was 12.7 days (range 2 to 51). Average age was 44.7 years (range 15 to 64). Thirteen patients had no vasospasm at initial angiography, in 5 it was localized, and in 1 diffuse. In only 1 of the 19 patients was an intracerebral hematoma found at operation; that patient survived.

Discussion

Pathological changes responsible for postoperative hemiparesis are likely due to the same mechanism as hemiplegia, albeit a less extensive or severe process. The frequency distribution of this postoperative event with respect to each aneurysm site was as follows: internal carotid group, 26.7%; middle cerebral group, 8.8%; anterior cerebral group, 12.7%. This distribution approximates closely the percentages in cases with postoperative hemiplegia. Virtually the same rationale applies to this complication as that given in the discussion on hemiplegia. Whereas 50% of patients with postoperative hemiplegia subsequently expired, only 26.5% (9 of 34) who had hemiparesis died during the 16-day postoperative period. Since the cause of death was essentially the same in the two groups, it appears that varying degrees of infarction, edema and/or ischemia are the factors underlying coma, hemiplegia and/or hemiparesis in the postoperative state.

Aphasia

In our opinion, the cause of this disorder is the same as for other postoperative events discussed previously. In all probability, vascular insufficiency to a strategic area(s) in the dominant hemisphere (usually the left) was due to small or large vessel occlusion, in conjunction with cerebral infarction and/or edema.

The overall incidence of this disorder was 12.3% (28 of 228). In all but 6 instances it remained permanent throughout hospitalization. Five patients were categorized as dysphasic after surgery, 23 as aphasic. Eight deaths (3.5% of 228) occurred within 14 days following operation. In 22 patients hemiplegia (11 cases) or hemiparesis (11 cases) was associated with aphasia, and in 6 no other complications were noted.

Internal Carotid Aneurysm

Analysis of each specific aneurysm site reveals that 20% (9 of 45) in the internal carotid group had postoperative aphasia, 4 cases were associated with hemiparesis and 5 with hemiplegia. Six patients were in Grade 2 preoperatively, and 1 each in Grades 3, 4 and 5. Six were in good medical condition; 3 were in fair condition. The average interval from last bleed to surgery was

13.3 days (range 2 to 41). There were 4 deaths in the 14-day postoperative period, all due to progressive deterioration. In all cases except 1, the deficits remained permanent until the end of hospitalization. The average age was 53.3 years (range 21 to 69). Six patients had no vasospasm at the time of initial angiography; in 1 it was localized, and in 2 it was diffuse.

Middle Cerebral Aneurysm

In the middle cerebral group, 3 of 34 patients (8.8%) had postoperative aphasia. Two had associated hemiparesis and hemiplegia, 1 had no other deficits. Two patients were in Grade 2, one in Grade 3. All 3 were in fair medical condition. The average interval from last bleed to surgery was 26.6 days (range 8 to 55). In 2 instances the aphasia remained permanent, and in 1 it cleared prior to discharge. Average age was 50 years (range 44 to 54). In 1 patient there was no vasospasm; in 1 it was localized, and in 1 diffuse.

Anterior Cerebral Complex

In the anterior cerebral group, postoperative aphasia was found in 16 patients (10.7% of 149). Four of this group were listed as "dysphasic." Five patients had associated hemiplegia, 6 had hemiparesis and 5 patients had no associated neurologic deficits. Eleven patients were in good neurologic condition (Grade 2), 4 were in Grade 3, 1 was in Grade 5. Six were in good medical condition, 9 in fair condition and 1 was in poor condition. The average interval from last bleed to surgery was 11.6 days (range 1 to 45). In 12 the aphasic or dysphasic disorder remained permanent; in 4 it cleared prior to discharge. Average age was 41.6 years (range 17 to 68). No vasospasm was noted at initial angiography in 12; localized spasm was present in 3 and diffuse in 1.

In summary, 20% of patients with internal carotid aneurysm had an aphasic deficit,

8.8% of the middle cerebral group and 10.7% of the anterior cerebral group. An aphasic deficit was associated with hemiparesis or hemiplegia in 78.6% (22 of 28). Therefore, in most instances aphasia was noted in association with other deficits, all of which are likely caused by the same pathological mechanisms.

Confusion and Dementia

Postoperative confusion and dementia were more difficult to analyze, but were of considerable significance in terms of the functional aspects of the patient. One can suspect that frontal lobe functions were compromised by the same pathological processes as discussed previously.

The frequency of confusion and dementia was 8.9% (4 of 45) for the internal carotid group, none for the middle cerebral group and 18.8% (28 of 149) for the anterior cerebral group, an overall incidence of 14% (32 of 228 operations). Two of 4 patients in the internal carotid group had postoperative hemiparesis, and 4 of 28 in the anterior cerebral group. All remaining patients (2 internal carotid and 24 anterior cerebral) were noted to have confusion and/or dementia as the only postoperative deficit. Two patients (6.3% of 32) died within 14 days after surgery following progressive deterioration; in 1 a gradual comatose condition developed and the other had immediate postoperative hemiparesis.

Analysis of this group of patients reveals that 27 (84.4% of 32) were in Grades 1 and 2, and 5 were in Grade 3 preoperatively. Sixteen (50%) were in good medical condition, 14 were in fair condition and 2 were in poor condition. The average interval from last bleed to surgery was 12.6 days (range 2 to 42). In 20 patients (62.5% of 32) the problem was temporary in that the mental derangement cleared by the time of discharge; in 12 (37.5% of 32) it remained permanent throughout hospitalization. Average

age was 49 years (range 18 to 65). Twenty patients (62.5%) had no vasospasm; in 8 (24.0%) vasospasm was localized, and in 4 (12.5%) diffuse.

Discussion

The most striking finding was the absence of patients in the middle cerebral group with difficulty in the form of dementia or confusion. This has been the trend for this group throughout the analysis of postoperative findings. The internal carotid group had only 4 patients, 2 with associated hemiparesis. Twenty percent of the internal carotid group had postoperative aphasia, hemiparesis (26.7%) or hemiplegia (22%). The higher number of cases with confusion and dementia among the anterior cerebral group (18.8%) implies that a considerable amount of vascular and/or edematous change occurs in the distribution of the frontal lobes and hypothalamus. The question arises of how much mechanical manipulation at the time of surgery was responsible for precipitating these changes in an already compromised brain. In all cases, preoperative mental derangement was not evident since patients in Grades 1 to 3 were alert and oriented in all spheres. In 57.1% confusion and dementia cleared prior to discharge.

Miscellaneous Complications

In addition to the neurologic dysfunctions associated with the surgical procedure as discussed in the preceding section, a number of additional events were noted to occur less frequently.

Internal Carotid Aneurysm

In this group of 45 operated patients, 1 had a blood transfusion reaction during the operation and died with subsequent anuria. During the postoperative period, 2 patients were treated for a scalp wound infection necessitating antibiotics and/or surgical drainage. In 1 additional patient, a subdural hematoma with encephalomalacia developed. In 1 instance each, diabetes insipidus, diabetes mellitus and fever of unknown origin for 4 days needed special attention.

Pulmonary infections were treated in 8 patients during the postoperative period. There were 4 who were treated for genitourinary tract infection. Four were treated for gastrointestinal hemorrhage of mild to moderate severity, and 3 had electrolyte imbalance sufficiently severe to necessitate administration of special intravenous fluids. There was 1 report of peripheral venous thrombosis in the postoperative state, but none of pulmonary emboli. Hydrocephalus requiring an internal shunt procedure occurred in 1 patient. In no instances were convulsions noted in the postoperative period. All of the above conditions occurred in 19 patients (42.2% of 45).

Middle Cerebral Aneurysm

During the operative procedure, a transfusion reaction developed in 1 patient. Severe vasospasm was noted in this same patient during the operation. Postoperatively, in 1 instance each the following conditions were treated: subdural hematoma, pneumothorax and later cardiac arrest, pulmonary infarction, myocardial infarction, peripheral venous thrombosis with a fatal pulmonary embolus, peripheral venous thrombosis without pulmonary embolus and 1 instance of electrolyte imbalance. Three patients were treated for a pulmonary infection, 5 for a genitourinary tract infection. None was treated for postoperative wound infection, gastrointestinal hemorrhage, hydrocephalus or convulsions. Two developed postoperative intracerebral hemorrhage, documented by reoperation. Among 34 patients with a middle cerebral aneurysm, 15 (44.1%) had these various postoperative events.

Anterior Cerebral Complex

In this group, 149 patients were operated upon. During the operative procedure difficulties such as cardiac or respiratory arrest, pneumothorax and rupture of the aneurysm during induction of anesthesia occurred respectively in these patients. Postoperatively, a wound infection at the surgical site was treated with drainage and antibiotics in 4 cases, evacuation of a subdural hematoma in 3 additional patients and an epidural hematoma in 1. Medical complications occurred in the form of pulmonary infections in 14, electrolyte imbalance requiring special intravenous therapy in 13, genitourinary tract infection in 10, gastrointestinal hemorrhage in 6, peripheral venous thrombosis with pulmonary embolus in 5 (2 fatal) and peripheral venous thrombosis without pulmonary embolus in 5. Hydrocephalus developed in 4 patients requiring an internal shunt procedure, 2 acquired a pneumothorax and in 1 instance each a myocardial infarction, cardiac arrest 24 hours postoperatively, a respiratory distress syndrome and convulsions occurred. All of the above were observed in 73 of the 149 patients (49%).

Rebleeding After Definitive Surgical Procedure

The primary reason for intracranial surgical repair for ruptured intracranial aneurysm is prevention of rebleeding. Yet in this group of 228 operations, there were 19 (8.3%) proved or suspected rebleeding episodes following surgery. There were 16 deaths (7%) from this cause. Rebleeding in these patients indicates that the aneurysm was not adequately treated. Table 9–49 shows that all patients were in satisfactory medical and neurologic conditions preoperatively, with one exception (case 9).

In the majority of instances, the aneurysm was wrapped, the clip was misplaced or

Table 9-49.   Proved and Suspected Rebleeding Episode After Intracranial Surgery.

Registry No.	Age/Sex	Neurologic Condition	Medical Condition	Surgical Procedure	Angio. Postop.	Interval Surgery to Rebleed	Vasospasm	Remarks
9*	49/F	4	2	Clip of neck	Internal carotid Malposition of clip	9 mo	Diffuse	Postmortem exam denied
44	56/F	2	2	Investment with EDH-adhesive	Middle cerebral Aneurysm smaller 95 day after SAH	6 mo	None	Rupture of aneurysm with 4 × 4 cm intracerebral hematoma at postmortem
854	37/M	2	1	Clip occl. of neck	None	8 day	Diffuse	Misplaced clip found at postmortem exam
62	58/F	2	1	Clip proximal to aneurysm	Anterior cerebral Tantalum clip spontaneously opened	8 mo	None	Recurrent hemorrhage and massive intraparenchymal hematoma at postmortem
64	48/M	2	1	Fundus clipped and wrapped	None	6 day	Localized	Partial obliteration of fundus found on postmortem
77	38/M	2	2	Investment of aneurysm with muslin	Aneurysm larger after rebleed	18 day	Localized	Recurrent bleed adjacent to edge of gauze wrap. Intracerebral and intraparenchymal hematoma at postmortem
194	51/F	2	1	Gauze wrap	None	11 day	None	Recurrent hemorrhage with intraventricular hematoma at postmortem
230	45/M	2	1	Muslin wrap	None	5 day	None	L. P. Evidence of rebleed; remained alive with no neurologic deficit
263	59/F	2	1	Muslin wrap	None	8 day	Localized	Recurrent hemorrhage through gauze wrap with intraventricular hematoma at postmortem
327*	62/F	2	2	Muslin wrap	Aneurysm enlarged	39 day	Diffuse	Postmortem exam denied
333	54/M	3	2	Proximal ligation of parent vessel	Aneurysm enlarged	46 day	Localized	Recurrent hemorrhage at dome of aneurysm; right frontal lobe hematoma and intraventricular hemorrhage
381	30/M	2	1	Clip across neck	Spontaneous opening of clip	6 day	None	Recovered from comatose condition. L. P. showed rebleed
383*	76/M	2	2	Muslin wrap	None	65 day	None	Postmortem report not available
397	47/M	2	1	Clipping of neck	Parent vessel filled	3 yr, 9 mo	None	Confirmed at postmortem
513	49/F	2	1	Gauze wrap	None	52 day	None	At postmortem, unwrapped portion of aneurysm rebled into frontal lobe with intraventricular hemorrhage
545	34/M	2	2	Trap procedure	Same size	12 day	Diffuse	Ligatures on rt. ant. cereb. artery. Aneurysm filled from left. At autopsy intraparenchymal and intraventricular hemorrhage
603	60/F	2	1	Gauze wrap	Same size	2 yr, 3 mo	None	Confirmed at postmortem
632*	44/F	2	2	Proximal ligation of parent vessel	Parent vessel did not fill	4 yr	None	Postmortem exam denied
900*	56/M	2	2	Clip occlusion of neck	Parent vessel filled	6 mo	None	Postmortem exam denied

* Suspected rebleed.

opened spontaneously. The interval between surgery and death was variable (8 days to 3 years, 9 months). In essence, recurrence of bleeding was due to technical failure of the method used for that particular aneurysm.

Rupture of Aneurysm During Operation

Introduction

Aneurysmal rupture during intracranial dissection has always been dreaded by the surgeon. Special attention must be given to this possibility because of its effect on the eventual outcome. The amount of extravasated blood, rate of ejection and specific location of rupture are variables which were extremely difficult to interpret. Characteristic descriptions in the protocols were "brisk bleeding," "a small jet of blood," "ruptured during dissection," "bleeding after clip applied" and a few cases of brief "uncontrolled bleeding."

Internal Carotid Aneurysm

Among the 45 operations in this group, in 17 patients (37.8%) bleeding occurred from rupture of the aneurysm during operation. The average age was 48.4 years (range 16 to 69); 7 were males and 10 were females. Average angiographic aneurysm size was 227.6 mm^3 (range 18 to 655 mm^3). Thirteen patients were in Grades 1 and 2, 2 in Grade 3 and 1 each in Grades 4 and 5. In no instance was a preoperative hematoma described. In 11 (64.7%) of the 17 there were postoperative complications: coma in 2; coma, hemiparesis or hemiplegia and aphasia in 3; hemiparesis or hemiplegia alone in 3; and hemiplegia and aphasia in 3. This compares with postoperative complicating events in 60% (27 of 45) for all operations. These two figures (64.7 and 60.0%) are not significantly different, and therefore rupture of

the aneurysm during surgery appeared to produce no change in the rate of postoperative neurologic deficits at this aneurysm site. Six of the 17 (35.3%) died within 14 days following operation, all attributed to progressive cerebral deterioration.

Middle Cerebral Aneurysm

There were 7 cases of aneurysm rupture (20.6%) in the 34 operations in the middle cerebral group. The average age was 48.8 years (range 37 to 59); 5 were males and 2 were females. Average angiographic aneurysm size was 609.4 mm^3 (range 15 to 2,520 mm^3). Two patients had a preoperative intracerebral hematoma. Preoperatively, 4 patients were in Grade 2, 1 in Grade 3 and 2 in Grade 4. Two patients had postoperative coma and died, and 1 had hemiparesis and remained alive. Total numbers involved are too small to draw any further conculsions, except to say that none of these variables was responsible for predisposition to aneurysm rupture. Four of the 7 died within 14 days following operation, 3 following progressive decline in cerebral functions and 1 due to a proved rebleed.

Anterior Cerebral Aneurysm

Aneurysmal rupture at this site occurred in 10.7% of the patients (16 of 149). Average age was 43.5 years (range 17 to 76); 10 were males and 6 were females. Angiographic aneurysm size averaged 460.4 mm^3 (range 210 to 1,248 mm^3). There were no preoperative hematomas. Preoperatively, 2 patients were in Grade 1, 12 were in Grade 2 and 2 in Grade 3. Five patients had postoperative coma and died; 3 had coma, hemiparesis and aphasia with 2 deaths; 5 had dementia or aphasia; and 1 had hemiplegia and aphasia. Two patients had no postoperative neurologic deficits. Five deaths (31.2% of 16) occurred within 14 days following operation, all following progressive clinical deterioration.

Discussion

Aneurysms on the internal carotid group had the highest incidence of rupture (37.8%), followed by middle cerebral (20.6%) and anterior cerebral (10.7%). However, the anterior cerebral group had the highest rate of postoperative neurologic deficits (87.5%, or 14 of 16). This was followed by the internal carotid group with 64.7%, and in the middle cerebral group with 42.8%. These percentages are based upon the total number of aneurysms that ruptured within each site. Of the 40 patients whose aneurysm ruptured during operation, 15 (37.5%) died within 14 days following the procedure.

Mortality in Various Centers

Of the 15 centers contributing to this study, 2 ceased participation. One contributed only 1 case; the other contributed none at the time of withdrawal from the study group. Because of the relatively large number of surgeons involved, one might expect that the mortality might be different for a variety of reasons. Such reasons might be related to the surgeon's experience in the intracranial surgery of aneurysms, the source and character of case material under his care, the physical facilities and personnel with which he had to work, and the surgical philosophies of the individual surgeon. In general, direct comparisons could not be exact because of differences in numbers of patients at various centers, as well as the differences in numbers of aneurysms treated at specific sites. One center, for example (No. 20), was unquestionably the largest contributor (74 cases). The next largest (Center 28) contributed about one third of this number (33), whereas the next in order (Center 27) entered 25 cases to the study. Six centers contributed between 12 and 17 cases to the study, whereas four contributed 7 or less. In only three centers was treatment accomplished in all instances, a total of 36. The one center

(No. 20) with the largest number of cases (74) treated only anterior cerebral complex aneurysms; all other centers submitted protocols for treatment of aneurysms at the three major sites. In general, the number of patients in each center that did not have treatment accomplished was distributed proportionately except for Centers 27 and 28, because patients were usually referred later after SAH than to the other centers. This would account for a relatively larger number referred in better condition. Conversely, a smaller number were included in poor condition or relegated to the "treatment not accomplished" category because of such condition. Because of these variations in numbers of patients treated in the different centers, it does not appear valid to make comparisons of gross mortalities. By the same token, the validity of comparing the results of treatment of the largest number of anterior cerebral complex aneurysms (Center 20) with the much smaller number from the other centers is open to question. The mortality for Center 20 (anterior cerebral aneurysms) was almost the same as for all other centers combined.

Discussion

Those patients who did not have intracranial surgery require little comment. We have previously alluded to this group, questioning the validity of including them in the overall morbidity and mortality because they did not undergo surgery. These patients were left untreated because in the judgment of the surgeon, a successful operation was precluded by their poor clinical state, usually following a recurrent SAH. It may be argued that there is nothing lost in operating upon such patients, so that operation should have been undertaken. On the other hand, experience has shown that operation in this type of patient has not been very fruitful. Whether it is wiser to attempt a surgical procedure to salvage a very small percentage of such patients who might survive in a vegetative state or whether one should not operate upon such patients whose neurologic fate is highly predictable is a matter of dispute. This is an unanswered philosophical question.

The average overall mortality in this large series of patients treated for aneurysms at the three major sites was 36.8%. For the anterior communicating complex, the mortality was 34.8% (all contributing centers). In the instance of the middle cerebral artery, the average mortality from 10 centers was 35.3%; for the internal carotid, 46.7% from 11 contributing centers.

The largest contributor (Center 20) of anterior cerebral complex aneurysms reported a mortality of 36.5% (27 of 74 patients). For all other centers it was, interestingly enough, about the same (32%, 24 of 75). One of the 27 from Center 20 who died was asymptomatic at the time of operation, 24 had only headache and signs of meningeal irritation, whereas 2 had major neurologic deficits. In Center 27, no deaths were recorded among 11 patients with anterior cerebral complex aneurysms. Four good-condition patients had surgery after the 16th day following SAH, 2 between 16 and 20 days, and 2 between 26 and 30 days. Of 4 others in good condition, 2 had surgery in the 6 to 10-day interval and 2 in the 11 to 15-day interval, respectively. Three with major deficits were operated in the 0 to 5, 11 to 15 and 30 + day periods, respectively.

Early surgery in the management of internal carotid artery aneurysms appeared particularly formidable. Twenty-six operations made within the first 2 weeks after SAH were associated with 15 deaths (57.7%). A prominent feature in these 15 deaths was a progressive deteriorating course in 12. Six of the 12 deaths were in patients who had major neurologic difficulty before the operative procedure. Two fatalities were unrelated to either the hemorrhage or operation, and in another the cause was due to a suspected rebleed.

Of the 45 patients in the internal carotid group, 17 were poor candidates for surgery, but the remainder were classified as favorable. The number of patients in each center is too small to make meaningful comparisons. Two centers had no deaths among 6 and 3 patients, respectively. In the former, 5 good-condition patients were operated on after day 16 following SAH, the other with a major deficit in the 11 to 15-day interval. In the latter, all were good-condition patients. One was operated on in the 6 to 10-day period, the other 2 after the 11th day following the bleed. The largest number (8) from one center was associated with a 50% mortality, 4 patients failing to improve following operation. Two were considered poor surgical candidates. Three had surgery before day 5 following the bleed, and of these, 2 died. Here again, patient condition and later operation appeared to be the keynote to a successful outcome.

Thus, the results of surgical treatment in this large series were not happy ones. This is at marked variance with the more glowing reports by authors such as Pool.[8] The difference is due, most likely, to selection of patients and later operation. Valid comparisons cannot be made. If these are attempted, they must be made with rigid analysis of factors which are known to influence surgical treatment. The surgeons engaged in this study were those with wide experience in the surgical management of intracranial aneurysms. Under the circumstances, it is difficult to relate the wide variation in success and failure to differences in surgical expertise alone. Even if one excludes the 40 patients who did not have intracranial operation, most of whom died following recurrent SAH, the outlook for this mode of treatment is still not favorable. In this review, it has been stressed that patients subjected to intracranial surgery were for the most part in "good" neurologic and medical condition "at the time of operation."

Whether or not a patient was operated on may have been determined by the surgical philosophy of the individual surgeon. For example, he may have been pressed to operate in order to rescue a patient whose originally good condition at the time of randomization deteriorated. The salvage rate under such circumstances is known to be low. On the other hand, the surgeon may have decided against operation because of the patient's initial poor condition, preferring to wait until this improved. Similarly, a patient originally in good condition may have deteriorated and failed to recover to his original state while awaiting operation. During this time, the optimal conditions for surgery were apparently lost. He was then ultimately operated upon under less than favorable circumstances. Operation in a patient in poor condition at the time of randomization may have been delayed for a variable period, during which he improved to the state where the surgeon considered him an acceptable but not ideal candidate for operation. All of these conditions obviously would influence the surgical result.

The remarkably low mortality of 2.4% (1 death among 41 patients) reported by Pool[8] in the surgical treatment of anterior communicating artery aneurysms among good (Grade 1) and fair (Grade 2) risk patients alone is challenging. Including 3 deaths in Grades 3 and 4 (poor-risk patients), the mortality among his 56 patients was 7.1%. In the 15 Grade 3 and 4 patients, the mortality was 20%. All 4 Grade 5 patients died. The total mortality for all grades of risk among his 60 patients was 13% (8 of 60). The 68% "excellent" results are all the more remarkable. Of the 4 "salvage" (Grade 5) patients, death in 2 was directly related to a "cerebral condition" that is, "massive cerebral edema" and subarachnoid hemorrhage from a second aneurysm which had been previously undetected. Eighteen of Pool's cases were operated on before the 7th day following SAH with 3 deaths accounting for a mortality of 16.6%, whereas only 1 death occurred among 38 patients operated on after the 8th day.

Krayenbühl et al.[9] report a similarly impressive series. There was no mortality among their 112 Grade 1 and 2 condition patients. The result of operation was described as good in 100% of Grade 1 and 96% of Grade 2 patients. Among 119 patients in

Grades 3, 4 and 5, there were 13 deaths, a mortality of only 10.9%. A good result was achieved in 66 of 74 Grade 3, 16 of 41 Grade 4 and in none of 6 Grade 5 patients. Twelve of 13 fatalities occurred in those operated on before the 14th day following SAH, 1 in the 1st and 5 in the 2nd week. A correlation between the timing of operation and clinical condition in these 13 is not defined. It is likely that these deaths occurred in patients who had early operation (before 2 weeks) and who were in Grades 3, 4 and 5.

These more favorable reports again point out that good-condition patients operated upon "late" after SAH have a greater chance of survival. Those operated upon earlier have usually been in good condition, but other unknown factors appear to influence the outcome unfavorably in a respectable number. Those in poor condition operated on early have a poor prognosis. Certainly technical advances (microtechniques) have helped to improve the operative results, but patient selection and late timing for operation obviously have influenced mortality figures to a great degree.

The high complication rate in this study should be noted. It has been mentioned above that in 75 patients with anterior cerebral complex aneurysms operated in all centers combined (excluding Center 20), there were 24 deaths and 51 survivors. Of the 51, 14 (27.4%) were not good surgical risks. Seven (50%) of the 14 poor-risk patients died, 6 having major preoperative neurologic deficits, the other being "seriously ill." Death was related among these 7 to proved recurrent SAH in 2, indicating clearly an unsatisfactory surgical management of the aneurysm; whereas in 4, death followed progressive postoperative regression. The role that condition and intraoperative events played in the final outcome is impossible to determine. It appears that both were important factors. The last patient died of an unrelated cause.

If the 17 patients who died but who were good surgical risks are analyzed in the same way, it is noted that in 3 instances the operation itself could be considered technically inadequate, as death followed a proved recurrent SAH in 1 and a suspected SAH in 2. In 11 of these 17, death occurred as progressive deterioration developed postoperatively, resulting from a host of operative complications which included, in particular, uncontrolled cerebral swelling related to operative manipulation, vasoconstriction and cerebral infarction. These 11 deaths must be related directly to the surgery since the patient had minimal symptoms at the time of the surgical procedure. Three of the 17 died of unrelated causes. The mortality among good-risk patients then in this series was 33.3% (17 of 51).

Since the mortality for anterior cerebral complex aneurysms at Center 20 was similar, with approximate numbers of patients treated as in the rest of the centers combined, a comparison of some factors involved points up some interesting facts. All but 6 patients in Center 20's group of 74 were in good condition at the time of operation. Two of these 6 died in progressive deterioration; 1 was operated on within 4 days, and the other 16 days after SAH. The other 4 survived. Sixty-eight (91.9%) were in good condition. Of these, 25 died (mortality 36.8%). Of those that died, more than one half (14) were operated upon within 10 days of the last SAH, 7 before and 7 after the 6th day; whereas 11 were operated on after the 10th day, 9 between 11 and 14 days, and the remaining 2 after the 15th day following the last SAH. Death was associated with a proved recurrent SAH in 7 and a suspected SAH in 2, indicating a failure in the technical aspects of operation to eliminate the aneurysm. Undoubtedly, technical success in some cases may have been precluded by adverse anatomical relationships of the aneurysm to parent vessels. In 9 cases, death followed progressive decline. In the remaining 7, it was due to factors not directly related to the operative procedure or the effects of SAH.

Eighteen of the 25 deaths must be considered to have resulted from operation and/or the effects of the bleed. However, since these patients were in good condition at the time of operation, it appears that the surgical

procedure was the more important factor in the mortality.

The mortality (all centers combined) for operation on and prior to the 11th day was 45% (54 of 120), 44.5% (65 of 146) for patients operated on and prior to 14 days from last bleed, and 23.2% for patients operated on after 14 days following the last bleed. Pool[8] reported no mortality among 24 patients operated upon 15 or more days after SAH. It is not clear if there is a "critical optimal time" for making a successful intracranial operation, other factors being equal. It is clear, however, that the longer one can wait after SAH to attack an aneurysm, assuming that another SAH does not occur, the greater is the possibility of carrying out the operation successfully. Whether operation is justified after a patient has survived 6 or more weeks, however, is open to differences in opinion. From the first Cooperative Study,[3] based on the natural history of SAH from a ruptured intracranial aneurysm, it was learned that if a patient survives 2 weeks, the chance of surviving 6 weeks is about 83%. If he survives 6 weeks, the chance of survival for 1 year is about 82%. A recurrent SAH after 1 year is rare. In the series of Troupp and af Björkesten[7] (comprising 92 unoperated patients), "the majority of the 9 fatal recurrences occured within the first month after hemorrhage." Death occurred in 5 instances between the 32nd and 49th day after the first SAH, in 3 instances in the 3rd or 4th month after the initial bleed. Only 1 death occurred later than 4 months after the initial hemorrhage from a recurrent one or "from diseases related to the original illness, for example, intracranial thrombosis after carotid ligature." This point has been emphasized by Troupp and af Björkesten[7] in their comparative analysis of surgical versus nonsurgical treatment of intracranial aneurysms. They point out the good prognosis for Grade 1 aneurysm patients who are left untreated, questioning the value of operation even late in the management of these lesions. There is little room for argument here. The risk of late (2 to 3 months) recurrent hemorrhage weighed against the risk of operation was notably low. From his studies of SAH patients in Finland, Pakarinen[10] indicated a late mortality of 5% annually for patients at risk during the 2nd through 5th years. This figure is at variance with the findings of Troupp and af Björkesten, who indicated a 10% mortality from recurrent SAH during a 3.5-year period. The difference is believed by the latter authors to be due to the inclusion in Pakarinen's study of "all types of aneurysms, single as well as multiple, operable as well as inoperable, as well as patients in all conditions." To us, it appears that only the presence of multiple aneurysms would be germane to the question of recurrent SAH after the first 2 or 3 months. It is evident that the Troupp and af Björkesten[7] study is one of an unusually select group of patients whose overall mortality was high (in the range of 50%) and excluded by the natural aspect of the disease process that portion of the population which they analyzed selectively. Under such circumstances, comparisons with the present study are not valid. Most investigators accept the statistics of Winn et al. reporting a 2.5 to 3% mortality per year. At this time, an accurate prediction of the course of an individual aneurysm which has ruptured once is not possible. Operation is made to prevent a recurrent hemorrhage. If there were some way of knowing if an aneurysm would rebleed and if it did, when it would do so, there would be no problem in making a decision as to whether the patient should or should not be operated upon. This is the crux of the matter.

Summary

1. During the interval from June 15, 1963, through February 15, 1970, 274 patients with a single intracranial aneurysm were randomly allocated to intracranial surgery. Fifty patients had the aneurysm located on the internal carotid artery, 38 on the middle cerebral artery, 180 on the anterior cerebral-anterior communicating complex and 6 on the vertebral-basilar system. In this group, 132 were males and 142 were females.

2. Forty patients had no surgical procedure. Thirty-two (80%) died. Due to paucity of cases, the analysis of patients with a vertebral-basilar aneurysm was suspended following an accumulation of 6 patients with an aneurysm at this site. The remaining 228 patients had an aneurysm on the anterior portion of the circle of Willis. Overall mortality during the 9.5-year period was 36.8%.

3. Among 84 deaths, 15 were unrelated to operation and in 2 the cause was unknown. In the remaining 67, 48 died with progressive cerebral deterioration following the surgical procedure, and 16 as a result of rebleeding. One each died following cerebral embolism, pneumonia and myocardial infarction, respectively, within 2 weeks of operation. These 67 deaths (29.4%) were considered failures of intracranial surgery.

4. Overall mortality for patients with an internal carotid aneurysm was 46.7%, 35.3% for the middle cerebral group, and 34.2% for the anterior cerebral complex.

5. Mortality in patients operated on within 14 days from last bleed was 44.5%; for those operated on beyond the 14-day interval it was 23.2%.

6. Neurologic condition was good (Grades 1 and 2) in 73.7% at the time of allocation to surgical treatment. Mortality was higher in relation to poor neurologic condition. Increased mortality was also associated with fair to poor preoperative medical conditions and advanced age. Pre-existing hypertension was the most frequent medical condition (21.1%). Patients in good medical condition had a 29.2% mortality; for those in fair condition it was 44%, and for those in poor condition 69.2%.

7. Fifty percent of patients with an internal carotid aneurysm had localized or diffuse vasospasm, whereas for those with

a middle cerebral aneurysm it was 44.7%, and 35.2% for those with an anterior cerebral aneurysm. Increased frequency of vasospasm was directly associated with severity of neurologic condition and interval from last bleed to the time of angiography. No significant relationship in frequency of vasospasm and level of systolic or mean blood pressure was observed.

8. The degree of cerebral vasospasm had no appreciable influence on mortality. Mortality among patients with no angiographic evidence of vasospasm was 38.7%, where vasospasm was localized it was 37%, and in the diffuse category, 29%.

9. Proved rebleeding prior to admission to the reporting hospital occurred 2 or more times in 24.4% of patients with an internal carotid aneurysm, 23.5% with middle cerebral aneurysm and 17.4% with anterior cerebral aneurysm.

10. Most patients (42.1%) had ligation or clip occlusion of the aneurysm neck, 17.1% had investment of the aneurysm by various materials, 10.1% had proximal ligation in continuity with the parent vessel. A group of 18% had more than one specific technical procedure done to the aneurysm at operation.

11. Mortality among patients in whom urea was used as a hyperosmolar surgical adjunct alone or in combination with other agents was 33.8%. Mortality in those who had other means of controlling intracranial pressure such as hyperventilation or mannitol was 11.4% and 14.1%, respectively. In those where no adjuncts were used, it was 14%.

12. Mortality in patients who received moderate hypothermia was 26.4%; in those with no hypothermia it was 14.2%. Postoperative mortality in those patients who received no drug-induced hypotension during surgery was 17.8%; in those who received hypotensive drugs it was 23.4%.

13. Postoperative events characterized by coma, stupor, behavioral disorder, confusion, convulsions, aphasia, hemiparesis or hemiplegia were found in 47.8%.

14. Postoperative complications such as infections, pulmonary or myocardial infarctions, diabetes insipidus and diabetes mellitus occurred in 42.2% of patients with an internal carotid aneurysm, 33.4% of the middle cerebral group and 49% with an aneurysm on the anterior cerebral complex.

15. Following 228 operations, 8.3% had a proved or suspected rebleeding episode. There were 16 deaths from a rebleed in this group (7%). One additional patient died later following progressive deterioration.

16. In 40 patients who had significant bleeding from the aneurysm during operation, 15 (37.5%) died within 14 days following operation.

References

1. Dandy, W.E.: Intracranial Arterial Aneurysms. Comstock Publishing Co., Inc., Ithaca, NY, 1944.
2. Graf, C.J.:Results of direct attack on nonfistulous intracranial aneurysms with remarks on statistics. J. Neurosurg 12:146–153, 1955.
3. Sahs, A.L., Perret, G., Locksley, H.B., et al. (eds): Intracranial Aneurysms and Subarachnoid Hemorrhage: A Cooperative Study. J.B. Lippincott Co., Philadelphia, 1969.
4. McKissock, W., Richardson, A., Walsh, L.: Middle cerebral aneurysms. Further results in the controlled trial of conservative and surgical treatment of ruptured intracranial aneurysms. Lancet 2:417–421, 1962.
5. McKissock, W., Richardson, A., Walsh, L.: "Posterior-communicating" aneurysms. A controlled trial of the conservative and surgical treatment of ruptured aneurysms of the internal carotid artery at or near the point of origin of the posterior communicating artery. Lancet 1:1203–1206, 1960.
6. McKissock, W., Paine, K.W.E., Walsh, L.: An analysis of the results of treatment of ruptured intracranial aneurysms; report of 772 consecutive cases. J. Neurosurg 17:762–776, 1960.
7. Troupp, H., af Björkesten, G.: Results of a controlled trial of late surgical versus conservative treatment of intracranial arterial aneurysms. J. Neurosurg 35:20–24, 1971.

8. Pool, J.: Bifrontal craniotomy for anterior communicating artery aneurysms. J. Neurosurg 30:212–220, 1972.

9. Krayenbühl, H.A., Yasargil, M.G., Flamm, E.S., et al.: Microsurgical treatment of intracranial saccular aneurysms. J. Neurosurg 37:678–685, 1972.

10. Pakarinen, S.: Incidence, aetiology, and prognosis of primary subarachnoid haemorrhage. Acta Neurol Scand (Suppl 29):1–128, 1967.

11. Winn, R.H., Richardson, A.E., Jane, J.A.: Late morbidity and mortality in cerebral aneurysms: a ten-year follow-up study of 364 conservatively treated patients with a single cerebral aneurysm. Trans Am Neurol Assoc 98:148–149, 1973.

Chapter 10

Cooperative Aneurysm Study. Long-term Follow-up Evaluation of Randomized Study

Carl J. Graf, M.D., James C. Torner, M.S., George E. Perret, M.D., Ph.D. and Donald W. Nibbelink, M.D., Ph.D.

Abstract

A 10-year follow-up evaluation was made of 972 patients who were treated for a single ruptured aneurysm on the anterior portion of the circle of Willis. The study was designed to compare mortality and rebleeding among patients allocated randomly to four treatments: (1) regulated bed rest, (2) drug-induced hypotension, (3) carotid ligation and (4) intracranial surgery.

The most common cause of death in the regulated bed rest and drug-induced hypotension groups was rebleeding. For patients who had intracranial operation, death was most commonly due to postoperative complications. In patients who had carotid ligation, the most common cause of death was early (3 months) recurrent hemorrhage.

The frequency of rebleeding was highest during the first 3 months of follow-up in all categories of treatment. The distribution was highest for regulated bed rest (34.3%) and lowest for intracranial operation (16.4%). It was 25.4% for carotid ligation and 28.5% for drug-induced hypotension. Beyond the 6-month interval, rebleeding and mortality remained nearly the same for all treatment categories.

Introduction

The original plan of the Cooperative Aneurysm Study (Phase I), "Report on the Cooperative Study on Intracranial Aneurysms and Subarachnoid Hemorrhage,"[11] was a collection of patients with a recently ruptured intracranial aneurysm treated by surgical and nonsurgical methods. It produced a comprehensive analysis of the problem of spontaneous subarachnoid hemorrhage. The best known reference on the natural history of subarachnoid hemorrhage, especially from a ruptured aneurysm, this monograph was analyzed in detail and has been quoted widely. It was hoped that the study would provide an answer to the question: How are aneurysms that have bled best managed? However, despite an intensive and discriminating analysis of a ponderous amount of information, the final answer was not obtained.

During the early phase of the Cooperative Aneurysm Study, strong opinions and biases were expressed on the "proper" or "best" treatment of ruptured intracranial aneurysms. Examination of the results revealed sobering facts on various methods of treatment. It soon became evident that closer cooperation among investigators and improved study design were necessary to achieve more conclusive results. Because the conditions under which this large number of patients were treated and the number of variables relating to the problem were not the same, a comparative treatment study was proposed to offer a solution to the problem of aneurysm therapy.

The purpose of the Randomized Study[4] was to compare the various available treatments for ruptured intracranial aneurysm at 1 month, 3 months, 6 months and yearly up to 5 years, with an optimal follow-up evaluation up to 10 years. This study, designated as Phase II of the Cooperative Study, was designed so that patients were allocated randomly to one of four treatment categories: (1) regulated bed rest, (2) drug-induced hypotension, (3) common carotid artery ligation and (4) intracranial operation.

Clinical Material

A total of 972 patients from 15 participating institutions comprised the four treatment groups. Two hundred and two patients were allocated to regulated bed rest and 309 to drug-induced hypotension. In the surgical category, 187 patients were allocated to carotid artery ligation and 274 to intracranial operation. The results of treatment by intracranial surgery and regulated bed rest have been published.[3,5]

The interval of follow-up and the number of patients in each category of treatment followed for 3 months to 10 years are shown in Table 10–1. It is evident that a greater number of patients were followed in the ear-

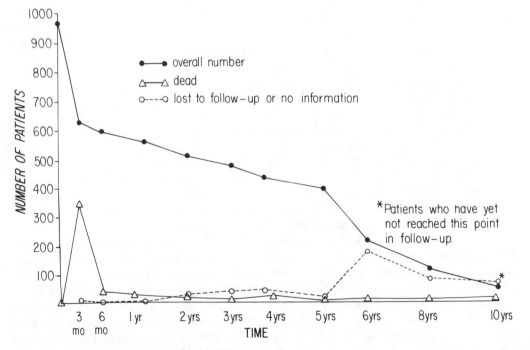

Fig. 10–1.   Total number of patients followed (10-yr period).

lier periods after treatment was completed. A fall-off of patients available for follow-up occurred at the 5-year interval.

In Figure 10–1, the distribution of all patients (972) in this study who were followed from 3 months to 10 years is represented. During the first 3 months, there was a sharp drop in the number of patients eligible for follow-up evaluation due to death in one third of the patients. This figure represents a gross mortality related to the effects of subarachnoid hemorrhage and/or treatment. During the interval between 3 months and 5 years, an average of 40 patients per year were lost by death or by failure of follow-up. Between the 5th and 10th (especially in the 6th) years, the largest number of patients was lost to follow-up (33% of the total number in the study). The outcome of 467 patients (48%) is not known, because one half of the participants withdrew from the study for one reason or another. One hundred and forty-four patients (14.8%) have not reached the 10-year point in the follow-up. For ready reference, the number of patients followed at specific time intervals is recorded in tabular form (Table 10–1).

Loss to Follow-up

Follow-up evaluations could not be obtained in 2% (12 of 643) of the surviving patients at the 3-month period; at 6 months, 3% (19 of 618) could not be evaluated; at 1 year, 5% (30 of 598); at 5 years, 27% (144 of 537); and at 10 years, 90% (467 of 519). This included 134 patients who have not reached a 10-year post-hemorrhage interval. In those patients treated by regulated bed rest (Fig. 10–2), outcome status is known at 3 months for 99%, at 6 months for 99%, at 1 year for 97%, at 5 years for 80% and at 10 years for 61%. For the group who had drug-induced hypotension (Figure 10–3),status is known for 99% (3 months), 97% (6 months), 97% (1 year), 85% (5 years) and 51% (10 years). Carotid ligation (Fig. 10–4) patients had complete follow-up of 98% at 3 months, 98% at 6 months, 97% at 1 year, 83% at 5 years and 47% at 10 years. Patients undergoing intracranial surgery (Fig. 10–5) were available for complete follow-up at the rates of 99% at 3 months, 98% at 6 months, 97% at 1 year, 85% at 5 years and 50% at 10 years.

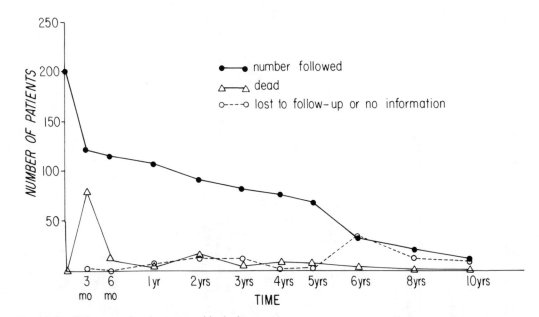

Fig. 10–2.   Follow-up of patients treated by bed rest.

Table 10–1. Number of Patients Followed.

		Follow-up Interval									
		3 months	6 months	1 year	2 years	3 years	4 years	5 years	6 years	8 years	10 years
Bed Rest (202)*	Followed	121	115	107	91	82	76	68	32	20	11
	Died	79‡	6	3	9	3	5	5	2	0	0
	Lost to follow-up or no information	2	0	5	7	6	1	3	34	12	9
Drug-Induced Hypotension (309)	Followed	202	192	182	168	152	131	125	57	38	14
	Died	104	5	9	5	6	7	1	4	1	1
	Lost to follow-up or no information	3	5	1	9	10	14	5	64	18	23
Carotid Ligation (187)	Followed	124	123	118	112	105	94	87	55	34	14
	Died	60	1	3	1	1	1	1	1	2	2
	Lost to follow-up or no information	3	0	2	5	6	10	6	31	19	18
Intracranial Surgery (274)	Followed	184	169	161	150	138	121	113	61	30	13
	Died	86	13	5	4	2	6	4	2	3	0
	Lost to follow-up or no information	4	2	3	7	10	11	4	50	28	17
Overall (972)	Followed	631	599	568	521	477	422	393	205	122	52
	Died	329	25	20	19	12	19	11	9	6	3
	Lost to follow-up or no information	12	7	11	28	32	36	18	179	77†	67†

* Number of patients randomized into the treatment category and not disqualified.
† Pertains to those who have not reached this point in this follow-up history.
‡ Deaths in this table include those dying during the period when a follow-up was due.

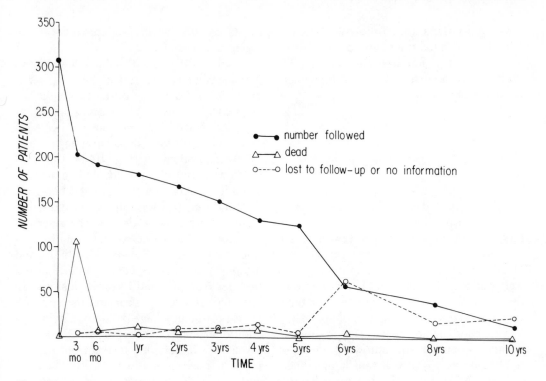

Fig. 10–3.   Follow-up of patients treated by drug-induced hypotension.

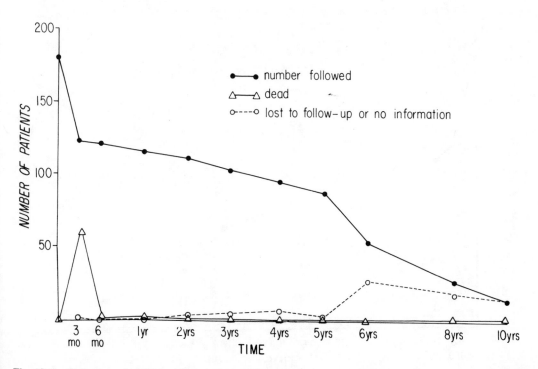

Fig. 10–4.   Follow-up of patients treated by carotid ligation.

Hence, comparable follow-up was obtained for each treatment group, but beyond 5 years after randomization, considerable dropout had occurred due to declining center participation.

Mortality

Death is reported in the analysis based on information provided by the reporting centers and verified by autopsy reports when postmortem examination was carried out. Death in the immediate treatment period was primarily the result of (1) a progressive deterioration of central nervous system functions associated with the pathology of the subarachnoid hemorrhage, (2) a progressive decline associated with untoward effects of treatment and (3) a recurrent hemorrhagic episode. After 6 months, recurrent hemorrhage remained a major cause of death, but causes of death unrelated to the aneurysm or its treatment became apparent in the group under study.

Death associated with subarachnoid hemorrhage can be characterized by two phases, early and late. The majority of deaths occurred within the initial 3 months post-hemorrhage. Thirty-three percent (323 of 972) of the patients were dead prior to the first follow-up evaluation (Fig. 10–1). Cause of death was primarily a recurrent hemorrhage in patients allocated to regulated bed rest, drug-induced hypotension and carotid artery ligation. Progressive decline characterized the mortality of those patients who had intracranial surgery. Between 3 months and 6 months another 31 deaths occurred, and between 6 months and 1 year 22 deaths were reported. Between 1 year and the end of 5 years post-hemorrhage (study-qualifying) 59 additional deaths were reported. Death after 1 year was largely due to recurrent hemorrhage in those patients who received bed rest and drug-induced hypotension, and to unrelated causes in those treated by carotid ligation and intracranial operation.

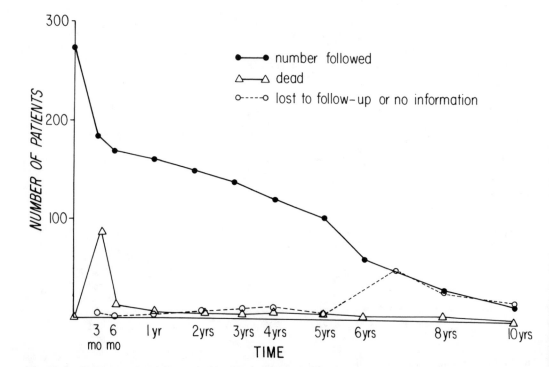

Fig. 10–5.   Follow-up of patients treated by intracranial operation.

Table 10–2. Long-Term Mortality Associated with Bed Rest Therapy.

Time from Bleed	No. of Deaths	Mortality Rate* for Each Interval	Cause of Death				
			Complications of Treatment	Proved Rebleed	Suspected Rebleed	Unrelated Event	Unknown
0–3 months	78	38.8%	13	54	7	2	2
3–6 months	7	5.8%	1	3	2	1	0
½–1 year	3	2.7%	1	1	0	0	1
1–2 years	10	9.7%	0	4	0	3	3
2–3 years	3	3.0%	0	2	0	1	0
3–4 years	5	6.1%	0	3	0	1	1
4–5 years	4	5.7%	0	1	2	1	0
	5-year rate	56.5%					
5–6 years	2	4.2%	1	0	0	1	0
6–8 years	0	0.0%	0	0	0	0	0
8–10 years	0	0.0%	0	0	0	0	0
	10-year rate	58.3%					

* Adjusted for loss-to-follow-up.

Bed Rest Therapy

Table 10–2 presents the mortality findings for the follow-up period. Proved rebleeds characterized the natural history of this group. Of the deaths occurring within 3 months after the hemorrhage for which the patient was admitted to the study, 78% were due to proved or suspected rebleeds (71% for those from 3 to 6 months, and 52% from 6 months through 5 years). Causes of death from unrelated or accessory events were (in sequence that patients died): bronchopneumonia, pneumonia, pulmonary edema, pneumonia, carcinoma of prostate, bronchopneumonia, other CNS disease, myocardial infarction and motor accident. The mortality rate for 5 years for this study group was 56.5% (adjusted by life table methods for loss-to-follow-up).

Drug-Induced Hypotension Therapy

Among patients allocated to drug-induced hypotension, death was generally associated with recurrent hemorrhage (Table 10–3). Seventy percent (70%) of deaths in the first 3 months were due to proved or suspected

Table 10–3. Long-Term Mortality Associated With Drug-Induced Hypotension Therapy.

Time from Bleed	No. of Deaths	Mortality Rate* for Each Interval	Cause of Death				
			Complications of Treatment	Proved Rebleed	Suspected Rebleed	Unrelated Event	Unknown
0–3 months	104	33.8%	19	59	14	7	5
3–6 months	5	2.5%	1	0	0	2	2
½–1 year	9	4.7%	1	4	2	2	0
1–2 years	6	3.4%	1	3	0	2	0
2–3 years	6	3.8%	0	2	1	2	1
3–4 years	6	4.2%	0	2	3	1	0
4–5 years	1	0.8%	0	1	0	0	0
	5-year rate	48.3%					
5–6 years	4	4.9%	0	0	2	2	0
6–8 years	1	2.5%	0	0	0	1	0
8–10 years	1	5.6%	0	0	0	1	0
	10-year rate	52.5%					

* Adjusted for loss-to-follow-up.

rebleeding. No deaths were recorded from the same causes between 3 and 6 months. However, rebleeding was indicated as the major cause of death for 65% of deaths in the 6-month to 5-year interval. Deaths due to separate events or those unrelated to subarachnoid hemorrhage in chronological order included: vertebral-basilar artery thrombosis, gastrointestinal bleeding, bilateral pulmonary embolism, myocardial infarction (2 patients), pneumonia, ventricular fibrillation during anesthesia, pneumonia, acute cardiac insufficiency, suicide, inanition, renal failure, acute pyelonephritis, multiple myeloma, lung cancer, and bronchitis-emphysema-heart failure. The 5-year mortality rate for this treatment-defined group was 48.3%.

Carotid Ligation Therapy

Mortality within the first 3 months for patients having carotid ligation was also predominantly from recurrent hemorrhage (62% of deaths). However, after the initial treatment period only 1 death due to a suspected rebleed was reported (Table 10-4). Causes of death for patients reported dying of accessory or unrelated events were pulmonary emboli, cardiopulmonary arrest, frontal lobe hematoma, bilateral pyoarthritis, hematuria-septicemia, hemolytic anemia, pneumonia, uremic encephalopathy, renal failure, systemic lupus erythematosus, myocardial infarction, suicide, coronary thrombosis, and myocardial infarction, respectively. The 5-year death rate for patients allocated to carotid ligation was 36.5%.

Intracranial Surgery Therapy

Death associated with progressive decline was reported in 50 patients (60% of 83 deaths in the first 3 months) (Table 10-5). Recurrent hemorrhage accounted for 30% of the deaths during the early period. Rebleeding continued as a major cause of death for patients allocated to this group throughout 4 years. Unrelated events were reported as follows (in sequence that patients died): respiratory arrest and cardiovascular collapse, primary hypertensive hemorrhage, myocardial infarction, bronchopneumonia, gastrointestinal bleeding, pneumonia, pulmonary embolism (3 patients), pyelonephritis, respiratory infection, diabetes, lung cancer, bronchopneumonia, cardiac arrest, cerebral embolism, metastatic cancer and congestive heart failure, myocardial infarction (3 patients), congestive heart failure, cerebral edema, pneumonia, lung cancer, bronchopneumonia, myocardial infarction (2 patients), gangrene of leg, bronchopneumonia and coronary thrombosis. The overall

Table 10-4.   Long-Term Mortality Associated With Carotid Ligation Therapy.

Time from Bleed	No. of Deaths	Mortality Rate* for Each Interval	Cause of Death				
			Complications of Treatment	Proved Rebleed	Suspected Rebleed	Unrelated Event	Unknown
0–3 months	58	31.3%	18	24	12	4	0
3–6 months	3	2.4%	1	0	0	1	1
½–1 year	5	3.3%	1	0	2	2	0
1–2 years	0	0.0%	0	0	0	0	0
2–3 years	1	0.9%	0	0	0	1	0
3–4 years	1	1.0%	0	0	0	1	0
4–5 years	1	1.1%	0	0	0	0	1
		5-year rate 36.5%					
5–6 years	1	1.5%	0	0	0	1	0
6–8 years	2	5.1%	0	0	0	2	0
8–10 years	2	10.8%	0	0	0	2	0
		10-year rate 47.0%					

* Adjusted for loss-to-follow-up.

Table 10–5. Long-Term Mortality Associated with Intracranial Surgery Therapy.

Time from Bleed	No. of Deaths	Mortality Rate* for Each Interval	Cause of Death				
			Complications of Treatment	Proved Rebleed	Suspected Rebleed	Unrelated Event	Unknown
0–3 months	83	30.4%	50	20	5	8	0
3–6 months	16	8.5%	7	1	1	6	1
½–1 year	6	3.6%	2	2	1	1	0
1–2 years	3	1.9%	0	0	2	1	0
2–3 years	3	2.1%	0	2	0	1	0
3–4 years	5	3.8%	0	1	1	3	0
4–5 years	4	3.6%	0	0	0	4	0
	5-year rate	45.3%					
5–6 years	2	2.6%	0	0	0	2	0
6–8 years	3	7.3%	0	2	0	0	1
8–10 years	1	5.6%	0	0	0	0	2
	10-year rate	53.4%					

* Adjusted for loss-to-follow-up.

5-year mortality rate for this group was 45.3%.

Recurrent Hemorrhage

The incidence of rebleeding was greatest in the first 3 months of follow-up. Eighty-seven percent of the rebleeds occurring in the first 5 years were reported during the initial time period (Table 10–6). Bed rest therapy was associated with the highest rebleed rate (34.3%) for the early period and intracranial surgery the lowest (16.4%). Recurrent hemorrhages for bed rest were approximately 3% per year, for drug-induced hypotension approximately 2% per year, for intracranial surgery approximately 1% per year and for carotid ligation 0% per year after the initial 3-month period. At the end of 5 years, 45% of the bed rest patients, 36% of drug-induced hypotension patients, 25% of carotid ligation patients and 19% of intracranial surgery patients had suffered a recurrent bleed.

Source of Information Related to Treatment and Credibility of Follow-up Information

Information regarding patients during the period of follow-up evaluation was derived from five sources. Information was either

Table 10–6. Long-Term Rates of Recurrent Hemorrhage for Each Treatment Category.

Time from Bleed to Treatment	Bed Rest		Drug-Induced Hypotension		Carotid Ligation		Intracranial Surgery	
	Proved Rebleeds	Rate*	Proved Rebleeds	Rate	Proved Rebleeds	Rate	Proved Rebleeds	Rate
0–3 months	65	34.3%	82	28.5%	44	25.4%	40	16.4%
3–6 months	2	1.8%	1	0.6%	0	0.0%	1	0.6%
½–1 year	2	2.0%	4	2.3%	0	0.0%	1	0.6%
1–2 years	4	4.3%	3	1.9%	0	0.0%	0	0.0%
2–3 years	2	2.5%	3	2.1%	0	0.0%	2	1.5%
3–4 years	3	4.0%	2	1.6%	0	0.0%	1	0.8%
4–5 years	2	3.2%	2	1.8%	0	0.0%	0	0.0%
5-year total	80	45.2%	97	35.6%	44	25.4%	45	19.3%

* Adjusted for loss-to-follow-up and loss-to-death.

"direct," that is, either from the patients themselves at the time of an examination at the reporting center, or it was "indirect," when the patient himself did not respond for some reason. This failure to respond may have been because of a physical or neurologic disability, e.g., he may have been unable to report for examination to the center at which he was treated, or he may have been unable to write or to talk. "Indirect" information came through a physician, a relative of the patient, a social worker or "other." Responses were sometimes from more than one source.

The greatest percentage of follow-up responses in all treatment categories was direct, i.e., from the patients themselves. Information was next highest from "other" sources, i.e., telephone or letter. At 3 months, information was supplied directly (examination at the reporting hospital), varying from a high of 88.7% for patients who had carotid ligation to a low of 81.5% for those who had intracranial operation. The percentages of responses from bed rest and drug-induced hypotension-treated patients were 87.6 and 85.6%, respectively. Information from "other" sources ranged from a high of 16.3% for the intracranial surgery group to a low of 8.1% for the carotid ligation group. The percentages for regulated bed rest and drug-induced hypotension patients were between these values. The source for "direct" (patient) information (from 3 months through 3 years) was in the 85% range for those treated by regulated bed rest, drug-induced hypotension and carotid ligation. At the 5-year follow-up, "direct" (patient) information was obtained in 77.9% of patients treated with bed rest, 75.2% by drug-induced hypotension and 79.3% by carotid ligation. The lowest percentage of "direct" information was noted among the intracranial surgery-treated patients, with a response rate of 81% at 3 months, dropping progressively to 73.5% at 5 years.

The trend of reference for "indirect" patient information was reversed from the 3rd month progressively through the 5-year period of evaluation. For bed rest-treated patients, it ranged from a low of 2.5% at 3 months to 21% at 5 years; for those who had drug-induced hypotension, from a low of 4% at 3 months to 19% at 5 years. The differences were less among those who had carotid ligation, with a low of 4.8% at 3 months to 9.2% at 5 years; whereas for patients who had an intracranial operation, the figure was 3.8% at 3 months and 13.3% at 5 years. The contribution of information from "other" sources was low among all treatments except for the intracranial surgery group. This information ranged from 2.5% at 3 months to 1.5% at 5 years in the bed rest-treated group and 3.5% at 3 months to 7.2% at 5 years among drug-induced hypotension-treated patients. For those who had carotid ligation, the figure was virtually the same—5.6% at 3 months to 5.7% at 5 years. For those who had an intracranial operation, the percentage ranged from a high of 16.3% at 3 months to a low of 9.7% at 5 years.

It appeared that as a patient's condition became stable, he declined to visit the examining center after the 3rd year and referred requests for follow-up information to his physician and "other" sources.

Results

Change in Condition from Previous Report Related to Treatment

A graphic demonstration of the change in the condition of bed rest-treated patients (121) at the time of the respective follow-up intervals is shown in Figure 10–6. The change in the condition of the patient ("improved," "unchanged," "worse") is illustrated in terms of the percentage of patients who were in the designated condition at the follow-up period. The trend for improvement declines from 3 months over the 5-year period of follow-up. There is a corresponding progressive rise in the percentage of patients who show no change, this rise peaking gradually at 3 years and remaining so thereafter. The rate of change to a worse condi-

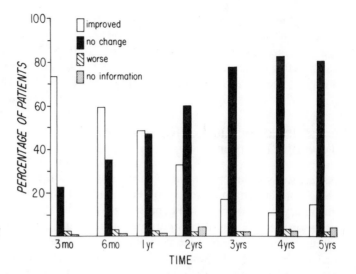

Fig. 10–6. Change in condition of
bed rest-treated patients.

tion remains essentially unchanged from
2.5% at 3 months to 1.5% at 5 years, with
a peak of 3.9% at 4 years.

Figure 10–7 depicts the change in condition in the 202 patients who were treated
with drug-induced hypotension. The trend
is substantially the same among the patients
in this category as in the bed rest-treated
group. The number who became worse during the 5 years is a little higher, reflecting,
it appears, the larger number of patients in
this category, although the percentage designated as "worse" was 5.4% at 3 months
and 5.6% at 5 years, with a lower (1.2 to
2.6%) percentage between these dates.

The picture is much the same in the 124
patients who had carotid ligation (Fig. 10–8).
The tendency for improvement falls off
rather sharply after the 2nd year of follow-
up, with corresponding rises in the percentage of patients who have reached a plateau
as far as neurologic improvement is concerned.

Patients available for follow-up in the intracranial surgery treatment category numbered 184. The pattern was similar to that
seen in the other treatment groups (Fig.
10–9). After 3 years, approximately 12 to
14% of the patients were described as showing some improvement, a trend noted also

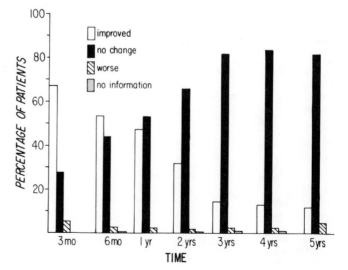

Fig. 10–7. Change in condition of
patients treated with drug-induced hypotension.

in the other treatment categories. The decline in the number showing improvement was conspicuous between 6 months and 2 years. After the 2nd, but especially after the 3rd year, there was little improvement.

Neurologic Evaluation Related to Type of Treatment

As this study is directed to the eventual outcome of treatment in patients who have had an aneurysmal subarachnoid hemorrhage, it is important to know their neurologic condition at various times following the hemorrhagic event that led to their hospital admission. The neurologic condition would reflect the complications of the initial hemorrhage, the result of a recurrent hemorrhage, the complications of a particular treatment or intercurrent neurologic disease, e.g., a "stroke." The neurologic condition of the patient was determined by the evaluation of basic sensory and motor activity, behavioral patterns and integrity of speech and memory (Table 10–7).

Bed Rest Therapy

At 3 months in the bed rest-treated patients, the findings listed as the first four items (Group A) were noted to be "normal," in the range of 98.3% of the patients (corneal protective response) to 94% (response to verbal stimuli), with the other two between these percentages. Specifically, it means that of 118 patients evaluated at this time (3 of the 121 in this group were not evaluated), 1.7% did not elicit a corneal protective response. Parenthetically, it should be noted that a patient designated as "not evaluated" was not actually examined by a physician, but that information regarding the follow-up findings was obtained via the specific center by telephone or letter. For Group B signs, the range of capability of speech reception and speech emission was 89.3 to 91.4%, respectively. In Group C, 93.6% were indicated as having no difficulty. Disturbed social behavior, however, was evident in 9.4%, and motor limb function indicated under E and G ranged between 90.5 to 97.2%, respectively. Stereognostic sense was preserved in 98% (right side) and 97.2% (left side).

At 6 months, the responses in Group A were normal in 97%; in B, normal in 92.8%; in C, 94.8%; in D, 92.9%. The range was 91 to 96.7% in E and G, respectively, and 93 to 100% in F.

When the 1-year evaluation was made, a similar percentage of "normal" examinations was observed as at the 6-month period. At 2 years there was no change in the percentage of patients with normal examinations for group A, a 2.7% greater percentage for B, 3.3% greater for C, and 2% greater

Table 10–7.   Definition of Assessment of Neurologic Condition.

A	B	C	D	E	F	G
Corneal protective response	Speech reception and speech emission	Recall and orientation	Propriety of social behavior	Crude involuntary limb power (right side)	Stereognosis (right side)	Prehension (right side)
Response to deep pain				Crude involuntary limb power (left side)	Stereognosis (left side)	Prehension (left side)
Response to limb drop						
Response to verbal stimuli						

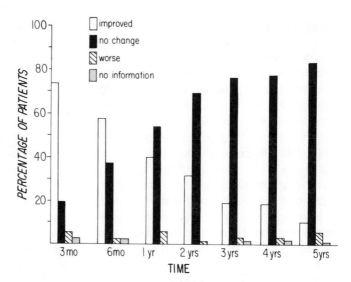

Fig. 10–8.   Change in condition of patients treated with carotid ligation.

for D neurologic signs. For group E, a 10% increase was noted whereas for F it was 1.6% less. Considering the variability regarding differences in numbers of patients examined, there was virtually no change at the end of 5 years. At that time, 100% of patients had normal examinations for group A signs, whereas in the other groups the percentage ranged from 2.1% to 6.4% in one or another of the modalities tested.

From 6 months to 5 years there was a very small increase (1% to 2%) in the number of patients who had normal examinations, so that at 5 years, 100% who were evaluated were described as "normal" for group A signs. Four tenths of 1% (0.4%) had less speech perception (97.9% were normal) than at 4 years, but 1.3% (97.9% were normal) had greater speech emission at 5 than at 4 years. These small differences, we believe, reflect differences in interpretation of the neurological examination and differences in the number of patients examined. The fact remains, however, that at 5 years, 100% of patients were not neurologically normal. At 8 years, 7 patients were evaluated, all of whom were considered to have normal examinations.

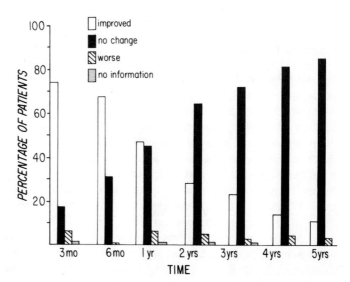

Fig. 10–9.   Change in condition of patients treated by intracranial operation.

Drug-Induced Hypotension

At the first (3 months) check, protocol information revealed that in the neurological examination, 40 patients (of 202 in the follow-up) did not have tests of stereognostic sense made of either side; as many as 38 were not tested for functions of orientation and recall. This indicates that an incomplete examination was made according to the protocol. It might also mean that the patient's mentation was so severely disturbed to interfere with such a specialized test; this may also be suggested by the failure of evaluation for recall and orientation in the 38 alluded to above. For Group A signs, there was a trend toward a normal examination in 4 to 8% during the ensuing 5 years. For Group B evaluation, the change was similar, but at 5 years 7 to 10% still had abnormal findings referable to the specific examination. Less difference was reported in examination of Group C signs, with a change from normal in 93.9% at 3 months to 96.4% at 5 years. In Group E, there was a fall for "crude limb movement—left side" from 91.6% with a normal examination at 3 months to 90.7% at 5 years; whereas "prehension—left hand" improved from 90.9% with a normal examination at 3 months to 94% of the patients at 5 years. The stereognosis category changed little.

Carotid Ligation

By and large, at the 3-month evaluation the percentage of normal examinations was little different for those patients treated by carotid ligation (2 to 3%) than in the other treatment categories. There was a slightly lower percentage with normal speech as compared to patients treated by bed rest, but it was higher than for drug-induced hypotension-treated patients (1.3%) and especially for those who had intracranial surgery (7 to 8%). Motor limb function was not quite as good as in the bed rest-treated group, about the same as in the drug-induced hypotension

group and considerably higher (4 to 8%) than in the intracranial surgery group of patients.

At 6 months, speech was improved in all treatment groups (10% greater for speech emission in those patients who had intracranial operation). At 1 year, all of the 98 patients evaluated had normal Group A symptom-sign examinations. In speech reception, the percentage of patients with normal function was about the same for all treatment groups (93 to 96%) and was about the same for intracranial surgery. However, for speech emission, the percent normal was greater for the medically treated than the carotid ligation-treated patients. The number of patients with normal voluntary limb function remained less than for prehensile activity, a finding which is difficult to reconcile. The recall and orientation percentage increased 4.2%, from 92.6% at 3 months to 96.8% at 1 year.

At 2 years, Group A responses were 100% normal in carotid ligation-treated patients, and neurologic function improved in all areas tested. After 2 years, there was little change; only small differences in the percentage of patients with normal neurologic examinations were observed. However, the percentage of disturbances in voluntary motor function remained about the same, whereas prehensile function improved and was disproportionately greater than voluntary motor activity. This is difficult to understand, because the inferences are that there was some degree of paresis which would be a measure of disturbed hand function.

Intracranial Surgery

One hundred and eighty-four patients who were treated by intracranial operation were available for the first (3 months) evaluation; 86 died from the time of randomization and 4 were lost to follow-up examination. There was a disturbingly high percentage of patients who did not have normal examinations. In the Group A portion of the neurologic evaluation, 8.1 and 12.1% of the patients had impaired response to deep pain and verbal stimuli, respectively. Speech difficulty was observed in 18 to 19%, and symptoms referable to frontal and temporal lobe function were shown to be similarly high in 17 to 18% of patients. There was a closer relationship of voluntary limb function to prehensile power in the patients treated by intracranial surgery; about 17 and 13%, respectively, did not have normal examinations. These findings imply a substantial impairment of cerebral function. Whether this was due primarily to the effects of the subarachnoid hemorrhage, the surgical procedure, or both, is not determined from the gross figures themselves, but they suggest that both are accountable.

At 6 months, improvement was noted in all aspects of the examination, especially in the percentage of patients with normal speech and limb function. There was an average 2 to 3% improvement rate at 1 year over the 6-month evaluation, and this rate continued until a relative plateau was reached at 2 years. At 5 years, approximately 6% of patients still did not have normal speech and about the same percentage had impaired social behavior. The disparity of patients with disturbed voluntary limb power (approximately 9%) in contrast to 100% with normal hand activity was again noted.

Generally, at the 3-month period the largest percentage of patients who did not have a normal neurologic evaluation was in the intracranial surgery treatment category. After 2 years only minor differences of the percentage of normal examinations among patients in the four treatment categories were evident. There were obvious differences in the number of patients evaluated, a situation which must be recognized as influencing the analysis. For example, at 5 years, 47 to 48 patients in the bed rest-treated category, 83 to 86 allocated to drug-induced hypotension, 56 to 59 delegated to carotid ligation and 64 to 70 to intracranial surgery were evaluated. The spread in the figures in each category may be a reflection of an incomplete examination.

Follow-up Neurologic Evaluation Related to Neurologic Grade at Time of Randomization

At the 3-month interval in the bed rest-treated patients, the percentage with normal neurologic evaluations was high (96% or more) for those who were in good condition (Grades 1 and 2) at the time of randomization, as compared to, and as expected for, patients in Grades 3, 4 and 5. Except for basic neurologic function (response to pain, response to verbal stimulation, etc.), trends to improvement in Grades 3, 4 and 5 patients were low. In testing higher cerebral function (speech and motor limb activity), the usual percentage of patients with normal function was in the 60 to 70% range. There was a progressive tendency during the next 5 years toward normal function in all patients. However, the percentage came progressively closer to 100% at the 5-year period in Grades 1 and 2 than in Grade 3, 4 and 5 patients. In Grade 3, 4 and 5 patients, it came within the 71 to 85% range for higher neurologic function, whereas the responses to Group A functions occurred in 100% of the patients examined. At 5 years, only 7 patients were evaluated. The state was much the same for the drug-induced hypotension and carotid ligation-treated groups. The ratio of good grade (1, 2) to poor grade (3, 4, 5) condition patients was 4 or 5 to 1 in the treatment categories listed above. For the intracranial surgery category, the percent normal at 3 months was distressingly low (80 to 92%), especially in the evaluation of speech, memory and motor activity, even among the patients in Grades 1 and 2, but particularly so in Grades 3, 4 and 5. The ratio of good grade (1, 2) to poor grade (3, 4, 5) patients was about 2.7 to 1. Among the Grade 1 and Grade 2 patients, the influence of a poor surgical result is evident; the poor condition at follow-up of patients in Grades 3, 4 and 5 indicates both the devastating effect of the hemorrhage and of operation. In Grade 1 and 2 patients, there was a progressive tendency to neurologic improvement, so that at the end of 5 years this reached the 95% level (basic responses were present in 100%). For patients in Grades 3, 4 and 5, a tendency to only slight improvement was apparent, again indicating the permanency of a neurologic deficit which resulted either from the hemorrhage, operation, or both. At that time, moreover, only 10 of the original 46 patients were available for examination.

Incidence of Intercurrent Disease

Following treatment of subarachnoid hemorrhage from a ruptured aneurysm, it is important to determine if the hemorrhage, its treatment, or both, can adversely affect the course of the patient. This will be considered on both a short-term and long-term basis.

During the first 3 to 6 months (short-term), it is expected that the incidence of adverse effects of the disease and its treatment would be greater than at a later date, during which time some degree of recovery is anticipated. The neurologic effects of a destructive intracerebral hematoma, of cerebral ischemia perhaps associated with vasospasm, and the circulatory complications that might attend operation by carotid ligation or intracranial surgery will be most numerous at that time.

In those patients treated "conservatively," that is, by bed rest and drug-induced hypotension over the short-term, the concern is that of recurrent subarachnoid hemorrhage and the complications of prolonged physical inactivity, e.g., thrombophlebitis, pulmonary thromboembolism, pulmonary and urinary tract infections, decubiti and so forth. On the long-term basis, the threat of recurrent subarachnoid hemorrhage is constantly present, since there is no assurance that adequate healing of the ruptured aneurysm has taken place to preclude another rupture. In patients who have had a serious immediate neurologic insult (hemiplegia, prolonged unconsciousness, etc.) as a result of an intracerebral clot or infarction, secondary complications of decubiti and urinary and pulmonary tract infections can be anticipated as short-term or as long-term complications. On a short-term basis in patients who have undergone operation, except for the immediate complications associated with operation, one expects few secondary complications that would tend to become chronic.

Aside from the complications relative to aneurysmal subarachnoid hemorrhage and its treatment (especially in the 3 to 6-month period), one would expect that the attrition from other diseases (cancer, cardiovascular disease, infection, metabolic disorders, etc.) would be much the same as among the general population. In reviewing the problems which beset the patients in this study, we have, therefore, tried to analyze them according to whether they were direct or indirect results of the subarachnoid hemorrhage and its treatment or were unrelated to them and occurring in the natural course of events. We have arbitrarily considered the "short term" as up to 6 months and "long term" as the period thereafter. This then resolves itself into residuals seen at the 3 and 6-month intervals as the direct result of the hemorrhage and/or its treatment. This list would include serious neurologic deficits such as hemiparesis, hemiplegia, speech disturbance, visual field loss, dementia, hydrocephalus, as well as the immediate temporary complications which frequently attend the bed-ridden, incontinent patient who is subject to bronchopneumonia, urinary tract infection and bed sores. Secondly, we attempted to determine the possible latent effects of carotid occlusion on the cerebral circulation. The difficulty in making interpretations or drawing conclusions from this, however, becomes evident. One may have only a very general impression of the degree of cerebrovascular disease that a patient may have had at the time of the original evaluation. The evaluation of progressive vascular disease is at best difficult and is made usually after a long follow-up. In the case of carotid occlusion, one can only speculate on its effects upon the cerebral circulation in a patient who incurred no cerebral insult at the time of operation, particularly if he should develop difficulty many years later.

The analysis of intercurrent illness in patients who incurred a subarachnoid hemorrhage was made upon two groups of disorders. One comprised specific disturbances and included major surgery, malignant disease, serious infection, acute heart disease, major trauma, postoperative hematoma, postoperative infection, transient and permanent cerebrovascular insult and convulsions. The other covered a wider spectrum of medical and surgical problems.

The proportion of patients with intercurrent illnesses was approximately the same in each treatment group (Table 10–8). Permanent cerebrovascular insults and seizures comprised a major portion of each treatment group. Serious infections and major surgery outside of the central nervous system were also characteristic of each group. No treatment group had an unexpected incidence of intercurrent illness which would lead one to suspect serious consequences of the primary treatment at the beginning of the study.

Other medical-surgical conditions or complaints affected 29 patients. Among the bed rest-treated group, this consisted of daily headache in 1, infection as bronchitis and cystitis in another, and renal hypertensive disease in a third. In the drug-induced hypotension group, 2 became alcoholic and 2 had poorly described spells of dizziness and "blackout" (the latter being considered to be of vasovagal nature). Transitory left leg paresthesia was noted in 1 and occasional "flashing lights" with headache in another.

Infections included a case of thrombophlebitis of the left leg. Huntington's chorea developed in 1 patient, another had recurrent severe nosebleeds, and a third required a prostatectomy. Among carotid ligation-treated patients, 2 had severe mental changes, 1 with features suggesting a senile state, the other having considerable deterioration, with disorientation, and disturbed gait and memory. One patient had recurrent dyspepsia, another complained of frequent headache and had a short course of treatment for hypertension. Another who became hypertensive was treated accordingly. One developed right saphenous vein thrombosis and an-

Table 10–8. Number of Reported Intercurrent Illnesses* over Five-Year Period.

	Bed Rest (Years)						Drug-Induced Hypotension (Years)						Carotid Ligation (Years)						Intracranial Surgery (Years)					
	½	1	2	3	4	5	½	1	2	3	4	5	½	1	2	3	4	5	½	1	2	3	4	5
Major surgery	2	0	1	2	3	0	2	1	2	1	2	1	0	1	4	2	0	0	5	0	3	4	4	2
Malignant disease	0	2	2	1	2	0	0	1	0	1	0	0	0	0	0	0	0	0	0	0	0	0	0	1
Serious infection	3	4	1	1	3	0	4	4	3	3	4	1	0	0	1	0	1	0	5	2	2	0	1	1
Acute heart disease	0	0	0	0	1	1	1	0	0	1	1	2	0	0	1	0	0	1	1	0	0	1	1	1
Major trauma	1	0	0	0	1	0	0	0	1	0	0	0	0	0	0	1	0	0	0	0	2	0	2	0
Postoperative hematoma	0	0	0	0	0	0	0	0	0	0	0	0	0	0	0	0	0	0	0	0	0	0	0	0
Postoperative wound infection	0	0	0	0	0	0	0	0	0	0	0	0	0	0	0	0	0	0	0	0	0	0	0	0
Transient cerebral ischemia	0	2	0	3	0	0	3	5	3	5	0	0	2	2	1	0	0	0	3	2	0	2	1	0
Permanent cerebrovascular insult	3	5	2	2	3	1	3	4	3	4	5	5	1	3	3	1	0	0	2	2	0	0	0	1
Seizures	0	1	1	2	0	0	3	5	2	3	1	1	5	5	5	6	4	5	9	7	4	4	3	3
Total	9	14	7	11	13	2	16	20	14	18	13	10	10	15	20	15	10	10	25	21	19	21	17	15

* Illnesses that were observed between follow-up intervals, including illnesses that were prevalent in early period but were unresolved.

other spondylosis. The protocol was deficient in information in 1. There were 3 patients who had intracranial surgery that were mentally impaired (psychosis, severe depression, gross mental incompetence with disorientation). Hypertension developed in 1 and angina in another. Occurring in 1 patient each were intermittent claudication, diabetes mellitus and recurrent epistaxis.

It is important to know the influence of a neurologic deficit resulting from a subarachnoid hemorrhage or its treatment upon the eventual outcome of the patient. Similarly, the effects of treatment of a disease must be weighed against the effects of the natural history of that disease. If any treatment offers no more improvement than can be expected in the natural course of the disease process, then there is no advantage in its use. An attempt. is made here to make such an appraisal, recognizing that we are dealing with groups of patients and that individual patients present special problems. It appeared reasonable to use patients who developed a permanent neurologic defect either from the subarachnoid hemorrhage or the treatment to make the analysis; the time of the insult to death (if it occurred) was considered to be the end point.

Among the 22 bed rest-treated patients who died in the follow-up period, 7 had permanent neurologic insults. One death occurred 8 months after randomization as a result of complications of the treatment. There were 14 deaths from recurrent subarachnoid hemorrhage. Such deaths occurred from 3 to 60 months after assignment to treatment, 5 in an approximate 1.5 to 2-year period, 4 within 10 months and 4 between 38 and 60 months. One death occurred at 51 months from a suspected rebleed. Four deaths were from causes unrelated to SAH and occurred between a 13 to 57-month interval. The cause of death in 2 patients who died at 12 and 18 months, respectively, was unknown. Four developed permanent cerebrovascular deficits during the interval of follow-up, 1 each from a proved and suspected subarachnoid hemorrhage and 2 from unrelated events.

The cause of death in the drug-induced hypotension-treated group of patients was also higher due to recurrent SAH in 12 instances; 4 occurring between 7 to 12 months and 3 between 18 to 23 months. Two deaths were noted between the 31st and 34th and 3 between the 39th and 54th months. Suspected SAH accounted for an additional 4 fatalities between 11 and 68 months after randomization. Deaths unrelated to SAH were noted 4 times in the 10 to 94-month interval, whereas there was 1 mortality, the result of complications of treatment, occurring at 14 months. Two patients in the drug-induced hypotension category developed permanent cerebrovascular insults between the 3-month and the 1-year follow-up, both from unrelated causes.

The absence of late recurrent hemorrhage (after 1 year) in the carotid ligation group of patients was an unexpected finding. Neither were there any late (after 1 year) deaths from complications of treatment. Two deaths were recorded from unrelated causes, 1 at 61 months and the other at 94 months. The cause of another death is not known. The etiology of a permanent neurologic deficit in 1 patient was undetermined.

The most common cause of death among patients treated by intracranial operation was recurrent subarachnoid hemorrhage. This befell 7 patients and involved 3 in the 3 to 7-month interval; the other 4 occurred at 28, 35, 46 and as late as 85 months after operation. A suspected rebleed in another occurred at 9 months. These deaths clearly represent a failure of treatment by intracranial operation, indicating that technically the aneurysm was not obliterated. A remote possibility is that the hemorrhage may have been due to rupture of another aneurysm which was not previously recognized, or from one that developed "de novo." Two deaths were the result of complications of treatment. Four patients died from unrelated causes. Three had developed permanent cerebrovascular deficits—1 with a suspected recurrent subarachnoid hemorrhage at the 3-month to 6-month interval; and 2 from unrelated causes, 1 at the 3-month and another at the 6-month interval. One should note that the surgical group of patients was generally in good medical and neurologic condition when treated. In the carotid ligation group, for example, 59.9% were in good and 26.2% in fair medical condition; neurologic condition was Grades 1 and 2 in 69.5% (4.3% were symptom-free and 65.2% had minor symptoms of headache, neck stiffness and the like). Seventy-four percent of patients treated by intracranial surgery were in Grades 1 or 2 neurologic condition (8.3% symptom-free, 65.5% with minor symptoms). Considering the factor of age, medical condition was good in 29.2% and fair in 44%. It appears, then, that the treatment rendered to patients had little influence as a causative factor on the death of patients in the follow-up period.

Relation of Treatment and Site of an Aneurysm to Capacity for Self-Care and Employability

The capability for self-management was used as the basis for determining a patient's immediate and long-term physical and neurologic recovery. The ability to work was coded according to six levels, as outlined in Table 10–9.

There may be difficulty in understanding the problem of the patient who is working, but doing so at a less strenuous job than usual. Because job definitions are not clearly spelled out, an analysis such as this probably means less than what is optimally desirable when considering working capacity, since it refers to groups of patients rather than the

Table 10–9. Definition of Employability.

1—Ability to work full-time at the same or an equivalent job
2—Ability to work part-time at the same or an equivalent job
3—Inability to work at one's usual occupation, but working at jobs requiring less strenuous activity
4—Inability to work at usual job, but at jobs consistent with the patient's neurologic deficit(s)
5—No gainful employment, but able to work
6—Unfit for gainful employment

individual. For example, the patient who makes his living as a professional (teacher, attorney, etc.), although physically able to be about, may have lost the intellectual capacity to function as before. The matter is substantially the same for the man who drives a truck or is a menial laborer. His mental capability may be sufficiently good to carry out this task, but he may not be able to do so because he has a physical defect in the form of hemiparesis, for example. The effect is the same, but the reason is different. There is a lesser problem in the case of the patient who works at a less strenuous activity than before his illness, or the one who works according to limitations imposed by his neurologic deficit. There is no difficulty with the patient who is "unfit for gainful employment." There is difficulty in assessing patients who are "not gainfully employed, but able to work." This information may point to relationships which are more socially than medically determined, and the information from a protocol is difficult to interpret. Numbers of patients in different occupations take on various significance. In some sectors of the social framework, the work of the housewife may not be considered "a job," one reason being that there is no direct or usual monetary compensation. Seasonal influences of work may bear upon the answers to questions in specific instances. For example, the farmer may consider his "working time" as being in the spring and the fall seasons. If he is examined or information is requested of him in the winter, he may well respond that he is "not working," "working a little," or the like. Information in the analysis indicates that there is little change in the number of patients who move from one to another category of working capability. This raises questions of socioeconomic rather than purely medical factors that determine where the patient rates in this scheme. It is apparent that things change little after the first year. The number of patients with disabilities of various types, especially the "unfit for gainful employment," is high in all treatment categories, especially at the 3-month follow-up interval. It remains relatively high and constant from the 6th month and thereafter. There is a fall-off between the first and second 3 months, the reason for which is not entirely clear. It suggests, however, that the fall-off is due to a failure of the follow-up, the lack of available information, or that there has been attrition by death due to disorders which complicate the subarachnoid hemorrhage or treatment. There is no noteworthy change in the condition of patients or in the number of patients in whom such changes may have occurred. The group "not gainfully employed, but able to work" raises a most interesting question, because the numbers remain much the same throughout the period of analysis.

The capacity for self-care according to the definitions of the protocol involves three states: (1) the ability of the patient to care for himself using no special aids other than a cane or crutches; (2) the ability of the patient to care for himself, but with the requirement of special devices, e.g., braces or a wheelchair, to get about; and (3) the inability of the patient to take care of himself. The follow-up information dealing with the status of the patient at specified time intervals directs itself to his working capacity at that time. Knowledge of this information was to determine whether he was the same as when previously examined, or whether he was improved, or worse.

Referring to Table 10–10, it is noted that the percentage figures in the various treatment groups are nearly the same at the end of 3 months, except for the intracranial surgery treatment category. At 3 months, especially in the self-care group, differences are approximately 10% lower for patients treated by intracranial operation. Similarly, the number of patients unable to care for themselves was about three times greater for those who had intracranial operation than for those who were treated by carotid ligation and about two times greater than those treated by bed rest or drug-induced hypotension. At 6 months, the capability for self-care was remarkably similar in all groups and remained so throughout the remainder of the follow-up.

The problem becomes more complicated, and it is difficult to draw conclusions, when the capacity for self-care related to a specific treatment for a ruptured aneurysm at a specific site is analyzed. It appears that this is so because of the large differences in the numbers of patients with aneurysms at different sites (Table 10–11). For example, 73 patients had anterior cerebral artery aneurysms compared to 5 vertebrobasilar, 8 middle cerebral and 17 internal carotid artery aneurysms. The ability for self-care and continued disability remains remarkably similar in patients with aneurysms at three different anatomical sites. In patients with vertebrobasilar aneurysms, 100% remained capable of self-care throughout the period of follow-up. However, they numbered only 5 and are therefore excluded from the analysis. Referring to Table 10–12, when comparing patients treated by drug-induced hypotension with those treated by bed rest at the 3-month interval, a markedly greater capacity for self-care (18%) is noted among patients who had a middle cerebral artery aneurysm. Even this figure is misleading, because there were 19 patients treated by drug-induced hypotension, whereas only 8 were treated with bed rest. No such marked differences were observed in patients with internal carotid artery and anterior cerebral artery aneurysms. In the latter group, percentages for the drug-induced hypotension and bed rest group were almost the same, although 37 more patients had drug-induced hypotension. This trend continues for the middle cerebral site from the 1st year and thereafter. In the 3rd and 4th years for patients with aneurysms at the internal carotid site, self-care rates at these times were, respectively, 12 and 11% higher than in the bed rest-treated group. However, the number of patients was similarly 3 and 2.5 times greater in the drug-induced hypotension group.

A review of Table 10–13, on the capacity for self-care following carotid ligation, reveals similar trends. Fifty percent more patients who had middle cerebral artery aneurysms were treated by carotid ligation than by bed rest (16 and 8, respectively), and

Table 10-10. Capacity for Self-Care Related to Type of Treatment.

		Follow-up Interval																		
		3 months		6 months		1 year		2 years		3 years		4 years		5 years		6 years		8 years		10 years	
		No.	%	No.	%	No.	%	No.	%	No.	%	No.	%	No.	%	No.	%	No.	%	No.	%
Bed Rest (202)	Self-care	103	85.1	104	90.4	95	88.8	87	95.6	79	96.3	72	94.7	65	95.5	28	87.5	19	95.0	11	100.0
	Self-care with aid	3	2.5	4	3.5	4	3.7	1	1.1	1	1.2	1	1.3	0	1.5	1	3.1	0	0.0	0	0.0
	Unable to care for self	14	11.6	7	6.1	6	5.6	2	2.2	1	1.2	2	2.6	0	0.0	1	3.1	0	0.0	0	0.0
Drug-induced hypotension (309)	Self-care	169	83.7	176	91.7	169	92.9	161	95.8	142	93.4	122	93.1	114	91.2	50	87.7	34	89.5	12	85.7
	Self-care with aid	5	2.5	4	2.1	4	2.2	3	1.8	5	3.3	3	2.3	3	2.4	2	3.5	1	2.6	1	7.1
	Unable to care for self	27	13.4	11	5.7	8	4.4	3	1.8	5	3.3	5	3.8	7	5.6	5	8.8	3	7.9	0	0.0
Carotid ligation (187)	Self-care	107	86.3	109	88.6	103	87.3	100	89.3	94	89.5	88	93.6	78	89.7	51	92.7	31	91.2	11	78.6
	Self-care with aid	6	4.8	9	7.3	7	5.9	7	6.3	6	5.7	3	2.3	2	2.3	1	1.8	1	2.9	0	0.0
	Unable to care for self	11	8.9	4	3.3	7	5.9	5	4.5	4	3.8	2	1.5	4	4.6	3	5.5	2	5.9	1	7.1
Intracranial surgery (274)	Self-care	130	70.7	133	78.7	135	83.9	130	86.7	126	91.3	114	94.2	103	91.2	56	91.8	27	90.0	12	92.3
	Self-care with aid	6	3.3	10	5.9	7	4.3	6	4.0	2	1.4	1	0.8	1	0.9	1	1.6	2	6.7	1	7.7
	Unable to care for self	48	26.1	24	14.2	18	11.2	12	8.0	9	6.5	6	5.0	5	4.4	4	6.6	0	0.0	0	0.0
Total	Self-care	509	80.7	522	87.1	502	88.4	478	91.7	441	92.5	396	93.8	360	91.6	185	90.2	111	91.0	46	88.5
	Self-care with aid	20	3.2	27	4.5	22	3.9	17	3.3	14	2.9	8	1.9	7	1.8	5	2.4	4	3.3	2	3.8
	Unable to care for self	100	15.8	46	7.7	39	6.9	22	4.2	19	4.0	15	3.6	16	4.1	13	6.3	5	4.1	1	1.9

Note: Table does not list incomplete observations. Percentages were determined from total number of patients followed, including those with incomplete information (Table 10–1).

Table 10-11.   Capacity for Self-Care Related to Site of Aneurysm for Bed Rest Therapy.

		Follow-up Interval																		
		3 months		6 months		1 year		2 years		3 years		4 years		5 years		6 years		8 years		10 years	
		No.	%	No.	%	No.	%	No.	%	No.	%	No.	%	No.	%	No.	%	No.	%	No.	%
Internal carotid	Self-care	17	89.5	18	94.7	16	94.1	15	100.0	12	100.0	12	100.0	9	90.0	8	80.0	6	100.0	3	100.0
	Self-care with aid	0	0.0	0	0.0	0	0.0	0	0.0	0	0.0	0	0.0	0	0.0	0	0.0	0	0.0	0	0.0
	Unable to care for self	1	5.3	1	5.3	1	5.9	0	0.0	0	0.0	0	0.0	0	0.0	1	10.0	0	0.0	0	0.0
Middle cerebral	Self-care	8	72.7	9	81.8	8	80.0	5	71.4	5	71.4	4	66.7	4	80.0	3	75.0	2	100.0	2	100.0
	Self-care with aid	1	9.1	1	9.1	1	10.0	1	14.3	1	14.3	1	16.7	1	20.0	1	25.0	0	0.0	0	0.0
	Unable to care for self	2	18.2	1	9.1	1	10.0	0	0.0	0	0.0	0	0.0	0	0.0	0	0.0	0	0.0	0	0.0
Anterior cerebral	Self-care	73	84.9	73	90.1	67	88.2	63	96.9	58	98.3	52	96.3	48	98.0	14	93.3	8	88.9	4	100.0
	Self-care with aid	2	2.3	3	3.7	3	3.9	0	0.0	0	0.0	0	0.0	0	0.0	0	0.0	0	0.0	0	0.0
	Unable to care for self	11	12.8	5	6.2	4	5.3	2	3.1	1	1.7	2	3.7	0	0.0	0	0.0	0	0.0	0	0.0
(Posterior) Vertebrobasilar	Self-care	5	100.0	4	100.0	4	100.0	4	100.0	4	100.0	4	100.0	4	100.0	3	100.0	3	100.0	2	100.0
	Self-care with aid	0	0.0	0	0.0	0	0.0	0	0.0	0	0.0	0	0.0	0	0.0	0	0.0	0	0.0	0	0.0
	Unable to care for self	0	0.0	0	0.0	0	0.0	0	0.0	0	0.0	0	0.0	0	0.0	0	0.0	0	0.0	0	0.0

Note: Table does not list incomplete observations.

Table 10-12.   Capacity for Self-Care Related to Site of Aneurysm for Drug-Induced Hypotension.

		Follow-up Interval																		
		3 months		6 months		1 year		2 years		3 years		4 years		5 years		6 years		8 years		10 years	
		No.	%	No.	%	No.	%	No.	%	No.	%	No.	%	No.	%	No.	%	No.	%	No.	%
Internal carotid	Self-care	48	80.0	53	93.0	46	88.5	43	91.5	36	87.8	31	88.6	28	87.5	22	88.0	14	82.4	3	100.0
	Self-care with aid	1	1.7	2	3.5	2	3.8	1	2.1	2	4.9	1	2.9	0	0.0	0	0.0	0	0.0	0	0.0
	Unable to care for self	11	18.3	1	1.8	3	5.8	2	4.3	3	7.3	2	5.7	4	12.5	3	12.0	3	17.6	0	0.0
Middle cerebral	Self-care	19	90.5	17	85.0	19	95.0	19	100.0	18	94.7	15	93.7	15	93.7	13	92.9	9	100.0	5	100.0
	Self-care with aid	0	0.0	0	0.0	0	0.0	0	0.0	1	5.3	1	6.3	1	6.3	1	7.1	0	0.0	0	0.0
	Unable to care for self	2	9.5	3	15.0	1	5.0	0	0.0	0	0.0	0	0.0	0	0.0	0	0.0	0	0.0	0	0.0
Anterior cerebral	Self-care	102	84.3	106	92.2	104	94.5	99	97.1	88	95.0	76	95.7	71	92.2	15	83.3	11	91.7	4	80.0
	Self-care with aid	4	3.3	2	1.7	2	1.8	2	2.0	2	2.2	1	1.3	2	2.6	1	5.6	1	8.3	1	20.0
	Unable to care for self	14	11.6	7	6.1	4	3.6	1	0.9	2	2.2	3	3.7	3	3.9	2	11.1	0	0.0	0	0.0

Note: Table does not list incomplete observations.

Table 10–13. Capacity for Self-Care Related to Site of Aneurysm for Carotid Ligation Therapy.

		Follow-up Interval																		
		3 months		6 months		1 year		2 years		3 years		4 years		5 years		6 years		8 years		10 years	
		No.	%	No.	%	No.	%	No.	%	No.	%	No.	%	No.	%	No.	%	No.	%	No.	%
Internal carotid	Self-care	54	85.7	57	90.5	54	87.1	49	86.0	47	87.0	43	93.5	37	88.1	32	91.4	17	85.0	5	62.5
	Self-care with aid	4	6.3	4	6.3	3	4.8	4	7.0	4	7.4	2	4.3	1	2.4	1	2.9	1	5.0	0	0.0
	Unable to care for self	5	7.9	2	2.3	4	6.5	4	7.0	3	5.6	1	2.2	3	7.1	2	5.7	2	10.0	1	12.5
Middle cerebral	Self-care	16	94.1	15	88.2	13	92.9	12	92.3	11	91.7	11	91.7	8	88.9	7	87.5	5	100.0	2	100.0
	Self-care with aid	0	0.0	0	0.0	0	0.0	0	0.0	0	0.0	0	0.0	0	0.0	0	0.0	0	0.0	0	0.0
	Unable to care for self	1	5.9	1	5.9	1	7.1	1	7.7	1	8.3	1	8.3	1	11.1	1	12.5	0	0.0	0	0.0
Anterior cerebral	Self-care	37	84.1	37	86.0	36	85.7	39	92.9	36	92.3	34	94.4	33	91.7	12	100.0	9	100.0	4	100.0
	Self-care with aid	2	4.5	5	11.6	4	9.5	3	7.1	2	5.1	1	2.8	1	2.8	0	0.0	0	0.0	0	0.0
	Unable to care for self	5	11.4	1	2.3	2	4.8	0	0.0	0	0.0	0	0.0	0	0.0	0	0.0	0	0.0	0	0.0

Note: Table does not list incomplete observations.

Table 10–14. Capacity for Self-Care Related to Site of Aneurysm for Intracranial Surgery Therapy.

		Follow-up Interval																		
		3 months		6 months		1 year		2 years		3 years		4 years		5 years		6 years		8 years		10 years	
		No.	%	No.	%	No.	%	No.	%	No.	%	No.	%	No.	%	No.	%	No.	%	No.	%
Internal carotid	Self-care	18	56.2	18	60.0	20	74.1	19	79.2	17	81.0	13	81.2	10	71.4	8	72.7	5	100.0	2	100.0
	Self-care with aid	1	3.1	3	10.0	1	3.7	1	4.2	0	0.0	0	0.0	0	0.0	0	0.0	0	0.0	0	0.0
	Unable to care for self	13	40.6	9	30.0	6	22.2	4	16.7	4	19.0	3	18.8	3	21.4	3	27.3	0	0.0	0	0.0
Middle cerebral	Self-care	18	66.7	19	82.6	19	90.5	18	90.0	18	94.7	18	94.7	16	94.1	13	92.9	8	88.9	2	100.0
	Self-care with aid	2	7.4	2	8.7	1	4.8	1	5.0	0	0.0	0	0.0	0	0.0	0	0.0	0	0.0	0	0.0
	Unable to care for self	7	25.9	2	8.7	1	4.8	1	5.0	1	5.3	1	5.3	1	5.9	1	7.1	0	0.0	0	0.0
Anterior Cerebral	Self-care	92	76.7	94	83.2	94	84.7	92	88.5	90	93.7	81	96.4	75	93.7	34	100.0	13	86.7	8	88.9
	Self-care with aid	3	2.5	5	4.4	5	4.5	4	3.8	2	2.1	1	1.2	1	1.2	0	0.0	2	13.3	1	11.1
	Unable to care for self	25	20.8	12	10.6	11	9.9	6	5.8	3	3.1	2	2.4	1	2.4	0	0.0	0	0.0	0	0.0
(Posterior) Vertebrobasilar	Self-care	2	4.0	2	66.7	2	100.0	1	50.0	1	50.0	2	100.0	2	100.0	1	50.0	1	100.0	0	0.0
	Self-care with aid	0	0.0	0	0.0	0	0.0	0	0.0	0	0.0	0	0.0	0	0.0	1	50.0	0	0.0	0	0.0
	Unable to care for self	3	60.0	1	33.3	0	0.0	1	50.0	1	50.0	0	0.0	0	0.0	0	0.0	0	0.0	0	0.0

Note: Table does not list incomplete observations.

three more (19) were treated by carotid ligation than by drug-induced hypotension (16). Seven percent more patients who had drug-induced hypotension were capable of self-care, whereas in the carotid ligation and bed rest groups the percentages were similar. However, the numbers in the drug-induced hypotension and carotid ligation groups were greater at the 3-month interval. This tendency persists throughout the follow-up period. Little differences were apparent at the internal carotid artery site when the number of patients in the drug-induced hypotension and carotid ligation groups were compared; this was especially the case after the 3-month interval. Despite a greater than 3 to 1 ratio in the number of patients with anterior cerebral aneurysm in the drug-induced hypotension and carotid artery ligation allocation, the percentages of patients able to take care of themselves were quite similar, except at 1 year when a 9% difference was present in favor of the drug-induced hypotension group.

In Table 10–14, one notes that for patients with aneurysms at the three sites designated on the anterior circulation the percentage of patients who had intracranial operation who were able to care for themselves was much lower than for those in the other treatment categories at the 3-month follow-up. The highest percentage, as well as the gross numbers of those requiring total help, was present at 3 months. This was particularly the case for patients with anterior cerebral artery aneurysms. The percentage of patients with internal carotid artery aneurysms treated by intracranial surgery who were capable of self-care (despite the smaller number treated) was very much lower at the 3-month evaluation. At that time, the percentage was much lower than for patients with aneurysms of the middle cerebral artery. Conversely, at 3 months, the number of patients completely disabled was 5 times greater for intracranial surgery-treated patients than those who had carotid artery ligation, 2 times greater than for those who had drug-induced hypotension and 8 times greater than for those who had regulated bed rest. This sug-

gests a high complication rate for intracranial operation. This trend continued throughout the follow-up period for the internal carotid artery site. However, for the anterior and middle cerebral sites, the percentage of patients who could care for themselves at 6 months and thereafter remained comparable. The results, then, generally do not appear to be as good for intracranial surgery at the internal carotid artery site than for the other treatment groups.

The degree of employability was defined according to six classes, as noted in Table 10–9. Table 10–15 indicates that at 3 months, a greater percentage of patients treated by carotid ligation than those in the other treatment categories were working full time. This table shows that 14% more patients were working full time following carotid ligation than following bed rest, 13% more than for intracranial surgery and 10% more than for drug-induced hypotension. The number of patients unfit for gainful employment was highest for those who had intracranial operations and approximately 20% lower for each of the other treatment categories. Although at the 2-year interval the trend for full employability in terms of percentages remained highest for carotid ligation patients, drug-induced hypotension was comparable. At 3 years, the percentage of patients with the capacity for full-time work in the drug-induced hypotension and carotid ligation groups was comparable, remaining lowest for the bed rest and intracranial surgery groups. At the 4-year interval, the figures are similar, except for the bed rest group which was 5 to 8% lower. At the 5-year evaluation, the carotid ligation group had the highest percentage of patients fully employed. Total disability remained high: 11.8% for patients allocated to bed rest, 18.4% for those who had drug-induced hypotension, 15% for those who had intracranial surgery and 9.2% for patients who had carotid ligation. Generally, employability and disability remained at similar relative levels throughout the follow-up period following the first 3 and 6-month observation period.

Table 10-15. Present Employment Related to Type of Treatment.

Treatment	Present Employment	3 months No.	%	6 months No.	%	1 year No.	%	2 years No.	%	3 years No.	%	4 years No.	%	5 years No.	%	6 years No.	%	8 years No.	%	10 years No.	%
Bed rest	1	27	22.3	52	45.2	54	50.5	52	57.1	50	61.0	42	55.3	36	52.9	15	46.9	13	65.0	6	54.5
	2	18	14.9	14	12.2	8	7.5	11	12.1	10	12.2	6	7.9	7	10.3	2	6.2	0	0.0	0	0.0
	3	7	5.8	4	3.5	5	4.7	6	6.6	5	6.1	1	1.3	1	1.5	2	6.2	1	5.0	0	0.0
	4	0	0.0	1	0.9	0	0.0	1	1.1	0	0.0	1	1.3	1	1.5	1	3.1	0	0.0	0	0.0
	5	45	37.2	29	25.2	25	23.4	12	13.2	10	12.2	15	19.7	12	17.6	6	18.8	4	20.0	3	27.3
	6	24	19.8	15	13.0	15	14.0	8	8.8	5	6.1	9	11.8	8	11.8	5	15.6	1	5.0	0	0.0
Drug-induced hypotension	1	54	26.7	91	47.4	112	61.5	107	63.7	96	63.2	79	60.3	71	56.8	31	54.4	21	55.3	4	28.6
	2	29	14.4	24	12.5	10	5.5	12	7.1	8	5.3	11	8.4	13	10.4	2	3.5	2	5.3	4	28.6
	3	4	2.0	4	2.1	7	3.8	6	3.6	7	4.6	4	3.1	3	2.4	2	3.5	0	0.0	0	0.0
	4	0	0.0	0	0.0	2	1.1	1	0.6	1	0.7	1	0.8	0	0.0	1	1.8	1	2.6	1	7.1
	5	70	34.7	40	20.8	28	15.4	26	15.5	19	12.5	17	13.0	15	12.0	7	12.3	5	13.2	1	7.1
	6	45	22.3	32	16.7	23	12.6	15	8.9	20	13.2	19	14.5	23	18.4	14	24.6	9	23.7	2	14.3
Carotid ligation	1	45	36.3	71	57.8	78	66.1	78	69.6	70	66.7	59	62.8	59	67.8	35	63.6	20	58.8	9	64.3
	2	7	5.6	12	9.8	9	7.6	9	8.0	11	10.5	11	11.7	5	5.7	5	9.1	5	14.7	1	7.1
	3	4	3.2	1	0.8	4	3.4	4	3.6	2	1.9	5	5.3	3	3.4	2	3.6	1	2.9	0	0.0
	4	4	3.2	1	0.9	2	1.7	2	1.8	5	4.8	1	1.1	1	1.1	0	0.0	0	0.0	0	0.0
	5	39	31.5	18	14.6	9	7.6	8	7.1	6	5.7	13	13.8	10	11.5	6	10.9	6	17.6	2	14.3
	6	25	20.2	17	13.8	14	11.9	11	9.8	11	10.5	5	5.3	8	9.2	7	12.7	2	5.9	2	14.3
Intracranial surgery	1	43	23.4	74	43.8	81	50.3	83	55.3	79	57.2	77	63.6	68	60.2	34	55.7	17	56.7	7	53.8
	2	13	7.1	13	7.7	10	6.2	9	6.0	6	4.3	5	4.1	6	5.3	4	6.6	3	10.0	2	15.4
	3	4	2.2	5	3.0	6	3.7	7	4.7	5	3.6	6	5.0	6	5.3	6	9.8	3	10.0	0	0.0
	4	0	0.0	0	0.0	0	0.0	2	1.3	3	2.2	4	3.3	5	4.4	3	4.9	2	6.7	1	7.7
	5	52	28.3	31	18.3	26	16.1	23	15.3	17	12.3	8	6.6	7	6.2	3	4.9	1	3.3	1	7.7
	6	72	39.1	45	26.6	38	23.6	26	17.3	28	20.3	21	17.4	17	15.0	10	16.4	3	10.0	2	15.4
Overall	1	169	26.8	288	48.1	325	57.2	320	61.4	295	61.8	257	60.9	234	59.5	115	56.1	71	58.2	26	50.0
	2	67	10.6	63	10.5	37	6.5	41	7.9	35	7.3	33	7.8	31	7.9	13	6.3	10	8.2	7	13.5
	3	19	3.0	14	2.3	22	3.9	23	4.4	19	4.0	16	3.8	13	3.3	12	5.9	5	4.1	0	0.0
	4	4	0.6	2	0.3	4	0.7	6	1.2	9	1.9	7	1.7	7	1.8	5	2.4	3	2.5	2	3.8
	5	206	32.6	118	19.7	88	15.5	69	13.2	52	10.9	53	12.6	44	11.2	22	10.7	16	13.1	7	13.5
	6	166	26.3	109	18.2	90	15.8	60	11.5	64	13.4	54	12.8	56	14.2	36	17.6	15	12.3	6	11.5

Note: Table does not list incomplete observations. See note under Table 10-10.

Capacity for Self-care and Employability Related to Treatment

The data to be presented refer to patients who were assigned to a particular treatment category according to the randomization procedure. The information, therefore, is post-randomization information.

Bed Rest

Referring to Tables 10–10 and 10–15, among the 202 patients in the bed rest-treated category, at 3 months following the subarachnoid hemorrhage 79 of the original group had died and there was no information obtainable in 2, leaving 121 whose progress could be assessed. Of these 121 patients, 103 (85%) were able to take care of themselves, 3 required aids (braces, wheelchair), 14 were totally dependent (i.e., unable to care for themselves) and 1 had no status reported. Usefulness of these patients to themselves and to society, translated into terms of employability, revealed a dismal picture. Only 27 (22.3%) were fully and 18 (14.9%) partly employed at the same or an equivalent occupation in which they were engaged before their subarachnoid hemorrhage. Seven were working at jobs less strenuous than their original ones. The most distressing figure was that 69 were not employed, 24 (19.8%) because they were unfit for work. It is not entirely clear why 45 (37.2%) were not working, although they were able to work.

At 6 months, 52 of 115 (45.2%) were fully employed, whereas 14 (12.2%) were at part-time usual job activity. Four (3.5%) were at less vigorous jobs and 1 was doing special work because of a neurologic problem. Forty-four (38.2%) were not working, 29 (25.2%) for various reasons not clearly noted and 15 (13%) because they were unfit for work. At this time, 90.4% (104) were capable of self-care. Four (3.5%) required aids such as braces or a wheelchair and 7 were unable to care for themselves.

At 1 year, 88.8% were able to care for themselves, 4 required aids and 6 were completely disabled. Fifty-four (50.5%) were working full time, 8 (7.5%) part time at their usual jobs. Five were occupied at less demanding work and 40 (37.4%) were not employed, 15 (14.0%) because they were unfit for gainful work.

Two years after allocation to bed rest treatment, 87 (95.6%) of the remaining 91 were capable of taking care of themselves, but 63 (69.2%) were at their original jobs—full-time for 52 (57.1%) and part-time for 11 (12.1%). One took care of himself but used a prosthesis to get about, whereas 2 required total care. Twelve patients in this category, although described as being able to work, were not doing so, and 8 were not fit for gainful work.

Eighty-two patients were available for evaluation at the 3-year period. Seventy-nine (96.3%) were capable of self-care, 1 could carry on with an aid, another was totally disabled. Of the 60 (73.2%) at full-time or part-time former working capacity, 50 (61%) were full-time, 10 (12.2%) were part time. Five were working but not at the same level and 5 (6.1%) were totally disabled. Ten (12.2%) were noted to be able to work but were not employed.

At 4 years, a little more than one half (76) of the original 121 were followed. Among the 76 known to be alive, 42 (55.3%) were at full working capacity and 6 (7.9%) were doing their original work on a part-time basis. Whereas 1 was carrying out less physical activity, another worked at a job commensurate with his neurologic deficit. A relatively high percentage (19.7%, 15 patients) said to be able to work were not employed. Nine at this time were unfit to earn a livelihood.

The follow-up at 5 years yielded 68 patients. Thirty-six (52.9%) were at their original and full-time employment; 7 were part time. Eight patients (11.8%) were totally disabled and 12 (17.6%) were not working, although they were said to be able to work. Two were at lesser activity jobs than their usual ones.

Only one quarter (32) of the original 121 patients in follow-up could be evaluated at the 6th year. Twenty-eight (87.5%) were caring fully for themselves, 1 required a physical appliance and 1 was unable to care for himself. Fifteen of these 32 (46.9%) were at their usual jobs, 2 were doing part-time work, 3 were at less demanding tasks, 5 were unfit for gainful employment, and 6, although said to be able to work, were not doing so.

Drug-induced Hypotension

Three hundred and nine patients were originally allocated according to the randomization process to treatment by drug-induced hypotension. This group comprised the largest number of patients. At the 3-month interval, 202 were available for evaluation of their progress. At that point, slightly more than one third (104) had expired. Of the 202 patients who were still living, 169 were able to care for themselves. Five did so with the aid of braces, a wheelchair or the like, whereas 27 (13.4%) were completely dependent upon others for care. Only 54 (26.7%) were capable of full-time work at their usual job, and 29 (14.4%), although at their usual job, worked only on a part-time basis. Four were doing less strenuous work. Even though slightly more than one third (70) were described as being able to work, they were not employed; the reasons for this are not clear. A relatively high percentage (22.3%, or 45) were completely disabled.

At the 6-month interval, 192 patients were followed. Five additional patients had died. At this time, 176 (91.7%) were capable of self-care while 4 required aids. Eleven were fully incapacitated. One hundred and fifteen were at their previous jobs—91 (47.4%) full-time and 24 (12.5%) part-time. Four were at less demanding work. Of the 70 patients who were able to work at 3 months but were not doing so, 30 had returned. Thirty-two (16.7%) remained unsuitable for gainful employment.

At 1 year, 182 patients were available for examination; 169 (92.9%) could take care of themselves unaided, 4 required mechanical aids and 8 were incapacitated. One hundred and twelve (61.5%) were doing the same or similar work on a full-time basis and 10 (5.5%) on a part-time basis. Seven (3.8%) were working less actively than before their illness and 2 worked at jobs limited by their neurologic deficiency. Of the 40 patients capable of but not working at 6 months, 28 became employed; 23 (12.6%) were unfit for employment.

Fourteen fewer patients could be followed at the 2-year time interval. Of the 168, 161 (95.8%) were capable of self-care, 3 were disabled and 3 required mechanical aids. One hundred and seven (63.7%) and 12 (7.1%), respectively, were at their usual full-time and part-time working capacity. Seven (4.2%) could not perform as before but were working within their capabilities. Twenty-six (15.5%), although able, were not working; 15 (8.9%) were fully disabled.

At 3 years, information was available on only 152 of the original 309 patients in the drug-induced hypotension treatment category. One hundred and forty-two (93.4%) were self-sufficient, 5 required aids for self-care and 5 were unable to care for themselves. Ninety-six (63.2%) were working full-time at their usual occupations and an additional eight (5.3%) part-time. Eight were working at limited tasks consistent with their disabilities. Twenty (13.2%) were totally disabled and, although capable, 19 were not working.

Four years after randomization, there were 131 patients available for analysis. One hundred and twenty-two of these patients (93.1%) were fully sufficient, 3 required mechanical assistance and 5 were disabled. While 79 (60.3%) were able to devote full time to their original work, 11 were able to do this only on a part-time basis. Five patients were functioning at limited activity and 19 (14.5%) were completely disabled. Seventeen (13%) were not gainfully employed but were able to work.

At 5 years, 125 patients were followed.

One hundred and fourteen (91.2%) were caring for themselves without help, whereas another 3 required mechanical assistance. Seven were incapable of self-care. Seventy-one (56.8%) were at full-time and 13 (10.4%) at part-time activity in their usual work. Three patients were limited in their working capacity and were occupied at less strenuous jobs, whereas 23 (18.4%) were totally dependent for their needs and were unfit for employment. Fifteen were described as being able to work but were not employed.

Fifty-seven of the 202 patients were available for follow-up at 6 years, an additional 64 having been lost in the 5 to 6-year interval. Fifty (87.7%) were self-sufficient, 2 needed help and 5 were incapable of self-care. Only 31 (54.4%) were at their original jobs on a full-time basis and only 2 (3.5%) were doing part-time work in their original activity. Two patients were at limited work, 14 (24.6%) were totally disabled and 7 (12.3%) were not employed.

Carotid Ligation

One hundred and eighty-seven patients were treated by carotid ligation. This procedure raises questions which are considered pertinent and common to several areas in the management of patients with aneurysmal subarachnoid hemorrhage. With this operation, there is deliberate occlusion of a major cerebral vessel in an attempt to alter the effect of the direct and indirect blood pressure head and blood flow through an aneurysm, hoping to obliterate the lesion by thrombosing it—or perhaps to promote the healing process at the point of rupture by the process of thrombosis. When employing deliberate carotid occlusion to treat an aneurysm, one must consider the immediate risk of compromising the cerebral circulation when depriving a portion of the brain of a major source of its blood supply. If occlusion of the vessel is tolerated without production of a neurologic deficit, one becomes concerned with (1) its long-term effect upon the cerebral circulation, especially in the age

group in which most subarachnoid hemorrhages occur, and (2) the risk of an ischemic episode at that time or within a few years thereafter when the development of atherosclerotic disease is expected. A major vessel has been "sacrificed." Does this affect the physiologic function of other major cerebral vessels? How much greater is the risk, if any, of an eventual cerebrovascular insult in the patient who has had a carotid artery deliberately occluded? These questions are unanswered. However, Winn et al.[8] found significant hypertension in their patients with carotid ligation (for carotid-posterior communicating artery aneurysms) on the average as compared to the blood pressures in those patients who were treated conservatively. It was their opinion that carotid ligation offered no protection against recurrent bleeding over the late follow-up period, although it appeared to be protective against rebleeding during the first 6 months. This is at variance with Perret's[7] data in which there was no recurrent hemorrhage after the 1st until the 8th year following the ligation. It is of interest that Winn et al.[8] found no episodes of ischemic cerebrovascular disease but found recurrent hemorrhage during the follow-up period.

Within the first 3 months following randomization to this treatment category, 58 of the 187 patients had died and 5 were lost to follow-up. One hundred and seven (86.3%) were able to care for themselves, 6 required help to function on their own and 11 were incapable of self-care. Forty-five (36.3%) were at their usual working capacity at the 3-month interval and 7 (5.6%) were working part-time at their usual jobs. Eight (6.4%) patients were engaged in less strenuous and special work. Twenty-five (20.2%) were incapable of working and 39 (31.5%) were noted as not working but able to do so.

The review at 6 months disclosed 123 patients for examination. One hundred and nine (88.6%) were capable of self-care, 9 required aid such as a wheelchair or the use of other appliances and 4 were incapable of self-care. Seventy-one (57.7%) were at full-time, 12 (9.8%) at part-time regular employment. Two worked at different jobs with the limitations imposed by their physical and neurologic condition. Eighteen were not working, although they were able to do so, and 17 (13.8%) were physically unable to work.

Between 6 and 12 months, 118 subjects were available for study. Of these, 103 (87.3%) were capable of self-care, 7 required aids and 7 were in need of total care. At this time, 78 (66.1%) were working full time at their previous or similar jobs and 9 (7.6%) were so engaged on a part-time basis. Six worked at different jobs without limitations and 14 (11.9%) were totally disabled. Nine (7.6%), although capable of working, were not employed.

At the 2-year interval, 112 patients were reviewed; there was no follow-up of 5. One hundred (89.3%) were capable of self-care, 7 were capable of self-care with aid and 5 were unable to care for themselves at all. Seventy-eight (69.6%) were working full time, as before their illness, and 9 (8%) part time. Six (5.4%) worked with the constraints of their physical and neurologic disabilities. Eleven (9.8%) were completely disabled, whereas 8 (7.1%) were not gainfully employed but were able to work.

The end of the 3-year interval allowed 105 patients for evaluation. Ninety-four (89.5%) were self-sufficient, 6 required aids and 4 were totally dependent. Seventy (66.7%) were at their usual full-time job; 11 (10.5%) were at their usual job but performing only part-time. Seven were limited to lesser endeavors and 11 (10.5%) were fully disabled. Six were not working but were said to be able to do so.

Eighty-eight (93.6%) of the 94 patients at 4 years cared for themselves, 3 required the aid of some type of appliance and 2 were unable to care for themselves at all. Seventy (74.5%) were at their usual jobs: 59 (62.8%) at full-time and 11 (11.7%) at part-time activity. Six were working with restrictions and 13 (13.8%) were unemployed for reasons that were not clear. Five were classified as having a total disability.

The 5-year interval left 87 patients for re-

view. Seventy-eight (89.7%) could care for themselves, 2 required mechanical aids and 4 were totally dependent. Fifty-nine (67.8%) and 5 (5.7%) were at their former work on a full-time or part-time basis, respectively. Four additional patients were limited to less strenuous and special work. Eight (9.2%) were at full disability, and although employable, 10 (11.5%) were not employed.

The number of patients lost to follow-up rose sharply at 6 years. Thirty-two of the 87 reviewed 1 year previously were not available. Fifty-one (92.7%) of 55 patients cared for themselves, 1 required an appliance and 3 were incapable of self-care. Thirty-five (63.6%) were at full-time and 5 at part-time work on their usual jobs, whereas seven (12.7%) were totally disabled and 6 (10.9%) were unemployed.

At the end of the 10th year, the records of only 14 patients were available. It appeared that the trend for self-care and partial self-care increased, as did working capacity. However, the marked loss of patients to follow-up examination raises doubt that this is true, but is rather a reflection of the small number available for analysis. What is most impressive in the carotid ligation group of patients is the absence of complications of treatment after the first year.

Intracranial Surgery

Of the 274 patients originally randomized to the intracranial surgery treatment category, 184 were available for follow-up at the 3-month period (Table 10–1). Forty patients in this group died before they had operation.[3] In other words, patients allocated to surgery were included in the surgical section whether or not they underwent operation. This produced an original list of 234 patients on whom intracranial surgery was carried out. During the 3-month interval, 86 patients had died and 4 were lost for follow-up analysis. At 3 months, 130 (70.7%) were capable of self-care but 26.1% were completely dependent. Six (3.3%) were able to move about in a wheelchair or with braces (Table

10–10). Although a good number of patients were capable of caring for themselves, less than one half (56) had returned to their original jobs. Of these, 23.4% (43 of 184) were at full-time and 7.1% (13 of 184) at part-time activity. Only 4 (2.2%) were at less strenuous activity at a different occupation. Seventy-two (39.1%) of the patients were totally disabled, whereas 52 (28.3%) were described as able but not working.

At the 6-month interval, 19 additional deaths had occurred. The number of patients capable of self-care increased by 3 (133, or 78.7%), 10 required aids and 24 (14.2%) remained totally disabled. At the 6-month period, however, 74 (43.8%) were back at their former work but 13 (7.7%) did this only on a part-time basis. Forty-five (26.6%) were unfit for employment and 31 (18.3%) were not gainfully employed even though they were noted as being able to work. Five were at a less strenuous job than their previous one.

The 1-year evaluation disclosed that there were 5 additional deaths; 2 patients were lost to follow-up and 161 completed the follow-up examination. Fifty percent (81) of the patients were then fully employed and 6.2% (10) partly so; 6 (3.7%) were at less vigorous working capacity. Thirty-eight (23.6%) were unemployable and 26 (16.1%) were not engaged in gainful activity. Despite this poor work record, 135 (83.9%) were caring for themselves, 18 (11.2%) were completely disabled and 7 (4.3%) were partly disabled but caring for themselves.

At 2 years, of the 161 patients available at 1-year, 4 had died and 7 were lost to follow-up. Of the 150 remaining for the 2-year follow-up analysis, 130 (86.7%) were self-sufficient, whereas 12 (8%) were unable to care for themselves and 6 (4%) needed physical appliances.

A slightly higher number (83, or 55.3%) than in the previous year were at their original jobs working full time; 9 (6%) were at part-time activity. Twenty-six (17.3%) remained unfit for work, 23 (15.3%) were not gainfully employed and 9 (6%) worked within the limits of their neurologic disabil-ities but at jobs different than their pre-illness ones.

Forty-six fewer patients (138) than the original 184 were reviewed at 3 years. At this time, 91.3% (126) were capable of self-care, 9 (6.5%) were completely dependent upon someone else and 2 required aid. Seventy-nine (57.2%) worked full-time and 6 (4.3%) part-time at their usual occupations. However, 28 (20.3%) were unemployable, 17 (12.3%) were not employed and 8 (5.8%) were at less strenuous or special work necessitated by their impairments.

Of 121 patients at 4 years, 114 (94.2%) were able to care for themselves, 6 (5%) were totally disabled and 1 needed mechanical aids. Seventy-seven (63.6%) were at full-time and 5 (4.1%) were at part-time working capacity. Ten were at less physically demanding jobs, 21 (17.4%) were unfit for work and 8 (6.6%) were unemployed.

At 5 years, the number of patients followed had dropped to 113. One hundred and three (91.2%) took care of themselves; there was incomplete information on 4 patients and 1 required a mechanical aid. Sixty-eight (69.2%) were back at their usual jobs, whereas another 6 (5.3%) were employed on a part-time basis. Eleven (9.7%) were at special jobs determined by their disabilities. Seventeen (15%) could not work and 7 (6.2%) were unemployed but were said to be able to work.

Average Mean Blood Pressure and Pulse Rate at Follow-up

Blood pressure measurements (supine position for 30 min) were taken at the scheduled follow-up for those patients reporting for examination. For regulated bed rest, 106 patients (52% of 202) had measurements taken at 3 months, 76 (38%) at 6 months, 70 (35%) at 1 year, 63 (31%) at 2 years, 59 (29%) at 3 years, 44 (22%) at 4 years and 32 (16%) at 5 years. Those patients completing follow-up blood pressures had averaged 1.5 mm Hg lower than the overall group (105.2 mm Hg) at their randomization evaluations. The average change in blood pressure was 1 mm Hg above randomization level at 3 months and 6 months, 2.5 mm Hg at 1 year, approximately 5 mm Hg at years 2, 3 and 4, and 2 mm Hg at the 5th year (Fig. 10–10).

For patients allocated to drug-induced hypotension, 160 (52% of 309) had 3-month follow-up blood pressures, 123 (40%) were observed at 6 months, 131 (42%) at 1 year, 115 (37%) at 2 years, 99 (32%) at 3 years, 77 (25%) at 4 years and 66 (21%) at 5 years. Average blood pressure at randomization was 1.1 mm Hg lower for those followed than for all patients in the drug-induced hypotension treatment group (108.7 mm Hg). A reduction of 8.1 mm Hg in mean blood pressure was observed in those completing the 3-month follow-up period (Fig. 10–10). Examination of the data for those who had not stopped antihypertensive medication showed that mean blood pressure reduction averaged from 6.7 to 9.6 mm Hg lower than randomization levels. Those who stopped medication exhibited a variable follow-up blood pressure. This suggests that those who had not continued on antihypertensive medications did not have routine blood pressures taken consistently at follow-up. Of note is the reduction in blood pressure among those who were still at maintenance levels in the post-treatment period. An average reduction of 12.1 to 17.4 mm Hg was found from initial levels (110.5 mm Hg). Those not maintaining blood pressure reduction had increased blood pressures over time ranging from 2.3 mm Hg at 3 months (from an initial average level of 105 mm Hg) to 7.0 mm Hg at 3 years.

Of 187 patients treated initially by carotid ligation, 51% had blood pressures taken at 3 months, 42% at 6 months, 42% at 1 year, 40% at 2 years, 32% at 3 years, 30% at 4 years and 26% at 5 years. The average initial mean blood pressure at randomization in the patients who were followed was 4.5 mm Hg lower than that for the overall group (106.3 mm Hg). Blood pressure change was observed to be 4.5 mm Hg greater than initial randomization levels at 3 months (Fig. 10–10). This increase remained between 4.3 and 5.8 mm Hg for the 6-month to 2-year period. At 3 years, an increase to 8.5 mm Hg above initial levels was observed. The change was equally as high at 4 years, but then dropped to 4.5 mm Hg at 5 years.

Patients allocated to intracranial surgery had a 50% blood pressure follow-up rate at 3 months, 40% at 6 months, 39% at 1 year, 31% at 2 years, 24% at 3 years, 19% at 4 years and 17% at 5 years. At randomization, those patients who would complete follow-up blood pressure examinations averaged 3 mm Hg lower than the overall initial group

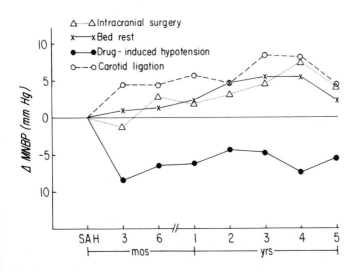

Fig. 10–10. Change in mean blood pressure from randomization level.

(104.5 mm Hg). After a decline in blood pressure of 1.1 mm Hg for the 3-month follow-up, average mean blood pressure rose to 2.9 mm Hg above initial levels at 6 months and up to 7.4 mm Hg at 4 years (Fig. 10–10). At 5 years, mean blood pressure had fallen but was still 4.2 mm Hg above initial levels.

Comparison blood pressures at the follow-up intervals showed that mean blood pressures were significantly lower for drug-induced hypotension patients than the other treatment categories (Fig. 10–11). The continued lower blood pressure in the drug-induced hypotension patients reflects the results of continued antihypertensive therapy. The rise in blood pressure post-carotid ligation appeared in the first 3-month period. This group had approximately 45% internal carotid aneurysms, 40% anterior cerebral-anterior communicating aneurysms and 15% in poor neurologic condition, while the other treatment groups had from 15 to 30% internal carotid aneurysms, 60 to 70% anterior cerebral aneurysms and approximately 20% in poor neurologic condition. Initial mean blood pressure for drug-induced hypotension patients followed at the 5th year was 2.5 mm Hg higher than for those followed in earlier intervals; for the other treatment categories, less than 1 mm Hg difference between initial levels was found.

Pulse rate measurements were taken in addition to blood pressures. No significant difference in average pulse rate level was observed, but drug-induced hypotension patients averaged 1 to 3 beats per minute slower than those in the other treatment groups. At 3 months, the average pulse ranged from 78.8 for drug-induced hypotension to 81.8 for bed rest. At 5 years, average pulse rates ranged from 76.6 for drug-induced hypotension and 80.3 for carotid ligation. No change in average pulse rate for patients in carotid ligation was observed over the follow-up period, while a decline of 1 to 3 beats per minute was observed for patients in other treatment groups followed at 5 years compared to those followed at 3 months.

Results Relating to Specific Treatments

Drug-induced Hypotension

Effective drug-induced hypotension was defined according to the degree of reduction of the systolic blood pressure compared to the level of the systolic pressure in the resting state. Reduction was considered "effective" or "satisfactory" if, according to definition, a systolic blood pressure of 140 mm Hg or lower was reduced by 20%. If the systolic blood pressure ranged between 140

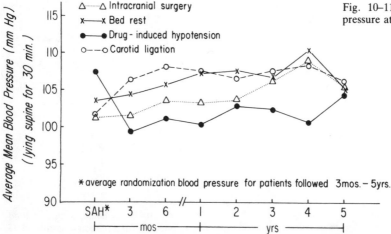

Fig. 10–11. Average mean blood pressure at follow-up intervals.

and 180 mm Hg, a reduction of 25% was defined as satisfactory; if blood pressure was more than 180 mm Hg, a 30% reduction was required.

Interesting facts emerged in the analysis of this group of patients relative to their adherence to the antihypertensive drug regimen and the effectiveness of drug therapy as it was carried out by the patient and the physician. One should note that the highest mortality (80%) was among that group of patients treated by drug-induced hypotension who did not have an adequate reduction of blood pressure as defined above. These patients died *before blood pressure was satisfactorily reduced.* Further, when such failure occurred, the blood pressure reduction had not been accomplished until after the second week of treatment.

Referring to the bar graph in Figure 10–12, one notes a progressively smaller number of patients who continued to take antihypertensive medication during the 5-year period of observation. The number who discontinued their medication showed little change from the first 3 months through the entire follow-up period. The number becomes greater in successive follow-up intervals, and thus the number of patients known to have continued to take medication dropped to one half of the original number (163 at 3 months to 75 at 5 years). During the 5-year period of observation, medication was discontinued by the patient himself because of

"annoying side-effects" in 23 instances. Discontinuance of the drug was spread quite uniformly at the particular follow-up intervals during the first 3 years. During the 5-year period, the drug was discontinued by the physician 36 times, in more than one half of the patients (21) within the first year. Drug treatment was discontinued in 127 patients for "other reasons" (patient was erratic about taking medication, got "tired" of taking it, etc.).

The 80% mortality from rebleeding in patients treated by drug-induced hypotension in whom an "adequate" (as defined) reduction of blood pressure was not achieved is sobering. It is important, then, to see what "effective" blood pressure had been accomplished and over what length of time.

Figure 10–13 depicts graphically the number of patients who had "effective" (as defined by protocol) drug-induced hypotension determined at the respective follow-up periods. At 3 months, a surprisingly low number of patients—a little less than two thirds (98, or 60%) of those who were actively treated—had maintained a reduced blood pressure. A similar figure (62, or 60%) was recorded until the 3-year interval. In the 4th and 5th years, it was 68 and 66%, respectively. It may be argued that more vigorous measures could have been utilized to obtain the desired lower blood pressure. From the observed data, however, it cannot be stated that such measures were not maximal.

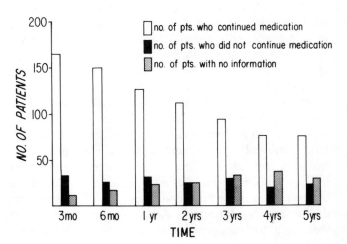

Fig. 10–12. Drug-induced hypotension treatment at follow-up.

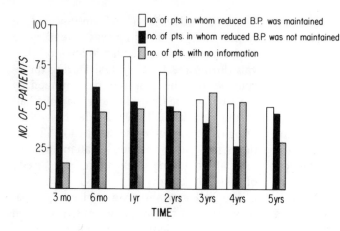

Fig. 10–13.   Maintenance of reduced blood pressure in patients treated by drug-induced hypotension.

Carotid Ligation at Follow-up

Among the original 187 patients followed during the 10-year period (and noting the fall-off in the last 5 years of that period), 20 complications were related to treatment. Sixteen of these occurred in the initial 30-day period and 2 in the 31 to 90-day interval. All of those patients died. Two additional complications took place from the 3rd to the 12th months. Within the first 90 days, 24 proven recurrent hemorrhages had taken place, 21 within the first 30-day period. There were no proved rebleeding episodes thereafter until the 8th year. Twelve patients were suspected of having had a rebleed, all in the initial 90-day period. During the second 6 months of the first year, another hemorrhage was suspected, but none thereafter. In the 3-month interval following randomization, 5 permanent cerebrovascular deficits were recorded. Permanent defects occurred in 2 patients with internal carotid artery aneurysms and in 3 with anterior cerebral artery aneurysms. At the 6-month follow-up, 1 patient had incurred a permanent and another a transient cerebrovascular insult. At 1 year, two instances of a transient deficit were noted in patients with middle and anterior cerebral artery aneurysms, respectively. A transient ischemic attack occurred in 2 patients with middle cerebral artery aneurysm and in 1 who had an aneurysm of the internal carotid artery. At the time of the 3-year analysis, permanent cerebrovas-

cular defects resulted in 2 patients, both of whom had internal carotid artery aneurysms. No new neurologic problems considered to be the consequences of protracted ischemia or of infarction were noted in the 4th year. However, in the 5th year, a permanent cerebrovascular accident occurred followed within 3 weeks by the patient's death, which was considered unrelated to the original hemorrhage.

Ophthalmodynamometry

The effectiveness of treating an intracranial aneurysm by carotid ligation is based on the concept that if the pressure within the vessel (aneurysm), the pulsatile flow and the "water-hammer" effect upon the aneurysm are reduced, thrombosis is promoted to allow healing of the rent in the aneurysm, thereby preventing rerupture. It is not known what degree of reduction in intravascular (aneurysm) pressure is necessary to accomplish this. Once the aneurysm is thrombosed, there would appear to be no further need for reduction. Postoperative studies by angiography to determine critical pressure reduction, vis-à-vis its effect upon obliteration of the aneurysm, have not been made. Adequate sealing of the rent in the aneurysm must have a variable function in terms of time. From this standpoint there have been no concerted studies to determine how long it takes to secure an aneurysm and to protect the patient against re-rupture by carotid ligation. Ecker and Riemenschneider[1] in 1951 reported on the deliberate thrombosis of an intracranial aneurysm under fluoroscopic control. There are no other accounts of similar studies although spontaneous thrombosis in an aneurysm of the carotid and posterior-inferior cerebellar artery was observed (personal experience) and thrombosis in an aneurysm following carotid ligation was reported by Logue in a personal communication to Ecker and Riemenschneider[1].

An indirect measure of carotid artery pressure at the level of the ophthalmic artery can be made by ophthalmodynamometry. Despite the requirements of the protocol, a disappointingly small number of patients had serial follow-up ophthalmodynamometry. The reasons for this are not apparent. The examiner may have reasoned that since the patient's progress was satisfactory, the test would add nothing since a carotid artery had already been "sacrificed." Angiography may have revealed the aneurysm to be no longer visible or smaller and because of this the need for further ophthalmodynamometric determination was considered superfluous. The examiner may have thought that no matter what the reading might be, nothing else could be done with the respective artery.

The procedure employed was the determination in each eye of the minimal pressure (in terms of grams) that would collapse the retinal arteries and the minimal pressure (grams) that would allow the earliest visible pulsation of the retinal arteries. The mean arterial pressure was then determined by adding to the latter pressure one-third the difference between the two. The difference (unoccluded minus occluded side) in the mean value was then divided by the mean value of the unoccluded side to determine the percentage drop of pressure on the occluded side.

In the first 3-month check, when reports from 124 patients were available, pressures were recorded in only 37 (29.8%). Only 22 of the 37 were noted to have a drop in pressure on the side of the occluded carotid artery. The average drop in mean pressure was 20.3%, being in the range from a low of 3.2% to a high of 55.6%. The drop was only between 3.2 and 13% in 7 patients, between 17.3 and 23.7% in 7 patients and between 25 and 55.6% in 8 patients.

At the 6-month follow-up, pressure measurements were made only in 24 of 123 patients. Among the 24, 18 were indicated as showing a drop in mean pressure which averaged 26.9%. The range of percentage drop was between 5 and 49.2%. Four measurements fell between 5 and 14.6%, 6 between 23.1 and 26.9% and the remainder (8) between 31.9 and 49.2%.

At 1 year, among the 118 patients that could be followed, the ophthalmodynamometric examination was made in 29 but significant recordings numbered only 12. The average fall in mean pressure on the side of the occluded carotid artery was 24.4%, ranging between 3 and 50%. Three patients had pressure drops of 3 to 5.2% and 1 of 11.1%. Four were in the range of 21.4 to 29% and 4 ranged between 35.9 and 50%.

The 2-year follow-up yielded 112 patients in whom 26 pressure determinations were made, with significant recordings in 10. The average mean pressure fall in these 10 patients was 22%, in the range of 3.9 and 45%. Five were between 3.9 and 20.6% and 5 between 22.1 and 45%.

In the 3-year follow-up, there were 105 patients. Ophthalmodynamometry was made in 21, with pertinent recordings in only 5. The average of the mean percentage reduction in pressure on the side of the occluded artery was 16.6%, the lowest being 1.4% and the highest 37.5%.

Among 94 patients at the 4-year evaluation, there were 15 pressure determinations, but only 4 were recorded. The average mean pressure drop was 10.7%, the lowest being 4.2% and the highest 21.7%.

At 5 years, the number of patients reported in the follow-up period was 87, of whom 14 had pressure measurements made. Six were recorded as significant tests. An average mean pressure reduction of 14.4% was noted, ranging between 2.7 and 44.1%.

The tendency for the degree of pressure

reduction tended to remain relatively the same where several determinations were made at the follow-up period. Information concerning a relationship of the degree of mean pressure drop in patients who developed a transient ischemic attack (TIA) or a permanent cerebrovascular insult was insufficient to suggest such a relationship. There were 7 patients with a TIA and 10 with a permanent cerebrovascular insult. Among these, the tests were not made regularly, not made at all, or made only once either at the time the episode was recorded or at a later date. For example, 2 patients with TIA did not have measurements at the time the TIA was recorded (at 3 months in 1, at 1 year in another) or in the subsequent follow-up. Six with permanent cerebrovascular insults had no measurements made, including 3 whose deficit was noted at 3 months, 1 recorded at 6 months and 2 recorded at 3 years. In 1 patient with a TIA at 6 months, a measurement at 1 year was evidently poorly performed. In another patient with a TIA noted at 3 months, the mean pressure fall was 25%. During the next 3 years, the value ranged between 49 and 37%. In another with a TIA at 3 months, no drop was noted at 3 months; a drop of 13% was observed at 6 months, but none thereafter in the 5-year follow-up when determinations were regularly made. One patient with a TIA at 2 years was noted at the 3-month evaluation to have had a 19% drop in pressure, but no determinations were made thereafter. A TIA was noted at 1 year in a patient. The mean pressure drop at 3 months was 65%; at 6 months and at 1 year, it was 27%. However, at 3, 4 and 5 years, no fall was measured. Three patients who were noted to have permanent cerebrovascular defects at 3 months showed no measured fall in pressure at that time or subsequently. One had had serial measurements over the 5-year follow-up period, another at 1 and at 2 years and the third had had but one determination made at 3 months. A permanent cerebrovascular insult was noted at 5 years in a patient in whom at 3 months to 4 years no pressure drop had been recorded. It is likely that ophthalmodynamometry

is of little value as a predictive tool in determining which patients with a carotid ligation will develop a transient or permanent cerebrovascular insult. In only 2 instances (both in patients with TIAs) were significant drops in pressure measured at 3 and 6 months. In 1, the reduction was greater at 3 months than at 6 months, while in the other, the reverse was true. After 6 months, no appreciable change had occurred.

Therapy-accomplished Patients

Eight hundred and twenty-five patients subsequently were treated as designated by the randomization process. Previous descriptions of the characteristics, mortality and rebleeding of these patients have been reported.[2-7]

Follow-up Completion

Knowledge of death or survival status was 97% complete at 1 year, 91% at 3 years, 84% at 5 years and only 48% at 10 years (Table 10–16). Carotid ligation patients were the lowest, with 83% at 4 years, 79% at 5 years and 29% at 10 years. Regulated bed rest had 88% follow-up at 5 years and 61% at 10 years. If only survivors are analyzed, follow-up percentages for all groups are 98% at 3 months, 96% at 1 year, 86% at 3 years, 74% at 5 years and only 10% at 10 years. Follow-up of survivors was equivalent for all therapy-accomplished treatment groups.

Mortality

Since the therapy-accomplished group includes only patients surviving from randomization to treatment, patients suitable for that therapy (in terms of medical condition) and patients who received the complete procedure (i.e., antihypertensive therapy, complete carotid clamp closure, definitive surgical procedure), the survival would be

Table 10–16.   Treatment-Accomplished Subgroups: Number of Patients Followed.

Treatment		SAH	Follow-up Interval						
			3 months	6 months	1 year	2 years	3 years	4 years	5 years
Bed rest	Followed	194	116	111	104	88	79	73	66
	Died		75	6	3	10	3	5	3
Drug-induced	Followed	273	185	175	166	156	142	124	118
hypotension	Died		85	5	8	4	6	6	1
Carotid	Followed	126	106	106	103	98	92	82	75
ligation	Died		17	1	3	0	1	1	1
Intracranial	Followed	232	172	158	153	143	133	116	108
surgery	Died		55	14	5	2	2	5	4
Overall	Followed	825	579	550	526	485	446	395	367
	Died		232	26	19	16	12	16	9

expected to be better than in the randomization-defined treatment group.

For regulated bed rest, the mortality rates are approximately equivalent to those of the overall group. Thirty-nine percent of patients having bed rest therapy were not alive at 3 months, 50% at 2 years and 57% at 5 years (Fig. 10–14). Proved or suspected rebleed accounted for 72% of all deaths in the 5-year period.

Of the 273 patients who received adequate bed rest and antihypertensive medication, 31% had not survived by the 3rd month. The overall drug-induced hypotension category had a 34% mortality rate for the same period. By the end of 5 years, a 43% rate in the treated group was demonstrated. The cause of death distribution was the same for the overall and actually treated groups.

The largest difference in mortality between the overall randomization group and the treatment-accomplished subgroup was in carotid ligation. The overall group experienced a 31% mortality rate by 3 months, while the ligation-accomplished subgroup suffered only a 14% mortality rate for the same interval. Over the remaining follow-up period, a 6% mortality rate produced a 5-year mortality experience of 20%, 17% lower than the total group. Perret and Nibbelink[7] have found that one third of the patients who did not have carotid ligation ac-

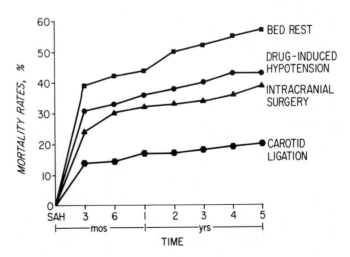

Fig. 10–14.   Cumulative mortality rates for treatment-accomplished patients.

Table 10-17. Condition Since Last Follow-up for Treatment-Accomplished Subgroups.*

Treatment	Condition	Follow-up Interval												
		3 months		6 months		1 year		2 years		3 years		4 years		5 years	
		No.	%	No.	%	No.	%	No.	%	No.	%	No.	%	No.	%
Bed rest	Improved	86	74.1	66	59.5	52	50.0	30	34.1	14	17.7	9	12.3	10	15.2
	Same	26	22.4	40	36.0	48	46.2	52	59.1	61	77.2	59	80.8	53	80.3
	Worse	5	4.3	3	2.7	3	2.9	2	2.3	2	2.5	3	4.1	1	1.5
Drug-induced hypotension	Improved	123	66.5	94	53.7	80	48.2	52	33.3	22	15.4	17	13.7	13	11.0
	Same	51	27.6	78	44.6	84	50.6	102	65.4	114	80.3	103	83.1	98	83.1
	Worse	11	5.9	3	1.7	2	1.2	1	0.6	4	2.8	3	2.4	7	5.9
Carotid ligation	Improved	80	75.5	57	53.8	38	36.9	29	29.6	15	16.3	15	18.3	9	12.0
	Same	22	20.8	44	41.5	58	56.3	68	69.4	73	79.3	64	78.0	60	80.0
	Worse	3	2.8	2	1.9	7	6.8	1	1.0	2	2.2	3	3.7	5	6.7
Intracranial surgery	Improved	130	75.6	108	68.3	74	48.4	42	29.4	32	24.1	16	13.8	12	11.1
	Same	27	15.7	49	31.0	67	43.8	93	65.0	96	72.2	96	82.8	93	86.1
	Worse	12	7.0	1	0.6	10	6.5	7	4.9	4	3.0	4	3.4	3	2.8
Overall	Improved	419	72.4	325	59.1	244	46.4	153	31.5	83	18.6	57	14.4	44	12.0
	Same	126	21.8	211	38.4	257	48.9	315	64.9	344	77.1	322	81.5	304	82.8
	Worse	29	5.0	9	1.6	22	4.2	11	2.3	12	2.7	13	3.3	16	4.4

* Note: Table does not list incomplete observations, which were included in calculating percentages.

Table 10–18. Capacity for Self-Care at Follow-up for Treatment Accomplished.*

Treatment	Capacity	3 months		6 months		1 year		2 years		3 years		4 years		5 years	
		No.	%	No.	%	No.	%	No.	%	No.	%	No.	%	No.	%
Bed rest	Self-Care	99	85.3	101	91.0	93	89.4	85	96.6	77	97.5	70	95.9	63	95.5
	Self-Care with aid	3	2.6	4	3.6	4	3.8	1	1.1	1	1.3	1	1.4	1	1.5
	Unable to care for self	13	11.2	6	5.4	5	4.8	1	1.1	0	0.0	1	1.4	0	0.0
Drug-induced hypotension	Self-care	156	84.3	162	92.6	156	94.0	150	96.2	133	93.7	116	93.5	108	91.5
	Self-care with aid	5	2.7	3	1.7	4	2.4	3	1.9	5	3.5	3	2.4	3	2.5
	Unable to care for self	24	13.0	10	5.7	5	3.0	2	1.3	4	2.8	4	3.2	6	5.1
Carotid ligation	Self-care	96	90.6	97	91.5	92	89.3	89	90.8	84	91.3	79	96.3	68	90.7
	Self-care with aid	3	2.8	6	5.7	4	3.9	4	4.1	3	3.3	1	1.2	1	1.3
	Unable to care for self	7	6.6	2	1.9	6	5.8	5	5.1	4	4.3	2	2.4	3	4.0
Intracranial surgery	Self-care	125	72.7	129	81.6	130	85.0	125	87.4	124	93.2	110	94.8	99	91.7
	Self-care with aid	5	2.9	9	5.7	6	3.9	6	4.2	1	0.8	1	0.9	1	0.9
	Unable to care for self	42	24.4	19	12.0	16	10.5	10	7.0	7	5.3	5	4.3	4	3.7
Overall	Self-care	476	82.2	489	88.9	471	89.5	449	92.6	418	93.7	375	94.9	338	92.1
	Self-care with aid	16	2.8	22	4.0	18	3.4	14	2.9	10	2.2	6	1.5	6	1.6
	Unable to care for self	86	14.9	37	6.7	32	6.1	18	3.7	15	3.4	12	3.0	13	3.5

Follow-up Interval

* Note: See note under Table 10–17.

complished died after randomization and before application and closure of the clamp. Winn et al.[8] reported that late bleeding in this group does occur in significant numbers.

The mortality of 232 intracranial surgery patients with treatment accomplished was 6% lower than the overall randomization group. At 3 months, 24% had died; by 5 years, 39%. The mortality experience difference can be accounted for by the number of patients having a recurrent hemorrhage. By 3 months, rebleeding accounted for 30% of all deaths for the randomization group, but 15% of the total for the surgery-performed group.

Condition Since Last Follow-up

Improvement from the previous evaluation for those reporting for follow-up evaluation was apparent up to 1 year post-hemorrhage and was similar to that of the overall randomization groups. Seventy-two percent of treatment-accomplished patients seen at follow-up improved from discharge to 3 months; 22% were the same (Table 10–17). At 6 months, 59% had improved while 38% remained the same. By 1 year, 46% were improved from their 6-month status and 49% were the same. Improvement in clinical condition declined successively to 32% at 2 years, 19% at 3 years, 14% at 4 years and 12% at 5 years, while stabilization of the patients' status became more predominant (65% at 2 years, 77% at 3 years, 82% at 4 years and 83% at 5 years).

Bed rest-treated patients followed a similar trend as the overall group, with 74% improved at 3 months, 50% at 1 year and 15% at 5 years. By 1 year, the patients' condition was the same in 46%; by 5 years, 80% had not changed.

Drug-induced hypotension patients showed less improvement up to 6 months from previous evaluations. Sixty-six percent of patients improved between discharge and 3 months and 54% between 3 months and 6 months. By the 3rd year, 80% of the patients did not change status from the 2nd-year assessment.

Carotid ligation patients followed a trend similar to the bed rest patients at 3 months, but more patients remained the same at subsequent intervals. By 2 years, 69% of these patients had no change in condition; by 3 years, 80% were the same.

Intracranial surgery patients improved at a 76% rate for the discharge to 3-month evaluation. The interval to the 6-month follow-up showed that 68% of the patients were still improving. By 2 years, 65% of patients had not changed from their 1-year level. By 5 years, 86% of the patients had not changed.

Capacity for Self-care

The ability to care for one's self varied according to the treatment-accomplished group. Patients having regulated bed rest and drug-induced hypotension had similar results (Table 10–18). Eighty-five percent of these patients could care for themselves by 3 months; 12% were unable to care for themselves. By 6 months, over 90% of those followed could perform self-care with no assistance; by 2 years, less than 5% required assistance. Carotid ligation patients had the highest level of self-care at 3 months: 91%. These patients remained at this level throughout the 5-year follow-up. This experience was better than that of the overall randomization group throughout the interval. Patients treated with intracranial surgery had the lowest level of self-care, 73%, and the greatest level of patients unfit for self-care, 24%, at 3 months. Eighty-two percent could perform self-care by 6 months, 6% required assistance and 12% were unfit for self-care. By 3 years, the patients with intracranial surgery had reached 93% total care and only 5% were unable to care for themselves.

Employment Capability

The ability to return to gainful employment varied not only by time from hemorrhage but also treatment (Table 10–19). At 3

Table 10-19. Present Employment Capability for Treatment-Accomplished Subgroups.

Treatment	Present Employment*	Follow-up Interval												
		3 months		6 months		1 year		2 years		3 years		4 years		5 years	
		No.	%	No.	%	No.	%	No.	%	No.	%	No.	%	No.	%
Bed rest	1	26	22.4	51	45.9	54	51.9	52	59.1	50	63.3	42	57.5	36	54.5
	2	17	14.7	12	10.8	6	5.8	9	10.2	8	10.1	4	5.5	5	7.6
	3	7	6.0	4	3.6	5	4.8	6	6.8	5	6.3	1	1.4	1	1.5
	4	0	0.0	1	0.9	0	0.0	1	1.1	0	0.0	1	1.4	1	1.5
	5	43	37.1	29	26.1	25	24.0	12	13.6	10	12.6	15	20.5	12	18.2
	6	23	19.8	14	12.6	14	13.5	7	8.0	4	5.1	8	11.0	8	12.1
Drug-induced hypotension	1	48	25.9	82	46.9	104	62.7	99	63.5	89	62.7	75	60.4	66	55.9
	2	29	17.7	24	13.7	9	5.4	11	7.1	8	5.6	10	8.1	13	11.0
	3	4	2.2	4	2.3	7	4.2	6	3.8	7	4.9	4	3.2	3	2.5
	4	0	0.0	0	0.0	2	1.2	1	0.6	1	0.7	1	0.8	0	0.0
	5	64	34.6	37	21.1	25	15.1	26	16.7	19	13.4	16	12.9	14	11.9
	6	40	21.6	28	16.0	19	11.4	12	7.7	17	12.0	18	14.5	22	18.6
Carotid ligation	1	42	39.6	66	62.3	70	68.0	70	71.4	63	68.5	53	64.6	53	70.7
	2	5	4.7	10	9.4	9	8.7	7	7.1	9	9.8	9	11.0	3	4.0
	3	4	3.8	1	0.9	4	3.9	4	4.1	2	2.2	5	6.1	3	4.0
	4	4	3.8	1	0.9	2	1.9	2	2.0	3	3.3	1	1.2	1	1.3
	5	36	34.0	16	15.1	7	6.8	7	7.1	6	6.5	10	12.2	7	9.3
	6	15	14.2	10	9.4	9	8.7	8	8.2	9	9.8	4	4.9	7	9.3
Intracranial surgery	1	42	24.4	70	44.3	77	50.3	80	55.9	77	57.9	76	65.5	67	62.0
	2	13	7.6	13	8.2	10	6.5	9	6.3	6	4.5	5	4.3	6	5.6
	3	4	2.3	5	3.2	6	3.9	7	4.9	5	3.8	6	5.2	6	5.6
	4	0	0.0	0	0.0	0	0.0	1	0.7	3	2.3	3	2.6	5	4.6
	5	48	27.9	31	19.6	26	17.0	23	16.1	17	12.8	7	6.0	7	6.5
	6	65	37.8	39	24.7	34	22.2	23	16.1	25	18.8	19	16.4	15	13.9
Overall	1	158	27.3	269	48.9	305	58.0	301	62.1	279	62.6	246	62.3	222	60.5
	2	65	11.2	59	10.7	34	6.5	36	7.4	31	7.0	28	7.1	27	7.4
	3	19	3.3	14	2.5	22	4.2	23	4.7	19	4.3	16	4.1	13	3.5
	4	4	0.7	2	0.4	4	0.8	5	1.0	7	1.6	6	1.5	7	1.9
	5	191	33.0	113	20.5	83	15.8	68	14.0	52	11.6	48	12.2	40	10.9
	6	143	24.7	91	16.5	76	14.4	50	10.3	55	12.3	49	12.4	52	14.2

* See Table 10–9.

months post-hemorrhage, 22% of bed rest patients were working full time at the same or equivalent occupation and 15% were working part time. Drug-induced hypotension patients demonstrated a 26 and 18% level, respectively. Forty percent of carotid ligation-treated patients were working full time and 5% part time. With intracranial surgery, 25% were at full-time and 8% at part-time jobs at 3 months. Only 14% of carotid ligation patients, 20% of bed rest patients, 22% of drug-induced hypotension patients and 38% of intracranial surgery patients were unable to work. By 1 year, 77% of carotid ligation patients, 68% of drug-induced hypotension patients, 58% of bed rest patients, and 57% of intracranial surgery patients were full time or part time. Continuing through the 5-year follow-up, carotid ligation patients had the highest level of employment capability (75% full time or part time at 5 years) and the lowest level of persons unfit for gainful employment.

Summary

A cooperative study was conducted to determine the best available treatment for subarachnoid hemorrhage from a ruptured intracranial aneurysm. The aneurysm was located at one of three sites on the anterior portion of the circle of Willis, namely, the internal carotid artery, the middle cerebral artery or the anterior cerebral-anterior communicating artery complex. Specific treatment was by allocation through a randomization process and according to a defined protocol.

Nine hundred and seventy-two patients allocated to one of four treatments were studied according to a detailed analysis of: (1) regulated bed rest, (2) drug-induced hypotension, (3) carotid artery ligation and (4) intracranial operation. The initial intent was to analyze a 10-year follow-up at specific intervals. However, between the 6th and 10th years (and especially in the 5 to 6-year period), 33% of the patients were lost to the follow-up process. The fate of 467 patients (48%) is therefore unknown. The loss of responders, especially during the last 5 years, was due to the fact that more than one half of the investigators withdrew from the study. It was therefore impossible to carry the complete analysis beyond the 5-year period because of inadequate information. Two hundred and two patients were delegated to treatment by bed rest, 309 by drug-induced hypotension, 187 by carotid ligation and 274 by intracranial operation. The overall 10-year mortality for patients in the bed rest-treated group who could be followed was 55% (112 of 202). At the end of 5 years, 110 patients (54%) had died; 55 (24%) had been lost to the follow-up process, the mortality among this latter number being unknown. For patients in the drug-induced hypotension category, the overall 10-year mortality was 46% (143 of 309). Until the end of the 5th year, 47 (15%) had been lost to the follow-up process; thereafter, the loss was 34% (105 of 309).

The carotid ligation group had an overall mortality for 10 years of 39% (73 of 187); 100 (53%) were lost to follow-up, 69 (37%) during the 5 to 10-year period.

The overall mortality among patients treated by intracranial operation was 45% (126 of 274). At the end of 5 years, 15% (41 of 274) were lost to follow-up. From the end of the 5th to the end of the 10th year, an additional 95 (35%) were lost, making a total of 136 over a 10-year period.

These high mortality rates are disturbing, but it should be emphasized that they represent a mortality from *all* causes of death during the 10-year period. More significant figures are those dealing with the mortality at the 3-month interval following randomization. It is necessary also to point out that allocation to a particular treatment did not necessarily mean that the treatment was accomplished. The 3-month interval gives a better idea of the mortality directly related to the subarachnoid hemorrhage. The figure is distorted, however, in that it includes the mortality from hemorrhage as well as the complications of treatment. At this time, the mortality was 39% (78 of 202) for bed rest, 34% (104 of 309) for drug-induced hypotension, 31% (58 of 187) for carotid ligation and 30% (83 of 274) for patients treated by intracranial operation.

The capacity for self-care among patients in the bed rest category at 3 months was 85% (103 of 121); 2.5% required assistance and 11.6% (14 of 121) were completely disabled. The percentage of those able to care for themselves rose to 95% at 5 years, but only about one half (68) were available for follow-up at that time. At the same interval there were no patients with total disability, whereas at 4 years 2.6% (2 of 76) were disabled.

For the 202 patients who were designated to drug-induced hypotension, 84% (169) were able to care for themselves at 3 months, whereas 13% (27) were totally disabled and 2.5% (5) required aids. By 5 years, the percentage able to care for themselves rose to 91% (114 of 125); 2.4% (3) required aids and 5.6% (7) remained totally disabled.

Among the carotid ligation patients, 86% (107 of 124) were capable of self-care at the 3-month interval, 4.8% (6) required assistance and 8.9% (11 of 124) were totally disabled. At the 5-year evaluation, 92.6% (78 of 87) cared for themselves, 2.3% (2) needed assistance and 4.6% (4) continued with total disability.

In the group of patients treated with intracranial operation, the 3-month evaluation disclosed 70.7% (130 of 184) capable of self-care, 3.3% (6) requiring assistance and 26.1% (48) completely disabled. The tendency for improvement was much greater in this category of patients, so that at 5 years 91.2% (103 of 113) were self-sufficient, 0.9% (1) required aids and 4.4% (5) remained totally disabled.

The percentage of patients capable of self-care fell from 96% at 3 months to 87.5% at 5 years for patients with internal carotid artery aneurysms and rose from 90 to 93.7% in patients with middle cerebral artery aneurysms. There was an 8% increase (84.3 to 92.2%) for those with anterior cerebral artery aneurysms. By 5 years, no patients were

totally disabled among the middle cerebral artery group, but 12.5 and 3.9% in the internal carotid and anterior cerebral artery groups, respectively, were totally disabled. In the carotid ligation patients, the tendency for the number capable of caring for themselves at 3 months was about the same for those with an internal carotid artery as with an anterior cerebral artery aneurysm—85.7 and 84.1%, respectively; it was 94.1% for the much smaller number who had aneurysms of the middle cerebral artery. The trend for self-care at 5 years increased from 85.5 to only 88.1% for those with internal carotid and from 84.1 to 91.7% for those with anterior cerebral artery aneurysms, but decreased from 94.1 to 88.9% for patients with middle cerebral artery aneurysms at the time of the 5-year evaluation. Total disability at 3 months was highest among those patients who were allocated to intracranial operation for aneurysms at all sites. The ability for self-care was 20% greater for those patients with anterior cerebral artery than for those with internal carotid and 10% greater than for those with middle cerebral artery aneurysms. However, the number of patients with an aneurysm of the anterior cerebral artery was 5 times greater than for those with an aneurysm of the middle cerebral artery or internal carotid artery. The disability was 5% lower for those patients with anterior cerebral artery than for middle cerebral artery aneurysms and 20% lower than for those with internal carotid artery aneurysms. At the end of 5 years (as compared to 3 months), there was a trend for a greater number of patients to be able to take care of themselves. In patients with aneurysms of the middle cerebral artery, for example, 27% more patients were capable of self-care at 5 years than at 3 months. For those with anterior cerebral artery aneurysms, 20% more cared for themselves at 5 years than at 3 months. The increase was 15% for those with internal carotid artery aneurysms. The small number of patients with internal carotid and middle cerebral artery aneurysms indicate, however, that this increase is only relative. Twenty percent fewer patients with aneurysms at the three major sites were totally disabled at 5 years than at 3 months.

For patients with bed rest, 52.9% were working full time at their usual jobs at the 5-year interval. This represented a decrease of 8% at 3 years (61%), but was 30% higher than at 3 months. The percentage of patients unfit for gainful employment at 5 years was 11.8%, 8% lower than at the 3-month evaluation.

For the drug-induced hypotension group, 56.8% were fully employed at 5 years, 30% more than at 3 months (26.7%). The percentage unable to work was 22.3% at 3 months and 18.4% at 5 years.

Among the patients with carotid artery ligation, 16% more were at usual working capacity at 5 years than at 3 months (52.2 vs 36.3%). The percentage disabled at 3 months was 20.2%; at 5 years, it was 7.1%.

At 5 years, the percentage of patients of the intracranial operation category who were at full-time original work was 60.2%, whereas at 3 months this was 23.4%. Total disability involved 39.1% of patients at 3 months and 15% at 5 years.

Ophthalmodynamometry is not a useful indicator in determining a patient's tolerance to carotid ligation.

Comment

The immediate prognosis for patients with a ruptured intracranial aneurysm is measured against time. The risk of subarachnoid hemorrhage from a ruptured intracranial aneurysm is both short- and long-term. The short-term risk resolves itself into the mortality of the first hemorrhage (10 to 15%); the long-term risk concerns the possibility of recurrent hemorrhage occurring on a day-to-day basis during the first 2 weeks after the initial one. The chance of recurrent hemorrhage rises from day to day until a peak at 7 to 10 days, after which it falls off rather abruptly. At a variable time, usually be-

tween the 5th and 8th days, secondary complications of the hemorrhage presumed to be ischemic and due to constriction of the cerebral arteries (vasospasm) take place in 40 to 50% of patients. There is then a plateau at the 12th day lasting for several days, and then a gradual decline.

Optimal treatment of an aneurysm is its exclusion from the circulation. This accomplishes but one thing: removal of the threat of a recurrent hemorrhage. Although exclusion of the aneurysm prevents recurrent bleeding, there is no evidence that it affects the unpredictable occurrence of vasospasm and its putative effect upon the brain. Although early (1 to 4 days) operation is desirable from the standpoint of controlling the aneurysm, it does not obviate the subsequent "natural" occurrence of vasospasm, as well as the effects of operative manipulation upon the brain which may produce or aggravate such spasm. Although it appears possible to operate early after subarachnoid hemorrhage more safely than in the past, especially in Grade 1, 2 and even Grade 3 patients, the specter of vasospasm occurring in the critical 4 to 7-day period persists. The reports of Sano and Saito[9] and Hori and Suzuki[10] in this regard are encouraging, however. The initial "known" 10 to 15% mortality (probably closer to 50% considering those patients who die before reaching hospital) from aneurysmal hemorrhage is clouded by the issue of the incidence of rebleeding, since it is frequently not certain whether a patient may have bled before the hemorrhage leading to admission to hospital. Our original impressions[2] were that recurrent hemorrhage from an aneurysm was rare after 1 year and particularly after 2 years. The long-term study of Kaste and Troupp,[12] however, which covered a mean period of 109 months, indicated that fatal rebleeding did occur at a significant rate after several years. In a controlled trial of late surgical versus conservative treatment for intracranial artery aneurysms, in which patients were allocated to a specific treatment on an average of 51 days after subarachnoid hemorrhage, they found that in 92 patients delegated to conservative (bed rest) treatment, 4 had recurrent hemorrhage in the 1st month and 2 in the 2nd month. Recurrent hemorrhage appeared in 10 others at 3, 4, 17, 57, 81, 85, 98, 104, 123 and 139 months. Among the 86 who had intracranial surgery, 6 rebled and died. Since the interval between hemorrhage and the decision for either operation or conservative treatment was from 15 to 127 days for those who had operation and 15 to 171 days for those who were to have conservative treatment, these groups, although comparable, were very selective. During the interval until a specific decision for specific treatment was made, a considerable number of patients who would have had complications (recurrent hemorrhage, an ischemic insult, and so forth) expected to occur early in the natural course of the disease were eliminated. The rate of recurrence then does represent an accurate appraisal of the rate of "late" rebleeding. Similarly, the study of Winn, Richardson, and Jane in their 10-year[13] and 15-year[14] follow-up of patients with aneurysmal subarachnoid hemorrhage indicated a rebleeding rate of about 3% per year. The figures in these series then approximate each other very closely: 3.5% by Kaste and Troupp,[12] 3% by Winn et al.[13,14]

Intracranial operation prevents rerupture if the aneurysm is accurately occluded. Occlusion of a carotid artery by ligation appeared to be protective against a rebleed in a study by Perret and Nibbelink[7]. Among 125 patients who had occlusion of the carotid artery, they found 13 (10.4%) who rebled— 9 within 6 days of complete occlusion and 4 (3.2%) between 13 and 26 days following occlusion. There was no recurrent hemorrhage then until 8 years later.

Among the four treatments discussed, rebleeding over both the short- and long-term is best prevented by operation, especially by intracranial operation. To be weighed against this is the risk of complications of the operative procedure.

Aneurysm surgery, like cardiac surgery, is not an exercise for the occasional operator. The best expertise and the most properly equipped operating room and experienced personnel should be made available. The time is long past for revision of the impressions that were depicted in the original Cooperative Aneurysm Project as to the results of intracranial operation that were considered "par for the course." This is being borne out by detailed papers being published by surgeons with a large experience in the field (Sano and Saito,[9] Yoshimoto et al.[15]). Unquestionably, greater care is being exercised in the selection of patients for operation. Along with this, it is evident that technical advances and experience have improved operative results, especially in good-condition patients. No longer does the surgeon struggle with a "tight" swollen brain that in the past frequently thwarted even exposure of the aneurysm before it ruptured. This has been accomplished by expert modern neuroanesthesia. The employment of deep barbiturate narcosis protection for the brain, controlled monitoring with the electroencephalogram, prolonged deep hypotension along with drainage techniques, and other methods for reducing brain bulk produce a slack, relaxed brain with open cerebrospinal fluid pathways which facilitate safer access to the aneurysm and its management. The operating microscope and microdissection techniques with sophisticated instrumentation have made operation appreciably safer even in the hands of the less adept surgeon. Early (1 to 3 days) operation following subarachnoid hemorrhage, therefore, is being re-evaluated because of these technical advances. It is much easier to remove a recent soft clot by gentle suction from about an aneurysm seen at that time in contrast to the difficult dissection of an aneurysm surrounded by a "tough" brain, fibrotic tissue and thickened arachnoid operated upon in the 2nd or 3rd week after the hemorrhage.

Early operation, however, does not solve the problem of "vasospasm"—the angiographic narrowing of cerebral vessels and its presumed effects which follow subarachnoid hemorrhage, especially from a ruptured aneurysm. Appearing about the 4th day following hemorrhage and reaching a peak incidence at the 7th to 10th days post-hemorrhage, it adds to operation the risk of an ischemic insult to a brain which, until that time, has been protected by adequate blood flow. A technical success of excluding an aneurysm from the circulation by early operation may be followed by disaster because of "spasm" which may develop at the critical 4 to 7-day period. There is further apprehension that early operation may make vasospasm worse or even produce it, despite the most gentle and expert manipulation of cerebral vessels.

Many questions relative to the role of "vasospasm" and its effect upon the brain remain elusive. Its anatomic pathology and pathophysiology are not clear. At present, the outstanding problem of the management of an intracranial aneurysm after the initial diagnostic features have been resolved appears to be that of vasospasm.

References

1. Ecker, A., Riemenschneider, P.: Deliberate thrombosis of intracranial arterial aneurysm by partial occlusion of the carotid artery with arteriographic control. J Neurosurg 8: 348–353, 1951.
2. Graf, C.: Prognosis for patients with non-surgically-treated aneurysms. Analysis of the cooperative study of intracranial aneurysms and subarachnoid hemorrhage. J Neurosurg 35:438–443, 1971.
3. Graf, C.J., Nibbelink, D.W.: Cooperative study of intracranial aneurysms and subarachnoid hemorrhage. Report on a randomized treatment study. III. Intracranial surgery. Stroke 5:557–601, 1974.
4. Nibbelink, D.W., Knowler, L.: Cooperative study of intracranial aneurysms and subarachnoid hemorrhage. Report on a randomized treatment study. II. Objectives and design of a randomized aneurysm study. Stroke 5:552–556, 1974.
5. Nibbelink, D.W., Torner, J.C., Henderson, W.G.. Intracranial aneurysms and subarachnoid hemorrhage. Report on a randomized treatment study. IV-A. Regulated bed rest. Stroke 8:202–218, 1977.
6. Nibbelink, D.W., Torner, J.C., Henderson, W.G.: Randomized treatment study. Drug-induced hypotension. In: Sahs, A.L., Nibbelink, D.W., Torner, J.C. et al: Aneurysmal Subarachnoid Hemorrhage, Urban & Schwarzenberg, Baltimore, 1981, Chapter 6, pp 77–106.
7. Perret, G.E., Nibbelink, D.W., Randomized treatment study. Carotid ligation. In: Sahs, A.L., Nibbelink, D.W., Torner, J.C., et al: Aneurysmal Subarachnoid Hemorrhage, Urban & Schwarzenberg, Baltimore 1981, Chapter 8, pp 121–143.
8. Winn, R.H., Richardson, A.E., Jane, J.A.: Late morbidity and mortality of common carotid ligation for posterior communicating aneurysms. A comparison to conservative treatment. J Neurosurg 47:727–736, 1977.
9. Sano, K., Saito, I.: Timing and indication of surgery for ruptured intracranial aneurysms with regard to vasospasm. Acta Neurochir 41:49–60, 1978.
10. Hori, S., Suzuki, J.: Early and late results of intracranial direct surgery for anterior communicating artery aneurysm. J Neurosurg 50:433–440, 1979.
11. Sahs, A.L., Perret, G.E., Locksley, H.B., Nishioka, H. (eds): Intracranial Aneurysms and Subarachnoid Hemorrhage: A Cooperative Study. J.B. Lippincott Co., Philadelphia, 1969.
12. Kaste, M., Troupp, H.: Subarachnoid haemorrhage: Long-term follow-up results of late surgical versus conservative treatment. Brit Med J 1:1310–1311, 1978.
13. Winn, H.R., Richardson, A.E., Jane, J.A.: Late morbidity and mortality in cerebral aneurysms: A ten-year follow-up of 364 conservatively treated patients with a single cerebral aneurysm. Trans Am Neurol Assoc 98:148–150, 1973.
14. Jane, J.A., Richardson, A.E., Winn, H.R.: Fifteen year late rebleed rate in 258 non-surgically treated patients with a single anterior communicating artery aneurysm. Presented at the Annual Meeting of the American Association of Neurological Surgeons. Paper #43, New Orleans, 1978.
15. Yoshimoto, T., Uchida, K., Kaneko, U., Kanyama, T., Suzuki, J.: An analysis of follow-up results of 1000 intracranial saccular aneurysms with definitive surgical treatment. J Neurosurg 50:152–157, 1979.

Chapter 11

Statistical Comparisons of End Results of a Randomized Treatment Study

James C. Torner, M.S., Donald W. Nibbelink, M.D., Ph.D. and Leon F. Burmeister, Ph.D.

Abstract

Between 1963 and 1970, 1,005 patients with a subarachnoid hemorrhage from a single intracranial aneurysm were randomized to four treatment groups: bed rest, drug-induced hypotension, carotid ligation and intracranial surgery. Excluding 33 disqualified patients and 13 patients with vertebral-basilar-posterior aneurysms, 959 patients were subsequently analyzed. Factors related to prognosis for mortality were: interval from hemorrhage to randomization, medical condition, neurologic condition, age of the patient, systolic blood pressure and size of the aneurysm. Factors related to recurrent hemorrhage were: interval to randomization, systolic blood pressure and size of the aneurysm. The location of the aneurysm was not consistently related to prognosis. The comparison of the randomized treatment groups demonstrated no significant difference in mortality in the first 6 months following hemorrhage. In the long-term period, both carotid ligation and intracranial surgery significantly reduced mortality. For recurrent hemorrhage, a significant reduction was found with intracranial surgery by the 3rd month following the pre-study hemorrhage, and with carotid ligation during the long-term period beginning at 6 months.

Introduction

The purpose of Phase II of the Cooperative Aneurysm Study (Randomized Treatment Study) was to determine which mode of treatment (regulated bed rest, drug-induced hypotension, carotid ligation or intracranial surgery) for a patient with a single intracranial aneurysm that bled within the previous 3 months from treatment produced the best results in terms of survival. Duration of acute illness, residual neurologic deficits related to treatment, and the capacity for self-care and gainful employment were some of the secondary objectives investigated in this study.

The design and the scope of the Randomized Treatment Study are presented in Chapters 2 and 3. Detailed descriptive reports of each treatment and its outcome are reported in Chapters 4 through 9. A detailed report of the long-term findings is presented in Chapter 10. Preliminary statistical analysis of the results was presented at the Eighth Princeton Conference of Cerebral Vascular Disease.[1] The purpose of the analysis in this report is to evaluate the comparability of the treatment groups, as well as to compare the end results of the randomized treatment groups and the end results of the treatment groups for patients who had therapy accomplished according to protocol.

Clinical Material

Between 1963 and 1970, 1,665 patients were registered into the Randomized Treatment Study. Six hundred and sixty patients were excluded because they did not satisfy eligibility criteria. Of the remaining 1,005, 214 patients were allocated to regulated bed rest, 315 to drug-induced hypotension, 191 to carotid ligation, 281 to intracranial surgery and 4 to a special study group (Fig. 11–1). Twenty-nine patients were disqualified due to protocol violation or refusal of the treatment program (Table 3–7, Chapter 3). The remaining 972 patients provided the data base for treatment comparison. As noted in the previous reports (Chapters 4,6,8,9), therapy as specified in the treatment protocol was not accomplished in all randomized patients. For regulated bed rest, 96% of patients (194 of 202) received therapy as specified. For drug-induced hypotension, 88% (273 of 309) of patients had antihypertensive medications and adequate bed rest carried out, but only 101 patients actually achieved the specified blood pressure reduction. Carotid ligation was completed in 126 of the 187 patients (67%), and intracranial surgery was performed in 232 of the 274 patients (85%) randomized to that category. Only 13 patients with vertebral-basilar aneurysms were randomized (7 to bed rest, 6

to intracranial surgery). These 13 patients were excluded from the statistical analysis.

Statistical Methods

Comparison of the distribution of patients with regard to randomization and other clinical variables between allocated and accomplished treatment groups was done by using chi-square tests for contingency tables and by analysis of variance procedures utilizing SAS1979 computer programs.

Estimates of survival and rebleeding probabilities were made using Kaplan-Meier product limit and Breslow maximum likelihood methods.[2,3] The prognostic factors and the comparison of treatments were determined by the proportional hazards model developed by D.R. Cox and adapted by Frank Harrell for SAS (see Appendix).[4,5] Logistic regression was performed to determine factors related to and treatment effects on the capacity for self-care and employability.

Results

Comparison of Randomized Treatment Groups

Distribution of Patients for Clinical Variables

Selected groups of patients were terminated at specific intervals of the study. These were patients with anterior cerebral-anterior communicating aneurysms allocated to carotid ligation, patients with internal carotid aneurysms admitted to bed rest and intracranial surgery within days 0–7, and patients with middle cerebral or anterior cerebral-anterior communicating aneurysms randomized to regulated bed rest. The distribution of patients by aneurysm site is significantly dif-

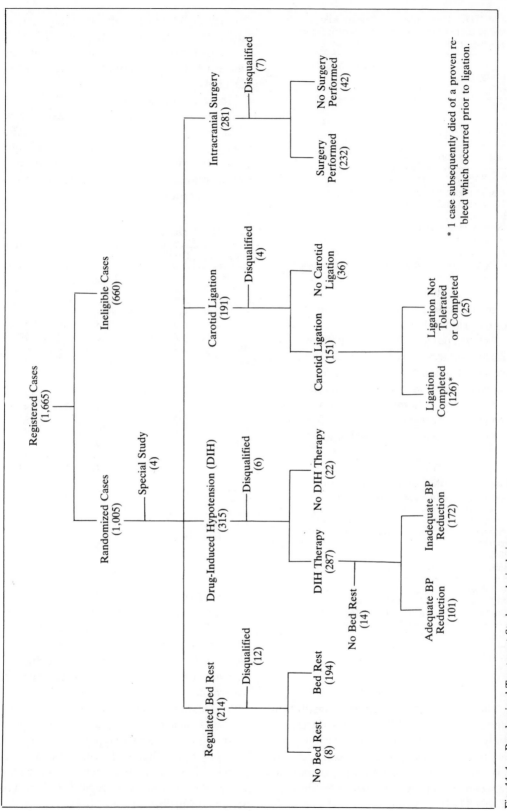

Fig. 11–1.   Randomized Treatment Study analysis design.

Table 11–1.   Distribution of Patients Allocated by Randomization to a Specified Treatment Group for Each Aneurysm Site.

Aneurysm Site†	Treatment Group*				
	BR	DIH	CL	ICS	Total
IC	37	82	88	50	257
MC	23	35	27	38	123
AC	135	192	72	180	579
Total	195	309	187	268	959

$X^2 = 60.574$, $P < 0.0001$
* BR = regulated bed rest
DIH = drug-induced hypotension
CL = carotid ligation
ICS = intracranial surgery
† IC = internal carotid
MC = middle cerebral
AC = anterior cerebral-anterior communicating

ferent between randomized treatment categories (Table 11–1).

Sixty-six percent of bed rest patients, 61% of drug-induced hypotension patients, 65% of carotid ligation patients and 56% of intracranial surgery patients entered in the first week post-hemorrhage (Table 11–2). No statistically significant difference for time of entry and treatment was found.

Table 11–2.   Distribution of Patients Allocated by Randomization to a Specified Treatment Group for Time to Randomization.

Interval from Last Bleed to Randomization	Treatment Group*				
	BR	DIH	CL	ICS	Total
0–7 days	128	190	122	151	591
8–21 days	51	88	49	87	275
22–92 days	16	31	16	30	93
Total	195	309	187	268	959

$X^2 = 5.650$, $P = 0.4635$
* See Table 11–1

The contribution by reporting institutions ranged from 12 to 308 patients during the study period. Although the contribution to the treatment categories by some centers was very small, the distribution of patients between centers was significantly different (Table 11–3).

Forty-eight percent of the patient population was male, for a ratio of 0.93 to 1.0 (male to female). The sex distribution was uniform between treatment categories (Table 11–4).

Medical condition (defined in Table 5–2) evaluated at the time of randomization was good in 55% of the patients, fair in 32%, poor in 10% and prohibitive in 3% (Table 11–4). Examination of the distribution between treatment groups revealed no significant differences.

Table 11–3.   Distribution of Patients Allocated by Randomization to a Specified Treatment Group for Participating Center.

Center	Treatment Group*				
	BR	DIH	CL	ICS	Total
12	9	17	8	16	50
19	12	23	18	17	70
20	74	95	45	94	308
22	6	4	1	1	12
24	8	12	10	17	47
25	10	19	16	15	60
26	14	21	18	16	69
27	17	29	11	25	82
28	22	48	32	33	135
29	8	6	9	7	30
30	9	11	7	12	39
31	2	5	3	7	17
32	1	5	4	3	13
33	3	14	5	5	27
Total	195	309	187	268	959

$X^2 = 42.586$, $P = 0.319$
* See Table 11–1

Neurologic condition (defined in Table 5–2) was assessed at the time of randomization. The majority of patients randomized were listed as Grade 2 (63%, 606 of 959). No significant difference in the distribution by neurologic condition was found between treatments (Table 11–4).

Pre-existing hypertension was noted on the basis of a previously diagnosed hypertensive state. Twenty-one percent of the patient population had had hypertension prior to their illness. Each treatment category had similar distributions with regard to their hypertension history (Table 11–4).

Table 11–4. Distribution of Patients Allocated by Randomization to a Specific Treatment for Categorical Nonrandomization Variables.

Variable	Category	Treatment Group*				
		BR	DIH	CL	ICS	Total
Sex	Male	88	152	92	131	463
	Female	107	157	95	137	496
		$X^2 = 0.980, P = 0.806$				
Medical condition	Good	107	171	111	138	527
	Fair	57	108	50	93	308
	Poor	27	22	23	26	98
	Prohibitive	4	8	3	11	26
		$X^2 = 14.145, P = 0.117$				
Neurologic condition	1	13	22	8	18	61
	2	121	198	122	165	606
	3	36	50	31	52	169
	4	17	24	16	17	74
	5	8	15	9	15	47
	6	0	0	1	1	2
		$X^2 = 6.948, P = 0.959$				
Pre-existing hypertension	Yes	39	74	38	53	204
	No	132	196	126	179	633
	Unknown	24	39	23	36	122
		$X^2 = 6.497, P = 0.689$				
Vasospasm	None	112	174	111	162	559
	Local	54	78	48	66	246
	Diffuse	28	57	28	39	152
	Unknown	1	0	0	1	2
		$X^2 = 5.141, P = 0.822$				

* See Table 11–1

Angiographically defined vasospasm was noted at the time of the first angiogram prior to randomization. The distribution of patients revealed that 58% had no vasospasm, 26% had localized vasospasm and 16% had diffuse vasospasm (2 patients had incomplete data). The distribution for each treatment regimen was similar (Table 11–4).

The average age of the study group was 47.5 years. Each of the treatment groups showed a similar average age (Table 11–5).

Systolic and diastolic blood pressure (BP) was measured in the hospital prior to randomization. The average of four readings taken four hours apart was used. Systolic BP ranged from 142.6 mm Hg for the intracranial surgery group to 149.2 mm Hg for the drug-induced hypotension study group (Table 11–5). Diastolic BP ranged from 85.7 mm Hg in the bed rest group to 89.5 mm Hg in the drug-induced hypotension group. Mean BP was calculated as two thirds the diastolic BP plus one third the systolic BP. The mean BP was highest in the drug-induced hypotension group (109.1 mm Hg). Two institutions were primarily responsible for this difference.

Size of aneurysm was determined by angiographic visualization and multiplication of the anterior-posterior and lateral projection measurements. The distribution by actual size was highly skewed due to several large aneurysms. The average was 598 mm³. Due to the wide variability in size, no statistically significant difference was found. Transformation of the size was made by taking the logarithm of the volume. The average $\log_{10}$ of the aneurysm size was 2.41. No difference was found between treatment groups (Table 11–5).

Table 11–5. Distribution of Patients Allocated by Randomization to a Specific Treatment for Continuous Nonrandomization Variables.

| Variable | BR | Treatment Group* | | | |
		DIH	CL	ICS	Total
Age (years)	$\bar{x} = 48.6$	47.6	46.3	47.5	47.5
		$F = 0.96, P = 0.411$			
Systolic BP (mm Hg)	$\bar{x} = 145.1$	149.2	143.8	142.6	145.5
		$F = 4.00, P = 0.008$			
Diastolic BP (mm Hg)	$\bar{x} = 85.7$	89.5	88.0	86.1	87.5
		$F = 4.54, P = 0.004$			
Mean BP (mm Hg)	$\bar{x} = 105.1$	109.1	106.3	104.6	106.5
		$F = 4.46, P = 0.004$			
Size of aneurysm (mm^3)	$\bar{x} = 525$	529	894	524	598
		$F = 1.78, P = 0.148$			
Size of aneurysm ($\log_{10}$[mm^3])	$\bar{x} = 2.39$	2.38	2.47	2.43	2.41
		$F = 1.04, P = 0.376$			

* See Table 11–1

Mortality

Analysis of end results stratified by aneurysm site in accordance with the study design revealed a statistically significant relationship between treatment groups and mortality for internal carotid aneurysms only (Table 11–6). Mortality at 1 month did not demonstrate a significant difference, but at 3 months and 6 months, bed rest therapy was inferior to both drug-induced hypotension and carotid ligation. For the periods of 1 year and 5 years post-subarachnoid hemorrhage (SAH), only carotid ligation was statistically superior. At 3 years and 5 years, carotid ligation was superior when compared to intracranial surgery. Aneurysms located on the middle cerebral or anterior cerebral-anterior communicating arteries did not show differences that were statistically significant, although intracranial surgery had consistently higher survival rates.

Table 11–6. Survival Rates* for Randomized Treatment Groups by Aneurysm Site.

| Site | Treatment Group† | No. | Time from SAH | | | | | |
			1 month	3 months	6 months	1 year	3 years	5 years
Internal carotid			[% ± SE]	[% ± SE]	[% ± SE]	[% ± SE]	[% ± SE]	[% ± SE]
	BR	37	65 ± 8	54 ± 8	51 ± 8	51 ± 8	48 ± 8	48 ± 8
	DIH	82	77 ± 5	73 ± 5	72 ± 5	67 ± 5	59 ± 6	58 ± 6
	CL	88	77 ± 4	76 ± 5	74 ± 5	74 ± 5	73 ± 5	71 ± 5
	ICS	50	70 ± 6	66 ± 7	60 ± 7	58 ± 7	56 ± 7	52 ± 7
Middle cerebral								
	BR	23	61 ± 10	52 ± 11	52 ± 11	52 ± 11	45 ± 11	38 ± 11
	DIH	35	63 ± 8	60 ± 8	60 ± 8	60 ± 8	60 ± 8	53 ± 9
	CL	27	70 ± 9	63 ± 9	63 ± 9	55 ± 10	55 ± 10	51 ± 10
	ICS	38	82 ± 6	74 ± 7	68 ± 8	62 ± 8	62 ± 8	62 ± 8
Anterior cerebral-anterior communicating								
	BR	135	75 ± 4	64 ± 4	61 ± 4	58 ± 4	50 ± 4	43 ± 4
	DIH	192	73 ± 3	64 ± 3	62 ± 4	59 ± 4	55 ± 4	52 ± 4
	CL	72	68 ± 5	62 ± 6	60 ± 6	58 ± 6	57 ± 6	57 ± 6
	ICS	180	75 ± 3	69 ± 3	64 ± 4	63 ± 4	60 ± 4	55 ± 4

* Kaplan-Meier Survival Rates with patient censored at loss-to-follow-up.
† See Table 11–1

Prognostic Factors

Factors significantly related to mortality from all causes varied for time following SAH (Table 11–7). The mortality rate was higher in the first 3 months. Hence, those factors related to early events (first 3 months) were prognostic in the cumulative 5-year period. Factors associated with early mortality included interval to randomization after SAH, medical condition, systolic blood pressure, neurologic condition and the presence of a middle cerebral aneurysm. At 3 months, vasospasm was related significantly to outcome while aneurysm site was not. From 6 months to 5 years, size of the aneurysm and patient's age were related to mortality.

For patients who survived the first 6 months following subarachnoid hemorrhage, mortality to 5 years was related to the patient's age (coeff. = 0.038), medical condition (coeff. = 0.511), interval to randomization (coeff. = −0.043), systolic blood pressure (coeff. = 0.012) and size ($\log_{10}$) of the aneurysm (coeff. = 0.662).

Death from a progressive decline in clinical condition was analyzed for prognostic factors for the period ending 6 months post-SAH. The neurologic condition (coeff. = 0.633), systolic blood pressure (coeff. = 0.017), interval to randomization (coeff. = −0.039) and patient's age (coeff. = 0.017) were found to significantly increase the risk for death from this cause.

For death from a proved or suspected rebleed, the factors of interval to randomization (coeff. = −0.054), medical condition (coeff. = 0.279), size of aneurysm (coeff. = 0.514), systolic blood pressure (coeff. = 0.008) and the presence of vasospasm (coeff. = 0.192) were prognostic. For 6-month survivors, the probability of death

Table 11–7. Factors Significantly Related to All-cause Mortality at Study Time Periods for Randomized Treatment Groups.

Factor	\multicolumn{6}{c}{Time from SAH}					
	1 month	3 months	6 months	1 year	3 years	5 years
Interval to randomization						
Coefficient	−.084	−.053	−.038	−.035	−.036	−.037
X^2	31.67	29.74	19.29	19.50	22.27	24.53
Medical condition						
Coefficient	.281	.264	.297	.275	.286	.287
X^2	9.49	10.12	12.71	11.32	13.24	14.11
Systolic blood pressure						
Coefficient	.014	.011	0.11	.010	.010	.010
X^2	30.39	24.51	21.79	18.15	18.53	22.76
Neurologic condition						
Coefficient	.301	.301	.281	.309	.300	.273
X^2	14.96	18.30	14.66	19.69	19.93	17.27
Middle cerebral aneurysm						
Coefficient	.278					
X^2	4.53					
Vasospasm						
Coefficient		.159				
X^2		4.32				
Size of aneurysm						
Coefficient			.232	.218	.249	.284
X^2			4.83	4.36	6.22	8.61
Age						
Coefficient				.011	.012	.013
X^2				5.64	7.39	8.60

Note: Coefficients estimated by proportional hazards method (see Appendix).

Table 11–8.   Coefficients and Standard Errors for Randomized Treatment Groups for All-Cause Mortality.

Treatment†	Time from SAH					
	1 month	3 months	6 months	1 year	3 years	5 years
DIH						
Coefficient	−.031	−.109	−.238	−.136	−.196	−.247
SE	.174	.151	.154	.151	.141	.136
X^2	0.03	0.52	2.39	0.82	1.93	3.29
CL						
Coefficient	−.007	−.173	−.188	−.123	−.283	−.356
SE	.194	.175	.174	.171	.165	.161
X^2	0.00	0.99	1.18	0.51	2.94	4.91*
ICS						
Coefficient	.036	−.118	−.125	−.087	−.216	−.228
SE	.182	.160	.158	.156	.148	.142
X^2	0.04	0.54	0.62	0.31	2.13	2.59

* $P < 0.05$
† See Table 11–1

from a proved or suspected rebleed by 5 years was related to size of the aneurysm (coeff. = 0.845) and the age of the patient (coeff. = 0.030).

Comparison with Bed Rest

Since bed rest therapy is most likely the closest to the natural history of patients with SAH, the comparison of treatment groups in relation to bed rest was done.

For mortality from all causes, no significant reduction in the number of deaths was found for patients with drug-induced hypotension or intracranial surgery (Table 11–8). Only at the 5th year was the cumulative survival probability significantly better for carotid ligation compared to bed rest.

For 6-month survivors only, the probability of 5-year mortality was significantly reduced for intracranial surgery (coeff. = −0.879, SE = 0.321, X^2 = 7.51) and for carotid ligation (coeff. = −1.587, SE = 0.462, X^2 = 11.82). No difference from bed rest in long-term outcome was found for drug-induced hypotension patients.

Analysis for cause of death demonstrated that patients in the intracranial surgery category had a significantly greater probability of death from complications of therapy than bed rest patients at 6 months following SAH (coeff. = 1.334, SE = 0.312, X^2 = 18.31). No difference for drug-induced hypotension or carotid ligation was found. However, for death due to proved and suspected rebleed, drug-induced hypotension (coeff. = −0.354, SE = 0.180, X^2 = 3.88), carotid ligation (coeff. = −0.531, SE = 0.218, X^2 = 5.94) and intracranial surgery (coeff. = −1.109, SE = 0.236, X^2 = 22.04) had significantly better outcome than bed rest.

For the period from 6 months to 5 years, drug-induced hypotension did not decrease mortality due to proved and suspected rebleeds. Both carotid ligation (coeff. = −2.667, SE = 1.045, X^2 = 6.51) and intracranial surgery (coeff. = −1.071, SE = 0.484, X^2 = 4.90) were related to a reduction in mortality in the long-term period.

Comparison of Intracranial Surgery and Carotid Ligation

Factors related to survival for patients only in the intracranial surgery and carotid ligation combined treatment group were also determined. For death in the first 6 months post-SAH, neurologic condition (coeff. = 0.534), systolic blood pressure (coeff. = 0.014), interval to randomization (coeff. = −0.027) and age (coeff. = 0.017) were significant. Factors related to long-term mortality in the 6-month to the 5-year interval were age (coeff. = 0.052), neurologic condition (coeff. = 0.806), systolic blood pressure (coeff. = 0.019) and vasospasm at first angiography (coeff. = -0.655). The inclusion of vasospasm may be due to the low number of observed deaths during the period and represents the composition of cases who were followed during this interval.

The addition of treatment variable did not add significantly to the proportional hazards model and hence represents no significant difference in mortality between carotid ligation and intracranial surgery for the initial 6-month period. For the long-term period, the addition of a variable for intracranial surgery showed a higher risk of death (coeff. = 0.849), but statistical significance was marginal ($X^2 = 3.37$, $P = 0.066$).

Rebleeding

Comparison of rates of recurrent subarachnoid hemorrhage by selected clinical parameters revealed that a significant difference between treatment categories occurred for each site (Table 11–9). In the initial 1-month period, rebleeding had its greatest impact. For internal carotid aneurysms rebleeding prior to surgery and in poor-risk patients, the intracranial surgery group experienced an initially high rate of rebleeding. By contrast, in the middle cerebral aneurysm group only 1 rebleed occurred during the initial period for the intracranial surgery group. During the initial 1-month period, the an-

terior cerebral-anterior communicating patients allocated to intracranial surgery had a rebleed rate no different from that of the other treatments. After the first 3 months, no rebleeds occurred in the internal carotid or middle cerebral aneurysms for patients allocated to carotid ligation and intracranial surgery. For anterior cerebral-anterior communicating aneurysms, less than 1% per year rebleeding occurred following intracranial surgery and no rebleeding occurred in the carotid ligation group.

Prognostic Factors

Factors determined by the proportional hazards model to be associated with early rebleeding included age, neurologic condition, medical condition, systolic blood pressure and time of entry into the study (Table 11–10). Systolic blood pressure and time of entry continued to be prognostic for the entire cumulative period. Size of aneurysm became significant at 6 months and increased in importance with time. At the 5-year period, patients with anterior cerebral-anterior communicating aneurysms demonstrated an increased risk of recurrent SAH.

For patients who survived and who did not rebleed during the first 6 months, the size of the aneurysm (coeff. = 1.305, X^2 = 13.02), the presence of an anterior cerebral-

Table 11–9. Rebleed Rates for Randomized Treatment Groups by Aneurysm Site.

Site	Treatment Group*	No.	1 month	3 months	6 months	1 year	3 years	5 years
			[% ± SE]	[% ± SE]	[% ± SE]	[% ± SE]	[% ± SE]	[% ± SE]
Internal carotid								
	BR	37	18 ± 7	29 ± 8	29 ± 8	29 ± 8	29 ± 8	29 ± 8
	DIH	82	24 ± 5	28 ± 5	28 ± 5	30 ± 5	35 ± 6	35 ± 6
	CL	88	16 ± 4	17 ± 4	17 ± 4	17 ± 4	17 ± 4	17 ± 4
	ICS	50	34 ± 3	34 ± 3	34 ± 3	34 ± 3	34 ± 3	34 ± 3
Middle cerebral								
	BR	23	38 ± 11	43 ± 11	43 ± 11	43 ± 11	43 ± 11	53 ± 13
	DIH	35	31 ± 8	31 ± 8	31 ± 8	31 ± 8	31 ± 8	31 ± 8
	CL	27	17 ± 8	26 ± 9	26 ± 9	26 ± 9	26 ± 9	26 ± 9
	ICS	38	3 ± 3	9 ± 5	9 ± 5	9 ± 5	9 ± 5	9 ± 5
Anterior cerebral-anterior communicating								
	BR	135	29 ± 4	35 ± 4	35 ± 4	37 ± 4	43 ± 5	48 ± 5
	DIH	158	22 ± 3	28 ± 3	29 ± 3	31 ± 4	33 ± 4	37 ± 4
	CL	72	30 ± 6	35 ± 6	35 ± 6	35 ± 6	35 ± 6	35 ± 6
	ICS	180	20 ± 3	21 ± 3	21 ± 3	22 ± 3	24 ± 3	25 ± 3

* See Table 11–1

Table 11–10. Factors Significantly Related to Recurrent Hemorrhage at Study Time Periods For Randomized Treatment Groups.

Factor	1 month	3 months	6 months	1 year	3 years	5 years
Interval to randomization						
Coefficient	− .056	− .064	− .062	− .062	− .061	− .059
X^2	28.57	25.91	23.34	23.95	25.09	24.41
Systolic blood pressure						
Coefficient	.012	.009	.008	.008	.008	.008
X^2	29.27	11.56	7.76	8.02	9.50	9.38
Medical condition						
Coefficient	.261					
X^2	11.67					
Neurologic condition						
Coefficient	.312					
X^2	24.48					
Age						
Coefficient	.011					
X^2	5.77					
Size of aneurysm ($\log_{10}$)						
Coefficient			.275	.292	.340	.381
X^2			4.85	5.63	8.19	10.52
Anterior cerebral-anterior communicating aneurysm						
Coefficient						.297
X^2						4.20

anterior communicating aneurysm (coeff. = 1.375, X^2 = 6.09) and systolic blood pressure (coeff. = 0.014, X^2 = 4.95) were related to recurrent hemorrhage in the long-term period from 6 months to 5 years.

Comparison with Bed Rest

No significant decline in rebleeding was found in the initial 1-month period (Table 11–11). Beginning at 3 months, intracranial surgery patients had the greatest protection against further hemorrhage. Not until 3 years following the pre-study SAH did carotid ligation become significant, and only at 5 years following SAH was drug-induced hypotension, demonstrating a significant cumulative lower rebleed rate.

For patients followed in the long-term period of 6 months to 5 years, the difference between bed rest and drug-induced hypotension was not significant. Patients who received carotid ligation (coeff. = −2.268, SE = 1.055, X^2 = 4.62) and intracranial surgery (coeff. = −1.597, SE = 0.587, X^2 = 7.41) showed a significant reduction in the probability of rebleeding.

Comparison of Intracranial Surgery and Carotid Ligation

Rebleeding in the first month following SAH for these combined patient groups was related to interval to randomization, systolic blood pressure, neurologic condition and age. No significant difference between treatments was demonstrated.

At 6 months, the factors associated with rebleeding were interval to randomization (coeff. = −0.055), anterior cerebral-anterior communicating aneurysm (coeff. = 0.831) and systolic blood pressure (coeff. = 0.010). At this time period, intracranial surgery had a significantly lower probability of rebleeding (coeff. = −0.620, X^2 = 7.35).

For the 6-month survivors who did not rebleed, the only factor related to recurrent hemorrhage in the 6-month to 5-year period was the presence of an anterior cerebral-anterior communicating aneurysm. No rebleeds occurred in the internal carotid or middle cerebral site for the intracranial surgery group, and no rebleeds occurred in the carotid ligation group.

Table 11–11. Coefficients and Standard Errors for Randomized Treatment Groups for Recurrent Hemorrhage.

Treatment‡	Time from SAH					
	1 month	3 months	6 months	1 year	3 years	5 years
DIH						
Coefficient	−.125	−.238	−.319	−.287	−.319	−.319
SE	.143	.168	.173	.170	.163	.160
X^2	0.76	2.01	3.41	2.86	3.82	3.98*
CL						
Coefficient	−.108	−.266	−.317	−.340	−.453	−.407
SE	.163	.197	.202	.201	.198	.203
X^2	0.44	1.84	2.45	2.84	5.24*	4.00*
ICS						
Coefficient	−.011	−.660	−.673	−.672	−.741	−.791
SE	.147	.203	.204	.202	.195	.192
X^2	0.01	10.60†	10.88†	11.10†	14.36†	16.97†

* $P < 0.05$
† $P \leq 0.001$
‡ See Table 11–1.

To assess whether there was a statistical difference between intracranial surgery and carotid ligation, a rebleed event was assigned to a patient at the 5-year time period. No statistically significant difference in the rate of rebleeding was found.

Capacity for Self-Care

The capacity for self-care was assessed at each routine follow-up (3 months, 6 months and yearly). Three classifications were specified: (1) able to care for self with special aids other than possibly cane or crutches, (2) able to care for self but requires the aid of specially constructed equipment or prosthetic devices, or (3) unable to care for self. The number of patients in these categories was presented in Chapter 10 (Table 10–10). Due to the low number of patients in the self-care with aid category and for the purpose of this analysis, these patients were grouped with those patients who had a capacity for self-care without physical aids. The analysis of the capacity for self-care was analyzed using the multiple logistic regression procedure where outcome is the likelihood of being able to care for oneself. The analysis was performed for two groups: (1) those patients who were alive and completed follow-up, and (2) for all patients

prior to lost-to-follow-up where death prior to the follow-up was considered as an inability to care for self.

Factors related to the ability to care for oneself were neurologic condition, medical condition, age and sex (Table 11–12). At the 5-year follow-up, the low number of cases unable to care for self in the follow-up group resulted in inability to estimate the function. Inclusion of deaths in the logistic model calculation showed that factors related to the likelihood of death predominated.

The addition of the treatment variables to the logistic model is presented in Table 11–13. Patients in the intracranial surgery group were significantly less in their likelihood for capacity for self-care in the follow-up group at 3 and 6 months. The inclusion of the mortality information showed no effect of intracranial surgery on outcome, and only at the 5-year interval did carotid ligation show a statistically significant better outcome.

Employability

Employment capability following SAH and treatment was assessed at various follow-up periods. The employment classification utilized is presented in Table 11–14. For the purpose of this analysis, categories 1 through

Table 11–12.   Logistic Regression Coefficients for Factors Related to the Capacity for Self-Care for Randomized Treatment Patients.

Factor	Time from SAH			
	3 months	6 months	1 year	5 years
Follow-up Group				
Neurologic condition	− .836	− .822	− .672	*
Medical condition	− .855	− .430	− .472	
Age	− .034	− .030	− .023	
Sex		− .655	− .893	
Follow-Up and Death Group				
Neurologic condition	− .581	− .525	− .516	− .502
Medical condition	− .627	− .498	− .526	− .570
Age	− .017	− .019	− .022	− .032
Interval to randomization	.039	.037	.042	.052
Vasospasm	− .297	− .249		
Systolic blood pressure	− .012	− .012	− .011	

* Function not able to be estimated due to low number of patients unable to care for self at this follow-up
Note age = years; sex: male = 1, female = 2

5 were combined and are considered to be patients who were employable whether or not they actually were working or at the same or similar previous occupations.

Employment capability was related to neurologic condition, medical condition, age, sex and the number of hemorrhages at the 3-month evaluation (Table 11–15). At

Table 11–13.   Logistic Regression Coefficients for Randomized Treatment Groups for the Capacity for Self-Care.

Treatment†	Time from SAH			
	3 months	6 months	1 year	5 years
Follow-up Group				
DIH				
Coefficient	− .205	− .081	.076	
X^2	0.25	0.02	0.02	
CL				
Coefficient	0.042	0.513	− .427	
X^2	0.01	0.55	0.49	
ICS				
Coefficient	−1.176	−1.091	−1.026	
X^2	9.19*	4.96*	3.78	
(Model intercept)	7.237	8.097	7.920	
Follow-up and Death Group				
DIH				
Coefficient	.185	.254	.243	.294
X^2	0.75	1.46	1.32	1.71
CL				
Coefficient	.402	.451	.326	.722
X^2	2.72	3.52	1.86	7.93*
ICS				
Coefficient	− .173	− .077	.028	.384
X^2	0.62	0.13	0.02	2.69
(Model intercept)	5.250	4.971	4.530	2.304

* $P < 0.05$
Note: Prognostic factors (coefficients from Table 11–12) included in logistic regression estimation.
† See Table 11–1.

Table 11–14.   Definition of Employability.

1—ability to work full-time at the same or an
    equivalent job
2—ability to work part-time at the same or an
    equivalent job
3—inability to work at one's usual occupation, but
    working at a job requiring less strenuous activity
4—inability to work at usual job, but at job
    consistent with the patient's neurological deficit(s)
5—no gainful employment, but able to work
6—unfit for gainful employment

Treatment Accomplished Groups

Of the 959 patients who were randomized
into the four treatment programs, 814 (85%)
received therapy as specified in the protocol.
As previously mentioned, bed rest had the
highest accomplishment rate (96%) while
carotid ligation had the lowest (67%, P
< 0.001).

A comparison of patients who had treatment accomplished with those who did not
demonstrated that those who did not receive
allocated therapy were in worse medical condition ($P < 0.001$), in worse neurologic condition ($P < 0.001$), had a history of pre-existing hypertension ($P < 0.04$), were older
($P<0.001$), had higher systolic ($P < 0.001$)
and diastolic BP ($P = 0.006$) and had larger
aneurysms ($P = 0.006$). No difference in site
distribution or interval to randomization between accomplished and not-accomplished
patient groups was found.

the 6-month and 1-year follow-up intervals,
the number of hemorrhages prior to treatment showed no relationship to employability. With the inclusion of deaths in the
analysis, the interval to randomization was
significant, but sex of the patient was not.

For the follow-up group, intracranial surgery was related to a lower capability for
employment at the 3-month, 6-month and
1-year follow-up than the other treatments
(Table 11–16). When deaths are included,
carotid ligation-treated patients showed a
significantly greater employment capability
at all time intervals; intracranial surgery also
showed a significantly higher employment
capability at the 5-year period. This relationship is probably related to the low mortality in these two groups during the follow-
up period.

Distribution of Patients for Clinical Variables

For the patients who had treatment accomplished, the difference in site distribution
between treatment categories was statistically significant (Table 11–17). The lower
percentage of anterior cerebral-anterior

Table 11–15.   Logistic Regression Coefficients for Factors Related to Employability for Randomized
Treatment Groups.

	Time from SAH			
Factor	3 months	6 months	1 year	5 years
Follow-up Group				
Neurologic condition	− .812	− .746	− .665	*
Medical condition	− .916	− .387	− .527	
Number of hemorrhages†	− .622			
Age	− .034	− .031	− .029	
Sex	− .317	− .858	−1.010	
Follow-up and Death Group				
Neurologic condition	− .510	− .430	− .369	− .358
Medical condition	− .725	− .547	− .582	− .478
Interval to randomization	.036	.035	.042	.046
Number of hemorrhages	− .377			
Age	− .019	− .022	− .025	− .032

* Function not able to be estimated due to low number of cases unfit for employment.
† Number of hemorrhages prior to study entry (minimum = 1).

Table 11–16.   Logistic Regression Coefficients for Randomized Treatment Groups for Employability.

Treatment†	Time from SAH			
	3 months	6 months	1 year	5 years
Follow-up Group				
DIH				
Coefficient	− .182	− .229	.286	
X^2	0.18	0.17	0.18	
CL				
Coefficient	.178	.771	− .622	
X^2	0.11	0.81	0.87	
ICS				
Coefficient	− 1.184	− 1.130	− 1.223	
X^2	8.33*	4.60*	4.50*	
(Model intercept)	8.603	8.351	8.707	
Follow-up and Death Group				
DIH				
Coefficient	.223	.239	.266	.412
X^2	1.07	1.29	1.56	3.27
CL				
Coefficient	1.070	1.163	0.852	1.336
X^2	13.15*	15.25	9.24*	18.81*
ICS				
Coefficient	− .009	.091	.145	.494
X^2	0.00	0.17	0.43	4.31*
(Model intercept)	3.706	2.863	2.940	2.027

* $P < 0.05$
† See Table 11–1

communicating aneurysm patients in the carotid ligation group was the principal reason for the difference.

No statistically significant difference in time to randomization was found between treatment-accomplished categories (Table 11–17). Sixty-one percent of the cases entered in the early (0 to 7-day) period. Reporting center differences in patient contribution did not reflect any significant difference between treatment subgroups.

A significant difference in medical condition was found between patients of the treatment-accomplished subgroups (Table 11–18). Seventy-four percent of the carotid ligation patients were in good medical condition, in contrast to 55% for bed rest, 56% for drug-induced hypotension and 57% for intracranial surgery. A greater percentage of poor or prohibitive patients were in the bed rest and drug-induced hypotension subgroups.

For continuous variables presented in Table 11–19, age and blood pressure were statistically significant between groups. Bed rest patients were older; carotid ligation patients were younger. Systolic blood pressure, diastolic blood pressure and mean blood pressure were highest in the subgroup who received drug-induced hypotensive medications. The carotid ligation and intracranial surgery groups had lower average systolic blood pressures.

Mortality

Prognostic Factors

Factors related to mortality were interval to randomization, medical condition, systolic blood pressure and middle cerebral aneurysm at the 1-month period (Table 11–20). Vasospasm at the time of first angiography was related to mortality for the 3-month and 6-month cumulative mortality rates. Age and initial neurologic condition were prognostic for the 6-month to 5-year intervals. Size of aneurysm was significant only at the 5-year period.

Table 11–17. Distribution of Patients Who Had Treatment Accomplished for Aneurysm Site, Interval to Randomization and Reporting Center.

Variable	BR	DIH	CL	ICS	Total
Aneurysm site					
IC	35	72	68	45	220
MC	22	32	16	34	104
AC	130	169	42	149	490

$X^2 = 63.289, P = 0.0001$

Last bleed to randomization					
0–7 days	124	173	79	124	500
8–21 days	49	74	36	75	234
22–92 days	14	26	11	29	80

$X^2 = 7.972, P = 0.240$

Reporting center					
12	9	16	8	16	49
19	12	21	13	13	59
20	73	85	30	74	262
22	6	3	0	1	10
24	6	8	8	15	37
25	9	16	10	15	50
26	13	14	7	14	48
27	15	25	8	23	71
28	22	48	22	29	121
29	8	4	7	6	25
30	9	10	4	9	32
31	1	4	3	6	14
32	1	5	2	2	10
33	3	14	4	5	26

$X^2 = 47.159, P = 0.173$

* See Table 11–1

For patients who survived the initial 6-month period, factors associated with mortality in the time period of 6-months post-SAH to 5-years post-SAH were size of the aneurysm (coeff. = 0.659), medical condition (coeff. = 0.321), systolic blood pressure (coeff. = 0.015) and age (coeff. = 0.033).

Mortality related to complications of therapy in the first 6-month period in the treatment-accomplished subgroups was associated with medical condition (coeff. = 0.281), age (coeff. = 0.034), interval to randomization (coeff. = 0.044) and neurologic condition (coeff. = 0.394).

Mortality due to a proved and suspected rebleed occurring in the first 6 months was related to interval to randomization (coeff. = −0.056), medical condition (coeff. = 0.308), vasospasm (coeff. = 0.281) and size of the aneurysm (coeff. = 0.338). For the

5-year period, medical condition (coeff. = 0.276), systolic blood pressure (coeff. = 0.005) and size of the aneurysm (coeff. = 0.458) were the factors predictive of death. For those patients surviving the first 6 months, only size of the aneurysm (coeff. = 0.822) and age of the patient (coeff. = 0.031) were significantly associated with death from a proved and suspected rebleed.

Comparison with Bed Rest

Given that the prognostic factors account for differences in patient outcome, the treatment effects were compared with bed rest. No difference was found for drug-induced hypotension, except at the 5-year period (Table 11–21). Intracranial surgery showed a significant effect on mortality from all causes in the 3-month, 3-year and 5-year evaluation periods. Carotid ligation was associated with a significant reduction in mortality events for all periods.

For the 6-month survivors, the 5-year event rates were significantly reduced for drug-induced hypotension (coeff. = −0.647, SE = 0.297, X^2 = 4.75), carotid ligation (coeff. = −1.640, SE = 0.499, X^2 = 10.79) and intracranial surgery (coeff. = −0.853, SE = 0.330, X^2 = 6.67).

Six-month mortality due to complications of therapy showed no difference for drug-induced hypotension or carotid ligation when compared to bed rest, but intracranial surgery was significantly related to greater mortality events (coeff. = 1.396, SE = 0.328, X^2 = 18.14).

For 6-month mortality due to proved and suspected rebleeding, all three treatment-accomplished groups had a significant lowering of mortality. Drug-induced hypotension (coeff. = −0.404, SE = 1.88, X^2 = 4.61) had the least reduction, intracranial surgery (coeff. = −2.154, SE = 0.378, X^2 = 32.44) had the greatest reduction, and carotid ligation (coeff. = −1.524, SE = 0.360, X^2 = 17.88) was in between. At 5 years, the same results were found as at 6 months (drug-induced hypotension: coeff. = −0.392, SE = 0.170, X^2 = 5.28; carotid ligation: coeff. = -1.692, SE $= 0.340$, X^2 = 24.75; intracranial surgery: coeff. = -1.835, SE $= 0.295$, $X^2 = 38.81$). For the 6-month survivors, 5-year mortality due to a proved or suspected rebleed was significantly reduced for carotid ligation (coeff. $= -2.556$, SE $= 1.046$, $X^2 = 5.97$) and for intracranial surgery (coeff. $= -1.188$, SE $= 0.508$, $X^2 = 5.47$). Hence, the reduction of deaths from this cause for drug-induced hypotension was during the initial 6-month period only.

Comparison of Intracranial Surgery and Carotid Ligation

Factors related to mortality in this study subgroup were neurologic condition, age, systolic blood pressure and interval to randomization. Mortality events were significantly higher for the intracranial surgery treatment group for each interval (1 month

through 5 years). However, for 6-month survivors whose prognostic factors were systolic blood pressure and absence of vasospasm, no significant difference was found between carotid ligation and intracranial surgery in the long-term period of 6 months to 5 years. This suggests that the initial mortality due to complications following intracranial surgery was responsible for the difference in the cumulative mortality found at 5 years.

Rebleeding

Prognostic Factors

Factors related to recurrent SAH in the treatment-accomplished groups were interval to randomization and systolic blood pressure for all time intervals (Table 11–22), neurologic condition and medical condition at

Table 11–18. Distribution of Patients Who Had Treatment for Sex, Medical Condition, Neurologic Condition, Pre-Existing Hypertension and Vasospasm.

Variable	Category	Treatment Group*				
		BR	DIH	CL	ICS	Total
Sex	Male	83	134	61	112	390
	Female	104	139	65	116	424
		$X^2 = 1.229, P = 0.746$				
Medical condition	Good	102	152	93	130	477
	Fair	56	94	26	84	260
	Poor	26	20	7	13	66
	Prohibitive	3	7	0	1	11
		$X^2 = 30.226, P = 0.0004$				
Neurologic condition	1	11	20	6	18	55
	2	117	177	93	150	537
	3	36	41	19	46	142
	4	16	23	6	11	56
	5	7	12	2	3	24
		$X^2 = 14.854, P = 0.249$				
Pre-existing hypertension	Yes	36	62	22	47	167
	No	127	175	93	156	551
	Unknown	24	36	11	25	96
		$X^2 = 7.956, P = 0.539$				
Vasospasm	None	106	156	80	142	484
	Local	54	69	29	54	206
	Diffuse	26	48	17	31	122
	Unknown	1	0	0	1	2
		$X^2 = 6.396, P = 0.670$				

* See Table 11–1

Table 11–19.   Distribution of Patients Who Had Treatment for Age, Systolic BP, Diastolic BP, Mean BP and Size of Aneurysm.

Variable	BR	DIH	CL	ICS	Total
			Treatment Group*		
Age (years)	$\bar{x} = 48.6$	47.4	44.4	46.3	46.9
			$F = 2.92, P = 0.033$		
Systolic BP (mm Hg)	$\bar{x} = 145.0$	149.2	139.4	140.8	144.3
			$F = 7.70, P = 0.0001$		
Diastolic BP (mm Hg)	$\bar{x} = 85.5$	89.7	85.6	85.6	87.0
			$F = 5.86, P = 0.0007$		
Mean BP (mm Hg)	$\bar{x} = 104.9$	109.2	103.2	103.7	105.7
			$F = 7.10, P = 0.0001$		
Size of aneurysm (mm³)	$\bar{x} = 543$	526	707	336	505
			$F = 2.30, P = 0.074$		
Size of aneurysm ($\log_{10}$[mm³])	$\bar{x} = 2.40$	2.38	2.47	2.36	2.39
			$F = 1.09, P = 0.354$		

* See Table 11–1

Table 11–20.   Factors Significantly Related to All Cause Mortality at Study Time Periods for Treatment Accomplished Groups.

Factor	1 month	3 months	6 months	1 year	3 years	5 years
			Time from SAH			
Interval to randomization						
Coefficient	−0.091	−0.052	−0.038	−0.034	−0.035	−0.034
X^2	23.85	20.82	16.20	15.74	17.52	17.19
Medical condition						
Coefficient	0.450	0.387	0.298	0.294	0.290	0.330
X^2	23.18	20.81	9.15	9.68	10.21	12.46
Systolic blood pressure						
Coefficient	0.011	0.008	0.008	0.008	0.008	0.008
X^2	11.95	8.49	7.61	9.40	10.53	11.08
Middle cerebral aneurysm						
Coefficient	0.454					
X^2	4.48					
Vasospasm						
Coefficient		0.218	0.182			
X^2		6.37	4.72			
Age						
Coefficient			0.011	0.014	0.015	0.013
X^2			4.19	6.62	9.20	6.49
Neurologic condition						
Coefficient			0.192	0.228	0.237	0.167
X^2			5.13	8.12	9.54	4.19
Size of aneurysm						
Coefficient						0.278
X^2						6.17

1 month only, and size of the aneurysm at 3 and 5 years only.

For patients who survived the first 6 months and who did not rebleed prior to 6 months, the size of the aneurysm (coeff. = 0.088) was the only prognostic factor for rebleeding in the chronic period in the treatment subgroups.

Comparison with Bed Rest

The rate of recurrent hemorrhage for the

Table 11–21.   Coefficients and Standard Errors for Treatment Accomplished Groups for All Cause Mortality.

Treatment**	Time from SAH					
	1 month	3 months	6 months	1 year	3 years	5 years
DIH						
Coefficient	−0.138	−0.229	−0.187	−0.139	−0.211	−0.336
SE	0.185	0.160	0.157	0.152	0.143	0.143
X^2	0.56	2.05	1.43	0.84	2.19	5.56*
CL						
Coefficient	−1.099	−1.061	−0.960	−0.867	−1.014	−1.057
SE	0.333	0.271	0.259	0.244	0.235	0.231
X^2	10.89†	15.35†	13.72†	12.68†	18.55†	20.99†
ICS						
Coefficient	−0.286	−0.411	−0.227	−0.221	−0.344	−0.452
SE	0.210	0.181	0.171	0.166	0.158	0.158
X^2	1.86	5.16*	1.77	1.77	4.72*	8.20*

* $P < 0.05$ ** See Table 11–1
† $P \leq 0.001$

treatment-accomplished patients (Table 11–23) was significantly reduced for those who received carotid ligation at all intervals, for intracranial surgery patients at all intervals beyond 1 month post-SAH, and for drug-induced hypotension patients at 3 months, 6 months, 3 years and 5 years (Table 11–23).

For patients surviving 6 months without a rebleed, the risk of a recurrent hemorrhage in the remaining 4.5 years was significantly reduced for intracranial surgery (coeff. = −1.903, SE = 0.652, X^2 = 8.52) and carotid ligation (coeff. = −2.681, SE = 1.046, X^2

= 6.57). To estimate the effect of carotid ligation, a sham rebleed was added to the carotid ligation group; hence, the estimated result is worse than what actually occurred in the study group.

Comparison of Intracranial Surgery and Carotid Ligation

For patients in the intracranial surgery and carotid ligation subgroups, factors relating to early rebleeding in the initial 1-month period were interval to randomization (coeff. = −0.054), systolic blood pressure (coeff.

Table 11–22.   Factors Significantly Related to Recurrent Hemorrhage at Study Time Periods for Treatment Accomplished Groups.

Factor	Time from SAH					
	1 month	3 months	6 months	1 year	3 years	5 years
Interval to randomization						
Coefficient	−0.059	−0.071	−0.071	−0.071	−0.066	−0.064
X^2	22.66	21.30	21.65	22.47	20.63	21.15
Systolic blood pressure						
Coefficient	0.012	0.006	0.006	0.007	0.006	0.006
X^2	22.85	4.19	4.13	4.53	3.84	4.24
Neurologic condition						
Coefficient	0.225					
X^2	8.17					
Medical condition						
Coefficient	0.336					
X^2	13.34					
Size of aneurysm						
Coefficient					0.284	0.331
X^2					4.42	6.26

Table 11–23.   Coefficients and Standard Errors for Treatment Accomplished Groups for Recurrent Hemorrhage.

	Time from SAH					
Treatment‡	1 month	3 months	6 months	1 year	3 years	5 years
DIH						
Coefficient	− 0.236	− 0.346	− 0.349	− 0.330	− 0.400	− 0.426
SE	0.151	0.176	0.175	0.171	0.170	0.166
X^2	2.45	3.86*	3.98*	3.72	5.55*	6.60*
CL						
Coefficient	− 0.819	− 0.908	− 0.928	− 0.976	− 1.024	− 1.105
SE	0.231	0.268	0.268	0.267	0.266	0.265
X^2	12.54†	11.45†	12.01†	13.36†	14.80†	17.42†
ICS						
Coefficient	− 0.173	− 0.991	− 1.011	− 1.015	− 1.091	− 1.133
SE	0.162	0.234	0.234	0.230	0.229	0.224
X^2	1.13	17.86†	18.67†	19.51†	22.72†	25.51†

* $P < 0.05$
† $P \leqslant 0.001$
‡ See Table 11–1

= 0.013), age (coeff. = 0.026), medical condition (coeff. = 0.306) and the number of previous hemorrhages (coeff. = 0.294). By 3 months, the only factor associated with the cumulative rebleeds was the presence of anterior cerebral-anterior communicating aneurysm (coeff. = 0.908). At 5 years, the factors found to be significantly associated with recurrent SAH were the presence of an anterior cerebral-anterior communicating aneurysm (coeff. = 0.871) and interval to randomization (coeff. = −0.307). Interestingly, if only 6-month survivors with no previous rebleed are considered, the only long-term factor significantly associated with recurrent hemorrhage was systolic blood pressure (coeff. = 0.037). The instability of these factors is related to the low number of events in the two treatment groups.

Only at the 1-month period was the rebleed rate significantly different between treatment groups; intracranial surgery had a higher recurrent hemorrhage rate (coeff. = 0.859, SE = 0.343, X^2 = 6.29). The cumulative rebleed rates, however, at subsequent intervals throughout the follow-up period showed no significant difference. In addition, no difference between carotid ligation and intracranial surgery was found for the 6-month to 5-year period for those patients surviving and not rebleeding during the initial 6 months.

Capacity for Self-Care

For treatment-accomplished groups, a logistic regression analysis was performed similar to the analysis for randomized treatment groups.

For patients who were followed at 3 months, 6 months and 1 year, factors relating to the probability of self-care were neurologic condition, medical condition, age, sex (at 6 months and 1 year) and number of previous hemorrhages (at 3 months only, Table 11–24). Only intracranial surgery patients showed a significant effect on the capacity for self-care (Table 11–25). The effect was most evident at 3 months, but a significantly lower capacity for self-care was also found at 6 months and 1 year.

When deaths were included in the analysis, the overall effect of intracranial surgery showed no detrimental or beneficial effect. Carotid ligation patients demonstrated a higher capacity for self-care in the study subgroup comparison.

Employability

Factors related to employability in the first 3 months following SAH include neurologic condition, medical condition, age and number of previous hemorrhages (Table 11–26). Medical condition and neurologic condition

Table 11–24. Logistic Regression Coefficients for Factors Related to the Capacity for Self-Care for Treatment-Accomplished Patients.

	Time from SAH			
Factor	3 months	6 months	1 year	5 years
Follow-up Group				
Neurologic condition	−0.812	−0.746	−0.665	
Medical condition	−0.916	−0.387	−0.527	
Number of hemorrhages	−0.622			
Age	−0.034	−0.031	−0.029	
Sex		−0.858	−1.010	
Follow-up and Death Group				
Neurologic condition	−0.510	−0.430	−0.369	−0.358
Medical condition	−0.725	−0.547	−0.582	−0.478
Interval to randomization	0.036	0.035	0.042	0.046
Number of hemorrhages	−0.376			
Age	−0.019	−0.022	−0.025	−0.033

* Logistic function not able to be estimated due to low number of cases

were related at longer periods, while the other factors were less consistent over time.

For the follow-up and death group, neurologic condition, systolic blood pressure, age and medical condition were consistent predictors. The number of previous hemorrhages and the presence of vasospasm

were related early to employability outcome, while sex and interval to randomization affected the long-term 5-year outcome.

Treatment effects were similar to the results of capacity for self-care. For the follow-up group only, a negative effect of intracranial surgery was found during the first

Table 11–25. Logistic Regression Coefficients for Treatment Accomplished Groups to the Capacity for Self-Care.

	Time from SAH			
Treatment‡	3 months	6 months	1 year	5 years
Follow-up Group				
DIH				
Coefficient	− 0.182	− 0.229	−0.286	
X^2	0.18	0.17	0.18	
CL				
Coefficient	0.178	0.771	−0.622	
X^2	0.011	0.81	0.87	
ICS				
Coefficient	− 1.184	− 1.130	−1.223	
X^2	8.33*	4.60*	4.50*	
(Model intercept)	8.603	8.351	8.707	
Follow-up and Death Group				
DIH				
Coefficient	0.223	0.239	0.266	0.412
X^2	1.07	1.29	1.56	3.27
CL				
Coefficient	1.070	1.163	0.852	1.336
X^2	13.15†	15.25†	9.24*	18.81†
ICS				
Coefficient	− 0.009	0.091	0.145	0.494
X^2	0.00	0.17	0.43	4.31*
(Model intercept)	3.706	2.863	2.940	2.027

* $P < 0.05$
† $P < 0.001$
‡ See Table 11–1

Table 11–26.   Logistic Regression Coefficients for Factors Related to Employability for Treatment Accomplished Groups.

Factor	Time from SAH			
	3 months	6 months	1 year	5 years
Follow-up Group				
Neurologic condition	−0.629	−0.712	−0.636	
Medical condition	−0.850	−0.762	−0.764	
No. of hemorrhages	−0.591	−0.479		
Age	−0.029			
Follow-up and Death Group				
Neurologic condition	−0.492	−0.551	−0.538	−0.540
Medical condition	−0.643	−0.600	−0.602	−0.420
Systolic blood pressure	−0.012	−0.013	−0.012	−0.012
Number of hemorrhages	−0.383	−0.336		
Vasospasm	−0.313	−0.272		
Age	−0.015	−0.013	−0.011	−0.027
Interval to randomization		0.030		0.032
Sex				0.490

year (Table 11–27). For the group including deaths as an untoward outcome, carotid ligation did significantly better at all intervals, while intracranial surgery showed benefit at the 5-year period only.

Discussion

The rationale for the analysis presented in this chapter is based on the realization that many factors other than site of the aneurysm

Table 11–27.   Logistic Regression Coefficients for Treatment Accomplished Groups to Employability.

Treatment‡	Time from SAH			
	3 months	6 months	1 year	5 years
Follow-up Group				
DIH				
Coefficient	−0.129	−0.402	0.092	
X^2	0.15	1.04	0.05	
CL				
Coefficient	0.097	0.070	0.212	
X^2	0.06	0.02	0.19	
ICS				
Coefficient	−1.081	−0.965	−0.815	
X^2	11.05†	6.34*	4.49*	
(Model intercept)	6.380	5.500	4.677	
Follow-up and Death Group				
DIH				
Coefficient	0.264	0.215	0.319	0.459
X^2	1.51	0.98	2.23	3.71
CL				
Coefficient	0.902	0.958	0.940	1.383
X^2	10.47†	11.06†	11.39†	21.11†
ICS				
Coefficient	−0.209	−0.156	0.025	0.546
X^2	0.89	0.48	0.01	4.95*
(Model intercept)	5.479	5.322	4.476	3.185

* $P < 0.05$
† $P \leq 0.001$
‡ See Table 11–1

and interval to treatment play a role in determining outcome. In this analysis, the determination of prognostic factors was carried out through recently developed multivariate methods for survival data. After adjustment for these factors, the comparison of treatments was made for their respective randomized groups and selected treatment-accomplished subgroups. The randomized group represents a population of patients whose treatment designation is based on a randomized distribution of an overall management philosophy, i.e., once a patient enters the hospital, a decision to select a given therapy is included in the outcome evaluation whether or not the treatment is actually received. The treatment-accomplished subgroups represent those patients who actually received the allocated treatment after randomization.

The original protocol for the Randomized Treatment Study comprised a stratified randomization procedure and analysis. The results of a sequential, pair-wise comparison of treatment groups were presented at the Eighth Princeton Conference in an introductory report.[1] The conclusions of the original analysis were that: (1) bed rest therapy was inferior in preventing mortality for all sites, (2) drug-induced hypotension and carotid ligation were the preferred therapies for internal carotid aneurysms, (3) no overall conclusions were drawn for middle cerebral aneurysms due to a small sample size, and (4) no treatment was consistently better for anterior cerebral-anterior communicating aneurysms, but intracranial surgery was favored at scattered time intervals.

The factors consistently related to early mortality in our analysis were early admission and randomization, poor medical condition and poor neurologic condition. The presence of a middle cerebral aneurysm was significantly related to higher mortality at 1 month only. Vasospasm was related only to overall mortality at the 3-month period. Vasospasm was correlated with neurologic condition, and its impact on outcome may be concealed in the relationship of neurologic condition and mortality. From 6 months

post-SAH to the end of the study period (5 years), the level of systolic blood pressure, the patient's age and the size of the aneurysm became important in determining mortality over this long-term period. Except at the 1-month interval, no significant difference in mortality was found among aneurysm sites during the 5-year period.

Locksley[6] reported in his review of the Phase I Study that aneurysm site, age, neurologic condition and time from SAH were important factors in patients treated with bed rest, carotid ligation or intracranial surgery. Other factors identified previously by Richardson et al.,[7] Stornelli and French,[8] and McKissock et al.[9] were systolic and diastolic blood pressures, the size and configuration of the aneurysm, the presence of cerebral vasospasm, and sex of the patient. Winn et al.[10] demonstrated that patients with anterior cerebral-anterior communicating aneurysms who survived 6 months had a long-term outcome related to neurologic condition, diastolic blood pressure, the presence of vasospasm and the presence of an intracranial clot. In our study, which also included internal carotid and middle cerebral aneurysms, the factors relating to death in the long-term period were age, medical condition, time to randomization, systolic blood pressure and size of the aneurysm.

Factors related to recurrent hemorrhage in the acute period were age, neurologic condition, medical condition, systolic blood pressure and time of study entry. Richardson et al.[11] found that for patients with anterior communicating aneurysms who were nonsurgically treated, factors of age, sex, systolic blood pressure, diastolic blood pressure, consciousness level, shape of the aneurysm and direction of the aneurysm were predictive. For posterior communicating aneurysm patients, sex, vasospasm, the presence of a hematoma and size of the aneurysm were prognostic for rebleeding.

For the period beyond 6 months, Winn et al.[12] found that for anterior communicating aneurysm patients, the time of admission was prognostic for late rebleeding, while for posterior communicating aneurysms, sex, systolic blood pressure and diastolic blood pressure were prognostic. Anterior communicating aneurysm patients had less late rebleeding than posterior communicating aneurysm patients. In our study population, patients with anterior cerebral-anterior communicating aneurysms had a significantly higher rebleed rate than aneurysms at internal carotid or middle cerebral sites in the long-term period. In addition, the size of the aneurysm and the level of systolic blood pressure were prognostic for rebleeding.

Differences in prognostic factors between those found in our report and previous reports are due to differences in the composition and size of the study groups. In the analysis presented in this report, we found no statistically consistent differences for separating patient groups by site. However, the neurosurgeon's approach to treatment has usually considered aneurysm site as a factor of utmost prognostic importance. The findings in this report do not include the surgical methods used for obliteration of the aneurysm, which may be of major importance in the determination of the best therapy for a given patient.

The comparison of treatments based on overall results as designated in the randomized treatment group analysis demonstrated no difference in mortality among the four groups in the first 6 months following subarachnoid hemorrhage. Beyond 6 months, both carotid ligation and intracranial surgery were superior in producing a lower mortality in the long-term period. In the comparison of carotid ligation and intracranial surgery, the results suggested a better long-term result for carotid ligation.

For rebleeding, no difference between treatments was found at the end of 1 month. At 3 months, only intracranial surgery significantly prevented rebleeding. However, beyond the initial 6-month period, rebleeding was significantly reduced for intracranial surgery and carotid ligation. No difference was found between intracranial surgery and carotid ligation in the occurrence of recurrent hemorrhage during the late period.

When capacity for self-care and employability were analyzed, intracranial surgery demonstrated a statistically poorer result than the other categories. With the addition of the death information, the better survival coupled with a poor capacity for self-care or employability produced equivalent results of intracranial surgery to bed rest and to drug-induced hypotension, while carotid ligation produced significantly better results.

The treatment-accomplished groups showed the effect of selection on outcome. Eighty-five percent of patients randomized to intracranial surgery actually had surgery performed, while only 67% of patients in the randomized carotid ligation group had a complete ligation carried out.

Carotid ligation showed a significant reduction in mortality at all periods. Only intracranial surgery was significant in the long-term period (post-6 months). The postoperative mortality associated with intracranial surgery was the reason for poor early results. Recurrent hemorrhage was significantly reduced for drug-induced hypotension, carotid ligation and intracranial surgery in comparision to bed rest. In the long-term period, no rebleed occurred for carotid ligation patients and only anterior cerebral-anterior communicating aneurysm patients rebled in the intracranial surgery group.

Comparison with findings of other studies is difficult since the criteria for selection of cases are different and the methods of analysis have varied.

McKissock et al.[9,13] recognized the influence of several prognostic factors and incorporated them in a randomized trial of conservative therapy versus surgical therapy for middle cerebral aneurysms and anterior communicating aneurysms. Their findings demonstrated a significantly better prognosis for men treated with surgery of middle cerebral aneurysms at 6 months post-SAH. For anterior communicating aneurysms, no difference between conservative and surgical therapies was found for both men and women.

Locksley[6] reviewed, retrospectively, the

results of patients treated with bed rest, carotid ligation and intracranial surgery in the Phase I data collection study of the Cooperative Aneurysm Study. The overall survival rate at 6 months showed that carotid ligation produced a 79% survival rate, intracranial surgery 66% and bed rest 53%.

In another study[14], 178 patients treated between 1964 and 1969 were matched for age, sex, blood pressure, state of consciousness and site of aneurysm. Surgical therapy produced a significant reduction in fatal rebleeding episodes but no difference in deaths from all causes at 1, 5 and 11 years of follow-up.

Based on the results of the previously cited studies and our own analysis, intracranial surgery, as performed during the 1960's, did not offer a satisfactory reduction in mortality when compared to conservative medical management. The favorable outcomes associated with carotid ligation must be considered in accordance with a 67% accomplishment rate and a 34% rate of ischemic cerebral complications (Chapter 8). The use of antihypertensive medications may be effective on a long-term basis for inoperable aneurysms, but as an acute treatment the difficulty in achieving a satisfactory reduction in blood pressure also precludes this therapy as a universal modality for prevention of mortality and morbidity.

The results of the Randomized Treatment Study have not shown the amount of improvement in the treatment of intracranial aneurysms that the retrospective analysis had produced in the Phase I Cooperative Aneurysm Study. However, the Phase II Study has established the baseline rates that could have been expected with treatment of intracranial aneurysms in the 1960's. The improvements in anesthesia and surgical procedures have changed the postoperative outcome of intracranial surgery. The use of antifibrinolytic medication has altered the acute therapeutic period in an attempt to reduce the risk of recurrent hemorrhage prior to surgery. These contemporary forms of therapy have comprised a major step in the success of treating patients with recently ruptured intracranial aneurysms.

Acknowledgment

The authors are grateful to Robert F. Woolson, Jerome A. Fleming and Adolph L. Sahs for their advice in the analysis and the content of this report.

References

1. Sahs, A.L., Nibbelink, D.W., Knowler, L.A.: Cooperative aneurysm project: Introductory report of a randomized treatment study. In: McDowell, F.H., Brennan, R.W.: Cerebral Vascular Diseases. Transactions of the Eighth Princeton Conference. Grune & Stratton, New York, 1973, pp 33–41.
2. Kaplan, E.L., Meier, P.: Nonparametric estimation from incomplete observations. J Am Stat Assoc 53:457–481, 1958.
3. Breslow, N.E.: Covariance analysis of censored survival data. Biometrics 30:89–100, 1974.
4. Cox, D.R.: Regression models and life tables (with discussion). J Roy Stat Soc (B) 34:187–220, 1972.
5. Harrell, F.: The PHGLM procedure. SAS Technical Report S–109, 1980.
6. Locksley, H.B.: Results of aneurysm treatment by intracranial surgery, carotid ligation and bed rest in defined groups of patients. In: Sahs, A.L., Per-

ret, G.E., Locksley, H.B., et al.: Intracranial Aneurysms and Subarachnoid Hemorrhage. A Cooperative Study. J. B. Lippincott Co, Philadelphia, 1969, pp 245–275.
7. Richardson, A.E., Jane, J.A., Payne, P.M.: Assessment of the natural history of anterior communicating aneurysms. J Neurosurg 21:266–274, 1964.
8. Stornelli, S.A., French, J.D.: Subarachnoid hemorrhage: Factors in prognosis and management. J. Neurosurg 21:769–780, 1964.
9. McKissock, W., Richardson, A.E., Walsh, L: Middle cerebral aneurysms. Lancet 2:415–421, 1962.
10. Winn, H.R., Richardson, A.E., O'Brien, W.O., et al.: The long-term prognosis in untreated cerebral aneurysms: II. Late morbidity and mortality. Ann Neurol 4:418–426, 1978.
11. Richardson, A.E., Jane, J.A., Yashon, D.: Prog-

nostic factors in the untreated course of posterior communicating aneurysms. Arch Neurol 14:172–176, 1966.

12. Winn, H.R., Richardson, A.E., Jane, J.A.: The long-term prognosis in untreated cerebral aneurysms. I. The incidence of late hemorrhage in cerebral aneurysm: a 10-year evaluation of 364 patients. Ann Neurol 1:358–370, 1977.

13. McKissock, W., Richardson, A.E., Walsh, L.: Anterior communicating aneurysms: A trial of conservative and surgical treatment. Lancet 1:873–876, 1965.

14. Kaste, M., Troupp, H.: Subarachnoid hemorrhage: Long-term follow-up results of late surgical versus conservative treatment. Br Med J 1:1310–1311, 1978.

Appendix

In the present report, the determination of prognostic factors and comparison of treatment effects was done utilizing the proportional hazards model developed by D.R. Cox.[1] This model incorporates a set of covariates, $Z = (Z_{il}, . . ., Z_{ip})$, which are related to the death probability for an individual at time t. This death probability ("hazard") is denoted as $\lambda(t;Z)$. Hence, for all persons in the study population, the hazard is equal to the following:

$$\lambda[t;(Z_1, . . ., Z_p)] = exp(\sum_{j=1}^{p} \beta_j Z_j) \lambda_0(t),$$

where β_j is the regression coefficient associated with the particular covariate and $\lambda_0(t)$ is the underlying hazard for the study group. The regression coefficients can be estimated by the maximum likelihood procedure developed by Breslow[2] and applied by Frank Harrell[3] for SAS. Detailed descriptions and applications of the proportional hazards model have been presented by Kalbfleisch and Prentice,[4] Anderson et al.,[5] and Woolson et al.[6]

In our application of the model, the time intervals of interest were suggested in the study objectives and are based on the natural history of subarachnoid hemorrhage. Since risk of death or recurrent hemorrhage is inversely related to the time from subarachnoid hemorrhage to randomization (treatment), the survival time contributed by each patient in our study was the interval from randomization to the time of death or follow-up. For analysis, a person was considered a

Table 11–A–1. Underlying Probability of Outcome.

Time from SAH	Survival		Rebleeding	
	Randomized	Therapy Accomplished	Randomized	Therapy Accomplished
1 month	77	82	81	84
3 months	70	74	77	81
6 months	67	72	76	80
1 year	65	70	76	80
3 years	60	66	73	77
5 years	56	62	72	76

Table 11–A–2.   Scales and Means for Variables.

Variable	Coding Scale	Groups Means	
		Randomized	Treatment Accomplished
Medical condition	1 = good, 2 = fair	1.61	1.52
	3 = poor, 4 = prohibitive		
Neurologic condition	1,2,3,4,5,6	2.42	2.33
Vasospasm	1 = none, 2 = local,	1.57	1.55
	3 = diffuse		
Interval to randomization	Days	9.5	9.5
Age	Years	47.6	47.0
Systolic blood pressure	mm Hg	145.5	144.3
Middle cerebral aneurysm	1 = yes, 0 = no	0.13	0.13
Anterior cerebral aneurysm	1 = yes, 0 = no	0.60	0.60
Drug-induced hypotension group	1 = yes, 0 = no	0.32	0.34
Carotid ligation group	1 = yes, 0 = no	0.20	0.15
Intracranial surgery group	1 = yes, 0 = no	0.28	0.28

death if the individual died prior to the designated interval and was considered "censored" if the patient was lost to follow-up or died at a later time. Hence, the survival time for an individual is only the time that an individual contributes to the study, and the likelihood of death in a specified interval is based on the time of entry into the study.

To estimate the survival probability for given patients or a group of patients, the following relationship is utilized:

$$S_1(t) = [S_0(t)]^\theta,$$

where $S_1(t)$ is the estimated survival probability, $S_0(t)$ the underlying survival distribution, and θ the hazard function. In the proportional hazards model, θ is equal to $exp(\Sigma\beta_j Z_j)$, where the Z_j's are the values of the covariates for the patient. To calculate the probability of survival, use the probabilities presented in Table 11–A–1 as the underlying survival function, the β_j's from the appropriate table presented in this report. The Z_j is the difference of the individual's covariate profile and that of the study population (Table 11–A–2). $S_0(t)$ will be estimated as in Breslow.[2] An example of a calculation of a 5-year probability of survival for a patient treated with carotid ligation would be as follows:

Patient profile:
   SAH to randomization of 5 days,
   Medical condition of Good (1),
   Systolic blood pressure of 150 mm Hg,
   Age of 55 years,
   Neurologic condition of 2.

$\Sigma\beta_j Z_j = [-.034(5-9.5) + .330(1-1.52) +$
$.008(150-144.3) + .013(55-47) +$
$.167(2-2.3) - 1.057(1-.15) - .336(0-.34)$
$- .452(0-.28)],$

$$S(5 \text{ years}) = .62^{e^{-.577}}$$
$$= .76$$

Hence, the likelihood of 5-year survival for this patient would be 76%.

In addition to the application of this model for determination of a patient's individual risk, the model can be applied to retrospective and prospective data. Instead of stratifying on several individual factors, a combined score can be calculated using the multivariate model. Then strata based on the risk probabilities could be identified and the comparison of groups between and across strata performed.[7] Also, for prospective studies the multivariate risk function could be calculated to provide strata in which randomization or matching could be done to achieve balance between treatment groups. These approaches provide useful alternatives when sample sizes are small relative to the number of influential factors related to outcome.

Appendix References

1. Cox, D.R.: Regression model and life tables (with discussion). J Roy Stat Soc (B) 34:187–220, 1972.
2. Breslow, N.E.: Covariance analysis of censored survival data. Biometrics 30:89–100, 1974.
3. Harrell, F.: The PHGLM procedure. SAS Technical Report S–109, 1980.
4. Kalbfleisch, J.D., Prentice, R.L.: The Statistical Analysis of Failure Time Data. John Wiley and Sons, New York, 1980.
5. Anderson, S., Auquier, A., Hauck, W.W., et al.: Statistical Methods for Comparative Studies. John Wiley and Sons, New York, 1980.
6. Woolson, R.F., Tsuang, M.T., Fleming, J.A.: Utility of the proportional-hazards model for survival analysis of psychiatric data. J Chron Dis 33:183–195, 1980.
7. Miettenin, O.S.: Stratification by a mulitvariate confounder score. Am J Epidemiol 104:609–620, 1976.

Chapter 12

Pathologic Results from Patients Who Died in Randomized Study (Phase II)

Pasquale A. Cancilla, M.D., James C. Torner, M.S. and
Donald W. Nibbelink, M.D., Ph.D.

Abstract

Of 453 patients who died during the follow-up period of treatment in the randomized study of the Cooperative Aneurysm Program, 206 had pathologic findings reported to the Central Registry. Eighty-five percent of the patients had a recently ruptured intracranial aneurysm. The majority of aneurysms (63%) were between 6 and 15 mm in greatest dimension. The site of rupture of the aneurysm sac was at the dome in 66%, at the body in 12%, at the neck in 3% and undetermined in 19% of patients. The location of hemorrhagic sequelae was in the subarachnoid space alone in 29% and intraparenchymal alone in 8%. When more than one anatomic location of hemorrhagic sequelae was identified, subarachnoid hemorrhage was observed 66% of the time and intraparenchymal hemorrhage was reported in 58% of the cases. Ischemic complications were identified in 46% of the patients. These sequelae consisted of a pale or hemorrhagic infarct in 39% of the autopsy specimens. There was a spread in the distribution of ischemic lesions by treatment group. The distribution of ischemic lesions ranged from a low of 31% for bed rest to a high of 57% for both the carotid artery ligation and intracranial surgery groups. Drug-induced hypotension was associated with a 42% incidence of ischemic complications. Eighteen patients had vascular thrombosis of major vessels. The location of the thrombi was: intracranial vessels, 4; extracranial vessels, 10; and both sites, 4. Nine of the cases of thrombosis were associated with carotid artery ligation and 5 were a complication following intracranial surgery. The cause of death was intracranial in 82% of the pathology reports with recent rupture of the aneurysm (85%). Of the extracranial causes of death (7%), pulmonary infection (8%) and pulmonary emboli (4%) were the major events.

Introduction

Patients in the randomized treatment program (Phase II) of the Cooperative Aneurysm Study were assigned to one of four groups: regulated bed rest, drug-induced

Table 12–1.   Deaths, Autopsies, and Protocols Received in Treatment Groups.

Treatment Group	Patients	Deaths	Autopsies	Pathology Reports Registered
Bed Rest	202 (21)*	112 (55)†	74 (66)‡	52 (70)‡
Drug-induced hypotension	309 (32)	143 (46)	90 (63)	66 (73)
Carotid Ligation	187 (19)	73 (39)	41 (56)	30 (73)
Intracranial Surgery	274 (28)	125 (46)	81 (65)	58 (72)
Total	972 (100)	453 (47)	286 (63)	206 (72)

* Number in parentheses denotes percent.   ‡ Percent of deaths
† Percent of patients in treatment group   ‡ Percent of autopsies

hypotension with regulated bed rest, carotid artery ligation or intracranial surgery.[1-3] A total of 972 completed protocols was available for detailed analysis of the comparative treatment groups. As part of this program, a protocol was developed and utilized to obtain data on all patients who died during the follow-up period of the study. From 453 patients who died, 206 (45%) patient data forms documenting the intracranial and extracranial postmortem findings were returned to the Central Registry. In this report, the neuropathologic features and the pertinent general autopsy findings from the 206 patient data forms are discussed and compared with the pathologic findings described with ruptured aneurysms reported from other studies available in the literature.

Clinical Parameters

Between 1963 and 1970, data forms on 972 patients treated in the Cooperative Aneurysm Study were registered. The patient distribution of treatment groups is as follows (Table 12–1): regulated bed rest (21%), drug-induced hypotension with regulated bed rest (32%), carotid artery ligation (19%) and intracranial surgery (28%). The technical approach to intracranial surgery and carotid ligation was at the discretion of the neurosurgeon. The allocation of patients with vertebral-basilar artery aneurysms was suspended because the number of patients with aneurysms on these vessels was insufficient for statistical purposes. Allocation of

Table 12–2.   Vital Data and Cause of Death in Treatment Group.

	Treatment Group				
	Bed Rest	Drug-induced Hypotension	Carotid Ligation	Intracranial Surgery	Total
No. of patients	52	66	30	58	206
Actively treated	49	59	20	41	169
Male	26	31	12	25	94
Female	26	35	18	33	112
Mean age (yr)	49.4	47.5	47.6	51.2	49
Age range (yr)	19–71	15–72	22–74	13–77	13–77
Mean time to death	118	49.5	27.1	41.5	61.3
4–30 days	35	54	27	38	154
31–90 days	11	8	1	12	32
91–180 days	2	0	1	4	7
> 181 days	4	4	1	4	13
Cause of death					
Treatment complication	8	14	11	30	63
Proved rebleed	41	44	10	17	112
Suspected rebleed	1	2	5	2	10
Unrelated	2	6	4	9	21

Table 12.3   Distribution of Aneurysm Site in Treatment Groups.

| Treatment Group | Aneurysm Site | | | | |
	Internal Carotid	Middle Cerebral	Anterior Cerebral-Anterior Communicating	Vertebral-Basilar	Total
Bed rest	5	7	38	2	52 (25)*
Drug-induced hypotension	17	7	42	0	66 (32)
Carotid ligation	12	4	14	0	30 (15)
Intracranial surgery	8	6	42	2	58 (28)
Total	42 (20)*	24 (12)	136 (66)	4 (2)	206 (100)

* Number in parentheses denotes percent.

carotid ligation for recently ruptured anterior cerebral-anterior communicating aneurysms was also suspended during the study. Table 12–1 shows the number of patients, deaths, autopsies and pathology data forms registered for each treatment group. There was an overall mortality of 47%. The mortality by treatment group was 55% for bed rest, 46% for drug-induced hypotension, 39% for carotid ligation and 46% for intracranial surgery. The percentage of autopsies performed in each treatment group was similar (56 to 65%), and the percentage of patients with pathology protocols registered was nearly the same in each treatment group (70 to 73%). In all, pathology reports were received for 45% of deaths. Table 12–2 shows the vital data and cause of death for each treatment group. There were more females (54%) than males (46%). The mean age for all treatment groups was 49 years, with a range of 13 to 77 years. The mean

time from diagnosis to death was: bed rest, 118 days; drug-induced hypotension, 49.5 days; carotid ligation, 27.1 days; and intracranial surgery, 41.5 days. The mean time to death in the bed rest group appears high because of long-term survival in some patients. Thus, the data on time to death are also displayed by intervals. The majority of deaths (75%) occurred between 4 and 30 days and were distributed as follows: bed rest, 67%; drug-induced hypotension, 82%; carotid artery ligation, 90%; and intracranial surgery, 65%.

Morphologic Features

The distribution of the aneurysm site is shown in Table 12–3. Aneurysms of the anterior cerebral-anterior communicating arteries were most frequent (66%), followed

Table 12–4.   Size of Ruptured Aneurysm in Treatment Groups.

| Size of Aneurysm (mm)* | Treatment Group | | | | |
	Bed Rest	Drug-Induced Hypotension	Carotid Ligation	Intracranial Surgery	Total
≤ 5	11	17	8	14	50 (24)
6–15	34	41	18	37	130 (63)
≥ 16	4	7	1	4	16 (8)
Unknown	3	1	3	3	10 (5)
Total	52	66	30	58	206 (100)

* Greatest dimension
† Number in parentheses denotes percent.

Table 12–5.   Site of Aneurysm Rupture in Treatment Groups.

| Site of Rupture | Treatment Group | | | | |
	Bed Rest	Drug-Induced Hypotension	Carotid Ligation	Intracranial Surgery	Total
Dome	32	44	20	40	136 (66)*
Body	7	11	2	4	24 (12)
Neck	4	1	0	1	6 (3)
Unknown	9	10	8	13	40 (19)
Total	52	66	30	58	206 (100)

* Number in parentheses denotes percent.

by internal carotid artery (20%), middle cerebral artery (12%) and vertebral-basilar arteries (2%). There was some variability in the representation of aneurysm site in the various treatment groups. With the exception of the vertebral-basilar location, all aneurysm sites were adequately represented in each group.

The size of the ruptured aneurysms for each treatment group is given in Table 12–4. The majority of aneurysms (63%) were between 6 and 15 mm in greatest diameter; 24% were 5 mm or less in diameter. The major site of rupture (66%) occurred in the dome of the aneurysm (Table 12–5). Rupture of the body of the aneurysm was the next most frequent location (12%), and only rarely was a rupture of the neck of the aneurysm (3%) described. There was evidence of recent rupture of the aneurysm in 85% of the patients (Table 12–6). Recent rupture was demonstrated in 83% of patients treated with bed rest, 94% of drug-induced hypotension, 83% of carotid ligation and 78% of the intracranial surgery patients.

Table 12–7 shows the distribution of hemorrhagic sequelae following rupture of the aneurysm. The major locations of the hemorrhagic sequelae were: subarachnoid alone (29%); intraventricular and intraparenchymal (18%); a combination of subarachnoid, intraparenchymal and intraventricular (18%), subarachnoid and intraparenchymal (10%); and intraparenchymal alone (8%). For the entire group, subarachnoid hemorrhage was identified in 66% of the cases and intraparenchymal hemorrhage was present in 58%.

The ischemic sequelae of aneurysm rupture are shown in Table 12–8. Recent infarcts of a pale or hemorrhagic type were present in 39% of the autopsy specimens. When alone, recent pale infarcts were more common than recent hemorrhagic infarcts. An old infarct was present in 7% of the specimens and accompanied recent infarcts in an additional 3%. The distribution of ischemic lesions among the various treatment groups was as follows: bed rest, 31%, drug-induced hypotension, 42%; carotid ligation, 57%; and intracranial surgery, 57%.

Table 12–6.   Integrity of Aneurysm at Postmortem.

| Integrity of Aneurysm | Treatment Group | | | | |
	Bed Rest	Drug-Induced Hypotension	Carotid Ligation	Intracranial Surgery	Total
Recently ruptured	43 (83)*	62 (94)	25 (83)	45 (78)	175 (85)*
Not recently ruptured	7	4	4	9	24 (12)
No information	2	0	1	4	7 (3)
Total	52	66	30	58	206

* Number in parentheses denotes percent.

Table 12–7.   Distribution of Hemorrhagic Sequelae of Aneurysm Rupture.

| Location of Hemorrhage | Treatment Group | | | | Total |
	Bed Rest	Drug Induced Hypotension	Carotid Ligation	Intracranial Surgery	
Subarachnoid	4	24	10	21	59 (29)*
Intraparenchymal	4	6	3	4	17 (8)
Intraventricular	3	1	1	0	5 (2)
Subarachnoid/ intraparenchymal	3	5	8	5	21 (10)
Subarachnoid/intraventricular	4	4	0	2	10 (5)
Subarachnoid/subdural	0	2	0	3	5 (2)
Intraventricular/ intraparenchymal	18	6	5	8	37 (18)
Subarachnoid/ intraparenchymal/ intraventricular	13	14	2	8	37 (18)
Subarachnoid/ intraparenchymal/ intraventricular/subdural	1	2	0	0	3 (1)
Subarachnoid/ intraparenchymal/subdural	0	0	0	1	1 (0)
Intraparenchymal/ intraventricular/subdural	0	1	0	2	3 (1)
No hemorrhage	2	1	1	4	8 (4)
Total	52	66	30	58	206 (100)

* Number in parentheses denotes percent.

Eighteen patients had vascular thrombosis of major vessels noted in the protocols. The distribution of the thrombi was: intracranial vessels, 4; extracranial vessels, 10; and both sites, 4. Nine of the cases of thrombosis were associated with carotid artery ligation and five were a complication of intracranial surgery.

The cause of death by treatment group is illustrated in Table 12–9. Intracranial causes accounted for death in 82% of patients. In this group, there was an association with recent rupture of the aneurysm in 85% of the cases (Table 12–6). The cause of death in the extracranial (7%) and combined intracranial and extracranial groups (9%) was

Table 12–8.   Ischemic Sequelae of Aneurysm Rupture in Treatment Groups.

| Ischemic Sequelae | Treatment Group | | | | Total |
	Bed Rest	Drug-Induced Hypotension	Carotid Ligation	Intracranial Surgery	
Recent pale infarct	5	15	8	12	40 (43)*
Recent hemorrhagic infarct	5	6	3	12	26 (28)
Old infarct	2	4	2	6	14 (15)
Recent pale and hemorrhagic infarct	2	2	3	1	8 (9)
Recent hemorrhagic and old infarcts	1	1	0	1	3 (3)
Recent pale and old infarcts	1	0	1	1	3 (3)
Total affected	16	28	17	33	94
Total in treatment group(s)	52	66	30	58	206
Percent affected	31	42	57	57	46

* Number in parentheses denotes percent.

Table 12–9. Cause of Death in Treatment Group.

Cause	Treatment Group				
	Bed Rest	Drug-Induced Hypotension	Carotid Ligation	Intracranial Surgery	Total
Intracranial	44	57	25	43	169 (82)*
Extracranial	2	4	1	8	15 (7)
Intracranial and extracranial	6	5	3	5	19 (9)
Unknown	0	0	1	2	3 (1)
Total	52	66	30	58	206

* Number in parentheses denotes percent.

reported in 34 patients. Bronchopneumonia was found in 17 (8%) patients, followed by pulmonary embolism (8 patients, 4%), pulmonary edema (4 patients, 2%), myocardial infarct (2 patients, 1%), perforated duodenum (1 patient) and pneumothorax (1 patient). In 3 instances (1%), no cause of death was identified.

Discussion

The study design of the overall Phase II program utilized regulated bed rest as the baseline treatment group in order to compare the difference in mortality and rebleeding in drug-induced hypotension with regulated bed rest, carotid artery ligation and intracranial surgery.[3] The numbers of patients registered in each treatment group and the prerandomized treatment variables were adequate for valid statistical comparisons. As reported in other series, there were slightly more female than male patients represented (54% compared to 46%).[4,5] The mean age (49 years) compared well to other series and the age range showed a similar spread from 13 to 77 years.[4–10] There were no aneurysms in the prepubertal age range. The mortality for all treatment groups was 46%, with a high of 55% in the regulated bed rest group to a low of 39% in the patients treated with carotid artery ligation. The finding of a 45% mortality with intracranial surgery was sur-

prising and raised many questions relating to patients assigned to this treatment group. These questions have been discussed by Sahs,[1] who pointed out that the data were similar to those found in the studies of Klafta and Hamby[11] and Paul and Arnold[12] and were higher than those reported by Pool[13] and by Krayenbühl et al.[14] Seventy-five percent of the deaths occurred within 30 days of the aneurysm rupture and 90% took place within 90 days.

The aneurysms were most frequently located on the anterior cerebral-anterior communicating arteries, a feature in common with reported series of symptomatic aneurysms. Sixty-three percent of the ruptured aneurysms were 6 to 15 mm in greatest diameter and the predilection for rupture of aneurysms of this size was constant between the treatment groups. Twenty-four percent of the ruptured aneurysms were 5 mm or less in diameter. In autopsy series which include symptomatic and asymptomatic aneurysms less than 5 mm in diameter,[15] it is unusual to find rupture of aneurysms less than 5 mm in diameter. Our study includes only patients with symptomatic aneurysms; however, the frequency of rupture of aneurysms of this size is higher than usual. While the cause of this difference is not evident, there were multiple observers involved, a situation which may have introduced some variability in measurement. Even with this consideration, there likely remains a group of patients with rupture of aneurysms of this size. The predilection for rupture of the dome, followed by rupture of the body of the aneurysm, was substantiated in our series.[9]

Eighty-five percent of the patients in our series had evidence of recent rupture of the aneurysm. The reference group treated by bed rest had an 83% incidence of recent rupture. The four treatment groups did not differ significantly from each other.

In our study, there was a 46% overall incidence of ischemic sequelae to the aneurysm rupture. The bed rest group had a 31% incidence, while the drug-induced hypotension with regulated bed rest group had a 42% incidence, and that for carotid ligation and intracranial surgery was 57%. McCormick[15] reported a 32% overall incidence of infarcts associated with ruptured aneurysms and noted that there is no obvious relationship to hypertension or to treatment in regard to this pathologic finding. Sakurai et al.[16] found an 18% incidence of infarcts in 827 operated cases of ruptured saccular cerebral aneurysms and noted that the infarcts occurred

5 to 15 days following the last bleed. No structural abnormalities were found regularly for the high incidence of ischemic complications following surgery, although vasospasm, a common complication of aneurysm rupture, may have been aggravated by the operative intervention. Drug-induced hypotension resulted in a 42% incidence of ischemic lesions. This incidence was midway between the bed rest and surgically treated groups. Again, no structural basis for ischemia was found. In these patients, reduced cerebral perfusion in combination with ischemia due to vasospasm may have augmented the higher incidence of infarcts.

Recent rupture of the aneurysm was the leading cause of death. Of the extracranial causes of death, bronchopneumonia (8%) and pulmonary embolism (4%) were the major entities. The overall incidence of pulmonary embolism in this series will be an important base for the evaluation of patients treated with antifibrinolytic therapy.

References

1. Sahs, A.L.: History of the Cooperative Aneurysm Study and Central Registry. Chapter 1. In: Sahs, A.L., Nibbelink, D.W., Torner, J.C., et al.: Aneurysmal Subarachnoid Hemorrhage. Report of the Cooperative Study. Urban & Schwarzenberg, Baltimore, 1981, pp 3–16.
2. Nibbelink, D.W.: Intracranial Hemorrhage. In: Siekert, R.G.: Cerebrovascular Survey Report (Revised), Whiting Press Inc., Rochester, MN, 1976, pp 172–182.
3. Nibbelink, D.W., Knowler, L.A.: Objectives and Design of Randomized Aneurysm Study. Ch 3. In: Sahs, A.L., Nibbelink, D.W., Torner, J.C., et al.: Aneurysmal Subarachnoid Hemorrhage. Report of the Cooperative Study. Urban & Schwarzenberg, Baltimore, 1981, pp 21–26.
4. Wilson, G., Riggs, H.E., Rupp, C.: The pathologic anatomy of ruptured cerebral aneurysms. J Neurosurg 11:128–134, 1954.
5. Locksley, G.G.: Natural History of Subarachnoid Hemorrhage, Intracranial Aneurysms and Arteriovenous Malformations. Based on 6368 Cases in the Cooperative Study. Parts I and II. In: Sahs, A.L., Perret, G.E., Locksley, H.B., et al.: Intracranial Aneurysms and Subarachnoid Hemorrhage. A Cooperative Study. J.B. Lippincott Company, Philadelphia, 1969, pp 37–108.
6. Housepean, E.M., Pool, J.L.: A systematic analysis of intracranial aneurysms from the autopsy file of the Presbyterian Hospital 1914–1956. J Neuropath Exp Neurol 17:409–423, 1958.
7. McCormick, W.F., Acosta-Rua, G.J.: The size of intracranial saccular aneurysms. An autopsy study. J Neurosurg 33:422–427, 1970.
8. Chason, J.L., Hindman, W.M.: Berry aneurysms of the circle of Willis: Results of a planned autopsy study. Neurology 8:41–44, 1958.
9. Stehbens, W.E.: Aneurysms and anatomical variations of cerebral arteries. Arch Path 75:45–64, 1973.
10. McCormick, W.F., Schochet, S.S.: Atlas of Cerebrovascular Disease. Ch 2. Aneurysms and Angiomas. W.B. Saunders Co., Philadelphia, 1976, pp 49–105.
11. Klafta, L.A., Hamby, W.B.: Significance of cerebrospinal fluid pressure in determining time for repair of intracranial aneurysms. J Neurosurg 31:217–219, 1969.
12. Paul, R.L., Arnold, J.G.: Operative factors influencing mortality in intracranial aneurysm surgery: Analysis of 186 consecutive cases. J Neurosurg 32:289–294, 1970.

13. Pool, J.L.: Bifrontal craniotomy for anterior communicating artery aneurysms. J Neurosurg 36:212–220, 1972.
14. Krayenbühl, H.A., Yasargil, M.G., Flamm, E.S., et al.: Microsurgical treatment of intracranial saccular aneurysms. J Neurosurg 37:678–686, 1972.
15. McCormick, W.F.: The natural history of intracranial saccular aneurysms. Neurol and Neurosurg 1(3):2–7, 1978.
16. Sakurai, Y., Oka, N., Suzuki, J.: Cerebral Infarction Due to Vasospasm Following Intracranial Aneurysm Rupture. In: Suzuki, J.: Cerebral Aneurysms. Neuron Publishing Co., Tokyo, 1979, pp 73–81.

Section III

Antifibrinolytic Therapy

Chapter 13

Antihypertensive and Antifibrinolytic Therapy Following Subarachnoid Hemorrhage from Ruptured Intracranial Aneurysm

Donald W. Nibbelink, M.D., Ph.D.

Abstract

From 1970 to 1972, the participants of the Cooperative Aneurysm Study conducted a randomized treatment study using antihypertensive and antifibrinolytic drugs alone and in combination. Of the 242 patients studied during a 2-week interval, 28.9% of those receiving drug-induced hypotension, 5.8% of those on antifibrinolytic therapy and 23.8% of those receiving a combination of the two drugs died.

Introduction

Morbidity and mortality associated with rebleeding from ruptured intracranial aneurysms occur with greatest frequency during the 14-day interval following the initial bleed.[1] Interest in the use of antifibrinolytic agents for prevention of rebleeding has continued,[2-4] following the reports of preliminary observations.[5,6] The participants of the Cooperative Aneurysm Study conducted a randomized comparative treatment program so formulated that antihypertensive and antifibrinolytic drugs were used alone and in combination through a prospective scheme of random allocation. Protocols were submitted with the Central Registry from March 1970 through July 10, 1972. From March 1970 through February 1972, the study was conducted as a "pilot project," with continuation of the identical plan from February 1972 through July 10, 1972. In February, only minor changes were made in the format of the protocols submitted with the Central Registry. The preliminary results of this "pilot project" have been reported.[4]

The aneurysm site distribution (Table 13–1) reveals that in a total of 246 patients, 52 had a single aneurysm on the intracranial portion of the internal carotid artery, 31 on the middle cerebral distribution, 91 on the anterior cerebral complex, 18 on the vertebral-basilar system and 54 had more than one intracranial aneurysm (multiple; see

Table 13–1.   Tabulation of Cases for Each Participating Center with Respect to Aneurysm Site.

Center Code No.	IC	MC	AC	VB	M	Total
05	5	3	10	1	5	24
12	10	4	9	3	8	34
19	7	5	6	2	3	23
20	0	0	13	2	17	32
24	0	0	3	0	2	5
25	1	0	0	0	0	1
26	3	1	3	0	1	8
27	7	6	16	8	9	46
28	11	8	17	1	3	40
31	4	0	4	0	1	9
33	4	4	9	1	4	22
37	0	0	1	0	1	2
Subtotal	52	31	91	18	54	246
				Disqualified		4
				Total		242

Abbreviations: IC, internal carotid; MC, middle cerebral; AC, anterior cerebral-anterior communicating; VB, vertebral-basilar; and M, multiple.

Table 13–2.   Definition of Aneurysm Site or Location.

I. Internal carotid—a single aneurysm located on the internal carotid artery distal to its emergence from the cavernous sinus to its terminal bifurcation, and including those aneurysms at the junction of the posterior communicating artery with the internal carotid artery. Infundibular dilatations 2 mm in diameter or less were not included.

II. Middle cerebral—a single aneurysm on middle cerebral artery and its branches.

III. Anterior cerebral-Anterior communicating—a single aneurysm on the anterior cerebral artery and its branches, the anterior communicating artery, and its junction with the anterior cerebral artery.

IV. Vertebral-basilar—a single aneurysm on the vertebral, basilar, posterior communicating-posterior cerebral artery junction; posterior cerebral artery, and all its branches.

V. Multiple—this category is designated to include all patients with more than one intracranial aneurysm, no matter if they are located on the same parent vessel or not.

Table 13–2 for definition). Four patients were disqualified; 1 required intracranial surgery during the 2-week interval and 3 patients were allocated to treatment incorrectly. Therefore, 242 patients remained for subsequent analysis.

In addition to those patients submitted for randomization, 38 were registered as excluded cases. The decision for certain pa-tients to be excluded was made by the at-tending physician at the investigating center. The reason for exclusion (Table 13–3) re-veals that most patients (17 of 38) were al-located to Condition A and operated upon, and the second most frequent reason for ex-clusion was the presence of an intracranial mass lesion requiring immediate surgery. None of these patients entered the random-ization process.

Mechanics of Randomization

The design of the study was formulated so that all patients with recent subarachnoid

Table 13–3.   Excluded Case Registrations.

No. of Patients	Reason for Exclusion
17	Patient allocated to Condition A, and operated upon
8	Intracranial mass lesion requiring immediate surgery
3	Complicating medical disease sufficiently severe to prevent admission to study
2	Previous treatment conflicting with proposed treatment program
2	Patient died before randomization
6	Miscellaneous
38	Total

hemorrhage due to ruptured intracranial aneurysm had their diagnostic evaluation completed within 7 days following the last bleed, and were randomized with respect to location of intracranial aneurysm, the interval from last bleed (day 0 through 7) to the day of diagnosis as confirmed by angiography, and the clinical condition of the patient.

Five major aneurysm sites (internal carotid, middle cerebral, anterior cerebral-anterior communicating, vertebral-basilar-posterior cerebral circulation, and multiple aneurysms), as defined in Table 13–2, were allocated into one of three treatment programs: (1) drug-induced hypotension (chlorothiazides, methyldopa, reserpine, and hydralazine alone or in combination),* (2) antifibrinolytic therapy (epsilon-aminocaproic acid (EACA), 24 to 36 g per day, oral or intravenous route of administration, or tranexamic acid†), or (3) drug-induced hypotension *and* antifibrinolytic therapy. Each treatment program was initiated within 7 days and continued through 14 days, following the last bleed. In this manner, some patients were treated a minimum of 7 days and others a maximum of 14 days.

All patients were randomized within one of four clinical conditions—Condition A, B, C or D. *Condition A* patients were alert, oriented, and appropriately responsive; good clinical risks with no pre-existing serious medical disease; no neurologic deficit except for related cranial nerve signs such as an isolated third cranial nerve paralysis, lumbar puncture pressure of 250 mm H_2O or below; no evidence of vasospasm by arteriography; and stable vital signs. Patients in *Condition B* had minor symptoms such as headache, meningeal irritation or diplopia and, in addition, could have a major neurologic deficit such as hemiparesis or hemiplegia , but were

fully responsive. *Condition C* patients had an impaired state of alertness but were capable of protective or other adaptive responses to noxious stimuli, or were poorly responsive but with stable vital signs. Patients in *Condition D* included such clinical signs as no response to verbal stimulation or shaking, nonadaptive response to noxious stimuli, or progressive instability of vital signs.

Figure 13–1 illustrates the mechanics of the randomization process by aneurysm location, clinical grade and interval from last bleed.

Each patient was treated from 7 to 14 days, depending upon the day of entry into the study. At the end of the 2-week interval, the extended treatment program remained exclusively with the decision of the physician in charge at each investigating center.

Results

Overall mortality at the end of the 2-week interval following the last bleed was one end point in the study; the second end point was the occurrence of rebleeding. During the 2-week interval, 28.9 % died (20 of 69) among those who received drug-induced hypotension (Table 13–4), 5.8% (5 of 85) died

RANDOMIZATION SCHEME

SITE (IC, MC, AC-AC, V-B, MULTIPLE)

CONDITION (A, B, C, D)

DAY (0, 1, 2, 3, 4, 5, 6, 7)

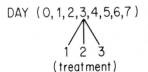

1   2   3
(treatment)

Fig. 13–1. Randomization scheme to allocation of treatment by site, condition and day. (See text for further description; see also Table 13–2 for description of aneurysm location). Treatment 1—drug-induced hypotension; Treatment 2—antifibrinolytic therapy; Treatment 3—drug-induced hypotension and antifibrinolytic therapy.

*This treatment category was defined as a 20% reduction in systolic blood pressure under 140 mm Hg, 25% reduction in pressure between 140 and 180 mm Hg and 30% reduction over 180 mm Hg, with respect to average of four prerandomization systolic values.

†Tranexamic acid is a more potent antifibrinolytic agent used exclusively by some overseas participants. The dosage given was 4 to 12 g per day, administered by the oral or intravenous route.

Table 13–4.   Tabulation of Mortality and Proved Rebleeds During the Two-week Period for Patients in Each Treatment Category.

Treatment	No. of Patients	Deaths	Proved Rebleeds
Drug-induced hypotension	69	20 (28.9%)	15 (21.7%)
Antifibrinolytic therapy	85	5 (5.8%)	5 (5.8%)
Drug-induced hypotension and antifibrinolytic therapy	88	21 (23.8%)	15 (17.0%)
Total	242	46 (19.0%)	35 (14.5%)

among the antifibrinolytic group and 23.8% (21 of 88) died in the combined therapy group (statistically significant at $P < 0.05$). The most frequent cause of death (tabulated with respect to interval in Table 13–5) was a proved rebleed in 8.3% (20 of 242), with the second most common cause being direct cerebral effects from the prerandomized bleed (15 of 242, or 6.2%). The distribution of deaths within each treatment program reveals 20 of the 46 deaths occurred 5 to 9 days following their last bleed (Table 13–5). One patient who died from "unrelated cause," upon postmortem examination was noted to have renal and splenic infarctions, and the single patient in the category designated "other" died following a cardiac arrest. Nine patients died following a suspected rebleed; that is, a comparatively abrupt clinical deterioration and death without evidence of rebleeding as determined by lumbar puncture or postmortem examination. Comparison of the number of deaths in Condition C and D patients was 31.3% (25 of 80; Table 13–6), while those in Conditions A and B had a mortality of 13.0% (21 of 162). These deaths occurred primarily in those who received drug-induced hypotension alone, and those who received the combination of drug-induced hypotension and antifibrinolytic medication.

Sex distribution among all treatment categories was 62% female (150 patients) and 38% male (92 patients). In the 92 males,

Table 13–5.   Tabulation of Cause of Death at Specified Intervals for Each Treatment Category.

Days	Proved Rebleed	Suspected Rebleed	Direct Cerebral Effects	Complications of Treatment	Unrelated Cause	Other	Total
			Drug-induced hypotension (69)*				
0–4	2	0	2	0	0	1	5
5–9	5	1	4	0	0	0	10
10–14	2	1	2	0	0	0	5
Subtotal	9	2	8	0	0	1	20
			Antifibrinolytic therapy (85)*				
0–4	0	2	1	0	0	0	3
5–9	1	0	0	0	0	0	1
10–14	0	0	1	0	0	0	1
Subtotal	1	2	2	0	0	0	5
		Drug-induced hypotension and antifibrinolytic therapy combined (88)*					
0–4	3	1	0	0	0	0	4
5–9	2	3	3	0	1	0	9
10–14	5	1	2	0	0	0	8
Subtotal	10	5	5	0	1	0	21
Total	20	9	15	0	1	1	46

* Total patients allocated to each treatment category.

Table 13–6.   Tabulation of Deaths (Numerator) for Total Patients (Denominator) in Each Condition and Treatment Category.

Treatment	A	B	C	D	Total	%
			Neurologic Condition			
Drug-induced hypotension	2/4	11/42	6/21	1/2	20/69	(28.9%)
Antifibrinolytic therapy	0/10	2/52	3/18	0/5	5/85	(5.8%)
Drug-induced hypotension and antifibrinolytic therapy	0/3	6/51	14/30	1/4	21/88	(23.8%)
Total	2/17	19/145	23/69	2/11	46/242	(19.0%)

there were 16 deaths (17.4 per cent) and 8 proved rebleeds (8.7%); in the 150 females, there were 30 deaths (20%) and 27 proved rebleeds (18%).

Neurologic Condition

A statistical analysis of factors directly applicable to the outcome in each therapeutic program revealed that neurologic condition (as defined in Table 13–7) had a marked

Table 13–7.   Definition of Neurologic Status.

Grade	Symptoms
1	Symptom-free
2	Minor symptoms (headache, meningeal irritation, diplopia)
3	Major neurologic deficit but fully responsive
4	Impaired state of alertness but capable of protective or other adaptive responses to noxious stimuli
5	Poorly responsive but with stable vital signs
6	No response to address or shaking, nonadaptive response to noxious stimuli and progressive instability of vital signs

influence upon mortality. Good-condition patients (Grades 1 and 2) had a 12.1% mortality within 14 days following last bleed, but poor-condition patients (Grades 3 to 6) had a 28.7% mortality. Proved rebleeds also occurred more frequently in poor-condition patients (20.8%) in comparison with those in good condition (9.9%, $P < 0.03$). When subdividing all patients into three subgroups (Table 13–8), the lower percentage of deaths remains significant ($P < 0.01$), but not for proved rebleeds ($P = 0.06$). Therefore, it appears that neurologic condition per se has a greater influence upon mortality than rebleed rate within the 14-day interval.

Systolic Blood Pressure

Death rate and rebleeding were also analyzed with respect to specified levels of systolic blood pressure. Average systolic pressures were calculated from four representative values taken at 4-hour intervals prior to beginning treatment. Patients were subdivided into three subgroups: one subgroup with sys-

Table 13–8.   Distribution of Deaths and Rebleeds for Patients into Neurologic Status.

Distribution	1 and 2	3 and 4	5 and 6	Total
		Neurologic Status		
Deaths/survivors	17/124 (12.1%)*	23/59 (28.0%)	6/13 (31.6%)	46/196
Rebleeds/no rebleeds	14/127	17/65	4/15	35/207
Total patients	141	82	19	242

* Percent mortality of total patients

Table 13–9. Distribution of Deaths and Rebleeds for All Patients with Average Systolic Blood Pressures Subdivided into Three Categories as Designed Below.

	Systolic Blood Pressure			
	≤120	≥121 ≤160	≥161	Total
Deaths/survivors	4/23 (14.8%)*	17/114 (13.0%)	25/59 (29.8%)	46/196
Rebleeds/no rebleeds	4/23 (14.8%)	12/119 (9.2%)	19/65 (22.6%)	35/207
Total patients	27	131	84	242

* Percent of total patients.

tolic values equal to or below 120 mm Hg, a second with values above 120 mm Hg and equal to or below 160 mm Hg, and a third with average values above 160 mm Hg. Significant differences among the three subgroups ($P < 0.01$) appear by virtue of the 29.8% mortality in those with systolic blood pressure equal to or above 161 mm Hg (Table 13–9). The number of proved rebleeds during this 14-day interval was also highest (22.6%) in patients with average systolic values equal to and above 161 mm Hg, but were lowest in the group with 121 to 160 mm Hg. By subdividing all patients into approximately equal groups (Table 13–10), mortality was highly significant ($P < 0.01$) among the specified levels of average systolic blood pressure. Death rate was lowest in the group with average pressures of 128 to 142 mm Hg, and highest in those with blood pressure equal to or over 176 mm Hg. A significant difference for proved rebleeds ($P < 0.05$) was also noted (Table 13–10). However, the highest rates were at the lowest and highest ranges of average systolic blood pressures. There was no evidence of gradual decline in death or rebleed rates at specific decrements in systolic blood pressure.

Cerebral Vasospasm

Angiographic visualization of arterial narrowing was measured at each investigating center. Those segments considered to be narrowed due to vasospasm were recorded in the protocol as localized, ipsilateral diffuse, and bilateral diffuse vasospasm (Table 13–11). Analysis of vasospasm with respect to age, sex, neurologic condition, systolic blood pressure and size of aneurysm revealed no statistically significant differences with regard to the presence or absence of vasospasm within each variable. Detailed analysis of patients who had their angiographic survey on each day following the last bleed (Fig. 13–2) revealed that from days 4 through 7, a greater percentage were likely to show some degree of vasospasm with comparison to those whose angiographic survey was done prior to day 4. Each aneurysm location manifested moderate variation in presence of vasospasm. Each site followed

Table 13–10. Distribution of Patients into Five Approximately Equal Groups to Show Mortality, Rebleeds and Range in Average Systolic Blood Pressure.

	Systolic Blood Pressure					
	≤127	≥128 ≤142	≥143 ≤158	≥159 ≤175	≥176	Total
Deaths/survivors	8/42 (16.0%)*	3/44 (6.4%)	7/42 (14.3%)	10/39 (20.4%)	18/29 (38.3%)	46/196
Rebleeds/no rebleeds	10/40 (20.0%)	4/43 (8.5%)	2/47 (4.1%)	7/42 (14.3%)	12/35 (25.5%)	35/207
Total patients	50	47	49	49	47	242

* Percent of total patients.

Table 13–11.   Definition of Cerebral Vasospasm as Characterized Angiographically.

None	No spasm
Localized	Narrowing of segmental portions of individual vessels
Diffuse (ipsilateral)	Main ipsilateral vessels
Diffuse (bilateral)	All major vessels

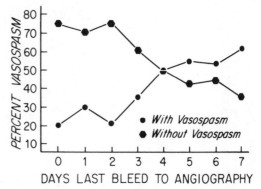

Fig. 13–2.   Distribution of patients with and without vasospasm.

by the percentage with vasospasm was as follows: internal carotid, 48.1%; middle cerebral, 25%; anterior cerebral, 30.2%; vertebral-basilar, 33.3%; and multiple, 40.7%.

Analysis of deaths and presence of vasospasm revealed no statistically significant correlation, although mortality was 10% more in those manifesting some degree of vasospasm (Table 13–12). Neither was proved rebleeding significantly greater in the group with vasospasm compared with those without vasospasm. However, it must be noted that there were 9.7% more rebleeds among the group with vasospasm.

Table 13–12.   Distribution of Deaths and Proved Rebleeds with and without Vasospasm.

Vasospasm	Deaths/Total	Rebleeds/Total
Yes	22/87 (25.3%)	18/87 (20.7%)
No	24/155 (15.5%)	17/155 (11.0%)

Death and Rebleeding Probabilities

In order to compare the probability of death or rebleeding at specified intervals within the 14-day period for each treatment program, the number of deaths every 3 days was subtracted from the number of survivors at the beginning of that interval. Calculations on a daily basis produced a very irregular pattern, but the 3-day interval was found to be most meaningful. The probability for death to occur increased sharply in the 3 to 5 day interval and continued to rise slowly during the remaining period in patients who received drug-induced hypotension (T–1) or the combined therapy program (T–3, Fig.

13–3). However, those patients who received antifibrinolytic medication alone had an average probability of 1% for death to occur during each 3-day period.

The risk for rebleeding, calculated on the basis of the number of patients alive at the beginning of each interval, showed maximum rates to occur during the 6 to 8 and 9 to 11-day intervals for those who received drug-induced hypotension (T–1) and the combined treatment program (T–3, Fig. 13–4). A slight rise to 3.5% was observed in the antifibrinolytic group during the 6 to 8-day interval only.

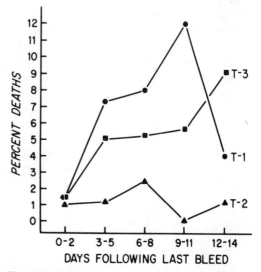

Fig. 13–3.   Mortality rate for patients at risk at three-day intervals. *T–1*, drug-induced hypotension; *T–2*, antifibrinolytic therapy; *T–3*, combined therapy group.

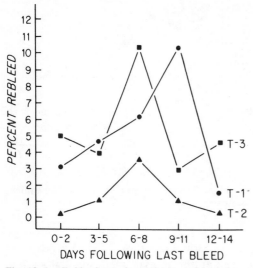

Fig. 13–4.   Rebleed rate for patients at risk at three-day intervals. *T–1*, drug-induced hypotension; *T–2*, antifibrinolytic therapy; *T–3*, combined therapy group.

Discussion

Epsilon-aminocaproic acid (EACA) is a known fibrinolytic inhibitor of the plasminogen-plasmin system.[7,8] Recent studies show that its mechanism may be mediated by plasminogen depletion.[9,10] The introduction of antifibrinolytic agents in acute subarachnoid hemorrhage with presentation of rationale and results of treatment in such patients has been reported.[2,3,5,6,11] Analysis of these reports reveals that in patients whose treatment began within 7 days, the number of rebleeds is low within the 2-week period. Total patients in the five series

(Table 13–13) show an overall 7.0% rate for rebleeding. In one series,[3] there were 3 rebleeds in 50 patients within 2 weeks, but these patients had drug-induced hypotension with EACA. Their mortality during the 2-week interval was not reported. In another series,[11] antihypertensive medication was also given, but in relatively low dosage. The data from Gibbs and O'Gorman[5] include only those patients who had EACA started within 7 days and continued at least 14 days whether or not they had "nondefinitive" surgery. The 5.8% mortality and 5.8% rebleed rate (see Table 13–4) in the present study is comparable to the reports discussed above. Only 1 patient in the antifibrinolytic group died during the 2-week interval following a proved rebleed; 2 following a suspected rebleed, and 2 following direct cerebral effects of the prerandomized bleed.

A surprising feature in this study was the 23.8% mortality and 17.0% proved rebleed rate in those who received the combined therapy of antifibrinolytic drugs with antihypertensive medication. Analysis of classification of drugs used, dosage and route of therapy revealed none of these to be responsible for this observation. Insufficient fibrinolytic studies were performed during administration of these medications; therefore, no pertinent laboratory evaluations are available to properly compare results with those given antifibrinolytic agents alone. So the questions arise, What pharmacologic influence does antihypertensive medication have on EACA? Are the antifibrinolytic properties of EACA by some mechanism

Table 13–13.   Distribution of Rebleeds and Deaths within Two Weeks in Patients Receiving Antifibrinolytic Therapy Beginning within Seven Days from Last Bleed.

Study	No. of Patients	Rebleeds	Deaths
Gibbs and O'Gorman (1967)[5]	19	5	5
Mullan and Dawley (1968)[6]	35	1	0
Norlen and Thulin (1969)[2]	7	0	0
Ranshoff et al. (1972)[3]	50	3	Unknown
Tovi (1972)[11]	32	1	2
Total	143	10 (7.0%)	7

inhibited at the molecular or cellular level? It is suggested that the answers may lie in the kinetics of drug interaction.

No tendencies were apparent toward increase in undesirable complications during antifibrinolytic therapy. Two patients experienced pulmonary embolism. One was demonstrated by pulmonary arteriography while the patient was receiving EACA and reserpine; the other patient had received EACA and methyldopa and the embolus was demonstrated at postmortem examination. One patient had EACA terminated because of electrocardiographic changes suggestive of myocardial ischemia.

All patients were followed with regard to proper systolic blood pressure maintenance at the desired level. These patients were kept under the closest surveillance, and if there was any interval of more than 48 hours that proper levels were not maintained, that patient was regarded as not being properly controlled. Blood pressures were taken every 4 hours and in many, recordings were made every hour. In the 64 patients who had "inadequate response to antihypertensive medication" during the 14-day interval (40.7%), 25.0% died, a percentage not appreciably different from the mortality of the entire group receiving drug-induced hypotension. These data are consistent with those of the previous investigations by the Cooperative Aneurysm Study. Although rebleeding, cerebral vasospasm, cerebral edema and other factors may be responsible for causing failure in designated decrease in systolic blood pressure, none of these was significantly more or less frequent than in the group who achieved prescribed blood pressure control.

Analysis of risk of rebleeding during the 14-day interval with respect to average systolic blood pressure soon after admission to the hospital (see Table 13–10) suggests that pressures in the lower ranges ($\leq$ 127 mm Hg) give no assurance that rebleeding is unlikely to occur. On the contrary, the lowest rebleed rate (4.1%) took place in the group with average systolic values in the range of 143 to 158 mm Hg. This suggests that there could be an "optimal" blood pressure level

where rebleeds tend to occur least often, rather than a "hypotensive" level. Further analysis of the group who received drug-induced hypotension alone and the combined therapy group whose average systolic blood pressure prior to treatment was between 143 and 158 mm Hg revealed 46.4% (13 of 28) had their blood pressure brought under control according to protocol. There were 1 rebleed and 2 deaths in this group. In the remaining 15, 1 had a proved rebleed and 2 a suspected rebleed. There were 5 deaths, 3 following progressive deterioration, and 2 following suspected rebleed. In the group whose average systolic values were 127 mm Hg or below (total of 28 patients who received drug-induced hypotension alone and the combined therapy program), 9 had a 20% decrease or more during the 14-day period and 4 of these rebled. Four additional patients received no antihypertensive drugs because the average systolic pressure was too low to safely administer such medication. One rebled and died and 1 died following progressive decline in his neurologic condition. Fifteen patients had less than 20% reduction in blood pressure during the 14-day interval; 3 rebled and 2 of them died within 14 days. Therefore, 8 rebleeds occurred among these 28 patients (28.6%) who were allocated to antihypertensive therapy. This percentage is higher than the 22.6% rebleed rate in the bed rest series in the previous randomized study.

Summary and Conclusions

This study, supported by the National Institute of Neurological Diseases and Stroke, summarizes the results of the randomized use of antihypertensive drugs alone, antifibrinolytic therapy alone, and their combination in 246 patients, 4 of whom were disqualified, leaving a residuum of 242 for analysis. This study included only those aneurysm patients whose treatment was initiated within 7 days following the last bleed.

Treatment was carried out during a period not in excess of 2 weeks after the ictus, but every patient was treated at least 7 days. Five major aneurysm sites were selected. Further stratification was made in terms of clinical condition of the patients.

The gross mortality of the group receiving antifibrinolytic therapy was impressive (5.8%). Parenthetically, it can be stated that this figure led to the temporary suspension of the other two types of therapy until further studies could be continued in the antifibrinolytic group to determine whether the mortality figure of 5.8% was a fortuitous accidental finding or whether more cases in that category would change the statistics.

Of the 242 patients, 155 (64%) had no vasospasm. Strangely, only 11% of this group rebled, while 21% of the group with diffuse and localized vasospasm rebled.

Attempts were made to correlate deaths and proved rebleeding episodes with various patient characteristics. Factors such as age, sex, aneurysm location, systolic blood pressure and size of aneurysm were analyzed. Poor neurologic condition and average systolic blood pressure above 160 mm Hg emerged as the most important determinants for death and rebleeding.

The possible mechanisms of action of antifibrinolytic treatment are discussed. EACA appears to be free from severe and frequent side effects. Further studies should elucidate the role of optimal blood pressure and other factors in protecting patients with ruptured aneurysms during the critical 2-week period after the bleeding episode.

References

1. Sahs, A.L., Perret, G.E., Locksley, H.B., Nishioka, H.: Intracranial Aneurysms and Subarachnoid Hemorrhage. A Cooperative Study. J.B. Lippincott, Philadelphia, 1969.
2. Norlen, G., Thulin, C.A.: The use of antifibrinolytic substances in ruptured intracranial aneurysms. Neurochirurgia (Stuttg.) 12:101–102, 1969.
3. Ransohoff, J., Goodgold, A., Benjamin, M.V.: Preoperative management of patients with ruptured intracranial aneurysms. J. Neurosurg 36:525–530, 1972.
4. Nibbelink, D.W., Sahs, A.L.: Antifibrinolytic therapy and drug-induced hypotension in treatment of ruptured intracranial aneurysms. (Preliminary Report.) Trans Am Neurol Assoc 97:145–147, 1972.
5. Gibbs, J.R., O'Gorman, P.: Fibrinolysis in subarachnoid hemorrhage. Postgrad Med J 43:779–784, 1967.
6. Mullan, S., Dawley, J.: Antifibrinolytic therapy for intracranial aneurysms. J Neurosurg 28:21–23, 1968.
7. Ablondi, F.B., Hagan, J.J., Philips, M., De Renzo, E.C.: Inhibition of plasmin, trypsin, and the streptokinase-activated fibrinolytic system by epsilon-aminocaproic acid. Arch Biochem Biophys 82:153–160, 1959.
8. Alkjaersig, N., Fletcher, A.P., Sherry, S.: Epsilon-aminocaproic acid: An inhibitor of plasminogen activation. J Biol Chem 234:832–837, 1959.
9. Rabiner, F.S., Goldfine, I.D., Hart, A., Summara, L., Robbins, K.C.: Radioimmunoassay of human plasminogen and plasmin. J Lab Clin Med 74:265–273, 1969.
10. Nibbelink, D.W., Jacobsen, C.D.: Plasminogen depletion during administration of epsilon-aminocaproic acid. Thromb Diath Haemorrh 29:598–602, 1973.
11. Tovi, D.: Studies of Fibrinolysis in the Central Nervous System. Centraltryckeriet, Umea, Sweden, 1972.

Chapter 14

Antifibrinolytic Therapy in Recent Onset Subarachnoid Hemorrhage

Donald W. Nibbelink, M.D., Ph.D., James C. Torner, M.S. and William G. Henderson, Ph.D.

Abstract

In this cooperative study among 13 institutions, 502 patients were treated with antifibrinolytic medication (epsilon-aminocaproic acid or tranexamic acid) within a 14-day period following rupture of an intracranial aneurysm. Mortality at the end of 14 days was 11.6%; the proved rebled rate was 12.7%. Patients with an internal carotid or anterior cerebral aneurysm had the highest mortality and rebleed rate. Most rebleeds occurred between the 6th and 11th days following the initial bleed. Significantly higher mortality was reported among patients with cerebral vasospasm, yet rebleed rate was no different among those patients with or without vasospasm. The same pattern was observed among patients with a mean blood pressure value above and below 110 mm Hg. We conclude that antifibrinolytic therapy provides beneficial treatment to patients with recent onset subarachnoid hemorrhage (SAH) following rupture of an intracranial aneurysm.

Introduction

Morbidity and mortality following rupture of an intracranial aneurysm have the highest frequency during the 14-day interval immediately following the day of the initial bleed.[1] Rebleeding alone has been the major cause of death among unoperated patients during this 2-week period. Patients operated upon within 2 weeks following the bleed also have the highest morbidity and mortality compared to those operated upon after that interval.[2-5] For protection against an early rebleed prior to surgery, previous reports have described the use of antifibrinolytic agents in the treatment of recent onset subarachnoid hemorrhage (SAH). From March 1970 through July 1972, the participants of the Cooperative Aneurysm Project pursued a study so formulated that antihypertensive and antifibrinolytic drugs were used randomly, either alone or in combination.[6,7] In that study, mortality and morbidity during the 14-day period were significantly improved with antifibrinolytic therapy alone as compared to the group treated with antihypertensive medication alone or the combination of antihypertensive and antifibrinolytic medication. Following that study, all patients from every participating institution who entered the study had antifibrinolytic therapy initiated within 7 days, a treatment which was continued until 14 days following the bleed. The primary objective was the prevention of rebleeding. With neurologic and medical conditions stabilized at 14 days, a decision was made for definitive surgical or continued medical therapy following that interval. The following report describes the preliminary results of that study.

Treatment Management

From October 1972 through June 1974, 471 patients were treated with epsilon-amino-caproic acid (EACA) or tranexamic acid during a period of 7 to 14 days following the bleed. Treatment was initiated following the clinical diagnosis of a ruptured intracranial aneurysm with the finding of grossly bloody spinal fluid as determined by lumbar puncture and with roentgenographic determination of one or more intracranial aneurysms. The protocol stipulated that laboratory studies such as a complete blood count, urinalysis, platelet determination, fibrinogen level and a serum biochemical profile be completed prior to treatment. Twenty-four or 36 g of EACA was given by continuous drip intravenously in 800 to 1,000 ml of 5% dextrose in water every 24 hours. The dosage of EACA was monitored by the streptokinase clot lysis time.[8,9] After 3 to 10 days of intravenous therapy, EACA was given or-

ally every 2 hours until the end of the 14-day interval following the last bleed. At that time, a decision was made for the patient to undergo surgery or be continued on medical therapy. Tranexamic acid, a more potent antifibrinolytic agent, was given by two participating centers in dosages of 8 to 16 g per 24 hours, initially by the intravenous route, followed by the oral preparation until the end of the treatment period. No antihypertensive medications were administered and no salicylates were prescribed. In instances where the blood pressure was excessively elevated, such patients were removed from the study. From a total of 502 protocols submitted to the Central Registry, 471 remained for detailed analysis.

Clinical Material

Among the 471 patients, 100 had an aneurysm on the intracranial portion of the internal carotid artery, 83 had one on the middle cerebral distribution, 171 on the anterior cerebral-anterior communicating complex and 27 on the vertebrobasilar system; in 90 patients, more than one aneurysm was seen in the cerebral angiogram (Table 14–1). Thirty-one patients were disqualified for various reasons (Table 14–2), which included those who had a craniotomy prior to the end of the 14-day treatment period.

Forty-eight percent of patients had antifibrinolytic therapy initiated within 2 days following the last bleed (87.4% within 5

Table 14–1.   Distribution of Patients for Each Aneurysm Site and Interval Following Last Bleed.

Last Bleed to Treatment	Aneurysm Site					
	Internal Carotid	Middle Cerebral	Anterior Cerebral	Vertebrobasilar	Multiple	Total
0–2 days	39	34	84	11	57	225
3–5 days	45	39	70	12	21	187
6–8 days	16	10	17	4	12	59
Total	100	83	171	27	90	471

Table 14–2. Reason for Disqualification.

Reason	No.
Craniotomy performed prior to end of 14-day period	20
Carotid ligation prior to day 14	2
No cerebral angiographic survey	2
Myocardial infarction after treatment started	1
Thrombocytosis and metastasis	1
Intracerebral hematoma requiring immediate surgery	1
Received drug-induced antihypertensive agents	1
No aneurysm found at surgery	1
Entered 9 days from bleed	1
Transferred from hospital	1
Total	31

days). On the day of entry into the study, the neurologic condition was specified for each patient (Table 14–3). The distribution of patients in these conditions was correlated with the degree of vasospasm as visualized by cerebral angiography. Twenty-six percent (82 of 317) who were in good neurologic condition (Grades 1 and 2) had localized and diffuse vasospasm, and 33% of those in poor condition (Grades 3 to 6) had vasospasm ($P = 0.09$).

Sixty-one percent of the patients were women. Interestingly, for all patients 50 years of age and over, 69% (166 of 240) were females, whereas in the group below age 50, 52.4% were women. The distribution of men above and below age 50 was nearly the same.

The majority of patients were women among three aneurysm sites, namely, internal carotid, vertebrobasilar and multiple locations (Table 14–4). Although the proportion of men and women with an aneurysm on the middle cerebral and anterior cerebral complex was similar, there were more women than men in the entire group. Among the 62 female patients with multiple aneurysms, 61.3% had one of their intracranial aneurysms on the internal carotid artery.

Overall medical condition was assessed on the day antifibrinolytic therapy was initiated. A total of 44.6% were in good condition, 45.4% in fair condition and 10% in poor and prohibitive condition (Table 14–5). For patients in fair, poor and prohibitive medical condition, 38% had mean blood pressures below 100 mm Hg; 66% had mean pressures above 100 mm Hg. In contrast, patients in good medical condition had

Table 14–4. Sex Distribution for Each Aneurysm Site.

Aneurysm Site	Sex Distribution		Total
	Men	Women	
Internal carotid	29	71	100
Middle cerebral	35	48	83
Anterior cerebral	82	89	171
Vertebrobasilar	9	18	27
Multiple	28	62	90
Total	183	288	471

Table 14–3. Distribution of Patients With Various Degrees of Vasospasm for Each Neurologic Condition.

Neurologic Condition (grade)*	Cerebral Vasospasm			Total
	None	Localized	Diffuse	
1	4	0	0	4
2	231	57	25	313
3	21	7	7	35
4	58	12	14	84
5	21	5	2	28
6	2	3	2	7
Total	337	84	50	471

* Definition of neurologic condition: 1 = symptom-free, 2 = minor symptoms (headache, meningeal irritation, diplopia), 3 = major neurologic deficit but fully responsive, 4 = impaired state of alertness but capable of protective or other adaptive responses to noxious stimuli, 5 = poorly responsive but with stable vital signs, 6 = no response to address or shaking, nonadaptive response to noxious stimuli, and progressive instability of vital signs.

Table 14–5.   Distribution of Patients in Various Medical Conditions with Mean Blood Pressures Above and Below 100 mm Hg.

| Mean BP Prior to Treatment | Medical Condition† | | | Total |
	Good	Fair	Poor and Prohibitive	
≥100 mm Hg	107	55	10	172
<100 mm Hg	102	158	37	297
Total	209	213	47	469*
%	44.6	45.4	10.0	

* 2 additional patients had insufficient blood pressure information
† Definition of medical condition: *good*—alert, normotensive, and good health prior to SAH; *fair*—patients with single underlying medical disorder such as hypertension, cirrhosis, anemia, atherosclerosis, or pulmonary disease; *poor*—patients with more than one adverse factor or one serious disorder; *prohibitive*—patients with one or more complicating illness which pre-existed onset of SAH.

nearly equal distribution of mean blood pressures above and below 100 mm Hg, whereas patients in fair to prohibitive medical condition had a higher association with elevated blood pressures ($P < 0.001$).

Results

Determination of mortality and proved rebleeds during the 14-day interval following the last bleed was the primary objective in this study. Mortality at the end of 14 days was 11.6%. Proved rebleed rate (as determined by lumbar puncture or postmortem examination) was 12.7%. A proved rebleed was the major cause of death in 27 patients (Table 14–6). The highest proportion of these deaths occurred during the second week after the bleeding event. Analysis of the interval to rebleed following the initial episode which prompted hospitalization reveals that 2.5% rebled within 5 days, 7.4% within 8 days and 10.4% within 11 days. A similar time distribution was observed for patients who died following progressive decline from the direct cerebral effects of the original bleed (14 of 17 deaths). Most recurrent hemorrhages (61.7%, or 37 of 60) occurred between the 6th and 11th days following the initial bleed (Table 14–7). This was the main reason for the high number of deaths reported during the 6 through 14-day

period. Following the initiation of treatment with antifibrinolytic medication, the interval required to reach a proper antifibrinolytic effect was usually 3 to 5 days.[8] Analysis of the interval between the beginning of antifibrinolytic medication and recurrent hemorrhage reveals that 45.4% of proved and suspected rebleeds occurred prior to the day proper antifibrinolytic effect was reached.

Analysis of Clinical Characteristics as Related to Mortality and Morbidity

Various characteristics in patients with SAH potentially influence the outcome (death and/or rebleeding from a ruptured intracranial aneurysm). For this discussion, several variables such as age, sex, aneurysm site, neurologic and medical conditions, blood pressure and vasospasm were correlated with mortality and proved rebleeds during the 14-day interval.

For patients below age 50, 9.2% died and 10.9% rebled. For those aged 50 or above, 13.7% died ($P > 0.05$) and 14.2% rebled ($P > 0.05$). Sex distribution revealed that 9.3% of deaths occurred in men and 13.2% in women ($P > 0.05$); the rebleed rate was 6.5% for men and 16.7% for women ($P < 0.001$). Mortality distribution for each aneurysm site was similar to the rebleed rate

Table 14–6. Distribution of Cause of Death During 14-Day Interval Following Last Bleed.

Cause of Death	Interval to Death Following Last Bleed (days)					
	0–2	3–5	6–8	9–11	12–14	Total
Proved rebleed	1	3	10	6	7	27
Progressive decline	1	1	5	7	3	17
Suspected rebleed	0	0	1	2	2	5
Complications not related to treatment	0	0	0	1	4	5
Complication of treatment	0	0	0	0	1	1
Total	2	4	16	16	17	55

with the exception of patients with an internal carotid aneurysm (Table 14–8). Among those patients, 21% rebled and 14% died. Patients with an aneurysm on the internal carotid or anterior cerebral distribution had the highest mortality and rebleed rate.

Neurologic condition on the day of allocation of treatment was clearly related to mortality. For patients with impaired state of mental alertness beyond a few days following the last bleed, mortality was proportionately greater than the rebleed rate (Table 14–9). Average mortality for patients in Grades 1 and 2 was 6.9% (22 of 317), whereas for patients in poor condition (Grades 3 through 6) mortality was 21.4% (33 of 154, $P < 0.001$). Average rebleed rate was 11.3% for the former group and 15.6% for the latter ($P > 0.05$).

Medical condition also was related to mortality and rebleed rate. Patients in poor and prohibitive medical condition had mortality and rebleed rates three times that seen in patients classified as being in good and fair condition. Those in good and fair condition

had a combined mortality of 9.4% (40 of 424), and a rebleed rate of 11.1% (Table 14–10). Mortality in poor and prohibitive conditions combined was 31.9% (15 of 47, $P < 0.001$) and had a proved rebleed rate of 27.7% (13 of 47, $P < 0.001$).

Cerebral vasospasm (as demonstrated by cerebral angiography) was categorized as localized or diffuse. Localized vasospasm was interpreted as a decrease in intra-arterial diameter of 1 to 3 cm over the proximal portions of the internal carotid, middle cerebral, anterior cerebral or vertebrobasilar arteries. Diffuse vasospasm was regarded as decreased diameter of the internal carotid artery and all its main branches, either ipsilateral or contralateral to the aneurysm.

Rebleed rate was unrelated to the degree of vasospasm. However, the proportion of deaths among patients with diffuse vasospasm was twice that among those without vasospasm (22 vs 9.2%, Table 14–11). This finding was highly significant ($P = 0.013$). Therefore, pathophysiologic changes associated with cerebral vasospasm can produce

Table 14–7. Distribution of Rebleeds During 14-Day Interval Following Last Bleed.

Interval from Last Bleed (days)	Rebleed	
	Proved	Suspected
0–2	1	0
3–5	11	2
6–8	23	5
9–11	14	3
12–14	11	2
Total	60	12

Table 14–8. Distribution of Mortality and Rebleed Rate for Aneurysm Site.

Aneurysm Site	No. Patients	Deaths	Rebleeds
Internal carotid	100	14 (14)*	21 (21)
Middle cerebral	83	7 (8.4)	5 (6)
Anterior cerebral	171	24 (14)	25 (14.6)
Vertebrobasilar	27	2 (7.4)	2 (7.4)
Multiple	90	8 (8.9)	7 (7.8)
Total	471	55 (11.6)	60 (12.7)

* Number in parentheses denotes percent.

Table 14–9.   Distribution of Mortality and Rebleed Rate by Neurologic Condition.

Neurological Condition* (grade)	No. Patients	Deaths	Proved Rebleeds
1	4	1 (25)†	1 (25)
2	313	21 (6.7)	35 (11.2)
3	35	5 (14.3)	2 (5.7)
4	84	15 (17.8)	12 (14.3)
5	28	9 (32.1)	7 (25)
6	7	4 (57.1)	3 (42.8)
Total	471	55 (11.6)	60 (12.7)

* Defined in table 14–3.
† Number in parentheses denotes percent.

sufficient structural and/or metabolic damage to cause severe degrees of localized or widespread deterioration in neuronal function.

Mortality and rebleed rates were directly related to increments in mean blood pressure as measured on the day of allocation to treatment. Patients with average mean blood pressures of 110 mm Hg or below had an average mortality of 8.3% (23 of 276) and a rebleed rate of 10.5% (Table 14–12). Patients with average mean blood pressures above 110 mm Hg had a mortality of 16.1% and rebleed rate of 16.1%. These results for mortality and rebleed rates below and above a mean blood pressure of 110 mm Hg were significant for mortality rate ($P = 0.015$) but not for rebleed rate ($P = 0.103$).

Signs and Symptoms Observed During the Treatment Period

Thirty items were monitored and recorded in the treatment protocol. The list of these

various conditions (Table 14–13) with the percent of total patients affected in each condition reveals the broad spectrum of medical disorders affecting patients with SAH. The most frequent condition was diarrhea (24.3%), which was drug-related (oral epsilon-aminocaproic or tranexamic acid). Patients who developed ischemic neurologic deficit acquired a hemiparesis, hemiplegia and/or aphasia. In our opinion, these were not drug-related events. All the remaining conditions also were considered to be unrelated to drug therapy with the exception of the dermatologic problems. These were

Table 14–11.   Distribution of Mortality and Rebleed Rate for Patients with Various Degrees of Vasospasm.

Cerebral Vasospasm*	No. Patients	Deaths	Rebleeds
None	337	31 (9.2)†	44 (13)
Localized	84	13 (15.5)	11 (13.1)
Diffuse	50	11 (22)	5 (10)
Total	471	55 (11.6)	60 (12.7)

* See text for definition (p 301).
† Number in parentheses denotes percent.

Table 4–10.   Distribution of Mortality and Rebleed Rate for Medical Condition.

Medical Condition*	No. Patients	Deaths	Rebleeds
Good	210	17 (8.1)†	24 (11.4)
Fair	214	23 (10.7)	23 (10.7)
Poor	44	14 (31.8)	12 (27.3)
Prohibitive	3	1 (33.3)	1 (33.3)
Total	471	55 (11.6)	60 (12.7)

* Defined in Table 14–5.
† Number in parentheses denotes percent.

Table 14–12.   Distribution of Mortality and Rebleed Rate for Mean Blood Pressure.

Mean BP (mm Hg)	No. Patients	Deaths	Rebleeds
≤90	67	2 (3)*	6 (8.9)
91–110	209	21 (10)	23 (11)
11–130	147	20 (13.6)	22 (15)
>130	46	11 (23.9)	9 (19.6)
Total	469†	54 (11.4)	60 (12.7)

* Number in parentheses denotes percent.
† Two additional patients had insufficient blood pressure information available.

difficult to delineate because of other analgesic and anti-inflammatory medications prescribed in conjunction with antifibrinolytic therapy.

Discussion

Hemorrhagic cerebrospinal fluid from a ruptured intracranial aneurysm is associated with a marked increase in fibrinolytic activity. This is caused by a rapid increase in the amount of fibrinolytic precursor (plasminogen).[10] Epsilon-aminocaproic acid and tranexamic acid are known fibrinolytic inhibitors. Recent studies suggest that the mechanism of these agents may be through inhibition of the synthesis in the plasminogen-plasmin system.[11,12] The mechanism for prevention of recurrent hemorrhage follow-

Table 14–13.   Distribution of Signs or Symptoms Observed During the Treatment Period for the 464 Protocols in which This Information Was Received at the Central Registry.

Sign or Symptom	Degree of Severity			%
	Mild	Moderate	Severe	
Anemia	29	8	0	8.0
Aphasia	4	13	21	8.2
Bleeding time abnormality	1	0	0	0.2
Clotting derangement	3	0	0	0.6
Coagulation factor abnormality	1	1	0	0.4
Conjunctival suffusion	1	0	1	0.4
Convulsions	7	0	2	1.9
Diarrhea	50	52	11	24.3
Dysphasia	7	15	19	8.8
Edema (extremities)	7	2	0	1.9
Electrolyte imbalance	39	20	3	13.4
Gastrointestinal hemorrhage	4	6	4	3.0
Genitourinary tract infection	23	21	3	10.1
Hemiparesis	22	20	37	17.0
Hemiplegia	11	13	28	11.2
Uric acid elevation	6	4	3	2.8
Ischemic neurologic deficit	23	18	37	16.8
Increased white blood count	21	12	2	7.5
Myocardial infarction	1	0	0	0.2
Nausea	25	6	0	6.7
Psychiatric disturbance	19	11	5	7.5
Pulmonary embolism	0	0	2	0.4
Rash (pruritic)	0	2	0	0.4
Rash (maculopapular)	4	4	1	1.9
Restlessness	36	18	10	13.8
Platelet increase	1	2	0	0.6
Uremia	8	3	5	3.4
Venous thrombosis (deep)	1	2	2	1.1
Venous thrombosis (superficial)	13	5	2	4.3
Vomiting	19	5	0	5.2

ing a recently ruptured intracranial aneurysm is assumed to be an inhibition of this fibrinolytic mechanism. The use of antifibrinolytic therapy with recently ruptured intracranial aneurysm has been associated with favorable results upon recurrent rebleed rate and mortality prior to definitive surgery. This combined medical-surgical approach toward treatment of recently ruptured intracranial aneurysms was pursued in this study.

Several clinical characteristics of patients with SAH were related to mortality and rebleed rates during the 2-week treatment period. Female patients with an internal carotid aneurysm had the poorest survival. Most rebleeds occurred between the 6th and 11th days following the last bleed. On the average, the rebleed rate was higher among women than men and, therefore, increased mortality was reported among women, although the differences did not reach statistical significance. Patients in poor neurologic condition had a higher mortality than those in good condition because they had more pulmonary or genitourinary tract infections and were more likely to die from the direct cerebral effects of the original bleed. No significant difference in *rebleed* rate was seen between patients in good and poor neurologic conditions. Rebleed rate was unrelated to vasospasm, but mortality was higher among those with severe localized and diffuse vasospasm. Vasospasm neither promoted nor improved the rebleed rate, yet the biochemical and structural changes were responsible for the production of edematous and/or ischemic changes to such a degree that mortality was appreciably higher in patients with vasospasm.

Patients with mean blood pressure above 110 mm Hg at the onset of therapy had increased mortality and rebleed rates during the 14-day period compared with those below 110 mm Hg. Mortality was particularly low (3%) in the group with mean blood pressure below 90 mm Hg. A number of factors may be responsible for elevated blood pressure, including stress, pre-existing essential hypertension, degree of increased intracranial pressure, fluid balance, drugs, and the extent of infarction or size of the hematoma.

In a previous investigation conducted by the participants of the Cooperative Aneurysm Study, patients with SAH were randomly allocated to one of four treatment programs: regulated bed rest, drug-induced hypotension, carotid ligation and intracranial surgery. For patients allocated to regulated bed rest within 7 days following the last bleed,[13] both mortality and rebleed rates at 14 days were 20.9%. Rebleed rate was similar between each aneurysm site. Twenty percent of the patients with an internal carotid aneurysm rebled, 16.7% with a middle cerebral aneurysm, and 21.8% with an aneurysm on the anterior cerebral complex. Mortality at 14 days was highest for the internal carotid group (36%). Patients with a middle cerebral or anterior cerebral aneurysm had 16.7 and 17.2% mortality rates, respectively. Overall mortality and rebleed rates were significantly higher ($P < 0.05$) in those patients compared with the group described in this report who received antifibrinolytic therapy. In a similar group of patients treated by intracranial surgery within 14 days following the last bleed, 44.5% died following operation. In those who were allocated to drug-induced hypotension, 21.7% died and 16.9% had a proved rebleed within the 14-day interval. Therefore, comparison of these groups of patients with those who were treated with antifibrinolytic therapy during a 14-day period reveals that the latter group had the best survival and rebleed rates.

Considerable attention has been devoted to the complicating events which are said to be attributed to the use of antifibrinolytic agents. Arteriopathic changes as visualized by cerebral angiography (without histologic verification),[14] and segmental thrombosis of cerebral vessels,[15,16] have been said to result from antifibrinolytic therapy. An extensive review of potential complications associated with the use of epsilon-aminocaproic acid in non-neurologic disorders has been reported.[17] A detailed list of potential conditions on symptoms was monitored in this study while antifibrinolytic therapy was administered. The treatment protocols provided especially for this information. The most frequent drug-related condition reported was diarrhea in 24.3% of the patients. In only 2.4% was this complication severe. Hemiparesis was reported in 17% and hemiplegia in 11.2%. Particular attention was given to certain hematologic factors such as clotting derangements, bleeding time abnormalities, evaluation of certain coagulation factors and occurrence of pulmonary embolism. So-called clotting derangements were reported in 3 patients; 1 had an elevated partial thromboplastin time of 88 sec (with a control of 37), 1 patient had a prothrombin time of 8 sec (with a control of 12) and in the third patient no information was specified. Coagulation factor abnormalities were classified as minor in each of 2 patients. These were manifested in 1 patient as a mild gastrointestinal hemorrhage; the other had marked increase in serum fibrinogen and platelet count without clinical manifestations. Two patients developed pulmonary emboli. One was subclinical, i.e., the pathologic report described multiple small lung emboli, and in the other patient cardiorespiratory difficulties alerted the attending physician to this diagnosis. The condition was confirmed by a radioactive lung scan. Both of these patients were poorly responsive as a result of the intracranial event, and 1 was excessively obese as well. Among the 464 patients, these reports show clearly that the necessary risk in the administration of antifibrinolytic drugs was minimal in comparison to its therapeutic effectiveness.

Included in the protocols was a question relating to the overall clinical course during therapy with regard to whether the clinical condition of the patient improved, remained the same, or deteriorated. Comparison of improvement rates in overall clinical condition in the previous Phase III study[7] revealed that among patients who received antifibrinolytic medication alone, 45.9% improved, whereas of those who received antihypertensive agents alone, 30.4% improved, and in the group treated with antifibrinolytic therapy and antihypertensive

medication, only 23.8% improved. In the present study, 42.3% improved, 30.6% became worse and the remainder had no change in their condition during antifibrinolytic therapy. Although these data were basically judgment decisions made by the attending physicians, the information is useful and practical. Rather than using one specific measurement in stating whether or not a patient improves or deteriorates, in this evaluation the global perspective of each patient's clinical status was reviewed.

Patients who received epsilon-aminocaproic acid intravenously in a dosage of 36 g per day appeared to do better than those who received a lower or similar dosage by the oral route. Unpublished preliminary observations[18] reveal there is considerable variability in absorption rates and urinary excretion patterns following the administration of EACA by the oral route. This factor by itself may have considerable effect upon the amount of antifibrinolytic activity present in the serum at a particular time in any one patient.

Since the introduction of antifibrinolytic agents in patients with recently ruptured intracranial aneurysm, the dosage of epsilon-aminocaproic acid has been increased from 4 g every 4 hours orally to 36 g per day by the intravenous route. The best results are achieved when patients are treated with 36 g per day intravenously (preferably through administration of 18 g of EACA in 400 ml of 5% dextrose in water every 12 hr in a continuous intravenous drip). This approach should be used for 10 days followed by oral therapy in the form of 3 g every 2 hours. This dosage may be maintained until surgery is performed. When a surgical procedure is not performed, antifibrinolytic therapy can be continued until 21 days following the last bleed, when the dosage should be decreased gradually over the next week, by decreasing the daily amount to 24 g per day (2 g every 2 hr) for 3 days, followed by 1 g every 2 hours for 3 days, and then discontinued. In the author's experience (D.W.N.), this schedule has been the most effective manner of administration of EACA for patients with recently ruptured intracranial aneurysm.

References

1. Sahs, A.L., Perret, G.E., Locksley, H.B., et al.: Intracranial Aneurysms and Subarachnoid Hemorrhage: A Cooperative Study. J.B. Lippincott Co., Philadelphia, 1969.
2. McKissock, W., Paine, K.W.E., Walsh, L.: An analysis of the results of treatment of ruptured intracranial aneurysms; Report of 772 consecutive cases. J. Neurosurg 17:762–776, 1960.
3. Pool, J.: Bifrontal craniotomy for anterior communicating artery aneurysms. J Neurosurg 30:212–220, 1972.
4. Krayenbühl, H.A., Yasargil, M.G., Flamm, E.S., et al.: Microsurgical treatment of intracranial saccular aneurysms. J Neurosurg 37:678–685, 1972.
5. Graf, C., Nibbelink, D.W.: Cooperative study of intracranial aneurysms and subarachnoid hemorrhage. III. Intracranial surgery. Stroke 5:559–601, 1974.
6. Nibbelink, D.W., Sahs, A.L.: Antifibrinolytic therapy and drug-induced hypotension in treatment of ruptured intracranial aneurysms. (Preliminary report.) Trans Amer Neurol Assoc 97:145–147, 1972.
7. Nibbelink, D.W.: Cooperative aneurysm study: Antifibrinolytic therapy following subarachnoid hemorrhage from ruptured intracranial aneurysm. In: Whisnant, J.P., Sandok, B.A. (eds): Cerebral Vascular Diseases. Ninth Princeton Conference. Grune & Stratton, New York, 1975, pp 155–165.
8. Nibbelink, D.W.: Antifibrinolytic activity during administration of epsilon-aminocaproic acid. Stroke 2:555–558, 1971.
9. Geronemus, R., Herz, D.A., Shulman, K.: Streptokinase clot lysis time in patients with ruptured intracranial aneurysms. J Neurosurg 40:499–503, 1974.
10. Wu, K.K., Jacobsen, C.D., Hoak, J.C.: Plasminogen in normal and abnormal human cerebrospinal fluid. Arch Neurol 28:64–66, 1973.
11. Rabiner, S.F., Goldfine, I.D., Hart, A., et al.: Radioimmunoassay of human plasminogen and plasmin. J Lab Clin Med 74:265–273, 1969.
12. Nibbelink, D.W., Jacobsen, C.D.: Plasminogen depletion during administration of epsilon-aminocaproic acid. Thromb Diath Haemorrh (Stuttgart) 29:598–602, 1973.
13. Nibbelink, D.W., Henderson, W.G., Torner, J.C.: Cooperative aneurysm study: IV. Regulated bedrest. Stroke 8:202–218, 1977.
14. Sonntag, V.K.H., Stein, B.M.: Arteriopathic complications during treatment of subarachnoid hemorrhage with epsilon-aminocaproic acid. J Neurosurg 40:480–485, 1974.
15. Norlen, G., Thulin, C.A.: The use of antifibrinolytic substances in ruptured intracranial aneurysms. Neurochirurgia 12:100–102, 1969.
16. Mullan, S., Dawley, J.: Antifibrinolytic therapy for intracranial aneurysms. J Neurosurg 28:21–23, 1968.
17. Bergin, J.J.: The complications of therapy with epsilon-aminocaproic acid. Med Clin N Amer 50:1669–1678, 1966.
18. Nibbelink, D.W., SteginK, L.: Serum levels and urinary excretion rates of epsilon-aminocaproic acid following oral and intravenous administration. (Unpublished data.).

Chapter 15

Fluid Restriction in Combination with Antifibrinolytic Therapy

Donald W. Nibbelink, M.D., Ph.D., James C. Torner, M.S. and Leon F. Burmeister, Ph.D.

Abstract

From 1974 to 1977, 601 patients were randomized into three treatment categories: antifibrinolytic therapy with fluid restriction (FR), antifibrinolytic therapy without fluid restriction (NFR) and glycerol with fluid restriction (GFR). Seventy-five patients did not satisfy eligibility criteria. GFR patients suffered a higher than expected rebleed rate and patient entry was suspended after 16 months. Fourteen-day mortality for the 245 NFR patients was 10.6%; for the 266 FR patients it was 9.4%. Rebleed rates for the same time period were 8.2% for the NFR group and 9.4% for the FR patients. A significant change in neurologic status was demonstrated, with more improvement occurring in patients in the FR category. Analysis of average fluid balance suggests that lower fluid intake may be associated with a lower rate of death as related to progressive effects of the initial hemorrhage.

Introduction

Interest in the natural history and treatment of subarachnoid hemorrhage (SAH) led to the formation of the Cooperative Aneurysm Study (CAS) with a Central Registry at the University of Iowa in 1957. The first phase of this multicenter study was a collection of 6,368 patients who contributed data to the natural history of the disease.[1] The second phase was a randomized study among four treatments: regulated bed rest, drug-induced hypotension, carotid ligation and intracranial surgery. The results of this phase demonstrated a distressing mortality for those undergoing early surgery,[2] and the documentation of an unsatisfactory risk of rebleeding and death during nonsurgical therapy (Chapter 6). Based on results of antifibrinolytic therapy by Gibbs and O'Gorman,[3] Mullan and Dawley,[4] and Norlen and Thulin,[5] the CAS began a randomized study comparing antifibrinolytic therapy and drug-induced hypotension. That study demonstrated a marked reduction in mortality and rebleeding with antifibrinolytic therapy alone during the 2-week treatment period [6] The fourth phase of the CAS con-

307

tinued with antifibrinolytic therapy only, to evaluate drug dosage, complications of therapy and differential treatment effects.[7]

The basis for the randomized study with fluid restriction comes from the mortality observed between centers and the experience of Nibbelink, reported in 1974.[8] Observational findings of the fourth phase indicated that low daily antifibrinolytic dosages (≤ 24 g orally) and high fluid intake had higher mortality and rebleeding. The case series Nibbelink reported showed a 2-week mortality of 19% in 63 non-fluid-restricted patients and 0% in 44 fluid-restricted patients ($P < 0.01$). Rebleeding was also significantly lower in the fluid-restricted group (2.3 vs 15.9%).

A plausible mechanism for the observed benefits was the marked water loss (up to 1,000 ml per day) associated with improvement in neurologic status. Epsilon-aminocaproic acid (EACA) appeared to act not only as an antifibrinolytic agent but also as a diuretic. It was concluded that the improvement in neurologic state might be due to reduction in cerebral edema. Subsequently, a randomized treatment program of fluid restriction of 1,200 ml/day with 36 g/day of EACA (intravenously and/or orally) was proposed.

Methods

Study Design

In 1974, a randomized clinical trial was proposed comparing antifibrinolytic therapy without fluid restriction (NFR), antifibrinolytic therapy with fluid restriction (FR) and glycerol with fluid restriction (GFR). The latter category provided a control for the possible beneficial effect of anti-edema therapy in combination with antifibrinolytic agents. Eleven institutions agreed to participate; however, only 5 (Centers 5, 12, 19, 27, 38) agreed to randomize to glycerol therapy (Table 15–1). Patients who were admit-

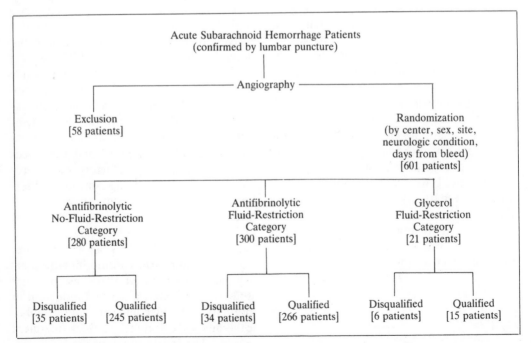

Fig. 15-1. Study Design.

Table 15–1. Antifibrinolytic-Fluid Restriction Program Participating Investigators and Centers.

Center Code	Investigators	Centers
05	Guy L. Odom, M.D. Wesley A. Cook, Jr., M.D.	Duke University Medical Center, Durham, North Carolina
12	Mark L. Dyken, M.D. Robert Campbell, M.D.	Indiana University Medical Center, Indianapolis, Indiana
19	Donald W. Nibbelink, M.D. Maurice Van Allen, M.D. Adolph L. Sahs, M.D. Andres Keichian, M.D. George E. Perret, M.D. Carl J. Graf, M.D. John VanGilder, M.D. Pasquala Cancilla, M.D. William Henderson, Ph.D. Leon Burmeister, Ph.D. James Torner, M.S.	University of Iowa Hospitals, Iowa City, Iowa
20	Lawrence S. Walsh, FRCS Alan E. Richardson, FRCS, MRCS David Uttley, FRCS, MB Ch B	Atkinson Morley's Hospital, London, England
26	Kenneth Shulman, M.D.	Albert Einstein College of Medicine, The Bronx, New York
27	Ladislau Steiner, M.D.	Karolinska Institute, Stockholm, Sweden
28	W. L. Elrick, FRCS, FRACS	Alfred Hospital, Prahran, Victoria, Australia
31	Edwin B. Boldrey, M.D.	University of California Medical Center, San Francisco, California
33	Orlando Andy, M.D. Robert R. Smith, M.D.	University of Mississippi, Jackson, Mississippi
37	John Riishede, M.D. Aage Harmsen, M.D.	University Hospital, Copenhagen, Denmark
38	S. Peerless, M.D., FRCS	University of British Columbia, Vancouver, British Columbia, Canada (discontinued August 1975)

ted within 7 days of the SAH from a ruptured intracranial aneurysm were eligible for randomization (Fig. 15–1). Patients with multiple aneurysms were also included. Randomization to the treatment program was carried out by sealed envelopes designated by center, aneurysm site, sex, neurologic condition and interval from bleed. The Central Registry registered all cases and maintained a check of the randomization procedures. Initial sample size estimates based on hypothesized outcome estimates of 5 and 20% mortality and a power of 90% suggested that a study size of 140 patients per group would be necessary. Periodic testing comparing 14-day mortality and rebleeding was carried out with decisions regarding continuation of treatment made by the participants based on statistical and ethical considerations.

Treatment Management

Antifibrinolytic therapy with EACA was recommended to be administered by continuous intravenous drip in a mixture of 18 g EACA in 400 ml of 5% dextrose in water every 12 hours. After 5 to 8 days of therapy, the dosage could be decreased to 24 g of EACA per day if the streptokinase clot lysis time was more than 24 hours. One participating institution (Center 20) used tranexamic acid (TA) in a dosage of 12 g/day given intravenously. Fluid restriction therapy consisted of a fluid intake of total intravenous and oral fluids not to exceed 1,200 ml per 24 hours. Diet without caffeinated or alcoholic beverages was recommended. This therapy usually produced a negative water balance of 300 to 500 ml per 24 hours within a few days with serum sodium, blood urea nitrogen and serum osmolality at the upper limits of normal. Fluid therapy was then to be adjusted such that fluid intake and output were equal. If fluid output was in such excess to cause dehydration, gradual fluid replenishment was suggested.

Non-fluid-restriction therapy was defined as a total of 2,000 ml of intravenous and oral fluids per 24 hours in addition to the patient's usual diet.

Glycerol and fluid restriction therapy consisted of fluid restriction with glycerol given orally in a dosage of 2 g/kg/day or intravenously at 0.3 g/kg in a 10% solution in divided doses.

On a daily basis, doses of antifibrinolytic medication, glycerol and fluid input and output were recorded. Supportive therapy included (1) maintenance of an adequate airway, (2) seizure prophylaxis, (3) daily nutrition of 1,000 calories per day, (4) sedation by phenobarbital or diazepam for restless-

Table 15–2.   Adequacy of Randomization—Overall Group.

Variable/Category	NFR No.	NFR %	FR No.	FR %	GFR* No.	GFR* %
Aneurysm site						
Internal carotid	60	(21.4)	69	(23.0)	7	(33.3)
Middle cerebral	40	(14.3)	38	(12.7)	2	(9.5)
Anterior cerebral-anterior communicating	92	(32.9)	96	(32.0)	5	(23.8)
Vertebral, basilar or posterior	23	(8.2)	24	(8.0)	1	(4.8)
Multiple	65	(23.2)	73	(24.3)	6	(28.6)
Sex						
Male	100	(35.7)	108	(36.0)	9	(42.9)
Female	180	(64.3)	192	(64.0)	12	(57.1)
Neurologic condition						
A or B	227	(81.1)	234	(78.0)	13	(61.9)
C or D	53	(18.9)	66	(22.0)	8	(38.1)
Interval to randomization						
0–3 days	143	(51.1)	145	(48.3)	13	(61.9)
4–7 +	137	(48.9)	155	(51.7)	8	(38.1)
Total	280	(100.0)	300	(100.0)	21	(100.0)

* Suspended after 13 months
+ Two cases were randomized in the 4 to 7 day category after 7 days post-bleed
NFR   Antifibrinolytic and no-fluid-restriction therapy
FR   Antifibrinolytic and fluid-restriction therapy
GFR   Glycerol and fluid-restriction therapy

Neurologic Condition:
A—alert, oriented and appropriately responsive; good clinical risk; no pre-existing serious medical disease; no neurologic deficit except for related cranial nerve signs; LP pressure of 250 mmH₂O or below; no evidence of spasm by arteriography; stable vital signs
B—minor symptoms (headache, meningeal irritation, diplopia, drowsiness) or major neurologic deficit such as hemiparesis or hemiplegia, but fully responsive upon arousal
C—impaired state of alertness but capable of protective or other adaptive responses to noxious stimuli, or poorly responsive but with stable vital signs
D—no response to address or shaking, nonadaptive response to noxious stimuli and instability of vital signs

ness, (5) proper urinary drainage and stool softening agents, (6) codeine or meperidine for severe pain, (7) appropriate antibiotics and (8) use of corticosteroids. No antihypertensive medication was allowed. Frequent observation of vital signs and neurologic status was recommended and was reported on the case report forms.

Clinical Material

Between July 1974 and March 1977, 601 patients entered the study. Patients were randomized into the GFR treatment group only until August 1975. The distribution of cases by aneurysm site, sex, neurologic condition and interval to randomization was uniform across the treatment categories (Table 15–2). Of the 601 patients, 22.6% (136) had internal carotid (IC) aneurysms, 13.3% (80) middle cerebral aneurysms (MC), 32.1% (193) anterior cerebral-anterior communicating aneurysms (AC), 8.0% (48) vertebral, basilar or posterior circulation aneurysms (VBP) and 24.0% (144) had multiple aneurysms

Table 15–3. Reasons for Disqualification from Comparative Analysis.

Reason	No.
Craniotomy performed prior to 12 days post-bleed	35
Incomplete treatment period information	15
Complicating medical conditions prior to treatment	5
Carotid ligation prior to 12 days post-bleed	3
No lumbar puncture	3
Conflicting therapy during treatment period	3
Complicating medical conditions requiring surgery	2
Discharged prior to the end of the treatment period	2
Randomized after 7 days post-bleed	2
MI after treatment started	1
No aneurysm found at autopsy	1
No aneurysm found at subsequent angiography	1
Uncooperative patient	1
Treatment started prior to randomization	1
Total	75

(MULT). Thirty-six percent of the patients were men, for a female to male ratio of 1.77:1. The majority of patients (78.9%, 474 of 601) entered in good neurologic condition and one half (301) entered within 3 days of the hemorrhage.

Of the 601 patients, 75 (12.5%) were disqualified from the comparative analysis. Reasons for disqualification are listed in Table 15–3. Fifty-one percent of those disqualified were considered suitable for early surgery and hence were removed from the study. Twenty percent had incomplete treatment information. Thirty-five disqualified cases were in the NFR group, 34 in the FR group and 6 in the GFR group.

The number of cases which satisfied the entry criteria was 245 in the NFR group, 266 in the FR group and 15 in the GFR treatment group. The number of cases admitted to each group by most participating centers was similar (Table 15–4). Center 20 contributed 34% of patients for analysis, Center 27 contributed 15% and the remaining 9 centers contributed 51%. Only 3 centers entered qualified patients to the GFR group.

Examination of the pretreatment randomization variables showed no disparity between treatments and no difference from the overall group. Patients with anterior cerebral-anterior communicating aneurysms comprised 33.7% of the cases, internal carotid aneurysms 22.7%, middle cerebral aneurysms 14.0%, vertebral-basilar-posterior aneurysms 7.8% and multiple aneurysm sites 24.6%. Sixty-five percent of the patients were female. Seventy-nine percent were in good neurologic condition (A and B), and 50% entered the study within 3 days of their hemorrhage.

Comparison of patient characteristics and clinical conditions not stratified in the randomization procedure also showed similarity between treatments (Tables 15–5 and 15–6). More cases were 60 years or older in the FR group, but no statistical difference in the distributions existed. Medical condition was not statistically different between the groups, although more poor-condition patients were included in the FR group. Pre-existing hy-

Table 15–4.   Distribution of Qualified Cases by Center.

| Center | Treatment Category | | | | | |
| | NFR | | FR | | GFR | |
	No.	%	No.	%	No.	%
05	11	(4.5)	10	(3.8)	0	
12	16	(6.5)	15	(5.6)	5	(33.3)
19	4	(1.6)	14	(5.3)	6	(40.0)
20	89	(36.3)	88	(33.1)	0	
26	12	(4.9)	17	(6.4)	0	
27	43	(17.6)	33	(12.4)	0	
28	24	(9.8)	31	(11.7)	0	
31	4	(1.6)	13	(4.9)	0	
33	15	(6.1)	13	(4.9)	0	
37	21	(8.6)	24	(9.0)	0	
38*	6	(2.4)	8	(3.0)	4	(26.7)
Total	245	(100.0)	266	(100.0)	15	(100.0)

* Ceased participation August 1975.

Table 15–5.   Distribution of Patient Characteristics and Conditions Not Included in Randomization for Qualifying Patients by Randomized Treatment Category.

| Variable/ Category | Treatment Category | | | | | |
| | NFR | | FR | | GFR | |
	No.	% of 245	No.	% of 266	No.	% of 15
Age						
<40 years	56	22.9	63	23.7	0	0.0
40–49	70	28.6	55	20.7	6	40.0
50–59	74	30.2	84	31.6	6	40.0
60+	45	18.4	64	24.1	3	20.0
Medical condition						
Good	118	48.2	131	49.2	9	60.0
Fair	110	44.9	113	42.5	3	20.0
Poor	17	6.9	22	8.3	3	20.0
Pre-existing hypertension						
Yes	55	22.4	75	28.2	2	13.3
No	164	66.9	172	64.7	10	66.7
Vasospasm at angiography						
Present	69	28.2	82	30.8	4	26.7
Absent	172	70.2	182	68.4	11	73.3
Size of aneurysm						
≤200 mm³	101	41.2	114	42.9	4	26.7
>200	123	50.2	134	50.4	7	46.7
Mean blood pressure						
≤110 mmHg	156	63.7	167	62.8	10	66.7
>110	89	36.3	98	36.8	5	33.3

Medical Condition:
   Good—alert, normotensive and good health prior to SAH
   Fair—patient with single underlying medical disorder such as hypertension, cirrhosis, anemia, atherosclerosis or pulmonary disease
   Poor—Patient with more than one adverse factor or one serious disorder
Mean Blood Pressure = 2/3 × diastolic + 1/3 × systolic
Note: Not all patients had information recorded for pre-existing hypertension, vasospasm, size of aneurysm and mean blood pressure.

Table 15–6.   Means and Standard Deviations of Patient Characteristics for Qualifying Patients by Randomized Treatment Category.

| | Treatment Category | | | | | |
| | NFR | | FR | | GFR | |
Variable	$\bar{x}$	SD	$\bar{x}$	SD	$\bar{x}$	SD
Age	48.2	12.1	49.1	12.8	53.7	9.7
Systolic BP	144.6	23.3	145.0	23.4	147.7	14.2
Diastolic BP	86.4	12.3	85.9	13.0	84.9	8.4
Mean BP	105.8	14.8	105.6	15.4	105.7	9.7
Size of aneurysm	724	2081	593	1185	540	788

pertension, presence of vasospasm, size of the aneurysm, and systolic, diastolic and mean blood pressures showed no statistically significant difference between randomized treatments.

Results

Primary outcome measures of 14-day post-bleed mortality and rebleeding were period-ically evaluated for the determination of statistical significance. Figures 15–2 and 15–3 demonstrate the differences in mortality and rebleeding between randomized treatment groups during the course of the study. The GFR randomization was terminated after 16 months of patient entry due to a high rebleed rate and low patient entry. Patient entry for the FR and NFR groups continued for a total of 33 months.

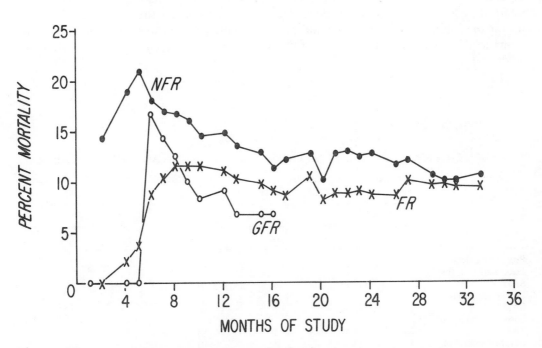

Fig. 15-2.   Cumulative 14-day mortality rates by months of study.

Mortality

Five months after initiating the study, the greatest difference between 14-day mortality for NFR and FR groups was observed (Fig. 15–2). Fifty NFR patients had a 20.9% mortality rate and 54 FR patients had a 3.7% mortality rate ($P = 0.02$). It was decided to continue the study for an additional month to assess the stability of these rates. By the 7th month the difference had diminished to 9.2%. Hence, the trial was continued. As the trial progressed, the difference between treatment groups became smaller. At the termination of the trial, mortality was 10.6% for the NFR patients and 9.4% for FR patients.

Examination of randomization variables demonstrated no statistical difference which would account for the time-related change in mortality. Analysis of medical condition, vasospasm status, blood pressure and dosage of antifibrinolytic drugs showed no imbalance with changes in mortality. Average daily fluid input during the treatment period was not found to be related to change in mortality. However, the average daily fluid input per group increased approximately 100 ml for the FR group and between 100 to 200 ml for the NFR group from the initial patients to the final patients admitted to the study.

No statistically significant differences in cause of death for the NFR and FR treatment categories were demonstrated. Progressive decline in clinical condition from the pre-study SAH occurred more in FR than NFR patients. Recurrent SAH occurred less often (Table 15–7). One patient each in the NFR group and in the FR group died within 14 days of infarction following the onset of vasospasm.

Recurrent SAH

Throughout the course of the study, proved rebleed rates (confirmed by lumbar puncture or postmortem examination) remained nearly the same between the NFR and FR groups (Fig. 15–3). At 30 months, the patient groups had equivalent rebleed rates; at the end of the study, NFR patients had an 8.2% rebleed rate and FR patients a 9.4% rate.

The distribution of time to rebleed for the NFR patients was uniform during the interval of 3 to 14 days (Table 15–8). FR patients, however, had the majority of rebleeds occur at the end of the first week (Table 15–8). The differences between NFR and FR groups in time of rebleeding were not statistically significant.

Table 15–7.   Cause of Death for Qualified Patients Who Died Within 14 Days After the Study-Qualifying SAH.

	Treatment Category					
	NFR		FR		GFR	
Cause	No.	(%)	No.	(%)	No.	(%)
Progressive decline associated with the SAH	12	(46.2)	14	(56.0)	0	
Proven recurrent SAH	12	(46.2)	9	(36.0)	1	(100.0)
Suspected recurrent SAH	1	(3.8)	1	(4.0)	0	
Cerebral infarction	1	(3.8)	1	(4.0)	0	
Total	26	(100.0)	25	(100.0)	1	(100.0)

Table 15–8.   14-Day Rebleed Events for Qualified Patients.

| Rebleed Status:* | Treatment Category | | | | |
| | NFR | | FR | | |
	Proved	Suspected	Proved	Suspected	Total
Totals	20	3	25	3	51
Days from SAH to rebleed					
0–2	1	1	0	0	2
3–5	4	1	4	0	9
6–8	5	1	13	1	20
9–11	6	0	5	2	13
12–14	4	0	3	0	7

* Proved: confirmed by lumbar puncture or postmortem examination.
  Suspected: clinically suggestive without confirmation.

Change in Clinical Condition

At the end of each patient's treatment period, the reporting investigators evaluated the overall clinical condition (medical and neurologic) in relation to the patient's status at the beginning of therapy. Of 245 NFR patients, 93 (38.0%) improved, 69 (28.2%) remained the same and 83 (33.9%) became worse. For the FR patients, 41.0% (109) improved, 27.8% (74) remained the same and 30.8% (82) worsened (1 patient did not have clinical condition recorded). These small differences were not statistically significant.

Change in Neurologic Status

At admission to the study and at the end of treatment, each patient was evaluated on the basis of neurologic function. The scale utilized for this assessment was the Cooperative

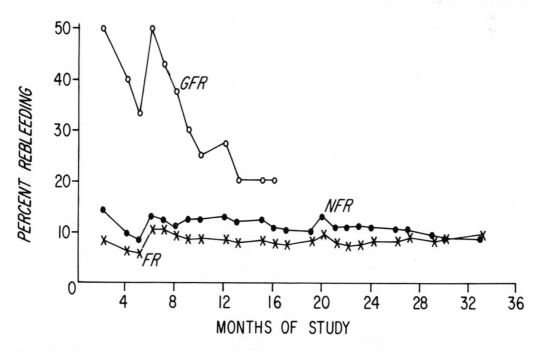

Fig. 15-3.   Cumulative 14-day rebleed rates by months of study.

Aneurysm Study Neurological Status Scale. Status 1 is defined as symptom-free. Status 2 includes minor symptoms (headache, diplopia, meningeal irritation). Status 3 represents major neurologic deficit but the patient is fully responsive. Status 4 records impaired state of alertness but the patient is capable of protective or other adaptive responses to noxious stimuli. Status 5 represents poor responsiveness but the patient has stable vital signs. Status 6 indicates no response to address or shaking, nonadaptive response to noxious stimuli and progressive instability of the vital signs. For assessment of neurologic outcome, Status 7 is death during the treatment period. The change in neurologic status represents the difference of the CAS Neurologic Status at the end of treatment and the CAS Neurologic Status at admission to the study. Hence, a negative score represents improvement, a zero score represents no change and a positive score represents decline in neurologic function. For patients in the NFR category, 15.5% improved, 46.9% remained stable and 37.1% declined in neurologic function (1 patient had incomplete information). For FR-category patients, 25.6% improved, 44.0% had no change and 30.4% became worse. The difference in neurologic function was statistically significant ($P = 0.017$). For patients surviving the 14-day period with complete information, FR patients exhibited statistically significant improvement compared to NFR patients ($P = 0.021$). For the 218 NFR patients, improvement was found in 17.4%, no change in 52.5% and decline in 29.7%. For the 241 FR patients, 28.2% improved, 47.7% remained the same and 24.1% worsened.

Table 15–9.   14-Day Mortality Rates for Randomization Variables for Each Randomized Treatment Group.

Randomization Variable	Treatment Group					
	NFR		FR		GFR	
Neurologic condition						
A–B	12/196	6.1%	10/207	4.8%	1/11	9.1%
C–D	14/49	28.6%	15/59	25.4%	0/4	0.0%
Interval to Randomization						
0–3 days	16/123	13.0%	17/126	13.5%	1/9	11.1%
4–7 days	10/122	8.2%	8/140	5.7%	0/6	0.0%
Sex						
Male	7/86	8.1%	6/97	6.2%	1/6	16.7%
Female	19/159	11.9%	19/169	11.2%	0/9	0.0%
Site						
IC	6/53	11.3%	6/60	10.0%	0/4	0.0%
MC	2/36	5.6%	2/35	5.7%	0/1	0.0%
AC	12/83	14.5%	8/86	9.3%	0/5	0.0%
VBP	1/20	5.0%	3/19	15.8%	0/1	0.0%
MULT	5/53	9.4%	6/66	9.1%	1/4	25.0%
Center						
5	0/11	0.0%	1/10	10.0%		
12	2/16	12.5%	1/15	6.7%	0/5	0.0%
19	0/4	0.0%	0/14	0.0%	0/6	0.0%
20	6/89	6.7%	5/88	5.7%		
26	1/12	8.3%	5/17	29.4%		
27	7/43	16.3%	6/33	18.2%		
28	4/24	16.7%	1/31	3.2%		
31	0/4	0.0%	2/13	15.4%		
33	2/15	13.3%	0/13	0.0%		
37	1/21	4.8%	4/24	16.7%		
38	3/6	50.0%	0/8	0.0%	1/4	25.0%

Analysis by Randomization Variables

Mortality at 14 days post-bleed was analyzed for each randomization variable category (Table 15–9). No significant differences were found between treatment groups. The largest differences were among patients with anterior communicating-anterior cerebral aneurysms (14.5% mortality rate for NFR vs 9.3% for FR) and vertebral-basilar-posterior aneurysms (5.0% mortality rate for NFR vs 15.8% for FR). Some differences within centers by treatment category were observed, particularly Centers 26, 28 and 38, but none of the differences was statistically significant.

Analysis of proved rebleeds also showed no subgroup differences to be statistically significant (Table 15–10). Patients with in-ternal carotid, vertebral-basilar-posterior, and multiple aneurysms did worse with FR therapy, while patients with middle cerebral and anterior communicating-anterior cerebral aneurysms did better. Small patient groups for each center produced considerable differences, with rebleeds occurring in one or two patients. None of the differences approached a level of statistical significance.

Comparison of change in clinical condition for each subgroup also showed no significant differences (Table 15–11). However, positive changes in clinical condition were observed for FR patients who entered the study 4 to 7 days post-bleed and those with middle cerebral aneurysms. Considerable center differences in outcome by treatment category were observed, especially Centers 28 and 37. Due to small patient numbers, none was statistically significant.

Table 15–10.   14-Day Rebleed Rates for Randomization Variables for Each Randomized Treatment Group.

Randomization Variable	Treatment Group					
	NFR		FR		GFR	
Neurologic condition						
A–B	11/196	5.6%	18/207	8.7%	2/11	18.2%
C–D	9/49	18.4%	7/59	11.9%	1/4	25.0%
Interval to randomization						
0–3 days	15/123	12.2%	16/126	12.7%	2/9	22.2%
4–7 days	5/122	4.1%	9/140	6.4%	1/6	16.7%
Sex						
Male	5/86	5.8%	6/97	6.2%	1/6	16.7%
Female	15/159	9.4%	19/169	11.2%	2/9	22.2%
Site						
IC	3/53	5.7%	6/60	10.0%	1/4	25.0%
MC	3/36	8.3%	1/35	2.9%	1/1	100.0%
AC	9/83	10.8%	7/86	8.1%	0/5	0.0%
VBP	2/20	10.0%	3/19	15.8%	0/1	0.0%
MULT	3/53	5.7%	8/66	12.1%	1/4	25.0%
Center						
5	2/11	18.2%	0/10	0.0%		
12	1/16	6.3%	1/15	6.7%	0/5	0.0%
19	0/4	0.0%	1/14	7.1%	1/6	16.7%
20	7/89	7.9%	7/88	8.0%		
26	1/12	8.3%	3/17	17.6%		
27	4/43	9.3%	5/33	15.2%		
28	2/24	8.3%	2/31	6.5%		
31	0/4	0.0%	2/13	15.4%		
33	0/15	0.0%	0/13	0.0%		
37	2/21	9.5%	2/24	8.3%		
38	1/6	16.7%	2/8	25.0%	2/4	50.0%

Table 15-11. Change in Clinical Condition for Randomization Variable for Each Randomized Treatment Group.

	Change in Clinical Condition											
	NFR Treatment Group						FR Treatment Group*					
	Improved		Same		Worse		Improved		Same		Worse	
Randomization Variable	No.	%	No.	%	No.	%	No.	%	No.	%	No.	%
Neurologic condition												
A-B	78	(39.8)	60	(30.6)	58	(29.6)	91	(44.2)	61	(29.6)	54	(26.2)
C-D	15	(30.6)	9	(18.4)	25	(51.0)	18	(30.5)	13	(22.0)	28	(47.5)
Interval to randomization												
0–3 days	47	(38.2)	33	(26.8)	43	(35.0)	51	(40.8)	24	(19.2)	50	(40.0)
4–7 days	46	(37.7)	36	(29.5)	40	(32.8)	58	(41.4)	50	(35.7)	32	(22.9)
Sex												
Male	37	(43.0)	23	(26.7)	26	(30.2)	40	(41.7)	27	(28.1)	29	(30.2)
Female	56	(35.2)	46	(28.9)	57	(35.8)	69	(40.8)	47	(27.8)	53	(31.4)
Site												
IC	22	(41.5)	13	(24.5)	18	(34.0)	32	(54.2)	10	(16.9)	17	(28.8)
MC	14	(38.9)	8	(22.2)	14	(38.9)	16	(45.7)	12	(34.3)	7	(20.0)
AC	28	(33.7)	23	(27.7)	32	(38.6)	29	(33.7)	26	(30.2)	31	(36.0)
VBP	8	(40.0)	8	(40.0)	4	(20.0)	9	(47.4)	5	(26.3)	5	(26.3)
MULT	21	(39.6)	17	(32.1)	15	(28.3)	23	(34.8)	21	(31.8)	22	(33.3)
Center												
5	1	(9.1)	6	(54.5)	4	(36.4)	2	(20.0)	4	(40.0)	4	(40.0)
12	3	(18.8)	7	(43.8)	6	(37.5)	6	(40.0)	4	(26.7)	5	(33.3)
19	2	(50.0)	2	(50.0)	0	(0.0)	6	(42.9)	6	(42.9)	2	(14.3)
20	30	(33.7)	35	(39.3)	24	(27.0)	36	(40.9)	35	(39.8)	17	(19.3)
26	5	(41.7)	0	(0.0)	7	(58.3)	6	(37.5)	1	(6.3)	9	(56.3)
27	23	(53.5)	3	(7.0)	17	(39.5)	16	(48.5)	1	(3.0)	16	(48.5)
28	12	(50.0)	4	(16.7)	8	(33.3)	11	(35.5)	12	(38.7)	8	(25.8)
31	2	(50.0)	2	(50.0)	0	(0.0)	6	(46.2)	3	(23.1)	4	(30.8)
33	6	(40.0)	3	(20.0)	6	(40.0)	7	(53.8)	4	(30.8)	2	(15.4)
37	8	(38.1)	7	(33.3)	6	(28.6)	11	(45.8)	2	(8.3)	11	(45.8)
38	1	(16.7)	0	(0.0)	5	(83.3)	2	(25.0)	2	(25.0)	4	(50.0)

* 1 incomplete observation.

Table 15-12. Change in Neurologic Status for Randomization Variables for Each Randomized Treatment Group.

	NFR Treatment Group						FR Treatment Group*					
	Improved		Same		Worse		Improved		Same		Worse	
Randomization Variable	No.	%	No.	%	No.	%	No.	%	No.	%	No.	%
Neurologic condition												
A-B	25	(12.8)	103	(52.6)	68	(34.7)	42	(20.3)	104	(50.2)	61	(29.5)
C-D	13	(26.5)	12	(24.5)	24	(49.0)	26	(44.1)	13	(22.0)	20	(33.9)
Interval to randomization												
0–3 days	18	(14.6)	55	(44.7)	50	(40.7)	27	(21.4)	49	(38.9)	50	(39.7)
4–7 days	20	(16.4)	60	(49.2)	42	(34.4)	41	(29.3)	68	(48.6)	31	(22.1)
Sex												
Male	9	(10.5)	47	(54.7)	30	(34.9)	23	(23.7)	48	(49.5)	26	(26.8)
Female	29	(18.2)	68	(42.8)	62	(39.0)	45	(26.6)	69	(40.8)	55	(32.5)
Site												
IC	9	(17.0)	23	(43.4)	21	(39.6)	21	(35.0)	25	(41.7)	14	(23.3)
MC	4	(11.1)	14	(38.9)	18	(50.0)	8	(22.9)	20	(57.1)	7	(20.0)
AC	11	(13.2)	37	(44.6)	35	(42.2)	17	(19.8)	35	(40.7)	34	(39.5)
VBP	1	(5.0)	14	(70.0)	5	(25.0)	5	(26.3)	10	(52.6)	4	(21.0)
MULT	13	(24.5)	27	(50.9)	13	(24.5)	17	(25.7)	27	(40.9)	22	(33.3)
Center												
5	2	(18.2)	5	(45.5)	4	(36.4)	1	(10.0)	5	(50.0)	4	(40.0)
12	3	(18.8)	6	(37.5)	7	(43.8)	6	(40.0)	3	(20.0)	6	(40.0)
19	3	(75.0)	1	(25.0)	0	(0.0)	6	(42.9)	5	(35.7)	3	(21.4)
20	17	(19.1)	43	(48.3)	29	(32.6)	25	(28.4)	44	(50.0)	19	(21.6)
26	0	(0.0)	2	(16.7)	10	(83.3)	4	(23.5)	3	(17.6)	10	(58.8)
27	2	(4.7)	26	(60.5)	15	(34.9)	1	(3.0)	21	(63.6)	11	(33.3)
28	4	(16.7)	11	(45.8)	9	(37.5)	8	(25.8)	15	(48.4)	8	(25.8)
31	1	(25.0)	1	(25.0)	2	(50.0)	2	(15.4)	8	(61.5)	3	(23.1)
33	2	(13.3)	7	(46.7)	6	(40.0)	5	(38.5)	4	(30.8)	4	(30.8)
37	3	(14.3)	12	(57.1)	6	(28.6)	9	(37.5)	6	(25.0)	9	(37.5)
38	1	(16.7)	1	(16.7)	4	(66.7)	1	(12.5)	3	(37.5)	4	(50.0)

Change in Neurologic Status

* 1 incomplete observation.

Change in neurologic status demonstrated larger differences than clinical condition for subgroups compared by treatment group. Statistically significant differences in the distribution of change in neurologic state were found in patients who entered the study 4 to 7 days after the bleed ($P = 0.017$) and in patients with middle cerebral aneurysms ($P = 0.027$) (Table 15–12). Close to significant results were found for males and for internal carotid aneurysms. Considerable center differences occurred, but only Center 37 had a distributional difference that was close to statistical significance.

Fluid Analyses

Total fluid intake and output were to be recorded for each patient from the date of entry into the study until 14 days post-hemorrhage. Notation of diarrhea, vomiting, fever, etc, was also included with the daily record, but quantitation of their contribution to fluid loss was most difficult; hence, fluid output on a daily basis was in some cases an underestimate.

Treatment Period Average Daily Fluid Input

Daily fluid inputs (IV and oral) from the day of randomization to the day of termination of the treatment program (rebleed, death or end of the treatment period) were averaged for determination of overall fluid balance. For patients randomized to fluid restriction, the mean of the average daily fluid input was 1,346 ml, with a standard deviation of 325 ml. NFR patients averaged 2,019 ml, with a standard deviation of 485 ml. The difference was statistically significant ($P < 0.001$). The distribution of average daily fluid input showed that 36.5% of the patients in the FR category had averaged less than 1,200 ml per day, 44.4% averaged between 1,200 and 1,499 ml per day and 18.4% had 1,500 ml or more per day (Fig. 15–4). Two patients had incomplete fluid information. In the NFR randomized patient group, 62% averaged fluid input of 1,800 ml or greater per day, 23.7% were between 1,799 and 1,500 ml and 10.6% had fluid input less than 1,500 ml per day. Nine patients in this group had insufficient information. In summary, 223 patients (44.6%) had average fluid input within the range of 1,200 to 1,800 ml, of which 65% were FR patients and 35% were NFR patients.

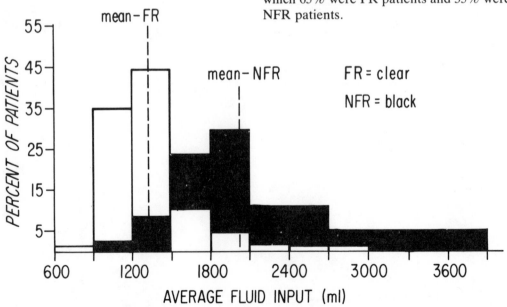

Fig. 15-4. Average daily fluid input for randomized treatment groups.

Randomization Variables

The distribution of average daily fluid input was examined to detect if variation in therapy occurred with regard to the randomization variables. For NFR and FR patients combined, a comparison of the means of fluid input demonstrated that patients who entered on days 4 to 7 averaged 1,602 ml and those who entered on days 0 to 3 averaged 1,728 ml ($P = 0.008$). Patients in Neurological Condition A-B averaged 1,643 ml and patients in Neurological Condition C-D averaged 1,744 ml fluid input ($P = 0.08$). Site of aneurysm and sex of the patient were not related to fluid input.

For NFR patients alone, the daily average level of fluid input was related to interval of entry. Patients entering in the first 3 days averaged 2,093 ml in the treatment period, while those patients entering the study in days 4 through 7 averaged 1,944 ml ($P = 0.02$). Condition C or D patients averaged 200 ml higher than Condition A or B patients, but the difference was not statistically significant. Aneurysm site and the patient's sex were not related to fluid therapy level. Center differences in average fluid input were statistically significant, and the range of fluid levels was from 1,462 to 2,589 ml, with a mean of 2,019 ml.

For FR patients, initial neurologic condition was related to average fluid input. Patients in Condition A-B averaged 1,317 ml fluid intake and patients in Condition C-D averaged 1,452 ml ($P = 0.005$). Time of entry into the study was also associated with fluid input. Early patients (days 0 to 3) averaged 1,386 ml per day, while later patients (days 4 to 7) averaged 1,310 ml per day ($P = 0.06$). Patients with anterior cerebral-anterior communicating aneurysms averaged higher fluid input (1,411 ml) than patients with aneurysms at the other sites; middle cerebral aneurysm patients averaged the lowest with 1,239 ml. The comparison of mean levels for the five site groups was not statistically significant ($P = 0.10$). Sex of the patient was not associated with fluid level. Considerable center variation in fluid levels was found in the average fluid input levels. The mean levels ranged from 1,217 to 1,640 ml, with an average of 1,346 ml for the entire FR group.

Mortality

Fourteen-day mortality for each randomized treatment category is contained in Table 15–13. For NFR patients, significantly higher mortality occurred in low fluid intake and in high fluid intake groups (2,100+ ml). For FR patients, significantly higher mortality occurred in high fluid intake groups only. Excluding the GFR patients, the overall 14-day mortality rates were 9.7% for patients with less than 1,200 ml, 8.0% for 1,200 to

Table 15–13. Mortality Rates by Average Daily Fluid Input and Randomized Treatment Category.

	Treatment Category							
	NFR		FR		GFR		Total	
Average Daily Fluid Input	P	%	P	%	P	%	P	%
<1200 ml	3/6	50.0	7/97	7.2	1/8	12.5	11/111	9.9
1200–1499	4/20	20.0	7/118	5.9	0/4	0.0	11/142	7.7
1500–1799	1/58	1.7	4/27	14.8	0/3	0.0	5/88	5.7
1800–2099	4/72	5.6	5/12	41.7			9/84	10.7
2100+	13/80	16.3	2/10	20.0			15/90	16.7
Total	25/236	10.6	25/264	9.5	1/15	6.7	51/515	9.9

11 cases without fluid data.
P = # of deaths/# at risk.

Table 15–14.   Cause of Death for Patients Who Died Within 14 Days by Average Daily Fluid Input and Randomized Treatment Category.

	NFR Treatment Category				FR Treatment Category				Total			
	PD*	PB	SB	OT	PD	PB	SB	OT	PD	PB	SB	OT
Average daily fluid input (ml)												
<1200	0	3			1	5		1	1	8		1
1200–1499	3	1			3	3	1		6	4	1	
1500–1799	1	0			3	1			4	1		
1800–2099	1	2		1	5	0			6	2		1
2100+	7	6			2	0			9	6		

* Cause of death: PD = progressive downhill course   SB = suspected rebleed
                           PB = proved rebleed   OT = other

1,499 ml intake, 5.9% for 1,500 to 1,799 ml, 10.7% for 1,800 to 2,099 ml, and 16.7% for 2,100 ml or more per day. In summary, the lowest 14-day mortality occurred in the 1,500 to 1,799 ml fluid intake category; the highest mortality observed in each treatment group occurred with average daily fluid input at the opposite level as proposed in the treatment protocol and in those patients exceeding 2,100 ml in both randomized treatment categories.

The distribution of cause of death by average fluid input demonstrated a statistically significant ($P = 0.046$) result (Table 15–14). Patients with low fluid intake had more deaths due to rebleeding than patients with higher fluid intake who died from a progressive downhill course. Examination by treatment category showed that this trend existed for the FR group but not the NFR group. For patients randomized to NFR and who received less than 1,500 ml of fluid, 3 died of progressive decline in clinical condition and 4 died of a proved rebleed. Of NFR patients who received ≥1,500 ml of fluid and died, 9 deaths were due to a progressive downhill course and 8 to a proved rebleed. For FR patients receiving <1,500 ml, 4 died due to a progressive decline and 8 due to rebleeding (excluding 1 death due to a suspected rebleed). For patients in the FR category who died after receiving an average of ≥1,500 ml, 10 deaths resulted from a progressive downhill course and 1 from a proved rebleed. Of note, 25% of the deaths

due to rebleeding in the NFR group occurred in patients who received less than 1,200 ml daily and 50% of those deaths due to progressive decline in the FR group occurred in patients receiving 1,800 ml or more per day.

Analysis of fluid input and cause of death was also performed, stratifying by initial neurologic condition. Table 15–15 shows that for Condition A-B patients, rebleeding was the major cause of death. Except for 6 deaths due to rebleeding in the <1,200 ml group, deaths from progressive decline and rebleeding were uniform across fluid groups. For Condition C-D patients, the major cause of death was progressive downhill course and was twice the rate of death due to rebleeding across fluid groups. In addition, mortality was lowest for patients given 1,500 to 1,799 ml fluids daily for both the A-B and C-D groups.

Rebleeding

The distribution of rebleed rates by average daily fluid input demonstrated a decline in the incidence of recurrent hemorrhage with larger levels of fluids. Overall, for NFR and FR groups combined, 14.6% of patients who received <1,200 ml per day during treatment rebled, 8.0% of those patients receiving 1,200 to 1,499 ml rebled, 7.1% of those patients receiving 1,500 to 1,799 ml rebled, 6.0% of those patients receiving 1,800 to

Table 15–15. Cause of Death for Patients Who Died Within 14 Days by Average Daily Fluid Input and Initial Neurologic Condition.

| Average daily fluid input (ml) | Neurologic Condition A–B* | | | | | Neurologic Condition C–D* | | | | |
| | Cause of Death‡ | | | | | Cause of Death‡ | | | | |
	PD	PB	SB	OT	Rate†	PD	PB	SB	OT	Rate†
<1200	0	6			7.4	1	2		1	18.2
1200–1499	2	2	1		4.3	4	2			27.3
1500–1799	2	1			4.2	2	0			14.3
1800–2099	2	1		1	6.4	4	1			23.8
2100+	2	2			6.1	7	4			45.8

* 403 patients were in Neurologic Condition A–B and 108 in Neurologic Condition C–D.
† = Percent mortality for all causes.
‡ = See Table 15–14 for definitions.

2,099 ml rebled and 7.8% of those patients who received 2,100 ml or more rebled. Examination of rebleed rates for the NFR group alone showed a similar trend of decreasing rates for increasing fluids (Table 15–16). The lowest rebleed rate occurred in patients who received 1,500 to 1,799 ml per day ($P < 0.01$). High rebleed rates characterized patients who were concurrently treated with fluids at levels opposite from that specified in the protocol for the NFR category. FR patients demonstrated their highest rebleed rates when fluid intake was less than 1,200 ml/day (12.4%). No rebleeding occurred in 22 patients who received more than 1,800 ml of fluids. The differences within the FR group were not statistically significant.

Analysis of 14-day rebleeding by sex distribution revealed that a 20.6% rate of re-

current hemorrhage occurred for female patients who received less than 1,200 ml (Table 15–17). For fluids less than 2,100 ml, females demonstrated greater rebleed rates than males. The rates for males were not significantly different between fluid groups. For

Table 15–17. Rebleed Rates by Average Daily Fluid Input by Sex of the Patient.

| Average Fluid Input | Male | | | Female | | |
	#Rebled/ #At Risk	%		#Rebled/ #At Risk	%	
<1200 ml	2/40	5.0		13/63	20.6	
1200–1499	2/43	4.7		9/95	9.5	
1500–1799	2/31	6.5		4/54	7.4	
1800–2099	1/29	3.4		4/55	7.3	
2100+	3/37	8.1		4/53	7.5	
Total	10/180	5.6		34/320	10.6	

Table 15–16. Rebleed Rates by Average Daily Fluid Input and Randomized Treatment Category.

| Average Daily Fluid Input | Treatment Category | | | | | | | |
| | NFR | | FR | | GFR | | Total | |
	P	%	P	%	P	%	P	%
<1200	3/6	50.0	12/97	12.4	1/8	12.5	16/111	14.4
1200–1499	2/20	10.0	9/118	7.6	1/4	25.0	12/142	8.5
1500–1799	3/58	5.2	3/27	11.1	1/3	33.3	7/88	8.0
1800–2099	5/72	6.9	0/12	0.0			5/84	6.0
2100+	7/80	8.8	0/10	0.0			7/90	7.8
Total	20/236	8.5	24/264	9.1	3/14	21.4	47/515	9.1

11 cases without fluid data.

Table 15–18.   Rebleed Rates by Average Daily Fluid Input by Interval to Randomization.

	Day of Randomization				
	0–3			4–7	
Average Fluid Input	#Rebled/ #At Risk	%		#Rebled/ #At Risk	%
<1200 ml	8/43	18.6		7/60	11.7
1200–1499	8/65	12.3		3/73	4.1
1500–1799	5/38	13.2		1/47	2.1
1800–2099	3/45	6.7		2/39	5.1
2100+	7/53	13.2		0/37	0.0
Total	31/244	12.7		13/256	5.1

Table 15–19.   Rebleed Rates by Average Daily Fluid Input by Neurologic Condition.

	Neurologic Condition				
	A–B			C–D	
Average Fluid Input	#Rebled/ #At Risk	%		#Rebled/ #At Risk	%
<1200	12/81	14.8		3/22	13.6
1200–1499	7/116	6.0		4/22	18.2
1500–1799	5/71	7.0		1/14	7.1
1800–2099	3/63	4.8		2/21	9.5
2100+	2/66	3.0		5/24	20.8
Total	29/397	7.3		15/103	14.6

females, the distribution in rebleeds approached statistical significance ($P = 0.07$).

Day of randomization in relation to the pre-study SAH also demonstrated differential rebleed rates. Patients who entered the study during days 0 to 3 had greater rebleed rates in every fluid group (Table 15–18). Rebleed rate differences were not statistically significant for fluid levels for those patients entering in the early period. For patients who entered the study during the 4 to 7-day period, the distribution of rebleeds was close to statistical significance ($P = 0.08$).

Patients who were in Neurologic Condition C or D prior to treatment had significantly greater rebleeding (14.6%) than patients in Condition A or B (7.3%). Analysis of average fluid intake demonstrated that although C-D patients had higher rebleed rates, the relationship was not consistent across all fluid groups (Table 15–19). For Condition C-D patients, fluid levels did not significantly affect rebleeding. For Condition A-B patients, however, a decreasing rebleed rate was found during higher fluid intake ($P = 0.05$).

In summary, rebleed rate was related to level of fluid input and the differential effect of fluids on rebleeding appeared to be greatest for: (1) female patients, (2) patients who entered 4 to 7 days post-SAH and (3) patients who were in Neurologic Condition A or B.

Change in Clinical Condition

For the 499 patients with complete observation of average fluid input and change in clinical condition at the end of the treatment period, 40% improved, 27% remained the

Table 15–20.   Average Fluid Input and Change in Clinical Condition.

	Change in Clinical Condition					
	Improved		Same		Worse	
Average Fluid Input	No.	%	No.	(%)	No.	(%)
<1200 ml	46	(45.1)	30	(29.4)	26	(25.5)
1200–1499	58	(42.0)	41	(29.7)	39	(28.3)
1500–1799	32	(37.6)	26	(30.6)	27	(31.8)
1800–2099	29	(34.5)	23	(27.4)	32	(38.1)
2100+	34	(37.8)	17	(18.9)	39	(43.3)
Total	199	(39.9)	137	(27.5)	163	(32.7)

Table 15–21. Average Fluid Input and Change in Neurologic Status.

Average Fluid Input (ml)	Change in Neurologic Status					
	Improved		Same		Worse	
	No.	%	No.	(%)	No.	(%)
<1200	27	(26.2)	49	(47.6)	27	(26.2)
1200–1499	31	(22.5)	67	(48.6)	40	(29.0)
1500–1799	21	(24.7)	35	(41.2)	29	(34.1)
1800–2099	17	(20.2)	35	(41.7)	32	(38.1)
2100+	9	(10.1)	39	(43.8)	41	(46.1)
Total	105	(21.0)	225	(45.1)	169	(33.9)

same and 33% became worse. The distribution of change in clinical condition between categorical fluid groups demonstrated a trend toward increased improvement with lower fluids and decline with higher fluids (Table 15–20).

Change in Neurologic Status

The difference in neurologic status between the start and the termination of the treatment period showed close to significant ($P = 0.055$) results for average fluid level (Table 15–21). Greatest improvement was demonstrated for lower fluid patients, while patients receiving higher fluids did worse. The worst outcome was found in patients with 2,100 ml or more average fluid input. Only 10% of these patients improved, 44% remained the same and 46% declined.

Analysis by initial neurologic condition (Table 15–22) showed that for patients initially in Neurologic Condition A–B, similar trends but smaller differences existed ($P = 0.49$). However, for Condition C–D patients, the differences in the distribution of change in neurologic status for fluid cate-

Table 15–22. Change in Neurologic Status for Levels of Average Fluid Input and Neurologic Condition.

Average Fluid Input (ml)	Neurologic Condition A–B					
	Change in Neurologic Status					
	Improved		Same		Worse	
	#	%	#	(%)	#	(%)
<1200	17	(21.0)	44	(54.3)	20	(24.7)
1200–1499	22	(19.0)	60	(51.7)	34	(29.3)
1500–1799	12	(16.9)	34	(47.9)	25	(35.2)
1800–2099	10	(15.9)	29	(46.0)	24	(38.1)
2100+	6	(9.2)	34	(52.3)	25	(38.5)
	Neurologic Condition C–D					
<1200	10	(45.5)	5	(22.7)	7	(31.8)
1200–1499	9	(40.9)	7	(31.8)	6	(27.3)
1500–1799	9	(64.3)	1	(7.1)	4	(28.6)
1800–2099	7	(33.3)	6	(28.6)	8	(38.1)
2100+	3	(12.5)	5	(20.8)	16	(66.7)

Table 15–23.   Distribution of Average Daily Fluid Input and Average Daily Fluid Balance.

Average Fluid Input	Average Fluid Balance (ml)							
	≤ −100		−99 to 100		101 to 500		>500	
	No.	(%)	No.	(%)	No.	(%)	No.	(%)
<1200 ml	22	(21)	23	(22)	54	(52)	4	(4)
1200–1499	26	(19)	51	(37)	53	(38)	8	(6)
1500–1799	7	(8)	14	(16)	39	(46)	25	(29)
1800–2099	2	(2)	9	(11)	35	(42)	38	(45)
+2100 ml	6	(7)	10	(11)	28	(31)	46	(51)
Total	63	(13)	107	(21)	209	(42)	121	(24)

gories were larger and significant (P = 0.04).

Fluid Water Balance

The average difference of fluid input and output was calculated as a measure of hydration of the patient over the treatment period. Thirty-four percent of the patients who received less than 1,200 ml fluid input had a negative or neutral fluid balance, while 56% of those receiving 1,200 to 1,499 ml had a fluid balance in the same range. For those patients who received over 1,500 ml fluid input, the average fluid balance was greater than 100 ml per day in 81% of the cases (Table 15–23).

Average fluid balance was not significantly related to mortality by 14 days (Table 15–24). Higher mortality (27%) was observed in the 11 patients that had averaged a negative water balance of over 500 ml. Rebleeding did show a significant relationship between fluid balance levels. Patients who had a negative water balance of 100 ml

Table 15–24.   14-Day Mortality and Rebleeding for Levels of Average Fluid Input and Water Balance.

	Mortality							
Average Water Balance (ml)	Average Fluid Input (ml)							
	≤1400		1401–1799		≥1800		Total	
≤ −500	2/8	(25%)	0/1	(0%)	1/2	(50%)	3/11	(27%)
−499 to −100	4/37	(11%)	1/9	(11%)	2/6	(33%)	7/52	(13%)
−99 to 100	3/60	(5%)	2/28	(7%)	6/19	(32%)	11/107	(10%)
101 to 500	7/88	(8%)	4/58	(7%)	6/63	(10%)	17/209	(8%)
> 500	2/9	(22%)	1/28	(4%)	9/84	(11%)	12/121	(10%)
Total	18/202	(9%)	8/124	(6%)	24/174	(14%)	50/500	(10%)
	Rebleeding							
Average Water Balance (ml)	Average Fluid Input (ml)							
	≥ 1400		1401–1799		≥ 1800		Total	
≤ −500	1/8	(13%)	0/1	(0%)	1/2	(50%)	2/11	(18%)
−499 to −100	11/37	(30%)	0/9	(0%)	1/6	(17%)	12/52	(23%)
−99 to 100	3/60	(5%)	3/28	(11%)	2/19	(11%)	8/107	(7%)
101 to 500	8/88	(9%)	4/58	(7%)	2/63	(3%)	14/209	(7%)
> 500	0/9	(0%)	4/28	(14%)	6/84	(7%)	10/121	(8%)
Total	23/202	(11%)	11/124	(9%)	12/174	(7%)	46/500	(9%)

Table 15–25. Treatment Period Change in Clinical Condition and Change in Neurologic Status for Levels of Average Fluid Input and Average Water Balance.

Average Water Balance	Average Fluid Input (ml)											
	≤ 1400			1401–1799			≥ 1800			Total		
	Change in Clinical Condition											
	I*	S	W	I	S	W	I	S	W	I	S	W
≤ − 500	4	2	2	1	0	0	1	0	1	6 (55%)	2 (18%)	3 (27%)
− 499 to − 100	11	10	16	4	2	3	2	0	4	17 (33%)	12 (23%)	23 (44%)
− 99 to 100	30	16	14	13	4	11	4	2	13	47 (44%)	22 (21%)	38 (36%)
101 to 500	41	32	15	17	18	23	27	16	20	85 (41%)	66 (32%)	58 (28%)
> 500	3	3	2	12	10	6	29	22	33	44 (37%)	35 (29%)	41 (34%)
Total	89 (44%)	63 (31%)	49 (24%)	47 (38%)	34 (27%)	43 (35%)	63 (36%)	40 (23%)	71 (41%)	199 (40%)	137 (27%)	163 (33%)
	Change in Neurologic Status											
≤ − 500	2	4	2	1	0	0	0	1	1	3 (27%)	5 (45%)	3 (27%)
− 499 to − 100	5	18	14	2	4	3	1	1	4	8 (15%)	23 (44%)	21 (40%)
− 99 to 100	19	27	14	7	12	9	3	3	12	29 (27%)	42 (40%)	35 (33%)
101 to 500	20	47	21	18	19	21	14	30	19	52 (25%)	96 (46%)	61 (29%)
> 500	3	3	3	2	17	9	8	39	37	13 (11%)	59 (49%)	49 (40%)
Total	49 (24%)	99 (49%)	54 (27%)	30 (24%)	52 (42%)	42 (34%)	26 (15%)	74 (43%)	73 (42%)	105 (21%)	225 (45%)	169 (34%)

* I = improved; S = remained the same; W = worsened

or more per day averaged a 22% rebleed rate, while patients with a neutral or positive balance suffered a 7% rate.

Change in clinical condition was not significantly affected by fluid balance levels (Table 15–25). However, change in neurologic status was significantly different for balance levels. Better outcome was observed in patients who maintained a fluid balance level in the ≤-500 ml and the -99 to +500 ml ranges.

Discussion

The purpose of this multiclinic study was to determine the therapeutic response of re-stricted fluid intake in patients with acute subarachnoid hemorrhage from ruptured intracranial aneurysm. The overall results show no clinical or statistically significant differences in mortality or rebleed rate between treatment groups. However, selected subgroups of patients experienced significant change in clinical response during the treatment period.

The lowest 14-day mortality occurred in patients with a daily fluid intake of 1,500 to 1,800 ml, whereas some of the highest mortalities were reported in patients with the lowest and highest amounts of daily fluid intake. For the fluid-restricted group, patients with low fluid intake had more deaths due to rebleeding than patients with high fluid intake. Patients in the latter group were more likely to die following a progressive decline in cerebral function. In the non-fluid-restricted group, the proportion of deaths between rebleeding and progressive downhill course remained nearly the same. For both treatment groups, good-condition patients had a high proportion of deaths due to rebleeding and poor-condition patients died from progressive downhill course. In both good and poor-condition patients, the mortality was lowest in the 1,500 to 1,800 ml daily fluid intake groups.

Noncompliance of fluid therapy (i.e., ≤1,400 ml in NFR and ≥1,800 in FR) was carried out in 22 FR and 14 NFR patients. Their clinical condition or abnormal laboratory results precluded continuation with the assigned randomized treatment. Reasons for noncompliance included severe vasospasm, fever and diarrhea, ischemic neurologic deficit, chronic renal disease, pretreatment electrolyte imbalance, elevated environmental temperature and poor hydration. Many of these conditions required special medical attention. An additional 124 patients who received 1,400 to 1,800 ml of average daily fluid intake in the NFR and FR treatment groups (67 and 57 patients, respectively) were also noncompliant to protocol specifications. The reasons for noncompliance cited above were also the reasons these patients were not given the designated fluid treatment. Therefore, a total of 163 patients (32% of 511) did not receive their treatment according to protocol.

The complications of fluid-restriction therapy depend on the amount of restriction carried out, degree of negative water balance and duration of therapy. The importance of closely supervised nursing care cannot be minimized. Most frequent adverse effects are dry mouth, thirst, superficial phlebothrombosis and elevated BUN and serum sodium value. When fluid restriction is allowed to continue beyond the level of a slightly elevated serum sodium determination and an approximate 10% rise in serum osmolarity occurs, the BUN will continue to rise, renal shut-down may occur, deep vein thrombosis develops and possibly

pulmonary embolism and/or pneumonia develop. Hypotension may appear under conditions of rapid diuresis or negative water balance, elevated body temperature from environmental factors or infection, or intractable diarrhea.

Realizing the complexity of fluid and electrolyte balance in brain-injured patients, detailed attention to patient care on a day-to-day basis is required for proper regulation of water balance and electrolyte concentrations. It became apparent during the study that body fluid metabolism and its monitoring requirements were greater than what most institutions were prepared to carry out in detail. The integration of all clinical laboratory parameters such as accurate intake and output, serum osmolarity, blood volume, body weight, serum sodium, blood urea nitrogen and hematocrit is required to maintain the optimum response to fluid-restriction therapy in subarachnoid hemorrhage. Under conditions of poor neurologic status, intracranial pressure monitoring, status of cerebral blood flow and blood volume are desirable. Such measurements were not available at most institutions at the time when this study was carried out.

Some patients not treated according to the protocol guidelines did worse than expected in both the NFR and FR treatment groups. From data supplied regarding the patients who died, it is apparent that an extremely high proportion of patients succumb with an edematous brain. The causes of brain edema in subarachnoid hemorrhage appear to be multiple, and it is clear that most patients with intracerebral and intraventricular hemorrhage do not respond to fluid-restriction therapy. When cerebral autonomic regulatory functions remain intact, such as in good-condition patients, this study shows that the overall clinical condition tends to improve.

The most favorable results in this study were obtained from good-condition patients who were maintained in approximately neutral fluid balance (-500 to 0 ml). In these patients, isometric concentration of intravascular volume and nearly normal serum osmolarity, serum sodium, and urea content were maintained. Fluid balance (intake minus output) remained slightly on the negative side, without regard to insensible loss. Therefore, it appears that modified fluid-restriction therapy is most applicable to selected patients where close monitoring practices are available. As additional data on fluid-restricted intake become available, and the dynamics of intravascular blood volume become more completely understood,[9,10] the preoperative treatment of ruptured intracranial aneurysms should reach a higher level of knowledge than was available during the period of this study.

Conclusions

1. Although early differences in mortality between antifibrinolytic therapy with fluid restriction and without fluid restriction were observed, at the end of 33 months of patient randomization and treatment the difference was 1.2% (10.6% for non-fluid restriction and 9.4% for fluid restriction).No statistically significant difference in the cause and/or rate of death at 14 days was found.
2. Rebleed rates at 14 days post-hemorrhage were similar for both randomized treatment groups during the course of the study. Fluid restriction with antifibrinolytic therapy had a 9.4% rebleed rate and non-fluid restriction with antifibrinolytic therapy had an 8.2% rebleed rate; a nonsignificant difference.
3. Due to a higher than expected rebleed rate in patients randomized and treated with glycerol and fluid restriction, patient entry was suspended after 16 months.
4. Change in clinical condition demon-strated little difference between randomized treatment groups during the 2-week study period.
5. Change in neurologic status was statistically significant at the 2-week interval, with 25.6% of fluid-restriction-with-antifibrinolytic-therapy patients improving and 44.0% remaining the same. In non-fluid-restriction patients, 15.5% improved and 46.9% remained stable.
6. Analysis by average fluid input per day indicated overlap of fluid levels between treatment groups. Average fluid level varied by time of entry, neurologic condition and reporting center. Mortality was less in the 1,500 to 1,800 ml fluid group, but no statistically significant relationship to fluid level was found. Cause of death, however, when analyzed by fluid level, indicated that more deaths due to proved rebleeding occurred at low fluid levels and more deaths due to progressive decline occurred at higher levels. Rebleed rates were observed to be higher at lower fluids also, but the rates were not statistically significant. A trend toward lower fluid level and improvement in clinical condition and neurologic status was observed, but only change in neurologic status was significant.

In summary, little improvement in overall 14-day mortality was found in this randomized study. The results suggest that lower fluids are associated with improvement in neurologic function and lower deaths due to progressive decline, presumably due to cerebral edema, but a greater rebleed rate may result. The difficulty in managing fluid intake by the cooperative group suggests that alternatives such as mannitol be studied with assessment measures such as serum osmolality, in an attempt to reduce death from cerebral edema without increasing the rate of recurrent hemorrhage.

References

1. Sahs, A.L., Perret, G.E., Locksley, H.B., et al.: Intracranial Aneurysms and Subarachnoid Hemorrhage: A Cooperative Study. J.B. Lippincott Co., Philadelphia, 1969.
2. Graf, C.J., Nibbelink, D.W.: Cooperative study of intracranial aneurysms and subarachnoid hemorrhage. III. Intracranial surgery. Stroke 5:559–601 (July-Aug), 1974.
3. Gibbs, J.R., O'Gorman, P.: Fibrinolysis in subarachnoid hemorrhage. Postgrad Med J 43:779–784, 1967.
4. Mullan, S., Dawley, J.: Antifibrinolytic therapy for intracranial aneurysms. J Neurosurg 28:21–23, 1968.
5. Norlen, G., Thulin, C.A.: The use of antifibrinolytic substances in ruptured intracranial aneurysms. Neurochirurgia 12:100–102, 1969.
6. Nibbelink, D.W.: Cooperative Aneurysm Study: Antifibrinolytic Therapy Following Subarachnoid Hemorrhage from Ruptured Intracranial Aneurysm. In Whisnant, J.P., Sandok, B.A., (eds): Cerebral Vascular Diseases. Ninth Princeth Conference. Grune & Stratton, New York, 1975, pp 155–165.
7. Nibbelink, D.W., Torner, J.C., Henderson, W.G.: Intracranial aneurysms and subarachnoid hemorrhage. A cooperative study. Antifibrinolytic therapy in recent onset subarachnoid hemorrhage. Stroke 6:622–629 (Nov.-Dec.), 1975.
8. Nibbelink, D.W.: The Role of Fluid Restriction in Treatment of Acute Subarachnoid Hemorrhage Following Ruptured Intracranial Aneurysms. Presented at American Academy of Neurology Annual Meeting, San Francisco, 1974.
9. Maroon, J.C., Nelson, P.B.: Hypovolemia in patients with subarachnoid hemorrhage: Therapeutic implications. Neurosurgery 4:223–225, 1979.
10. Shenkin, H.A., Pezier, H.S., Bouzarth, W.F.: Restricted fluid intake. Rational management of the neurosurgical patient. J Neurosurg 45:432–436, 1976.

Chapter 16

Antifibrinolytic Therapy in Patients With Aneurysmal Subarachnoid Hemorrhage

Harold P. Adams, Jr., M.D., Donald W. Nibbelink, M.D., Ph.D., James C. Torner, M.S. and A. L. Sahs, M.D.

Abstract

This paper includes a summary of 1,114 patients who had aneurysmal subarachnoid hemorrhage (SAH) and who were treated with antifibrinolytic therapy by the 13 institutions of the Cooperative Aneurysm Study. Patients were started on treatment within 1 week after the SAH occurred, and therapy was discontinued 14 days after the ictus. Rebleeding occurred in 10% of the treated patients. Overall mortality among the treated patients during the 2 weeks following hemorrhage was 10.7%. Although some minor and a few major side effects occurred, serious complications of therapy were infrequent.

Introduction

Unlike other forms of acute cerebrovascular disease, the frequency of subarachnoid hemorrhage (SAH) has not declined in the last decade. At the reported incidence of 11 per 100,000 population, at least 20,000 persons in the United States suffer aneurysmal SAH annually.[1] The actual number is probably higher by 6,000. During the first 2 weeks after SAH, patients die of the acute consequences of the hemorrhage, of cerebral vasospasm and infarction and of recurrent hemorrhage. Treatment of acute SAH must include amelioration of cerebral edema and increased intracranial pressure, correction of fluid and electrolyte level disturbances, avoidance of cerebral infarction and prevention of recurrent hemorrhage.

Among patients treated within 7 days of SAH with bed rest only, 22.6% suffered recurrent hemorrhage and 21.0% died within 2 weeks after the inital hemorrhage.[2] Among patients treated within 7 days of SAH with drug-induced hypotension, 18.0% had rebleeding and 22.6% died within 14 days after the initial hemorrhage. While reducing the frequency of rebleeding, hypotensive therapy does not reduce the early mortality from SAH. Vigorous blood pressure reduction tends to aggravate the development of cerebral ischemia, presumably by reducing the effective cerebral perfusion pressure. Past attempts to treat the aneurysm by an intracranial operation within 7 days of SAH were associated with a 20.9% mortality at 2 weeks after the initial SAH.[3] Because early operation has been associated with a high mortality and because bed rest and drug-induced hypotension have been complicated by frequently recurring hemorrhage, attention has been focused on the usefulness of antifibrinolytic therapy in the management of a patient within the first 2 weeks after SAH.

After rupture of the aneurysm, the rent in the sac is rapidly occluded by perianeurysmal clot, which helps prevent recurrent hemorrhage. The fibrinolytic activity of the cerebrospinal fluid (CSF) markedly increases during the first hours after the hemorrhage.[4] Blood in the CSF activates the conversion of plasminogen to plasmin, inducing lysis of the clot. Aminocaproic acid inhibits the conversion of plasminogen to plasmin and also affects the direct action of plasmin.[5] Tranexamic acid has an antifibrinolytic potency about 10 times that of aminocaproic acid. Both drugs cross the blood-brain barrier and thus presumably help to maintain the integrity of the perianeurysmal clot.[6] The goal of treating patients with aneurysmal SAH with antifibrinolytic agents is to preserve the naturally occurring clot in the aneurysm's rent, thus avoiding recurrent SAH while allowing the patient's condition to improve before operation on the aneurysm.

Patient Population

This review summarizes the clinical data from several studies carried out by 13 institutions of the Cooperative Aneurysm Study (CAS) on the effectiveness of antifibrinolytic therapy in patients with SAH. In the 7-year period from March 1970 to March 1977, 1,114 patients were treated with antifibrinolytic agents. The randomized clinical trial, which compared induced blood pressure reduction with antifibrinolytic therapy, was performed from the initiation of the study until July 1972 (132 patients), and was

reported in 1975.[7] Randomization was discontinued when the results among patients treated with antifibrinolytic agents were found to be statistically superior to drug-induced hypotension. From July 1972 to July 1974, a data collection study evaluated the therapy in regard to drug dosage, clinical condition and blood pressure (471 patients).[8] The final phase included antifibrinolytic therapy combined with randomized restriction of fluids (511 patients). The results of this trial demonstrated no significant difference between fluid groups.

Patients included in this analysis comprised 419 men and 695 women who suffered aneurysmal SAH within 7 days before entry into the study. The 3rd day after hemorrhage was the average point of admission to the study; 276 patients were admitted within the first 2 days, 362 on days 2 or 3, 298 on days 4 or 5 and 178 on days 6 or 7 post-SAH. The patients' ages ranged from 11 to 78 years, with a mean of 48 years. The aneurysm arose from the internal carotid artery in 241 patients, from the middle cerebral artery in 172, from the anterior cerebral artery in 383 and from the vertebrobasilar system in 76. Multiple aneurysms were discovered in 242 patients. Single hemorrhages occurred in 864 patients, while 212 patients were treated after a 2nd hemorrhage and 38 had 3 or more hemorrhages before antifibrinolytic therapy. On admission to the study, the neurologic status of the patients (according to the CAS grading scale[8]) was as follows: Grade 1, 26 patients; Grade 2, 733 patients; Grade 3, 94 patients; Grade 4, 197 patients; Grade 5, 52 patients; and Grade 6, 12 patients.

Treatment was begun after a ruptured aneurysm was confirmed by the presence of bloody CSF as determined by lumbar puncture and by roentgenographic demonstration of one or more aneurysms. Complete blood cell counts, fibrinogen levels and biochemical studies were obtained prior to and during the treatment period. Adjunctive therapies, such as fluid restriction, antihypertensive drugs, anticonvulsant drugs, anticerebral edema agents, sedatives and analgesics, were employed as needed. Epsilon-aminocaproic acid (EACA) was administered to 729 patients. The dosage varied, with most patients receiving between 24 and 36 g daily. Initial therapy was effected by a continuous intravenous (IV) infusion of EACA in 800 to 1,000 ml of 5% dextrose in water every 24 hours. After three to 10 days, if practical or possible, the drug was administered orally every 2 hours until the end of the 14-day interval after the hemorrhage. The dosage of EACA was to be monitored by the streptokinase clot lysis time.[9] Tranexamic acid was given to 385 patients. The dosage in most patients was 10.5 to 12 g daily. The drug was initially administered intravenously with conversion to the oral form to complete the treatment period. On the 14th day after the SAH, a decision was made to perform an operation or to continue medical therapy. Rebleeding, death (and its cause) and the development of neurologic or systemic complications during the first 14 days of the SAH were recorded. When rebleeding was suspected, confirmation was sought by CSF examination or at autopsy. Any complications requiring cessation of antifibrinolytic therapy were specifically noted.

Results of Treatment

Mortality

By the end of the 14-day interval following the SAH, 119 deaths had occurred (10.7% mortality) (Table 16–1). The mortality was similar throughout the 7 years of the data collection. In the period 1970 to 1972, the 2-week mortality was 9.8%; from 1972 to 1974, the mortality was 11.6%; and in the years 1974 to 1977, the mortality was 10.0%. Death from all causes was 12.1% (88/729) among those patients treated with EACA and 8.1% (31/385) in those given tranexamic acid. During the first 14 days after SAH, fatal rebleeding developed in 4.4% (17/385) of the patients treated with tranexamic acid and in 4.5% (33/729) of those given EACA. Another 11 deaths were from "suspected" new hemorrhages (Table 16–1). An additional 11 persons rebled in the initial 14 days after the SAH and subsequently died after the period of observation. The deaths of 50 patients were associated with a progressive decline in neurologic function following hospitalization. Gradual deterioration in level of consciousness or development of focal neurologic deficits were attributed to the effects of the initial hemorrhage, including intracerebral hematoma, vasospasm, hydrocephalus or cerebral edema. Thirty-four of these cases were examined at necropsy. Twenty-one persons died from an intracerebral hemorrhage in the frontal, parietal or temporal lobes. Eight patients died of cerebral edema as shown by flattened gyri, uncal grooving or tonsillar herniation. Five patients died with recent nonhemorrhagic infarctions in the distribution of a major artery; all but one had flattened gyri and uncal or tonsillar herniation. In the single patient without edema, the infarction extended

Table 16–1. Cause of Death (by 14 Days After Subarachnoid Hemorrhage) for Drug Used.

Cause of Death	Aminocaproic Acid	Tranexamic Acid	Total
Proved rebleeding	33 (4.5)*	17 (4.4)*	50 (4.5)*
Suspected rebleeding	8 (1.1)	3 (0.8)	11 (1.0)
Progressive downhill course	43 (5.9)	7 (1.8)	50 (4.5)
Complications of treatment	2 (0.3)	0 (0.0)	2 (0.2)
Other	2 (0.3)	4 (1.0)	6 (0.5)
Total	88 (12.1)	31 (8.1)	119 (10.7)

729 patients were treated with aminocaproic acid, 385 with tranexamic acid.
* Percent of patients at risk.

throughout the distribution of the anterior and middle cerebral arteries on one side of the brain. During the first 2 weeks after SAH, a fatal, progressive, downhill course developed in 1.8% (7/385) of the patients given tranexamic acid and in 5.9% (43/729) of those treated by EACA. Two patients (1 with a pulmonary embolus and the other with a cerebral infarction) died of complications attributed to EACA treatment. Three patients died of complications following arteriography, 1 of complications following severe gastrointestinal hemorrhage, and 1 from a pulmonary embolism that was believed not to be secondary to therapy, while the exact cause of the third patient's sudden death was not ascertained.

Recurrent Hemorrhage

In the initial 2 weeks, 111 patients had proven rebleeding (10% incidence). The rebleeding rate was 9.4% (36/385) among all patients given tranexamic acid and 10.2% among those administered EACA. Documented rebleeding developed in 4.5% of patients treated during 1970 to 1972, in 12.7% of those treated from 1972 to 1974 and in 8.8% of those treated from 1974 to 1977. In the years 1972 to 1974, the optimal dosage of antifibrinolytic therapy was being studied. Though the frequency of rebleeding was lowest in those patients treated with daily doses of approximately 36 g of EACA or 12 g of tranexamic acid, an optimal dosage has not been established.

Neurologic Status

Comparison of neurologic status at the beginning of treatment and at the end of the 14th day after the SAH showed that 17.8% of the patients initially in good neurologic condition improved, while 50.8% remained stable and 31.3% deteriorated or died (Table 16–2). However, 79.5% (677 patients) of those initially in good neurologic condition remained in CAS Grades 1, 2 or 3, and only

6.8% died. Of patients initially in poor condition, 37.7% improved to a better status, 25.8% were unchanged and 36.5% were worse or died. Improvement to a good neurologic condition by 14 days after the beginning of bleeding was noted in 33.1% of the patients initially in poor condition. The mortality among patients in poor condition was 23.5% by 14 days after SAH. The 14-day mortality of 6.8% among initially good-condition patients and of 23.5% for patients in poor condition was statistically significant ($X^2 = 56.09$, $P < 0.0001$).

Interval to Treatment

The number of days from the hemorrhage until onset of treatment was inversely related to the 14-day rebleed incidence and mortality (Table 16–3). Early entry posed a greater risk for rebleeding, independent of neurologic condition on admission ($X^2 = 19.13$, $P = 0.004$). Among those patients who did not die or suffer rebleeding within 7 days of SAH, rebleed rates in the day 8 to 14 interval were 8.3% for patients who entered on day 0 or 1, 6.5% for entry on day 2 or 3, 3.2% for entry on day 4 or 5 and 4.5% for entry on days 6 through 8 ($X^2 = 7.357$, $P = 0.061$).

Aneurysm Site

The location of the aneurysm did not significantly alter the outcome. Patients with internal carotid artery aneurysms (241) had a 12.9% rebleed rate and 11.6% mortality at 2 weeks; patients with middle cerebral artery aneurysms (172) had a 5.2% rebleed rate and 7% mortality; patients with anterior cerebral aneurysms (383) had an 11.0% rebleed rate and 12.3% mortality; patients with vertebrobasilar system aneurysms (76) had a 9.2% rebleed rate and 7.9% mortality; and patients with multiple aneurysms (242) had a 9.1% rebleed rate and 10.7% mortality.

Table 16–2.   Change in Neurologic Status from Onset of Treatment to 14 Days after Hemorrhage.

Initial Neurologic Status*	No. of patients	No. Improved	No. Unchanged	No. Worse	No. Deaths
Good condition (Grades 1–3)	852	152 (17.8%)	433 (50.8%)	267 (31.3%)‡	[58]
Poor condition (Grades 4–6)	260	98 (37.7%)	67 (25.8%)	95 (36.5%)‡	[61]
Total	1112†	250 (22.5%)	500 (45.0%)	362 (32.5%)‡	[119]

* Cooperative Aneurysm Study (CAS) Neurological Status Scale:
Grade 1—symptom-free.
Grade 2—minor symptoms (headache, meningeal irritation, diplopia).
Grade 3—major neurologic deficit but fully responsive.
Grade 4—impaired state of alertness but capable of protective or other adaptive responses to noxious stimuli.
Grade 5—poorly responsive but with stable vital signs.
Grade 6—no response to address or shaking, nonadaptive response to noxious stimuli, and progressive instability of the vital signs.
† There were 2 incomplete observations
‡ Includes deaths.

Medical and Neurologic Complications

Table 16–4 lists the symptoms and signs that appeared during the observation period. We were particularly interested to determine possible complications of antifibrinolytic therapy. Focal neurologic signs developed in 310 patients; in 206, the signs were believed to be of ischemic origin. The most common deficits were aphasia and hemiparesis. These signs were of similar frequency in patients treated with EACA or with tranexamic acid. Other neurologic conditions included restlessness, convulsions and psychiatric disturbances. Diarrhea was the most frequent side effect, and was a particular problem in those patients given oral tranexamic acid. An abnormal bleeding time, clotting derangement or coagulation factor disorder occurred in 21 patients. Deep vein thrombosis was noted in 12 patients, while 47 had superficial vein thrombosis (usually at the site of IV administration). Seven persons suffered pulmonary embolism.

Comment

Reports by Gibbs and O'Gorman[10] and by Mullan and Dawley[11] have drawn attention to the clinical usefulness of antifibrinolytic therapy in the preoperative management of

Table 16–3.   Interval from Last Hemorrhage to Treatment by Initial Clinical Condition and Outcome at 14 Days after Hemorrhage.

Interval from Last Hemorrhage until Treatment	No. of Patients	Mortality		Rebleeding Rate	
		Good Condition*	Poor Condition	Good Condition	Poor Condition
0–1 days	276	9.7%	30.0%	14.5%	21.1%
2–3 days	362	5.4%	23.5%	8.7%	15.3%
4–5 days	298	7.9%	20.9%	6.3%	11.6%
6–8 days	178	3.7%	11.9%	3.7%	4.8%
Total	1114	6.8%	23.5%	8.4%	15.0%

* See Table 16–2 for definition.

Table 16–4. Symptoms or Conditions Developing During Antifibrinolytic Therapy.

Symptom or Condition	Tranexamic Acid No.	%	Amino-caproic Acid No.	%	Total No.	%
Neurologic-Psychiatric						
Focal neurologic deficit*	103	(28.5)†	207	(33.4)	310	(31.6)
Convulsions	21	(5.7)	15	(2.4)	36	(3.6)
Psychiatric disturbances	43	(11.6)	56	(8.1)	99	(9.9)
Restlessness	52	(14.1)	104	(16.7)	156	(15.6)
Hematologic-Thrombotic						
Anemia	17	(4.6)	57	(9.1)	74	(7.4)
Coagulation factor disorder	0	(0.0)	5	(0.8)	5	(0.5)
Clotting derangement	1	(0.3)	9	(1.5)	10	(1.0)
Abnormal bleeding time	1	(0.3)	5	(0.8)	6	(0.6)
Leukocytosis	32	(8.7)	51	(8.3)	83	(8.3)
Purpura	0	(0.0)	2	(0.3)	2	(0.2)
Thrombocytopenia	1	(0.3)	6	(1.0)	7	(0.7)
Deep vein thrombosis	3	(0.8)	9	(1.4)	12	(1.2)
Superficial vein thrombosis	0	(0.0)	47	(7.5)	47	(4.7)
Pulmonary embolism	2	(0.5)	5	(0.8)	7	(0.7)
Gastrointestinal						
Diarrhea	210	(56.6)	64	(10.2)	274	(27.4)
Gastrointestinal hemorrhage	6	(1.6)	19	(3.0)	25	(2.5)
Nausea	88	(23.9)	48	(7.8)	136	(13.7)
Vomiting	44	(12.0)	39	(6.3)	83	(8.4)
Other						
Angina pectoris	1	(0.3)	5	(0.8)	6	(0.6)
Myocardial infarction	0	(0.0)	4	(0.6)	4	(0.4)
Conjunctival suffusion	2	(0.5)	3	(0.5)	5	(0.5)
Peripheral edema	1	(0.3)	16	(2.6)	17	(1.7)
Electrolyte imbalance	56	(15.3)	77	(12.4)	133	(13.3)
Genitourinary infection	21	(5.7)	94	(15.1)	115	(11.5)
Hyperuricemia	3	(0.8)	24	(4.0)	27	(2.8)
Elevated blood urea nitrogen	20	(5.4)	31	(5.0)	51	(5.1)
Rash	3	(0.8)	19	(3.0)	22	(2.2)

* Presence of at least one of the following conditions:
aphasia, dysphasia, hemiplegia, hemiparesis, ischemic neurologic deficit.
† Percent of patients observed for each symptom or condition.

patients with aneurysmal SAH. Gibbs and O'Gorman treated 32 patients with different doses of EACA for various treatment periods, noting 6 instances of rebleeding in comparison with 7 instances in 10 control patients. Ransohoff et al. gave oral or IV EACA to 85 patients for a period of 26 days or less and observed 6 instances of rebleeding.[12] Similar favorable results have been reported by Sengupta et al.,[13] Schisano,[14] Maurice-Williams[15] and Fodstad et al.[16]

Girvin compared 39 patients treated with EACA with 17 control patients, noting 14 instances of rebleeding (6 fatal) among treated patients and 4 deaths and 3 rebleeding events in the control patients.[17] While he did not mention the daily administered dosage of EACA, he concluded that the drug was of no therapeutic benefit. Van Rossum et al. compared 26 patients treated with tranexamic acid for 10 days with 25 other patients in a double-blind, randomized study.[18] They found similar rebleed rates and mortality in both groups. However, they evaluated patients with a variety of causes of SAH, including those with bleeding secondary to anticoagulant agents, and the dosage of tranexamic acid administered was only 4 g/day. Tovi randomized 21 patients treated with tranexamic acid with 19 control patients.[19] Both groups did well, and the only fatality was a control patient. Another randomized study compared 82 patients treated with standard supportive therapy with 83 patients treated with EACA; recurrent hemorrhage developed in 22 control and in 3 EACA-treated patients.[20] The randomized, double-blind study of Chandra also reported a lower mortality and rebleed rate in the patients treated with antifibrinolytic therapy.[21] In a critical review of antifibrinolytic therapy in subarachnoid hemorrhage caused by ruptured intracranial aneurysm, Ramirez-Lassepas[21a] concluded that the data failed to demonstrate the efficacy of this preparation.

In our series, recurrent hemorrhage occurred in 111 of the 1,114 patients treated with aminocaproic acid or tranexamic acid during the first 14-day period after the initial SAH. A 10% incidence of rebleeding in the first 2 weeks of the SAH is lower than the frequency of this complication in patients in the previously reported randomized studies who were treated with bed rest (22.6%)[2] or with drug-induced hypotension (18%). The recurrent hemorrhage was fatal in about half of our patients. Most clinical studies have not isolated those patients treated soon after the hemorrhage. In our series, rebleed rate and mortality were highest among those patients admitted within the first 3 days after the initial hemorrhage (Table 16–3). Selection by a difference in initially observed conditions and effect of change in neurologic status over time might explain this; however, these results reflect the critical nature of this illness in the first few days after the SAH and are similar to those reported by Ransohoff et al.[12] It is important that time of entry be considered in determining the prognosis of patients treated with antifibrinolytic therapy. Mortality was greatest in those patients with a poor initial neurologic condition.

We found that the most beneficial dosage of EACA was approximately 36 g/day. The other studies demonstrating the therapeutic benefit of EACA have used a daily dosage of 24 to 36 g.[12,13,20] The administered dose of EACA was not included in the report of Girvin.[17] The daily dosage of tranexamic acid of approximately 12 g produced the greatest protection. This dose is greater than the amount administered in other clinical studies. The optimal dose or duration of therapy has not been established. We concentrated on the initial 2 weeks after the hemorrhage, although others have extended therapy to 6 weeks.[15] Antifibrinolytic therapy was used in the CAS as a preoperative modality rather than as a substitute for operation.

Fifty of our patients died of complications following the initial hemorrhage, as manifested by a progressive neurologic decline attributed to the effects of an intracranial hematoma, vasospasm, cerebral ischemia or hydrocephalus. An equal number of patients in our series died from this group of disorders as died after rebleeding. The use of antifibrinolytic drugs will not prevent the death of such patients. Cerebral ischemia, vasospasm and hydrocephalus are known complications of aneurysmal SAH and have been the major reason for delaying operative repair of the aneurysm for 2 weeks after the initial hemorrhage.

Whether antifibrinolytic therapy potentiates the development of neurologic complications has been of concern. Using echoencephalography, Knibestöl et al. found ventricular dilation more frequently among patients given tranexamic acid than untreated patients.[22] Park recently reported ventricular enlargement in 17% of patients after SAH and in 43% of those also given antifibrinolytic medications.[23] In several other series, the authors did not find hydrocephalus to be more common in those patients receiving antifibrinolytic therapy than in control patients.[13,14,17] We did not specifically investigate the development of hydrocephalus in our patients.

The role of vasospasm in the development of cerebral ischemia has been controversial. Recently, Fisher et al. attributed 25 instances of new, ischemia-induced neurologic deficits to vasospasm among 50 patients with fresh aneurysmal SAH.[24] In an autopsy series performed prior to the use of antifibrinolytic agents, Schneck discovered cerebral infarction in 55% of the cases.[25] Kågström and Palma reported more frequent ischemia-

Chapter 17

Pathologic Review of Deaths in Patients with Antifibrinolytic Therapy

Pasquale A. Cancilla, M.D., James C. Torner, M.S. and Donald W. Nibbelink, M.D., Ph.D.

Abstract

1,098 patients were treated with epsilon-aminocaproic acid (EACA) or tranexamic acid (TXA) up to 14 days following subarachnoid hemorrhage from a ruptured aneurysm. Of the 367 patients who died during the one-year follow-up period, 188 had pathology data forms reported to the Central Registry. Seventy percent of the patients had a recently ruptured intracranial aneurysm. The overall mortality was 33%. The majority of aneurysms (67%) were between 6 and 15 mm in diameter. The site of rupture of the aneurysm sac was at the dome in 57%, at the body in 6%, at the neck in 2% and unidentified in 35% of the patients. The major locations of the hemorrhagic sequelae of aneurysm rupture were: subarachnoid only, 34%; subarachnoid, intraparenchymal and intraventricular, 21%; subarachnoid, intraparenchymal, 14%; and subarachnoid, intraventricular, 7%. Ischemic complications were found in 36% of the patients. The vascular supply to the ischemic areas followed major vascular distributions. The cause of death was intracranial in 78% of the pathology data forms. Of the extracranial causes of death, pulmonary emboli (10%) and bronchopneumonia (4%) were the major events.

Introduction

The antifibrinolytic agents, epsilon-aminocaproic acid (EACA) and tranexamic acid (TXA), inhibit the conversion of plasminogen to plasmin and directly affect the action of plasmin.[1] The use of these drugs could help to maintain the integrity of a perianeurysmal blood clot which develops after rupture of an aneurysm, thereby preventing a recurrence of the subarachnoid hemorrhage and its associated complications. The third phase of the Cooperative Aneurysm Program was designed to evaluate the effect on mortality and rebleeding of antifibrinolytic therapy given within 7 days of the onset of subarachnoid hemorrhage from a ruptured aneurysm.[2] A group of 1,098 patients received antifibrinolytic therapy.

As a part of this study, data forms were prepared on patients who died within a year

Table 17–1. Deaths, Autopsies and Data Forms Received for Antifibrinolytic Study.

Study Phase	Patients		Deaths*		Autopsies		Data Forms Registered	
	No.	(%)	No.	(%)	No.	(%)	No.	(%)
III–B†	116	(11)	41	(35)‡	28	(68)‡‡	26	(93)‡‡‡
IV	471	(43)	163	(35)	101	(62)	80	(79)
V	511	(47)	163	(32)	105	(64)	82	(78)
Total	1098	(100)	367	(33)	234	(64)	188	(80)

* 1-year follow-up

† Patients who received antifibrinolytic therapy; Phase III–A patients and patients treated with drug-induced hypotension are excluded

‡ Percent of patients   ‡‡ Percent of deaths   ‡‡‡ Percent of autopsies

of rupture of the aneurysm. There were 367 deaths, 234 autopsies and 188 pathology protocols registered. This report will analyze the neuropathologic and general postmortem findings described in the 188 data forms and will compare the data with those derived from pathology protocols in earlier phases of the aneurysm program.

Clinical Parameters

The clinical study of the effectiveness of antifibrinolytic therapy in patients with sub-arachnoid hemorrhage evolved in three stages between 1970 and 1977 (Table 17–1). The initial phase (III–B) compared patients treated with antifibrinolytic agents to patients with drug-induced hypotension.[3] This study was discontinued in favor of a study (Phase IV) evaluating drug dosage, clinical condition and blood pressure in a series of patients receiving antifibrinolytic therapy. The final stage (Phase V) compared patients receiving antifibrinolytic therapy in combination with randomized restriction of fluid.

In the three studies, 1,098 patients received antifibrinolytic therapy within 7 days of onset of subarachnoid hemorrhage. There

Table 17–2. Vital Data and Cause of Death.

	Study Phase			
	III–B	IV	V	Total
No. of patients	26	80	82	188
Sex				
Male	12	24	22	58 (31%)
Female	14	56	60	130 (69%)
Age				
Mean (years)	49.9	52	51.8	51.4
SD	11.3	12.4	11.6	12.4
Range	24–70	13–78	23–53	13–78
Days to death				
Mean	20.6	26.6	30.6	27.4
1–14	8	37	33	78 (42%)
15–30	11	25	22	58 (31%)
31–90	7	15	24	46 (24%)
91–365	0	3	3	6 (3%)
Cause of death				
Progressive decline	6	18	27	51 (27%)
Proved rebleed	9	35	35	79 (42%)
Suspected rebleed	1	6	5	12 (6%)
Treatment complication	0	0	7	7 (4%)
Complications other than treatment	4	16	3	23 (12%)
Other causes	6	5	5	16 (9%)

were 367 deaths (33%) during a 1-year follow-up period. Data forms from 188 patients were available in the Central Registry from the total group of 234 patients who had an autopsy examination. Table 17–2 shows the vital data and cause of death in the 188 patients. There were 58 men and 130 women. The mean age was 51.4 years, with a standard deviation of 12.4 years and a range of 13 to 78 years. The mean time to death was 27.4 days, with the following distribution: 1 to 14 days, 42%; 15 to 30 days, 31%; 31 to 90 days, 24%; and 91 to 365 days, 3%. The cause of death of these patients included: progressive decline, 27%; proved rebleed, 42%; suspected rebleed, 6%; treatment complication, 7%; complications other than treatment, 12%; and other unrelated disorders, 9%.

Morphologic Features

The anatomical location of the aneurysms (Table 17–3) revealed that aneurysms of the anterior cerebral-anterior communicating arteries were most common (46%), followed by internal carotid artery (23%), middle cerebral artery (18%) and posterior circulation arteries (including the posterior cerebral arteries) (13%). The size of the ruptured aneurysm was between 5 and 15 mm in greatest diameter in the majority (67%) of instances (Table 17–4). Ruptured aneurysms 5 mm or less in diameter were demonstrated in 21% of the patients, while aneurysms greater than 15 mm were found in only 3% of the patients. The size of the aneurysm was not

Table 17–4. Size of Ruptured Aneurysm at Postmortem in Patients Receiving Antifibrinolytic Therapy.

Maximal Size (mm)	No. (%)
< 5	39 (21)
5–15	126 (67)
> 15	6 (3)
Unknown	17 (9)
Total	188 (100)

known in 9%. The aneurysm had recently ruptured in 70% of the patients (Table 17–5). There was no evidence of recent rupture in 15% of the patients, and in an additional 15% the integrity of the aneurysm was not identified. The major site of rupture of the aneurysm was the dome (57%) (Table 17–6). The body was the location of the rupture in 6%, the neck in 2%; the site was unidentified in 35%.

Table 17–5. Integrity of Aneurysm at Postmortem in Patients Receiving Antifibrinolytic Therapy.

Integrity of Aneurysm	No. (%)
Recently ruptured	131 (70)
Not recently ruptured	29 (15)
Unknown	28 (15)
Total	188 (100)

Table 17–6. Site of Aneurysm Rupture in Patients Receiving Antifibrinolytic Therapy.

Site of Rupture	No. (%)
Dome	107 (57)
Body	12 (6)
Neck	4 (2)
Unknown	65 (35)
Total	188 (100)

Table 17–3. Location of Aneurysm in Patients Receiving Antifibrinolytic Therapy.

Location of Aneurysm	No. (%)
Internal carotid	44 (23)
Middle cerebral	33 (18)
Anterior cerebral-anterior communicating	86 (46)
Posterior circulation	25 (13)
Total	188 (100)

The major locations of the hemorrhagic sequelae of aneurysm rupture were subarachnoid only, 34%; subarachnoid, intraparenchymal and intraventricular, 21%; subarachnoid, intraparenchymal, 14%; and subarachnoid, intraventricular, 7% (Table 17–7). There was no evidence of recent hemorrhage in 7% of the autopsy examinations.

Table 17–7.   Distribution of Hemorrhagic Sequelae of Aneurysm Rupture in Patients Receiving Antifibrinolytic Therapy.

Location of Hemorrhage	No. (%)
Subarachnoid	64 (34)
Subarachnoid/intraparenchymal	27 (14)
Subarachnoid/intraparenchymal/ intraventricular	39 (21)
Subarachnoid/intraventricular	13 (7)
Subarachnoid/intraparenchymal/ intraventricular/subdural	5 (3)
Subarachnoid/subdural	4 (2)
Subarachnoid/intraparenchymal/subdural	6 (3)
Intraparenchymal/intraventricular	5 (3)
Subarachnoid/intraventricular/subdural	2 (1)
Intraparenchymal	2 (1)
Intraventricular	3 (2)
Subdural	1 (1)
No evidence of recent hemorrhage	13 (7)
Unknown	4 (2)
Total	188 (100)

Subarachnoid hemorrhage was identified 85% of the time and intraparenchymal hemorrhage was present in 45% of the cases. The dimensions of the intraparenchymal hemorrhage were available in 67 patients (Table 17–8). The mean dimensions were 4.4 cm anterior-posterior, 3.3 cm medial-lateral and 2.9 cm dorsal-ventral, with ranges of 1 to 12 cm, 1 to 10 cm and 1 to 6 cm, respectively.

Table 17–8.   Dimensions of Intraparenchymal Hemorrhage in 67 Patients Receiving Antifibrinolytic Therapy.

	Antero-Posterior (cm)	Medial-Lateral (cm)	Dorsal-Ventral (cm)
Mean	4.4	3.3	2.9
Range	1–12	1–10	1–6

The ischemic sequelae after aneurysm rupture are shown in Table 17–9. Recent infarcts of a pale or hemorrhagic type were present in 31% of the autopsy specimens. Recent pale infarcts (23%) were more common than recent hemorrhagic infarcts (8%). Old infarcts were present in 5% of the specimens. The vascular supply to the recent and

Table 17–9.   Ischemic Sequelae After Aneurysm Rupture.

Type of Ischemic Lesion	No. (%)
Recent pale infarct	43 (23)
Recent hemorrhagic infarct	15 (8)
Old infarct	9 (5)
No infarct	100 (53)
Unknown	21 (11)
Total	188 (100)

old ischemic lesion was: middle cerebral, 30%; anterior cerebral, 25%; anterior cerebral and middle cerebral, 13%; posterior cerebral, 8%; middle cerebral and posterior cerebral or vertebral-basilar, 6%; and vertebral-basilar alone, 3% (Table 17–10). In 7% of the cases, the ischemic lesions were diffuse; in 3% of the cases, the distribution of the lesions was not known.

The cause of death was primary intracranial in 78% of patients. There was an association with recent rupture of the aneurysm in 70% of the cases. A proved rebleed (42%) and progressive decline in the condition of the patient (27%) were the two major complicating situations. The cause of death in the extracranial (7%) and combined intracranial and extracranial groups (12%) was reported in 37 patients (20%). Pulmonary emboli were found in 18 (10%), followed by bronchopneumonia (3 patients, 2%), pulmonary edema (4 patients, 2%), arteriosclerosis (3 patients, 2%), a combination of pulmonary emboli and broncho-

Table 17–10.   Vascular Supply to Ischemic Lesion.

Vascular Distribution	No. (%)
Anterior cerebral	17 (25)
Middle cerebral	20 (30)
Posterior cerebral	8 (12)
Anterior cerebral/middle cerebral	9 (13)
Middle cerebral/posterior cerebral or vertebral basilar	4 (6)
Vertebral basilar	2 (3)
Diffuse	5 (7)
Unknown	2 (3)
Total	67 (100)

pneumonia (2 patients, 1%), and tubular nephritis, pneumothorax, progressive decline, carcinoma of lung, septicemia, bleeding duodenal ulcer and cardiopulmonary arrest (1 patient each). In 5 patients (3%), no cause of death was listed.

Discussion

The third phase of the Cooperative Aneurysm Program was designed to evaluate the effect on mortality and rebleeding of antifibrinolytic therapy given within 7 days of the onset of subarachnoid hemorrhage from aneurysmal rupture.[3] Adams et al. reported on the results of antifibrinolytic therapy in 1,114 patients treated at the collaborating institutions.[2] The patients were treated with either EACA or TXA within 1 week following subarachnoid hemorrhage and therapy was stopped 14 days after the ictus. Rebleeding occured in 10% of the treated patients. The overall mortality among treated patients during the 2-week interval following hemorrhage was 10.7%. These authors concluded that antifibrinolytic therapy was a useful mode of treatment in the preoperative management of patients with subarachnoid hemorrhage and that the treatment was not accompanied by frequent, severe neurologic or medical complications. The patients studied in our pathology data forms are derived from essentially the same group as those reported in the clinical studies by Adams et al.[2] For the pathology studies, we have chosen to compare the data in the protocol forms with those reported earlier for patients treated with regulated bed rest alone, since regulated bed rest patients have been considered the baseline group in other studies.[4] In both groups, there are adequate numbers of patients for valid comparisons.

When these comparisons are made, there are no essential differences in the following (bed rest/antifibrinolytic therapy): autopsy percentage (66/64); mean age of patients (49.4/51.4 yr); percent of autopsied patients who died within 30 days of onset of subarachnoid hemorrhage (67/73); size of aneurysm (5mm or less—21/21, 5 to 15 mm—65/67, 16 mm or greater—8/3 and unknown—6/9%); site of aneurysm rupture (dome—62/57, body—13/6, neck—8/2 and unknown—17/35%); and percent distribution of cause of death by location (intracranial—85/78, extracranial—4/7, combination of intracranial and extracranial—12/12 and unknown—0/3). Some differences were evident in an evaluation of the following (bed rest/antifibrinolytic therapy): percent of pathology data forms registered (70/80); percent of female patients in the study (50/69); integrity of aneurysm (recently ruptured—83/70, not recently ruptured—13/15 and no information—4/15%); overall mortality (55/33); percent with intracranial ischemic sequelae (46/36, with 11% unknown in the antifibrinolytic therapy group); and percent distribution of major extracranial causes of death (bronchopneumonia—8/4 and pulmonary emboli—4/10).

Are any of these differences due to the antifibrinolytic therapy? These studies were begun on the premise that antifibrinolytic therapy with EACA or TXA would reduce mortality and the rebleed rate by preventing the lysis of the perianeurysmal blood clot with its attendant complications.[1,2] Thus, the decrease in the overall mortality from 55% in the bed rest group to 33% in the patients receiving antifibrinolytic therapy is of interest. However, antifibrinolytic therapy was used only up to 14 days after onset of subarachnoid hemorrhage, and the death rate in the first 30 days after aneurysmal rupture was essentially the same in the two groups of patients (67% in the bed rest group and 73% in patients receiving antifibrinolytic therapy). The rebleed rate as indicated by the integrity of aneurysm in the pathology data forms was less in the group receiving antifibrinolytic therapy (70%) compared with the patients treated with bed rest alone (83%). Unfortunately, no data were known in 15% of the treated group. Thus, there may be no significant effect on rebleeding in the patients studied at autopsy. Since pathology data forms were available only in 51% of the patients who died in the antifibrinolytic therapy group, and since these patients represent only 17% of the entire treated group, the clinical data showing a 10% rebleed rate in the first 2 weeks after hemorrhage are probably more representative.[2]

One finding that warrants further evaluation, both clinically and at autopsy, is the presence of pulmonary emboli as a cause of death in 10% of the patients examined at autopsy from the antifibrinolytic group. Adams et al. described pulmonary emboli as a complication in 0.7% of all patients in the clinical studies of EACA and TXA.[2] However, Sahs, in his review of the history of the Cooperative Aneurysm Study, notes that some investigations have suggested that pulmonary emboli occur 2 to 3 times more frequently than expected when EACA is administered.[3] Our data would tend to support the latter view.

References

1. Nibbelink, D.W., and Jacobsen, D.D.: Plasminogen depletion during administration of epsilon-aminocaproic acid. Thrombos Diathes Haemorrh (Stuttgart) 29:598–602, 1973.
2. Adams, H.P., Nibbelink, D.W., Torner, J.C., and Sahs, A.L.: Antifibrinolytic therapy in patients with aneurysmal subarachnoid hemorrhage. In: Sahs, A.L., Nibbelink, D.W., Torner, J.C., et al.: Aneurysmal Subarachnoid Hemorrhage. Report of the Cooperative Study. Urban and Schwarzenberg, Baltimore, MD, 1981, pp 331–339.
3. Sahs, A.L.: History of the Cooperative Aneurysm Study and Central Registry. In: Sahs, A.L., Nibbelink, D.W., Torner, J.C., et al.: Aneurysmal Subarachnoid Hemorrhage. Report of the Cooperative Study. Urban and Schwarzenberg, Baltimore, MD, 1981, pp 3–16.
4. Cancilla, P.A., Torner, J.C., and Nibbelink, D.W.: Randomized Treatment Study. Pathologic results from patients who died in randomized study (Phase II). In: Sahs, A.L., Nibbelink, D.W., Torner, J.C., et al.: Aneurysmal Subarachnoid Hemorrhage. Report of the Cooperative Study. Urban and Schwarzenberg, Baltimore, MD, 1981, pp 277–284.

Section IV

Patients with Severe Neurologic Deficit

Chapter 18

Subarachnoid Hemorrhage: Patients with Severe Neurologic Deficit

John C. VanGilder, M.D. and James C. Torner, M.S.

Abstract

Sixty-three patients with a severe neurologic deficit were evaluated in a pilot study to assess the relationship of intracranial pressure (ICP) to neurologic condition and outcome. All patients were admitted to the study within 14 days of subarachnoid hemorrhage and had ICP measurements for at least 2 days. Seventy-seven percent of the patients had an ICP equal to or greater than 20 torr. Level of ICP was related to the neurologic condition of the patient. All patients with diffuse vasospasm had an elevated ICP ($\geq$ 20 torr). Treatments for elevated ICP included mannitol, controlled respiration, fluid restriction, cerebrospinal fluid drainage and surgical decompression. Fifty-eight percent of the patients with initially elevated ICP had a reduction of ICP to normal levels and suffered a 15% mortality by 28 days posthemorrhage. Patients with elevated ICP whose pressure remained elevated suffered a 58% mortality. No significant difference in overall mortality was found when compared to a historical control of nonmonitored patients. Computerized axial tomography results demonstrated a negative relationship of blood around the midbrain and ICP. The presence of an intraventricular hemorrhage and the presence of blood around the midbrain were related to 28-day mortality.

Introduction

The prognosis of subarachnoid hemorrhage secondary to ruptured intracranial aneurysm has been enhanced by increased knowledge of cerebral physiology, medical therapy and improved surgical technique. However, there remains a population of patients with a poor prognosis who have a severe neurologic deficit and decreased levels of consciousness following ruptured intracranial aneurysm. One day following the initial ictus, 44.7% of patients with subarachnoid hemorrhage attributed to ruptured intracranial aneurysms are seriously ill or moribund.[1] At the time of first angiography, 22.1% of these patients are responsive only to noxious stimuli or are unresponsive.[1] The natural history of this population at 1 year is a predicted survival rate of 25 to 29%. Surgical intervention in this population has been unrewarding. The mortality in patients with disturbance of consciousness but responding, unresponsive or moribund on the day of intracranial surgery for the treatment of recently ruptured intracranial aneurysms is 55.1%.[2] Delay of surgical intervention until patients achieve a good neurologic condition significantly decreases the operative mortality and morbidity,[2-4] but increases the risk of rebleeding.

The use of antifibrinolytic medication has significantly reduced the incidence of rebleeding during the initial 2 weeks following rupture of an intracranial aneurysm. The present 8.8% rebleed rate in patients starting epsilon-aminocaproic acid (EACA) treatment within 7 days compares to 22.6% in patients without EACA therapy (regulated bed rest).[5,6] Administration of EACA in patients in Condition C (impaired state of alertness but capable of protective or other adaptive responses to noxious stimuli, or poorly responsive but with stable vital signs) and patients in Condition D (no response to verbal stimulation or shaking, nonadaptive response to noxious stimuli, or progressive instability of vital signs) resulted in a mortality of 27.7% within the 2-week treatment period.[7] Sixty percent of this group succumbed to a progressive downhill course.

Several studies suggest that the majority of patients with significant neurologic deficit and altered levels of consciousness (Grade 3)[3,8] have associated increased intracranial pressure.[9-13] Increased intracranial pressure may be specifically the result of cerebral edema, hydrocephalus, intracerebral and intraventricular hemorrhage, infarction, increased intracerebral blood volume and/or a combination of these factors. The subsequent neurologic status and intracranial pressure measurements are determined by volume and site of extravasated blood, the vasomotor reaction and intracranial pressure compensatory buffering capacity. Cerebral blood flow, cerebral perfusion pressure, cerebral edema, cerebral metabolic rate of oxygen utilization and amount of PCO_2 accumulation are the prime factors requiring control for optimum neurologic function.

There is a large volume of literature elucidating the physiology of the nutrient supply to the brain with increased intracranial pressure.[14-16] In general, the concepts relate to a functioning cerebral autoregulation. With modest increase in intracranial pressure, there is a decrease in intracranial perfusion pressure. Cerebral blood flow remains constant while cerebral blood volume increases secondary to vasodilatation. With further increase in intracranial pressure or drop in perfusion pressure, the bounds of autoregulation are exceeded, with decrease in cerebral blood flow and subsequent development of ischemia.

As determined by cerebral angiography, the role of cerebral vasospasm and its contribution to the neurologic state following subarachnoid hemorrhage is subject to considerable controversy. Statistically and clinically, spasm may or may not be related to the frequency of neurologic complications.[17-20] More recent experimental studies suggest arterial spasm in the presence of increased intracranial pressure results in decreased blood flow in the involved vasculature with subsequent ischemia of brain.[21]

Provided that increased intracranial pressure is the most commonly present variable in Condition C and D patients following subarachnoid hemorrhage from ruptured intracranial aneurysms, reduction of increased intracranial pressure with presumed subsequent increase in perfusion pressure and blood flow should significantly reduce the mortality and morbidity in this patient population. Exclusive of operation for massive intracerebral hemorrhage, the three most effective therapies for increased intracranial pressure are osmotic diuretics, controlled ventilation and change in cerebrospinal fluid volume. Osmotic diuretics remove fluid from those parts of the central nervous system where the blood-brain barrier is intact. Controlled ventilation reduces intracranial blood volume secondary to vasoconstriction of intracranial vessels in the presence of intact autoregulation. Drainage of cerebrospinal fluid directly reduces intracranial volume. In addition, administration of corticosteroids and regulation of serum osmolality have proved to be effective adjunctive agents in the control of increased intracranial pressure.

The specific aims of this study were to determine if increased intracranial pressure was a common denominator in patients with poor neurologic condition (C and D) following a ruptured intracranial aneurysm. Does reduction of increased intracranial pressure lower the morbidity and mortality in poor-neurologic-condition patients following subarachnoid hemorrhage from a ruptured aneurysm when compared to present levels using EACA and dexamethasone as a standard? Is there a temporal relationship in patient prognosis associated with reduction of increased intracranial pressure? Is there a relationship of vasospasm to increased intracranial pressure, and is this combination a detriment to mortality? What is the relationship of computerized tomographic findings to presence or absence of increased intracranial pressure in Condition C and D patients?

Clinical Material

From May 1977 to October 1978, 63 patients were entered into the Cooperative Aneurysm Study from 10 participating institutions, with data forms submitted to the Central Registry for analysis. Patients admitted to the study were those with subarachnoid hemorrhage from ruptured intracranial aneurysm confirmed by lumbar puncture and cerebral angiography. An additional diagnostic study performed on each patient was computerized axial tomography. Only patients with a neurologic level of Condition C or D were acceptable. The Condition C patient is defined as having an impaired state of alertness but is capable of protective or other adaptive responses to noxious stimuli, or is poorly responsive but has stable vital signs. The Condition D patient has no response to address or shaking, a nonadaptive response to noxious stimuli and instability of vital signs.

Each patient had his or her intracranial pressure measured and subsequently monitored with a polygraph write-out of data for a permanent record. A measurement of 20 torr or above was selected to represent increased intracranial pressure. The intracranial pressure monitoring apparatus included an epidural or subarachnoid screw, intraventricular or lumbar subarachnoid catheter measurements, as preferred by the individual investigator. Each patient was included in the study for 14 days from commencement of therapy. In those patients with C or D condition having intracerebral pressure less than 20 torr intracranial pressure, monitoring was continued for no more than 2 days. Pressure determination was calculated as the average of the 4 highest intracranial pressure readings (torr) during a 4-hour period of each 24 hours. In those patients with intracranial pressure greater than 20 torr, monitoring was continued until the patient: (1) improved in neurologic state to A or B condition* and remained in the latter condition for 48 hours, (2) died or (3) showed no change in neurologic condition after 2 weeks of monitoring.

Condition A or B patients were excluded unless they deteriorated to Condition C or D, at which time they were entered into the study. The time of entry into the study was within the first 2 weeks following subarach-

---

*Condition A patients have the following characteristics:
  (1) Alert, oriented and appropriately responsive;
  (2) good clinical risk; no pre-existing serious medical disease
  (3) no neurologic deficit except for related cranial nerve signs;
  (4) lumbar puncture pressure of 250 mm H_2O or below;
  (5) no evidence of spasm by arteriography;
  (6) stable vital signs.

Condition B patients include those with:
  (1) Minor symptoms, e.g., headache, meningeal irritation, diplopia, drowsiness;
  (2) major neurologic deficit such as hemiparesis or hemiplegia, but fully responsive upon arousal.

noid hemorrhage. Patients with single or multiple intracranial aneurysms at all anatomical sites were eligible. Patients in good, fair or poor medical condition were included providing the necessary treatment for such conditions did not interfere with the treatment.*

Exclusive of those patients with massive intracerebral hemorrhage, which was surgically evacuated at the discretion of the surgeon, patients with intracranial pressure greater than 20 torr were treated to maintain the intracranial pressure less than 20 torr by the following therapies:

1. Mannitol (20% solution in Volutrol) administered as an initial dose between 0.75 and 1.5 g/kg intravenously as a bolus with subsequent administration up to 10 g every 2 hours contiguous upon the monitored intracranial pressure reading and serum osmolality.

2. Controlled or assisted ventilation as required. The patient was either sedated (morphine sulfate) or paralyzed, depending upon the ability to control respiratory cycling. The $PaCO_2$ was maintained between 20 and 30 mm Hg, measured every 12 hours and/or following change in ventilatory volume-rate ratios, or if indicated by electrolyte abnormality.

3. Drainage of cerebrospinal fluid either by ventricular or lumbar catheter.

4. The combination of any of the above techniques.

All patients received dexamethasone (20 to 60 mg/day) in divided doses, EACA (36 g/day) for a 14-day period and fluids bal-

---

* Patients in *good* medical condition were defined as those who were alert, normotensive, with no more than a degree of fever and in good health prior to subarachnoid hemorrhage. Patients in *fair* condition had a single underlying medical problem such as hypertension, cirrhosis of the liver, advanced age, anemia, poor nutrition, generalized atherosclerosis or chronic pulmonary disease. Patients in *poor* condition were those with more than one adverse factor or one medical condition which was particularly severe. *Prohibitive* condition was defined as patients with a complicated illness with one or more undesirable conditions.

anced to maintain a serum osmolality of 300 ± 10 mOs. Antihypertensive medication was administered as necessary when the diastolic arterial pressure exceeded 110 mm Hg. Antihypertensive medications included hydrochlorothiazide (100 mg/day), hydralazine (25 to 150 mg/day), methyldopa (500 to 1,000 g/day) or propranolol (titrated).

Results

Patient Characteristics

The distribution of the intracranial aneurysm locations was: internal carotid (37%), anterior cerebral-anterior communicating (23%), middle cerebral (14%), vertebral-basilar (10%) and multiple aneurysms (16%). Forty-three patients were female and 20 were male. The age of patients with subarachnoid hemorrhage was between 5 and 80 years, with a peak (25 patients) presenting with subarachnoid hemorrhage in the 5th decade. The distribution of aneurysm site, sex and age when subarachnoid hemorrhage occurred was consistent with previous observations.[22] Fifteen patients were in good medical condition at entry into the study, 37 in fair condition and 11 were in poor-prohibitive condition. The mean blood pressure (1/3 systolic plus 2/3 diastolic) at entry into the study was below 100 mm Hg in 30 patients (48% of 63). Vasospasm was present as demonstrated by angiography in 30 patients (48%). Eighteen patients had localized vasospasm (segmental or involving an individual vessel) and 12 had diffuse vasospasm (narrowed main ipsilateral vessels or all major vessels). Thirty-one patients had no evidence of vasospasm and 2 were of unknown status. Neurologic condition at the time of entry into the study included 49 patients in Condition C and 14 patients in Condition D. These can be further subdivided into neurologic state. Forty-five patients had impaired state of alertness, but were capable of protective or other adaptive responses to

Table 18–1.   Comparison of Intracranial Pressure Groups.

Neurologic* Condition	Normal ICP No. (% of 14)	Elevated ICP No. (% of 48)
C	13 (93)	36 (75)
D	1 (7)	12 (25)

* See p. 350.

noxious stimuli (Neurologic Status 4); 10 patients were poorly responsive, but with stable vital signs (Neurologic Status 5); and 8 patients had no response to address or shaking, nonadaptive response to noxious stimuli and progressive instability of vital signs (Neurologic Status 6; see Table 18–7).

Intracranial pressure measurements were reported in 62 patients. The first measurement was made during the first 3 days following initial subarachnoid hemorrhage in 33 patients, during days 4 to 7 in 18 patients, during days 8 to 11 in 10 patients and during day 14 in 1 patient. The average intracranial pressure (ICP) level for the first 2 days of measurement was equal to or greater than 20 torr in 48 patients (77% of 62) (Table 18–1). A test for the hypothesis that the percentage of C-D condition patients with increased intracranial pressure is equal to 50% of the population demonstrated a statistically significant level of $P < 0.0001$. Hence, a C-D condition patient is more likely to have elevated intracranial pressure than not.

Each of the aforementioned patient characteristics, including site of aneurysm, sex, age, medical condition, neurologic condition, neurologic status, mean blood pressure and interval from subarachnoid hemorrhage to entry into the study, was compared when these patients were subdivided into groups with normal and elevated intracranial pres-

sure. Chi-square tests for these variables demonstrated no statistical significance between these characteristics whether they had increased intracranial pressure or normal pressure. Although not statistically significant, observational differences that were found for the group with increased intracranial pressure included a predominance of patients with internal carotid aneurysm, more females, more Condition D patients, more Neurologic Status 6 patients and patients with mean blood pressure exceeding 110 mm Hg. The presence, absence and type of vasospasm demonstrated no statistical difference comparing patients with increased and normal intracranial pressure. However, patients with normal intracranial pressure usually had no vasospasm and all those with diffuse vasospasm had increased intracranial pressure. In contrast, the percentage of patients with local vasospasm showed no difference when one compared the two intracranial pressure groups (Table 18–2).

The distribution of intracranial pressure level was significantly different between Condition C and D patients. Eight percent of Condition D patients (1 of 13) had an intracranial pressure level under 20 torr on the 2nd day, 15% (2 of 13) were between 20 and 30 torr, 31% (4 of 13) were between 30 and 40 torr and 46% (6 of 13) were over 40 torr. In Condition C patients, 27% (13 of 49) had an intracranial pressure level under 20 torr, 45% (22 of 49) had a level between 20 and 30 torr, 14% (7 of 49) were between 30 and 40 torr and 14% (7 of 49) were over 40 torr. Hence, 73% of Condition C patients had an intracranial pressure level above 20 torr, whereas 92% of Condition D patients were included in the above 20 torr range. Only 14% of Condition C patients had ex-

Table 18–2.   Comparison of Intracranial Pressure Groups.

Vasospasm	Normal ICP No. (% of 14)	Elevated ICP No. (% of 48)	Significance (P value)
None	10 (72)	21 (44)	0.063
Local	3 (21)	14 (29)	
Diffuse	0 (0)	12 (25)	
Not reported	1 (7)	1 (2)	

Table 18–3. Interval to Normal ICP for Initially Elevated ICP Patients.

	Days from Study Entry* to Normal ICP						
	0–2	3–5	6–8	9–11	12–14	15–28	
Returned to Normal							
Condition C		9	10	2	2	0	$\bar{x}$ = 6.4 days
Condition D		2		1			$\bar{x}$ = 5.7 days
Total	0	11	10	3	2	0	$\bar{x}$ = 6.3 days

* 1st ICP measurement.

cessively increased intracranial pressure above 40 torr, as compared to 46% of Condition D patients.

Treatment

Therapies utilized for the reduction of elevated intracranial pressure consisted of the use of mannitol in 75% of patients, controlled respiration in 60%, fluid restriction in 48%, cerebrospinal fluid drainage in 38%, surgical decompression in 3% and all other therapies (glycerol, Lasix, low-molecular-weight Dextran, Nembutal) in 8%. Eight of the 14 patients with normal intracranial pressure also received one of the aforementioned treatments considered useful for reducing intracranial pressure.

Measurement of intracranial pressure during the treatment period as specified previously was performed in 45 patients who had elevated pressure levels on day 2 of measurement. Nineteen of the 45 patients (42%) remained at greater than 20 torr for the duration of their intracranial pressure monitoring. The average time until a normal intracranial pressure was achieved was 6.3 days in the 26 patients who had intracranial pressure reduction. Eleven patients (24% of 45) had their intracranial pressure reduced to normal between 3 and 5 days of intracranial pressure monitoring. Only 3 of 10 Condition D patients had a reduction in intracranial pressure to normal, while 23 of 35 (66%) Condition C patients were observed to have their intracranial pressure levels return to normal (Table 18–3).

Mortality

Mortality was assessed at 2 and 4 weeks following subarachnoid hemorrhage. A comparison of mortality rates between patients

Table 18–4. Number of Deaths and Mortality Rates for Patient Groups.

Neurologic Condition	Days from Bleed	Normal ICP	Elevated ICP	Total ICP Study	Antifibrinolytic Studies*
C	0–14	3 (25%) P = 0.049†	5 (14%)	8 (17%) X^2 = 0.565, P = 0.452	55 (23%)
	0–28	5 (42%) P = 0.049†	8 (22%)	13 (27%) X^2 = 0.673, P = 0.412	83 (34%)
D	0–14	0 (0%) P = 0.872†	8 (73%)	8 (62%) X^2 = 2.150, P = 0.143	10 (32%)
	0–28	1 (50%) P = 0.461†	8 (73%)	9 (69%) X^2 = 0.061, P = 0.805	22 (71%)
Total	0–14	3 (21%) P = 0.535†	13 (28%)	16 (26%) X^2 = 0.048, P = 0.827	65 (24%)
	0–28	6 (43%) P = 0.178†	16 (34%)	22 (36%) X^2 = 0.050, P = 0.824	105 (39%)

with normal intracranial pressure and those with elevated intracranial pressure revealed a lower mortality for Condition C patients at both the 2 and 4-week intervals in the elevated intracranial pressure group (Table 18–4).

In order to compare patients treated with fluid restriction, steroids and EACA, but without knowledge of intracranial pressure, the mortality was compared to those Condition C and D patients in Phases III to V of the Cooperative Study (Table 18–5).[5–7,20] This comparison demonstrated a lower mortality for Condition C patients in the increased intracranial pressure group. There was a higher mortality at 2 weeks in the Condition D patients with increased intracranial pressure, but no difference at 4 weeks. Comparison of the overall group showed very little difference.

The average interval to death in those patients with increased intracranial pressure was 6.5 days for those dying during the treatment period. For the 19 patients whose intracranial pressure remained elevated, the average time of death was 4.7 days, with 9 of 11 deaths occurring by day 6. The average time of death in those patients who had reduction of their intracranial pressure to less than 20 torr was 11.5 days, 2 of the 4 patients dying in the initial 2 weeks and the other 2 dying between days 14 and 28. In Condition C patients, the mortality was 9% for the 23 patients who had return of increased intracranial pressure to normal, in contrast to 42% (5 of 12 patients) in those with persistent intracranial pressure. Two of 3 Condition D patients died despite return of increased intracranial pressure to normal, and 6 of 7 with persistent increased intracranial pressure were dead by 28 days (Table 18–5).

When comparing the intracranial pressure level and mortality, the lowest mortality in the 2-week and 4-week period occurred in the patient group with an initial intracranial pressure level of 20 to 30 torr (5 of 24 patients, 21%). The highest mortality occurred in patients with intracranial pressure levels of 40 torr or more (7 of 12, 58%). For Condition C patients, mortality was significantly different in patients with various levels of increased intracranial pressure. Those patients with intracranial pressure between 20 and 29 torr and 30 to 39 torr ranges fared

Table 18–5.   Relationship of ICP Level and Outcome.

ICP level	Elevated ICP Group			
	Alive	Dead by 28 Days*	Total	% Dead
Remained elevated	8	11	19	58
Returned to normal	22	4	26	15
Total	30	15	45	33
	Elevated ICP Group—Condition C			
Remained elevated	7	5	12	42
Returned to normal	21	2	23	9
Total	28	7	35	20
	Elevated ICP Group—Condition D			
Remained elevated	1	6	7	86
Returned to normal	1	2	3	67
Total	2	8	10	80

* Post-SAH-ICP measure.

Table 18–6.   Relationship of ICP Level on Day 2 of Measurement and Mortality in the Treatment Period.

ICP Level	No. of Patients	Mortality Period			
		14 Days No.	(%)	28 Days No.	(%)
1–19	13*	3	(23)	5	(38)
20–29	24	3	(13)	5	(21)
30–39	11	4	(36)	4	(36)
40+	12*	6	(50)	7	(58)
		Condition C			
1–19	12*	3	(25)	5	(42)
20–29	22	2	(9)	4	(18)
30–39	7	0	(0)	0	(0)
40+	7	3	(43)	4	(57)
		Condition D			
1–19	1	0	(0)	0	(0)
20–29	2	1	(50)	1	(50)
30–39	4	4	(100)	4	(100)
40+	5*	3	(60)	3	(60)

* One patient in each group with incomplete follow-up.

better than those in Condition C levels in the 1 to 19 or over 40 torr range (Table 18–6).

Considerable loss to follow-up occurred in the 3-month and 1-year evaluation. Thirty-eight percent (24 patients) did not have 3-month status report completed. At 1 year, an additional 3 patients did not have a follow-up report completed. Several requests for follow-up information did not improve the completion rate. Of the 39 patients whose status was known at 3 months, 30 died (77%), 5 had major deficits on neurologic examination (Neurological Status 3—major

Table 18–7.   Neurologic Status at Follow-up.

Neurologic Status*	3-Month Follow-up						1-Year Follow-up					
	Normal ICP		Elevated ICP		Total		Normal ICP		Elevated ICP		Total	
	No.	%	No.	%	No.	%	No.	%	No.	%	No.	%
1	0		3	6	3	5	1	7	2	4	3	5
2	0		1	2	1	2	0		0		0	
3	3	20	2	4	5	8	0		2	4	2	3
4	0		0		0		0		0		0	
5	0		0		0		1	7	0		1	2
6	0		0		0		0		0		0	
No Information	5	33	19	40	24	38	6	40	21	44	27	43
Died Prior to Follow-up	7	47	23	48	30	48	7	47	23	48	30	48

* Neurologic Status:
1—Symptom free
2—minor symptoms (headache, meningeal irritation, diplopia)
3—major neurologic deficit but fully responsive
4—impaired state of alertness but capable of protective or adaptive responses to noxious stimuli
5—poorly responsive but with stable vital signs
6—no response to address or shaking, nonadaptive response to noxious stimuli and progressive instability of the vital signs

Table 18–8.   Vasospasm, ICP Group and 28-Day Mortality.

Vasospasm	Normal ICP	Elevated ICP	Total
None	4/10 (40%)*	8/21 (38%)	12/31 (39%)
Local	1/3 (33%)	6/13 (46%)	7/16 (44%)
Diffuse		1/12 (8%)	1/12 (8%)

* No. of deaths/no. of patients (% mortality).

neurologic deficit but fully responsive), 1 had minor symptoms and 3 were symptom-free. At 1 year, the only change observed was that 1 patient had deteriorated to a poorly responsive state (Table 18–7).

Disability status at the 3-month follow-up showed a similar result as neurologic status. Three patients had no related symptoms, 1 had annoying symptoms, and 1 was unable to perform the previous occupation but was able to work. Two patients were unable to work but cared for themselves, and 2 patients required nursing care. The 1-year follow-up showed no difference from the 3-month report.

Cause of death was progressive neurologic deterioration in 11 patients (50%), proven rebleed in 3 patients (14%), suspected rebleed in 1 patient (4%), complication of treatment in 3 patients (14%) and "other" in 4 patients (18%), for a total of 22 patients. The etiology of the deaths was not unlike that encountered in the antifibrinolytic studies.[5,6]

Vasospasm

No difference was observed between normal ICP and elevated ICP for 14-day or 28-day mortality in patients with no vasospasm or local vasospasm (Table 18–8). Only elevated ICP patients had diffuse vasospasm observed on the initial angiogram. This subgroup of patients had only 1 death in the 4-week treatment period. However, the low mortality in this group was not statistically significant from that of the "no vasospasm" and "local vasospasm" patients. For those patients with vasospasm, ICP and outcome in-

Table 18–9.   Treated ICP Level and Spasm Status.

	Elevated Group	
Vasospasm	Returned to Normal	Remained Elevated
None	11 (3)*	10 (5)
Local	5	7 (6)
Diffuse	10 (1)	2

* Deaths in parentheses.

formation, only 1 death in the treatment period occurred in patients with vasospasm (local and diffuse) who had their ICP level reduced (Table 18–9). Six of 7 patients with local vasospasm died while their ICP levels were elevated. There were no deaths in the 2 patients with diffuse vasospasm.

Computerized Axial Tomography Findings

Forty-eight patients had computerized axial tomography (CAT scan) performed as part of their initial diagnostic evaluation. The most common findings were: cerebral edema (42%), blood around the midbrain (40%), intracerebral hematoma (27%), enlarged lateral ventricles (27%) and midline displacement (21%) (Table 18–10). Observed differences in the number of patients with elevated ICP compared to those with normal ICP were found with the presence of an intracerebral hematoma, cerebral edema, an ischemic infarction, a midline displacement and blood around the midbrain. Only blood around the midbrain demonstrated a statistically significant difference ($P < 0.05$) of 75% of normal ICP patients and 32% of elevated ICP patients.

Table 18–10.   Comparison of CAT Scan Findings for the ICP Groups.

CAT Scan Findings	Normal ICP		Elevated ICP		Total	
	No.	(% of 8)	No.	(% of 40)	No.	(% of 48)
Intracerebral hematoma	1	(12)	12	(30)	13	(27)
Cerebral edema	1	(12)	19	(47)	20	(42)
Localized	0	(0)	12	(30)	12	(25)
Generalized	0	(0)	5	(12)	5	(10)
Unspecified	1	(12)	2	(5)	3	(6)
Intraventricular hemorrhage	2	(25)	6	(15)	8	(17)
Hemorrhagic infarction	0	(0)	2	(5)	2	(4)
Ischemic infarction	0	(0)	6	(15)	6	(12)
Midline displacement	0	(0)	10	(25)	10	(21)
Enlarged lateral ventricles	3	(37)	10	(25)	13	(27)
Blood in 4th ventricle	1	(12)	2	(5)	3	(6)
Blood around midbrain	6	(75)	13	(32)	19	(40)
Subdural hematoma	1	(12)	3	(7)	4	(8)

An observed relationship of mortality to CAT scan findings was found for the presence of intracerebral hematoma, cerebral edema, intraventricular hemorrhage, midline displacement, blood in the fourth ventricle, blood around the midbrain and subdural hematoma. The presence of an intraventricular hemorrhage and blood around the midbrain was significantly related to mortality in the 28-day period ($P < 0.05$). Seventy-five percent of patients with intraventricular hemorrhage and 63% of patients who had blood around the midbrain died in the 28-day period.

CAT scan findings were compared for patients with vasospasm demonstrated on the first post-subarachnoid hemorrhage angiogram (Table 18–11). Lower percentages of patients with local or diffuse vasospasm were observed when compared to patients with no vasospasm for findings of an intraventricular hemorrhage, enlarged lateral ventricles, blood in the fourth ventricle and blood around the midbrain area. Only the latter finding was statistically significant. Higher percentages for vasospasm patients were observed for cerebral edema and midline displacement, but neither was statistically significant. More

Table 18–11.   Presence of Vasospasm at First Angiography and CAT Scan Findings.

CAT Scan Finding	Vasospasm					
	None		Local		Diffuse	
	No.	(% of 25)	No.	(% of 13)	No.	(% of 10)
Intracerebral hematoma	6	(24)	4	(31)	3	(30)
Cerebral edema	9	(36)	7	(54)	4	(40)
Localized	4	(16)	5	(38)	3	(30)
Generalized	2	(8)	1	(8)	2	(20)
Intraventricular hemorrhage	7	(28)	1	(8)	0	(0)
Hemorrhagic infarction	0	(0)	1	(8)	1	(10)
Ischemic infarction	4	(16)	1	(8)	1	(10)
Midline displacement	2	(8)	5	(38)	3	(30)
Enlarged lateral ventricles	10	(40)	2	(15)	1	(10)
Blood in 4th ventricle	3	(12)	0	(0)	0	(0)
Blood around midbrain	17	(68)	2	(15)	0	(0)
Subdural hematoma	1	(4)	1	(8)	2	(20)

Condition D patients were observed in the study to have an intracerebral hematoma, intraventricular hemorrhage and blood around the midbrain (Table 18–12). Lower percentages of CAT scan findings of cerebral edema and subdural hematoma were observed for the Condition D patients. Only for blood in the midbrain area was there a statistically significant difference between levels of neurologic condition.

Complications of ICP Measurements

During the 2-week monitoring period, 5 infections were reported. Three patients developed meningitis, 1 developed a wound infection and 1 had an unspecified infection. Two of the 5 patients died, 1 at 11 days following a progressive downhill course and 1 at 56 days with pneumonia and septicemia. Both patients were Condition D at the time of entry into the study.

Discussion

Although the total number of patients in this study is small, it is representative of a certain population of subarachnoid hemorrhage sec-

ondary to ruptured intracranial aneurysms in reference to location of aneurysms, age and sex distribution.[22] The majority of patients were in good or fair general medical condition, an observation which suggests that any possible underlying systemic pathology had little influence in the prognosis of the more important primary intracranial pathology.

The majority of patients (77%) had associated increased intracranial pressure greater than 20 torr. Increased intracranial pressure was a more common finding than either diffuse or local angiographic vasospasm, a condition which was present in 48% of the population studied. Abnormalities demonstrated by computerized tomography in Condition C and D patients included cerebral edema, hemorrhagic and ischemic infarction, and intracerebral, intraventricular and subdural hemorrhage, either alone or in combination. There were no patient characteristics or specific findings on computerized tomography to predict which patient would or would not have increased intracranial pressure. However, those patients in Condition D were more likely to have increased pressure than those in Condition C.

The 28-day mortality in Condition C patients was less than that for patients with Condition D. However, there was no significant difference in mortality when com-

Table 18–12. Neurologic Condition at Admission and CAT Scan Findings.

CAT Scan Finding	Neurologic Condition			
	C		D	
	No.	(% of 37)	No.	(% of 11)
Interacerebral hematoma	9	(24)	4	(36)
Cerebral edema	16	(43)	4	(36)
Localized	11	(30)	1	(9)
Generalized	4	(11)	1	(9)
Intraventricular hemorrhage	4	(11)	4	(36)
Hemorrhagic infarction	2	(5)	2	(18)
Midline displacement	7	(19)	3	(27)
Enlarged lateral ventricles	9	(24)	4	(36)
Blood in 4th ventricle	2	(5)	1	(9)
Blood around midbrain	11	(30)	8	(73)
Subdural hematoma	4	(11)	0	(0)
Ischemic infarction	4	(11)	2	(18)

paring those patients with and without increased intracranial pressure in the two groups. Examination of the pressure distribution curve demonstrated a trend for those Condition D patients to have higher intracranial pressure levels than those in Condition C. In general, survival in patients with pressures between 20 to 40 torr was better than in those with intracranial pressure greater than 40 torr. The overall mortality in this study was no different when compared to previous studies which excluded monitoring of intracranial pressure.[5-7,20].

The records of those patients with increased intracranial pressure were examined further to determine the response to treatment. In those 26 patients with increased pressure returning to normal levels (less than 20 torr), 21 (81%) had pressure reduced within 8 days following entry into the study. In Condition C patients, the 28-day mortality was 9% in those cases who responded to treatment as shown by return of pressure to normal, in contrast to a 42% mortality in those identically graded patients who had no elevated pressure. Analysis of Condition D patients, comparing the aforementioned parameters, showed no difference in mortality. Thus, a population of 23 of 63 patients (37%) was identified in neurologic Condition C with increased intracranial pressure which had a better prognosis using the treatment parameters outlined in this study.

Although all patients with diffuse vasospasm demonstrated increased intracranial pressure, the presence or absence of vasospasm showed no statistical significance when correlated with normal or increased intracranial pressure in the small number of patients available. Similarly, of the 26 patients with increased intracranial pressure whose pressure readings returned to normal following treatment, there was no correlation with the presence or absence of vasospasm. The low mortality (7%) in these patients suggests a better prognosis in this subgroup of patients when compared to those in the overall study.

Computerized tomographic observations showed no specific abnormality associated with increased intracranial pressure. Blood around the midbrain and intraventricular hemorrhage was significantly related to increased mortality, and blood in the midbrain was associated with patients seriously ill without increased intracranial pressure.

Although the loss to follow-up in this study at the 3-month and 1-year intervals was 38% and 42%, respectively, the 39 patients with completed protocols showed a 77% mortality at 3 months and 1 year. There is no difference when comparing this mortality to the natural history of this seriously ill population derived from the Cooperative Study, which has a predicted mortality of 71 to 75% at the end of 1 year.[1] Only 3 patients were symptom-free, 1 patient had minor symptoms and 5 patients had major neurologic deficit. Although a select group of patients with improved prognosis was identified at 28 days, long-term follow-up suggests little has been accomplished by this type of intervention to improve the prognosis in the seriously ill patients secondary to ruptured intracranial aneurysms. Management of these seriously ill patients remains a most challenging problem.

References

1. Locksley, H.B.: Natural history of subarachnoid hemorrhage, intracranial aneurysms, and arteriovenous malformations. Section V, Part II. Based on 6,368 cases in the Cooperative Study. J Neurosurg 25:321–368, 1966.
2. Skultety, F.M., Nishioka, H.: The results of intracranial surgery in the treatment of aneurysms. J Neurosurg 25:683–704, 1966.
3. Hunt, W.E., Hess, R.M.: Surgical risk as related to time of intervention in the repair of intracranial aneurysms. J Neurosurg 28:14–20, 1968.
4. Graf, C.J., Nibbelink, D.W.: Cooperative study of intracranial aneurysms and subarachnoid hemorrhage. Report on a randomized study. III. Intracranial surgery. Stroke 5:557–601, 1974.
5. Nibbelink, D.W., Torner, J.C., Henderson, W.G.:

Intracranial aneurysms and subarachnoid hemorrhage. A cooperative study. Antifibrinolytic therapy in recent onset subarachnoid hemorrhage. Stroke 6:622–629, 1975.

6. Nibbelink, D.W.: Cooperative aneurysm study: Antihypertensive and antifibrinolytic therapy following subarachnoid hemorrhage from ruptured intracranial aneurysm. In: Whisnant, J.P., and Sandok, B.A.: Cerebral Vascular Diseases. Grune & Stratton, Inc, New York, 1975, pp 155–165.

7. Nibbelink, D.W., Torner, J., Burmeister, L.: Fluid restriction in combination with antifibrinolytic therapy. In: Sahs, A.L., Nibbelink, D.W., Torner, J.C., et al.: Aneurysmal Subarachnoid Hemorrhage. Urban & Schwarzenberg, Baltimore, 1981, Chapter 15, pp 307–330.

8. Botterell, E.H., Lougheed. W.M., et al.: Hypothermia and interruption of carotid, or carotid and vertebral circulation in the surgical management of intracranial aneurysms. J Neurosurg 13:1–42, 1956.

9. Klafta, L.A., Hamby, W.B.: Significance of cerebrospinal fluid pressure in determining time for repair of intracranial aneurysms. J Neurosurg 31:217–219, 1969.

10. Nornes, H., Magnaes, B.: Intracranial pressure in patients with ruptured sacular aneurysm. J Neurosurg 36:537–547, 1972.

11. Nornes, H.: The role of intracranial pressure in the arrest of hemorrhage in patients with ruptured intracranial aneurysm. J Neurosurg 39:221–234, 1973.

12. Stornelli, S.A., French, J.D.: Subarachnoid hemorrhage—Factors in prognosis and management. J Neurosurg 21:769–780, 1964.

13. Kaufmann, G.E., Clark, K.: Continuous simultaneous monitoring of intraventricular and cervical subarachnoid cerebrospinal fluid pressure to indicate development of cerebral or tonsillar herniation. J Neurosurg 33:145–150, 1970.

14. Forbes, H.S.: The cerebral circulation 1. Observation and measurement of pial vessels. Arch Neurol Psychiat 19:751–761, 1928.

15. Langfitt, T.S., Kassell, N.F., et al.: Cerebral blood flow with intracranial hypertension. Neurology 15:761–773, 1965.

16. Grubb, R.L., Raichle, M.D., et al.: Effects of increased intracranial pressure on cerebral blood volume, blood flow, and oxygen utilization in monkeys. J Neurosurg 43:385–398, 1975.

17. Nibbelink, D.W., Torner, J.C., Henderson, W.G.: Intracranial aneurysms and subarachnoid hemorrhage—Report on a randomized treatment study. IV-A. Regulated bed rest. Stroke 8:202–218, 1977.

18. Nibbelink, D.W., Torner, J.C., Henderson, W.G.: Randomized treatment study. Drug-induced hypotension. In: Sahs, A.L., Nibbelink, D.W., Torner, J.C., et al.: Aneurysmal Subarachnoid Hemorrhage. Urban & Schwarzenberg, Baltimore, 1981, Chapter 6, pp 77–106.

19. Fisher, C.M., Roberson, G.H., Ojemann, R.G.: Cerebral vasospasm after ruptured aneurysm. Second Joint Meeting on Stroke and Cerebral Circulation, February 25–26, 1977. Stroke 8:11, 1977.

20. Nibbelink, D.W., Sahs, A.L., Knowler, L.A.: Antihypertensive and antifibrinolytic medications in subarachnoid hemorrhage and their relation to cerebral vasospasm. A report of the Cooperative Aneurysm Study. In: Smith, R.R., Robertson, J.T.: Subarchnoid Hemorrhage and Cerebrovascular Spasm. Charles C Thomas, Springfield, Ill, 1975, pp 177–205.

21. Farrar, J.K., Jr.: Chronic cerebral arterial spasm. The role of intracranial pressure. J Neurosurg 43:408–417, 1975.

22. Locksley, H.B.: Report on the cooperative study of intracranial aneurysms and subarachnoid hemorrhage. Section V, Part I. Natural history of subarachnoid hemorrhage, intracranial aneurysms and arteriovenous malformations. J Neurosurg 25:219–239, 1966.

Index

363

PRE-ALGEBRA

An Accelerated Course

Mary P. Dolciani
Robert H. Sorgenfrey
John A. Graham

Editorial Advisers

Richard G. Brown
Robert B. Kane

HOUGHTON MIFFLIN COMPANY · Boston

Atlanta   Dallas   Geneva, Ill.   Palo Alto   Princeton   Toronto

AUTHORS

Mary P. Dolciani formerly Professor of Mathematical Sciences, Hunter College of the City University of New York

Robert H. Sorgenfrey Professor of Mathematics, University of California, Los Angeles

John A. Graham Mathematics Teacher, Buckingham Browne and Nichols School, Cambridge, Massachusetts

Editorial Advisers

Richard G. Brown Mathematics Teacher, Phillips Exeter Academy, Exeter, New Hampshire

Robert B. Kane Dean of the School of Education and Professor of Mathematics Education, Purdue University, Lafayette, Indiana

Teacher Consultants

John E. Mosby Instructional Coordinator, Dixon School, Chicago, Illinois

William Voligny Mathematics Teacher, Olympia Junior High School, Auburn, Washington

ISBN: 0-395-59123-6

FGHIJ–VH–987654

Contents

Reading Mathematics

This page shows many of the metric measures and symbols that are used in this book. Use this page as a reference when you read the book.

Symbols

		Page			Page
$\cdot$	times	3	AB	the length of $\overline{AB}$	169
$\approx$	is approximately equal to	14	$\cong$	is congruent to	169
$^{-}1$	negative one	46	$\angle$	angle	173
$|^{-}3|$	absolute value of $^{-}3$	46	$60°$	sixty degrees	173
$>$	is greater than	47	$m\angle A$	measure of angle A	173
$<$	is less than	47	$\perp$	is perpendicular to	173
$\neq$	is not equal to	47	$\triangle ABC$	triangle ABC	178
$\geq$	is greater than or equal to	47	π	pi	188
$\leq$	is less than or equal to	47	$1:5$	1 to 5	210
$-b$	the opposite of b	59	$\%$	percent	227
$0.4\overline{36}$	36 repeats without end	117	$(5, 4)$	ordered pair 5, 4	312
$\overleftrightarrow{PQ}$	line PQ	164	$\sqrt{a}$	positive square root of a	394
$\overrightarrow{BA}$	ray BA	164	$\sim$	is similar to	406
$\overline{PQ}$	segment PQ	164	$3!$	3 factorial	453
$\parallel$	is parallel to	165	$P(E)$	probability of event E	461

Metric Measures

Prefixes

Prefix	kilo	centi	milli
Factor	1000	0.01	0.001
Symbol	k	c	m

Base Units

Length: **meter** (m)

Mass: **kilogram** (kg)

Capacity: **liter** (L)

Temperature **Degree Celsius** (°C)

Length 1 mm = 0.001 m   1 cm = 0.01 m   1 km = 1000 m
1 m = 1000 mm   1 m = 100 cm   1 cm = 10 mm

Mass 1 kg = 1000 g   1 mg = 0.001 g   1 g = 0.001 kg

Capacity 1 mL = 0.001 L   1 L = 1000 mL   1 L = 1000 cm³

Time 60 s = 1 min   60 min = 1 h   3600 s = 1 h

Examples of compound units   kilometers per hour: km/h
square centimeters: cm²   cubic meters: m³

Diagnostic Test of Whole Number and Decimal Skills

This test reviews the skills of addition, subtraction, multiplication, and division necessary to begin Chapter 1. More practice of these skills can be found on pages 480–483.

Addition

Add.

1. 142
    + 237

2. 374
    + 213

3. 103
     19
    + 42

4. 1007
     285
    + 59

5.   246
       9
    1064
     842
    + 83

6. 5.246
    + 6.38

7. 16.439
    + 28.32

8. 3.84
    2.07
    + 9.39

9. 72.8
    6.349
    + 0.76

10.   0.16
      54.3
     119.057
    +   2.0918

11. 32 + 56

12. 693 + 105

13. 34 + 17 + 25

14. 2306 + 19 + 429 + 1443

15. 18.7 + 5.394

16. 0.06 + 19.803

17. 11.882 + 6.49 + 0.083

18. 583.117 + 72.5 + 3.76824

19. 35.402 + 17.6 + 5.28 + 0.314

20. 3.4289 + 5.005 + 31 + 8.57

Subtraction

Subtract.

1. 864
    − 231

2. 9748
    − 2635

3. 4693
    − 2758

4. 801
    − 543

5. 3004
    − 2567

6. 6.75
    − 3.81

7. 14.90
    − 7.88

8. 388.6
    − 97.86

9. 705.56
    − 314.6

10. 0.986
    − 0.097

11. 768 − 654

12. 925 − 713

13. 853 − 432

14. 2670 − 357

15. 5323 − 789

16. 4803 − 567

Subtract.

17. 9.5 − 4.8

18. 46.71 − 22.52

19. 0.039 − 0.0271

20. 0.8743 − 0.33591

21. 0.039 − 0.0271

22. 5.04876 − 229

Multiplication

Multiply.

1. 63
× 21

2. 42
× 34

3. 131
× 25

4. 214
× 37

5. 381
× 206

6. 473
× 0.3

7. 846
× 2.5

8. 127.3
× 6.6

9. 67.05
× 2.39

10. 99.7
× 10.06

11. 51 × 73

12. 92 × 34

13. 732 × 24

14. 947 × 62

15. 4023 × 570

16. 9108 × 6027

17. 18.7 × 16

18. 0.08 × 58.6

19. 0.75 × 0.69

20. 27.9 × 33.3

21. 6.0810 × 148.3

22. 5.62 × 83.109

Division

Divide.

1. $7\overline{)91}$

2. $4\overline{)64}$

3. $8\overline{)296}$

4. $29\overline{)522}$

5. $74\overline{)3478}$

6. $607\overline{)6677}$

7. $5\overline{)37.60}$

8. $81\overline{)108.54}$

9. $5.4\overline{)3348}$

10. $1.6\overline{)99.68}$

11. $2.86\overline{)247.39}$

12. $1.13\overline{)1006.83}$

Divide. Round to the nearest tenth.

13. 56 ÷ 3

14. 49 ÷ 8

15. 319 ÷ 15

16. 628 ÷ 20

17. 948 ÷ 48

18. 9963 ÷ 542

19. 0.851 ÷ 0.33

20. 0.909 ÷ 1.35

21. 0.284 ÷ 7.31

22. 486 ÷ 0.391

23. 5.005 ÷ 0.095

24. 43.761 ÷ 27.515

1

Introduction to Algebra

All of the many pieces of information handled by computers are stored and processed by means of tiny microchips, such as the one shown at the right. Each microchip is about 2 mm square and is made up of thin layers of silicon crystals. Each layer is treated chemically and etched photographically with different patterns containing tens of thousands of microscopic switches. Information on the microchip is represented by a code made up of a series of "on" or "off" switches.

Although we use words and numbers to communicate with a computer, the machine does not work directly with those words and numbers. A program within the computer automatically translates the information that we use into the special code that the machine understands. In a similar way, when we work with algebra, we translate our words and ideas into the language of mathematics. In this chapter, you will learn many of the symbols that we use to express mathematical ideas.

Career Note

Consider how intricate the design of a single microchip is. Electrical engineers are involved in designing and testing new electrical equipment such as the microchip. Electrical engineers must therefore be qualified in both mathematics and science. Most, in fact, specialize in a major field such as communications, industrial equipment, or computers.

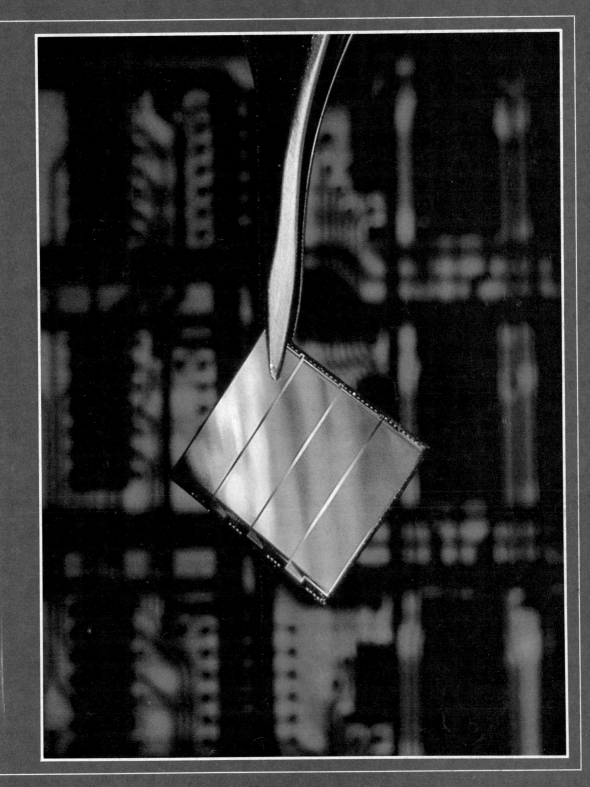

1-1 Mathematical Expressions

A **numerical expression** is simply a name for a number. For example,

4 + 6 is a numerical expression for the number 10.

Since 4 + 6 and 10 name the same number, we can use the equals sign, =, and write

$$4 + 6 = 10.$$

We **simplify the numerical expression** 4 + 6 when we replace it with its simplest name, 10.

EXAMPLE 1   Simplify each numerical expression.
      a. 400×4 **b.** $37 - 19$ **c.** $5.1 \div 3$

Solution   **a.** $400 \times 4 = 1600$ **b.** $37 - 19 = 18$ **c.** $5.1 \div 3 = 1.7$

If a computer can do 100 million arithmetic computations in one second, the table below shows how many million computations the computer can do in two, three, and four seconds.

Number of Seconds	Millions of Computations
1	100×1
2	100×2
3	100×3
4	100×4

Each of the numerical expressions 100×1, 100×2, 100×3, and 100×4 fits the pattern

$$100 \times n$$

where n stands for 1, 2, 3, or 4. A letter, such as n, that is used to represent one or more numbers is called a **variable.** The numbers are called the **values of the variable.**

An expression, such as $100 \times n$, that contains a variable is called a **variable expression.** When we write a product that contains a variable, we usually omit the multiplication sign.

$100 \times n$ may be written $100n$.

$x \times y$ may be written xy.

In a numerical expression for a product, such as 100×4, we must use a multiplication sign to avoid confusion.

A raised dot is also a multiplication sign.

$$100 \times 4 \text{ may be written } 100 \cdot 4.$$

When we replace each variable in a variable expression by one of its values and simplify the resulting numerical expression, we say that we are **evaluating the expression** or **finding the value of the expression.**

When the value of n is 4, the value of $100n$ is 400.

EXAMPLE 2   Evaluate each expression when $a = 6$ and $b = 2$.
a. $9 + a$ **b.** $a \div b$ **c.** $3ab$

Solution   **a.** Substitute 6 for a. $9 + a = 9 + 6 = 15$
b. Substitute 6 for a and 2 for b. $a \div b = 6 \div 2 = 3$
c. Substitute 6 for a and 2 for b. $3ab = 3 \times 6 \times 2 = 36$

In the expression $9 + a$, 9 and a are called the **terms** of the expression because they are the parts that are separated by the $+$. In an expression such as $3ab$, the number 3 is called the **numerical coefficient** of ab.

Reading Mathematics: *Vocabulary*
Look back at this first lesson. Notice the words in heavier type throughout the text. They are important new words and ideas, such as the following:

numerical expression	simplify a numerical expression
variable	value of a variable
variable expression	evaluate a variable expression
terms	numerical coefficient

When you see a word in heavier type, look near it for an explanation or example to help you understand the new word. For an unusual new word, look up the definition in the glossary to help you understand and remember it.

Class Exercises

Simplify the numerical expression.

1. $24 + 18 + 32$ **2.** $125 \div 5$ **3.** $3.6 + 5.1$ **4.** 0.25×10

Evaluate the variable expression when $x = 4$.

5. $x + 7$ **6.** $5x$ **7.** $28 \div x$ **8.** $13 - x$

9. What is another way to write $17 \times x$?

10. In the variable expression $12a$, the numerical coefficient is __?__ and the variable is __?__ .

Written Exercises

Simplify the numerical expression.

A
1. $16 \cdot 3$
2. $37 + 12$
3. $114 - 9$
4. $918 \div 6$

5. $1.65 + 12.5$
6. $1.05 + 9.7$
7. 0.5×9
8. $2.53 \div 11$

Evaluate the expression when $y = 2$.

9. $y + 23$
10. $6y$
11. $8 \div y$
12. $4 + y + 7$

Evaluate the expression when $q = 3$.

13. $36 \div q$
14. $q \div 3$
15. $q \times 9$
16. $q - q$

Evaluate the expression when $a = 5$.

17. $a - 3$
18. $a \times a$
19. $42 + a$
20. $a + a$

Evaluate the expression when $m = 8$.

21. $6 + 9 + 3 + m$
22. $m \times 3$
23. $m \times m \times m$
24. $m \div m$

Evaluate the expression when $x = 8$ and $y = 1$.

B
25. $x + y$
26. $x - y - 2$
27. $3x$
28. $x \div y$

Evaluate the expression when $c = 7.5$ and $d = 3$.

29. $c \div d$
30. $c + d + 20$
31. $c \times 15$
32. $4cd$

Evaluate the expression when $s = 12.3$ and $t = 6.15$.

33. $9st$
34. $s \div t$
35. $s - t - 3$
36. $73.8 \div s$

C
37. Find the value of a for which the expressions $2a$ and $2 + a$ have the same value.

38. Find a value of x for which $x \div 7$ and $7 \div x$ are equal.

Review Exercises

Perform the indicated operation.

1. $43.8 + 8.07$
2. 51×3.4
3. $80.47 - 34.54$
4. $6.29 + 0.124$

5. $11.61 \div 43$
6. 6.328×0.729
7. $32.004 \div 5.08$
8. $2403 - 976.8$

4   *Chapter 1*

1-2 Order of Operations

The expression

$$2 + (6 \times 3)$$

involves both addition and multiplication. The parentheses indicate that the multiplication is to be done first.

$$2 + (6 \times 3) = 2 + 18 = 20$$

For the expression

$$(2 + 6) \times 3$$

the parentheses indicate that the addition is to be done first.

$$(2 + 6) \times 3 = 8 \times 3 = 24$$

Parentheses used to indicate the order of the arithmetic operations are called **grouping symbols.** Operations within grouping symbols are to be done first.

We usually write a product such as $4 \times (3 + 5)$ without the multiplication symbol as $4(3 + 5)$. We may also use parentheses in any one of the following ways to indicate a product such as 4×8:

$$4(8) \qquad \text{or} \qquad (4)8 \qquad \text{or} \qquad (4)(8).$$

A fraction bar is both a division symbol and a grouping symbol. Recall that $18 \div 2$ may be written as $\frac{18}{2}$. When operation symbols appear above or below the fraction bar, those operations are to be done before the division. For example, to simplify

$$\frac{6 + 15}{3},$$

we add first:

$$\frac{6 + 15}{3} = \frac{21}{3} = 7.$$

EXAMPLE 1   Evaluate each expression when $n = 8$.

         a. $4(n - 3)$ **b.** $\dfrac{45 - 15}{n + 7}$

Solution   Substitute 8 for n in each expression.

         a. $4(n - 3) = 4(8 - 3) = 4(5) = 20$

         b. $\dfrac{45 - 15}{n + 7} = \dfrac{45 - 15}{8 + 7} = \dfrac{30}{15} = 2$

If there are no grouping symbols in an expression, we agree to perform the operations in the following order.

Rule for Order of Operations

When there are no grouping symbols:

1. Perform all multiplications and divisions in order from left to right.

2. Perform all additions and subtractions in order from left to right.

EXAMPLE 2   Simplify $392 + 637 \div 49$.

Solution $392 + \underbrace{637 \div 49}$

$\underbrace{392 + \quad 13}$

405

When a product of two numbers or of a number and a variable is written without a multiplication symbol, as in 5(7) or 4n, we perform the multiplication before the other operations.

EXAMPLE 3   Evaluate the expression when $x = 6$.

   a. $27 \div 2x$ **b.** $\dfrac{3x - 2}{4}$

Solution   Substitute 6 for x in each expression.

   a. $27 \div 2x = 27 \div 2(6) = 27 \div 12 = 2.25$

   b. $\dfrac{3x - 2}{4} = \dfrac{3(6) - 2}{4} = \dfrac{18 - 2}{4} = \dfrac{16}{4} = 4$

Class Exercises

Tell in which order the operations should be performed to simplify the expression.

   1. $6 + 14 \times 3$ **2.** $(6 + 14)3$ **3.** $18 - 12 \div 3 + 1$

   4. $18 - 12 \div (3 + 1)$ **5.** $23 - 9 \div 5 + 2$ **6.** $(9 + 16) \div (4 + 1)$

Evaluate the expression when $m = 4$.

7. $(m + 6)2$ **8.** $5m + 8$ **9.** $3(m - 1)$

10. $8 \div m + 7$ **11.** $m(2 + m)$ **12.** $\dfrac{3m}{18 - 6}$

Written Exercises

Simplify the expression.

A   **1.** $35 - 14 \div 2 + 64$ **2.** $54 \div 6 + 18 \times 2$ **3.** $44 + 17 - 5 \times 2$

     4. $(45 - 19)(8 + 7)$ **5.** $(12 + 18) \div (19 - 4)$ **6.** $\dfrac{9 + (4 \times 3)}{7}$

Evaluate the expression when $n = 7$.

     7. $(14 + n)6$ **8.** $36 \div (n - 3)$ **9.** $(n + 28) \div 5$

     10. $(27 - n)3$ **11.** $12(n - 4)$ **12.** $\dfrac{94 - 38}{n}$

Evaluate the expression when $t = 10$.

     13. $5t \div (14 - 9)$ **14.** $\dfrac{25 - t}{10 - 5}$ **15.** $(t + 6 - 9)t$

     16. $2(t + 5) - t$ **17.** $(t - 4)(t - 4)$ **18.** $50 \div (t + 15) + t$

Evaluate the expression when $s = 16$.

     19. $7(s + 12)$ **20.** $5(s - 4)$ **21.** $(s + 32) \div s$

     22. $(3s - 6) \div 7$ **23.** $18(6s - 12)$ **24.** $4s \div (s - 8)$

Evaluate the expression when $b = 6$ and $c = 7$.

B   **25.** $(b + c)c$ **26.** $3c \div (b - 4)$ **27.** $2bc \div (c - b)$

Evaluate the expression when $m = 4$ and $n = 9$.

     28. $5n \div (m + 5)$ **29.** $(n + m) \div (35 - n)$ **30.** $m(n - m) \div 8$

Evaluate the expression when $a = 3.6$ and $b = 8.2$.

     31. $ab \div 2a$ **32.** $(b - a)(3a + 6)$ **33.** $7ab(3b + a)$

Evaluate the expression when $e = 5$, $f = 8$, and $g = 13$.

34. $(e + f)(g + e)$ **35.** $f \div (g - f) + g$ **36.** $f(e + g) - e$

Copy the expression as shown. Add grouping symbols so that the value of the expression is 24 when $x = 3$, $y = 7$, and $z = 21$.

C **37.** $2x \times y - 4 + 2x$ **38.** $y + z \div 4 \times x + x$ **39.** $x \times y + z \div 3 + 1 - z$

Review Exercises

Evaluate the expression when $x = 2$, $y = 1$, and $z = 4$.

1. $2x + y$ **2.** $3z - 3x$ **3.** $5xy - z$ **4.** $4xyz - xz$

5. $6yz \div 4x$ **6.** $12z \times 3y$ **7.** $7z \times 3x$ **8.** $8xy \div z$

▮▮▮ Calculator Key-In

To use your calculator to simplify an expression with more than one operation, you must keep in mind the order in which you want the operations to be performed. Try to simplify $2(6 + 4)$ by entering the following on your calculator exactly as it is shown.

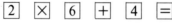

Although the correct answer is 20, your calculator will perform the operations in the order in which you entered them and will display 16 for the answer.

To obtain the correct answer, you must enter the expressions in the order in which you want them to be performed. Enter the following exactly as it is shown.

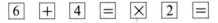

Now your calculator should display the correct answer, 20. By entering = after entering the expression in parentheses, you complete the operation inside the parentheses before doing the next operation. Some calculators will complete the operation for you even if you do not enter = between operations. Check to see if your calculator will.

Use your calculator to simplify the expression.

1. $12(15 + 9)$ **2.** $57 \div (36 - 17)$ **3.** $(437 + 322) \div 46$

4. $(108 + 63) \div (9 - 6)$ **5.** $(55 + 8) \times (2 + 94)$ **6.** $(56 - 32) \div (4 + 16) \times 5$

1-3 Exponents and Powers of Ten

When two or more numbers are multiplied together, each of the numbers is called a **factor** of the product. For example, in the multiplication

$$3 \times 5 = 15,$$

3 and 5 are the factors of 15.

A product in which each factor is the same is called a **power** of that factor. For example, since

$$2 \times 2 \times 2 \times 2 = 16,$$

16 is called the *fourth power* of 2. We can write this as

$$2^4 = 16.$$

The small numeral 4 is called an **exponent** and represents the number of times 2 is a factor of 16. The number 2 is called the **base.**

EXAMPLE 1   Simplify 4^3.

Solution $4^3 = 4 \times 4 \times 4 = 16 \times 4 = 64$

The second and third powers of a number have special names. The second power is called the **square** of the number and the third power is called the **cube.**

EXAMPLE 2   Read, then simplify.

   a. 12^2 **b.** 9^3

Solution   **a.** 12^2 is read "twelve squared."
              $12^2 = 12 \times 12 = 144$

          b. 9^3 is read "nine cubed."
              $9^3 = 9 \times 9 \times 9 = 81 \times 9 = 729$

Powers of 10 are important in our number system. Here is a list of the first five powers of 10.

First power: 10^1 (exponent usually not written) $= 10$
Second power: $10^2 = 10 \times 10$ $= 100$
Third power: $10^3 = 10 \times 10 \times 10$ $= 1000$
Fourth power: $10^4 = 10 \times 10 \times 10 \times 10$ $= 10,000$
Fifth power: $10^5 = 10 \times 10 \times 10 \times 10 \times 10$ $= 100,000$

If you study the preceding list carefully, you can see that the general rules below apply.

> ## *Rules*
>
> **1.** The exponent in a power of 10 is the same as the number of zeros when the number is written out.
> **2.** The number of zeros in the product of powers of 10 is the sum of the numbers of zeros in the factors.

EXAMPLE 3   Write 10,000 as a power of 10.

Solution   Because there are 4 zeros in 10,000, the exponent is 4.

$$10,000 = 10^4$$

EXAMPLE 4   Multiply 100×1000.

Solution   Since there are 2 zeros in 100 and 3 zeros in 1000, the product will have $2 + 3$, or 5, zeros.

$$100 \times 1000 = 100,000$$

Can we give an expression such as 7^0 a meaning? When the powers of any base are listed in order, we may recognize a pattern. Study the example below.

$$7^4 = 7 \times 7 \times 7 \times 7 = 2401$$
$$7^3 = 7 \times 7 \times 7 = 343$$
$$7^2 = 7 \times 7 = 49$$
$$7^1 = 7$$

Notice that in increasing order each power of 7 is seven times the preceding power. Conversely, in decreasing order, each power of 7 is the quotient of the preceding power divided by a factor of 7. That is, $7^3 = 7^4 \div 7$, $7^2 = 7^3 \div 7$, and so on. This decreasing pattern suggests that 7^0 (read *7 to the zero power*) is $7^1 \div 7$. Study the example below to verify that the expression $7^0 = 1$.

$$7^0 = 7^1 \div 7 = 7 \div 7 = 1$$

In general,

Class Exercises

Name the exponent and the base.

1. 8^3 **2.** 9^7 **3.** 3^5 **4.** 6^4

Write as a power of 10.

5. 1000   **6.** 100   **7.** 100,000   **8.** 100,000,000

Tell the number of zeros in the number or product.

9. 10^4 **10.** 10^8 **11.** 1000×1000 **12.** $100 \times 1,000,000$

Read the following, then simplify each.

13. 7^2 **14.** 9^2 **15.** 13^0 **16.** 6^2

17. 4^3 **18.** 8^0 **19.** 2^7 **20.** 13^2

Written Exercises

Use exponents to write each of the following expressions.

A   **1.** $5 \times 5 \times 5 \times 5 \times 5 \times 5$ **2.** $12 \times 12 \times 12 \times 12$

3. $8 \times 8 \times 8 \times 8 \times 8 \times 8 \times 8 \times 8 \times 8$ **4.** $20 \times 20 \times 20 \times 20 \times 20$

5. $7 \times 7 \times 7 \times 7 \times 7 \times 7 \times 7$ **6.** $9 \times 9 \times 9 \times 9$

7. $4 \times 4 \times 4 \times 4 \times 4 \times 4$ **8.** $3 \times 3 \times 3 \times 3 \times 3$

Write as a power of 10.

9. 10   **10.** 10,000,000   **11.** 1,000,000   **12.** 1,000,000,000

Multiply.

13. 1000×1000 **14.** $10 \times 10,000$ **15.** 100×100 **16.** $100 \times 100,000$

Simplify.

17. 4^2	18. 11^3	19. 16^2	20. 15^2
21. 20^2	22. 5^4	23. 15^3	24. 2^5
25. 80^2	26. 40^3	27. 2^8	28. 12^3
29. 6^4	30. 5^5	31. 16^3	32. 3^5
33. 5^3	34. 4^6	35. 13^2	36. 11^2

Multiply.

EXAMPLE $3^4 \times 2^3$

Solution

$$3^4 \times 2^3 = (3 \times 3 \times 3 \times 3) \times (2 \times 2 \times 2)$$
$$= 81 \times 8$$
$$= 648$$

B

37. $2^4 \times 5^2$	38. $1^3 \times 16^2$	39. $70^2 \times 7^3$	40. $3^4 \times 10^5$
41. $0^4 \times 15^8$	42. $15^2 \times 10^3$	43. $31^2 \times 1^5$	44. $20^5 \times 3^2$
45. $2^8 \times 1^5$	46. $5^3 \times 3^4$	47. $12^3 \times 2^2$	48. $200^3 \times 3^2$
49. $2^3 \times 3^2 \times 10^3$	50. $8^2 \times 5^3 \times 1^4$	51. $119^2 \times 2^5 \times 0^8$	52. $50^4 \times 2 \times 1^5$
53. $3^3 \times 2^0$	54. $2^5 \times 3^2$	55. $3^2 \times 10^4$	56. $10^5 \times 11^0$

Evaluate when $a = 3$ and $b = 5$.

C

57. a^3	58. b^3	59. $a^5 - b^2$	60. $a^3 + b^2$
61. $50 - b^2$	62. $20a^2$	63. $(ab)^2$	64. a^2b^3
65. a^3b^3	66. $(ab)^3$	67. $b^2 - a^2$	68. $(a - b)^2$

Review Exercises

Simplify the expression.

1. $48 + 20 \div 4 + 7$

2. $72 \div 9 + 3 \times 8$

3. $50 + 35 \div 7 + 2$

4. $105 - 30 \times 2 \div 5$

5. $36 - 24 \div (3 + 1)$

6. $60 + 40 \div (2 + 8)$

7. $\frac{28 + 20}{4} + 12$

8. $\frac{78 - 18 \div 3}{4} - 8$

1-4 The Decimal System

Our number system uses the powers of 10 to express all numbers. This system is called the **decimal system** (from the Latin word *decem,* meaning *ten*). Using the digits 0, 1, 2, . . . , 9, we can write any number. The **value** of each digit depends on the position of the digit in the number. For example, the 2 in 312 means 2 ones, but the 2 in 298 means 2 hundreds. The decimal system is a system with **place value.**

The chart below shows place values for some of the digits of a **decimal number,** or **decimal.**

Place-Value Chart

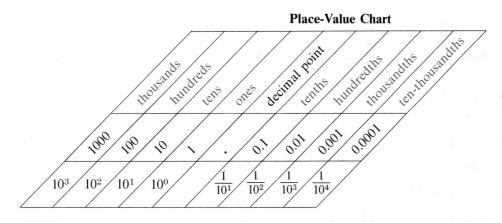

Moving left to right, place values decrease. As illustrated below, each place value is one tenth, or 0.1, of the place value to its left.

$$1000 \times 0.1 = 100 \qquad 10 \times 0.1 = 1 \qquad 0.01 \times 0.1 = 0.001$$

We can see from the place-value chart that values to the left of the decimal point are greater than or equal to 1, while values to the right are less than 1. If a digit is zero, then the product is zero and is usually not written.

When a decimal number is written, the value of the number is the sum of the values of the digits. To illustrate this, we can write decimal numbers in **expanded form,** that is, as a sum of products of each digit and its place value.

EXAMPLE 1   Write the decimal in expanded form.

           a. 3053   **b.** 16.9   **c.** 0.074

Solution   **a.** $3053 = (3 \times 1000) + (5 \times 10) + 3$

                b. $16.9 = (1 \times 10) + 6 + (9 \times 0.1)$

                c. $0.074 = (7 \times 0.01) + (4 \times 0.001)$

Decimals and whole numbers can be pictured on a number line. The **graph** of a number is the point paired with the number on the number line. The number paired with a point is called the **coordinate** of the point. The graphs of the whole numbers 0 through 8 are shown on the number line below. The coordinates of the points shown are 0, 1, 2, 3, 4, 5, 6, 7, and 8.

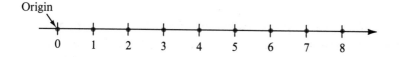

Starting with the graph of 0, which is called the **origin,** the graphs of the whole numbers are equally spaced. The greater a number is, the farther to the right its graph is.

The number line can be used to develop a method for **rounding** numbers. For example, we can see that 6.7 is closer to 7 than to 6 by graphing 6.7 on the number line. First we divide the portion of the number line between 6 and 7 into ten equal parts. Then we graph 6.7 on the number line as shown.

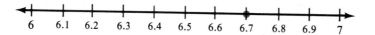

Because 6.7 is closer to 7 than to 6, we say that 6.7 rounded to the nearest whole number is 7. We write 6.7 $\approx$ 7. The symbol $\approx$ means *is approximately equal to.*

The rule for rounding decimal numbers can be stated as follows:

Rule

1. Find the decimal place to which you wish to round, and mark it with a caret ( ). Look at the digit to the right.

2. If the digit to the right is 5 or greater, add 1 to the marked digit. If the digit to the right is less than 5, leave the marked digit unchanged.

3. If the marked digit is to the left of the decimal point, replace each digit to the right of the marked place with "0," and drop all digits to the right of the decimal point.
   If the marked digit is to the right of the decimal point, drop all digits to the right of the marked place.

EXAMPLE 2 Round 16.0973 to the nearest

           a. ten   **b.** tenth   **c.** hundredth

Solution   **a.** 16.0973   **b.** 16.0973   **c.** 16.0973
                        ^   ^   ^
                  20   16.1   16.10

            16.0973 $\approx$ 20   16.0973 $\approx$ 16.1   16.0973 $\approx$ 16.10

    Rounding is often used as a quick check on calculations. In general, we **estimate** by rounding to the highest place value of the smaller number for all operations. As a result, our estimated answer should be reasonably close to the exact answer.

EXAMPLE 3   Find an estimated answer for each operation.

    a.   386   **b.**   2.849   **c.**   32.9   **d.** 12)253
           + 54   − 0.154   × 8.7

Solution   **a.**   386   →   390   **b.**   2.849   →   2.8
              + 54   + 50   − 0.154   − 0.2
                         440   2.6

                                                                    25
    c.   32.9   →   33   **d.** 12)253   → 10)250
           × 8.7   × 9
                    297

Class Exercises

Read the number.

  1. 5496   **2.** 0.51   **3.** 28.7   **4.** 0.0317   **5.** 8.026

Give the value of the digit 6 in the number.

  6. 657.3   **7.** 0.062   **8.** 8.1416   **9.** 6.023   **10.** 408.6

Round to the place underlined.

  11. 8.0<u>3</u>9   **12.** 2<u>9</u>4.65   **13.** 7<u>5</u>.452   **14.** 1<u>0</u>.988

  15. 0.9<u>9</u>6   **16.** 1.35<u>4</u>7   **17.** <u>3</u>19.84   **18.** 0.3<u>8</u>28

Round to the highest place value.

19. 43   **20.** 127.14   **21.** 0.036   **22.** 0.8981

23. 1986   **24.** 532.3   **25.** 0.073   **26.** 0.0249

Written Exercises

Write the decimal in expanded form.

A   **1.** 38   **2.** 256   **3.** 8091   **4.** 5   **5.** 0.47

     6. 28.4   **7.** 0.063   **8.** 9.070   **9.** 0.187   **10.** 5.5

Write as a decimal.

11. $(5 \times 10) + 4 + (5 \times 0.1) + (7 \times 0.01)$

12. $(4 \times 100) + (7 \times 0.01) + (3 \times 0.001) + (2 \times 0.0001)$

13. $(9 \times 1000) + 2 + (1 \times 0.1) + (4 \times 0.01) + (6 \times 0.001)$

14. $(1 \times 100) + (9 \times 10) + 3 + (2 \times 0.01) + (3 \times 0.001)$

Write as a decimal.

15. 7 and 43 hundredths   **16.** 11 and 4 tenths

17. 19 and 5 thousandths   **18.** 37 ten-thousandths

19. 48 ten-thousandths   **20.** 5 and 6 hundredths

21. 6 and 25 thousandths   **22.** 94 and 7 ten-thousandths

Round to the nearest ten.

23. 27.5149   **24.** 82.604   **25.** 293.4   **26.** 70.76

27. 648.01   **28.** 108.3   **29.** 159.62344   **30.** 97.23

Round to the nearest hundredth.

31. 72.459   **32.** 26.804   **33.** 0.0643   **34.** 12.395

35. 0.0103   **36.** 8.142   **37.** 18.1657   **38.** 0.70605

Round to the nearest thousandth.

39. 0.0006   **40.** 12.3568   **41.** 401.0904   **42.** 30.0317

43. 250.3407   **44.** 7.0063   **45.** 8.0995   **46.** 0.9996

Write in expanded form using exponents by writing each number as a sum of multiples of powers of 10.

EXAMPLE 367.04

Solution $(3 \times 10^2) + (6 \times 10^1) + (7 \times 10^0) + \left(4 \times \frac{1}{10^2}\right)$

47. 5280	**48.** 64.7	**49.** 183.08	**50.** 0.043
51. 0.091	**52.** 12.931	**53.** 7.482	**54.** 0.806
55. 204.5	**56.** 0.306	**57.** 38.003	**58.** 10.009

Select the most reasonable estimated answer.

B **59.** $89.6 + 13.5$ **a.** 90   **b.** 100   **c.** 70

    60. $35 + 12 + 26 + 11$ **a.** 70   **b.** 110   **c.** 90

    61. $65.43 - 8.92$ **a.** 56   **b.** 60   **c.** 90

    62. $2196 - 924$ **a.** 1300   **b.** 1000   **c.** 3100

    63. 6.82×4.7 **a.** 24   **b.** 35   **c.** 28

    64. $54 \div 2.5$ **a.** 30   **b.** 20   **c.** 18

    65. $36\overline{)283}$ **a.** 10   **b.** 3   **c.** 7

Review Exercises

Simplify.

1. $5.7 + (1.3 + 2.4)$ **2.** $(5.7 + 1.3) + 2.4$

3. $12 \times (10 \times 8)$ **4.** $(12 \times 10) \times 8$

5. $6 \times (4.7 + 5.3)$ **6.** $(6 \times 4.7) + (6 \times 5.3)$

7. $3.7 \times (7.9 - 3.9)$ **8.** $(3.7 \times 7.9) - (3.7 \times 3.9)$

Challenge

Write 100 using four 5's and any operation symbols you need.

Write 100 using the numbers 1 through 9 and any operation symbols you need.

Write 100 using four 9's and any operation symbols you need.

1-5 Basic Properties

Decimals and whole numbers share a number of properties which are used frequently in algebra.

Changing the order of the addends in a sum or the factors in a product does not change the sum or product. For example,

$$9.2 + 4.7 = 4.7 + 9.2 \qquad\qquad 3.5 \times 8.4 = 8.4 \times 3.5$$

Commutative Property

For all numbers a and b,

$$a + b = b + a \qquad \text{and} \qquad a \times b = b \times a$$

Changing the grouping of addends in a sum or of factors in a product does not change the sum or product. For example,

$5.6 + 0.8 + 11.2$	$4.1 \times 2.3 \times 7.2$
$(5.6 + 0.8) + 11.2 = 17.6$	$(4.1 \times 2.3) \times 7.2 = 67.896$
$5.6 + (0.8 + 11.2) = 17.6$	$4.1 \times (2.3 \times 7.2) = 67.896$

Associative Property

For all numbers a, b, and c,

$$(a + b) + c = a + (b + c)$$

$$\text{and} \qquad (a \times b) \times c = a \times (b \times c)$$

We can use these properties to find the easiest way to add or multiply a long list of numbers.

EXAMPLE 1 Use the properties to simplify the expression.

a. $4.8 + 1.1 + 0.2 + 3.9 + 7$ **b.** $2 \times 6 \times 5 \times 3$

Solution One possible way to rearrange the numbers is shown.

a. $4.8 + 1.1 + 0.2 + 3.9 + 7$ **b.** $2 \times 6 \times 5 \times 3$

$(4.8 + 0.2) + (1.1 + 3.9) + 7$ $(2 \times 5) \times (6 \times 3)$

$5 + 5 + 7$ 10×18

$10 + 7$ 180

17

The numbers 0 and 1 are called the **identity elements** for addition and multiplication respectively. The word *identity* comes from the Latin word *idem,* which means *the same*. The result of adding 0 to a number or subtracting 0 from a number is the same as the original number. The result of multiplying a number by 1 or dividing a number by 1 is the same as the original number. Study the following examples.

$$4.53 + 0 = 4.53 \qquad 29.7 \times 1 = 29.7$$
$$4.53 - 0 = 4.53 \qquad 29.7 \div 1 = 29.7$$

Addition and Subtraction Properties of Zero

For every number a,
$$a + 0 = a \qquad a - 0 = a$$
$$0 + a = a \qquad a - a = 0$$

Multiplication and Division Properties of One

For every number a,
$$a \times 1 = a \qquad a \div 1 = a$$
$$1 \times a = a \qquad a \div a = 1$$

The product of any number and 0 is 0. Similarly, 0 divided by any number is 0.

$$3.784 \times 0 = 0 \qquad 0 \div 3.784 = 0$$

Can we divide by 0? Recall that multiplication and division are inverse operations. Thus, if we were to divide 3.784 by 0, we would have the following.

$$3.784 \div 0 = x \qquad 3.784 = x \times 0$$

We cannot accept the equation at the right because any number times 0 is 0. So it makes no sense to divide by 0.

Multiplication and Division Properties of Zero

For every number a,
$$a \times 0 = 0 \qquad \text{and} \qquad 0 \times a = 0$$
For every number a, $a \neq 0$,
$$0 \div a = 0$$

The distributive property is different from the other properties because it involves two operations. The example below illustrates how we may distribute a multiplier over each term in an addition expression.

$$7 \times (8.2 + 1.8) \qquad\qquad (7 \times 8.2) + (7 \times 1.8)$$
$$7 \times 10 \qquad\qquad\qquad\qquad 57.4 + 12.6$$
$$70 \qquad\qquad\qquad\qquad\qquad 70$$

Therefore $7 \times (8.2 + 1.8) = (7 \times 8.2) + (7 \times 1.8)$.

We may also distribute a multiplier over each term in a subtraction expression.

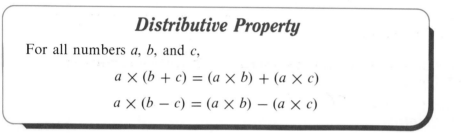

Distributive Property

For all numbers a, b, and c,

$$a \times (b + c) = (a \times b) + (a \times c)$$

$$a \times (b - c) = (a \times b) - (a \times c)$$

EXAMPLE 2 Use the distributive property to simplify the expression.
  a. $(4 + 6.2)5$ **b.** $(13 \times 2.7) - (13 \times 1.3)$

Solution   **a.** $(4 + 6.2)5 = (4 \times 5) + (6.2 \times 5) = 20 + 31 = 51$

             b. $(13 \times 2.7) - (13 \times 1.3) = 13(2.7 - 1.3) = 13(1.4) = 18.2$

EXAMPLE 3 What value of the variable makes the statement true?
  a. $6 + 5 = 5 + m$ **b.** $3.7 \times 4 = 4t$ **c.** $3(14 + 20) = 42 + b$

Solution   **a.** $6 + 5 = 5 + m$ **b.** $3.7 \times 4 = 4t$
               $6 + 5 = 5 + 6$, so $m = 6$ $3.7 \times 4 = 4 \times 3.7$, so $t = 3.7$

             c. $3(14 + 20) = 42 + b$
               $3(14 + 20) = (3 \times 14) + (3 \times 20) = 42 + 60$, so $b = 60$

Class Exercises

Name the property illustrated.

1. $7.6 + 0 = 0 + 7.6$

2. $(19 \times 3)6.2 = 19(3 \times 6.2)$

3. $11.9 \times 1 = 11.9$

4. $5(9 + 8.2) = (5 \times 9) + (5 \times 8.2)$

5. $138.6 \times 7.4 = 7.4 \times 138.6$

6. $6(1.2 + 0.8) = (1.2 + 0.8)6$

Use the properties of addition and multiplication to simplify the expression. Name the property or properties used.

7. 0.4×0

8. $3.02 \times 5 \times 2$

9. 1×12.87

10. $2.4 + 13 + 2.6$

11. $(8 \times 13) + (8 \times 7)$

12. 5.93×0

What value of the variable makes the statement true?

13. $25 + 37 = m + 25$

14. $(7 \times 6) + (5 \times 6) = (7 + 5)q$

15. $(17 + 12) + 8 = b + (12 + 8)$

16. $9(w - 20) = (9 \times 35) - (9 \times 20)$

Written Exercises

Use the properties to simplify the expression. Name the property or properties used.

A **1.** $2.6 + 11.5 + 0.5$

2. 0×23.15

3. $4(2.5 + 1.06)$

4. $8(40 - 12)$

5. $7.24 + 8.97 + 2.76$

6. $(22 \times 8) + (22 \times 2)$

7. $0.5 \times 2.1 \times 0.2$

8. $11.5 + 2.6 + 0.5 + 0.4$

True or false?

9. $7.386 + 0 = 0$

10. $(3 + 12)6 = (3 \times 6) + (12 \times 6)$

11. $(19.7 + 36 + 41.5)0 = 0$

12. $15(2 + 7.4) = (15 + 2) \times (15 + 7.4)$

What value of the variable makes the statement true?

13. $6 + n = 6$

14. $7.02 \times 23 = t \times 7.02$

15. $6.4 + t = 3.2 + 6.4$

16. $3r = 3$

17. $5w = w$

18. $2.43 \times 0 = f$

19. $(15.9 \times 3)4.2 = g(3 \times 4.2)$

20. $(13 - 11.7)8 = (13 \times 8) - (r \times 8)$

21. $(2 + 4.8)3 = (2n) + (4.8n)$

22. $(3.02 + 4.9)1 = b$

23. $5(11.7 + 313) = 58.5 + d$

24. $(7 \times 1.2) + (7 \times 3.8) = 7m$

25. $(8.31 + 2.73)t = t$

26. $2.59 + 7.03 + 18.61 + 3.97 = a + 11$

Use the properties to simplify the expression.

B **27.** $116 \times 3.7 \times 0 \times 4.93 \times 1.47 + 3.88$

28. $(78 \times 1) + (1.36 \times 0) + (92 + 0)$

29. $(18 + 46) + (12 + 4) + (8 \times 17) + (23 \times 8)$

30. $(12 \times 7) + (56 \div 8) + (13 \times 12)$

31. $5(81 \div 3) + 5(63 \div 1) + 450$

32. $(18 + 9)4 + (12 + 11)4$

33. $6(13 + 3) - 4(13 + 3)$

34. $1.4(2.61 + 7.39)$

Find values for *a*, *b*, and *c* that show that the equation is not true for all numbers.

C **35.** $(a \times b) + (b \times c) = b(a \times c)$

  36. $(a + b)(b + c) = b(a + c)$

  37. $(b + c)(a + c) = c(b \times a)$

  38. $a + (b \times c) = (a + b) \times (a + c)$

Self-Test A

Evaluate the expression when $k = 4$ and $m = 6$.

  1. $184 \div k$ **2.** $8 + m + 1$ **3.** $7km$ [1–1]

Evaluate the expression when $s = 12$ and $t = 18$.

  4. $\frac{s}{4} + 6$ **5.** $(t + 2) \div 5$ **6.** $2s - t$ [1–2]

Simplify.

  7. 2^4 **8.** 8^3 **9.** 9^1 **10.** 1000×100 **11.** $10 \times 10{,}000$ [1–3]

Round to the place specified.

12. tens: 84.307   **13.** hundredths: 3.176   **14.** hundreds: 293.84   [1–4]

Use the properties of addition and multiplication to simplify the expression. Name the property used.

15. $12(15 - 8) + 6 \times 3$ **16.** $(31 \times 4) + (15 \times 4) - 91$ [1–5]

17. $7(56 \div 8) - 7(24 \div 6)$ **18.** $9(0.36 \times 4) + 55$

Self-Test answers and Extra Practice are at the back of the book.

1-6 Equations

A **number sentence** indicates a relationship between two mathematical expressions. A sentence, such as the one below, that indicates that two expressions name the same number is called an **equation.**

$$4 \times 3 = 12$$

The expressions to the left and to the right of the equals sign are called the **sides** of the equation. In the example above, 4×3 is the left side of the equation, and 12 is the right side of the equation.

A number sentence may be *true* or *false*. For example, $3 + 9 = 12$ is a true equation, but $3 + 9 = 13$ is a false equation.

A number sentence that contains one or more variables is called an **open number sentence,** or simply an **open sentence.** Frequently a set of intended values, called the **replacement set,** for a variable is specified. An open sentence may be true or false when each variable is replaced by one of the values in its replacement set.

When a value of the variable makes an open sentence a true statement, we say that the value is a **solution** of, or **satisfies,** the sentence. We can **solve** an open sentence in one variable by finding all the solutions of the sentence. An open sentence may have one solution, several solutions, or no solutions.

EXAMPLE 1 Solve $x + 6 = 13$ for the replacement set $\{5, 6, 7\}$.

Solution Substitute each value in the replacement set for the variable x.

$5 + 6 = 13$	$6 + 6 = 13$	$7 + 6 = 13$
$11 = 13$	$12 = 13$	$13 = 13$
false	false	true

The solution of the equation is 7.

EXAMPLE 2 Solve $a - 1.2 = 0.7$ for the replacement set $\{1.8, 1.9, 2.0\}$.

Solution Substitute each value in the replacement set for the variable a.

$1.8 - 1.2 = 0.7$	$1.9 - 1.2 = 0.7$	$2.0 - 1.2 = 0.7$
$0.6 = 0.7$	$0.7 = 0.7$	$0.8 = 0.7$
false	true	false

The solution of the equation is 1.9.

EXAMPLE 3 The replacement set for q is the set of whole numbers. Find all solutions of

$$2q = 9.$$

Solution The replacement set for q is $\{0, 1, 2, 3, \ldots\}$, so $2q$ must be one of the numbers $2 \times 0, 2 \times 1, 2 \times 2, 2 \times 3, \ldots$, or $0, 2, 4, 6, \ldots$. Because 9 is not one of these numbers, the equation $2q = 9$ has no solution in the given replacement set.

Notice that in the solution to Example 2, we used three dots, read *and so on,* to indicate that the list of numbers continues without end.

Class Exercises

Tell whether the equation is true or false for the given value of the variable.

1. $20 - y = 17$; $y = 3$ **2.** $n \times 7 = 42$; $n = 8$

3. $144 \div r = 46$; $r = 3$ **4.** $156 + q = 179$; $q = 23$

5. $13.56 + p = 21.87$; $p = 6.31$ **6.** $8.91 \div c = 2.97$; $c = 3$

Solve the equation for the given replacement set.

7. $m + 6 = 72$; $\{50, 60, 70, 80\}$ **8.** $x \div 12 = 7$; $\{81, 82, 83, 84\}$

9. $r - 23 = 19$; $\{40, 41, 42, 43\}$ **10.** $b \times 8 = 64$; $\{2, 4, 6, 8\}$

11. $3.69 - n = 1.31$; $\{2.36, 2.37, 2.38\}$ **12.** $1.91 \times z = 9.55$; $\{4, 5, 6\}$

Written Exercises

Tell whether the equation is true or false for the given value of the variable.

A **1.** $x + 9 = 35$; $x = 26$ **2.** $r - 15 = 40$; $r = 55$

3. $10m = 130$; $m = 10$ **4.** $9 + y = 100$; $y = 91$

5. $44 - q = 11$; $q = 55$ **6.** $t \times 7 = 84$; $t = 91$

7. $n \div 8 = 104$; $n = 832$ **8.** $26 \div d = 2$; $d = 52$

9. $x + 6.71 = 10.82$; $x = 4.11$ **10.** $4.16a = 29.12$; $a = 8$

11. $m - 26 = 59$; $m = 85$ **12.** $q + 113 = 789$; $q = 901$

Solve the equation for the given replacement set.

13. $5d = 145$; $\{29, 30, 31\}$

14. $t - 53 = 67$; $\{13, 14, 15\}$

15. $b \times 14 = 112$; $\{6, 8, 10\}$

16. $c \div 12 = 228$; $\{17, 19, 21\}$

17. $98 - h = 21$; $\{75, 80, 85\}$

18. $38f = 912$; $\{24, 25, 26\}$

19. $e \div 19 = 152$; $\{8, 18, 28\}$

20. $46 + n = 99$; $\{50, 52, 54\}$

21. $q \div 23 = 66$; $\{1516, 1517, 1518\}$

22. $b \div 41 = 77$; $\{287, 288, 289\}$

23. $t + 1.21 = 2.47$; $\{1.25, 1.26, 1.27\}$

24. $y \div 1.2 = 3$; $\{3.3, 3.6, 3.9\}$

B 25. $4n + 7 = 51$; $\{10, 11, 12\}$

26. $58 - 3a = 10$; $\{16, 17, 18\}$

27. $4(b - 5) = 28$; $\{10, 11, 12\}$

28. $17(k + 4) = 170$; $\{4, 6, 8\}$

29. $(t + 18) \div 3 = 9$; $\{9, 10, 11\}$

30. $56 \div (d + 8) = 4$; $\{5, 6, 7\}$

31. $5(2c - 4) = 0$; $\{0, 1, 2\}$

32. $(3f + 7) \div 4 = 4$; $\{3, 4, 5\}$

Solve the equation. The replacement set is all even whole numbers.

33. $x + 1 = 10$

34. $5x = 35$

35. $4x = 16$

36. $x - 1 = 20$

Write an equation with the given solution if the replacement set is all whole numbers.

C 37. 10

38. 15

39. 100

40. Write an equation with no solution if the replacement set is all whole numbers.

Replace __?__ with $+$, $-$, $\times$, or $\div$ so the equation has the given solution.

41. x __?__ 17 __?__ $13 = 24$; 20

42. n __?__ 12 __?__ $8 = 11$; 36

43. 14 __?__ t __?__ $9 = 17$; 27

44. y __?__ 12 __?__ $6 = 10$; 8

45. d __?__ $(16$ __?__ $4)$ __?__ $8 = 8$; 12

46. 27 __?__ $(q$ __?__ $9)$ __?__ $15 = 45$; 18

47. 21 __?__ $(19$ __?__ $8)$ __?__ $b = 12$; 3

48. 11 __?__ $(16$ __?__ $a)$ __?__ $4 = 59$; 11

Review Exercises

Perform the indicated operation.

1. $7.81 + 3.86$

2. $11.65 - 8.58$

3. 1.18×23

4. $16.74 \div 2.79$

5. 2.53×2.9

6. $10.49 + 9.52$

7. $13.27 - 10.43$

8. $24.84 - 4.14$

1-7 Inverse Operations

Addition and subtraction are related operations, as shown by the following facts.

$$5 + 6 = 11$$
$$5 = 11 - 6$$

We say that adding a number and subtracting the same number are **inverse operations.**

The relationship between addition and subtraction holds when we work with variables, as well. Thus we can write the following related equations.

$$n + 6 = 11$$
$$n = 11 - 6$$

We can use this relationship to solve equations that involve addition or subtraction. Throughout the rest of the chapter if no replacement set is given for an open sentence, assume that the solution can be any number.

EXAMPLE 1   Use the inverse operation to write a related equation and solve for the variable.

   a. $x + 9 = 35$ **b.** $y - 12 = 18$

Solution   **a.** $x = 35 - 9$ **b.** $y = 18 + 12$
                              $x = 26$ $y = 30$
                  The solution is 26.   The solution is 30.

To check each solution, substitute the value of the variable in the original equation.

   a. $x + 9 = 35$ **b.** $y - 12 = 18$
         $26 + 9 = 35$ $\checkmark$ $30 - 12 = 18$ $\checkmark$

Multiplying by a number and dividing by the same number are inverse operations.

$$4 \times 6 = 24$$
$$6 = 24 \div 4$$

We can use this relationship to help solve equations that involve multiplication and division.

EXAMPLE 2   Use the inverse operation to write a related equation and solve for the variable.

   a. $6r = 30$ **b.** $x \div 7 = 12$

Solution   a. Recall that $6r$ means $6 \times r$.

$6 \times r = 30$

$r = 30 \div 6$

$r = 5$

The solution is 5.

Check: $6 \times 5 = 30$ ✓

b. $x \div 7 = 12$

$x = 12 \times 7$

$x = 84$

The solution is 84.

Check: $84 \div 7 = 12$ ✓

EXAMPLE 3   Use inverse operations to write a related equation and solve for the variable.

a. $x + 8.21 = 12.64$

b. $2.47a = 12.35$

Solution   a.

$x = 12.64 - 8.21$

$x = 4.43$

The solution is 4.43.

Check: $4.43 + 8.21 = 12.64$ ✓

b.

$a = 12.35 \div 2.47$

$a = 5$

The solution is 5.

Check: $(2.47)(5) = 12.35$ ✓

We can use inverse operations to solve equations that contain two operations.

EXAMPLE 4   Use inverse operations to solve the equation

$$3n + 25 = 61.$$

Solution   First write the related subtraction equation to find the value of $3n$.

$$3n = 61 - 25$$
$$3n = 36$$

Then write the related division equation to find the value of n.

$$n = 36 \div 3$$
$$n = 12$$

The solution is 12.

Check: $3(12) + 25 = 61$

$36 + 25 = 61$ ✓

Class Exercises

Use the inverse operation to state a related equation and solve for t.

1. $t + 6 = 15$

2. $t - 4 = 7$

3. $6t = 48$

4. $t \div 8 = 7$

5. $t + 24 = 60$

6. $13t = 78$

7. $t - 26 = 59$

8. $t \div 32 = 8$

9. $t + 3.19 = 5.26$

10. $t - 21.06 = 31.14$

11. $3.14t = 12.56$

12. $t \div 1.16 = 12$

Written Exercises

Use the inverse operation to write a related equation and solve for the variable.

A
1. $x + 8 = 15$
2. $a + 6 = 11$
3. $f + 38 = 74$
4. $t + 46 = 91$

5. $y - 9 = 14$
6. $n - 7 = 9$
7. $b - 25 = 32$
8. $r - 55 = 87$

9. $3c = 27$
10. $5g = 45$
11. $9m = 108$
12. $4d = 88$

13. $n \div 6 = 9$
14. $s \div 8 = 4$
15. $g \div 16 = 7$
16. $w \div 9 = 14$

17. $a + 17 = 17$
18. $j - 54 = 61$
19. $14n = 42$
20. $e + 26 = 61$

21. $h \div 11 = 297$
22. $b + 45 = 256$
23. $d - 87 = 110$
24. $18b = 18$

25. $31q = 465$
26. $k \div 17 = 527$
27. $p + 208 = 358$
28. $f - 11 = 523$

29. $c + 511 = 536$
30. $18r = 414$
31. $g - 19 = 401$
32. $m \div 4 = 216$

33. $x + 1.6 = 31.9$
34. $p - 1.9 = 18.4$
35. $1.6c = 2.56$
36. $m \div 3.27 = 6$

Use inverse operations to solve.

B
37. $3q + 9 = 27$
38. $4a + 19 = 39$
39. $7d - 12 = 37$

40. $5b - 16 = 39$
41. $3r + 24 = 63$
42. $2s - 30 = 62$

43. $9x - 84 = 69$
44. $6w + 81 = 486$
45. $(z \div 3) + 22 = 30$

46. $(l \div 7) - 4 = 4$
47. $(c \div 5) - 13 = 11$
48. $(v \div 3) + 15 = 36$

49. $4s + 7.41 = 9.57$
50. $6c + 3.60 = 9.72$
51. $7t - 8.43 = 14.67$

52. $9c - 8.32 = 7.61$
53. $(x \div 3.21) + 9 = 13$
54. $(y \div 1.67) + 5 = 12$

Replace __?__ with +, −, ×, or ÷ so the equation has the given solution.

C
55. $4 \underline{\ ?\ } a \underline{\ ?\ } 5 = 25;\ 5$
56. $7 \underline{\ ?\ } n \underline{\ ?\ } 4 = 14;\ 8$

57. $3 \underline{\ ?\ } c \underline{\ ?\ } 11 = 22;\ 11$
58. $5 \underline{\ ?\ } y \underline{\ ?\ } 3 = 7;\ 2$

59. $24 \underline{\ ?\ } x \underline{\ ?\ } 15 = 18;\ 8$
60. $60 \underline{\ ?\ } m \underline{\ ?\ } 2 = 15;\ 2$

Review Exercises

Evaluate the expression when $m = 2$, $n = 1$, and $p = 4$.

1. $2n^2$
2. $(m + n)^0$
3. $3p^2 + m^2$
4. $n^2 + m^3$

5. $p^3 - (mn)^2$
6. $2p^2 - n^0$
7. $4m^3 - n^3$
8. $(2mn^2)^0$

1-8 A Plan for Solving Problems

What we know about mathematics enables us to solve many problems. Problems, however, are not usually as neatly organized as the information in the expressions with which we have been working. We must sort out and organize the facts of a problem before we begin to solve. A plan such as the one below can be useful in solving many kinds of problems.

Plan for Solving Word Problems

1. Read the problem carefully. Make sure that you understand what it says. You may need to read it more than once.

2. Use questions like these in planning the solution:
What is asked for?
What facts are given?
Are enough facts given? If not, what else is needed?
Are unnecessary facts given? If so, what are they?
Will a sketch or diagram help?

3. Determine which operation or operations can be used to solve the problem.

4. Carry out the operations carefully.

5. Check your results with the facts given in the problem. Give the answer.

EXAMPLE 1 On Saturday, the Nizel family drove 17 mi from Topsfield to Newton and 22.5 mi from Newton to Harbor Bluffs. The trip took 50 min. On the way back, the Nizels took the same route, but they stopped for lunch after driving 9.5 mi. If they continue on the same route after lunch, how much farther will they have to drive to return to Topsfield?

Solution

• The problem asks for the number of miles to return to Topsfield.

• The following facts are given in the problem:

>   17 mi from Topsfield to Newton
>   22.5 mi from Newton to Harbor Bluffs
>   drove 9.5 mi back toward Topsfield

(The solution is continued on the next page.)

- We have enough facts to solve the problem since we know the distance between the cities and the distance driven toward Topsfield.

- We do not need to know that the trip took 50 min.

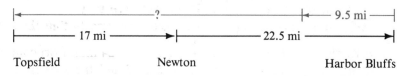

Topsfield   Newton   Harbor Bluffs

- The sketch shows that we subtract the distance driven back toward Topsfield from the distance between Topsfield and Harbor Bluffs.

$$(17 + 22.5) - 9.5 = 30$$

- Check: If they drive 9.5 mi and 30 mi farther, will the Nizels have driven the distance from Harbor Bluffs to Topsfield?

$$9.5 + 30 = 17 + 22.5 \checkmark$$

The Nizels must drive 30 mi to return to Topsfield.

EXAMPLE 2   Records at the Howard City Weather Bureau show that it rained on a total of 17 days during the months of July through September and on twice as many days during the months of October through December. During October through December, how many days did not have rain?

Solution

- The problem asks for the number of days without rain during October, November, and December.

- Given facts: 17 days of rain in July through September
  twice as many days of rain in October through December

- We need to supply these facts:
  31 days in October, 30 days in November, 31 days in December

- To find the number of days without rain, subtract the number of days that did have rain from the total number of days.
  $$(31 + 30 + 31) - (2 \times 17) = 92 - 34 = 58$$

- Check: Are 34 days twice as many as 17? $34 \div 2 = 17 \checkmark$
  Do 58 days without rain and 34 days with rain total the number of days in the three months?
  $$58 + 34 = 31 + 30 + 31 \checkmark$$

During October through December, 58 days did not have rain.

Class Exercises

For each problem, answer the following questions.
a. What number or numbers does the problem ask for?
b. Are enough facts given? If not, what else is needed?
c. Are unneeded facts given? If so, what are they?
d. What operation or operations would you use to find the answer?

1. Kevin completed the bicycle race in 2 h 24 min, Lori completed the race in 2 h 13 min, and Helen completed the race in 2 h 54 min. How much faster than Kevin's time was Lori's time?

2. Steve bought 1 lb of Swiss cheese, 12 oz of mild cheddar cheese, and 6 oz of sharp cheddar cheese. How much cheese did he buy in all?

3. Elise bought a record for $5.69, another record for $4.88, and a record cleaning kit for $12.75. How much more than the cost of the records was the cost of the kit?

4. The eighth-grade classes are holding a hobbies and crafts fair on Saturday. Maurice plans to help out at the stamp-collecting booth from 9 A.M. to 11 A.M. and at the model-airplane booth from 2 P.M. to 5 P.M. How many hours does he plan to spend helping?

Problems

Solve, using the five-step plan.

A 1. Mimi is buying weather-stripping tape for some windows. How much should she buy for a window that needs 4.85 m, a window that needs 4.25 m, and a window that needs 2.55 m?

2. Irene Lanata pays $235.40 each month to repay her automobile loan. How much will she pay in one year?

3. Hill School plans to buy 4 computers for each of 12 classrooms. The cost of each computer is $865. What will the total cost be?

4. An 8 mm camera shoots 24 frames of film each second. How many frames will it shoot in 5 min?

5. A package of 2 paintbrushes is on sale for $2.40. How much will 3 packages cost?

6. Roy paid $81.88 for a new jacket and sweater. He then exchanged the sweater, which cost $23.00, for another sweater that cost $19.99. What was the final cost for Roy's jacket and sweater?

Solve, using the five-step plan.

7. There are 38 rows with 2 dozen seats each in the Little Theater. An additional 24 people are allowed to stand during a performance. What is the total number of people that can attend a performance?

8. Yesterday it took Jeff Holland 1 h to get to work. This morning, Jeff drove to the train station in 20 min, waited for the train for 7 min, rode the train for 12 min, and then walked for 15 min to get to work. How long did it take Jeff to get to work this morning?

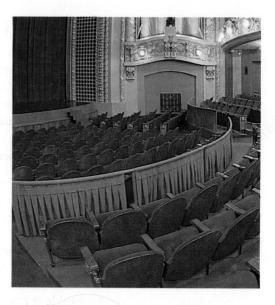

B 9. Tickets for the drama club's performance last weekend cost $2.50 for adults and $2.00 for students. Four hundred twenty adults attended the performance, and 273 students attended. What was the total amount of money collected from tickets for the performance last weekend?

10. Sarah Holness had her car tuned up for $60 and she purchased 4 new tires for $37 each. She gave the cashier 11 twenty-dollar bills. How much change did Sarah receive?

C 11. Joy and David Kramer had $30 to spend on dinner, a movie, and parking. Dinner cost $15.50 and parking cost $4. The Kramers had $2 left after paying for everything. What was the cost of one movie ticket?

12. The museum charges $4.50 per person for a 2 h tour with fewer than 20 people. If 20 or more people take the tour, the charge is $3.75 per person. Of the 23 people in today's tour, 17 had paid $4.50 in advance. How much money will the museum return as a refund?

Review Exercises

Estimate the answer using rounding.

1. 267 + 73	**2.** 941 − 189	**3.** 82.7 + 91.8	**4.** 261.6 − 131.9
5. 24 × 18	**6.** 36 × 41	**7.** 21.3 × 19.6	**8.** 18.7 × 29.3

1-9 Solving and Checking Problems

The five-step plan shown in the preceding lesson can be used to solve many problems. It is also useful to have methods for checking answers to problems. For example, when planning your solution to a problem, you may find that there is more than one way to proceed. When there is more than one method for solving a problem, you may find it helpful to use one method to obtain an answer and to use the other method to check your results. Study the following example.

EXAMPLE 1   The Treble Clef celebrated Heritage Day with a two-week sale on the Flexwood turntables. Twelve turntables were sold during the first week of the sale and 17 were sold during the second week of the sale. The sale price for each turntable was $74.90. How much money did the Treble Clef receive for the turntables sold?

Solution
- The problem asks for the amount of money received from the sale of the turntables.

- Given facts: 12 turntables sold the first week
17 more sold the second week
$74.90 received for each turntable

- There are two ways to solve this problem.

Method 1
First multiply the sale price by the number sold each week to find the amount of money received each week.

$$12 \times 74.90 = 898.80 \qquad 17 \times 74.90 = 1273.30$$

Then add the amounts of money received to find the total amount of money received from the sale of the turntables.

$$898.80 + 1273.30 = 2172.10$$

Method 2
First add to find the total number of turntables sold during the sale.

$$12 + 17 = 29$$

Then multiply the sale price by the total number sold to find the amount of money received from the sale of the turntables.

$$29 \times 74.90 = 2172.10$$

- By either method, the Treble Clef received $2172.10 from the sale of the turntables.

Another way to check an answer is to use rounding to find an estimated answer. If the answer and the estimate are close, then the estimate leads us to accept our answer.

EXAMPLE 2   Last summer Elka and David drove from Los Angeles to Boston. Along the way they stopped in Albuquerque, Kansas City, Atlanta, and Washington, D.C. They recorded the distance they traveled, as shown below.

Los Angeles–Albuquerque	806 mi
Albuquerque–Kansas City	790 mi
Kansas City–Atlanta	810 mi
Atlanta–Washington, D.C.	630 mi
Washington, D.C.–Boston	437 mi

How many miles did Elka and David travel?

Solution

• The problem asks for the total distance traveled.

• Given facts: traveled 806 mi, 790 mi, 810 mi, 630 mi, 437 mi

• To find the total distance traveled, we add.

$$806 + 790 + 810 + 630 + 437 = 3473$$

• Elka and David traveled 3473 miles on their trip.

To check the answer, we round the distances and add. In this case, round to the nearest hundred miles.

$$800 + 800 + 800 + 600 + 400 = 3400$$

The estimate, 3400 mi, and the answer, 3473 mi, are quite close, so the actual answer seems reasonable.

Class Exercises

State the operations you would use to solve the problem and the order in which you would use them.

1. The Dreyer Trucking Company moved 453 cartons one day, and then 485 the next day. On the third day they moved twice as many as on the first two days. What is the total number of cartons moved during those three days?

2. In January, Judy made the following deposits to her savings account: $107.50, $29.35, and $43.20. In February, she deposited twice as much money as in January. How much money did she deposit each month?

State two methods that you could use to solve the problem.

3. Three friends went out to dinner. The bill was $41.10, and they left a $6.15 tip. If they divide the total three ways, how much did each person pay?

4. Jay Elder took some clothes to Spotless Drycleaning. He was charged $4.00 for a jacket, $2.50 for a sweater, and $2.25 for a pair of slacks. Jay had coupons that allowed him to deduct $.50 from each item. How much will Jay pay for his drycleaning?

Estimate the answer to the problem.

5. Frank is in the check-out line at the grocery store. He has a gallon of milk ($1.83), a bag of flour ($2.15), a box of oatmeal ($1.15), a package of cheese ($1.57), and a dozen eggs ($1.05). How much is the bill?

6. Breda wants to buy a four-door sedan that has a base price of $5624.95, factory-installed options totalling $1213.50, and a destination charge of $183.00. How much does the car cost?

Problems

Solve. Check to be sure you have answered the question.

A **1.** The August electric bill for $75.80 was twice as much as the July bill. What was the total cost of electricity for July and August?

2. Alvin has $1863.50 in his savings account. His sister Alvis has $756 more in her account. Geoffrey borrowed $257 from each person. How much money do Alvin and Alvis have left in each of their accounts after making the loans?

3. Gregory ordered the following items from the Huntington Gardens catalog: a watering can for $15.80, a trowel for $4.49, and 6 packages of seeds for $.75 each. What is the total cost of the items?

4. Nancy's mobile needs 3 separate pieces of wire that measure 8 cm, 11 cm, and 15 cm. Nina's mobile needs two times the length of wire that Nancy's mobile needs. How much wire is needed for each mobile?

Solve. Check by using an alternate method.

5. Each member of the Best Buy Book Club receives 2 bonus points for every book ordered through the club. So far Chris has ordered 3 books in March, 2 in April, and 6 in May. How many bonus points has Chris accumulated so far?

6. The admission ticket to Tyler Amusement Park is $1.25 per person. A total of 815 tickets were sold on Saturday. The attendance decreased by 96 on Sunday. How much money did the park receive from ticket sales in all?

Solve. Check by estimating the answer to the problem.

7. Bonnema Brothers recently purchased four beach front lots of land. The areas of the two smaller lots are 2015 ft² and 2248 ft². The areas of the two larger lots are 8730 ft² and 7890 ft². What is the total area of the two smaller lots and the total area of the two larger lots?

8. Lake Tana in Africa has an elevation of 1829 m. Lake Tangra Tso in Tibet is situated 4724 m above sea level. In Europe, Lake Sevan has an elevation of 1915 m. What is the total height of the three lakes?

9. During one game at a bowling tournament the five-member Bright Team scored the following points: 169, 152, 187, 174, and 193. What is the difference between the highest and the lowest scores?

10. Jackie is taking an inventory of the furniture going on sale next week.

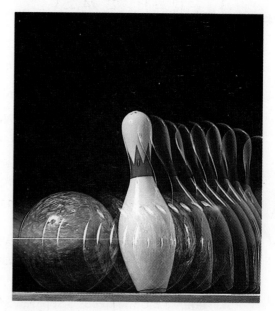

sofas, 128	platform beds, 250
love seats, 105	stereo cabinets, 83
lamps, 216	bookcases, 45

How many items are going on sale?

Solve.

B 11. The Hillview School Band held a car wash on Friday and Saturday. The charge was $2.25 per car on Friday and $2.50 per car on Saturday. On Friday, 87 cars were washed. On Saturday, 117 cars were washed. What was the total amount of money collected?

12. A photograph is enlarged so that its new dimensions are four times its original dimensions. If the new dimensions are 19.2 cm by 25.6 cm, what were the original dimensions?

13. Today the firm of Beckman and Beckman bought three types of stocks: 4780 shares of utility stocks, 1389 shares of commodity stocks, and 3542 shares of energy-related stocks. This is exactly three times the number of shares the firm bought yesterday. How many shares of stock did the firm buy in the past two days?

14. Yukio bought traveler's checks in the following denominations: five $50 checks, thirty $20 checks, five $10 checks, and twenty $5 checks. What is the total value of the checks bought?

15. A direct dial call from Boston to Australia costs $3.17 for the first minute and $1.19 for each additional minute. A station-to-station operator-assisted call costs $9.45 for the first 3 minutes and $1.19 for each additional minute. How much money would you save by dialing direct for a 5-minute call?

Self-Test B

Solve for the given replacement set.

1. $72 - m = 43$; $\{19, 29, 31\}$ 2. $6r = 48$; $\{6, 7, 8\}$ [1-6]

3. $t \div 12 = 11$; $\{23, 24, 25\}$ 4. $4d + 16 = 28$; $\{3, 4, 5\}$

Use inverse operations to solve.

5. $g - 32 = 12$ 6. $7d = 112$ 7. $5a + 4 = 49$ [1-7]

Solve, using the five-step plan.

8. Laura bought a hammer for $12.95, 5 lb of nails for $5.20, and 8 sheets of plywood for $12 each. What was her total bill?   [1-8]

9. Between the hours of 6 A.M. and 9 P.M., 8 buses that were filled to capacity left the terminal. If the capacity of each bus is the same and 392 tickets were sold, how many passengers were on each bus?

Solve. Check by estimating.

10. Jeremy and his roommate share the monthly utility bills evenly. For November the cost of electricity was $87.90, gas was $24.35, heating fuel was $215.80, and water was $36.43. How much did each person pay that month?   [1-9]

Self-Test answers and Extra Practice are at the back of the book.

The Development of Computers

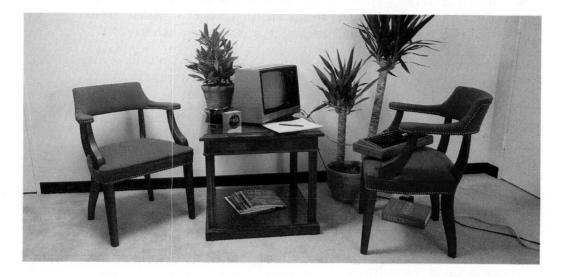

The development of the modern computer began in 1946 with the completion of the ENIAC computer. It weighed 30 tons, contained 18,000 vacuum tubes and 6000 switches, and filled a room 30 feet by 50 feet. Since that time computers have become steadily more compact, powerful, and inexpensive.

Today's large computer systems, called **mainframes,** can process large amounts of data at very fast speeds. **Minicomputers** are smaller and somewhat slower, meeting the needs of colleges and small businesses at lower cost. The smallest of today's computers, such as the computer shown in the photo above, are the **microcomputers.** These computers are often called personal computers because they are inexpensive enough and small enough to go into classrooms and homes. The processing unit of these small computers is the **microprocessor,** a one-quarter-inch-square integrated circuit chip. This tiny chip is more powerful than the ENIAC with its 18,000 vacuum tubes.

The microprocessor controls the microcomputer and performs arithmetic operations. But other parts are needed to make the computer a useful tool. The computer has two kinds of **memory. ROM** (read only memory) permanently stores information needed for the computer to work properly. It cannot be changed by the user. **RAM** (random access memory) is available to the user and can store the user's programs and data. Memory size is measured in **bytes** or K. One K is about 1000 bytes. Each byte can store one character (letter or digit), so an 8K memory can store about 8000 typed characters.

The **keyboard** is used to input programs and data, and the **CRT** screen displays input, results, and graphics. A **disk drive** can be used to read programs and data into the computer from a disk, or to save programs on disk. A **printer** will save output in printed form. A **modem** can connect you to a network of other computers over your telephone line.

As computers have evolved, people have invented programming languages to help users program the computer to solve problems. Some of the more common languages are **BASIC,** which is available on almost all microcomputers, **FORTRAN,** often used for scientific problem solving, and **COBOL,** a business-oriented language. **Pascal** and **Logo** are two languages finding increasing application in education.

The development of computers has opened many new careers. Systems analysts use computers to analyze and solve problems for business and government. Programmers write the programs, or software, that help users apply the computer to their needs. Installation and maintenance of a computer's physical components, or hardware, are done by field engineers.

1. The fastest modern computers can do 100 million arithmetic operations in a second. Estimate how long it would take you to do this many additions. Suppose you are adding two four-digit numbers each time.

2. Each byte of memory will hold one typed character. About how many K of memory would it take to store these two pages? A disk for a microcomputer holds 160 K. About how many pages of this book could you store on one disk?

3. Ask your librarian to help you find out about the Mark I, IBM 360, and UNIVAC 1 computers. Find out about the size of each computer, the number of its components, its purpose, its inventors.

4. The computer language ADA was named after Ada Byron Lovelace (1815–1852). See what you can find out about Ada Lovelace and the computer language.

Career Activity

Look in the Help Wanted section of a newspaper and make a list of the job openings for systems analysts and programmers. Include in your list education requirements, what computers or computer languages the candidate should be familiar with, and the salary range.

Chapter Review

1-21 all

1 4
over

Match.

1. 22×8 2. $52.6 - 9.95$ **A.** 32   **B.** 10^8 [1–1]

3. $9 \times (3 + 1) - 4$ 4. $\dfrac{4 + (6 \times 2 \times 5)}{(14 - 12)5}$ **C.** 42.65   **D.** 64   [1–2]

5. 4^3 6. $100,000,000$ **E.** 6.4   **F.** 176   [1–3]

True or false?

7. 21.09 to the nearest whole number is 20.   [1–4]

8. 124.4 to the nearest hundred is 100.

9. 83.415 to the nearest hundredth is 83.42.

10. 0.959 to the nearest tenth is 1.0.

11. $(17.2 + 1.8)4 = (1.8 + 17.2)4$ illustrates the commutative property.   [1–5]

12. $(8 + 7.9)2.3 = (8 \times 2.3) + (7.9 \times 2.3)$ illustrates the distributive property of multiplication with respect to subtraction.

13. $1.3(7 + 4) = (7 + 4)1.3$ illustrates the associative property.

Is the equation true or false for the given value of the variable?

14. $9y = 108$; $y = 12$ 15. $k \div 4 = 28$; $k = 7$ [1–6]

True or false?

16. If $k + 5 = 140$, $k = 140 - 5$.   17. If $p \div 21 = 14$, $p = 21 - 14$.   [1–7]

18. If $9b = 162$, $b = 162 \div 9$.   19. If $t - 87 = 87$, $t = 87 - 87$.

Write the letter of the correct answer.

20. Julia Carmona hired 3 people to landscape her yard. They each received the same hourly rate and it took them 5 h to do the job. If her bill was $60, how much did each person earn an hour?   [1–8]
    a. $6   **b.** $12   **c.** $3   **d.** $4

21. To raise money for a local charity, the 26 students of the eighth-grade class participated in a bike-a-thon. Each of the sponsors agreed to pay the students $.35 for each mile they rode their bicycles. If 20 students ride 20 mi each and the rest of the students ride 30 mi each, for how many miles will the students be paid?   [1–9]
    a. $203   **b.** 50 mi   **c.** $17.50   **d.** 580 mi

Chapter Test

Evaluate the expression when $a = 4$ and $b = 12$.

1. $91 + a$ **2.** $27 - b - a$ **3.** $5b$ **4.** $36 \div a$ [1–1]

Evaluate the expression when $m = 14$ and $n = 16$.

5. $n - 4 \times 3$ **6.** $3 \times \frac{m}{7}$ **7.** $2mn - 9$ **8.** $(m + n) \div 3$ [1–2]

Evaluate.

9. 3^4 **10.** 10^3 **11.** 2^5 [1–3]

Write as a single power of 10.

12. $10^4 \times 10^7$ **13.** $10^6 \times 10^6$ **14.** 10,000

Round to the place specified.

15. tenths: 7.49   **16.** tens: 423.6   **17.** hundredths: 4.283   [1–4]

What value of the variable makes the statement true?

18. $2.4 + (r + 9.5) = 2.4 + (9.5 + 7.8)$ **19.** $19.2k = k$ [1–5]

20. $62d - 19d = (62 - 19)4$ **21.** $1(3.4 + 1.3) = a$

Solve for the given replacement set.

22. $d - 9 = 27$; $\{3, 18, 35\}$ **23.** $14r = 70$; $\{3, 4, 5\}$ [1–6]

24. $9(x + 4) = 63$; $\{1, 2, 3\}$ **25.** $3k + 1 = 13$; $\{4, 5, 6\}$

Use inverse operations to solve.

26. $6g = 72$ **27.** $b \div 9 = 44$ **28.** $3f - 1 = 53$ [1–7]

Solve, using the five-step plan.

29. The tickets for the theater cost $7.50 each. Miles bought 4 of them and gave the cashier a fifty dollar bill. What was the cost of the tickets?   [1–8]

Solve and check your answer.

30. For the trip, Kari bought 3 stocking caps for $6.75 each and 3 scarfs for $8.50 each. How much money did she spend?   [1–9]

Cumulative Review

Exercises

Simplify.

1. $28 + 781$

2. $630 - 52.1$

3. $65.1 \div 21$

4. 1.2×3.64

5. $48 + 303.9$

6. 0.042×0.8

7. $3(14 - 5)$

8. $(6 + 3) \div 9$

9. $4 \times 5 + 5$

10. $16 - 2 \times 3 - 1$

11. $(8 + 2) \div (12 - 7)$

12. $(14 + 36) \times (54 - 8)$

Evaluate the expression when $a = 2$, $b = 5$, and $c = 3$.

13. $5b + 18$

14. $9c - 12$

15. $3b + c \div 2$

16. $4ab - 8$

17. $30 \div (a + c)$

18. $a(12 - c)b$

Simplify.

19. 3^3

20. 4^3

21. 2^6

22. 6^4

23. 5^6

24. 11^4

Select the most reasonable estimated answer.

25. $43.6 - 2.79$ **a.** 41   **b.** 20   **c.** 45

26. 9.6×53.66 **a.** 500   **b.** 450   **c.** 540

27. $22.7 + 18.9 + 7.38$ **a.** 49   **b.** 37   **c.** 110

28. $165.7 + 38.21 + 6.44$ **a.** 1300   **b.** 210   **c.** 246

True or false?

29. $16 \div 8 + 2 = 16 \div (8 + 2)$

30. $99.5 - (6 + 7) = (99.5 - 6) + 7$

31. $(43 \times 0) + (43 \times 1) = 0$

32. $11.89 + (426 \div 2) = (11.89 + 426) \div 2$

Find the solution of the equation for the given replacement set.

33. $k + 16 = 23$; $\{5, 6, 7\}$

34. $58 - d = 31$; $\{39, 38, 37\}$

35. $7x - 1 = 20$; $\{1, 2, 3\}$

36. $8(y - 3) = 32$; $\{7, 8, 9\}$

37. $5a = 2a + 57$; $\{19, 20, 21\}$

38. $(c + 6) \div 6 = 1$; $\{0, 1, 2\}$

Use inverse operations to solve.

39. $18 + g = 20$

40. $a \div 9 = 18$

41. $5z = 65$

42. $20d + 8 = 68$

43. $7f - 1 = 13$

44. $3h + 2 = 26$

Problems

Solve.

1. Merry and Sandy rented an apartment for $645 each month and shared the rent equally. After 4 months, Tess moved in and the rent was divided three ways. How much was Merry's rent for the year?

2. Hungarian paprika costs $1.30 for 2 oz, $4.00 for $\frac{1}{2}$ lb, and $6.00 for a pound. What is the cost of each ounce if you buy a pound? How much do you save per ounce if you buy a pound?

3. Mal ordered a set of 6 steak knives for $35.00. Additional costs included $4.95 for shipping, $1.25 for a gift box, and $1.75 for tax. What was the total cost of the order?

4. "I can save $19.50 if I buy a half dozen glasses on sale," said Ellis. How much is saved on each glass? If Ellis pays $30.00 for 6 glasses on sale, what was the original price of each glass?

5. House numerals that are 4 in. high cost $4.00 each. Numerals that are 7 in. high cost $10.00 each. How much will it cost to buy numerals that are 4 in. high for your house if your address is 16332 Long Meadow Road?

6. In 1918, a sheet of 100 airmail stamps was mistakenly printed with an airplane upside down. A stamp collector bought the sheet for $.24 per stamp and later sold the sheet for $15,000. How much did the collector make on his lucky buy?

7. A membership to the Science Center costs $53 per year and includes a subscription to a monthly magazine. If the magazine costs $3 per issue, what are the annual dues for membership alone?

8. Dale took advantage of the gas company's offer to make average monthly payments. The payments were based on the average of the two highest and the two lowest bills for the past 12 months. If these bills were $135.50, $142.71, $68.29, and $56.30, what is Dale's average monthly payment?

2

Positive and Negative Numbers

Lightning, as seen in the photograph, is a dramatic, electrical reaction that is usually associated with thunderclouds. It occurs as a result of a sudden, powerful exchange between the positive and negative centers within a cloud, between several clouds, or between a cloud, the air, and the ground. The long flash of light we see is part of the interaction. The positive and negative charges move through the atmosphere so rapidly that a tremendous amount of heat is generated, which warms up the surrounding air so quickly that a thunderous explosion results.

In this chapter you will study operations with positive and negative numbers.

Career Note

Earthquakes are similar to lightning in that they are sudden, dramatic natural events. Geologists study earthquakes as part of their study of the earth. By studying the structure and history of the rocks beneath the earth's surface, geologists may be able to predict future earthquakes. Geologists can also specialize in locating oil and other raw materials.

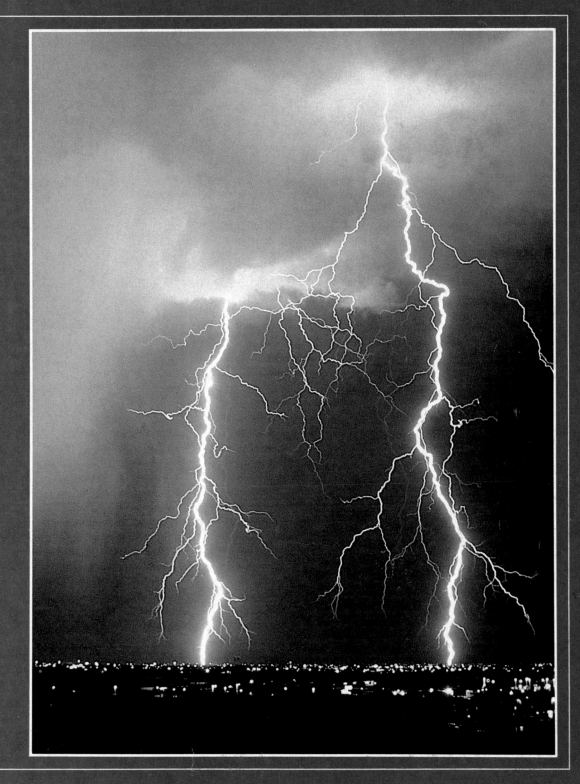

2-1 The Integers

When we measure temperature, we use a scale that has 0 as a reference point. We use *positive numbers* to indicate temperatures above 0°, and we use *negative numbers* to indicate temperatures below 0°.

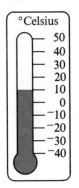

We often have occasion to measure quantities on different sides of a zero reference point, such as distances above and below sea level, time before and after a rocket launch, increases and decreases in stock prices, and deposits and withdrawals in a bank account. Positive and negative numbers help us to measure these quantities.

We may graph both positive and negative numbers on a horizontal number line by extending the number line to the *left* of the origin as shown below. Like the positive whole numbers, the negative whole numbers are equally spaced, but they are positioned to the left of 0.

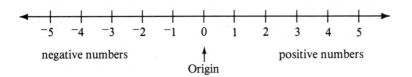

We read $^-1$ as *negative one.* We may read 1 as *positive one,* or simply *one.* For emphasis, we may use the symbol $^+1$ for positive one.

Any pair of numbers, such as 3 and $^-3$, that are the same distance from the origin but in opposite directions are called **opposites.** The opposite of 3 is $^-3$ and the opposite of $^-3$ is 3. The opposite of 0 is 0.

We use the symbol $|^-3|$, read *the absolute value of $^-3$,* to represent the distance between $^-3$ and 0. Because $^-3$ is 3 units from the origin, $|^-3| = 3$. In general, $|n|$ (read *the absolute value of n*) represents the distance between the number n and the origin.

The whole numbers, 0, 1, 2, 3, . . . , together with their opposites, 0, $^-1$, $^-2$, $^-3$, . . . , form the set of numbers called the **integers:**

$$. . . , \ ^-3, \ ^-2, \ ^-1, 0, 1, 2, 3, ...$$

The **positive integers** are the numbers 1, 2, 3, . . . , and the **negative integers** are the numbers $^-1$, $^-2$, $^-3$, ... Although 0 is an integer, it is neither positive nor negative.

EXAMPLE 1   Express as an integer.

       a. $|^-5|$ **b.** $|0|$

Solution   **a.** $|^-5|$ represents the distance between 0 and the number $^-5$. Thus $|^-5| = 5$.

       b. $|0|$ represents the distance between 0 and 0. Thus $|0| = 0$.

EXAMPLE 2   Arrange $^-3$, 1, $^-4$, 0, $^-1$ in order from least to greatest.

Solution   We can graph the numbers on a number line, with 1 at the right of 0.

Reading the coordinates of the points from left to right will order the numbers from least to greatest. $^-4$, $^-3$, $^-1$, 0, 1

Positive and negative numbers may be compared using inequality symbols as well as on the number line. The inequality symbols $>$ and $<$ are used to compare mathematical expressions. The use of these symbols in inequalities is shown below.

           $8 > 6$ $6 < 8$

Eight is greater than six.   Six is less than eight.

To avoid confusing these symbols, think of them as arrowheads whose small ends point toward the smaller numbers.

We can indicate that one number is between two others by combining two inequalities. We know that $5 < 6$ and $6 < 8$; thus we can write

             $5 < 6 < 8$ or $8 > 6 > 5.$

Other inequality symbols that we use are shown below with their meanings.

           $\neq$ *is not equal to*
           $\geq$ *is greater than or equal to*
           $\leq$ *is less than or equal to*

We can use inequality symbols to write open sentences. The open sentence $n \leq 6$ means $n < 6$ or $n = 6$.

EXAMPLE 3   Replace __?__ with $<$ or $>$.

       a. 14 __?__ 2   **b.** 1 __?__ 11   **c.** 8 __?__ 3 __?__ 0

Solution   **a.** $14 > 2$ **b.** $1 < 11$ **c.** $8 > 3 > 0$

Class Exercises

Name an integer that represents each of the following.

1. 15 s before blastoff of a rocket

2. A gain of 6 yd in a football play

3. A withdrawal of 90 dollars from a bank account

4. An elevation of 350 ft below sea level

5. The opposite of 80   6. The opposite of $^-2$

7. The absolute value of $^-14$ 8. The absolute value of 27

9. Name two integers, each of which is 12 units from 0.

10. If $|n| = 15$, then $n = \underline{\ ?\ }$ or $n = \underline{\ ?\ }$.

Replace $\underline{\ ?\ }$ with > or < to make a true statement.

11. **a.** $^-6 \underline{\ ?\ } ^-2$ **b.** $|^-6| \underline{\ ?\ } |^-2|$ 12. **a.** $4 \underline{\ ?\ } ^-5$ **b.** $|4| \underline{\ ?\ } |^-5|$

True or false?

13. $7 > 7$ 14. $18 \leq 20$ 15. $15 > 5$

16. $14 > 6 > 2$ 17. $20 < 18 < 16$ 18. $33 \geq 24 \geq 11$

Written Exercises

Graph the integers in each exercise on the same number line.

A   1. $0, 1, ^-1, 3, ^-3$ 2. $0, 2, ^-2, 5, ^-5$ 3. $6, 0, ^-4, ^-9, 7$ 4. $^-1, 3, ^-8, 4, ^-6$

Graph the number and its opposite on the same number line.

5. 3   6. 10   7. $^-7$ 8. $^-2$ 9. 0   10. $^-4$

Replace $\underline{\ ?\ }$ with =, >, or < to make a true statement.

11. $21 \underline{\ ?\ } 14$ 12. $18 \underline{\ ?\ } 35$ 13. $76 \underline{\ ?\ } 67$

14. $104 \underline{\ ?\ } 104$ 15. $265 \underline{\ ?\ } 256$ 16. $390 \underline{\ ?\ } 309$

17. $17 + 82 \underline{\ ?\ } 93$ 18. $47 - 31 \underline{\ ?\ } 61$ 19. $25 \div 5 \underline{\ ?\ } 10$

20. $26 \times 4 \underline{\ ?\ } 52$ 21. $19 \times 11 \underline{\ ?\ } 208$ 22. $84 \div 3 \underline{\ ?\ } 24$

23. $^-3 \underline{\ ?\ } ^-4$ 24. $^-2 \underline{\ ?\ } 1$ 25. $7 \underline{\ ?\ } ^-8$

26. $0 \underline{\ ?\ } ^-2$ 27. $^-11 \underline{\ ?\ } 0$ 28. $^-7 \underline{\ ?\ } 10$

Use > or < to write a true statement with the given numbers.

29. 18, 46, 32   **30.** 29, 5, 31   **31.** 103, 130, 310

32. 256, 652, 526   **33.** 986, 689, 698   **34.** 717, 177, 771

Express as an integer.

35. $|^-3|$ **36.** $|^-6|$ **37.** $|0|$ **38.** $|12|$ **39.** $|9|$ **40.** $|^-7|$ **41.** $|^-8|$ **42.** $|^-1|$

Write the numbers in order from least to greatest.

43. 6, $^-15$, 0, $^-2$ **44.** $^-3$, 1, 0, $^-7$

45. $^-12$, 7, $^-8$, 1, $^-1$ **46.** 0, 2, $^-5$, $^-9$, 10

47. $^-10$, 4, 14, $^-14$, 8   **48.** 3, 9, $^-13$, 11, $^-15$

49. $^-6.4$, 0.6, 3.1, $^-2.7$ **50.** 7.1, $^-0.9$, $^-3.6$, $^-9.4$

For Exercises 51–62, (a) list the integers that can replace n to make the statement true, and (b) graph the integers on a number line.

B **51.** $|n| = 6$ **52.** $|n| = 3$ **53.** $|n| = 4$

 54. $|n| = 5$ **55.** $|n| = 0$ **56.** $|n| = 14$

 57. $|n| < 2$ **58.** $|n| < 5$ **59.** $|n| \le 4$

 60. $|n| \le 7$ **61.** $2 < |n| < 8$ **62.** $0 < |n| < 3$

Complete with the word *positive* or *negative*.

C **63.** If an integer is equal to its absolute value, then the integer must be
    a ___?___ integer or 0.

 64. If an integer is equal to the opposite of its absolute value, then the
    integer must be a ___?___ integer or 0.

 65. Explain why there is no number that can replace n to make the
    equation $|n| = {}^-3$ true.

Review Exercises

Graph the number on a number line.

1. 4   **2.** 6   **3.** 3   **4.** 0   **5.** 2.4

6. 1.3   **7.** $3\frac{1}{2}$ **8.** $1\frac{1}{3}$ **9.** 3.7   **10.** 4.5

2-2 Decimals on the Number Line

The graphs of the *positive decimal* 2.5 and its opposite, the *negative decimal* ⁻2.5, are shown on the number line below. We graph 2.5 by locating the point that is 2.5 units to the *right* of 0, and we graph ⁻2.5 by locating the point that is 2.5 units to the *left* of 0.

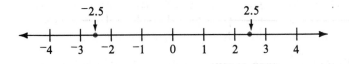

The positive decimals together with the negative decimals and 0 form the set of *decimal numbers*. The set of decimal numbers includes all of the whole numbers and all of the integers.

EXAMPLE 1   Write the following numbers in order from least to greatest.

$$^-2, 4.1, 0.2, ^-2.6, ^-1.34$$

Solution   We can graph the given numbers on a number line.

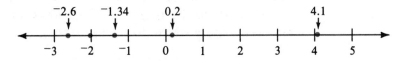

Reading the coordinates from left to right will give the numbers in order from least to greatest.

$$^-2.6, ^-2, ^-1.34, 0.2, 4.1$$

We have been representing decimals by their graphs, that is, by dots on a number line. We can also use directed line segments or arrows to illustrate decimals. Arrows that point to the *left* (the negative direction) represent negative numbers. Arrows that point to the *right* (the positive direction) represent positive numbers.

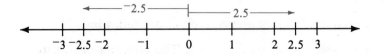

Notice in the diagram above that both the arrow representing ⁻2.5 and the arrow representing 2.5 have length 2.5.

An arrow representing a number may have any point on the number line as its starting point, as long as it has length and direction indicated by that number. The length of the arrow is the absolute value of the number that the arrow represents. The direction of the arrow is determined by the sign of the number.

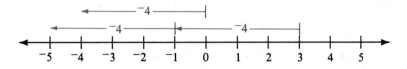

On the number line above, each arrow represents the decimal number ⁻4, for each has length 4 and points to the left.

EXAMPLE 2   What number is represented by the arrow above the number line below?

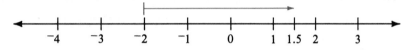

Solution   The starting point of the arrow is ⁻2 and the endpoint is 1.5. The arrow points to the right and is 3.5 units long. Thus, the arrow represents the positive decimal number 3.5.

EXAMPLE 3   An arrow representing the number ⁻7 has starting point 3. What is its endpoint?

Solution   Draw a number line. Starting at 3, draw an arrow 7 units long in the negative direction (left). The endpoint of the arrow is ⁻4.

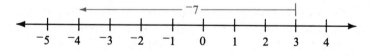

Class Exercises

Name a decimal number that represents each of the following.

1. The opposite of 8.71

2. The opposite of ⁻10.16

3. A discount of fifty-nine cents −.59

4. A rise in body temperature of 0.6°C
+0.6

5. The absolute value of ⁻67.5

6. The absolute value of 9.07

7. Name the letter written above the graph of the given number.

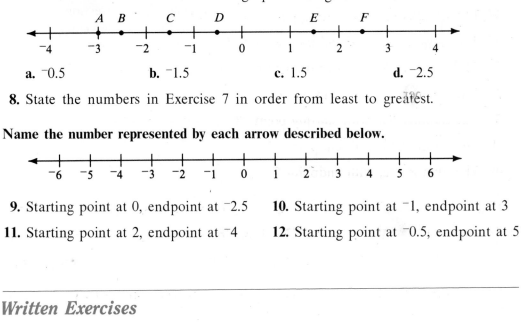

a. ⁻0.5   **b.** ⁻1.5   **c.** 1.5   **d.** ⁻2.5

8. State the numbers in Exercise 7 in order from least to greatest.

Name the number represented by each arrow described below.

9. Starting point at 0, endpoint at ⁻2.5   **10.** Starting point at ⁻1, endpoint at 3

11. Starting point at 2, endpoint at ⁻4   **12.** Starting point at ⁻0.5, endpoint at 5

Written Exercises

Graph the numbers in each exercise on the same number line.

A   **1.** ⁻2, ⁻3.5, 0   **2.** 3.2, ⁻4, ⁻3.2   **3.** ⁻1.5, ⁻7, ⁻3.25   **4.** ⁻0.9, ⁻1, ⁻4.1

Graph the number and its opposite on the same number line.

5. 2.25   **6.** 1.9   **7.** ⁻0.5   **8.** ⁻3.1

9. ⁻4.2   **10.** 0.75   **11.** 0.3   **12.** 5.5

Write the decimal number that is equal to each of the following.

13. |⁻2.36| **14.** |1.921| **15.** |⁻16| **16.** |⁻100| **17.** |3.03| **18.** |⁻0.2|

Replace $\underline{\ ?\ }$ **with < or > to make a true statement.**

19. ⁻2.93 $\underline{\ ?\ }$ 1.1   **20.** 4 $\underline{\ ?\ }$ ⁻0.5   **21.** ⁻8.1 $\underline{\ ?\ }$ 2.3

22. ⁻1.95 $\underline{\ ?\ }$ ⁻1.96   **23.** ⁻5.01 $\underline{\ ?\ }$ ⁻4.99   **24.** ⁻2.99 $\underline{\ ?\ }$ ⁻2.98

25. 0.1 $\underline{\ ?\ }$ ⁻18.25   **26.** 12.2 $\underline{\ ?\ }$ ⁻13.3   **27.** ⁻3.7 $\underline{\ ?\ }$ 3.07

Write the numbers in order from least to greatest.

28. ⁻2.72, ⁻3, 0.03, ⁻3.5, 0.2   **29.** 6.3, ⁻8, ⁻7.6, ⁻1.75, 6.03

30. 0, 2.99, ⁻10, ⁻0.1, ⁻0.01   **31.** ⁻100.5, ⁻2, 3.11, ⁻2.1, ⁻46.8

32. ⁻0.5, ⁻0.05, ⁻5, ⁻50, 500   **33.** ⁻0.3, 30.3, ⁻0.33, ⁻3.3, 33

Draw an arrow to represent each decimal number described below.

34. The number 3, with starting point ⁻1

35. The number 2.5, with starting point ⁻0.5

36. The number ⁻5, with starting point 1.5

37. The number ⁻3, with starting point ⁻0.5

38. The number 5.5, with starting point ⁻3

39. The number ⁻4, with endpoint ⁻2

40. The number ⁻2, with endpoint 5

List the decimal numbers that can replace x to make the statement true.

B **41.** $|x| = 4.1$ **42.** $|x| = 0.001$ **43.** $|x| = 26.3$

    44. $|x| = 0$ **45.** $|x| = |{}^-1.19|$ **46.** $|x| = |{}^-2.2|$

Copy and complete the chart so that the two arrows represent the same decimal number.

	Arrow 1		Arrow 2	
	Starting Point	**Endpoint**	**Starting Point**	**Endpoint**
47.	⁻2.5	⁻7	0	?
48.	?	4	1.5	⁻1.5
49.	⁻0.5	8.5	?	⁻3
50.	4	⁻6.25	?	⁻2

For Exercises 51–54, (a) list the *integers* that can replace n to make the statement true, and (b) show their graphs on a number line.

51. $|n| < 4.3$ **52.** $|n| < 2.99$ **53.** $|n| \leq 5.001$ **54.** $|n| \leq 0.08$

Review Exercises

Use the properties to simplify the expression. Name the property or properties used.

  1. $2(4.5 + 1.07)$ **2.** $3.7 + 12.5 + 0.5$ **3.** 1×27.18

  4. $8.69 + 4.78 + 2.31$ **5.** $7(30 - 11.1)$ **6.** $(44 \times 0.3) + (44 \times 0.7)$

  7. $6.25 \times 43 \times 4$ **8.** $0.2 \times 3.7 \times 0.5$ **9.** $17.6 \times 283 \times 0$

2-3 Adding Positive and Negative Numbers

We can use arrows on the number line, as shown below, to add two positive numbers or to add two negative numbers. We draw a solid arrow with starting point 0 to represent the first addend. We draw another solid arrow with *starting point at the endpoint of the first arrow* to represent the second addend. To represent the sum, we draw a dashed arrow from the starting point of the first arrow to the endpoint of the second arrow.

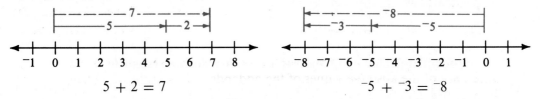

$$5 + 2 = 7 \qquad\qquad {}^-5 + {}^-3 = {}^-8$$

In each case, if we add the absolute values of the addends, we obtain the absolute value of the sum. The sum has the same sign as the addends.

Rules

The sum of two positive numbers is positive.

The sum of two negative numbers is negative.

EXAMPLE 1   Find the sum.   **a.** $2.5 + 4.3$ **b.** ${}^-7 + {}^-1.5$

Solution   **a.** Since the addends are positive, the sum is positive.
$$2.5 + 4.3 = 6.8$$

b. Since the addends are negative, the sum is negative.
$${}^-7 + {}^-1.5 = {}^-8.5$$

We can also use arrows on the number line to add a positive and a negative number. The sum of a positive and a negative number may be positive, negative, or zero, as shown in the following illustrations.

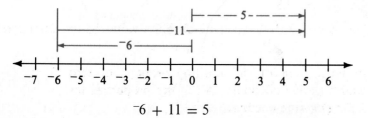

The positive number 11 has greater absolute value than the negative number ${}^-6$. Thus the sum is positive.

$${}^-6 + 11 = 5$$

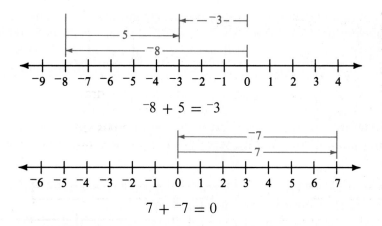

$$^-8 + 5 = ^-3$$

$$7 + ^-7 = 0$$

The negative number $^-8$ has greater absolute value than the positive number 5. Thus the sum is negative.

The positive number 7 and the negative number $^-7$ are opposites and thus have the same absolute value. The sum is zero.

Notice that, in each case, the absolute value of the sum is the *difference* of the absolute values of the addends. The sum has the same sign as the addend with the greater absolute value.

> ## Rules
>
> The sum of a positive number and a negative number is
>
> **1.** positive if the positive number has the greater absolute value.
> **2.** negative if the negative number has the greater absolute value.
> **3.** zero if the numbers have the same absolute value.

EXAMPLE 2 Find the sum.

    a. $3.5 + ^-10.5$ **b.** $^-7.6 + 12.2$ **c.** $^-4.8 + 0$ **d.** $^-6.7 + 6.7$

Solution **a.** The negative addend has the greater absolute value, so the sum is negative.

$$3.5 + ^-10.5 = ^-7$$

b. The positive addend has the greater absolute value, so the sum is positive.

$$^-7.6 + 12.2 = 4.6$$

c. Think of adding 0 as *moving no units* on the number line. Thus, $^-4.8 + 0 = ^-4.8$.

d. The numbers have the same absolute value, so the sum is zero.

$$^-6.7 + 6.7 = 0$$

As shown in Example 2, part (c), the addition property of zero holds for the positive and negative decimals. All of the properties for positive decimals hold for negative decimals as well.

EXAMPLE 3   Sally Wright bought some stock in ABC Computer Company. The stock went down $2.50 per share in the first week, went up $3.00 in the second week, and went down $1.25 in the third week. If Sally paid $30.50 per share for the stock, did she gain or lose money?

Solution   • The question asks if Sally gained or lost money.

• Given information: Sally paid $30.50 per share
   price went down $2.50, went up $3.00, went down $1.25

• First, find the new price per share. Express the given information as a sum of positive and negative decimals.

$$30.50 + {}^-2.50 + 3 + {}^-1.25 = (30.50 + 3) + ({}^-2.50 + {}^-1.25)$$
$$= 33.50 + {}^-3.75$$
$$= 29.75$$

To find whether Sally gained or lost money, compare the new price per share to the price paid per share.
$$29.75 < 30.50$$

• Because the new price per share is less than the price paid per share, Sally lost money.

Problem Solving Reminder
Many problems involve *more than one step,* but the steps may not always involve operations. In Example 3, we used addition in the first step, but in the second step we compared the answer to the first step with an amount given in the problem.

Class Exercises

State the addition fact illustrated by the diagram.

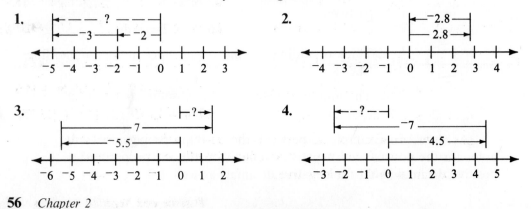

Without computing the exact sum, state whether the sum is positive, negative, or 0.

5. $-3.4 + {}^-2.6$ **6.** $25.7 + {}^-8.6 + {}^-25.7$ **7.** $2.37 + {}^-9.99$ **8.** ${}^-6.8 + 11.5$

Written Exercises

Find the sum by using arrows on a number line.

A   **1.** ${}^-3 + {}^-8$ **2.** $10.7 + {}^-10.7$ **3.** ${}^-12.5 + 22$ **4.** $2.9 + {}^-6.9$

Find the sum.

5. ${}^-2 + {}^-17$ **6.** ${}^-8 + {}^-9$ **7.** $8.3 + {}^-21.3$ **8.** ${}^-4.6 + 38.6$

9. ${}^-0.1 + {}^-0.2$ **10.** ${}^-1.82 + {}^-3.68$ **11.** $16.5 + {}^-16.5$ **12.** ${}^-8.7 + 3.4$

13. $16.9 + {}^-0.7$ **14.** ${}^-51.3 + 51.3$ **15.** $12.37 + {}^-8.2$ **16.** ${}^-85 + {}^-41$

17. $81.9 + {}^-81.9$ **18.** $32.8 + {}^-36$ **19.** $0 + {}^-0.12$ **20.** ${}^-7.9 + 0$

21. ${}^-4.2 + {}^-6.5 + 17$ **22.** $7.1 + {}^-9 + 2.3$ **23.** $5 + {}^-16.9 + 1.1$

24. ${}^-8.6 + {}^-17.1 + {}^-4.3$ **25.** ${}^-3.3 + {}^-7.25 + 3.3$ **26.** $0.98 + {}^-13.4 + {}^-0.98$

What value of the variable makes the statement true?

27. ${}^-8 + x = 4$ **28.** $x + 4 = {}^-9$ **29.** ${}^-41 + x = {}^-53$

30. ${}^-19 + x = 0$ **31.** $18.5 + x = 0$ **32.** ${}^-6 + x = {}^-1$

B   **33.** ${}^-4.3 + x = {}^-6.7$ **34.** $x + {}^-5.6 = {}^-37$ **35.** $x + 18.6 = {}^-1.2$

36. ${}^-0.66 + x = 0.10$ **37.** $12.9 + x = {}^-13$ **38.** $x + 20.2 = {}^-5.1$

Replace __?__ with =, >, or < to make a true statement.

39. $({}^-25.3 + {}^-8.8)$ __?__ $({}^-12.4 + {}^-19.7)$ **40.** $(6.24 + {}^-15.9)$ __?__ $({}^-6.24 + 15.9)$

41. $({}^-34.9 + 27.5)$ __?__ $(9.7 + {}^-18.4)$ **42.** $(14.4 + {}^-18.6)$ __?__ $({}^-3.2 + {}^-0.98)$

C   **43. a.** $|{}^-3 + {}^-19|$ __?__ $|{}^-3| + |{}^-19|$ **b.** $|{}^-4.6 + 4.6|$ __?__ $|{}^-4.6| + |4.6|$

     c. $|{}^-8.7 + 12.6|$ __?__ $|{}^-8.7| + |12.6|$ **d.** $|{}^-18.6 + 4.9|$ __?__ $|{}^-18.6| + |4.9|$

     e. $|53.5 + 3.7|$ __?__ $|53.5| + |3.7|$ **f.** $|{}^-4 + 13.75|$ __?__ $|{}^-4| + |13.75|$

     g. On the basis of your answers to parts (a)–(f), write a general rule for $|x + y|$ __?__ $|x| + |y|$ that holds for all numbers x and y. Explain why this rule is true.

Problems

Solve Problems 1–3 by first expressing the given data as a sum of positive and negative numbers. Then, compute the sum of the numbers and answer the questions.

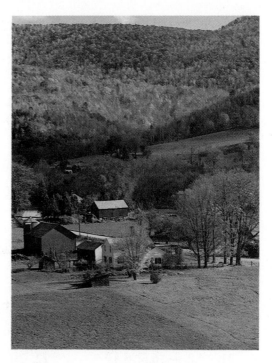

A　**1.** The temperature in Lynn at 7:00 A.M. was ⁻7°C. By 12:00 noon, the temperature had increased by 13°C, but it then decreased by 3°C between noon and 5:00 P.M. What was the temperature reading at 5:00 P.M.?

2. From the Andersons' farm, Bonnie drove 20.4 km due east to Fairvale. From Fairvale, she drove 33.7 km due west to Ward City. How far was she then from the farm and in what direction?

3. The Tigers football team gains 3.5 yd on a first down, loses 11 yd on the second down, and gains 2 yd on the third down. Do the Tigers gain or lose total yardage in these three plays? What is the total number of yards gained or lost?

B　**4.** For a summer job, Tom plans to clean the Wilsons' house. He estimates that each week he will spend $1.25 and $3.80 on cleaning supplies. How much should he charge the Wilsons if he wishes to make a profit of $6.50 each week?

5. Carl purchased stock in the Dependable Equipment Company. The price per share of the stock fell by $4.30 in the first month, rose by $2.50 in the second month, and rose by $2.60 in the third month. Carl sold the stock for $22.00 per share at the end of the third month. Did he gain or lose money?

Review Exercises

Evaluate the expression when $s = 2.7$ and $t = 8.4$.

1. $(25 - s)7$

2. $102 \div (t + 12)$

3. $11(7s - 13)$

4. $(t + 6 - 4.4)t$

5. $(s + 4)(s + 4)$

6. $10st \div (t - 4.2)$

7. $st \div 2s$

8. $(s + t) \div (t + 13.8)$

9. $(t - s)(5t + 8)$

2-4 Subtracting Positive and Negative Numbers

You know that $7.5 - 3 = 4.5$. In the preceding lesson, you learned that $7.5 + {}^-3 = 4.5$. Thus, $7.5 - 3 = 7.5 + {}^-3$. This example suggests the following general rule.

Rule

For any numbers a and b,

$$a - b = a + \text{(the opposite of } b\text{)}$$

or

$$a - b = a + (-b)$$

Note the lowered position of the minus sign in the expression $(-b)$, above. We use an *unraised* minus sign to mean *the opposite of*. For example,

$-3 = {}^-3$, read *the opposite of three equals negative three*

$-({}^-5) = 5$, read *the opposite of negative five equals five*

Because the numerals -3 and ${}^-3$ name the same number, one may be used in place of the other. From now on, we will use an unraised minus sign to denote subtraction, a negative number, and the opposite of a number.

EXAMPLE 1 Find the difference.

    a. $5 - 13$ **b.** $12.4 - (-8)$ **c.** $-10.9 - (-3.4)$

Solution   **a.** $5 - 13 = 5 + (-13) = -8$

           b. $12.4 - (-8) = 12.4 + 8 = 20.4$

           c. $-10.9 - (-3.4) = -10.9 + 3.4 = -7.5$

It is important to read a variable expression such as $-n$ as *the opposite of* n because n may denote a negative number, a positive number, or 0.

EXAMPLE 2 Evaluate the expression when $m = -5.2$.

    a. $m - 14$ **b.** $-m - 14$

Solution   **a.** $m - 14 = -5.2 - 14 = -5.2 + (-14) = -19.2$

           b. $-m - 14 = -(-5.2) - 14 = 5.2 - 14 = 5.2 + (-14) = -8.8$

Reading Mathematics: *Using Examples*

The worked-out examples in each lesson show you how the general statements in the lesson can be applied to specific situations. If you need help as
you work on the exercises, look back at the examples for models to follow or
for ideas on how to begin your solutions.

Class Exercises

Complete.

1. $6 - 12 = 6 + \underline{\ ?\ }$

2. $-10 - 8 = -10 + \underline{\ ?\ }$

3. $6.7 - (-1.5) = 6.7 + \underline{\ ?\ }$

4. $-26.01 - (-8.2) = -26.01 + \underline{\ ?\ }$

**Without computing the exact difference, state whether the difference is
positive, negative, or 0.**

5. $-4.2 - 4.2$ **6.** $4.2 - (-4.2)$ **7.** $4.2 - 4.2$ **8.** $-4.2 - (-4.2)$

Find the difference.

9. $3 - (-6)$ **10.** $-2 - (-3.5)$ **11.** $-1.8 - 5.8$ **12.** $2.25 - 4$

Written Exercises

Write the difference as a sum.

A   **1.** $7 - 19$ **2.** $-21 - 42$ **3.** $6.2 - (-8.3)$ **4.** $-2.9 + (-11.6)$

5-8. Find each difference in Exercises 1–4 above.

Find the difference.

9. $4 - 10$ **10.** $25 - 34$ **11.** $-3 - 24$ **12.** $-12 - 5$

13. $9 - (-33)$ **14.** $14 + (+46)$ **15.** $-2 - (-17)$ **16.** $-6 - (+5)$

17. $0 - 43$ **18.** $0 - 101$ **19.** $0 - (-20)$ **20.** $0 + (-14)$

21. $44 - 0$ **22.** $-16 + 0$ **23.** $6.9 - 8$ **24.** $12 + 20.5$

25. $4.3 - 2.1$ **26.** $23.4 - 6.8$ **27.** $-16.1 - 8.5$ **28.** $-0.4 - 8.9$

29. $-19 - 5.6$ **30.** $-41.1 + 2.9$ **31.** $0 - (-3.37)$ **32.** $0 - 12.8$

33. $12.4 - (-12.4)$ **34.** $-18.1 + (+25)$ **35.** $-52.9 - (-11.6)$

36. $(6 - 9.7) + 8.8$ **37.** $(-2.5 - 8.1) - (-12.4)$ **38.** $(0 - 8.3) - (-24.1)$

Evaluate the expression when $a = -4.5$ and $b = -6.2$.

39. $-a$ **40.** $-b$ **41.** $-|b|$ **42.** $-|a|$

43. $a - b$ **44.** $b - a$ **45.** $-a - b$ **46.** $-b - a$

47. $a - (-b)$ **48.** $b - (-a)$ **49.** $-b - (-a)$ **50.** $-a - (-b)$

What value of the variable makes the statement true?

B   **51.** $2 - d = -6$ **52.** $d - 5 = -13$ **53.** $-3 - d = -11$

    54. $8 - d = 13$ **55.** $-7 - d = 12$ **56.** $d - (-6) = -7$

    57. $-d - 4 = 14$ **58.** $-d - 5 = -9$ **59.** $7 - (-d) = 14$

    60. $d - (-8) = 17$ **61.** $-8 - (-d) = -16$ **62.** $-4 - (-d) = 10$

C   **63.** Replace __?__ with $=$, $>$, or $<$ to make a true statement.
      a. $|13.6 - 8.9|$ __?__ $|13.6| - |8.9|$ **b.** $|-8.9 - (-13.6)|$ __?__ $|-8.9| - |-13.6|$
      c. $|8.9 - 13.6|$ __?__ $|8.9| - |13.6|$ **d.** $|-8.9 - 13.6|$ __?__ $|-8.9| - |13.6|$
      e. Based on your answers to parts (a)-(d), write a general rule for
        $|x - y|$ __?__ $|x| - |y|$, where x and y are any decimal numbers.

Problems

Solve Problems 1-7 by first expressing the given data as a difference of positive and negative numbers. Then, compute the difference of the numbers and answer the question.

A   **1.** On a winter day, the temperature dropped from $-3°C$ to $-11°C$. Find the change in temperature.

    2. Find the difference in the ages of two people if one was born in 27 B.C. and the other was born in 16 A.D.

    3. The elevation of the highest point in a region is 1226 m above sea level. If the difference between the highest point and lowest point in the region is 1455 m, find the elevation of the lowest point.

    4. Two stages of a rocket burn for a total of 114.5 s. If the first stage burns for 86.8 s, how long does the second stage burn?

    5. Jan Miller purchased 140 shares of stock in the ABC Company at a price of $18.75 per share. During the next three days, the value declined by $1.00, $1.75, and $1.50. What was the value of a share of ABC stock at the end of three days?

6. A parachutist jumped from an airplane flying at an altitude of 1100 m, dropped 200 m in the first 25 s, and then dropped 350 m in the next 35 s. What was the altitude of the parachutist 60 s after jumping?

7. In Summit City, 78 cm of snow fell on Sunday. The snow melted approximately 5.8 cm on Monday, approximately 7.5 cm on Tuesday, and approximately 12 cm on Wednesday. Approximately how much snow remained?

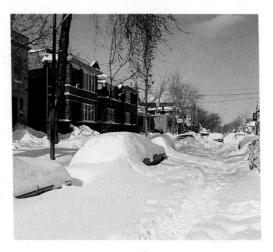

B   **8.** Donna receives an allowance every 2 weeks that includes $20 for school lunches. During the past 4 weeks, she spent $7.50, $8.25, $5.25, and $8.75 on lunches. How much did Donna have left from the money allowed for lunches for the 4 weeks?

9. Eric Chung had $65.10 in his checking account on June 1. He wrote two checks in June, one for $42.99. Eric forgot to write down the amount of the other check. At the end of the month, he received a notice that his account was overdrawn by $22.11. What was the amount of Eric's second check?

Self-Test A

Replace __?__ with =, >, or < to make a true statement.

1. 4 __?__ 7   **2.** 2 __?__ 1   **3.** $^-$8 __?__ 9   **4.** |$^-$7| __?__ 7   **5.** |0| __?__ 0   [2–1]

Write the numbers in order from least to greatest.

6. 0, 5.4, $^-$4.52, $^-$0.25, $^-$54   **7.** $^-$3.79, 37, $^-$7.3, $^-$0.37, $^-$0.09   [2–2]

Find the sum or difference.

8. $^-$9.3 + 42.3   **9.** 17.8 + $^-$17.8   **10.** 8.76 + $^-$10.2   [2–3]

11. 8 − (−27)   **12.** −5.1 − (−5.1)   **13.** 0 − 36   [2–4]

Evaluate the expression when $a = -6.4$ and $b = -5.2$.

14. $-b - a$ **15.** $a - (-b)$ **16.** $b - |a|$

Self-Test answers and Extra Practice are at the back of the book.

2-5 Multiplying Positive and Negative Numbers

To find a product such as $5(-2)$, we can think of the product as the sum of five identical addends.

$$5(-2) = -2 + (-2) + (-2) + (-2) + (-2)$$

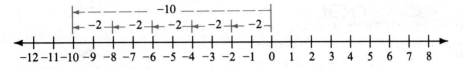

The diagram shows that $-2 + (-2) + (-2) + (-2) + (-2) = -10$. Thus $5(-2) = -10$.

To find the product $-7(2)$, we may use the commutative property of multiplication to write

$$-7(2) = 2(-7).$$

We know that $2(-7) = -7 + (-7) = -14$, so $-7(2) = -14$.

Notice that in the two examples above, the product is the opposite of the product of the absolute values of the numbers. The examples suggest the following rule.

Rule

The product of a positive number and a negative number is a negative number.

We may use other properties that we have learned for addition and multiplication of positive decimals to determine what a product of negative numbers, such as $-5(-3)$, must be. The multiplication property of zero states that the product of any number and 0 is 0. Thus,

$$-5(0) = 0.$$

Since we know that $3 + (-3) = 0$, we may write

$$-5[3 + (-3)] = 0.$$

By the distributive property, we may write the following.

$$-5(3) + (-5)(-3) = 0$$

$$-15 + (-5)(-3) = 0$$

But we know that $-15 + 15 = 0$, so $-5(-3)$ must equal 15.

Notice that the product of $-5(-3)$ is the product of the absolute values of the factors. The example suggests the following rule.

> ## Rule
>
> The product of two negative numbers is a positive number.

EXAMPLE 1 Find the product.
  a. $-4.5(8.6)$ **b.** $5.32(-1)$ **c.** $-1(-14.7)$ **d.** $-9.2(-3.1)$

Solution
  a. One number is negative and one number is positive, so the product is negative.
$$-4.5(8.6) = -38.7$$

  b. One number is positive and one number is negative, so the product is negative.
$$5.32(-1) = -5.32$$

  c. Both numbers are negative, so the product is positive.
$$-1(-14.7) = 14.7$$

  d. Both numbers are negative, so the product is positive.
$$-9.2(-3.1) = 28.52$$

Notice in Example 1, parts (b) and (c), that when one of the factors is -1, the product is the opposite of the other factor.

> ## Rule
>
> The product of -1 and any number equals the opposite of that number.

We may use the rules for products of positive and negative numbers to multiply any number of positive and negative numbers.

EXAMPLE 2 Find the product.
  a. $-3.7(2.5)(-4.8)$ **b.** $-11.1(-7)(6.5)(-3.2)$

Solution   **a.** $-3.7(2.5)(-4.8) = [-3.7(2.5)](-4.8) = (-9.25)(-4.8) = 44.4$

  b. $-11.1(-7)(6.5)(-3.2) = [-11.1(-7)][(6.5)(-3.2)]$
$$= 77.7(-20.8) = -1616.16$$

Example 2, on the preceding page, illustrates the following rules.

> ## *Rules*
>
> For a product with no zero factors:
> **1.** if the number of negative factors is odd, the product is negative.
> **2.** if the number of negative factors is even, the product is positive.

Class Exercises

Without computing the exact product, state whether the product is positive, negative, or 0.

1. $-3(-4.2)$ **2.** $2.1(-0.8)$ **3.** $-5(1.6)(-7)$ **4.** $-4.5(3.7)(0)$

Find the product.

5. $3(-16)$ **6.** $-7(-12)$ **7.** $13(-1)(-5)$ **8.** $-2(-8)(-5)(0)$

2-44 even

Written Exercises

Find the product.

A   **1.** $-3(-9)$ **2.** $4(-6)$ **3.** $-8(7)$ **4.** $-7(-11)$

5. $2(-8)(-6)$ **6.** $-3(5)(-6)$ **7.** $-2(0)(-12)$ **8.** $14(-1)(0)$

9. $-1.5(8)$ **10.** $0.6(-9)$ **11.** $-3.4(-1.5)$ **12.** $-0.4(-0.7)$

13. $2.9(-1)$ **14.** $-1(7.84)$ **15.** $-8.8(-1.75)$ **16.** $-1.11(70)$

17. $-20(0.25)$ **18.** $12(-1.2)$ **19.** $-15(-30.6)$ **20.** $0.24(-100)$

21. $3.9(-17.1)$ **22.** $-5.6(80.1)$ **23.** $-13.7(0)$ **24.** $16.7(0)$

25. $-1.8(-1.9)$ **26.** $-0.125(-8.1)$ **27.** $-5.4(20.6)$ **28.** $-8.9(30.9)$

29. $10.1(3.75)$ **30.** $4.25(20.4)$ **31.** $-3.72(-16.5)$ **32.** $0.78(-42)$

33. $-1.7(-0.2)(-3.1)$ **34.** $-9(-2.7)(-80)$ **35.** $3.25(-17)(0)$

36. $-1.21(0)(-1.1)$ **37.** $9.4(-3.5)(-11)$ **38.** $18(-5.75)(6.2)$

Simplify the expression.

B **39.** $(-1.2 - 6.5)(-1.2 + 6.5)$

40. $18 + 3 - (-12 - 7)$

41. $(-7)(2.4)(0)(-9.3)(-1) + (-8.2)$

42. $(14.4 - 200)(14.4 + 200)$

43. $-4[27 - (-9)] + (-4)(-2 - 9)$

44. $(-20 + 12)7 + (-2 + 20)7$

Find the integer n that will make the statement true.

45. $-3(n) = 6$

46. $4(n) = -28$

47. $-9(-n) = -18$

48. $3(n) = 6(-3)$

49. $-n(-7) = -14(0)$

50. $-5(n) = 25(2)$

C **51.** $-3(-1.5)(-n) = -18(-1)(-0.5)$

52. $-1.2(30)(-n) = -9(-0.4)(-100)$

53. $-1.5(n)(-0.8) = -12(-1.5)(-2)$

54. $-0.6(-n)(-1.9) = -18(-1.3)(0)$

55. $n(-3.7 + 61.4) = 0$

56. $-n(-1.1 - 30.6) = 0$

Review Exercises

Use the inverse operation to solve for the variable.

1. $f + 27 = 83$ **2.** $n - 13 = 54$ **3.** $g + 364 = 518$ **4.** $w - 216 = 435$

5. $6c = 78$ **6.** $x \div 17 = 6$ **7.** $14j = 364$ **8.** $y \div 37 = 142$

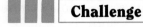 **Calculator Key-In**

Use your calculator to solve this problem: One day you tell a secret to a friend. The next day your friend tells your secret to two other friends. On the third day, each of the friends who was told your secret the day before tells it to two other friends. If this pattern continues from day to day, how many people will be told your secret on the fourteenth day?

Challenge

Using the first nine counting numbers, fill in the boxes so you get the same sum when you add vertically, horizontally, or diagonally. Can you do this with any nine consecutive counting numbers?

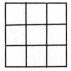

2-6 Dividing Positive and Negative Numbers

Recall that multiplication and division are inverse operations for positive numbers. For example, because we know that $4 \times 8 = 32$, we also know that $8 = 32 \div 4$. We can use the relationship between multiplication and division to find quotients of positive and negative numbers. Consider the following examples.

$$4 \times (-8) = -32 \qquad -8 = -32 \div 4$$
$$-4 \times 8 = -32 \qquad 8 = -32 \div -4$$
$$-4 \times (-8) = 32 \qquad -8 = 32 \div -4$$

Notice that in the examples above, the quotient of two numbers with differing signs is the opposite of the quotient of the absolute values of the numbers. The quotient of two numbers with the same sign is the quotient of the absolute values of the numbers.

The examples suggest the following rules for dividing positive and negative numbers.

Rules

The quotient of two positive or two negative numbers is positive.

The quotient of a positive number and a negative number is negative.

By the multiplication property of zero, we know that $-4 \times 0 = 0$ and thus $0 = 0 \div (-4)$. Remember that we cannot divide by 0.

EXAMPLE Find the quotient.

    a. $-3.06 \div 0.9$ **b.** $36.8 \div (-2.3)$ **c.** $-4.046 \div (-1.7)$

Solution **a.** Since -3.06 is negative and 0.9 is positive, the quotient will be negative.

$$-3.06 \div 0.9 = -3.4$$

b. Since 36.8 is positive and -2.3 is negative, the quotient will be negative.

$$36.8 \div -2.3 = -16$$

c. Since -4.046 and -1.7 are both negative, the quotient will be positive.

$$-4.046 \div (-1.7) = 2.38$$

Class Exercises

Without computing the exact quotient, state whether the quotient is positive, negative, or 0.

1. $-3.6 \div (-40)$ **2.** $-0.216 \div 400$ **3.** $0 \div (-17.5)$ **4.** $850 \div (-0.05)$

Find the quotient.

5. $-28 \div 7$ **6.** $33 \div (-1)$ **7.** $0 \div -50$

8. $-51 \div (-3)$ **9.** $-22 \div 4$ **10.** $-75 \div 15$

Written Exercises

Find the quotient.

A **1.** $-18 \div 3$ **2.** $25 \div (-5)$ **3.** $-21 \div (-7)$

4. $-54 \div (-18)$ **5.** $0 \div (-7)$ **6.** $0 \div (-24)$

7. $144 \div (-12)$ **8.** $-100 \div 25$ **9.** $22.5 \div (-3)$

10. $-42 \div 4$ **11.** $-3.6 \div (-1)$ **12.** $-1.01 \div (-1)$

13. $-1.75 \div 0.05$ **14.** $-69.3 \div 3.3$ **15.** $-32.86 \div 6.2$

16. $-17.05 \div (-1.1)$ **17.** $-0.48 \div (-0.06)$ **18.** $0.06 \div (-0.3)$

19. $0 \div (-14.7)$ **20.** $0 \div (-0.25)$ **21.** $-0.9 \div 1.8$

22. $-0.042 \div (-0.6)$ **23.** $-38 \div 4$ **24.** $-45 \div (-6)$

25. $9.9 \div (-4.5)$ **26.** $46.2 \div (-6)$ **27.** $-13.8 \div (-1)$

28. $0.003 \div (-1)$ **29.** $-9.27 \div (-60)$ **30.** $0.25 \div (-40)$

31. $13.23 \div (-2.1)$ **32.** $-2.6 \div 0.52$ **33.** $-14.57 \div (-3.1)$

34. $-0.53 \div (-0.1)$ **35.** $-18.5 \div 10$ **36.** $3.84 \div (-9.6)$

Evaluate the expression when $a = -8$ and $b = 2.5$.

37. $a \div b$ **38.** $b \div a$ **39.** $2b \div (-a)$ **40.** $-3a \div b$

41. $(a - b) \div b$ **42.** $2ab \div a$ **43.** $-9a \div 3ab$ **44.** $-5b \div (-2a)$

Use inverse operations to solve for the variable.

B **45.** $-3n = 6$ **46.** $d \div 5 = -7$ **47.** $b \div (-8) = 9$

48. $-15x = -30$ **49.** $-2y - 8 = 8$ **50.** $4c + 12 = -36$

C **51.** Explain why $\left|\dfrac{x}{y}\right| = \dfrac{|x|}{|y|}$ for all decimal numbers for which it is possible to find the quotient $\dfrac{x}{y}$.

52. Replace __?__ with $=$, $>$, or $<$ to make a true statement.

a. 0.10 __?__ 2.5

$\dfrac{0.10}{0.5}$ __?__ $\dfrac{2.5}{0.5}$

$\dfrac{0.10}{-0.5}$ __?__ $\dfrac{2.5}{-0.5}$

b. -0.21 __?__ 0

$\dfrac{-0.21}{70}$ __?__ $\dfrac{0}{70}$

$\dfrac{-0.21}{-70}$ __?__ $\dfrac{0}{-70}$

c. -3.6 __?__ -1.5

$\dfrac{-3.6}{3}$ __?__ $\dfrac{-1.5}{3}$

$\dfrac{-3.6}{-3}$ __?__ $\dfrac{-1.5}{-3}$

Use your answers to parts (a)–(c) to answer parts (d) and (e).

d. If $x < y$ and if k is a positive number, then $\dfrac{x}{k}$ __?__ $\dfrac{y}{k}$.

e. If $x < y$ and if j is a negative number, then $\dfrac{x}{j}$ __?__ $\dfrac{y}{j}$.

Write examples similar to those in parts (a)–(c) to answer parts (f) and (g).

f. If $x > y$ and if k is a positive number, then $\dfrac{x}{k}$ __?__ $\dfrac{y}{k}$.

g. If $x > y$ and if j is a negative number, then $\dfrac{x}{j}$ __?__ $\dfrac{y}{j}$.

Review Exercises

Evaluate the expression when $x = 3$, $y = 7$, and $z = 4$.

1. y^2
2. $5x^2$
3. $(7z)^2$
4. z^0
5. $7z^2$
6. $(6x)^2$
7. $(yz)^0$
8. xy^0
9. $z^3 - x^3$
10. $8x^3y$

███ **Calculator Key-In**

Does your calculator have a change-sign key? The key may look like this: ⊬. If you press this key after entering a number or doing a calculation, the sign of the number displayed on your calculator will change. For example, if you enter 116 ⊬, your calculator will change 116 to -116.

Solve with a calculator that has a change-sign key, if possible.

1. $20.7 + (-19.6)$
2. $-55.59 + 438.2$
3. $-0.86 + (-27.341)$
4. $-426.38 - (-25.004)$
5. $-83.5(-61.09)$
6. $6.8(-4.17)(-1.61)$

2-7 Using Positive Exponents

In Chapter 1, exponents were introduced. Recall that in the expression 3^5 (called a *power*), 3 is called the *base* and 5 is called the *exponent*.

If a product contains powers of the same base, the product may be written as a single power of that base. For example, $13^2 \times 13^3$ can be written as a single power of 13.

$$13^2 \times 13^3 = (13 \times 13) \times (13 \times 13 \times 13)$$
$$= 13 \times 13 \times 13 \times 13 \times 13$$
$$= 13^5$$

Notice that the exponent in the product is the sum of the exponents in the factors, that is, $2 + 3 = 5$.

In general,

> ## Rule
>
> For every number a ($a \neq 0$) and all whole numbers m and n,
>
> $$a^m \times a^n = a^{m+n}$$

Notice that the bases must be the same.

EXAMPLE 1 Write $15^3 \times 15^4$ as a single power of 15.

Solution $15^3 \times 15^4 = 15^{3+4} = 15^7$

EXAMPLE 2 Evaluate the expression if $n = 3$.

  a. n^2 **b.** $4n^2$ **c.** $(4n)^2$ **d.** $n^2 \times n^2$

Solution Replace n with 3 in each expression and simplify.

  a. $n^2 = 3^2 = 3 \times 3 = 9$

  b. $4n^2 = 4(3^2) = 4 \times 9 = 36$

  c. $(4n)^2 = (4 \times 3)^2 = 12^2 = 12 \times 12 = 144$

  d. $n^2 \times n^2 = n^{2+2} = n^4 = 3^4 = 3 \times 3 \times 3 \times 3 = 81$

Notice in parts (b) and (c) of Example 2 how grouping symbols change the values of expressions that have the same numbers.

Reading Mathematics: *Study Helps*
Look back at this lesson. Notice that the information in the blue box on page 70 summarizes important ideas from the lesson. The box gives a definition that is applied in the examples. Throughout the book, boxes are used to help you identify important definitions, rules, properties, facts, and formulas. Use them as reminders when you do the exercises and when you review the lesson.

Class Exercises

Read each expression.

1. 4^5 **2.** 9^1 **3.** 15^2 **4.** 3^7 **5.** 10^3 **6.** 2^8

Write using exponents.

7. 9 to the third power   **8.** 15 cubed   **9.** 4 squared

10. 6 to the fifth power   **11.** 216 is the third power of 6.

Express the number as a power of 3.

12. 9   **13.** 27   **14.** 3   **15.** 243   **16.** 1

Simplify the expression.

17. 8^2 **18.** 2^3 **19.** 1^{11} **20.** 18^0 **21.** 83^1

Written Exercises

Simplify the expression.

A   **1.** 2^6 **2.** 5^4 **3.** 10^2 **4.** 6^3 **5.** 14^1

6. $3^2 + 5^2$ **7.** $(3 \times 5)^2$ **8.** $2^4 + 3^2$ **9.** $(5 + 12)^0$ **10.** $(5 + 12)^1$

Which is greater?

11. 2^3 or 3^2 **12.** 5^2 or 2^5 **13.** 9×2 or 9^2

14. 3×10 or 10^3 **15.** $(16 \times 4)^2$ or $2 \times 16 \times 4$ **16.** $(10 + 2)^0$ or $10 + 2$

Write as a single power of the given base.

17. $2^3 \times 2^4$ **18.** $3^2 \times 3^5$ **19.** 10×10^4 **20.** $5^5 \times 5^6$ **21.** $n^3 \times n^8$

Evaluate the expression when $m = 5$, $n = 3$, and $p = 2$.

22. p^2 **23.** $4m^2$ **24.** $(9n)^2$ **25.** $9n^2$ **26.** n^0

27. $(8n)^2$ **28.** np^0 **29.** $(mn)^0$ **30.** $m^3 - n^3$ **31.** $5m^3 n$

B **32.** $(7n)^n$ **33.** $(3m)^p$ **34.** $6^2 \times 6^n$ **35.** $(8 + m)^{n-3}$ **36.** $(15^n)^{p-1}$

37. $p^n m^n$ **38.** $(7 + n)^n$ **39.** np^m **40.** $(p^m p^n) + 4$ **41.** $m^p + n^n$

42. $(m^p)^n$ **43.** $(m - n)^p$ **44.** $\dfrac{m^n}{m^p}$ **45.** $\dfrac{3p^n}{6p^m}$ **46.** $\dfrac{(m - 1)^{n+1}}{p}$

C **47.** Find a value of n such that $(5 + 2)^n = 5^n + 2^n$.

48. Is the equation true?

a. $4^4 \div 4^3 = 4^1$ b. $5^3 \div 5^1 = 5^2$ c. $2^7 \div 2^4 = 2^3$

d. Using your answers from parts (a)–(c), state a general rule to describe what appears to be true for division of powers of the same base.

Review Exercises

Solve using inverse operations.

1. $8 + x = 6$ **2.** $y + 4 = 1$ **3.** $n + 6 = 8$ **4.** $y + 10 = 6$

5. $-7 + a = 5$ **6.** $t + 3 = -8$ **7.** $-2 + c = -1$ **8.** $-13 + x = 0$

▮▮▮ Calculator Key-In

Use a calculator to simplify the expressions.

1. $15^2 - 13^2$ and $(15 + 13)(15 - 13)$

2. $47^2 - 21^2$ and $(47 + 21)(47 - 21)$

3. $82^2 - 59^2$ and $(82 + 59)(82 - 59)$

4. $104^2 - 76^2$ and $(104 + 76)(104 - 76)$

Do you recognize a pattern?
Write two expressions that will result in the same pattern.

2-8 Negative Integers as Exponents

You know by the rule of exponents that you learned for multiplying powers of the same base that

$$10^1 \times 10^2 = 10^{1+2} = 10^3.$$

Since we want to apply the same rule to negative exponents, we must have

$$10^1 \times 10^{-1} = 10^{1+(-1)} = 10^0 = 1$$

$$10^2 \times 10^{-2} = 10^{2+(-2)} = 10^0 = 1$$

and so on. We know that

$$10^1 \times \frac{1}{10} = 10 \times 0.1 = 1 \text{ and } 10^2 \times \frac{1}{10^2} = 100 \times 0.01 = 1,$$

so 10^{-1} should equal $\frac{1}{10}$ and 10^{-2} should equal $\frac{1}{10^2}$. These examples suggest the following general rule.

Rule

For all numbers $a(a \neq 0)$, m, and n,

$$a^{-m} = \frac{1}{a^m}$$

EXAMPLE Write the expression without exponents.
   a. 5^{-2} **b.** $(-3)^{-2}$ **c.** $(-4)^{-1}(-4)^{-2}$

Solution   **a.** $5^{-2} = \dfrac{1}{5^2} = \dfrac{1}{5 \times 5} = \dfrac{1}{25}$

b. $(-3)^{-2} = \dfrac{1}{(-3)^2} = \dfrac{1}{(-3)(-3)} = \dfrac{1}{9}$

c. $(-4)^{-1} \times (-4)^{-2} = (-4)^{-1+(-2)} = (-4)^{-3}$

$$= \dfrac{1}{(-4)^3} = \dfrac{1}{(-4)(-4)(-4)} = \dfrac{1}{-64}$$

Class Exercises

Use the rules for exponents to state the expression without exponents.

   1. 3^{-4} **2.** $(-6)^{-2}$ **3.** $10^4 \times 10^{-4}$ **4.** $3^5 \times 3^{-7}$ **5.** $(-2)^3(-2)^{-1}$

Use exponents to state as a power of 2.

6. 8   **7.** $\frac{1}{8}$ **8.** 64   **9.** $\frac{1}{64}$ **10.** $\frac{1}{512}$

Written Exercises

Write the expression without exponents.

A

1. $(-2)^{-5}$ **2.** 3^{-3} **3.** 10^{-3} **4.** $(-3)^{-5}$ **5.** 1^{-4}

6. $(-1)^{-6}$ **7.** $(-5)^{-2}$ **8.** 4^{-5} **9.** 2^{-6} **10.** $(-4)^{-2}$

11. $7^4 \times 7^{-6}$ **12.** $10^3 \times 10^{-2}$ **13.** $5^{10} \times 5^{-10}$

14. $6^{-23} \times 6^{23}$ **15.** $3^{-3} \times 3^0$ **16.** $2^{-3} \times 2^{-4}$

17. $(-4)^{-2} \times (-4)^{-2}$ **18.** $(-7)^{-1} \times (-7)^{-1}$ **19.** $(-2)^{-6} \times (-2)^3$

20. $(-8)^{-2} \times (-8)^0$ **21.** $6^{-1} \times 6^3 \times 6^{-2}$ **22.** $9^{-5} \times 9^{-1} \times 9^7$

What value of the variable makes the statement true?

23. $5^n = \frac{1}{125}$ **24.** $4^{-n} = \frac{1}{256}$ **25.** $3^{-n} = \frac{1}{243}$

26. $4^2 \times 4^{-2} = 4^n$ **27.** $7^3 \times 7^{-5} = 7^n$ **28.** $9^{-4} \times 9^3 = \frac{1}{9^n}$

B   **29.** $3^7 \times 3^n = 3^5$ **30.** $2^{-3} \times 2^n = 2^{-11}$

31. $(2)^{-5} \times (2)^n = 8$ **32.** $(-10)^3 \times (-10)^{-n} = -10$

33. $144 \times 12^{-2} = 12^n$ **34.** $5^{-3} \times 25 = 5^{-n}$

35. $4^n \times 4^{-3} = \frac{1}{16}$ **36.** $6^{-n} \times 6^3 = \frac{1}{216}$

37. $9^{-7} \times 9^{-n} = \frac{1}{729}$ **38.** $8^{-4} \times 8^{-n} = \frac{1}{64}$

39. $(-5)^{-n} \times (-5)^{-3} = 1$ **40.** $(-3)^{+n} \times (-3)^{-8} = \frac{1}{-243}$

Simplify. Write the expression with nonnegative exponents.

41. x^{-5} **42.** n^{-9} **43.** $a^{-3} \times a^{-2}$

44. $b^7 \times b^{-7}$ **45.** $w^{-10} \times w^3 \times w^{-1}$ **46.** $v^4 \times v^{-12} \times v^3$

C   **47.** Explain why $a^m = (-a)^m$ if m is any even integer.

48. Explain why $(-a)^n = -1(a)^n$ if n is any odd integer.

Self-Test B

Simplify.

1. $4.2(-11.3)$ **2.** $-6.7(20.4)$ **3.** $7.5(-4.2)(-12)$ [2-5]

4. $121 \div (-11)$ **5.** $-68.2 \div 2.2$ **6.** $-0.56 \div (-0.07)$ [2-6]

Evaluate the expression when $a = 2$, $b = 5$, and $c = 3$.

7. a^3 **8.** $(bc)^2$ **9.** $(2c)^4$ [2-7]

Write the expression without exponents.

10. 4^{-2} **11.** $(-6)^{-3}$ **12.** $7^5 \times 7^{-8}$ **13.** $(-9)^{-2} \times (-9)^0$ [2-8]

Self-Test answers and Extra Practice are at the back of the book.

Challenge

We use the symbol $[x]$ (read *the greatest integer in x*) to represent the greatest integer less than or equal to x.

EXAMPLE   **a.** $[5.4]$ **b.** $[^-3.2]$

Solution   **a.** There is no integer equal to 5.4, so we must find the greatest integer that is less than 5.4.

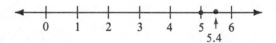

As shown on the number line, the greatest integer that is less than 5.4 is 5. Thus the greatest integer in 5.4 is 5.

     b. There is no integer equal to $^-3.2$, so we must find the greatest integer that is less than $^-3.2$.

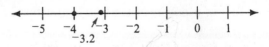

As shown on the number line, the greatest integer that is less than $^-3.2$ is $^-4$. Thus the greatest integer in $^-3.2$ is $^-4$.

Find the value.

1. $[6.2]$ **2.** $[1.23]$ **3.** $[3]$ **4.** $[45]$

5. $[^-12]$ **6.** $[^-1]$ **7.** $[^-4.89]$ **8.** $[^-0.36]$

Scientific Notation

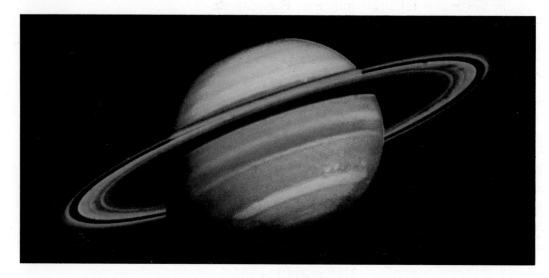

Scientists frequently deal with data that range from very small to very large magnitudes. For example, when Saturn is closest to Earth, it is about 1,630,000,000 km away. The diameter of a hydrogen atom is approximately $\frac{1}{100,000,000}$ cm. To cope with numbers such as these, a method for writing numbers, called **scientific notation,** has been adopted.

Scientific notation makes use of positive exponents to write large numbers and negative exponents to write small numbers. For example,

$$4800 = 4.8 \times 1000 = 4.8 \times 10^3$$

$$0.000507 = 5.07 \times \frac{1}{10,000} = 5.07 \times 10^{-4}$$

Rule

To express any positive number in scientific notation, write it as the product of a power of ten and a number between 1 and 10.

In addition to being a convenient method for expressing very large or very small numbers, scientific notation provides an exact gauge of the precision of a measurement, based on the smallest unit of calibration on the measuring instrument. Each digit in a number that specifies the degree of precision of measurement is called a **significant digit.**

Zeros that appear to the right of nonzero digits, and to the right of the decimal point, are significant. For example,

0.50 has two significant digits,

40,521 has five significant digits.

The zeros in a measurement such as 41,500 km, however, may be misleading since it is unclear whether the number is rounded to the nearest hundred or is an exact measurement. Scientific notation provides a means of avoiding this confusion. For example, when we write 40,500 as 4.05×10^4, it means that the measurement is precise to three significant digits. When we write 40,500 as 4.050×10^4, it means that the measurement is precise to four significant digits.

In general, to write a number in scientific notation, shift the decimal point to just after the first nonzero digit. Then multiply by 10^n, when n is the number of places the decimal point was shifted. As an example,

$$3165 = 3.165 \times 10^3.$$

Note that 7.46 is written as 7.46 since $10^0 = 1$. Also, 1,000,000 is usually written simply as 10^6 rather than 1×10^6.

Write the number in scientific notation.

1. 5798   2. 30,090   3. 8,915,673   4. 2,175,000,000

5. 1.75   6. 0.003   7. 0.0501   8. 0.0333

5.01×10^3

Write the number in decimal form.

9. 3.79×10^3 10. 4.86×10^4 11. 3.01×10^5 12. 6×10^9

13. 5.6×10^{-2} 14. 7.09×10^{-3} 15. 3.99×10^{-8} 16. 2.0111×10^{-6}

17. The diameter of a red blood cell is about 0.00074 cm. Write this number in scientific notation with two significant digits.

18. An atom of gold is about 0.0000000025 m in diameter. Write this number in scientific notation with two significant digits.

19. The radius of Earth's orbit is 150,000,000,000 m. Write this number in scientific notation with two significant digits.

20. A communications satellite was orbited at an altitude of 625,000 m. Write this number in scientific notation with three significant digits.

Chapter Review

Complete. Use =, >, or < to make a true statement.

1. 2 _?_ 11   2. 5 _?_ 3   3. 3 _?_ ⁻4   [2-1]

4. 0 _?_ ⁻1   5. |⁻9| _?_ 9   6. |2| _?_ ⁻2

7. ⁻8.7 _?_ ⁻0.87   8. ⁻42 _?_ 2.4   9. 3.05 _?_ −3.55   [2-2]

10. 0.4 _?_ ⁻4.3   11. |⁻5.6| _?_ ⁻5.6   12. |4.93| _?_ |⁻4.93|

True or false?

13. $0 + {}^-14.2 = 0$

14. $16.8 + {}^-16.8 = 33.6$ [2-3]

15. ${}^-13.2 + {}^-7.8 = {}^-21$

16. $7.6 + {}^-10.5 = 2.9$

17. ${}^-33 + 20.2 = {}^-12.8$

18. $19.5 + {}^-14.3 = {}^-5.2$

19. $37.2 - (-9.6) = 25.6$

20. $-5.8 - (-5.8) = 11.6$ [2-4]

21. $-12.2 - 13.1 = -25.3$

22. $0 - (-0.5) = -0.05$

23. If $a = -7$, $-a = -7$

24. If $b = -2.4$, $-|b| = -2.4$

25. $-40(0.33) = -1.42$

26. $1.2(-6.2) = -7.4$ [2-5]

27. $-17(-24.2) = 411.4$

28. $7(-8.3)0 = -58.1$

29. $-5(2.8)(-20) = 280$

30. $-12(-1)(-8.6) = 103.2$

31. $75.5 \div (-5) = -15.1$

32. $-0.006 \div (-1) = 0.006$ [2-6]

33. $-115.2 \div (-2.4) = 48$

34. $-5.04 \div 3.6 = 1.4$

35. $0 \div (-19.8) = 0$

36. $-6.21 \div (-0.23) = -27$

What value of the variable makes the statement true? Write the letter of the correct answer.

37. $2^n = 32$ a. 16   b. −5   c. 5   d. 30   [2-7]

38. $5^6 \times 5^2 = 5^n$ a. 4   b. 8   c. 12   d. 36

39. $7^n = 1$ a. 7   b. −6   c. 6   d. 0

40. $3^n = \dfrac{1}{81}$ a. 4   b. 81   c. −4   d. 9   [2-8]

41. $4^{-n} = \dfrac{1}{64}$ a. 16   b. −16   c. 4   d. 3

42. $7^{-6} \times 7^6 = 7^n$ a. −36   b. 0   c. 12   d. −12

Chapter Test

Replace ? with =, >, or < to make a true statement.

1. 7 _?_ 10 **2.** 6 _?_ 1 **3.** 0 _?_ ⁻6 **4.** ⁻2 _?_ ⁻3 [2-1]

Express as an integer.

5. |⁻3| **6.** |7| **7.** |⁻12| **8.** |0|

Write the numbers in order from least to greatest.

9. ⁻6.5, ⁻56, 6.05, ⁻556, ⁻0.6 **10.** 3.02, ⁻3.2, ⁻23, 0.32, ⁻333 [2-2]

Find the sum.

11. ⁻8.4 + 36.8 **12.** ⁻6.3 + ⁺0.12 **13.** 13.2 + ⁻13.2 [2-3]

14. 14.6 + 23.1 **15.** 0 + ⁻11.5 **16.** 0.89 + ⁻16.1 + ⁻0.94

Find the difference.

17. 26.5 − 8.3 **18.** −4.3 − 20.6 **19.** 0 − 13.6 [2-4]

20. −14.2 + (+9.5) **21.** 41 − (−11.67) **22.** −6.4 + (+6.4)

Evaluate the expression when $a = -5$ and $b = -3.6$.

23. $-a - b$ **24.** $-a - (-b)$ **25.** $-|b|$

Find the product.

26. 12(−6.37) **27.** −30(0.45) **28.** −0.37(−20.8) [2-5]

29. −1(−14.27) **30.** 5.4(−8.2)(−3) **31.** −6.11(−9)(−5.5)

Find the quotient.

32. 69.3 ÷ (−3) **33.** −18 ÷ (−2.5) **34.** −19.2 ÷ 10 [2-6]

35. −0.004 ÷ (−1) **36.** 0 ÷ (−15) **37.** −0.08 ÷ (−0.2)

Write the expression without exponents.

38. 5^3 **39.** 20^0 **40.** $4^2 \times 4^3$ **41.** 2^6 [2-7]

42. 6^{-2} **43.** $(-5)^{-3}$ **44.** $8^{-9} \times 8^7$ **45.** $(-3) \times (-3)^{-2}$ [2-8]

3

Rational Numbers

Hummingbirds, like the Violet-Capped Woodnymph Hummingbird shown at the right, can fly forward, vertically, and even backward. Perhaps their most unusual feat is their ability to hover apparently motionless in the air while sipping nectar from a flower. This ability comes from their specialized wing structure and its unique movement. The hummingbird pictured lives in the forests of Brazil. It is only $4\frac{1}{2}$ in. long and has a wing beat of 33 beats per second. To photograph the hummingbird so that its wings appear motionless, an electronic flash time of about $\frac{1}{1000}$ of a second was used. Exposure times of $\frac{1}{100,000}$ of a second have been used to study the precise motion of some hummingbirds' wings and to learn exactly how the wings enable hummingbirds to remain at a fixed point with great ease. In this chapter on rational numbers, you will learn about fractions and decimals and their relationship to each other.

Career Note

Understanding the relationship between animals and their environments is the job of the ecologist. Ecologists study the influence that factors such as temperature, humidity, rainfall, and altitude have on the environment. They monitor levels of pollutants and predict their long term effects on the life cycles of plants and animals.

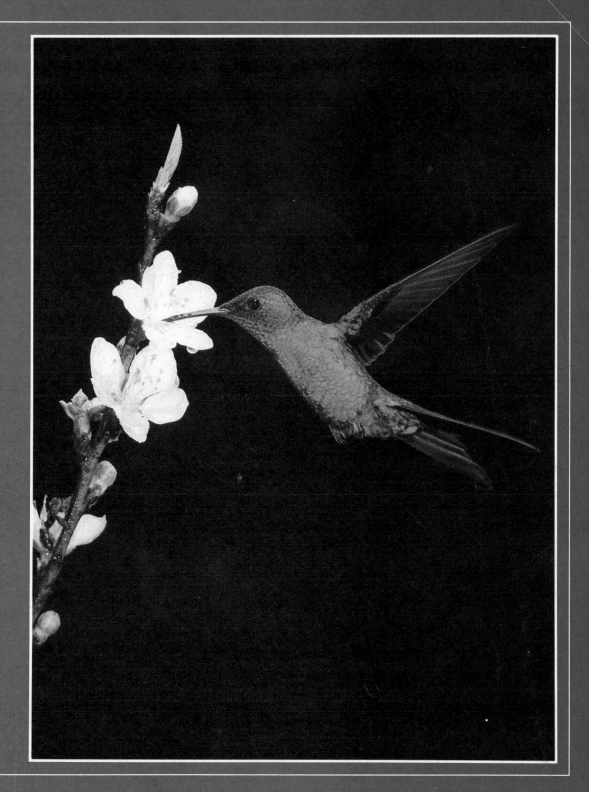

3-1 Factors and Divisibility

A **multiple** of a whole number is the product of that number and any whole number. You can find the multiples of a given whole number by multiplying that number by 0, 1, 2, 3, 4, and so on. For example, the first four multiples of 7 are 0, 7, 14, and 21, since:

$$0 \cdot 7 = 0 \qquad 1 \cdot 7 = 7 \qquad 2 \cdot 7 = 14 \qquad 3 \cdot 7 = 21$$

Any multiple of 2 is called an **even number.** A whole number that is not an even number is called an **odd number.** Notice that since

$$0 = 0 \cdot 2,$$

0 is a multiple of 2 and is therefore an even number.

In general, any number is a multiple of each of its factors. For example, 21 is a multiple of 7 and of 3.

You know that 60 can be written as the product of 5 and 12. Whenever a number, such as 60, can be written as the product of two whole numbers, such as 5 and 12, these two numbers are called **whole number factors** of the first number. A number is said to be **divisible** by its whole number factors. Thus, 60 is divisible by the factors 5 and 12.

To find out if a smaller whole number is a factor of a larger whole number, we divide the larger number by the smaller. If the remainder is 0, then the smaller number is a factor of the larger number. If the remainder is *not* 0, then the smaller number is *not* a factor of the larger number.

EXAMPLE 1 State whether or not the smaller number is a factor of the larger.

    a. 6; 138   **b.** 8; 154

Solution **a.** Divide 138 by 6.   **b.** Divide 154 by 8.

    $138 \div 6 = 23 \text{ R } 0$ $154 \div 8 = 19 \text{ R } 2$

    Since the remainder is 0,   Since the remainder is not 0,
    6 is a factor of 138.   8 is not a factor of 154.

EXAMPLE 2 Find all the factors of 24.

Solution Try each whole number as a divisor, starting with 1.

    $24 \div 1 = 24$ Thus, 1 and 24 are factors.
    $24 \div 2 = 12$ Thus, 2 and 12 are factors.
    $24 \div 3 = 8$ Thus, 3 and 8 are factors.

$24 \div 4 = 6$ Thus, 4 and 6 are factors.

$24 \div 5 = 4 \text{ R } 4$ Thus, 5 is not a factor.

Since $24 \div 6 = 4$, the factors begin to repeat, and we do not have to try any whole number greater than 5 as a divisor. Thus, the factors of 24 are 1, 2, 3, 4, 6, 8, 12, and 24.

Sometimes it may be possible to find the factors of a number by an inspection of the digits of the number. For example, let us

consider multiples of 2: 0, 2, 4, 6, 8, 10, 12, 14, 16, . . .

consider multiples of 5: 0, 5, 10, 15, 20, . . .

consider multiples of 10: 0, 10, 20, 30, 40, . . .

From the patterns we see in the last digits of the sets of multiples above, we can devise the following tests for divisibility.

> Divisibility by 2: A whole number has 2 as a factor if its last digit has 2 as a factor.
>
> Divisibility by 5: A whole number has 5 as a factor if its last digit is 5 or 0.
>
> Divisibility by 10: A whole number has 10 as a factor if its last digit is 0.

Suppose we want to check whether a number, such as 712, is divisible by 4. Since any multiple of 100 is divisible by 4, we know that 700 is divisible by 4. To test 712, then, we simply look at the last two digits. Since 12 is a multiple of 4, the number 712 is also a multiple of 4 ($712 \div 4 = 178$). A similar inspection shows that 950 is not a multiple of 4, since the number represented by the last two digits, 50, is not a multiple of 4 ($950 \div 4$ gives 237 R 2). This suggests the following test for divisibility.

> Divisibility by 4: A whole number has 4 as a factor if its last two digits represent a multiple of 4.

EXAMPLE 3   Test each number for divisibility by 2, 4, 5, and 10.

          a. 35   **b.** 150   **c.** 7736   **d.** 920

Solution
    a. 35: Since the last digit is 5 and is odd, 2 and 10 are not factors. Since 35 is not a multiple of 4, 4 is not a factor. Since the last digit is 5, 5 is a factor.

    b. 150: Since 0 is the last digit, 2, 5, and 10 are factors. 4 is not a factor, since 50 is not a multiple of 4.

    c. 7736: 2 is a factor, since the last digit, 6, is even. 4 is a factor, since 36 is a multiple of 4. 5 and 10 are not factors, since the last digit is not 5 or 0.

    d. 920: 2, 5, and 10 are all factors, since the last digit is 0. 4 is a factor, since the last two digits, 20, represent a multiple of 4.

    Rules for recognizing numbers divisible by 3 or 9 are a bit more difficult to discover. The rules relate to the sum of the digits of the number. Study the following numbers.

	Divisible by 3	Divisible by 9	Sum of digits
393	yes $393 \div 3 = 131$	no $393 \div 9$ gives 43 R 6	15
394	no $394 \div 3$ gives 131 R 1	no $394 \div 9$ gives 43 R 7	16
395	no $395 \div 3$ gives 131 R 2	no $395 \div 9$ gives 43 R 8	17
396	yes $396 \div 3 = 132$	yes $396 \div 9 = 44$	18

Notice that when the sum of the digits of the number is divisible by 3 (15 or 18), the number (393 or 396) is divisible by 3. Notice also that when the sum of the digits is divisible by 9 (18), the number (396) is divisible by 9. This illustrates the following tests.

> **Divisibility by 3:** A whole number has 3 as a factor if the sum of the digits of the number is a multiple of 3.
>
> **Divisibility by 9:** A whole number has 9 as a factor if the sum of the digits of the number is a multiple of 9.

EXAMPLE 4 Test each number for divisibility by 3 and 9.

   a. 714   **b.** 6291   **c.** 4813

Solution   **a.** 7 + 1 + 4 = 12. Since 12 is a multiple of 3 but not a multiple of 9, 714 is divisible by 3, but not by 9.

   b. 6 + 2 + 9 + 1 = 18. Since 18 is a multiple of 3 and of 9, 6291 is divisible by 3 and by 9.

   c. 4 + 8 + 1 + 3 = 16. Since 16 is not a multiple of 3 or of 9, 4813 is not divisible by 3 or by 9.

Class Exercises

State all the factors of each number.

1. 6   **2.** 10   **3.** 20   **4.** 18   **5.** 30

6. What number is a factor of every whole number?

Write the first five multiples of each number.

7. 9   **8.** 14   **9.** 15   **10.** 18

Test each number for divisibility by 2.

11. 130   **12.** 4681   **13.** 105   **14.** 3576

Test each number for divisibility by 4.

15. 8310   **16.** 712   **17.** 86,222   **18.** 5732

Test each number for divisibility by 5 and 10.

19. 8325   **20.** 7602   **21.** 870   **22.** 6395

Test each number for divisibility by 3 and 9.

23. 175   **24.** 288   **25.** 651   **26.** 8766

Written Exercises

List all the factors of each number.

A **1.** 42   **2.** 45   **3.** 32   **4.** 40   **5.** 56

   6. 31   **7.** 84   **8.** 51   **9.** 41   **10.** 112

State which of the numbers 2, 3, 4, 5, 9, and 10 are factors of the given number. Use the tests for divisibility.

11. 132   **12.** 150   **13.** 195   **14.** 4280   **15.** 567

16. 8155   **17.** 43,260   **18.** 720   **19.** 1147   **20.** 78,921

For each number, determine whether (a) 2 is a factor, (b) 3 is a factor, and (c) 6 is a factor. What appears to be true in order for 6 to be a factor?

21. 1316   **22.** 2,817,000   **23.** 31,027,302

24. 1224   **25.** 2,147,640   **26.** 36,111,114

Supply the missing digit of the first number if it is known to have the other two numbers as factors.

B **27.** 35?; 2, 3   **28.** 876?; 2, 5   **29.** 910?; 3, 5

30. 472?; 3, 4   **31.** 61?2; 4, 9   **32.** 47?2; 4, 9

33. Any multiple of 1000 is divisible by 8. Use this fact to devise a test for divisibility by 8.

34. The total number of pages in a book must be a multiple of 32. If the book consists of 10 chapters, each 24 pages long, and 8 pages of introductory material, how many blank pages will be left?

C **35.** Devise a test for divisibility by 25.

36. A **perfect number** is one that is the sum of all of its factors except itself. The smallest perfect number is 6, since $6 = 1 + 2 + 3$. Find the next perfect number.

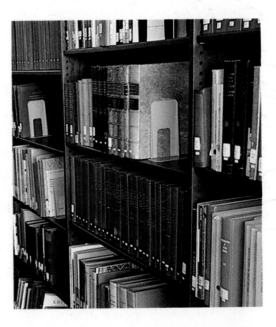

Review Exercises

Complete with <, >, or =.

1. 80 _?_ 800   **2.** 136 _?_ 119   **3.** 21.6 _?_ 2.29   **4.** 0.87 _?_ 0.0941

5. 3.081 _?_ 3.101   **6.** 48.88 _?_ 49.17   **7.** 3^3 _?_ $(2 + 1)^2$ **8.** $2^3 + 1$ _?_ $(2 + 1)^3$

3-2 Prime Numbers and Composite Numbers

Consider the list of counting numbers and their factors given at the right. Notice that each of the numbers 2, 3, 5, 7, and 11 has *exactly* two factors: 1 and the number itself. A number with this property is called a **prime number.** A counting number that has more than two factors is called a **composite number.** In the list 4, 6, 8, 9, 10, and 12 are all composite numbers. Since 1 has exactly one factor, it is neither prime nor composite.

Number	Factors
1	1
2	1, 2
3	1, 3
4	1, 2, 4
5	1, 5
6	1, 2, 3, 6
7	1, 7
8	1, 2, 4, 8
9	1, 3, 9
10	1, 2, 5, 10
11	1, 11
12	1, 2, 3, 4, 6, 12

About 230 B.C. Eratosthenes, a Greek mathematician, suggested a way to find prime numbers in a list of all the counting numbers up to a certain number. Eratosthenes first crossed out all multiples of 2, except 2 itself. Next he crossed out all multiples of the next remaining number, 3, except 3 itself. He continued crossing out multiples of each successive remaining number except the number itself. The numbers remaining at the end of this process are the primes.

```
      1    2    3    4    5    6    7    8    9
 10   11   12   13   14   15   16   17   18   19
 20   21   22   23   24   25   26   27   28   29
 30   31   32   33   34   35   36   37   . . .
```

The method just described is called the **Sieve of Eratosthenes,** because it picks out the prime numbers as a strainer, or sieve, picks out solid particles from a liquid.

Every counting number greater than 1 has at least one prime factor, which may be the number itself. You can factor a number into prime factors by using either of the following methods.

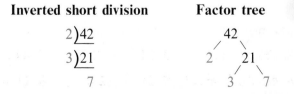

Inverted short division

$$2\overline{)42}$$
$$3\overline{)21}$$
$$7$$

Factor tree

42
2   21
3   7

Another factor tree for the number 42 is shown at the right. Notice that the prime factors of 42 are the same in either factor tree except for their order. Every whole number is similar to 42 in this respect. This fact is expressed in the following theorem.

$$\begin{array}{ccc} & 42 & \\ \diagup & & \diagdown \\ 3 & & 14 \\ & \diagup & \diagdown \\ & 7 & 2 \end{array}$$

Fundamental Theorem of Arithmetic

Every whole number greater than 1 can be written as a product of prime factors in exactly one way, except for the order of the factors.

When we write 42 as $2 \cdot 3 \cdot 7$, this product of prime factors is called the **prime factorization** of 42.

EXAMPLE Give the prime factorization of 60.

Solution

Method 1

$$\begin{array}{r} 2\overline{)60} \\ 2\overline{)30} \\ 3\overline{)15} \\ 5 \end{array}$$

Method 2

$$\begin{array}{ccc} & 60 & \\ \diagup & & \diagdown \\ 2 & & 30 \\ & \diagup & \diagdown \\ & 2 & 15 \\ & & \diagup \diagdown \\ & & 3 \quad 5 \end{array}$$

Using either method, we find that the prime factorization of 60 is $2 \cdot 2 \cdot 3 \cdot 5$, or $2^2 \cdot 3 \cdot 5$.

Class Exercises

State whether each number is prime or composite.

1. 7   **2.** 9   **3.** 15   **4.** 23   **5.** 22   **6.** 19

Name the prime factors of each number.

7. 21   **8.** 10   **9.** 18   **10.** 26   **11.** 30   **12.** 70

Name the number whose prime factorization is given.

13. $3^2 \cdot 5$ **14.** $2^2 \cdot 3^2$ **15.** $2^3 \cdot 3$

16. $2 \cdot 7^2$ **17.** $3^2 \cdot 11$ **18.** $2^2 \cdot 5^2$

Written Exercises 1-20

State whether each number is prime or composite.

A
1. 39　　2. 41　　3. 51　　4. 111　　5. 124　　6. 321
7. 641　　8. 753　　9. 894　　10. 1164　　11. 2061　　12. 3001

Give the prime factorization of each whole number.

13. 12　　14. 50　　15. 24　　16. 28　　17. 39　　18. 56
19. 66　　20. 51　　21. 54　　22. 63　　23. 84　　24. 90
25. 196　　26. 360　　27. 308　　28. 693　　29. 114　　30. 1150

B
31. Explain why 2 is the only even prime number.

32. Write the prime factorizations of the square numbers 16, 36, 81, and 144 by using exponents. What do you think must be true of the exponents in the prime factorization of a square number?

33. Explain why the sum of two prime numbers greater than 2 can never be a prime number.

34. Explain how you know that each of the following numbers must be composite: 111;　111,111;　111,111,111;　. . .

35. List all the possible digits that can be the last digit of a prime number that is greater than 10.

C
36. Choose a six-digit number, such as 652,652, the last three digits of which are a repeat of the first three digits. Show that 7, 11, and 13 are all factors of the number you chose.

37. Since 7, 11, and 13 are factors of any number of the type defined in Exercise 36, what is the largest composite number that is always a factor of such a number? What is the other factor?

38. Give an example to show that the Fundamental Theorem of Arithmetic would be false if 1 were defined to be a prime number.

Review Exercises

Simplify.

1. $-4 + 6$　　2. $8 + (-12)$　　3. $3 - 4$　　4. $10 - (-15)$
5. $-12 \cdot (-20)$　　6. $7 \cdot (-3)$　　7. $-48 \div (-24)$　　8. $-72 \div 8$

3-3 Positive and Negative Fractions

In any fraction the number above the fraction bar is called the **numerator** and the number below the bar is called the **denominator.** Since the fraction bar indicates division,

$$\tfrac{3}{5} \text{ means } 3 \div 5.$$

A study of fractions on a number line shows some important properties of fractions.

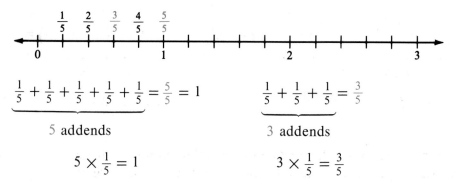

$$\tfrac{1}{5} + \tfrac{1}{5} + \tfrac{1}{5} + \tfrac{1}{5} + \tfrac{1}{5} = \tfrac{5}{5} = 1 \qquad\qquad \tfrac{1}{5} + \tfrac{1}{5} + \tfrac{1}{5} = \tfrac{3}{5}$$

$$\underbrace{}_{\text{5 addends}} \qquad\qquad\qquad \underbrace{}_{\text{3 addends}}$$

$$5 \times \tfrac{1}{5} = 1 \qquad\qquad\qquad 3 \times \tfrac{1}{5} = \tfrac{3}{5}$$

We can state these properties in general terms that apply to all positive fractions.

Properties

For all whole numbers a and b ($a > 0, b > 0$),

$$\underbrace{\tfrac{1}{b} + \tfrac{1}{b} + \cdots + \tfrac{1}{b}}_{b \text{ addends}} = \tfrac{b}{b} = 1 \qquad\qquad \underbrace{\tfrac{1}{b} + \tfrac{1}{b} + \cdots + \tfrac{1}{b}}_{a \text{ addends}} = \tfrac{a}{b}$$

$$b \times \tfrac{1}{b} = 1 \qquad\qquad\qquad\qquad a \times \tfrac{1}{b} = \tfrac{a}{b}$$

$$1 \div b = \tfrac{1}{b} \qquad\qquad\qquad\qquad a \div b = \tfrac{a}{b}$$

Just as the negative integers are the opposites of the positive integers, the negative fractions are the opposites of the positive fractions. For every fraction $\tfrac{a}{b}$ there is a fraction denoted by $-\tfrac{a}{b}$ that is said to be the **opposite** of $\frac{a}{b}$. On the number line the graphs of $\frac{a}{b}$ and $-\frac{a}{b}$ are on opposite sides of 0 and at equal distances from 0. For example, $\frac{3}{5}$ and $-\frac{3}{5}$ are opposites. They are shown on the number line below.

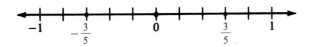

Properties similar to those for positive fractions apply to negative fractions.

$$-\frac{1}{5} + \left(-\frac{1}{5}\right) + \left(-\frac{1}{5}\right) + \left(-\frac{1}{5}\right) + \left(-\frac{1}{5}\right) = -1 \qquad -\frac{1}{5} + \left(-\frac{1}{5}\right) + \left(-\frac{1}{5}\right) = -\frac{3}{5}$$

$$\underbrace{\phantom{-\frac{1}{5} + \left(-\frac{1}{5}\right) + \left(-\frac{1}{5}\right) + \left(-\frac{1}{5}\right) + \left(-\frac{1}{5}\right)}}_{\text{5 addends}} \qquad \underbrace{\phantom{-\frac{1}{5} + \left(-\frac{1}{5}\right) + \left(-\frac{1}{5}\right)}}_{\text{3 addends}}$$

$$5 \times \left(-\frac{1}{5}\right) = -1 \qquad\qquad 3 \times \left(-\frac{1}{5}\right) = -\frac{3}{5}$$

In an earlier section you learned that the quotient of two numbers of opposite sign is negative. Using this rule we can write the following:

$$1 \div (-4) = \frac{1}{-4} = -\frac{1}{4} \qquad\qquad (-1) \div 4 = \frac{-1}{4} = -\frac{1}{4}$$

Therefore, we can write the opposite of $\frac{1}{4}$ as $-\frac{1}{4}$, or as $\frac{-1}{4}$, or as $\frac{1}{-4}$. In general, for $b \neq 0$, $-\frac{a}{b} = \frac{-a}{b} = \frac{a}{-b}$.

EXAMPLE 1   Express $-\frac{3}{8}$ in two other ways.

Solution $-\frac{3}{8} = \frac{-3}{8} = \frac{3}{-8}$

EXAMPLE 2   Complete.

        a. $\left(-\frac{1}{3}\right) + \left(-\frac{1}{3}\right) + \left(-\frac{1}{3}\right) = \underline{}$ **b.** $3 \times \underline{} = -1$

        c. $2 \times \left(-\frac{1}{5}\right) = \underline{}$ **d.** $-\frac{2}{5} = \underline{} \div 5$

Solution   **a.** $\left(-\frac{1}{3}\right) + \left(-\frac{1}{3}\right) + \left(-\frac{1}{3}\right) = -1$ **b.** $3 \times \left(-\frac{1}{3}\right) = -1$

        c. $2 \times \left(-\frac{1}{5}\right) = -\frac{2}{5}$ **d.** $-\frac{2}{5} = \frac{-2}{5} = -2 \div 5$

When we work with fractions having numerators and denominators that are integers, we are working with a new set of numbers called *rational numbers.* Any number that can be represented by a fraction $\frac{a}{b}$, where a and b are integers and b is not 0, is a **rational number.** Notice that the integers themselves are rational numbers. For example, -9 can be written as $\frac{-9}{1}$, 0 as $\frac{0}{1}$, and 26 as $\frac{26}{1}$.

Class Exercises

Name the rational numbers whose graphs are shown.

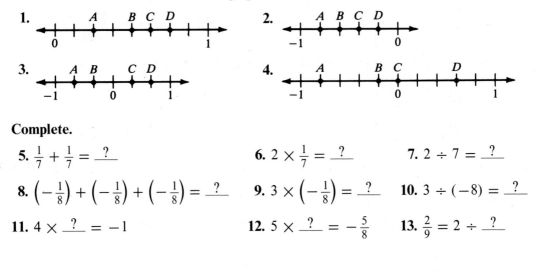

Complete.

5. $\frac{1}{7} + \frac{1}{7} = \underline{\quad?\quad}$

6. $2 \times \frac{1}{7} = \underline{\quad?\quad}$

7. $2 \div 7 = \underline{\quad?\quad}$

8. $\left(-\frac{1}{8}\right) + \left(-\frac{1}{8}\right) + \left(-\frac{1}{8}\right) = \underline{\quad?\quad}$

9. $3 \times \left(-\frac{1}{8}\right) = \underline{\quad?\quad}$

10. $3 \div (-8) = \underline{\quad?\quad}$

11. $4 \times \underline{\quad?\quad} = -1$

12. $5 \times \underline{\quad?\quad} = -\frac{5}{8}$

13. $\frac{2}{9} = 2 \div \underline{\quad?\quad}$

Written Exercises

Graph each set of rational numbers on a number line.

A **1.** $-1, -\frac{1}{3}, 0, \frac{1}{3}, 1$

2. $-1, -\frac{1}{4}, 0, \frac{1}{4}, 1$

3. $0, \frac{1}{5}, \frac{5}{5}, \frac{6}{5}$

4. $-\frac{4}{3}, -\frac{3}{3}, -\frac{2}{3}, 0$

5. $-\frac{5}{4}, -\frac{3}{4}, \frac{3}{4}, \frac{5}{4}$

6. $-\frac{5}{3}, -\frac{4}{3}, \frac{4}{3}, \frac{5}{3}$

Express in two other ways.

7. $-\frac{1}{2}$

8. $\frac{-1}{3}$

9. $\frac{-1}{11}$

10. $\frac{-1}{6}$

11. $\frac{2}{-9}$

12. $\frac{-9}{10}$

13. $-\frac{13}{6}$

14. $\frac{5}{-8}$

15. $-\frac{3}{4}$

16. $\frac{5}{-9}$

Complete.

17. $\underline{\ ?\ } \times \left(-\frac{1}{6}\right) = -1$

18. $4 \times \underline{\ ?\ } = \frac{4}{7}$

19. $3 \times \underline{\ ?\ } = \frac{3}{4}$

20. $5 \div 6 = \underline{\ ?\ }$

21. $2 \div \underline{\ ?\ } = \frac{2}{3}$

22. $4 \times \underline{\ ?\ } = -\frac{4}{9}$

Evaluate the expression when $a = 4$, $b = -3$, **and** $c = 5$.

B 23. $\frac{a+c}{b}$

24. $\frac{a-c}{a}$

25. $\frac{2b-1}{8}$

26. $\frac{2c-b}{a}$

27. $\frac{a^2-c^2}{2a+c}$
$\frac{\ \ }{\ \ }$

What value of the variable makes the statement true?

28. $x \times \frac{1}{5} = 1$

29. $3y = -1$

30. $\frac{1}{b} = -\frac{1}{8}$

31. $-\frac{3}{4} = \frac{c}{4}$

32. $-\frac{3}{5} = d \div 5$

33. $\frac{-5}{9} = \frac{5}{m}$

Write the expression as a positive or a negative fraction.

EXAMPLE   **a.** $3(7)^{-1}$ **b.** $(-5)^{-1}$

Solution   **a.** $3(7)^{-1} = 3 \times \frac{1}{7} = \frac{3}{7}$ **b.** $(-5)^{-1} = \frac{1}{-5} = -\frac{1}{5}$

C 34. $2(3)^{-1}$ **35.** $7(6)^{-1}$ **36.** $5^{-1} + 5^{-1}$ **37.** $7^{-1} + 7^{-1} + 7^{-1}$

38. $(-2)^{-1}$ **39.** $(-9)^{-1}$ **40.** $3(-5)^{-1}$ **41.** $2(-7)^{-1}$

42. $(-3)^{-1} + (-3)^{-1}$ **43.** $(-8)^{-1} + (-8)^{-1} + (-8)^{-1}$

Review Exercises

Complete.

1. Factors of 72: 1, 2, $\underline{\ ?\ }$, $\underline{\ ?\ }$, 6, $\underline{\ ?\ }$, 9, 12, $\underline{\ ?\ }$, 24, $\underline{\ ?\ }$, 72

2. What is the prime factorization of 72?

3. Factors of 90: $\underline{\ ?\ }$, 2, 3, $\underline{\ ?\ }$, $\underline{\ ?\ }$, 9, $\underline{\ ?\ }$, $\underline{\ ?\ }$, 18, $\underline{\ ?\ }$, $\underline{\ ?\ }$, 90

4. What is the prime factorization of 90?

5. $18x^2y = 3 \times \underline{\ ?\ } \times x \times \underline{\ ?\ } \times y$

6. $24ab^3 = 4 \times \underline{\ ?\ } \times \underline{\ ?\ } \times \underline{\ ?\ } \times b \times b$

3-4 Equivalent Fractions

The number line shows the graphs of several fractions.

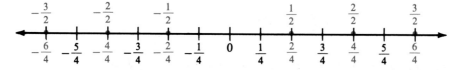

Since $-\frac{1}{2}$ and $-\frac{2}{4}$ have the same graph, they are two names for the same number. Fractions that represent the same number are called **equivalent** fractions. Thus,

$$-\frac{3}{2} \text{ is equivalent to } -\frac{6}{4}; \frac{3}{2} \text{ is equivalent to } \frac{6}{4}.$$

Notice that $\frac{3}{2} = \frac{3 \times 2}{2 \times 2} = \frac{6}{4}$ and $\frac{6}{4} = \frac{6 \div 2}{4 \div 2} = \frac{3}{2}$.

We may state the following general rule.

> ## Rule
>
> For all numbers a, b, and c ($b \neq 0$, $c \neq 0$),
>
> $$\frac{a}{b} = \frac{a \times c}{b \times c} \qquad \text{and} \qquad \frac{a}{b} = \frac{a \div c}{b \div c}$$

EXAMPLE 1   Write as an equivalent fraction with a denominator of 12.

   a. $\frac{5}{6}$ **b.** $-\frac{32}{48}$

Solution   **a.** Since $6 \times 2 = 12$, we write $\frac{5}{6} = \frac{5 \times 2}{6 \times 2} = \frac{10}{12}$.

   b. *Method 1*
   Since $48 \div 4 = 12$, we write

   $$-\frac{32}{48} = \frac{-32}{48} = \frac{-32 \div 4}{48 \div 4} = \frac{-8}{12}, \text{ or } -\frac{8}{12}.$$

   Method 2
   $$-\frac{32}{48} = -\frac{32 \div 4}{48 \div 4} = -\frac{8}{12}$$

Notice that we usually write our answers with the minus sign in front of the fraction.

Sometimes we simply show the results of dividing a numerator and denominator by the same number. In Example 1, we can think of dividing by 4 as we write

$$-\frac{\overset{8}{\cancel{32}}}{\underset{12}{\cancel{48}}} = -\frac{8}{12}.$$

A fraction is in **lowest terms** when the numerator and denominator have no common factor other than 1. To write a fraction in lowest terms, we can divide numerator and denominator by a common factor as many times as needed until they have no common factor other than 1.

$$\frac{45}{75} = \frac{45 \div 5}{75 \div 5} = \frac{9 \div 3}{15 \div 3} = \frac{3}{5}$$

Another way to write a fraction in lowest terms is to use the greatest common factor method. The **greatest common factor** (GCF) of two numbers is the greatest whole number that is a factor of each number. To find the GCF of two numbers, we write the prime factorizations of the two numbers, and find the greatest power of each prime factor that occurs in *both* factorizations. The product of these powers is the GCF.

EXAMPLE 2 Find the GCF of 84 and 120.

Solution
$$84 = 2 \times 2 \times 3 \times 7 = 2^2 \times 3 \times 7$$
$$120 = 2 \times 2 \times 2 \times 3 \times 5 = 2^3 \times 3 \times 5$$
$$GCF = 2^2 \times 3 = 12$$

To write a fraction in lowest terms, we divide the numerator and the denominator by their GCF.

EXAMPLE 3 Write $\frac{72}{80}$ in lowest terms.

Solution
$$72 = 2 \times 2 \times 2 \times 3 \times 3 = 2^3 \times 3^2$$
$$80 = 2 \times 2 \times 2 \times 2 \times 5 = 2^4 \times 5$$
$$GCF = 2^3 = 8$$

$$\frac{72}{80} = \frac{72 \div 8}{80 \div 8} = \frac{9}{10}$$

When two numbers have no common factor other than 1, they are said to be **relatively prime.** For example, 9 and 10 are relatively prime. A fraction is in lowest terms when its numerator and denominator are relatively prime.

A **common fraction** is a fraction whose numerator and denominator are both integers; for example, $\frac{2}{5}$ or $-\frac{12}{7}$. A **proper fraction** is a positive fraction whose numerator is less than its denominator, or the opposite of such a fraction; for example, $\frac{3}{8}$ or $-\frac{7}{9}$. A fraction that is not a proper fraction, such as $\frac{9}{4}$ or $-\frac{9}{4}$, is called an **improper fraction.** A number, such as $1\frac{1}{4}$, consisting of a whole number plus a fraction, is called a **mixed number.** Mixed numbers may be written as improper fractions, and improper fractions may be written as mixed numbers. A mixed number is in simple form if the fractional part is in lowest terms.

$$7\frac{15}{27} \text{ in simple form is } 7\frac{5}{9}.$$

EXAMPLE 4 Write as a mixed number in simple form.

a. $\frac{12}{8}$ b. $-\frac{12}{8}$

Solution   a. $\frac{12}{8} = 12 \div 8$, which gives 1 R4.

Therefore $\frac{12}{8} = 1\frac{4}{8} = 1\frac{1}{2}$.

b. $-\frac{12}{8}$ is *the opposite of* $\frac{12}{8}$, so $-\frac{12}{8} = -1\frac{1}{2}$.

EXAMPLE 5 Write $7\frac{2}{5}$ as an improper fraction.

Solution $7\frac{2}{5} = \frac{7}{1} + \frac{2}{5} = \frac{7 \times 5}{1 \times 5} + \frac{2}{5} = \frac{(7 \times 5) + 2}{5} = \frac{37}{5}$

Class Exercises

For each fraction, state the GCF of the numerator and denominator. Then state an equivalent fraction in lowest terms.

1. $\frac{4}{24}$ 2. $\frac{5}{20}$ 3. $\frac{-12}{16}$ 4. $-\frac{8}{12}$ 5. $\frac{-9}{12}$

State an equivalent improper fraction.

6. $3\frac{2}{5}$ 7. $-4\frac{1}{8}$ 8. $-7\frac{2}{3}$ 9. $9\frac{3}{4}$ 10. $-5\frac{1}{6}$

State an equivalent mixed number in simple form.

11. $\frac{13}{5}$ 12. $-\frac{14}{4}$ 13. $\frac{-24}{5}$ 14. $\frac{19}{3}$ 15. $\frac{-32}{10}$

Written Exercises

Complete.

A **1.** $\frac{2}{3} = \frac{?}{6}$ **2.** $\frac{5}{7} = \frac{?}{21}$ **3.** $1 = \frac{5}{?}$ **4.** $4 = \frac{?}{2}$ **5.** $-\frac{14}{32} = -\frac{?}{16}$

6. $\frac{42}{-54} = \frac{?}{-9}$ **7.** $\frac{18}{27} = \frac{2}{?}$ **8.** $-7 = -\frac{?}{3}$ **9.** $\frac{-7}{25} = \frac{-35}{?}$ **10.** $-\frac{3}{4} = -\frac{?}{16}$

Write as a proper fraction in lowest terms or as a mixed number in simple form.

11. $\frac{21}{35}$ **12.** $\frac{24}{40}$ **13.** $\frac{11}{4}$ **14.** $\frac{25}{7}$ **15.** $-\frac{9}{81}$

16. $\frac{54}{81}$ **17.** $-\frac{17}{3}$ **18.** $-\frac{56}{72}$ **19.** $\frac{-34}{85}$ **20.** $-\frac{29}{5}$

21. $\frac{125}{12}$ **22.** $\frac{49}{63}$ **23.** $-\frac{79}{13}$ **24.** $\frac{32}{10}$ **25.** $\frac{-300}{7}$

Write as an improper fraction.

26. $3\frac{1}{4}$ **27.** $2\frac{1}{8}$ **28.** $5\frac{3}{7}$ **29.** $6\frac{3}{16}$ **30.** $5\frac{3}{8}$

31. $-4\frac{3}{8}$ **32.** $-3\frac{7}{8}$ **33.** $-16\frac{1}{3}$ **34.** $-7\frac{2}{9}$ **35.** $-8\frac{3}{10}$

What value of the variable makes the statement true?

B **36.** $\frac{b}{4} = \frac{6}{12}$ **37.** $\frac{x}{16} = \frac{9}{48}$ **38.** $\frac{a}{6} = \frac{10}{60}$ **39.** $\frac{d}{5} = \frac{-3}{15}$

40. $\frac{1}{x} = \frac{4}{16}$ **41.** $\frac{0}{6} = \frac{n}{12}$ **42.** $\frac{5}{-1} = \frac{20}{n}$ **43.** $\frac{1}{3} = \frac{8}{n}$

Simplify by writing an equivalent fraction in which the numerator and denominator have no common factors.

EXAMPLE $\dfrac{15x^2y}{20xy^2} = \dfrac{3 \times \overset{1}{\cancel{5}} \times \overset{1}{\cancel{x}} \times x \times \overset{1}{\cancel{y}}}{4 \times \underset{1}{\cancel{5}} \times \underset{1}{\cancel{x}} \times \underset{1}{\cancel{y}} \times y} = \dfrac{3x}{4y}$

44. $\frac{2a}{6a}$ **45.** $\frac{4b}{20}$ **46.** $\frac{c}{c^2}$ **47.** $\frac{d^2e}{de^2}$

48. $\frac{3x}{15y}$ **49.** $\frac{6n^2}{18n}$ **50.** $\frac{4h}{6hk}$ **51.** $\frac{uv^2}{3u^2v}$

Review Exercises

Simplify.

1. 7^2 **2.** 11^3 **3.** 6^4 **4.** 2^8 **5.** 1^5

6. $5^2 \times 3^2$ **7.** $4^3 \times 9^2$ **8.** $2^4 \times 6^2$ **9.** $3^3 \times 3^2$ **10.** $8^2 \times 2^4$

3-5 Least Common Denominator

In calculations and comparisons, we work with more than one fraction. It is sometimes necessary to replace fractions with equivalent fractions so that all have the same denominator, called a *common denominator*. For example, in the addition $\frac{1}{6} + \frac{3}{4}$ we may write $\frac{1}{6}$ as $\frac{2}{12}$ and $\frac{3}{4}$ as $\frac{9}{12}$, using 12 as a common denominator. We may also use 24, 36, 48, or any other multiple of both denominators as a common denominator.

The **least common denominator** (LCD) is the most convenient denominator to use. The LCD is the least common multiple (LCM) of the denominators. The LCD is found using the prime factorizations of the denominators. For each prime factor of any of the denominators, find the highest power of that factor that occurs in *any* prime factorization. The product of these powers is the LCD.

EXAMPLE 1   Write equivalent fractions with the LCD: $\frac{5}{48}$, $\frac{11}{120}$.

Solution   The LCD is the least common multiple of 48 and 120. Use prime factorization to find the LCM.

Prime factorization of 48: $2 \times 2 \times 2 \times 2 \times 3$, or $2^4 \times 3$
Prime factorization of 120: $2 \times 2 \times 2 \times 3 \times 5$, or $2^3 \times 3 \times 5$

The LCM is the product of the highest powers of each factor. The LCM $= 2^4 \times 3 \times 5 = 240$, so the LCD $= 240$.

$$\frac{5}{48} = \frac{5 \times 5}{48 \times 5} = \frac{25}{240} \qquad\qquad \frac{11}{120} = \frac{11 \times 2}{120 \times 2} = \frac{22}{240}$$

EXAMPLE 2   Replace $\underline{\ ?\ }$ with $<$, $>$, or $=$ to make a true statement.

     a. $\frac{5}{6} \underline{\ ?\ } \frac{6}{7}$ **b.** $-\frac{5}{8} \underline{\ ?\ } -\frac{9}{14}$

Solution   First rewrite each pair of fractions as equivalent fractions with the LCD. Then compare the fractions.

a. The LCD is the LCM of 6 and 7, or 42.

$$\frac{5}{6} = \frac{5 \times 7}{6 \times 7} = \frac{35}{42} \qquad\qquad \frac{6}{7} = \frac{6 \times 6}{7 \times 6} = \frac{36}{42}$$

$$\frac{35}{42} < \frac{36}{42}, \text{ so } \frac{5}{6} < \frac{6}{7}.$$

b. The LCD is the LCM of 8 and 14, or 56.

$$-\frac{5}{8} = -\frac{5 \times 7}{8 \times 7} = -\frac{35}{56} \qquad\qquad -\frac{9}{14} = -\frac{9 \times 4}{14 \times 4} = -\frac{36}{56}$$

$$-\frac{35}{56} > -\frac{36}{56}, \text{ so } -\frac{5}{8} > -\frac{9}{14}.$$

When fractions have variables in their denominators, we may obtain a common denominator by finding a common multiple of the denominators.

EXAMPLE 3   Write as equivalent fractions with a common denominator: $\frac{2}{a}, \frac{3}{b}$.

Solution $\frac{2}{a} = \frac{2 \times b}{a \times b} = \frac{2b}{ab}$ $\frac{3}{b} = \frac{3 \times a}{b \times a} = \frac{3a}{ab}$

Class Exercises

State the LCM of the pair of numbers.

1. 6, 18   **2.** 11, 4   **3.** 10, 8   **4.** 15, 12   **5.** 32, 48

State the LCD of the pair of fractions.

6. $\frac{1}{2}, \frac{3}{4}$ **7.** $\frac{5}{6}, \frac{1}{2}$ **8.** $\frac{3}{4}, -\frac{1}{3}$ **9.** $-\frac{2}{9}, \frac{1}{6}$ **10.** $\frac{1}{16}, \frac{5}{12}$

Written Exercises

Write the fractions as equivalent fractions with the least common denominator (LCD).

A   **1.** $\frac{1}{3}, \frac{1}{12}$ **2.** $\frac{1}{4}, \frac{1}{12}$ **3.** $\frac{3}{4}, \frac{5}{8}$ **4.** $\frac{3}{8}, \frac{3}{16}$

5. $\frac{2}{9}, -\frac{1}{27}$ **6.** $-\frac{1}{7}, \frac{1}{49}$ **7.** $\frac{10}{21}, \frac{2}{49}$ **8.** $\frac{7}{18}, \frac{5}{36}$

9. $-\frac{2}{3}, \frac{7}{30}$ **10.** $\frac{5}{12}, -\frac{6}{11}$ **11.** $\frac{4}{75}, \frac{7}{100}$ **12.** $\frac{9}{56}, \frac{4}{63}$

13. $-\frac{3}{7}, -\frac{7}{112}$ **14.** $-\frac{4}{17}, -\frac{9}{16}$ **15.** $\frac{5}{42}, \frac{5}{49}$ **16.** $\frac{5}{84}, \frac{7}{12}$

B   **17.** $\frac{7}{8}, \frac{5}{16}, \frac{21}{40}$ **18.** $\frac{1}{4}, \frac{1}{9}, \frac{1}{5}$ **19.** $\frac{3}{7}, \frac{7}{4}, \frac{4}{9}$ **20.** $\frac{11}{18}, \frac{1}{54}, \frac{2}{27}$

21. $\frac{1}{65}, \frac{3}{5}, \frac{9}{26}$ **22.** $-\frac{7}{8}, \frac{9}{28}, \frac{2}{49}$ **23.** $-\frac{5}{6}, \frac{2}{9}, -\frac{7}{8}$ **24.** $\frac{11}{12}, \frac{1}{72}, -\frac{7}{8}$

25. $\frac{a}{3}, \frac{b}{6}$ **26.** $\frac{m}{25}, \frac{n}{15}$ **27.** $\frac{h}{25}, \frac{h}{100}, \frac{h}{125}$ **28.** $\frac{a}{2}, \frac{b}{3}, \frac{c}{4}$

Write the fractions as equivalent fractions with a common denominator.

29. $\frac{1}{c}, \frac{2}{3c}$ **30.** $\frac{1}{x}, \frac{1}{y}$ **31.** $\frac{3}{x}, \frac{1}{y}, \frac{5}{z}$ **32.** $\frac{-1}{r}, \frac{2}{rs}, \frac{r}{s}$

Replace ? with <, >, or = to make a true statement.

33. $\frac{1}{3}$? $\frac{3}{6}$

34. $\frac{3}{4}$? $\frac{5}{8}$

35. $-\frac{2}{3}$? $-\frac{7}{12}$

36. $-\frac{5}{8}$? $-\frac{5}{16}$

37. $-\frac{3}{5}$? $-\frac{5}{7}$

38. $-\frac{2}{4}$? $-\frac{3}{5}$

C **39.** Let $\frac{a}{b}$ and $\frac{c}{d}$ be fractions with $b > 0$ and $d > 0$. Write $\frac{a}{b}$ and $\frac{c}{d}$ as equivalent fractions with a common denominator. How do $\frac{a}{b}$ and $\frac{c}{d}$ compare when $ad < bc$? when $ad = bc$? when $ad > bc$? Give two examples to illustrate each of your conclusions.

Self-Test A

State which of the numbers 2, 3, 4, 5, 9, and 10 are factors of the given number. Use the tests for divisibility.

1. 756

2. 7821

3. 11,340

4. 34,447

[3–1]

Find out whether each number is prime or composite. If it is composite, give its prime factorization.

5. 108

6. 79

7. 87

8. 109

[3–2]

Complete.

9. $3 \times \underline{} = -1$

10. $7 \div 9 = \underline{}$

11. $-\frac{2}{3} = \frac{-2}{3} = \underline{}$

[3–3]

Write as a proper fraction in lowest terms or as a mixed number in simple form.

12. $\frac{16}{64}$

13. $-\frac{72}{30}$

14. $\frac{32}{42}$

15. $\frac{-71}{48}$

16. $\frac{68}{16}$

[3–4]

Write as an improper fraction.

17. $2\frac{1}{5}$

18. $-3\frac{2}{3}$

19. $6\frac{4}{15}$

20. $1\frac{7}{12}$

21. $-8\frac{5}{8}$

Write as equivalent fractions with the least common denominator.

22. $\frac{7}{10}, \frac{7}{8}$

23. $-\frac{10}{49}, \frac{2}{21}$

24. $\frac{3}{50}, \frac{6}{225}$

25. $-\frac{8}{15}, \frac{-1}{30}$

[3–5]

Self-Test answers and Extra Practice are at the back of the book.

3-6 Adding and Subtracting Common Fractions

You have added fractions having a common denominator by adding the numerators and writing the result with the same denominator. We can illustrate the reasoning for this rule using the sum $\frac{2}{13} + \frac{5}{13}$. The reason for each statement at left below is given on the same line at right. All of the properties for addition, subtraction, multiplication, and division of positive and negative numbers hold for the rational numbers.

$$\frac{2}{13} + \frac{5}{13} = \left(2 \times \frac{1}{13}\right) \times \left(5 \times \frac{1}{13}\right) \qquad \text{By the rule } \frac{a}{b} = a \times \frac{1}{b}$$

$$= (2 + 5) \times \frac{1}{13} \qquad \text{By the distributive property}$$

$$= (7) \times \frac{1}{13} \qquad \text{Substitution of 7 for } 2 + 5$$

$$= \frac{7}{13} \qquad \text{By the rule } a \times \frac{1}{b} = \frac{a}{b}$$

The methods for adding and subtracting positive fractions apply as well to adding and subtracting negative fractions.

Rules

For all numbers a, b, and $c(c \neq 0)$,

$$\frac{a}{c} + \frac{b}{c} = \frac{a + b}{c} \quad \text{and} \quad \frac{a}{c} - \frac{b}{c} = \frac{a - b}{c}$$

EXAMPLE 1 Add or subtract. Write the answers in lowest terms.

a. $-\frac{3}{8} + \frac{1}{8}$ **b.** $\frac{23}{60} - \left(-\frac{17}{60}\right)$

Solution **a.** $-\frac{3}{8} + \frac{1}{8} = \frac{-3}{8} + \frac{1}{8}$ **b.** $\frac{23}{60} - \left(-\frac{17}{60}\right) = \frac{23}{60} + \frac{17}{60}$

$$= \frac{-3 + 1}{8} \qquad\qquad = \frac{23 + 17}{60}$$

$$= \frac{-2}{8} \qquad\qquad = \frac{40}{60}$$

$$= \frac{-1}{4}, \text{ or } -\frac{1}{4} \qquad\qquad = \frac{2}{3}$$

When two fractions have different denominators, write the fractions as equivalent fractions with a common denominator before adding or subtracting.

EXAMPLE 2 Add or subtract. Write the answer in lowest terms.

$$\text{a. } \frac{1}{4} - \frac{7}{12} \qquad\qquad \text{b. } -\frac{1}{10} + \left(-\frac{5}{6}\right)$$

Solution

a. $\dfrac{1}{4} - \dfrac{7}{12} = \dfrac{3}{12} - \dfrac{7}{12}$

$$= \frac{3-7}{12}$$

$$= \frac{-4}{12}$$

$$= \frac{-1}{3}, \text{ or } -\frac{1}{3}$$

b. $-\dfrac{1}{10} + \left(-\dfrac{5}{6}\right) = -\dfrac{3}{30} + \left(-\dfrac{25}{30}\right)$

$$= \frac{-3}{30} + \frac{-25}{30}$$

$$= \frac{-3 + (-25)}{30}$$

$$= \frac{-28}{30}$$

$$= \frac{-14}{15}, \text{ or } -\frac{14}{15}$$

Class Exercises

Add or subtract. Write the answer as a whole number or as a common fraction in lowest terms.

1. $\dfrac{3}{16} + \dfrac{8}{16}$
2. $\dfrac{7}{10} - \dfrac{3}{10}$
3. $\dfrac{7}{11} + \dfrac{8}{11}$
4. $\dfrac{4}{6} - \dfrac{11}{6}$

5. $-\dfrac{8}{5} + \dfrac{4}{5}$
6. $\dfrac{12}{5} - \dfrac{16}{5}$
7. $-\dfrac{14}{3} + \dfrac{20}{3}$
8. $-\dfrac{9}{4} - \dfrac{13}{4}$

9. $-\dfrac{1}{7} + \left(-\dfrac{3}{7}\right)$
10. $\dfrac{11}{15} - \left(-\dfrac{2}{15}\right)$
11. $-\dfrac{4}{21} - \left(-\dfrac{2}{21}\right)$
12. $-\dfrac{7}{10} - \left(-\dfrac{3}{10}\right)$

Written Exercises

Add or subtract. Write the answer as a whole number or as a common fraction in lowest terms.

A 1. $\dfrac{2}{15} + \dfrac{8}{15}$
2. $\dfrac{9}{20} - \dfrac{7}{20}$
3. $-\dfrac{8}{17} + \dfrac{4}{17}$
4. $\dfrac{17}{8} - \dfrac{9}{8}$

5. $\dfrac{3}{4} + \left(-\dfrac{3}{4}\right)$
6. $-\dfrac{11}{15} - \dfrac{16}{15}$
7. $-\dfrac{9}{10} + \left(-\dfrac{13}{10}\right)$
8. $-\dfrac{7}{16} - \left(-\dfrac{23}{16}\right)$

9. $\dfrac{3}{7} + \dfrac{1}{3}$
10. $\dfrac{5}{4} - \dfrac{1}{2}$
11. $-\dfrac{7}{6} + \dfrac{14}{3}$
12. $-\dfrac{17}{7} - \dfrac{7}{3}$

13. $\frac{15}{4} + \left(-\frac{33}{8}\right)$ **14.** $-\frac{17}{5} - \frac{11}{3}$ **15.** $-\frac{23}{10} + \left(-\frac{14}{5}\right)$ **16.** $-\frac{21}{4} - \left(-\frac{32}{5}\right)$

17. $\frac{11}{12} + \frac{12}{13}$ **18.** $-\frac{5}{6} + \frac{7}{20}$ **19.** $-\frac{5}{8} + \frac{1}{18}$ **20.** $\frac{2}{15} + \frac{6}{21}$

B   **21.** $\frac{1}{3} + \frac{1}{6} + \frac{1}{12}$ **22.** $\frac{2}{15} + \frac{1}{5} + \frac{2}{3}$ **23.** $\frac{7}{10} + \left(-\frac{1}{2}\right) + \frac{2}{5}$

24. $\frac{11}{12} + \frac{2}{7} + \left(-\frac{1}{2}\right)$ **25.** $-\frac{5}{6} + \frac{2}{9} + \left(-\frac{1}{3}\right)$ **26.** $\frac{8}{14} - \left(-\frac{1}{7}\right) + \frac{3}{2}$

27. $\frac{3}{2} + \frac{7}{4} + \left(-\frac{5}{3}\right)$ **28.** $-\frac{7}{3} + \frac{2}{3} + \frac{9}{5}$ **29.** $\frac{9}{15} + \left(-\frac{2}{3}\right) - \left(-\frac{1}{6}\right)$

C   **30.** Show that $\frac{a}{c} + \frac{b}{c} = \frac{a+b}{c}$ $(c \neq 0)$ by applying the rule or property that justifies each statement.

$$\frac{a}{b} + \frac{b}{c} = \left(a \times \frac{1}{c}\right) + \left(b \times \frac{1}{c}\right) \qquad \text{Why?}$$

$$= (a + b) \times \frac{1}{c} \qquad \text{Why?}$$

$$= \frac{a + b}{c} \qquad \text{Why?}$$

31. As in Exercise 30, show that $\frac{a}{c} - \frac{b}{c} = \frac{a-b}{c}$ $(c \neq 0)$.

Review Exercises

Write each fraction as a mixed number.

1. $\frac{11}{8}$ **2.** $\frac{15}{11}$ **3.** $\frac{23}{7}$ **4.** $\frac{31}{6}$

5. $\frac{71}{12}$ **6.** $\frac{83}{9}$ **7.** $\frac{121}{13}$ **8.** $\frac{169}{16}$

▮▮▮ Challenge

Write a fraction whose value is between the given fractions.

1. $\frac{2}{5} < \underline{\ ?\ } < \frac{3}{5}$ **2.** $-\frac{2}{3} < \underline{\ ?\ } < -\frac{1}{3}$ **3.** $\frac{1}{8} < \underline{\ ?\ } < \frac{1}{4}$

4. $-\frac{2}{7} < \underline{\ ?\ } < -\frac{3}{14}$ **5.** $\frac{1}{6} < \underline{\ ?\ } < \frac{1}{4}$ **6.** $-\frac{5}{6} < \underline{\ ?\ } < -\frac{7}{9}$

3-7 Adding and Subtracting Mixed Numbers

The rules for adding and subtracting fractions also apply to mixed numbers. Before mixed numbers are added or subtracted, convert them to improper fractions.

EXAMPLE 1 Add or subtract. Write the answer as a proper fraction in lowest terms or as a mixed number in simple form.

a. $3\frac{7}{8} + 2\frac{3}{8}$

b. $2\frac{3}{5} - 1\frac{4}{5}$

Solution

a. $3\frac{7}{8} + 2\frac{3}{8} = \frac{31}{8} + \frac{19}{8}$

$= \frac{50}{8}$

$= 6\frac{2}{8} = 6\frac{1}{4}$

b. $2\frac{3}{5} - 1\frac{4}{5} = \frac{13}{5} - \frac{9}{5}$

$= \frac{4}{5}$

It is sometimes necessary to write mixed numbers as improper fractions having a common denominator before adding or subtracting.

EXAMPLE 2 Add or subtract. Write the answer as a proper fraction in lowest terms or as a mixed number in simple form.

a. $5\frac{1}{4} + \left(-2\frac{1}{3}\right)$

b. $\frac{5}{6} - 2\frac{3}{8}$

Solution

a. $5\frac{1}{4} + \left(-2\frac{1}{3}\right) = \frac{21}{4} + \left(-\frac{7}{3}\right)$

$= \frac{63}{12} + \left(-\frac{28}{12}\right)$

$= \frac{35}{12}$

$= 2\frac{11}{12}$

b. $\frac{5}{6} - 2\frac{3}{8} = \frac{5}{6} - \frac{19}{8}$

$= \frac{20}{24} - \frac{57}{24}$

$= -\frac{37}{24}$

$= -1\frac{13}{24}$

Mixed numbers can be added or subtracted using a vertical format.

EXAMPLE 3 Add or subtract. Write the answer as a proper fraction in lowest terms or as a mixed number in simple form.

a. $2\frac{3}{10} + 4\frac{1}{10}$

b. $4\frac{7}{8} - 2\frac{1}{5}$

Solution   a. $2\frac{3}{10}$

$$+4\frac{1}{10}$$

$$6\frac{4}{10} = 6\frac{2}{5}$$

b. $4\frac{7}{8} = 4\frac{35}{40}$

$$-2\frac{1}{5} = -2\frac{8}{40}$$

$$2\frac{27}{40}$$

Class Exercises

Add or subtract. Write the answer as a proper fraction in lowest terms or as a mixed number in simple form.

1. $1\frac{1}{3} + 3\frac{1}{3}$

2. $2\frac{7}{10} - 1\frac{5}{10}$

3. $4\frac{13}{15} + 5\frac{4}{15}$

4. $5\frac{5}{12} - 4\frac{7}{12}$

5. $-6\frac{1}{4} + 2\frac{3}{4}$

6. $5\frac{3}{8} - 6\frac{7}{8}$

7. $-8\frac{7}{11} + 9\frac{8}{11}$

8. $-6\frac{3}{5} - 8\frac{4}{5}$

9. $-1\frac{5}{6} + \left(-3\frac{1}{6}\right)$

10. $2\frac{4}{7} - \left(-7\frac{6}{7}\right)$

11. $-10\frac{1}{9} - \left(-8\frac{7}{9}\right)$

12. $-3\frac{7}{10} - \left(-1\frac{3}{10}\right)$

Written Exercises

Add or subtract. Write the answer as a proper fraction in lowest terms or as a mixed number in simple form.

A

1. $5\frac{2}{5} + 3\frac{2}{5}$

2. $9\frac{7}{10} - 6\frac{3}{10}$

3. $-6\frac{4}{11} + 7\frac{3}{11}$

4. $-8\frac{3}{4} - 4\frac{1}{4}$

5. $1\frac{5}{6} + 4\frac{5}{6}$

6. $-3\frac{3}{8} - 9\frac{5}{8}$

7. $-10\frac{3}{7} + \left(-9\frac{5}{7}\right)$

8. $-2\frac{4}{15} - \left(-7\frac{7}{15}\right)$

9. $2\frac{1}{2} + 1\frac{1}{3}$

10. $5\frac{3}{5} - 2\frac{1}{4}$

11. $-2\frac{1}{6} + 4\frac{2}{3}$

12. $-5\frac{3}{7} - 2\frac{1}{3}$

13. $10\frac{3}{8} + \left(-12\frac{7}{12}\right)$

14. $-5\frac{2}{5} - 6\frac{5}{6}$

15. $-1\frac{9}{10} + \left(-1\frac{2}{3}\right)$

16. $-3\frac{7}{9} - \left(-5\frac{11}{15}\right)$

17. $5 + \frac{3}{4}$

18. $7 - \frac{1}{5}$

19. $-3 - \frac{7}{8}$

20. $-2 - \frac{7}{10}$

21. $5\frac{2}{3} + 6$

22. $3\frac{9}{10} - 7$

23. $-10\frac{1}{5} + (-9)$

24. $-7 - \left(-8\frac{1}{9}\right)$

B

25. $3\frac{1}{2} + 2\frac{1}{3} + 4\frac{1}{12}$

26. $8\frac{3}{5} + 2\frac{1}{2} - 11\frac{1}{10}$

27. $-4\frac{1}{3} + 2\frac{1}{4} - 6\frac{1}{6}$

28. $10\frac{1}{8} + \left(-6\frac{3}{4}\right) - 9\frac{11}{24}$

29. $-4\frac{1}{7} + 3\frac{1}{2} + \left(-7\frac{9}{14}\right)$

30. $-8\frac{9}{10} + 6\frac{2}{5} - 3\frac{1}{2}$

31. $-1\frac{2}{3} - \left(-2\frac{1}{5}\right) + 3\frac{7}{15}$ **32.** $-6\frac{7}{10} - \left(-3\frac{2}{5}\right) - \left(-3\frac{3}{10}\right)$ **33.** $3 + 2\frac{1}{3} - 5\frac{1}{5}$

34. $4\frac{7}{8} + (-3) - 2\frac{1}{4}$ **35.** $1\frac{1}{5} + \frac{3}{10} - 1\frac{1}{4}$ **36.** $-4\frac{9}{16} + \frac{3}{32} + \frac{1}{2}$

Problems

Solve.

A **1.** Joan Kent bought $15\frac{3}{4}$ yd of drapery material for $63 at a sale. If she used all except $1\frac{1}{16}$ yd, how much material did she actually use?

2. Carl is 6 ft tall. If he grew $1\frac{1}{8}$ in. during the past year and $\frac{3}{4}$ in. the year before, how tall was he one year ago?

3. On Monday Kim jogged $1\frac{1}{2}$ mi in $\frac{1}{4}$ h. On Wednesday she jogged $2\frac{1}{3}$ mi in $\frac{1}{3}$ h. How much farther did Kim jog on Wednesday?

4. The gas tank of a popular compact car holds $15\frac{2}{5}$ gal of gasoline. How much gas has been used if $10\frac{1}{3}$ gal remain in the tank?

B **5.** Last year, total rainfall for April and May was $7\frac{1}{4}$ in. This year 3 in. of rain fell in April and $2\frac{5}{8}$ in. fell in May. How much less rain fell this year than last year during April and May?

6. Each share of stock in Unified Electronics had a value of $34\frac{3}{4}$ on Monday. The value of the stock declined by $1\frac{5}{8}$ on Tuesday and by $\frac{7}{8}$ on Wednesday. What was the value of the stock after Wednesday?

7. A 512-page book has pages that are 7 in. wide and 9 in. high. The printed area measures $5\frac{3}{8}$ in. by $7\frac{3}{4}$ in. The left margin is $\frac{5}{16}$ in. and the top margin is $\frac{9}{16}$ in. How wide are the margins at the right and at the bottom of the page?

Review Exercises

Complete.

1. $-\frac{2}{7} = \frac{-2}{7} = \underline{\quad?\quad}$ **2.** $-\frac{4}{11} = \frac{4}{-11} = \underline{\quad?\quad}$ **3.** $-\frac{5}{9} = \frac{-5}{9} = \underline{\quad?\quad}$

4. $\frac{7}{-20} = -\frac{7}{20} = \underline{\quad?\quad}$ **5.** $7 \times \underline{\quad?\quad} = -1$ **6.** $6 \times \left(-\frac{1}{7}\right) = \underline{\quad?\quad}$

7. $-\frac{4}{11} = \underline{\quad?\quad} \div (-11)$ **8.** $\frac{-1}{4} = 1 \div \underline{\quad?\quad}$ **9.** $3 \div \underline{\quad?\quad} = 1$

3-8 Multiplying Fractions

To develop a method for multiplying fractions, we begin by showing that $\frac{7}{3} \times 3 = 7$.

$$\frac{7}{3} \times 3 = \left(7 \times \frac{1}{3}\right) \times 3 \qquad \text{By the rule: } \frac{a}{b} = a \times \frac{1}{b}$$

$$= 7 \times \left(\frac{1}{3} \times 3\right) \qquad \text{By the associative property}$$

$$= 7 \times \left(3 \times \frac{1}{3}\right) \qquad \text{By the commutative property}$$

$$= 7 \times 1 \qquad \text{By the rule: } b \times \frac{1}{b} = 1$$

$$= 7 \qquad \text{By the multiplication property of one}$$

In a similar way, it can be shown that $-\frac{7}{3} \times 3 = -7$. It is possible to prove the following general rule for all fractions.

Rule

For all numbers a and b $(b \neq 0)$,

$$\frac{a}{b} \times b = a$$

The rule tells us how to find the product of a fraction and a whole number. Using the rule on page 92, we can arrive at another rule for finding the product of two fractions such as $\frac{1}{5} \times \frac{1}{2}$. We begin by showing that $10 \times (\frac{1}{5} \times \frac{1}{2}) = 1$.

$$10 \times \left(\frac{1}{5} \times \frac{1}{2}\right) = (2 \times 5) \times \left(\frac{1}{5} \times \frac{1}{2}\right) \qquad \text{Substitution of } 2 \times 5 \text{ for } 10$$

$$= \left(2 \times \frac{1}{2}\right) \times \left(5 \times \frac{1}{5}\right) \qquad \text{By the associative and commutative properties}$$

$$= 1 \times 1 \qquad \text{By the rule: } b \times \frac{1}{b} = 1$$

$$= 1 \qquad \text{By the multiplication property of one}$$

We have shown that $10 \times (\frac{1}{5} \times \frac{1}{2}) = 1$ and we know that $10 \times \frac{1}{10} = 1$, so we conclude that $\frac{1}{5} \times \frac{1}{2} = \frac{1}{10}$. Similarly, we may prove the general rule shown on the following page.

EXAMPLE 1 Multiply $\frac{1}{-3} \times \frac{1}{4}$.

Solution $\quad \frac{1}{-3} \times \frac{1}{4} = \frac{1}{-3 \times 4} = \frac{1}{-12}$, or $-\frac{1}{12}$

The preceding rules are used to prove the following rule for multiplying two fractions.

EXAMPLE 2 Multiply. Write the answers to parts (a) and (b) as proper fractions in lowest terms or as mixed numbers in simple form.

$$\textbf{a.} \ \frac{5}{6} \times \frac{7}{3} \qquad \textbf{b.} \ \frac{3}{2} \times \left(-\frac{5}{7}\right) \qquad \textbf{c.} \ -\frac{7}{a} \times \left(-\frac{4}{b}\right)$$

Solution $\quad \textbf{a.} \ \frac{5}{6} \times \frac{7}{3} = \frac{5 \times 7}{6 \times 3} = \frac{35}{18}$, or $1\frac{17}{18}$

$\textbf{b.} \ \frac{3}{2} \times \left(-\frac{5}{7}\right) = \frac{3}{2} \times \frac{-5}{7} = \frac{3 \times (-5)}{2 \times 7} = \frac{-15}{14}$, or $-1\frac{1}{14}$

$\textbf{c.} \ -\frac{7}{a} \times \left(-\frac{4}{b}\right) = \frac{-7}{a} \times \frac{-4}{b} = \frac{-7 \times (-4)}{a \times b} = \frac{28}{ab}$

Sometimes it is easier to divide by common factors of the numerator and denominator before multiplying.

EXAMPLE 3 Multiply $\frac{-3}{5} \times \frac{15}{16} \times \frac{-2}{3}$.

Solution $\quad \frac{-3}{5} \times \frac{15}{16} \times \frac{-2}{3} = \frac{\overset{-1}{\cancel{-3}}}{\underset{1}{\cancel{5}}} \times \frac{\overset{3}{\cancel{15}}}{\underset{8}{\cancel{16}}} \times \frac{\overset{-1}{\cancel{-2}}}{\underset{1}{\cancel{3}}} = \frac{-1 \times 3 \times (-1)}{1 \times 8 \times 1} = \frac{3}{8}$

To multiply mixed numbers, first write each mixed number as an
improper fraction.

EXAMPLE 4   Multiply. Write the answer as a proper fraction in lowest terms or
as a mixed number in simple form.

a. $3\frac{1}{2} \times \left(-\frac{1}{4}\right)$ b. $5\frac{1}{4} \times 1\frac{3}{7}$

Solution   a. $3\frac{1}{2} \times \left(-\frac{1}{4}\right) = \frac{7}{2} \times \frac{-1}{4} = \frac{-7}{8}$, or $-\frac{7}{8}$

b. $5\frac{1}{4} \times 1\frac{3}{7} = \frac{\overset{3}{\cancel{21}}}{\underset{2}{\cancel{4}}} \times \frac{\overset{5}{\cancel{10}}}{\underset{1}{\cancel{7}}} = \frac{15}{2}$, or $7\frac{1}{2}$

Class Exercises

Multiply.

1. $\frac{5}{6} \times 6$ 2. $-\frac{3}{5} \times (-5)$ 3. $-4 \times \frac{7}{4}$ 4. $9 \times \left(-\frac{8}{9}\right)$

5. $\frac{1}{8} \times \frac{1}{3}$ 6. $-\frac{1}{4} \times \frac{1}{5}$ 7. $\frac{1}{15} \times \left(-\frac{1}{2}\right)$ 8. $-\frac{1}{10} \times \left(-\frac{1}{10}\right)$

9. $\frac{5}{8} \times \frac{3}{11}$ 10. $\frac{2}{5} \times \left(-\frac{3}{7}\right)$ 11. $1\frac{1}{2} \times 2$ 12. $-3 \times 1\frac{1}{5}$

Written Exercises

**Multiply. Write the answer as a proper fraction in lowest terms or as a
mixed number in simple form.**

A   1. $\frac{7}{12} \times 12$ 2. $-6 \times \frac{3}{6}$ 3. $3 \times \left(-\frac{2}{3}\right)$ 4. $-14 \times \left(-\frac{5}{14}\right)$

5. $-\frac{1}{4} \times \left(-\frac{1}{7}\right)$ 6. $\frac{1}{8} \times \left(-\frac{1}{20}\right)$ 7. $-\frac{1}{10} \times \frac{1}{6}$ 8. $-\frac{1}{15} \times \frac{1}{2}$

9. $\frac{2}{3} \times \frac{5}{9}$ 10. $\frac{6}{7} \times \frac{2}{5}$ 11. $\frac{3}{8} \times \left(-\frac{2}{3}\right)$ 12. $\frac{5}{6} \times \left(-\frac{2}{5}\right)$

13. $-\frac{1}{3} \times \frac{2}{9}$ 14. $-\frac{3}{8} \times \frac{2}{9}$ 15. $\frac{-5}{8} \times (-1)$ 16. $\frac{-2}{5} \times \left(-\frac{15}{16}\right)$

Multiply.

17. $-\frac{1}{4} \times 0$ **18.** $-\frac{3}{4} \times 0$ **19.** $\frac{5}{16} \times \frac{30}{40}$ **20.** $\frac{9}{8} \times \frac{24}{27}$

B **21.** $3\frac{1}{4} \times \frac{4}{13}$ **22.** $5\frac{2}{5} \times \frac{5}{9}$ **23.** $4\frac{1}{4} \times 10\frac{1}{3}$ **24.** $10\frac{1}{2} \times 2\frac{3}{4}$

25. $-4\frac{2}{7} \times 5\frac{1}{6}$ **26.** $3\frac{1}{8} \times \left(-4\frac{1}{5}\right)$ **27.** $-2\frac{1}{3} \times \left(-1\frac{4}{9}\right)$ **28.** $-6\frac{1}{4} \times \left(-5\frac{2}{5}\right)$

29. $\frac{1}{4} \times \frac{1}{3} \times \frac{1}{2}$ **30.** $\frac{5}{16} \times \frac{1}{2} \times \frac{1}{5}$ **31.** $\frac{3}{4} \times \frac{1}{6} \times \frac{1}{9}$

32. $-\frac{5}{8} \times \left(-\frac{3}{25}\right) \times \left(-\frac{1}{9}\right)$ **33.** $-2\frac{1}{4} \times 6\frac{1}{2} \times \frac{12}{39}$ **34.** $-5\frac{1}{8} \times \frac{24}{25} \times 10\frac{1}{2}$

Multiply. Simplify the answer.

EXAMPLE $\frac{3}{5} \times 15a = \frac{3}{\overset{1}{\cancel{5}}} \times \frac{\overset{3a}{\cancel{15a}}}{1} = \frac{3 \times 3a}{1 \times 1} = 9a$

35. $\frac{2}{3} \times 9n$ **36.** $5 \times \frac{3x}{10}$ **37.** $-3 \times \frac{y}{6}$ **38.** $-5 \times \left(\frac{-7a}{10}\right)$

39. $\frac{2r}{5} \times \frac{1}{r}$ **40.** $\frac{-6}{s} \times \frac{s}{2}$ **41.** $\frac{3c}{5} \times \frac{5}{c}$ **42.** $\frac{2m}{7} \times \frac{14}{m}$

C **43.** Let $\frac{a}{b}$ be any fraction ($b \neq 0$). Show that $\frac{a}{b} \times b = a$ by supplying the rule or property that justifies each statement.

$\frac{a}{b} \times b = \left(a \times \frac{1}{b}\right) \times b$ Why?

$= a \times \left(\frac{1}{b} \times b\right)$ Why?

$= a \times \left(b \times \frac{1}{b}\right)$ Why?

$= a \times 1$ Why?
$= a$ Why?

44. Let $\frac{a}{b}$ and $\frac{c}{d}$ represent any two fractions ($b \neq 0$, $d \neq 0$). Show as in Exercise 43 that $\frac{a}{b} \times \frac{c}{d} = \frac{ac}{bd}$.

Review Exercises

Evaluate the expression when $x = -8$ and $y = 12$.

1. $5 \times y$ **2.** $7x \div 4$ **3.** $3x - y$ **4.** $x + 8y$

5. $2(x + y)$ **6.** $x \div (y - 6)$ **7.** $(2y + 4) \div (x - 1)$ **8.** $(x \div 4) \times (y \div 3)$

3-9 Dividing Fractions

To develop a method for dividing fractions, recall that multiplication and division are inverse operations. If $2 \times n = 10$, then $n = 10 \div 2$. Similarly, if $\frac{7}{5} \times x = \frac{2}{3}$, then $x = \frac{2}{3} \div \frac{7}{5}$. We can show by substitution that the multiplication equation is true when the value of x is $(\frac{2}{3} \times \frac{5}{7})$.

$$\frac{7}{5} \times \left(\frac{2}{3} \times \frac{5}{7}\right) = \frac{\overset{1}{\cancel{7}} \times 2 \times \overset{1}{\cancel{5}}}{\underset{1}{\cancel{5}} \times 3 \times \underset{1}{\cancel{7}}} = \frac{2}{3}$$

Therefore, the related division equation must also be true when the value of x is $(\frac{2}{3} \times \frac{5}{7})$. That is,

$$\frac{2}{3} \times \frac{5}{7} = \frac{2}{3} \div \frac{7}{5}.$$

Two numbers, like $\frac{5}{7}$ and $\frac{7}{5}$, whose product is 1 are called **reciprocals.** The reciprocal of $\frac{c}{d}$ is $\frac{d}{c}$ because $\frac{c}{d} \times \frac{d}{c} = 1$. Every nonzero rational number has exactly one reciprocal.

We may state the following general rule.

Rule

For all numbers a, b, c, and d ($b \neq 0, c \neq 0, d \neq 0$),

$$\frac{a}{b} \div \frac{c}{d} = \frac{a}{b} \times \frac{d}{c}$$

To divide by a fraction, multiply by its reciprocal.

EXAMPLE 1 Name the reciprocal, if any.

  a. $\frac{2}{3}$ **b.** $-\frac{5}{8}$ **c.** 2   **d.** 0

Solution

a. The reciprocal of $\frac{2}{3}$ is $\frac{3}{2}$ since $\frac{2}{3} \times \frac{3}{2} = 1$.

b. The reciprocal of $-\frac{5}{8}$ is $-\frac{8}{5}$ since $-\frac{5}{8} \times \left(-\frac{8}{5}\right) = 1$.

c. The reciprocal of 2 is $\frac{1}{2}$ since $2 \times \frac{1}{2} = 1$.

d. The equation $0 \times n = 1$ has no solution since 0 times any number is 0. Therefore, 0 has no reciprocal.

EXAMPLE 2 Divide. Write the answer as a proper fraction in lowest terms or as a mixed number in simple form.

$$\textbf{a. } -\frac{4}{3} \div \frac{5}{8} \qquad \textbf{b. } 2\frac{1}{3} \div 1\frac{3}{8} \qquad \textbf{c. } \frac{\frac{2}{5}}{\frac{1}{4}}$$

Solution

$$\textbf{a. } -\frac{4}{3} \div \frac{5}{8} = -\frac{4}{3} \times \frac{8}{5} = -\frac{32}{15}, \text{ or } -2\frac{2}{15}$$

$$\textbf{b. } 2\frac{1}{3} \div 1\frac{3}{8} = \frac{7}{3} \div \frac{11}{8} = \frac{7}{3} \times \frac{8}{11} = \frac{56}{33}, \text{ or } 1\frac{23}{33}$$

$$\textbf{c. } \frac{\frac{2}{5}}{\frac{1}{4}} = \frac{2}{5} \div \frac{1}{4} = \frac{2}{5} \times \frac{4}{1} = \frac{8}{5}, \text{ or } 1\frac{3}{5}$$

EXAMPLE 3 Ann bought 2 packages of ground beef. One package was $2\frac{1}{2}$ lb, and the other package was $3\frac{1}{8}$ lb. Ann divided the total amount of beef into 5 equal packages for the freezer. How many pounds were in each package?

Solution

- The problem asks for the number of pounds in each of the 5 packages.

- Given facts: $2\frac{1}{2}$ lb and $3\frac{1}{8}$ lb of beef
  total divided into 5 equal packages

- To solve, first add to find the total amount of beef, and then divide to find the amount in each package.

$$2\frac{1}{2} + 3\frac{1}{8} = 2\frac{4}{8} + 3\frac{1}{8} = 5\frac{5}{8}$$

$$5\frac{5}{8} \div 5 = \frac{\overset{9}{\cancel{45}}}{8} \times \frac{1}{\underset{1}{\cancel{5}}} = \frac{9 \times 1}{8 \times 1} = \frac{9}{8}, \text{ or } 1\frac{1}{8}$$

Each package contained $1\frac{1}{8}$ lb of beef.

Problem Solving Reminder

When solving a problem, *review the problem solving strategies and tips* that you have learned. As you work through the problems in the lesson, remember that you may need to supply additional information, eliminate extra information, or plan more than one step. Remember to reread the problem to be sure your answer is complete.

Class Exercises

State the reciprocal.

1. 4   2. -5 3. $\frac{3}{4}$ 4. $-\frac{5}{8}$ 5. $\frac{2}{7}$ 6. $\frac{11}{3}$

7. $-\frac{2}{3}$ 8. $-\frac{6}{5}$ 9. $\frac{11}{12}$ 10. $\frac{3}{16}$ 11. $-\frac{4}{7}$ 12. $\frac{14}{5}$

Complete.

13. $\frac{2}{3} \div 5 = \frac{2}{3} \times \underline{\ ?\ }$ 14. $\frac{2}{3} \div \frac{1}{5} = \frac{2}{3} \times \underline{\ ?\ }$

15. $\frac{6}{5} \div (-10) = \underline{\ ?\ } \times \left(-\frac{1}{10}\right)$ 16. $-\frac{3}{4} \div \frac{3}{10} = \underline{\ ?\ } \times \underline{\ ?\ }$

Written Exercises

Divide. Write the answer as a proper fraction in lowest terms or as a mixed number in simple form.

A   1. $\frac{2}{5} \div \frac{3}{5}$ 2. $\frac{7}{8} \div \frac{3}{8}$ 3. $5 \div \frac{1}{5}$ 4. $10 \div \frac{1}{2}$

5. $\frac{5}{8} \div \frac{9}{5}$ 6. $\frac{3}{4} \div \frac{7}{8}$ 7. $\dfrac{\frac{5}{9}}{\frac{1}{7}}$ 8. $\dfrac{\frac{2}{3}}{\frac{3}{8}}$

9. $-\frac{21}{4} \div \left(-\frac{7}{8}\right)$ 10. $-\frac{4}{5} \div \left(-\frac{36}{25}\right)$ 11. $3\frac{1}{4} \div \frac{5}{8}$ 12. $10\frac{1}{2} \div \frac{8}{9}$

13. $-5\frac{5}{8} \div 10$ 14. $11\frac{1}{9} \div 100$ 15. $-6\frac{1}{3} \div \left(-\frac{19}{21}\right)$ 16. $-10\frac{1}{3} \div \left(-\frac{31}{33}\right)$

B   17. $6\frac{1}{8} \div \left(\frac{8}{3} \times \frac{3}{7}\right)$ 18. $-7 \div \left(\frac{21}{4} \times \frac{3}{7}\right)$ 19. $\left(-1\frac{2}{3} \times \frac{18}{5}\right) \div 3$

20. $-\left(\frac{35}{4} \times \frac{2}{7}\right) \div \left(-\frac{4}{3}\right)$ 21. $-\left(3\frac{1}{5} \times \frac{5}{2}\right) \div \frac{8}{9}$ 22. $\left(-2\frac{1}{6} \div \frac{1}{9}\right) \times \frac{1}{13}$

23. $-\left(4\frac{1}{6} \div 5\right) \times \left(-\frac{2}{5}\right)$ 24. $-3\frac{1}{8} \div 4 \div \left(-\frac{5}{4}\right)$ 25. $5\frac{1}{3} \div 2\frac{2}{3} \div (-4)$

Problems

Solve.

A   1. To the nearest million, the number of households in the United States having television sets was 4 million in 1950 and 76 million in 1980. Express the first number as a fraction of the second.

2. A gasoline tank with a capacity of 15 gal is $\frac{3}{4}$ full. How many gallons will it take to fill the tank?

3. A town has raised $\frac{3}{8}$ of the $12,000 it needs to furnish its new library. How much more is it hoping to raise?

4. How many packages will $5\frac{1}{2}$ lb of raisins fill if each package holds 9 oz?

5. Karen Northrup worked $12\frac{1}{2}$ h last week and earned $50. What was her hourly rate of pay?

6. A television station released 300 balloons at an outdoor celebration. Of these, $\frac{3}{4}$ were orange. How many were orange?

7. Leo Delray earns $2 an hour for babysitting. If he works $3\frac{1}{4}$ h one evening, how much does he earn?

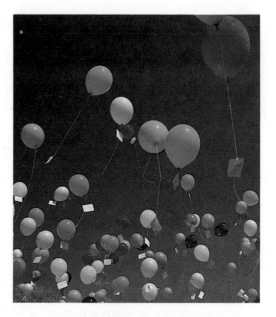

8. In a recent year there were 32,000 persons in the United States who had celebrated their 100th birthday. Of these, $\frac{3}{4}$ were women. How many were men?

B 9. One half of the class voted to have a picnic. One third of the class voted to hold a dinner instead. What fraction of the class wanted neither a picnic nor a dinner?

10. A picture measures $8\frac{3}{4}$ in. by 8 in. When framed it measures $10\frac{3}{4}$ in. by 10 in. How wide is each side of the frame?

C 11. Only $\frac{1}{5}$ of the downtown workers drive to work. Of those who do not drive, $\frac{3}{16}$ ride bicycles to work. What fraction of the workers ride bicycles to work?

12. Kevin's regular rate of pay is $4 per hour. When he works overtime, he earns $1\frac{1}{2}$ times as much per hour. How much will Kevin earn for $5\frac{1}{2}$ h of overtime work?

Review Exercises

Use the inverse operation to write a related equation. Solve for the variable.

1. $n + 135 = 240$ 2. $x - 45 = 52$ 3. $4y = 156$ 4. $9t = 504$

5. $12x = 432$ 6. $r \div 17 = 27$ 7. $38m = 418$ 8. $a \div 22 = 33$

3-10 Fractions and Decimals

Any fraction can be represented as a decimal. You may recall that a fraction such as $\frac{3}{4}$ can be easily written as an equivalent fraction whose denominator is a power of 10, and then as a decimal. To represent $\frac{3}{4}$ as a decimal, we first write it as an equivalent fraction with denominator 100.

$$\frac{3}{4} = \frac{3 \times 25}{4 \times 25} = \frac{75}{100} = 0.75$$

For most fractions, however, we use the fact that $\frac{a}{b} = a \div b$ and divide numerator by denominator.

EXAMPLE 1   Write as a decimal: **a.** $-\frac{5}{16}$ **b.** $\frac{24}{55}$

Solution   **a.** First find $5 \div 16$.

$$\begin{array}{r} 0.3125 \\ 16\overline{)5.0000} \\ \underline{4\,8} \\ 20 \\ \underline{16} \\ 40 \\ \underline{32} \\ 80 \\ \underline{80} \\ 0 \end{array}$$

Therefore, $-\frac{5}{16} = -0.3125$.

The decimal -0.3125 is called a **terminating decimal** because the final remainder is 0 and the division ends.

b. Find $24 \div 55$.

$$\begin{array}{r} 0.43636 \\ 55\overline{)24.00000} \\ \underline{22\,0} \\ 2\,00 \\ \underline{1\,65} \\ 350 \\ \underline{330} \\ 200 \\ \underline{165} \\ 350 \\ \underline{330} \\ 20 \end{array}$$

Therefore, $\frac{24}{55} = 0.43636\ldots$.

The digits 36 continue to repeat without end. The decimal $0.43636\ldots$ is called a **repeating decimal.** We often write $0.43636\ldots$ as $0.4\overline{36}$, with a bar over the block of digits that repeats.

To say that $\frac{24}{55} = 0.43636\ldots$ means that the successive decimals 0.436, 0.4363, 0.43636, and so on, will come closer and closer to the value $\frac{24}{55}$.

We can predict when a fraction will result in a terminating decimal because the fraction in lowest terms has a denominator with no prime factors other than 2 and 5. Thus, the fraction $\frac{24}{55}$ does not result in a terminating decimal because its denominator has 11 as a prime factor.

When working with a mixed number, such as $-1\frac{5}{16}$ or $1\frac{24}{25}$, we may consider the mixed number as a sum of a whole number and a fraction, or we may rewrite the mixed number as an improper fraction and then divide.

If a and b are integers and $b \neq 0$, the quotient $a \div b$ is either a terminating decimal or a repeating decimal. The reason for this is that, for any divisor, the number of possible remainders at each step of the division is limited to the whole numbers less than the divisor. Sooner or later, either the remainder is 0 and the division ends, as in part (a) of Example 1, or one of the remainders reappears in the division as in part (b) of Example 1. Then the same block of digits will reappear in the quotient.

Property

Every rational number can be represented by either a terminating decimal or a repeating decimal.

You already know how to write a terminating decimal as a fraction. Rewrite the decimal as a fraction whose denominator is a power of 10.

EXAMPLE 2 Write -0.625 as a fraction in lowest terms.

Solution $$-0.625 = -\frac{625}{1000} = -\frac{625 \div 125}{1000 \div 125} = -\frac{5}{8}$$

The next example shows a method for writing a repeating decimal as a fraction.

EXAMPLE 3 Write $-1.\overline{21}$ as a fraction in lowest terms.

Solution Let $n = 1.\overline{21}$.

Multiply both sides of the equation by a power of 10 determined by the number of digits in the block of repeating digits. Since there are

2 digits that repeat in the number $1.\overline{21}$, we multiply by 10^2, or 100.

$$100n = 121.\overline{21}$$
Subtract: $\quad\quad n = 1.\overline{21}$
$$99n = 120$$
$$n = \frac{120}{99} = \frac{40}{33}$$

Thus, $-1.\overline{21} = -\frac{40}{33}$, or $-1\frac{7}{33}$.

Property

Every terminating or repeating decimal represents a rational number.

Some decimals, such as those below, neither terminate nor repeat.

$$0.01001000100001\ldots \quad\quad\quad 1.234567891011121314\ldots$$

The two decimals shown follow patterns, but they are not repeating patterns. The decimal on the right is made up of consecutive whole numbers beginning with 1.

Decimals that neither terminate nor repeat represent **irrational numbers.** Together, the rational numbers and the irrational numbers make up the set of **real numbers.** The number line that you have studied is sometimes called the **real number line.** For every point on the line, there is exactly one real number and for every real number there is exactly one point on the number line.

Class Exercises

Tell whether the decimal for the fraction is terminating or repeating. If the decimal is terminating, state the decimal.

1. $\frac{1}{4}$ **2.** $\frac{5}{6}$ **3.** $2\frac{2}{5}$ **4.** $-\frac{9}{10}$ **5.** $-1\frac{1}{2}$ **6.** $\frac{13}{30}$

State as a fraction in which the numerator is an integer and the denominator is a power of 10.

7. 0.13 **8.** -0.9 **9.** 1.4 **10.** -0.007 **11.** 3.03 **12.** -5.001

State the repeating digit(s) for each decimal.

13. $6.666\ldots$ **14.** $0.0444\ldots$ **15.** $6.050505\ldots$ **16.** $0.1666\ldots$

17. $5.1\overline{5}$ **18.** $0.\overline{422}$ **19.** $1.0\overline{6}$ **20.** $0.3\overline{64}$

Written Exercises

Write as a terminating or repeating decimal. Use a bar to show repeating digits.

A

1. $\frac{1}{4}$ **2.** $\frac{1}{5}$ **3.** $\frac{2}{9}$ **4.** $\frac{3}{16}$ **5.** $\frac{9}{10}$ **6.** $-\frac{1}{18}$

7. $-\frac{2}{3}$ **8.** $\frac{4}{9}$ **9.** $-\frac{3}{8}$ **10.** $\frac{3}{5}$ **11.** $-\frac{3}{25}$ **12.** $\frac{7}{15}$

13. $1\frac{1}{10}$ **14.** $5\frac{2}{5}$ **15.** $\frac{7}{12}$ **16.** $-\frac{3}{11}$ **17.** $\frac{4}{15}$ **18.** $-4\frac{7}{8}$

19. $-1\frac{7}{18}$ **20.** $2\frac{1}{9}$ **21.** $\frac{3}{20}$ **22.** $\frac{17}{36}$ **23.** $3\frac{2}{7}$ **24.** $\frac{5}{13}$

Write as a proper fraction in lowest terms or as a mixed number in simple form.

25. 0.05 **26.** 0.005 **27.** -0.6 **28.** -2.1 **29.** 2.07

30. -0.62 **31.** 5.125 **32.** 4.3 **33.** -1.375 **34.** -10.001

35. 12.625 **36.** 10.3 **37.** 0.225 **38.** 0.8375 **39.** -1.826

B

40. $0.444\ldots$ **41.** $-0.555\ldots$ **42.** $0.0\overline{3}$ **43.** $-1.0\overline{1}$ **44.** $5.\overline{9}$

45. $0.1515\ldots$ **46.** $-1.\overline{20}$ **47.** $0.\overline{35}$ **48.** $0.7\overline{2}$ **49.** $-1.\overline{12}$

50. $1.3\overline{62}$ **51.** $2.13\overline{4}$ **52.** $-8.0\overline{16}$ **53.** $0.\overline{123}$ **54.** $-5.\overline{862}$

Tell whether the number is rational or irrational.

55. $\frac{-13}{17}$ **56.** $1.515151\ldots$ **57.** -3.72 **58.** $2.121121112\ldots$

Arrange the numbers in order from least to greatest.

59. $3.0,\ 3.\overline{09},\ 3.00\overline{9},\ 3.1$ **60.** $0.182,\ 0.182\overline{5},\ 0.18\overline{2},\ 0.1\overline{8}$

a. Express the first number as a fraction or mixed number.
b. Compare the first number with the second.

C   **61.** $0.\overline{9};\ 1$ **62.** $0.4\overline{9};\ \frac{1}{2}$ **63.** $-1.24\overline{9};\ -\frac{5}{4}$ **64.** $2.3\overline{9};\ 2\frac{2}{5}$

Self-Test B

Perform the indicated operation. Write the answer as a proper fraction in lowest terms or as a mixed number in simple form.

1. $\frac{1}{3} + \frac{1}{4}$ **2.** $\frac{2}{15} + \left(-\frac{5}{6}\right)$ **3.** $\frac{1}{5} - \frac{1}{3}$ [3-6]

4. $17\frac{1}{3} + 5\frac{1}{9}$ **5.** $-6\frac{3}{8} - 3\frac{2}{3}$ **6.** $16\frac{5}{8} - \left(-\frac{3}{4}\right)$ [3-7]

7. $\frac{3}{4} \times 5$ **8.** $\frac{1}{8} \times \left(-\frac{1}{3}\right)$ **9.** $-2\frac{4}{7} \times 3\frac{1}{6}$ [3-8]

10. $\frac{5}{8} \div \frac{10}{24}$ **11.** $-\frac{11}{16} \div \frac{44}{8}$ **12.** $4\frac{1}{3} \div \left(-\frac{26}{27}\right)$ [3-9]

Write as a decimal. Use a bar to show repeating digits.

13. $\frac{5}{8}$ **14.** $\frac{2}{11}$ **15.** $-\frac{1}{80}$ **16.** $\frac{7}{6}$ [3-10]

Write as a proper fraction in lowest terms or as a mixed number in simple form.

17. 0.875 **18.** $1.\overline{6}$ **19.** -2.213 **20.** $0.2\overline{3}$

Self-Test answers and Extra Practice are at the back of the book.

▌▌▌ Computer Byte

The following program will find the least common multiple of two numbers.

```
10  PRINT "TO FIND LCM:"
20  PRINT "INPUT A, B";
30  INPUT A,B
40  FOR X = 1 TO B
50  LET A1 = A * X
60  LET Q = A1 / B
70  IF Q = INT (Q) THEN 90
80  NEXT X
90  PRINT "LCM(";A;",";B;") = ";A1
100 END
```

RUN the program to find the least common multiple of the following.

1. 12, 25 **2.** 72, 84 **3.** 34, 60 **4.** 45, 80 **5.** 110, 240 **6.** 235, 180

BASIC, A Computer Language

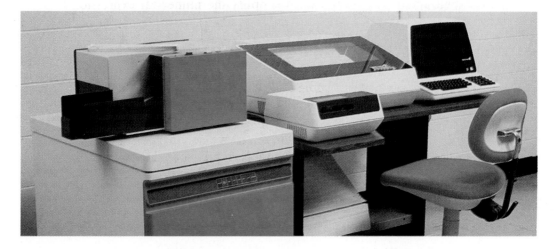

Computers are very powerful tools, but issuing an order such as "Do problem 12 on page 46 of my math book" will produce no results at all. There are many things computers can do more quickly and efficiently than people, but we need to communicate with computers in a special way to get them to work for us.

To tell a computer what to do, we write a set of instructions, called a *program,* using a *programming language.* Since most microcomputers use some version of BASIC (with slight differences), that is the language that we will use in this book. A BASIC program is made up of a set of *numbered lines* that provide step-by-step instructions for the computer. We can use any numbers from 1 to 99999 for line numbers, but we often use numbers in intervals of 10 so that we can insert other lines later if we need to.

A *statement* that tells the computer what to do follows each line number in a program. In the BASIC language, we use the symbols shown below to tell the computer to perform arithmetic operations.

+	addition	−	subtraction
*	multiplication	/	division

The symbol ↑ (or some similar symbol) is used to indicate exponentiation. Thus $3 \uparrow 6$ means 3^6. When a statement contains more than one operation, the computer will perform all operations in parentheses first and will follow the order of operations that you learned in Chapters 1 and 2.

We use a **PRINT** statement to tell the computer to perform the operations listed in a statement and to print the result. We use an **END** statement to tell the computer that the program is over. The program shown below tells the computer to simplify the numerical expression and print the answer.

```
10    PRINT 5↑3 * (16 - 8 / 2)
20    END
```

After you have typed in this program (press RETURN or ENTER after each line), you type the *command* **RUN** to tell the computer to run (or *execute*) the program. The result, or *output,* is 1500.

A computer handles variables much as we do. We can ask it, for example, to give us the value of a variable expression when we give it a value of the variable in it. One way of doing this is to use an **INPUT** statement. This causes the computer to print a question mark and wait for the value to be typed in. Here is a simple program with a RUN shown at the right below.

```
10    INPUT X                           RUN
20    PRINT X↑2 + 2 * X + 4             ?10
30    END                               124
```

As you can see, we need some statement to tell the person using this program what is expected after the question mark. We do this by enclosing a descriptive expression in quotation marks in a PRINT statement, as in line 5 below. The semicolon at the end of line 5 will cause the question mark from line 10 to be printed right after the quoted expression. We have also inserted lines 12 and 15. After typing lines 5, 12, and 15, we can type the command **LIST** to see the revised program. A RUN is shown at the right below.

```
5   PRINT "WHAT IS YOUR VALUE OF X";
10    INPUT X                           RUN
12    PRINT "FOR X = ";X                WHAT IS YOUR VALUE OF X?10
15    PRINT "X↑2 + 2X + 4 = ";          FOR X = 10
20    PRINT X↑2 + 2 * X + 4             X↑2 + 2X + 4 = 124
30    END
```

1. Change lines 15 and 20 in the program above to evaluate another variable expression, with x as the variable, that involves the operation or operations listed.
   a. subtraction   b. multiplication
   c. division   d. multiplication and addition
   e. division and subtraction

2. Change the program above to evaluate a variable expression using m as the variable.

Chapter Review

Complete.

1. 1, 2, 3, __?__, __?__, __?__, __?__, and __?__ are factors of 24. [3-1]

2. 40 is divisible by __?__, __?__, __?__, __?__, __?__, __?__, __?__, and __?__.

Write the letter of the correct answer.

3. What is the next prime number after 47? [3-2]

    a. 49   **b.** 51   **c.** 53   **d.** 57

4. What is the prime factorization of 72?

    a. $1 \cdot 72$ **b.** $6^2 \cdot 2$ **c.** $2^3 \cdot 3^2$ **d.** $3^3 \cdot 2^2$

True or false?

5. $8 \times \frac{1}{9} = \frac{9}{8}$ 6. $4 \times \left(-\frac{1}{5}\right) = -\frac{4}{5}$ 7. $\frac{-7}{11} = -\frac{7}{11}$ [3-3]

8. $-\frac{24}{148}$ in lowest terms is $-\frac{12}{74}$.   9. $7\frac{3}{8} = \frac{29}{8}$ [3-4]

10. The LCD of $\frac{2}{3}$ and $\frac{5}{11}$ is 33.   11. The LCD of $\frac{7}{30}$ and $-\frac{3}{35}$ is 150. [3-5]

Match.

12. $\frac{5}{12} + \frac{11}{18}$ 13. $\frac{1}{8} - \frac{3}{8}$ **A.** $-2\frac{11}{18}$ **B.** $-8\frac{17}{18}$ [3-6]

14. $-\frac{9}{16} - \left(-\frac{3}{4}\right)$ 15. $\frac{2}{5} + \frac{3}{10}$ **C.** $\frac{37}{36}$ **D.** $\frac{3}{16}$

16. $-2\frac{1}{6} + \left(-\frac{4}{9}\right)$ 17. $1\frac{3}{7} - \frac{5}{8}$ **E.** $\frac{27}{28}$ **F.** $-\frac{1}{4}$ [3-7]

18. $\frac{1}{4} \times \frac{1}{9}$ 19. $\frac{4}{5} \times \frac{3}{8}$ **G.** $\frac{7}{10}$ **H.** $\frac{1}{36}$ [3-8]

20. $-7\frac{2}{3} \times 1\frac{1}{6}$ 21. $\frac{2}{3} \times 5$ **I.** $3\frac{1}{3}$ **J.** $-1\frac{19}{30}$ [3-9]

22. $\frac{3}{14} \div \frac{2}{9}$ 23. $1\frac{2}{5} \div \left(-\frac{6}{7}\right)$ **K.** $\frac{45}{56}$ **L.** $\frac{3}{10}$

Complete. Use a bar to show repeating digits.

24. $\frac{4}{3}$ written as a decimal is __?__. [3-10]

Chapter Test

State which of the numbers 2, 3, 4, 5, 9, and 10 are factors of each number. Use the tests for divisibility.

1. 822   **2.** 410   **3.** 315   **4.** 660   [3–1]

Give the prime factorization of each number.

5. 168   **6.** 96   **7.** 53   **8.** 111   [3–2]

Complete.

9. $5 \times \underline{\ ?\ } = \frac{5}{7}$ **10.** $6 \times \frac{1}{6} = \underline{\ ?\ }$ **11.** $\frac{-1}{4} = \frac{1}{-4} = \underline{\ ?\ }$ [3–3]

Write as a fraction in lowest terms or as a mixed number in simple form.

12. $\frac{14}{40}$ **13.** $-\frac{26}{52}$ **14.** $-\frac{136}{160}$ **15.** $\frac{15}{4}$ **16.** $\frac{-83}{9}$ [3–4]

Write each pair of fractions as equivalent fractions with the least common denominator.

17. $\frac{3}{7}, \frac{5}{14}$ **18.** $\frac{1}{9}, \frac{6}{11}$ **19.** $\frac{5}{8}, \frac{13}{36}$ **20.** $\frac{7}{12}, \frac{5}{24}$ [3–5]

Perform the indicated operations. Write the answer as a proper fraction in lowest terms or as a mixed number in simple form.

21. $\frac{3}{8} + \frac{1}{7}$ **22.** $-\frac{3}{10} + \left(-\frac{1}{4}\right)$ **23.** $\frac{1}{2} - \frac{5}{12}$ [3–6]

24. $1\frac{3}{4} + \left(-2\frac{1}{2}\right)$ **25.** $1\frac{1}{3} - \left(-2\frac{3}{4}\right)$ **26.** $-2\frac{7}{10} - \left(4\frac{9}{11}\right)$ [3–7]

27. $\frac{4}{7} \times \left(-\frac{4}{11}\right)$ **28.** $8\frac{1}{8} \times 2\frac{3}{5}$ **29.** $-\frac{1}{4} \times \left(-\frac{1}{6}\right)$ [3–8]

30. $\frac{2}{3} \div \frac{7}{9}$ **31.** $-\frac{6}{19} \div \frac{9}{38}$ **32.** $-1\frac{1}{6} \div \left(-4\frac{2}{3}\right)$ [3–9]

Write as a decimal. Use a bar to show repeating digits.

33. $\frac{6}{25}$ **34.** $\frac{5}{33}$ **35.** $\frac{9}{16}$ **36.** $\frac{4}{9}$ [3–10]

Write as a fraction in lowest terms or as a mixed number in simple form.

37. 0.04   **38.** -0.375 **39.** 6.125   **40.** $0.\overline{7}$

Cumulative Review (Chapters 1–3)

Exercises

Give the solution of the equation for the given replacement set.

1. $x - 12 = 46$; {58, 59, 60}

2. $8d = 2$; $\left\{\frac{1}{3}, \frac{1}{4}, \frac{1}{5}\right\}$

3. $3(6 + y) = 39$; {7, 14, 21}

4. $(5 - a) \div (a + 7) = \frac{1}{5}$; {1, 2, 3}

5. $16r - 11 = 69$; {0, 5, 10}

6. $m^2(7 + m) = 176$; {3, 4, 5}

Evaluate the expression if $a = 3$, $b = 2$, and $c = 5$.

7. ab^2 **8.** $a^2 + b^2$ **9.** a^2c^2 **10.** bc^2 **11.** $2b^2$

12. a^2b^3 **13.** $(a + b)^2$ **14.** $c(a^2 + b)$ **15.** bc^3 **16.** $\frac{10b^2}{c^2}$

Use the symbol $>$ to order the numbers from greatest to least.

17. 75.70, 75.40, 75.06

18. 19.05, 19.18, 19.50

19. 0.03, 0.30, 0.33

20. 105.07, 10.507, 1050.7

List the integers that can replace x to make the statement true.

21. $|x| = 7$ **22.** $|x| = 18$ **23.** $|x| \geq 5$ **24.** $|x| < 7.3$

25. $4 < |x| < 6$ **26.** $6 > |x| > 0$ **27.** $31 < |x| < 40$ **28.** $17 \leq |x| \leq 25$

What value of the variable makes the statement true?

29. $-7 + y = 11$ **30.** $-3n = 51$ **31.** $-6(-b) = 72$

32. $17 - x = -5$ **33.** $8(-n) = 32$ **34.** $-a \div 15 = 3$

Evaluate the expression when $x = 5$, $y = -7$, and $z = -5$.

35. $\frac{y + 3}{x}$ **36.** $\frac{xy}{z}$ **37.** $\frac{x + y}{z}$ **38.** $\frac{yz}{x}$ **39.** $\frac{x - z}{y}$

40. $\frac{x^2 + y^2}{z^2}$ **41.** $\frac{x}{7} + \frac{y}{7}$ **42.** $\frac{2x}{15} + \frac{z}{3}$ **43.** $\frac{-y + z}{x}$ **44.** $\frac{-z - x}{-y}$

Solve. Write the answer as a proper fraction in lowest terms or as a mixed number in simple form.

45. $-5 \times \left(\frac{3}{8} \div \frac{1}{3}\right)$ **46.** $2\frac{1}{2} \div \left(\frac{5}{8} \times 1\frac{3}{4}\right)$ **47.** $7\frac{3}{8} + \left[-4\frac{1}{2} \div \left(-5\frac{2}{3}\right)\right]$

Problems

Solve.

1. The Maxwell children have hired a caterer to provide food for an anniversary party for their parents. The caterer has quoted a price of $15.75 per person and is asking for an advance payment of $\frac{1}{4}$ of the total bill. If the estimated number of guests is 50, how much is the advance payment?

2. The Clean-as-a-Whistle Company provides a matching service for people looking for home cleaners and people wishing to clean homes. The fees include $6.50 per hour for the cleaner, plus $1.50 per hour for the agency. If you hire a cleaner from the company for 5 h, how much will you pay?

3. As a general rule for brick work, masons estimate 6.5 bricks per square foot. Based on this estimate, will 2500 bricks be enough for a patio that is 396 ft^2?

4. The controller of a hospital found that laundry fees for a four-month period totaled $8755. Based on this total, what would be the estimated fee for an entire year?

5. Store owners at the Wagon Wheel Mall pay a monthly rental fee plus a maintenance fee. The maintenance fee is determined by the number of square feet occupied by the shop. The entire mall is 200,000 ft^2 and the annual fee for the entire mall is $63,000. What is the annual share of the maintenance fee for a store that occupies 2500 ft^2?

6. An investor bought 12 acres of land for $70,000. She later subdivided the land into 22 lots that she sold for $4500 apiece. What was her profit on the sale?

7. Douglas bought 75 shares of Health Care Company (HCC) stock and 150 shares of Bowwow Brands (BWB) stock. Last year HCC paid a dividend of $1.85 per share and BWB paid a dividend of $2.04 per share. What was the total of the dividends that Douglas received?

4

Solving Equations

NASA (National Aeronautics and Space Administration) is the government agency responsible for space exploration and experiments. The photograph shows a rocket about to be fired into space. It is carrying the space shuttle Columbia.

Aboard the shuttle is the Spacelab research station, where astronauts and other scientists will conduct in-flight scientific experiments. Much of the research will take months to analyze, but we know from earlier flights that the results will be of enormous importance in many fields, such as astronomy and medicine. For example, many of the experiments concern the effect of weightlessness on the human body.

Career Note

Space scientists require a strong background in mathematics, physics, and related sciences. The work is demanding but exciting. The men and women who perform experiments in the Spacelab are selected because of their specialized knowledge in various fields, for example, in biology, chemistry, or medicine.

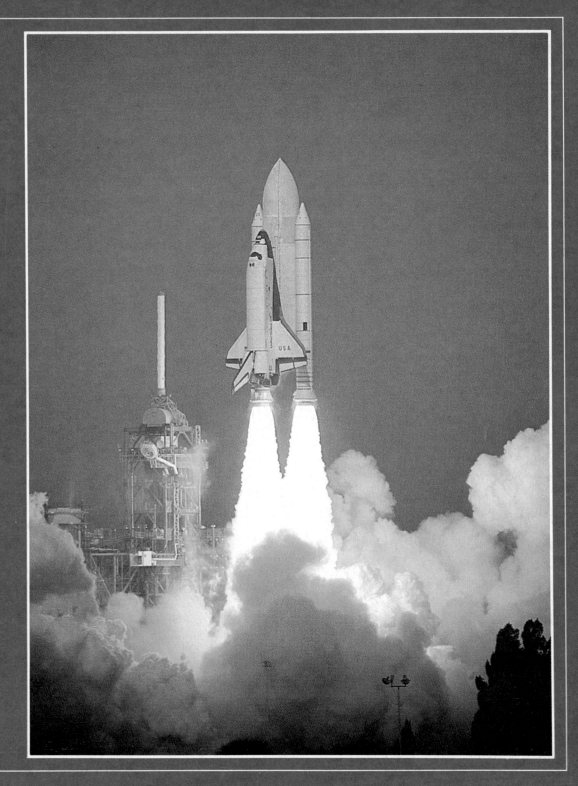

4-1 Equations: Addition and Subtraction

You have learned that an *equation* is a sentence that states that two expressions name the same number. A *replacement set,* consisting of values which may be substituted for the variable, is always stated or understood. For example, the equation

$$2x + 9 = 15$$

may have the replacement set $\{1, 3, 5\}$.

When a number from the replacement set makes an equation a true statement, it is called a *solution* of the equation. To determine whether a value in the replacement set $\{1, 3, 5\}$ is a solution of $2x + 9 = 15$, substitute it into the equation.

$2x + 9 = 15$	$2x + 9 = 15$	$2x + 9 = 15$
$2(1) + 9 = 15$	$2(3) + 9 = 15$	$2(5) + 9 = 15$
$2 + 9 = 15$	$6 + 9 = 15$	$10 + 9 = 15$
$11 = 15$	$15 = 15$	$19 = 15$
false	true	false

Thus, 3 is a solution of the equation $2x + 9 = 15$.

If the replacement set for an equation is the set of whole numbers, it is not practical to use substitution to solve the equation. Instead, we **transform,** or change, the given equation into a simpler, **equivalent equation,** that is, one that has the same solution. When we transform the given equation, our goal is to arrive at an equivalent equation of the form

$$\text{variable} = \text{number}.$$

For example:

$$n = 5$$

The number, 5, is then the solution of the original equation. The following transformations can be used to solve equations.

> Simplify numerical expressions and variable expressions.
>
> *Transformation by addition:* Add the same number to both sides.
>
> *Transformation by subtraction:* Subtract the same number from both sides.

EXAMPLE 1   Solve $x = 3 + 5$.

Solution   Simplify the numerical expression $3 + 5$.

$$x = 3 + 5$$
$$x = 8$$

The solution is 8.

EXAMPLE 2   Solve $x - 2 = 8$.

Solution   Our goal is to find an equivalent equation of the form

$$x = \text{a number}.$$

The left side of the given equation is $x - 2$. Recall that addition and subtraction are inverse operations. If we add 2 to both sides, the left side simplifies to x.

$$x - 2 = 8$$
$$x - 2 + 2 = 8 + 2$$
$$x = 10$$

The solution is 10.

EXAMPLE 3   Solve $x + 6 = -8$.

Solution   Subtract 6 from both sides of the equation to get an equivalent equation of the form $x = $ a number.

$$x + 6 = -8$$
$$x + 6 - 6 = -8 - 6$$
$$x = -14$$

The solution is -14.

In equations involving a number of steps, it is a good idea to check your answer. This can be done quite easily by substituting the answer in the original equation. Checking is illustrated in Example 4.

EXAMPLE 4   Solve $5 + x + 4 = 17$.

Solution
$$5 + x + 4 = 17$$
$$5 + 4 + x = 17$$
$$9 + x = 17$$
$$9 + x - 9 = 17 - 9$$
$$x = 8$$

Check: $5 + x + 4 = 17$
$5 + 8 + 4 \stackrel{?}{=} 17$
$13 + 4 = 17$ ✓

The solution is 8.

The following example shows how to solve an equation, such as $34 - x = 27$, in which the variable is being subtracted.

EXAMPLE 5   Solve $34 - x = 27$.

Solution   Add x to both sides.
$$34 - x = 27$$
$$34 - x + x = 27 + x$$
$$34 = 27 + x$$

Subtract 27 from both sides.
$$34 - 27 = 27 + x - 27$$
$$7 = x$$

The solution is 7.

Reading Mathematics: *Study Skills*
Review the worked-out examples if you need help in solving any of the exercises. When doing so, be certain to read carefully and to make sure that you understand what is happening in each step.

You may be able to solve some of the equations in the exercises without pencil and paper. Nevertheless, it is important to show all the steps in your work and to make sure you can tell which transformation you are using in each step.

Throughout the rest of this chapter, if no replacement set is given for an equation, you should assume that the replacement set is the set of all numbers in our decimal system.

Class Exercises

State which transformation was used to transform the first equation into the second.

1. $x - 3 = 5$
     $x - 3 + 3 = 5 + 3$

2. $x = 8 + 7$
     $x = 15$

3. $-3 - 1 = 3 - x$
     $-4 = 3 - x$

4. $x - 5 = 9$
     $x - 5 + 5 = 9 + 5$

Complete each equation. State which transformation has been used.

5. $x = 11 + 17$
   $x = \underline{\ ?\ }$

6. $x - 11 = 12$
     $x - 11 + 11 = 12 + \underline{\ ?\ }$

7. $x + 7 = 13$
     $x + 7 - 7 = 13 \underline{\ ?\ } 7$

8. $4 - x = -2$
     $4 - x + x = -2 \underline{\ ?\ } x$

Written Exercises

Use transformations to solve each equation. Write down all the steps.

A 1. $x + 15 = 27$

2. $x - 8 = 21$

3. $x - 6 = -7$

4. $19 + x = 35$

5. $8 + (-12) = x$

6. $3 + 16 = x$

7. $x = 38 - 15$

8. $x = -24 + 15$

9. $x + 7 = 3(6 + 2)$

10. $34 = 4(3 - 1) + x$

11. $23 = 30 - x$

12. $42 - x = -4$

B 13. $5(2 + 7) - x = 33$

14. $6(8 - 3) = 48 - x$

15. $9 + 12 = (3 \times 5) + x$

16. $3(72 \div 12) - x = 5$

17. $4(10 - 7) = x + 4$

18. $22 + x = 4(39 \div 3)$

19. $-\frac{3}{5} + n = -1$

20. $n - \frac{3}{4} = 3$

21. $5 = 8\frac{2}{3} - a$

22. $-4\frac{1}{5} + c = -2$

23. $n - 0.76 = 0.34$

24. $n + 0.519 = 0.597$

25. $0.894 - y = 0.641$

26. $0.321 + r = 0.58$

27. $x - 0.323 = 0.873$

28. $-0.187 + t = 0.67$

29. $3\frac{1}{2} + 5\frac{1}{4} = n - 1$

30. $4\frac{1}{3} - 1\frac{5}{6} = b + 1$

31. $n + 3\frac{1}{6} + 4\frac{1}{4} = 10$

32. $n + 5\frac{7}{8} - 1\frac{1}{6} = 7$

33. $n + 0.813 - 0.529 = 0.642$

34. $a + 0.952 - 0.751 = 0.7$

C 35. $8\left(4\frac{1}{10} - 3\frac{1}{4}\right) = y + 3$

36. $3\left(2\frac{1}{9} + 4\frac{5}{6}\right) = 25 - c$

37. $7(0.34 - 0.21) = b - 0.82$

38. $4(0.641 + 0.222) = n + 0.357$

Review Exercises

Complete.

1. $5x \div \underline{\ ?\ } = x$

2. $y \times 8 \div 8 = \underline{\ ?\ }$

3. $3z \div \underline{\ ?\ } = z$

4. $\frac{x}{4} \times \underline{\ ?\ } = x$

5. $\frac{x}{9} \times \underline{\ ?\ } = x$

6. $\frac{z}{7} \times 7 = \underline{\ ?\ }$

4-2 Equations: Multiplication and Division

If an equation involves multiplication or division, the following transformations are used to solve the equation.

> *Transformation by multiplication:* Multiply both sides of the
> equation by the same nonzero number.
>
> *Transformation by division:* Divide both sides of the equation
> by the same nonzero number.

EXAMPLE 1   Solve $3n = 24$.

Solution   Our goal is to find an equivalent equation of the form
$$n = \text{a number.}$$
Use the fact that multiplication and division are inverse operations
and that $3n \div 3 = n$.
$$3n = 24$$
$$\frac{3n}{3} = \frac{24}{3}$$
$$n = 8$$
The solution is 8.

EXAMPLE 2   Solve $-5x = 53$.

Solution   Divide both sides by 5.
$$-5x = 53$$
$$\frac{-5x}{-5} = \frac{53}{-5}$$
$$x = -10\frac{3}{5}$$
The solution is $-10\frac{3}{5}$.

EXAMPLE 3   Solve $\frac{n}{4} = 7$.

Solution   Multiply both sides by 4.
$$\frac{n}{4} = 7$$
$$\frac{n}{4} \times 4 = 7 \times 4$$
$$n = 28$$
The solution is 28.

Class Exercises

a. State the transformation you would use to solve each equation.
b. Solve the equation.

1. $2n = 26$ **2.** $\frac{n}{2} = -5$ **3.** $\frac{n}{3} = 12$ **4.** $-3n = 12$

5. $5n = 35$ **6.** $33 = 11n$ **7.** $-7 = \frac{n}{4}$ **8.** $\frac{n}{5} = 20$

9. $4 + x = 7$ **10.** $4x = -24$ **11.** $28 = \frac{x}{7}$ **12.** $-11 = x - 2$

Written Exercises

Use the transformations given in this chapter to solve each equation.
Show all steps. Check your solution.

A   **1.** $5n = 75$ **2.** $-87 = 3n$ **3.** $\frac{n}{3} = 6$ **4.** $-3n = 15$

     5. $7n = 42$ **6.** $\frac{n}{4} = -8$ **7.** $\frac{n}{6} = 9$ **8.** $-\frac{n}{5} = 6$

     9. $\frac{n}{4} = -21$ **10.** $10 = \frac{n}{6}$ **11.** $4 = \frac{n}{7}$ **12.** $5n = 55$

     13. $9n = 45$ **14.** $\frac{n}{8} = 9$ **15.** $11n = -110$ **16.** $8n = 96$

     17. $\frac{n}{13} = 7$ **18.** $\frac{n}{16} = -6$ **19.** $12n = 132$ **20.** $17n = -289$

B   **21.** $6x = 45$ **22.** $18x = 12$ **23.** $\frac{x}{17} = -13$ **24.** $\frac{x}{15} = 11$

     25. $-\frac{x}{21} = 12$ **26.** $\frac{x}{27} = 23$ **27.** $24x = -20$ **28.** $12x = 76$

     29. $9x = 80 + 7$ **30.** $-64x = 100 - 48$ **31.** $\frac{x}{26} = 2(3 + 4)$

     32. $42 + x = 179$ **33.** $x - 193 = 54$ **34.** $296 - x = -51$

C   **35.** $7x = \frac{14}{19}$ **36.** $11x = \frac{13}{20}$ **37.** $\frac{x}{16} = \frac{21}{32}$ **38.** $\frac{x}{9} = \frac{13}{84}$

Review Exercises

Multiply or divide.

1. $\frac{5}{8} \times \frac{12}{35}$ **2.** $\frac{14}{30} \div \frac{2}{15}$ **3.** $\frac{17}{9} \times \frac{6}{85}$

4. $3\frac{2}{3} \times 5\frac{9}{11}$ **5.** $3\frac{5}{8} \div 1\frac{3}{16}$ **6.** 0.09×3.74

4-3 Equations: Decimals and Fractions

Sometimes the variable expression in an equation may involve a decimal. When this occurs, you can use the transformations that you have learned in the previous lessons.

EXAMPLE 1 Solve the equation $0.42x = 1.05$.

Solution   Divide both sides by 0.42.

$$0.42x = 1.05$$

$$\frac{0.42x}{0.42} = \frac{1.05}{0.42}$$

$$x = 2.5$$

The solution is 2.5.

EXAMPLE 2 Solve the equation $\frac{n}{0.15} = 92$.

Solution   Multiply both sides by 0.15.

$$\frac{n}{0.15} = 92$$

$$0.15 \times \frac{n}{0.15} = 0.15 \times 92$$

$$n = 13.80$$

The solution is 13.80.

The variable expression in an equation may also involve a fraction. To see how to solve an equation such as $\frac{2}{3}x = 6$, think how you would solve an equation such as $2x = 6$. (You would divide both sides by 2, getting $x = 3$.) Thus, to solve $\frac{2}{3}x = 6$, you would divide both sides by $\frac{2}{3}$. This is the same as multiplying by the reciprocal of $\frac{2}{3}$, or $\frac{3}{2}$. Therefore, we solve equations involving fractions in the following way.

> If an equation has the form
>
> $$\frac{a}{b}x = c,$$
>
> where both a and b are nonzero,
>
> multiply both sides by $\frac{b}{a}$, the reciprocal of $\frac{a}{b}$.

EXAMPLE 3 Solve the equation $\frac{1}{3}y = 18$.

Solution Multiply both sides by 3, the reciprocal of $\frac{1}{3}$.

$$\frac{1}{3}y = 18$$

$$3 \times \frac{1}{3}y = 3 \times 18$$

$$y = 3 \times 18$$
$$y = 54$$

The solution is 54.

EXAMPLE 4 Solve the equation $\frac{6}{7}n = 8$. Check.

Solution Multiply both sides by $\frac{7}{6}$, the reciprocal of $\frac{6}{7}$.

$$\frac{6}{7}n = 8 \qquad\qquad \text{Check:} \qquad \frac{6}{7}n = 8$$

$$\frac{7}{6} \times \frac{6}{7}n = \frac{7}{6} \times 8 \qquad\qquad \frac{6}{7} \times \frac{28}{3} \overset{?}{=} 8$$

$$n = \frac{7}{\underset{3}{\cancel{6}}} \times \overset{4}{\cancel{8}} \qquad\qquad \frac{\overset{2}{\cancel{6}}}{\underset{1}{\cancel{7}}} \times \frac{\overset{4}{\cancel{28}}}{\underset{1}{\cancel{3}}} \overset{?}{=} 8$$

$$n = \frac{28}{3} \qquad\qquad\qquad \frac{2}{1} \times \frac{4}{1} = 8$$

The solution is $\frac{28}{3}$, or $9\frac{1}{3}$.

Class Exercises

a. State what number you would multiply or divide both sides of each equation by in order to solve it.
b. Solve the equation.

1. $\frac{3}{4}x = 15$ **2.** $0.2x = 6$ **3.** $\frac{x}{0.4} = 1.7$ **4.** $\frac{x}{1.3} = 2.4$

5. $\frac{1}{8}x = 7$ **6.** $\frac{17}{12}x = 34$ **7.** $\frac{8}{3}x = 24$ **8.** $\frac{1}{9}x = 14$

9. $\frac{x}{1.8} = 2.9$ **10.** $\frac{x}{2.3} = 5$ **11.** $0.35x = 10.5$ **12.** $0.55x = 2.20$

13. $0.28x = 2.24$ **14.** $0.67x = 6.03$ **15.** $\frac{x}{2.6} = 3.7$ **16.** $\frac{x}{5.9} = 14.2$

Written Exercises

Solve each equation.

A
1. $\frac{1}{8}x = 11$
2. $-\frac{1}{3}x = 13$
3. $0.4x = 8$
4. $0.6x = 24$

5. $\frac{x}{0.3} = -5$
6. $\frac{x}{0.7} = 4$
7. $-\frac{2}{3}x = 16$
8. $\frac{3}{4}x = 21$

9. $0.25x = 15$
10. $0.44x = -22$
11. $\frac{x}{1.5} = 13$
12. $-\frac{x}{2.2} = 22$

13. $\frac{3}{2}x = 27$
14. $\frac{5}{9}x = -65$
15. $\frac{12}{5}x = 48$
16. $\frac{12}{7}x = 60$

17. $-1.3x = 39$
18. $3.2x = 128$
19. $\frac{x}{4.5} = -11$
20. $\frac{x}{6.2} = 17$

B
21. $\frac{4}{3}n = 18$
22. $-\frac{6}{5}n = 20$
23. $\frac{8}{3}n = 28$
24. $\frac{6}{7}n = -21$

25. $3.9 = 0.6n$
26. $3.6 = 1.6n$
27. $-1.5n = 1.2$
28. $1.25n = 3.5$

29. $\left(2\frac{2}{5}\right)n = \frac{-4}{15}$
30. $\frac{3}{11} = \frac{9}{5}n$
31. $-\frac{7}{9} = \frac{14}{15}n$
32. $1\frac{5}{7}n = \frac{16}{35}$

33. $\frac{n}{2.45} = 3.1$
34. $\frac{n}{6.31} = -2.12$
35. $\frac{n}{5.37} = 0.004$
36. $-\frac{n}{0.09} = 2.79$

C
37. $\frac{2}{3}x = 3.8$
38. $\frac{3}{4}x = -6.93$
39. $\frac{3}{5}x = 9.36$

40. $\frac{x}{6.4} = \frac{5}{8}$
41. $\frac{x}{2.7} = \frac{11}{9}$
42. $\frac{x}{4.2} = \frac{17}{6}$

Review Exercises

Solve.

1. $x + 17 = 47$
2. $55 + x = 75$
3. $96 - x = 41$

4. $82 - x = 37$
5. $x - 45 = 58$
6. $5x = 95$

7. $3x = 51$
8. $7x = 91$
9. $4x = 76$

Calculator Key-In

Using a calculator can greatly simplify the computations involved in solving an equation with decimals. Use a calculator to solve the following equations.

1. $0.32x = 0.096$
2. $3.02x = 1.84$
3. $2.11x = 5.74$

4. $\frac{x}{0.79} = 1.08$
5. $\frac{x}{1.91} = 1.77$
6. $\frac{x}{4.002} = 0.107$

4-4 Combined Operations

Many equations may be written in the form

$$ax + b = c,$$

where a, b, and c are given numbers and x is a variable. To solve such an equation, it is necessary to use more than one transformation.

EXAMPLE 1 Solve the equation $3n - 5 = 10 + 6$.

Solution Simplify the numerical expression.

$$3n - 5 = 10 + 6$$
$$3n - 5 = 16$$

Add 5 to both sides.

$$3n - 5 + 5 = 16 + 5$$
$$3n = 21$$

Divide both sides by 3.

$$\frac{3n}{3} = \frac{21}{3}$$
$$n = 7$$

The solution is 7.

Example 1 suggests the following general procedure for solving equations.

> **1.** Simplify each side of the equation.
>
> **2.** If there are still indicated additions or subtractions, use the inverse operations to undo them.
>
> **3.** If there are indicated multiplications or divisions involving the variable, use the inverse operations to undo them.

It is important to remember that in using the procedure outlined above you must *always perform the same operation on both sides of the equation*. Also, you must use the steps in the procedure in the order indicated. That is, you first simplify each side of the equation, then undo additions and subtractions, and then undo multiplications and divisions.

EXAMPLE 2 Solve the equation $\frac{3}{2}n + 7 = -8$.

Solution Subtract 7 from both sides.

$$\frac{3}{2}n + 7 = -8$$

$$\frac{3}{2}n + 7 - 7 = -8 - 7$$

$$\frac{3}{2}n = -15$$

Multiply both sides by $\frac{2}{3}$, the reciprocal of $\frac{3}{2}$.

$$\frac{2}{3} \times \frac{3}{2}n = \frac{2}{3} \times (-15)$$

$$n = \frac{2}{\underset{1}{3}} \times (-\overset{5}{15})$$

$$n = -10$$

The solution is -10.

EXAMPLE 3 Solve the equation $40 - \frac{5}{3}n = 15$.

Solution Add $\frac{5}{3}n$ to both sides.

$$40 - \frac{5}{3}n = 15$$

$$40 - \frac{5}{3}n + \frac{5}{3}n = 15 + \frac{5}{3}n$$

$$40 = 15 + \frac{5}{3}n$$

Subtract 15 from both sides.

$$40 - 15 = 15 + \frac{5}{3}n - 15$$

$$25 = \frac{5}{3}n$$

Multiply both sides by $\frac{3}{5}$.

$$\frac{3}{5} \times 25 = \frac{3}{5} \times \frac{5}{3}n$$

$$\frac{3}{\underset{1}{5}} \times \overset{5}{25} = n$$

$$15 = n$$

The solution is 15.

Class Exercises

State the two transformations you would use to find the solution of each equation. Be sure to specify which transformation you would use first.

1. $3n + 2 = -10$

2. $4n - 1 = 19$

3. $\frac{1}{2}n - 6 = 1$

4. $\frac{1}{3}n + 5 = 7$

5. $\frac{2}{3}n - 6 = -12$

6. $\frac{5}{2}n + 2 = 13$

7. $3n - 6 = 15$

8. $7n + 21 = -63$

9. $\frac{3}{4}n - 8 = 12$

10. $\frac{1}{2}n + 2 = -5$

11. $2\frac{1}{3}n - 2 = 8$

12. $1\frac{2}{3}n + 15 = -21$

Written Exercises

Solve each equation.

A

1. $2n - 5 = 17$

2. $3n + 6 = -24$

3. $5n + 6 = 41$

4. $4n - 15 = 9$

5. $6n + 11 = 77$

6. $8n - 13 = 51$

7. $50 - 3n = 20$

8. $42 - 5n = 7$

9. $29 - 6n = 11$

10. $-79 - 8n = -15$

11. $\frac{1}{4}n + 5 = 25$

12. $\frac{1}{8}n - 11 = 21$

13. $\frac{1}{2}n + 3 = 18$

14. $\frac{1}{3}n - 7 = -11$

15. $\frac{1}{5}n - 2 = 9$

16. $\frac{1}{4}n + 3 = 8$

17. $\frac{2}{3}n + 12 = 28$

18. $\frac{3}{5}n + 11 = -7$

19. $6n - 7 = 19$

20. $10n - 6 = -39$

21. $\frac{6}{5}n - 7 = 20$

22. $\frac{15}{4}n + 7 = -68$

23. $2\frac{2}{5}n + 5 = 23$

24. $1\frac{1}{7}n - 9 = 27$

B

25. $\frac{3}{5}n + \frac{2}{3} = \frac{8}{3}$

26. $\frac{2}{3}n - \frac{5}{6} = -\frac{1}{8}$

27. $\frac{3}{4}n - \frac{11}{15} = \frac{3}{5}$

28. $\frac{5}{6}n + \frac{1}{10} = \frac{29}{30}$

29. $\frac{7}{8}n - \frac{5}{6} = \frac{3}{4}$

30. $\frac{1}{3}n - \frac{11}{25} = \frac{3}{10}$

31. $\frac{2}{5}n + \frac{3}{7} = \frac{11}{5}$

32. $\frac{1}{6}n + \frac{3}{5} = \frac{7}{11}$

33. $1\frac{1}{3}n + \frac{5}{12} = \frac{3}{4}$

34. $2\frac{2}{3}n - \frac{4}{7} = \frac{8}{9}$

35. $\frac{11}{3}n - \frac{5}{9} = \frac{5}{6}$

36. $\frac{7}{2}n - \frac{11}{12} = \frac{5}{9}$

37. $1\frac{3}{8}n + \frac{1}{4} = \frac{7}{8}$

38. $\frac{3}{4}n - \frac{1}{12} = \frac{7}{3}$

39. $\frac{3}{7}n + \frac{4}{5} = \frac{6}{7}$

C **40.** Solve $C = 2\pi r$ for r if $C = 220$ and $\pi \approx \frac{22}{7}$.

41. Solve $P = 2l + 2w$ for w if $P = 64$ and $l = 5$.

42. Solve $d = rt$ for r if $d = 308$ and $t = 3.5$.

Self-Test A

Use transformations to solve each equation.

1. $y + 7 = -17$ **2.** $x - 6 = 4$ [4-1]

3. $x + 6 = 27 - 12$ **4.** $5(7 + 2) = x - 11$

5. $7a = -91$ **6.** $-\frac{c}{4} = 17$ [4-2]

7. $-4t = -68$ **8.** $\frac{p}{3} = -11$

9. $\frac{1}{6}z = 25$ **10.** $-\frac{13}{3}y = 10$ [4-3]

11. $0.35a = -28$ **12.** $\frac{x}{0.03} = -58$

13. $8n - 40 = 180$ **14.** $\frac{2}{3}n + 18 = 98$ [4-4]

15. $\frac{1}{3}x + 4 = 6$ **16.** $5x - 2 = -17$

Self-Test answers and Extra Practice are at the back of the book.

▌▌▌ **Calculator Key-In**

Do the following on your calculator.

1. Press any 3 digits.	852
2. Repeat the digits.	852,852
3. Divide by 7.	?
4. Divide by 11.	?
5. Divide by 13.	?

What is your answer? Now multiply your answer by 1001. Try again using three different digits. Explain your results.

4-5 Writing Expressions for Word Phrases

In mathematics we often use symbols to translate word phrases into mathematical expressions. The same mathematical expression can be used to translate many different word expressions. Consider the phrases below.

Three more than a number n The sum of three and a number n

Written as a variable expression, each of the phrases becomes

$$3 + n.$$

Notice that both the phrase *more than* and the phrase *the sum of* indicate addition.

    The following are some of the word phrases that we associate with each of the four operations.

+	−	×	÷
add	subtract	multiply	divide
sum	difference	product	quotient
plus	minus	times	
total	remainder		
more than	less than		
increased by	decreased by		

EXAMPLE 1   Write a variable expression for the word phrase.
         a. A number t increased by nine   **b.** Sixteen less than a number q
         c. A number x decreased by twelve, divided by forty
         d. The product of sixteen and the sum of five and a number r

Solution   **a.** In this expression, the phrase *increased by* indicates that the operation is addition. $t + 9$

         b. In this expression, the phrase *less than* indicates that the operation is subtraction. $q - 16$

         c. In this expression, the phrases *decreased by* and *divided by* indicate that two operations, subtraction and division, are involved. $(x - 12) \div 40$

         d. In this expression, the words *product* and *sum* indicate that multiplication and addition are involved.
            $16 \times (5 + r),$ or $16(5 + r)$

Often a word expression contains more than one phrase that indicates an operation. Notice in Example 1 parts (c) and (d), on page 143 how parentheses were needed to represent the word phrase accurately. When translating from words to symbols, be sure to include grouping symbols if they are needed to make the meaning of an expression clear.

Many words that we use in everyday speech indicate operations or relationships between numbers. *Twice* and *doubled*, for example, indicate multiplication by 2. *Consecutive* whole numbers are whole numbers that differ by 1. The *preceding* whole number is the whole number *before* a particular number, and the *next* whole number is the whole number *after* a particular number.

EXAMPLE 2 If $2n$ is a whole number, represent (a) the preceding whole number and (b) the next four consecutive whole numbers.

Solution **a.** The preceding whole number is 1 less than $2n$, or $2n - 1$.

b. Each of the next whole numbers is 1 more than the whole number before.

$$2n + 1, \ 2n + 2, \ 2n + 3, \ 2n + 4$$

Class Exercises

Match.

1. A number x multiplied by fourteen   **A.** $14 - x$

2. The quotient of fourteen and a number x **B.** $2(x + 7)$

3. Fourteen less than a number x **C.** $14 \div (7 - x)$

4. Seven increased by a number x **D.** $7 + 14x$

5. A number x subtracted from fourteen   **E.** $14 \div x$

6. Fourteen more than a number x **F.** $7(14 + x)$

7. Seven more than the product of fourteen and a number x **G.** $x - 14$

8. Twice the sum of a number x and seven   **H.** $7 + x$

9. The product of seven and the sum of fourteen and a number x **I.** $14x$

    J. $x + 14$

10. Fourteen divided by the difference between seven and x

Written Exercises

Write a variable expression for the word phrase.

A 1. The product of eight and a number b

2. A number q divided by sixteen

3. A number d subtracted from fifty-three

4. Four less than a number f

5. Thirty increased by a number t

6. Five times a number c

7. The sum of a number g and nine

8. A number k minus twenty-seven

9. Seventy-eight decreased by a number m

10. A number y added to ninety

11. Nineteen more than a number n

12. Sixty-two plus a number h

13. The quotient when a number d is divided by eleven

14. The difference when a number a is subtracted from a number b

15. The remainder when a number z is subtracted from twelve

16. The total of a number x, a number y, and thirteen

17. Fifteen more than the product of a number t and eleven

18. The quotient when a number b is divided by nine, decreased by seven

19. The sum of a number m and a number n, multiplied by ninety-one

20. Forty-one times the difference when six is subtracted from a number a

21. A number r divided by the difference between eighty-three and ten

22. The total of a number p and twelve, divided by eighteen

23. The product of a number c and three more than the sum of nine and twelve

24. The sum of a number y and ten, divided by the difference when a number x is decreased by five

25. The total of sixty, forty, and ten, divided by a number d

26. The product of eighteen less than a number b and the sum of twenty-two and forty-five

B **27.** The greatest of four consecutive whole numbers, the smallest of which is b

28. The smallest of three consecutive whole numbers, the greatest of which is q

29. The greatest of three consecutive even numbers following the even number x

30. The greatest of three consecutive odd numbers following the odd number y

31. The value in cents of q quarters

32. The number of inches in f feet

33. The number of hours in x minutes

34. The number of dollars in y cents

C **35.** The difference between two numbers is ten. The greater number is x. Write a variable expression for the smaller number.

36. One number is six times another. The greater number is a. Write a variable expression for the smaller number.

Review Exercises

Use the inverse operation to solve for the variable.

1. $x + 32 = 59$ **2.** $2y = 68$ **3.** $a \div 8 = 72$ **4.** $q - 14 = -23$

5. $-7c = 105$ **6.** $y - 11 = 21$ **7.** $n - 6 = 13$ **8.** $p + 3 = -39$

▌▌▌ Challenge

In the set of whole numbers, there are two different values for a for which this equation is true.

$$a + a = a \times a$$

What are they?

4-6 Word Sentences and Equations

Just as word phrases can be translated into mathematical expressions, word sentences can be translated into equations.

EXAMPLE 1 Write an equation for the word sentence.

a. Twice a number x is equal to 14.
b. Thirty-five is sixteen more than a number t.

Solution

a. First, write the phrase *twice a number* x as the variable expression $2x$. Use the symbol $=$ to translate *is equal to*.

$$2x = 14$$

b. Use the equals sign to translate *is*. Write *sixteen more than a number* as $t + 16$.

$$35 = t + 16$$

A word sentence may involve an unknown number without specifying a variable. When translating such a sentence into an equation, we may use any letter to represent the unknown number.

EXAMPLE 2 Write an equation for the word sentence.
a. The sum of a number and seven is thirteen.
b. A number increased by six is equal to three times the number.

Solution

a. Let n stand for the unknown number. $n + 7 = 13$
b. Let x stand for the unknown number. $x + 6 = 3x$

Class Exercises

Write a problem that each equation could represent. Use the words in parentheses as the subject of the problem.

1. $x + 16 = 180$ (number of students in the eighth grade)

2. $0.59x = 2.36$ (buying groceries)

3. $48x = 630$ (traveling in a car)

4. $x - 25 = 175$ (number of cars in a parking lot)

5. $256 - x = 219$ (price reduction in a department store)

6. $10x = 26$ (running race)

7. $25x = 175$ (fuel economy in a car)

Written Exercises

Write an equation for the word sentence.

A 1. Five times a number d is equal to twenty.

2. A number t increased by thirty-five is sixty.

3. Seven less than the product of a number w and three equals eight.

4. The difference when a number z is subtracted from sixteen is two.

5. Five divided by a number r equals forty-two.

6. The sum of a number and seven is equal to nine.

7. A number decreased by one equals five.

8. Twelve equals a number divided by four.

9. Twice a number, divided by three, is fifteen.

10. The product of a number and eight, decreased by three, is equal to nine.

B 11. The quotient when the sum of four and x is divided by two is thirty-four.

12. The sum of n and twenty-two, multiplied by three, is seventy-eight.

13. Fifty-nine minus x equals the sum of three and twice x.

14. Two increased by eight times c is equal to c divided by five.

C 15. The quotient when the difference between x and 5 is divided by three is 2.

16. Twice a number is equal to the product when the sum of the number and four is multiplied by eight.

Review Exercises

Write a mathematical expression for each word phrase.

1. Four less than a number

2. Five times a number

3. A number divided by seven

4. Ten more than a number

5. Forty minus a number

6. Twelve plus a number

7. A number times two

8. Ninety divided by a number

4-7 Writing Equations for Word Problems

In order to represent a word problem by an equation, we first read the problem carefully.

Next, we decide what numbers are being asked for. We then choose a variable and use it with the given conditions of the problem to represent the number or numbers asked for.

Now, we write an equation based on the given conditions of the problem. To do this, we write an expression involving the variable and set it equal to another variable expression or a number given in the problem that represents the same quantity.

The following example illustrates this procedure.

EXAMPLE 1   Write an equation for the following word problem.

Fran spent 3 times as long on her homework for English class as on her science homework. If she spent a total of 60 min on homework, how long did she spend on her science homework?

Solution   • The problem asks how long Fran spent on her science homework.

• Let t = time spent on science. Since Fran spent 3 times as long on her English homework, she spent $3t$ on English. Therefore, the expression $t + 3t$ represents the amount of time spent on the two assignments. We are given that the total amount of time was 60 min.

• An equation that represents the conditions is

$$t + 3t = 60$$

Class Exercises

a. Name the quantity you would represent by a variable.
b. State an equation that expresses the conditions of the word problem.

1. Jennifer bought 5 lb of apples for $3.45. What was the price per pound?

2. After Henry withdrew $350 from his account, he had $1150 left. How much money was in his account before this withdrawal?

3. A road that is 8.5 m wide is to be extended to 10.6 m wide. What is the width of the new paving?

4. In the seventh grade, 86 students made the honor roll. This is $\frac{2}{5}$ of the entire class. How many students are in the seventh grade?

a. Name the quantity you would represent by a variable.
b. State an equation that expresses the conditions of the word problem.

5. A 25-floor building is 105 m tall. What is the height of each floor if they are all of equal height?

6. A 150 L tank in a chemical factory can be filled by a pipe in 60 s. At how many liters per second does the liquid enter the tank?

Problems

Choose a variable and write an equation for each problem.

A 1. On one portion of a trip across the country, the Oates family covered 1170 miles in 9 days. How many miles per day is this?

2. Carey's car went 224 km on 28 L of gas. How many kilometers per liter is this?

3. Marge has purchased 18 subway tokens at a total cost of $13.50. What is the cost per token?

4. After $525 was spent on the class trip, there was $325 left in the class treasury. How much was in the treasury before the trip?

5. By the end of one month a hardware store had 116 socket wrench sets left out of a shipment of 144. How many sets were sold during the month?

6. After depositing his tax refund of $350, Manuel Ruiz had $1580 in his bank account. How much money was in the account before the deposit?

7. If Mary Ling follows her usual route to work, she travels 12 km on one road and 18 km on another. If she takes a short cut her total distance to work is 19 km. How many kilometers does she save by taking the short cut?

8. A department store's total receipts from a sale on pillowcases were $251.64. If 36 pillowcases were sold, what was the price of each?

9. An investor has deposited $2000 into a special savings account. Two years later, the balance in the account is $2650. How much interest has been earned?

10. Deane's account in the company credit union had a balance of $3155. After she made a withdrawal to pay for car repairs, her balance was $2855. How much money did Deane withdraw?

B 11. In a school election $\frac{4}{5}$ of the students voted. There were 180 ballots. How many students are in the school?

12. In a heat-loss survey it was found that $\frac{3}{10}$ of the total wall area of the Gables' house consists of windows. The combined area of the windows is 240 ft². What is the total wall area of the house?

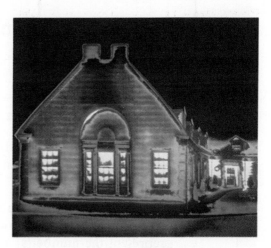

13. The difference between twice a number and thirty is 20. What is the number?

14. A bookstore received a shipment of books. Twenty were sold and $\frac{2}{5}$ of those remaining were returned to the publisher. If 48 books were returned, how many books were in the original shipment?

C 15. By mass, $\frac{1}{9}$ of any quantity of water consists of hydrogen. What quantity of water contains 5 g of hydrogen?

16. The balance in Peter Flynn's savings account is $6800. A withdrawal of $1000 is made, and the balance is to be withdrawn in 40 equal installments. What is the amount of each installment?

Review Exercises

Write an equation for each word sentence.

1. Eight less than a number is forty-three.

2. Twelve times a number is one hundred eight.

3. Fourteen more than a number is seventy.

4. A number divided by nine is twenty-two.

5. A number minus seventeen is thirty-four.

6. Five times a number is sixty-five.

 Challenge

A thoroughbred is 80 m ahead of a quarter horse, and is running at the rate of 27 m/s. The quarter horse is following at the rate of 31 m/s. In how many seconds will the quarter horse overtake the thoroughbred?

4-8 Solving Word Problems

The following five-step method will be helpful in solving word problems using an equation.

Solving a Word Problem Using an Equation

Step 1 Read the problem carefully. Make sure that you understand what it says. You may need to read it more than once.

Step 2 Decide what numbers are asked for. Choose a variable and use it with the given conditions of the problem to represent the number(s) asked for.

Step 3 Write an equation based on the given conditions.

Step 4 Solve the equation and find the required numbers.

Step 5 Check your results with the words of the problem. Give the answer.

EXAMPLE 1   An evergreen in Sam's yard is now 78 in. tall. If it grows 6 in. each year, how many years will it take to grow to a height of 105 in.?

Solution
- The problem says
  present tree height, 78 in.
  tree growth per year, 6 in.
  future tree height, 105 in.

- The problem asks for
  number of years for tree to grow to 105 in.

  Let n = number of years for tree to grow to 105 in.

  Since the tree grows 6 in. per year:
  height after 1 year, $78 + 6$
  height after 2 years, $78 + (6 \times 2)$
  height after 3 years, $78 + (6 \times 3)$
  height after n years, $78 + 6n$

- We now have two expressions for the height of the tree after n years. We set them equal to each other.

$$78 + 6n = 105$$

- Solve.

$$78 + 6n = 105$$
$$78 + 6n - 78 = 105 - 78$$
$$6n = 27$$
$$\frac{6n}{6} = \frac{27}{6}$$
$$n = 4\frac{1}{2}$$

- Check: If the tree grows 6 in. each year, in $4\frac{1}{2}$ years it will grow $4\frac{1}{2} \times 6$, or 27 in. The tree is now 78 in. tall. $78 + 27 = 105$. The result checks.

In $4\frac{1}{2}$ years the tree will grow to 105 in.

EXAMPLE 2 Two fifths of the members of the Riverview Sailing Club have signed up in advance for a club-wide race. On the day of the race, seven more members sign up, bringing the total of 41. How many members does the club have?

Solution

- The problem says
    two fifths of the members have signed up in advance
    the sum of this number and 7 is 41

- The problem asks for
    number of members in the club.

    Let n = number of members in the club.
    Two fifths of the members, or $\frac{2}{5}n$, have signed up in advance.
    The sum of this number and 7, or $\frac{2}{5}n + 7$, is 41.

- We now have two expressions for the same number. We set them equal to each other.

$$\frac{2}{5}n + 7 = 41$$

- Solve.

$$\frac{2}{5}n + 7 = 41$$
$$\frac{2}{5}n + 7 - 7 = 41 - 7$$
$$\frac{2}{5}n = 34$$
$$\frac{5}{2} \times \frac{2}{5}n = \frac{5}{2} \times 34$$
$$n = 85$$

- Check: Two fifths of 85 is 34, and $34 + 7 = 41$. The result checks.

The club has 85 members.

Problems

Solve each problem using the five-step method.

A **1.** A mineralogist has learned that $\frac{2}{5}$ of a certain ore is pure copper. If a quantity of this ore yields 100 lb of pure copper, how large is the quantity?

2. Three tenths of the seats in a college's football stadium are reserved for alumni on Homecoming Weekend. This amounts to 4800 seats. What is the capacity of the stadium?

3. Three fourths of all the books in a school library are nonfiction. There are 360 nonfiction books. How many books are in the school library altogether?

4. Charles has $800 in a savings account. If he decides to deposit $40 into the account each week, how many weeks will it take for the account balance to reach $2000?

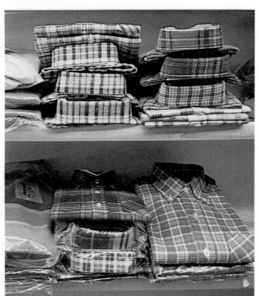

5. A department store received five cartons of shirts. One week later 25 shirts had been sold and 95 shirts were left in stock. How many shirts came in each carton?

6. The four walls in Fran's room have equal areas. The combined area of the doors and windows of the room is 12 m². If the total wall area (including doors and windows) is 68 m², what is the area of one wall?

B **7.** Three fifths of those attending a club picnic decided to play touch football. After one more person decided to play, there were 16 players. How many people attended the picnic?

8. Four fifths of the athletic club treasury was to be spent on an awards banquet. After $450 was paid for food, there was $150 left out of the funds designated for the banquet. How much money had been in the treasury originally?

9. After using $\frac{2}{3}$ of a bag of fertilizer on his garden, Kent gave 8 lb to a neighbor. If Kent had 42 lb left, how much had been in the full bag?

10. Marcie biked to a point 5 km from her home. After a short rest, she then biked to a point 55 km from her home along the same road. If the second part of her trip took 4 hours, what was Marcie's speed, assuming her speed was constant?

C **11.** When the gas gauge on her car was on the $\frac{3}{8}$ mark, Karen pumped 15 gal of gas into the tank in order to fill it. How many gallons of gas does the tank in Karen's car hold?

Self-Test B

Write a variable expression for the word phrase.

1. The product of twelve and a number x [4–5]

2. A number d subtracted from sixty

Match each problem with one of the following equations.

a. $x - 18 = 72$ **b.** $18x = 72$ **c.** $x + 18 = 72$ **d.** $72x = 18$

3. At 72 km/h how many hours would it take a car to travel 18 km?   [4–6]

4. Seth bought 18 more model cars for his collection. If he now has 72 cars, how many did he have before?

5. After the first day, 18 people were eliminated from the tournament. If 72 people were still playing, how many people started the tournament?

Choose a variable and write an equation for each problem.

6. Luann's car gets 21 miles per gallon. How many gallons of gasoline will Luann use to drive 189 miles?   [4–7]

7. John Silver made a withdrawal of $450 from his bank account. If there is $1845 left in the account, how much did he have in the bank before the withdrawal?

Solve.

8. At a recent tennis tournament, $\frac{3}{4}$ of the new balls were used. If 309 balls were used, how many new balls were there at the start of the tournament?   [4–8]

Self-Test answers and Extra Practice are at the back of the book.

Balancing Equations in Chemistry

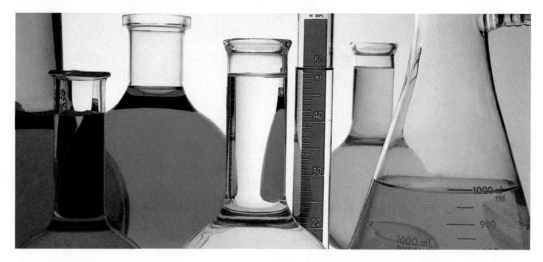

The basic chemical substances that make up the universe are called **elements.** Scientists often use standard symbols for the names of elements. Some of these symbols are given in the table below.

Element	Symbol	Element	Symbol	Element	Symbol
Hydrogen	H	Helium	He	Carbon	C
Nitrogen	N	Oxygen	O	Sodium	Na
Aluminum	Al	Sulfur	S	Potassium	K
Chlorine	Cl	Copper	Cu	Iron	Fe

The smallest particle of an element is called an **atom.** A pure substance made of atoms of two or more different elements is called a **compound.** In a compound the numbers of atoms of the elements always occur in a definite proportion. The formula for a compound shows this proportion. For example, the formula for water, H_2O, shows that in any sample of water there are twice as many hydrogen atoms as oxygen atoms.

In some elements and compounds, the atoms group together into **molecules.** The formula for a molecule is the same as the formula for the compound. The formula for oxygen is O_2 because a molecule of oxygen is made of two oxygen atoms. A molecule of water is made of two hydrogen atoms and one oxygen atom, so its formula is H_2O.

When compounds change chemically in a chemical reaction, we can describe this change by means of what chemists call an equation, although the equals sign is replaced by an arrow. An example of such a chemical equation is the following.

$$N_2 \quad + \quad 3\,H_2 \quad \longrightarrow \quad 2\,NH_3$$
nitrogen $\qquad$ hydrogen $\qquad\qquad$ ammonia

This equation indicates that a molecule of nitrogen (2 atoms) can combine with 3 molecules of hydrogen (2 atoms each) producing 2 molecules of ammonia.

Notice in the example that each side of the equation accounts for

$$\text{2 atoms of nitrogen: } N_2 \ldots \quad \longrightarrow \quad 2\,N \ldots$$

and $\qquad$ 6 atoms of hydrogen: $\ldots 3\,H_2 \longrightarrow 2 \ldots H_3$

A chemical equation in which the same number of atoms of each element appears on both sides is said to be **balanced.** What number should replace the _?_ in order to balance the following equation?

$$S \quad + \quad 2\,H_2SO_4 \longrightarrow \underline{\ ?\ } SO_2 \quad + \quad 2\,H_2O$$
sulfur $\qquad$ sulfuric $\qquad\qquad$ sulfur $\qquad\quad$ water
$\qquad\qquad$ acid $\qquad\qquad\qquad$ dioxide

To answer this question, let n represent the unknown number. Then by equating the number of oxygen atoms on each side, we have

$$2 \times 4 = (n \times 2) + (2 \times 1)$$
or $\qquad\qquad\qquad 8 = 2n + 2.$

Solving for n, we find that $n = 3$.

Replace each _?_ with a whole number to produce a balanced equation.

1. _?_ NO_2 $\qquad + \qquad$ H_2O $\quad \longrightarrow \quad$ $2\,HNO_3$ $\qquad + \qquad$ NO
$\quad$ nitric oxide $\qquad\qquad\qquad$ water $\qquad\qquad$ nitric acid $\qquad\qquad$ nitrous acid

2. $4\,FeS_2$ $\qquad + \qquad$ _?_ O_2 $\longrightarrow$ $2\,Fe_2O_3$ $\qquad + \qquad$ $8\,SO_2$
$\quad$ iron sulfide $\qquad\qquad\qquad$ oxygen $\qquad$ iron oxide $\qquad\qquad$ sulfur dioxide

3. $Al(OH)_3$ $\qquad + \qquad$ $3\,HCl$ $\longrightarrow$ $AlCl_3$ $\qquad + \qquad$ _?_ H_2O
$\quad$ aluminum $\qquad\qquad\qquad$ hydrochloric $\quad$ aluminum $\qquad\qquad$ water
$\quad$ hydroxide $\qquad\qquad\qquad$ acid $\qquad\qquad$ chloride

4. C_2H_5OH $\qquad + \qquad$ _?_ O_2 $\longrightarrow$ $2\,CO_2$ $\qquad + \qquad$ $3\,H_2O$
$\quad$ ethanol $\qquad\qquad\qquad\qquad$ oxygen $\qquad$ carbon dioxide $\qquad$ water

5. _?_ C_2H_6 $\qquad + \qquad$ _?_ O_2 $\longrightarrow$ $4\,CO_2$ $\qquad + \qquad$ $6\,H_2O$
$\quad$ ethane $\qquad\qquad\qquad\qquad$ oxygen $\qquad$ carbon dioxide $\qquad$ water

Chapter Review

Complete.

1. An equivalent equation for $2x - 4 = 16$ is $2x = \underline{\ ?\ }$. [4–1]

2. The solution to $5(11 - 3 + 12) = 2x$ is $\underline{\ ?\ }$.

3. To solve $4x = 82$, you would $\underline{\ ?\ }$ both sides by 4. [4–2]

4. The solution to $\frac{n}{9} = 27$ is $\underline{\ ?\ }$.

Write the letter of the correct answer.

5. Solve $\frac{4}{3}x = 60$.

    a. 45   **b.** 80   **c.** $60\frac{3}{4}$

6. Solve $\frac{n}{0.15} = 15$. [4–3]

    a. 1   **b.** 2.25   **c.** 22.5

7. Solve $\frac{3}{2}n - 5 = 70$.

    a. 40   **b.** $112\frac{1}{2}$ **c.** 50

8. Solve $\frac{n}{6} + 9 = 10.5$. [4–4]

    a. 9   **b.** 120   **c.** 96

9. Which expression represents the word phrase "the difference be- [4–5]
tween seven and a number n"?
    a. $n - 7$ **b.** $7 - n$ **c.** $7n - 7$ **d.** $7 + n$

10. Which equation represents the problem? [4–6]

    Luis bought 3 records on sale. The original cost of the records had
been \$29.85, but Luis paid only \$23.25 for all three. How much did
Luis save on each record?
    a. $29.85 + 3x = 23.25$ **b.** $23.25 - 3x = 29.85$ **c.** $29.85 - 3x = 23.25$

11. Write an equation for the following problem. [4–7]

    A rectangle has a perimeter of 84 cm. Find the length if the width is
15 cm.
    a. $2l + 2w = 84$ **b.** $2l + 30 = 84$ **c.** $2l + 15 = 84$ **d.** $2l = 99$

12. Use the five-step method to solve the following problem. [4–8]

    Tanya and Sara went biking. When they returned, they found that
they had gone 18 km in 0.75 h. What was their speed on the trip?
    a. 13.5 km/h   **b.** 32 km/h   **c.** 12 km/h   **d.** 24 km/h

Chapter Test

1-13

Use transformations to solve each equation.

1. $x - 18 = 11$ **2.** $3(7 - 2) + x = 19$ [4–1]

3. $9n = 1$ **4.** $\frac{n}{11} = 13$ **5.** $15n = 12$ [4–2]

6. $\frac{2}{3}x = 24$ **7.** $0.55x = 11$ **8.** $\frac{x}{1.2} = 8.6$ [4–3]

9. $4n - 16 = 32$ **10.** $\frac{3}{4}n + 18 = 51$ **11.** $30 - \frac{1}{2}n = 11$ [4–4]

Write an expression for each word phrase.

12. The product of a number n and twenty-one   [4–5]

13. Nine times the quotient of a number n and 3

Which equation represents the problem?

14. Toby Baylor wrote a check for $12 to pay a bill. Two days later he   [4–6]
deposited $20 in his checking account. If Toby had $88 in his account after these transactions, how much did he have originally?

     a. $20x - 12 = 88$ **b.** $x - 12 + 20 = 88$ **c.** $x - 88 = 12 + 20$

Write an equation for the following problem.

15. Annette Loo's car gets 23 miles per gallon. She is planning a trip to   [4–7]
San Diego. If Annette lives 345 miles from San Diego, how many gallons of gasoline will she use driving to San Diego?

Solve the following problem by the five-step method.

16. Bill and Roberta are shipping boxes to their new house. It costs $35   [4–8]
to ship each box and there is also a charge of $50 for the entire shipment. If the cost of shipping the boxes, including the $50 charge, comes to $610, how many boxes are being shipped?

Cumulative Review (Chapters 1–4)

Exercises

Evaluate the expression when $x = 2$, $y = 4$, and $z = 1$.

1. $x + y - z$

2. $6(x + y) - 5z$

3. $10y \div (3x + 2z)$

4. $-x - y$

5. $-y - (-3z)$

6. $y + 5z - (-2x)$

7. x^5

8. $3y^3$

9. y^x

Replace __?__ with $=$, $>$, or $<$ to make a true statement.

10. 31 __?__ 24

11. 206 __?__ 260

12. 581 __?__ 519

13. -4.68 __?__ 3.2

14. 0.6 __?__ -15.23

15. -8.99 __?__ -8.98

16. $\frac{1}{2}$ __?__ $\frac{4}{6}$

17. $-\frac{3}{7}$ __?__ $-\frac{4}{9}$

18. $\frac{11}{35}$ __?__ $-\frac{9}{40}$

What value of the variable makes the statement true?

19. $-6 + x = 2$

20. $x + 5 = -3$

21. $-11 + x = -31$

22. $-5.1 + x = -7.4$

23. $17.5 + x = -1$

24. $x + 28.3 = -4.7$

25. $3 - x = -2$

26. $x - 7 = -11$

27. $x - (-9) = -3$

Simplify.

28. $\frac{2}{3} + \left(-\frac{1}{6}\right)$

29. $-1\frac{1}{4} + \left(-2\frac{1}{3}\right)$

30. $\frac{5}{8} + (-6)$

31. $\frac{11}{8} - \frac{11}{4}$

32. $-2\frac{2}{3} - 1\frac{1}{5}$

33. $-11\frac{3}{4} - \left(-12\frac{9}{10}\right)$

34. $\frac{1}{7} \times \left(-\frac{1}{12}\right)$

35. $-12 \times 1\frac{3}{4}$

36. $-\frac{11}{16} \times \left(\frac{-9}{20}\right)$

37. $-11\frac{1}{9} \div 100$

38. $2\frac{1}{3} \div \left(-\frac{3}{7}\right)$

39. $-10\frac{1}{3} \div \left(-3\frac{1}{5}\right)$

Use transformations to solve each equation.

40. $y + 11 = 31$

41. $n - 8 = 12$

42. $29 = 5(6 - 3) + x$

43. $\frac{2}{3}x = 16$

44. $36 = 9y$

45. $-13n = 182$

46. $\frac{4}{3}t = -40$

47. $1.6c = 1.2$

48. $-1.5x = -22.5$

49. $4p - 7 = 37$

50. $\frac{1}{6}y - 7 = 14$

51. $\frac{-2}{3}n - 11 = -7$

Problems

Solve.

1. Calculator batteries are being sold at 2 for 99¢. How much will 6 batteries cost?

2. "My new camera cost a fortune," boasted Frank. "Mine cost twice as much as yours," returned Eddie. If together the two cameras cost $545.25, how much did Frank's camera cost?

3. A newspaper with a circulation of 1.1 million readers estimates $\frac{1}{5}$ of its readers have subscriptions. About how many readers have subscriptions?

4. Amos Ellingsworth earns $455 per week. About $\frac{1}{4}$ of his pay is deducted for taxes, insurance, and Social Security. To the nearest dollar, how much does Amos take home each week?

5. Sally Gray takes home $378.50 per week. She will get a $50 per week raise in her next weekly check. If Sally takes home $\frac{4}{5}$ of her raise, what will be her new take-home pay?

6. The population of Elmwood was 26,547 in 1950, 31,068 in 1960, 30,327 in 1970, and 29,598 in 1980. What was the total increase in population between 1950 and 1980?

7. The Carpenters make annual mortgage payments of $6430.56 and property tax payments of $1446.00. What are the combined monthly payments for mortgage and taxes?

8. Cormo Corporation stock sells for $13\frac{5}{8}$ dollars a share. If Lorraine has $327, how many shares can she buy?

9. At a recent job fair, there were $\frac{2}{3}$ as many inquiries about jobs in health care as in electronics. A reported 250 inquires were made about both fields. How many inquiries were made about health care?

5

Geometric Figures

The three fields shown in the center of the photograph are irrigated using the center-pivot irrigation system. Long arms, or booms, revolve around center pivots and distribute water over circular areas of land, such as those visible in the photograph. Although the booms miss the corners of the fields, traveling sprinklers would be much more expensive to use. The booms have the advantage of being able to control the amounts of water delivered with a minimum of labor.

Farmers have used irrigation for centuries, at least as far back as the Egyptians in 5000 B.C. Today we could not hope to feed the huge world population without the extension of water supplies by irrigation. According to a recent estimate, there are about 155,700,000 hectares of land under irrigation.

Career Note

The demand for a greater variety of farm products, for improved farming methods and machinery, and for more careful environmental planning has led to an increase in the demand for agricultural engineers. Manufacturers of farm equipment look for engineers to design systems and machinery. Engineers also participate in research, production, sales, and management.

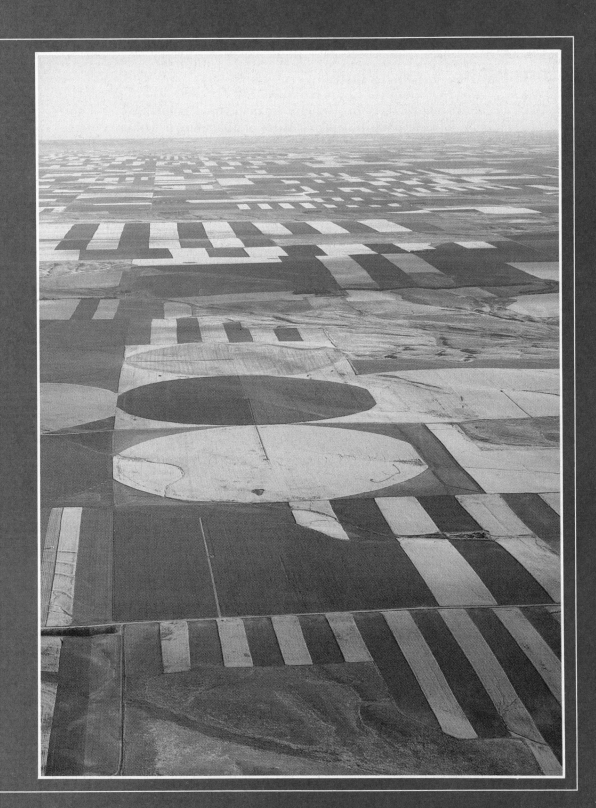

5-1 Points, Lines, Planes

All of the figures that we study in geometry are made up of **points.** We usually picture a single point by making a dot and labeling it with a capital letter.

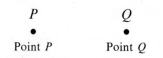

Point *P*   Point *Q*

Among the most important geometric figures that we study are straight lines, or simply **lines.** You probably know this important fact about lines:

> Two points determine exactly one line.

This means that through two points *P* and *Q* we can draw one line, and only one line, which we denote by $\overleftrightarrow{PQ}$ (or $\overleftrightarrow{QP}$).

Line *PQ*: $\overleftrightarrow{PQ}$, or $\overleftrightarrow{QP}$

Notice the use of arrowheads to show that a line extends without end in either direction.

Three points may or may not lie on the same line. Three or more points that do lie on the same line are called **collinear.** Points not on the same line are called **noncollinear.**

If we take a point *P* on a line and all the points on the line that lie on one side of *P*, we have a **ray** with **endpoint** *P*. We name a ray by naming first its endpoint and then any other point on it.

Ray *PQ*: $\overrightarrow{PQ}$ Ray *BA*: $\overrightarrow{BA}$

It is important to remember that the endpoint is always named first. $\overrightarrow{AB}$ is *not* the same ray as $\overrightarrow{BA}$.

If we take two points *P* and *Q* on a line and all the points that lie between *P* and *Q*, we have a **segment** denoted by $\overline{PQ}$ (or $\overline{QP}$). The points *P* and *Q* are called the **endpoints** of $\overline{PQ}$.

Segment *PQ*: $\overline{PQ}$, or $\overline{QP}$

EXAMPLE 1   Name (a) one line, (b) two rays, (c) three segments, (d) three collinear points, and (e) three noncollinear points in the given diagram. (Various answers are possible.)

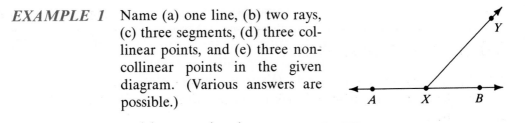

Solution   **a.** $\overleftrightarrow{AB}$ **b.** $\overrightarrow{XY}$, $\overrightarrow{AB}$ **c.** $\overline{AX}$, $\overline{XB}$, $\overline{XY}$ **d.** A, X, B **e.** A, Y, B

Just as two points determine a line, three noncollinear points in space determine a flat surface called a **plane.** We can name a plane by naming any three noncollinear points on it. Because a plane extends without limit in all directions of the surface, we can show only part of it, as in the figure below.

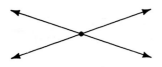

Plane *ABC*

Lines in the same plane that do not intersect are called **parallel lines.** Two segments or rays are parallel if they are parts of parallel lines. "$\overleftrightarrow{AB}$ is parallel to $\overleftrightarrow{CD}$" may be written as $\overleftrightarrow{AB} \parallel \overleftrightarrow{CD}$.

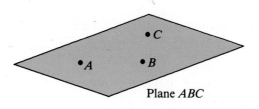

Intersecting lines
intersect in a point.

Parallel lines
do not intersect.

Planes that do not intersect are called **parallel planes.**

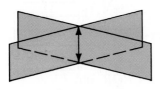

Intersecting planes
intersect in a line.

Parallel planes
do not intersect.

EXAMPLE 2   Use the box to name (a) two parallel lines, (b) two parallel planes, (c) two intersecting lines, (d) two intersecting planes, and (e) two nonparallel lines that do not intersect. (Various answers are possible.)

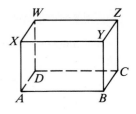

Solution

a. $\overleftrightarrow{AX}$ and $\overleftrightarrow{BY}$ b. plane ABC and plane XYZ

c. $\overleftrightarrow{AB}$ and $\overleftrightarrow{AX}$ d. plane ABC and plane ABY

e. $\overleftrightarrow{AD}$ and $\overleftrightarrow{BY}$

Two nonparallel lines that do not intersect, such as $\overleftrightarrow{AD}$ and $\overleftrightarrow{BY}$ in Example 2, are called **skew lines.**

Class Exercises

Tell how many endpoints each figure has.

1. a segment   **2.** a line   **3.** a plane   **4.** a ray

Exercises 5–9 refer to the diagram at the right in which $\overleftrightarrow{AB}$ and $\overleftrightarrow{CD}$ are parallel lines.

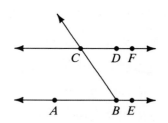

5. Name three collinear points.

6. Name two parallel rays.

7. Name two parallel segments.

8. Name two segments that are not parallel.

9. Name two rays that are not parallel.

Exercises 10–14 refer to the box at the right. Classify each pair of planes as parallel or intersecting. If the planes are intersecting, name the line of intersection.

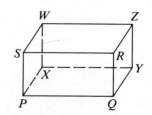

10. planes QRY and WSP **11.** planes PQR and PSW

12. planes SPW and XYQ **13.** planes PQR and WXY

14. In the box are $\overleftrightarrow{WX}$ and $\overleftrightarrow{RS}$ parallel, intersecting, or skew?

Written Exercises

In Exercises 1–4, give another name for the indicated figure.

A **1.** $\overline{XY}$ X ●————————————● Y

2. $\overleftrightarrow{BC}$ ◄——●——●————————●——► A B C

3. $\overrightarrow{PR}$ P ●——●————————●——► Q   R

4. $\overrightarrow{VU}$ ◄————●————————————●——● T   U V

5. Name one line and three rays in the diagram below.

6. Name three rays and three segments in the diagram below.

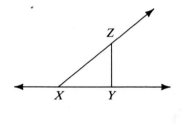

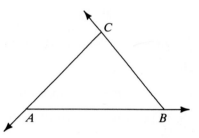

Exercises 7–20 refer to the diagram at the right. $\overleftrightarrow{PQ}$ **and** $\overleftrightarrow{ST}$ **are parallel. (There may be several correct answers to each exercise.)**

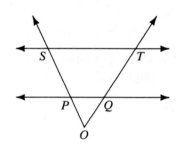

7. Name three collinear points.

8. Name three noncollinear points.

9. Name three segments that intersect at P.

10. Name two parallel rays.

11. Name two parallel segments.

12. Name two nonparallel segments that do not intersect.

13. Name two nonparallel rays that do not intersect.

14. Name two segments that intersect in exactly one point.

15. Name two rays that intersect in exactly one point.

16. Name a ray that is contained in $\overrightarrow{OT}$.

17. Name a ray that contains $\overline{SP}$.

18. Name the segment that is in $\overrightarrow{PQ}$ and $\overrightarrow{QP}$.

19. Name four segments that contain O.

20. Name two rays that intersect in more than one point.

Exercises 21–24 refer to the box at the right. (There may be several correct answers to each exercise.)

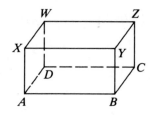

21. Name two intersecting lines and their point of intersection.

22. Name two intersecting planes and their line of intersection.

23. Name two parallel lines and the plane that contains them both.

24. Name two skew lines.

In Exercises 25–32, tell whether the statement is true or false.

B **25.** Two lines cannot intersect in more than one point.

26. Two rays cannot intersect in more than one point.

27. Two segments cannot intersect in more than one point.

28. If two rays are parallel, they do not intersect.

29. If two rays do not intersect, they are parallel.

30. If two points of a segment are contained in a line, then the whole segment is contained in the line.

31. If two points of a ray are contained in a line, then the whole ray is contained in the line.

32. If two points of a segment are contained in a ray, then the whole segment is contained in the ray.

C **33.** Draw $\overleftrightarrow{AB}$ and a point P not on $\overleftrightarrow{AB}$. Now draw a line through P parallel to $\overleftrightarrow{AB}$. How many such lines can be drawn?

34. Draw four points A, B, C, and D so that $\overline{AB}$ is parallel to $\overline{CD}$ and $\overline{AD}$ is parallel to $\overline{BC}$. Do you think that $\overline{AC}$ and $\overline{BD}$ must intersect?

35. We know that two points determine a line. Explain what we mean by saying that two nonparallel lines in a plane determine a point.

Review Exercises

Round to the nearest tenth.

1. 2.87　　　　**2.** 6.32　　　　**3.** 4.56　　　　**4.** 7.08

5. 2.98　　　　**6.** 11.753　　　　**7.** 9.347　　　　**8.** 6.482

5-2 Measuring Segments

In Washington, D.C., Jill estimated the length of a jet to be about 165 feet. When the plane landed in Paris, Jacques guessed the jet's length to be about 50 meters. Although the numbers 165 and 50 are quite different, the two estimates are about the same. This is so because of the difference in the units of measurement used.

The metric system of measurement uses the **meter (m)** as its basic unit of length. For smaller measurements we divide the meter into 100 equal parts called **centimeters (cm).**

We can measure a length to the nearest centimeter by using a ruler marked off in centimeters, as illustrated below.

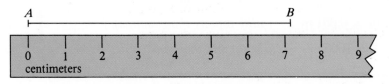

We see that the length of $\overline{AB}$ is closer to 7 cm than to 8 cm. The length of $\overline{AB}$ is written AB. The symbol $\approx$ means *is approximately equal to.* Therefore, $AB \approx 7$ cm.

The drawing at the right shows that the length of $\overline{XY}$ is about 3 cm.

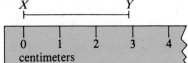

$$XY \approx 3 \text{ cm}$$

Measurements made with small units are more precise than those made with larger units. We can measure lengths more precisely by using a ruler on which each centimeter has been divided into ten equal parts called **millimeters (mm).** We see that to the nearest millimeter the length of $\overline{AB}$ is 73 mm.

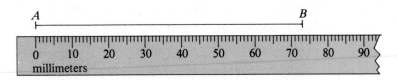

The drawing at the right shows that the length of $\overline{XY}$ is 28 mm and the lengths of $\overline{XM}$ and $\overline{MY}$ are 14 mm each. A point, such as M, that divides a segment into two other segments of equal length is called the **midpoint** of the segment. Thus, M is the midpoint of $\overline{XY}$. Segments of equal length are called **congruent segments.** The symbol $\cong$ means *is congruent to.* Since $XM = MY$, $\overline{XM} \cong \overline{MY}$.

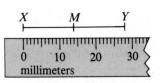

Usually centimeters and millimeters are marked on the same ruler, as shown below.

To measure longer lengths, such as distances between cities, we use **kilometers (km).** A kilometer is 1000 meters.

1 m = 100 cm = 1000 mm   1 cm = 10 mm

1 cm = 0.01 m   (*centi* means *hundredths*)

1 mm = 0.001 m   (*milli* means *thousandths*)

1 km = 1000 m   (*kilo* means *thousand*)

Never mix metric units of length. For example, do not write 3 m 18 cm; write 3.18 m or 318 cm instead.

Class Exercises

Copy and complete these tables.

	1.	**2.**	**3.**	**4.**
Number of meters	4	?	?	?
Number of centimeters	?	60	52	?
Number of millimeters	?	?	?	36

	5.	**6.**	**7.**	**8.**
Number of meters	3500	?	475	?
Number of kilometers	?	4.2	?	0.034

9. Estimate the length and width of your desk top to the nearest centimeter.

10. Estimate the length and width of this book to the nearest centimeter.

11. Estimate the height of the classroom door to the nearest centimeter.

12. Estimate your height to the nearest centimeter.

13. Estimate the thickness of your pencil to the nearest millimeter.

14. Estimate the distance from your home to school in meters and in kilometers.

In Exercises 15 and 16, M is the midpoint of $\overline{AB}$. Draw a sketch to help you complete these sentences.

15. If $AB = 18$ cm, then $AM = \underline{\ ?\ }$ cm and $MB = \underline{\ ?\ }$ cm.

16. If $AM = 4$ mm, then $MB = \underline{\ ?\ }$ mm and $AB = \underline{\ ?\ }$ mm.

In Exercises 17 and 18, P is a point of $\overline{XY}$. Draw a sketch to help you complete these sentences.

17. If $XP = YP$, then $\overline{XP}$ is $\underline{\ ?\ }$ to $\overline{YP}$.

18. If $\overline{XP} \cong \overline{YP}$, then P is the $\underline{\ ?\ }$ of $\overline{XY}$.

Written Exercises

Measure each segment (a) to the nearest centimeter and (b) to the nearest millimeter. (If you do not have a metric ruler, mark each segment on the edge of a piece of paper and use the ruler pictured earlier.)

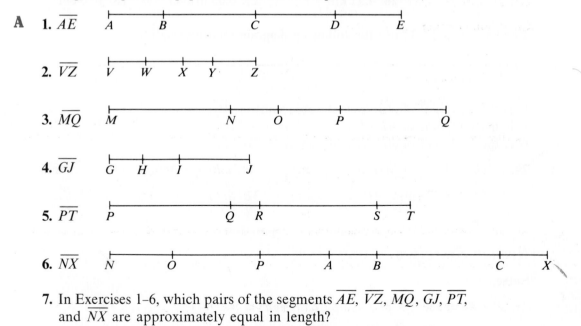

A **1.** $\overline{AE}$

2. $\overline{VZ}$

3. $\overline{MQ}$

4. $\overline{GJ}$

5. $\overline{PT}$

6. $\overline{NX}$

7. In Exercises 1–6, which pairs of the segments $\overline{AE}$, $\overline{VZ}$, $\overline{MQ}$, $\overline{GJ}$, $\overline{PT}$, and $\overline{NX}$ are approximately equal in length?

8. In Exercises 1–6, name the midpoints of $\overline{AE}$, $\overline{VZ}$, $\overline{MQ}$, $\overline{GJ}$, $\overline{PT}$, and $\overline{NX}$ given that the midpoint is named in each diagram.

Copy and complete these tables.

	9.	10.	11.	12.	13.	14.
Number of meters	4.5	1.63	?	?	?	?
Number of centimeters	?	?	250	82.6	?	?
Number of millimeters	?	?	?	?	60,000	368

	15.	16.	17.	18.	19.	20.
Number of meters	2000	20	625	?	?	?
Number of kilometers	?	?	?	3	4.5	0.25

Small units are often used to avoid decimals. However, it is sometimes easier to think about lengths given in meters. Change the following dimensions to meters.

B **21.** 374 cm by 520 cm   **22.** 425 cm by 650 cm

23. 4675 mm by 7050 mm   **24.** 5925 mm by 8275 mm

Rewrite each measurement using a unit that will avoid decimals.

25. 2.7 cm   **26.** 4.32 km   **27.** 0.65 m   **28.** 10.6 cm

For Exercises 29–32 use the following diagram and information.

C is the midpoint of $\overline{AB}$; D is the midpoint of $\overline{AC}$;
E is the midpoint of $\overline{AD}$; F is the midpoint of $\overline{AE}$;
G is the midpoint of $\overline{AF}$; H is the midpoint of $\overline{AG}$.

C **29.** If $AB = 140$ mm, $AH = \underline{\ ?\ }$ mm.   **30.** If $BC = 70$ mm, $AF = \underline{\ ?\ }$ mm.

31. If $AG = 4.375$ mm, $AD = \underline{\ ?\ }$ mm.   **32.** If $FE = 8.75$ mm, $DC = \underline{\ ?\ }$ mm.

Review Exercises

Solve.

1. $x + 90 = 180$ **2.** $x + 20 = 90$ **3.** $x + 35 = 75$

4. $100 - x = 45$ **5.** $180 - x = 40$ **6.** $90 - x = 30$

7. $75 + x = 180$ **8.** $180 - x = 115$ **9.** $25 + x = 90$

5-3 Angles and Angle Measure

An **angle** is a figure formed by two rays with the same endpoint. The common endpoint is called the **vertex,** and the rays are called the **sides.**

We may name an angle by giving its vertex letter if this is the only angle with that vertex, or by listing letters for points on the two sides with the vertex letter in the middle. We use the symbol ∠ for *angle*. The diagram at the right shows several ways of naming an angle.

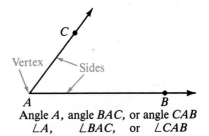

Angle *A*, angle *BAC*, or angle *CAB*
∠*A*,   ∠*BAC*,   or   ∠*CAB*

To measure segments we used a ruler marked off in unit lengths. To measure angles, we use a **protractor** that is marked off in units of angle measure, called **degrees.** To use a protractor, place its center point at the vertex of the angle to be measured and one of its zero points on a side. In the drawing at the left below we use the outer scale and read the measure of ∠*E* to be 60 degrees (60°). We write m ∠*E* = 60°.

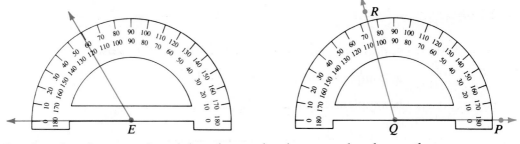

In the drawing on the right above the inner scale shows that m∠*PQR* = 105°.

We often label angles with their measures, as shown in the figures. Since ∠*A* and ∠*B* have equal measures we can write m∠*A* = m∠*B*. We say that ∠*A* and ∠*B* are **congruent angles** and we write ∠*A* ≅ ∠*B*.

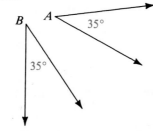

If two lines intersect so that the angles they form are all congruent, the lines are **perpendicular.** We use the symbol ⊥ to mean *is perpendicular to.* In the figure $\overline{WY} \perp \overline{XZ}$.

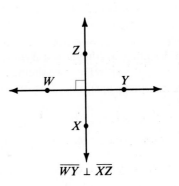

$\overline{WY} \perp \overline{XZ}$

Angles formed by perpendicular lines each have measure 90°. A 90° angle is called a **right angle.** A small square is often used to indicate a right angle in a diagram.

An **acute angle** is an angle with measure less than 90°. An **obtuse angle** has measure between 90° and 180°.

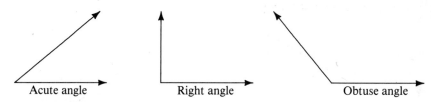

Acute angle   Right angle   Obtuse angle

Two angles are **complementary** if the sum of their measures is 90°. Two angles are **supplementary** if the sum of their measures is 180°.

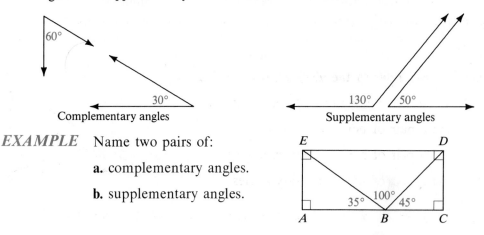

Complementary angles   Supplementary angles

EXAMPLE   Name two pairs of:

   a. complementary angles.

   b. supplementary angles.

Solution   **a.** Since $\angle AEB$ and $\angle BED$ form a right angle, they are complementary. Similarly, $\angle CDB$ and $\angle BDE$ are complementary.

   b. Since the sum of $\mathrm{m}\angle ABE$ and $\mathrm{m}\angle EBC$ is 180°, they are supplementary. Similarly, $\angle ABD$ and $\angle DBC$ are supplementary.

Although the sides of angles are rays, we often show the sides as segments, as in the figure for the example.

Reading Mathematics: *Symbols*

When you read a mathematical sentence, be sure to give each symbol its complete meaning. For example:

$\overleftrightarrow{AB} \perp \overleftrightarrow{CD}$ is read as *line AB is perpendicular to line CD.*

$\overline{AB} \cong \overline{CD}$ is read as *segment AB is congruent to segment CD.*

$AB \approx 6$ cm is read as *the length of $\overline{AB}$ is approximately equal to six centimeters.*

$\mathrm{m}\angle A = 10°$ is read as *the measure of angle A is equal to ten degrees.*

Class Exercises

1. If an angle is named ∠EFG, its vertex is __?__.

2. If an angle is named ∠GEF, its vertex is __?__.

Give three names for each angle.

3.

4.

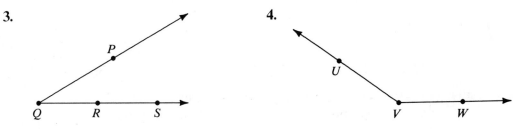

5. Use a protractor to find the measures of the angles in Exercises 3 and 4.

Exercises 6–9 refer to the diagram at the right.

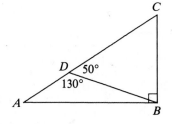

6. Name five acute angles and one obtuse angle.

7. Name a pair of perpendicular segments.

8. Name a pair of complementary angles.

9. Name a pair of supplementary angles.

State the measures of the complement and supplement of each angle.

10. m∠F = 70°   11. m∠G = 15°   12. m∠H = 45°   13. m∠J = 60°

Written Exercises

Use a protractor to draw an angle having the given measure.

A   1. 75°   2. 20°   3. 120°   4. 155°

Use a protractor to measure the given angle. State whether the angle is acute or obtuse.

5.

6.

Measure the given angle. Is the angle acute or obtuse?

7.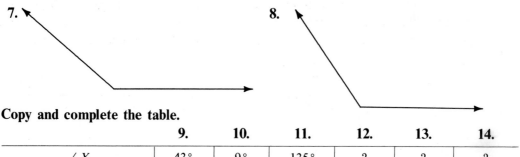

8.

Copy and complete the table.

	9.	10.	11.	12.	13.	14.
∠X	43°	9°	135°	?	?	?
Complement of ∠X	?	?	✕	12°	71°	?
Supplement of ∠X	?	?	?	?	?	150°

Use a protractor to draw an angle congruent to the angle in each given exercise.

15. Exercise 5   16. Exercise 6   17. Exercise 7   18. Exercise 8

Exercises 19–22 refer to the diagram at the right.

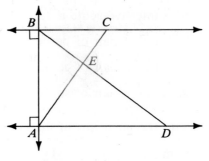

19. Name two pairs of perpendicular lines.

20. Name two pairs of complementary angles.

21. Name two pairs of supplementary angles.

22. What is the sum of the measures of the four angles having vertex *E*?

Angles that share a common vertex and a common side, but with no common points in their interiors, are called *adjacent angles*.

B 23. Draw two adjacent complementary angles, one of which has measure 65°.

24. Draw two adjacent supplementary angles, one of which has measure 105°.

25. Draw two congruent adjacent supplementary angles. What is the measure of each?

26. Draw two congruent adjacent complementary angles. What is the measure of each?

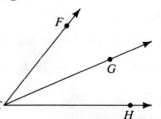

∠ *FEG* is adjacent to ∠ *GEH*
∠ *FEG* is *not* adjacent to ∠ *FEH*

True or false?

27. The supplement of an obtuse angle is acute.

28. The complement of an acute angle is obtuse.

C **29.** Measure the angles labeled 1, 2, 3, and 4. What general fact do your results suggest about angles formed by intersecting lines?

30. Measure the angles labeled 1, 2, 3, and 4. What general facts do your results suggest about two parallel lines intersected by a third line?

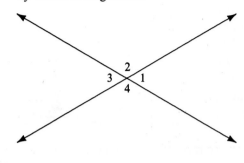

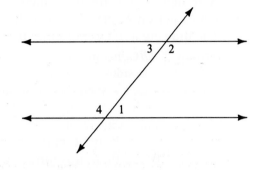

Self-Test A

Draw a sketch to illustrate each of the following.

1. $\overline{CD}$ **2.** $\overleftrightarrow{AX}$ **3.** $\overrightarrow{RS}$ [5–1]

Exercises 4–7 refer to the diagram below.

4. Name two parallel lines.

5. Name two parallel planes.

6. Name two intersecting lines.

7. Name two intersecting planes.

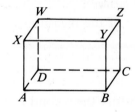

Complete each statement.

8. 4000 m = __?__ km   **9.** 87 cm = __?__ m   [5–2]

10. 785 mm = __?__ m   **11.** 109 mm = __?__ cm

12. If M is the midpoint of $\overline{AB}$, then $AM =$ __?__ and $\overline{AM} \cong$ __?__.

13. A right angle has measure __?__.   [5–3]

14. Two angles with the same measures are __?__.

15. ⊥ is the symbol for __?__.

16. A 37° angle is a(n) __?__ angle.

17. The complement of a 42° angle has measure __?__°.

18. The supplement of a 107° angle has measure __?__°.

Self-Test answers and Extra Practice are at the back of the book.

5-4 Triangles

A **triangle** is the figure formed when three points not on a line are joined by segments. The drawing at the right shows triangle *ABC*, written $\triangle ABC$, having the segments $\overline{AB}$, $\overline{BC}$, and $\overline{CA}$ as its **sides**. Each of the points *A*, *B*, and *C* is called a **vertex** (plural: *vertices*) of $\triangle ABC$. Each of the angles $\angle A$, $\angle B$, and $\angle C$ is called an **angle** of $\triangle ABC$.

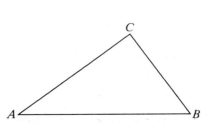

Suppose *A*, *B*, and *C* in the triangle above represent three points on a map. Do you think it is farther to travel from *A* to *B* and then to *C* or to travel directly from *A* to *C*? Measure to check. This illustrates the first fact about triangles stated below.

In any triangle:

1. The sum of the lengths of any two sides is greater than the length of the third side.

2. The sum of the measures of the angles is 180°.

You can verify the second fact by tearing off the corners of any paper triangle and fitting them together as shown at the right.

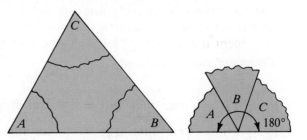

EXAMPLE 1   One angle of a triangle measures 40° and the other two angles have equal measures. Find the measures of the congruent angles.

Solution   The sum of the measures of the angles of a triangle is 180°. The sum of the measures of the congruent angles must be 180° − 40°, or 140°. Therefore each of the two congruent angles has measure 70°.

Problem Solving Reminder

Some problems do not give enough information. Sometimes you must *supply previously learned facts*. In the example above, you need to supply the additional information about the sum of the measures of the angles of a triangle.

There are several ways to name triangles. One way is by angles.

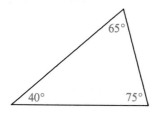

Acute Triangle
Three acute angles

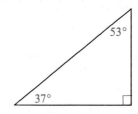

Right Triangle
One right angle

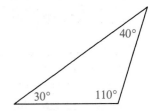

Obtuse Triangle
One obtuse angle

Triangles can also be classified by their sides.

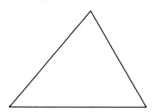

Scalene Triangle
No two sides
congruent

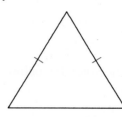

Isosceles Triangle
At least two sides
congruent

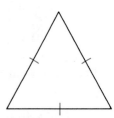

Equilateral Triangle
All three sides
congruent

As you might expect, the longest side of a triangle is opposite the largest angle, and the shortest side is opposite the smallest angle. Two angles are congruent if and only if the sides opposite them are congruent.

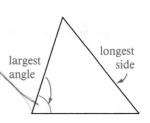

EXAMPLE 2   Classify each triangle by sides and by angles.

a.

b.

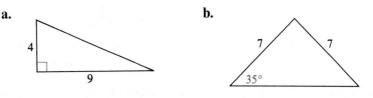

Solution

a. No two sides are congruent; the triangle is scalene.
There is one right angle; the triangle is a right triangle.
Scalene right triangle

b. Two sides are congruent; the triangle is isosceles.
The angles opposite the congruent sides are congruent; thus, the third angle has a measure of 110°; the triangle is obtuse.
Isosceles obtuse triangle

Class Exercises

How do you know, without measuring, that these triangles are labeled incorrectly?

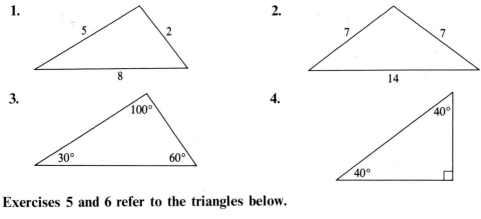

1. triangle with sides 5, 2, 8

2. triangle with sides 7, 7, 14

3. triangle with angles 100°, 30°, 60°

4. triangle with angles 40°, 40°, and a right angle

Exercises 5 and 6 refer to the triangles below.

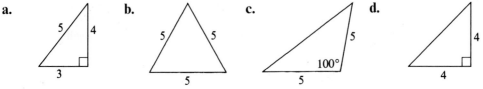

a. right triangle with sides 5, 4, 3

b. triangle with sides 5, 5, 5

c. triangle with side 5, angle 100°, side 5

d. right triangle with sides 4, 4

5. Classify each triangle by sides.

6. Classify each triangle by angles.

7. Explain how you know that a triangle with two congruent angles is isosceles.

8. Explain how you know that a triangle with three congruent angles is equilateral.

Exercises 9–13 refer to the diagram at the right.

9. What segment is a common side of △ADC and △BCD?

10. What segment is a common side of △ABC and △BCD?

11. What angle is common to △ABC and △CAD?

12. Name two right triangles.

13. Name an obtuse triangle.

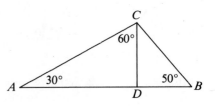

Written Exercises

The measures of two angles of a triangle are given. Find the measure of the third angle.

A   **1.** 40°, 60°   **2.** 15°, 105°   **3.** 35°, 55°   **4.** 160°, 10°

Classify each triangle by its sides.

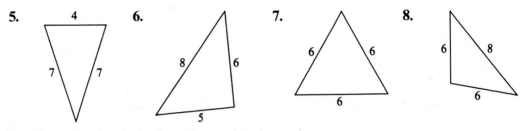

5.   **6.**   **7.**   **8.**

Classify each triangle by its sides and by its angles.

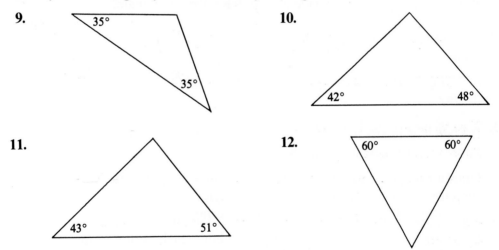

9.   **10.**

11.   **12.**

Exercises 13–16 refer to the diagram at the right.

13. Name three right triangles.

14. Name an isosceles triangle.

15. Name an acute scalene triangle.

16. Name an obtuse triangle.

17. Use a ruler and a protractor to draw (a) a scalene acute triangle and (b) an isosceles obtuse triangle.

18. Use a ruler and a protractor to draw (a) a scalene obtuse triangle and (b) an isosceles acute triangle.

B **19.** What measures do the angles of an equilateral triangle have?

20. One of the congruent angles of an isosceles triangle has measure 40°. What measures do the other angles have?

21. One of the acute angles of a right triangle measures 75°. What measure does the other acute angle have?

22. What measures do the angles of an isosceles right triangle have?

23. An isosceles triangle has a 96° angle. What are the measures of its other angles?

24. An isosceles triangle has a 60° angle. What are the measures of its other angles?

25. One acute angle of a right triangle is 45°. What relationship, if any, is there between the two shorter sides?

26. Why is it not possible to have an equilateral right triangle?

C **27.** In $\triangle ABC$, $AB = 8$ and $BC = 5$. Then (a) $AC < \underline{\ ?\ }$, and (b) $AC > \underline{\ ?\ }$.

28. In $\triangle PQR$, $PR = 10$ and $RQ = 7$. Then (a) $PQ < \underline{\ ?\ }$, and (b) $PQ > \underline{\ ?\ }$.

29. Explain why in any triangle the difference of the lengths of any two sides cannot be greater than the length of the third side.

30. Draw a triangle. Draw rays that divide each of its angles into two congruent angles. Do this for several triangles of different shapes. What seems always to be true of the three rays?

31. Draw a triangle. Then draw segments joining each vertex to the midpoint of the opposite side. (These segments are called **medians** of the triangle.) Do this for several triangles of different shapes. What seems always to be true?

Review Exercises

Add.

1. $3.75 + 4.92 + 6.41$

2. $7.83 + 6.91 + 5.29$

3. $8.36 + 4.95 + 2.21$

4. $5.3 + 6.21 + 7.3$

5. $8.02 + 5.1 + 7.21$

6. $3.07 + 4 + 5.93$

7. $11.27 + 6.513 + 4.09$

8. $10.03 + 5.7 + 4.93$

9. $12.004 + 4.9 + 7.864$

5-5 Polygons

A **polygon** is a closed figure formed by joining segments (**sides** of the polygon) at their endpoints (**vertices** of the polygon). We name polygons according to the number of sides they have.

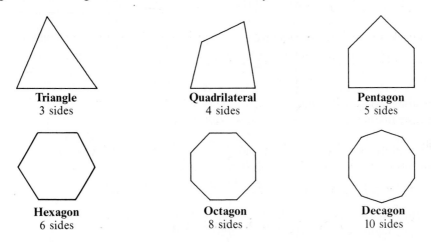

Triangle	**Quadrilateral**	**Pentagon**
3 sides	4 sides	5 sides
Hexagon	**Octagon**	**Decagon**
6 sides	8 sides	10 sides

A polygon is **regular** if all its sides are congruent and all its angles are congruent. As drawn above, the hexagon, the octagon, and the decagon are regular while the triangle, the quadrilateral, and the pentagon are not.

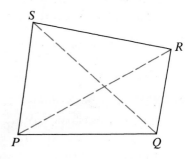

To name a polygon, we name its consecutive vertices in order. The quadrilateral shown at the right may be named quadrilateral *PQRS*.

A **diagonal** of a polygon is a segment joining two nonconsecutive vertices. Thus, $\overline{PR}$ and $\overline{QS}$ are the diagonals of quadrilateral *PQRS*.

Certain quadrilaterals have special names.

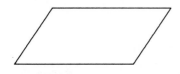

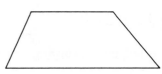

A **parallelogram** has its opposite sides parallel and congruent.

A **trapezoid** has just one pair of parallel sides.

Certain parallelograms also have special names.

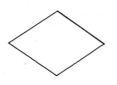

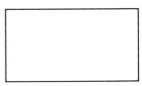

A **rhombus** has all its sides congruent.

A **square** has congruent sides and congruent angles.

A **rectangle** has all its angles congruent.

Reading Mathematics: *Vocabulary*
Many terms in mathematics have definitions with more than one condition. Be certain to read and learn the full definition. For example, a polygon is regular if (1) all its sides are congruent and (2) all its angles are congruent. Because the rhombus shown above does not meet condition 2, it is not a regular polygon. The square meets both conditions, so it is regular.

The **perimeter** of a figure is the distance around it. Thus, the perimeter of a polygon is the sum of the lengths of its sides.

EXAMPLE Find the perimeter of each polygon.

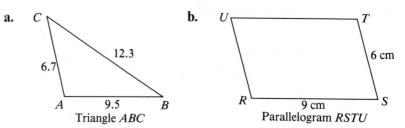

a.
Triangle *ABC*

b.
Parallelogram *RSTU*

Solution **a.** Perimeter = 9.5 + 12.3 + 6.7 = 28.5

b. Because opposite sides of a parallelogram are congruent, the unlabeled sides have lengths 9 cm and 6 cm. Therefore:
Perimeter = (9 + 6 + 9 + 6) cm = 30 cm

Class Exercises

Name each polygon according to the number of sides.

1.

2.

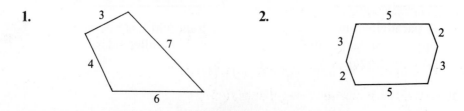

Name each polygon according to the number of sides.

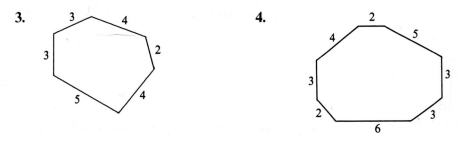

3.

4.

5-8. Find the perimeter of each polygon in Exercises 1-4.

9-12. State the number of diagonals that can be drawn from any one vertex of each figure in Exercises 1-4.

Give the most special name for each quadrilateral.

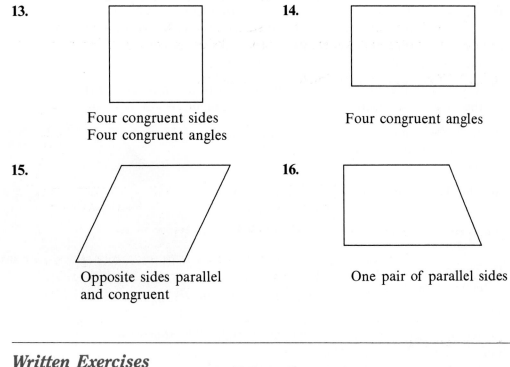

13.

Four congruent sides
Four congruent angles

14.

Four congruent angles

15.

Opposite sides parallel
and congruent

16.

One pair of parallel sides

Written Exercises

Name the polygon having the given number of sides.

A **1.** 5 **2.** 4 **3.** 6 **4.** 10 **5.** 3 **6.** 8

7. What is another name for a regular quadrilateral?

8. What is another name for a regular triangle?

Find the perimeter of each pentagon.

9.

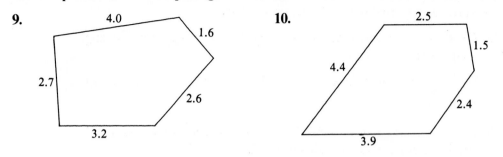

4.0
1.6
2.7
2.6
3.2

10.

2.5
1.5
4.4
2.4
3.9

Find the perimeter of a regular polygon whose sides have the given length.

11. Hexagon, 52 cm

12. Pentagon, 43 mm

13. Triangle, 24.2 mm

14. Quadrilateral, 16.5 m

15. Decagon, 135.6 m

16. Octagon, 4.25 m

17. The sum of the measures of the angles of a pentagon is 540°. Find the measure of each angle of a regular pentagon.

18. The sum of the measures of the angles of a hexagon is 720°. Find the measure of each angle of a regular hexagon.

19. A STOP sign is a regular octagon 32 cm on a side. Express its perimeter in meters.

20. The Pentagon building in Washington, D.C., is in the form of a regular pentagon 276 m on a side. Express its perimeter in kilometers.

21. The perimeter of a regular pentagon is 60 m. How long is each side?

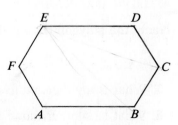

Exercises 22–24 refer to the hexagon at the right. The shorter sides are half as long as the longer sides.

22. Each shorter side is 3.2 cm long. What is the perimeter?

23. How many diagonals can be drawn from vertex *A*?

B 24. How many diagonals are there in all?

E   *D*
F   *C*
A   *B*

186 *Chapter 5*

Use a protractor and a ruler for Exercises 25 and 26. The sum of the measures of the angles of a hexagon is 720°.

25. Draw a hexagon that is not regular, but has all its angles congruent.

26. Draw a hexagon that is not regular, but has all its sides congruent.

27. In the diagram below, $ABDE$ is a rhombus and $\angle DBC \cong \angle DCB$. Find the perimeter of trapezoid $ACDE$.

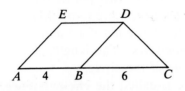

For Exercises 28 and 29 draw several polygons with different numbers of sides. Pick a vertex and draw all the diagonals from this vertex.

28. Count the number of triangles formed by the diagonals. How does the number of triangles compare to the number of sides of each polygon?

29. If the sum of the measures of the angles of the triangles formed equals the sum of the measures of the angles of the polygon, find the sum of the measures of the angles of the following.
   a. quadrilateral   **b.** decagon   **c.** trapezoid   **d.** octagon

C **30.** Write a general formula for the sum of the measures of the angles of any polygon with n sides. (*Hint:* See Exercises 28 and 29.)

31. Every pentagon has the same number of diagonals. How many? (*Hint:* First decide how many diagonals can be drawn from one vertex.)

32. Every octagon has the same number of diagonals. How many? (See the hint for Exercise 31.)

Review Exercises

Evaluate if $a = 7$, $b = 3.2$, and $c = 5.45$.

1. ab **2.** ac **3.** a^2 **4.** $15b$

5. $2c$ **6.** $2bc$ **7.** $2ab$ **8.** abc

5-6 Circles

A **circle** is the set of all points in a plane at a given distance from a given point O called the **center.** The drawing at the right shows how to use a **compass** to draw a circle with center O.

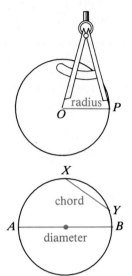

A segment, such as $\overline{OP}$, joining the center to a point on the circle is called a **radius** (plural: *radii*) of the circle. All radii of a given circle have the same length, and this length is called **the radius** of the circle.

A segment, such as $\overline{XY}$, joining two points on a circle is called a **chord,** and a chord passing through the center is a **diameter** of the circle. The ends of a diameter divide the circle into two **semicircles.** The length of a diameter is called **the diameter** of the circle.

The perimeter of a circle is called the **circumference.** The quotient

$$\text{circumference} \div \text{diameter}$$

can be shown to be the same for all circles, regardless of their size. This quotient is denoted by the Greek letter π (pronounced "pie"). No decimal gives π exactly, but a fairly good approximation is 3.14.

If we denote the circumference by C and the diameter by d, we can write

$$C \div d = \pi.$$

This formula can be put into several useful forms.

Formulas

Let C = circumference, d = diameter, and r = radius ($d = 2r$). Then:

$$C = \pi d$$
$$C = 2\pi r$$

EXAMPLE 1 The diameter of a circle is 6 cm. Find the circumference.

Solution We are given d and asked to find C. We use the formula $C = \pi d$.

$$C = \pi d$$
$$C \approx 3.14 \times 6 = 18.84$$
$$C \approx 18.8 \text{ cm, or } 188 \text{ mm}$$

When using the approximation $\pi \approx 3.14$, give your answer to only three digits (as in Example 1) because the approximation is good only to three digits. That is, we round to the place occupied by the third digit from the left.

EXAMPLE 2 The circumference of a circle is 20. Find the radius.

Solution To find the radius, use the formula $C = 2\pi r$.

$$C = 2\pi r$$
$$20 \approx (2 \times 3.14)r$$
$$20 \approx 6.28r$$
$$\frac{20}{6.28} \approx r$$
$$3.1847 \approx r$$

Since the third digit from the left is in the hundredths' place, round to the nearest hundredth. Thus, $r \approx 3.18$.

A polygon is **inscribed** in a circle if all of its vertices are on the circle. The diagram at the right shows a triangle inscribed in a circle.

It can be shown that three points *not on a line* determine a circle. This means that there is one circle, and only one circle, that passes through the three given points.

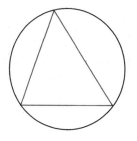

Class Exercises

Exercises 1–5 refer to the diagram below. B **is the center of the circle. Name each of the following.**

1. a diameter   **2.** three radii

3. five chords   **4.** two inscribed triangles

5. two isosceles triangles

Exercises 6–8 refer to the diagram above.

6. If $BE = 8$, find AC.   **7.** If $AC = 10$, find AB.

8. If $BC = 20$, find the circumference of the circle.

Draw a circle and an inscribed polygon of the specified kind.

9. a pentagon   **10.** a hexagon   **11.** an octagon

Written Exercises

Use $\pi \approx 3.14$ and round to three digits unless otherwise specified.

Find the circumference of each circle with the given diameter or radius.

A
1. diameter = 8 cm
2. diameter = 20 km
3. radius = 450 mm
4. radius = 16 cm
5. diameter = 42.6 m
6. radius = 278 mm

Find the diameter of each circle.

7. circumference = 283 m
8. circumference = 175 cm
9. circumference = 450 km
10. circumference = 468 mm
11. circumference = 625 m
12. circumference = 180 km

Find the radius of each circle.

13. circumference = 10 mm
14. circumference = 20 m
15. circumference = 23.5 km
16. circumference = 33.3 km
17. circumference = 17.5 cm
18. circumference = 27.2 m

19. The equator of Earth is approximately a circle of radius 6378 km. What is the circumference of Earth at the equator? Use the approximation $\pi \approx 3.1416$ and give your answer to five digits.

20. A park near Cristi's home contains a circular pool with a fountain at the center. Cristi paced off the distance around the pool and found it to be 220 m. What is the radius of the pool?

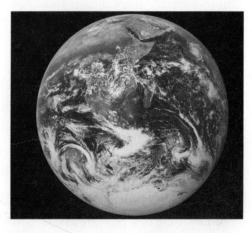

21. The diameter of a circular lake is measured and found to be 15 km. What is the circumference of the lake?

22. It is 45 m from the center of a circular field to the inside edge of the track surrounding it. The distance from the center of the field to the outside edge is 55 m. Find the circumference of each edge.

B 23. One circle has a radius of 15 m and a second has a radius of 30 m. How much larger is the circumference of the larger circle?

The curves in the diagrams below are parts of circles, and the angles are right angles. Find the perimeter of each figure.

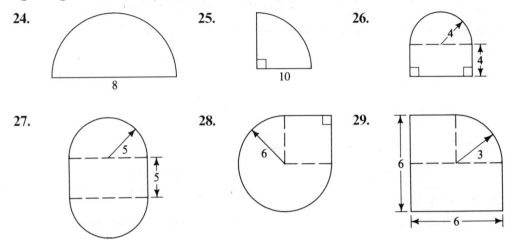

24.

8

25.

10

26.

4

4

27.

5

5

28.

6

29.

6

3

6

30. Find a formula that expresses the length, S, of a semicircle in terms of the radius, r.

31. Find a formula that expresses the length, S, of a semicircle in terms of the diameter, d.

In Exercises 32 and 33 use the fact that three points not on a line determine a circle.

32. Every triangle can be inscribed in some circle. Explain why this is so.

33. Explain how to draw a quadrilateral that cannot be inscribed in any circle.

C　**34.** What is the radius of the semicircle that forms the curve of a 400 meter track if each straightaway is 116 m long?

35. Draw a circle and one of its diameters, $\overline{AB}$. Then draw and measure $\angle APB$, where P is a point on the circle. Repeat this for several positions of P. What does this experiment suggest?

Review Exercises

Simplify.

1. $6 + 4 \times 3$　　　**2.** $16 \div 2 + 2$　　　**3.** $3(4 + 5)$　　　　**4.** $8(7 - 3)$

5. $64 \div (2 + 6)$　　**6.** $(18 + 3)2$　　　**7.** $14 + 3 \times 2 - 6$　　**8.** $52 - 18 \div 3 + 16$

5-7 Congruent Figures

Two figures are **congruent** if they have the same size and shape. Triangles *ABC* and *XYZ* shown below are congruent.

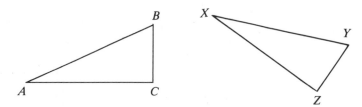

If we could lift △*ABC* and place it on △*XYZ*, *A* would fall on *X*, *B* on *Y*, and *C* on *Z*. These matching vertices are called **corresponding vertices.** Angles at corresponding vertices are **corresponding angles,** and the sides joining corresponding vertices are **corresponding sides.**

> Corresponding angles of congruent figures are congruent.
>
> Corresponding sides of congruent figures are congruent.

When we name two congruent figures, we list corresponding vertices in the same order. Thus, when we see

$$\triangle ABC \cong \triangle XYZ \quad \text{or} \quad \triangle CAB \cong \triangle ZXY,$$

we know that:

$$\angle A \cong \angle X, \qquad \angle B \cong \angle Y, \qquad \angle C \cong \angle Z$$
$$\overline{AB} \cong \overline{XY}, \qquad \overline{BC} \cong \overline{YZ}, \qquad \overline{CA} \cong \overline{ZX}$$

EXAMPLE 1   pentagon *PQUVW* ≅ pentagon *LMHKT*

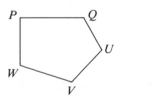
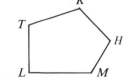

Complete these statements:

$$\angle W \cong \angle \underline{\ ?\ } \qquad \overline{QU} \cong \underline{\ ?\ } \qquad \angle H \cong \angle \underline{\ ?\ } \qquad \overline{TL} \cong \underline{\ ?\ }$$

Solution $\angle W \cong \angle T$ $\overline{QU} \cong \overline{MH}$ $\angle H \cong \angle U$ $\overline{TL} \cong \overline{WP}$

If two figures are congruent, we can make them coincide (occupy the same place) by using one or more of these basic **rigid motions:**

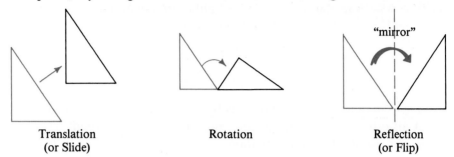

Translation
(or Slide)

Rotation

Reflection
(or Flip)

Consider the congruent trapezoids in panel (1) below. We can make *ABCD* coincide with *PQRS* by first reflecting *ABCD* in the line $\overleftrightarrow{BC}$ as in panel (2), and then translating this reflection as shown in panel (3).

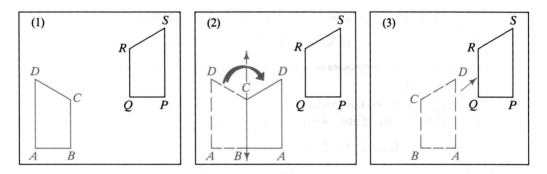

EXAMPLE 2   What type of rigid motion would make the red figure coincide with the black one?

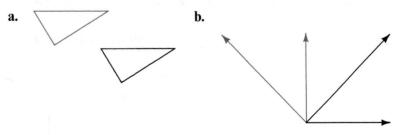

a.

b.

Solution   **a.** a translation: sliding the red triangle down and to the right would make it coincide with the black triangle

b. a rotation or a reflection: rotating the red angle around the vertex would make it coincide with the black angle; flipping the red angle over a line passing through the vertex would also make it coincide with the black angle

When working with triangles, we do not need to check all sides and all angles to establish congruence. Suppose that in the two triangles below, the sides and the angles marked alike are congruent.

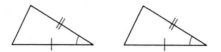

If we were to match the congruent parts by using translation, we would find that all other corresponding sides and angles are congruent also. Thus we can use the following method to establish congruence in two triangles.

The side-angle-side (SAS) test for congruence
If two sides of one triangle and the angle they form (the *included angle*) are congruent to two sides and the included angle of another triangle, then the two triangles are congruent.

Two other methods that we can use to establish congruence in triangles are:

The angle-side-angle (ASA) test for congruence
If two angles and the side between them (the *included side*) are congruent to two angles and the included side of another triangle, then the two triangles are congruent.

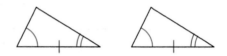

The side-side-side (SSS) test for congruence
If three sides of one triangle are congruent to the three sides of another triangle, then the two triangles are congruent.

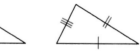

EXAMPLE 3 In the diagram, triangle ABC is isosceles, with $\overline{AB} \cong \overline{CB}$. $\overline{BD}$ bisects $\angle ABC$. Explain why $\triangle ABD \cong \triangle CBD$.

Solution We know that $\overline{AB} \cong \overline{CB}$.
Since $\overline{BD}$ bisects $\angle ABC$, $\angle 1 \cong \angle 2$.
Also, $\overline{BD}$ is a side of both triangles.
Therefore, by the SAS test,
$\triangle ABD \cong \triangle CBD$.

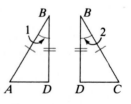

Class Exercises

Each figure in Exercises 1–8 is congruent to one of the figures _A – E_. State which one.

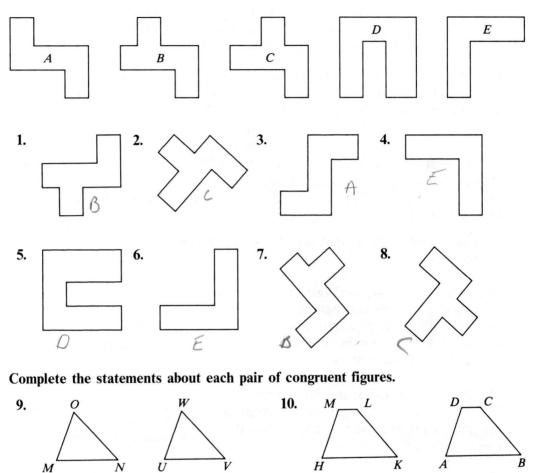

Complete the statements about each pair of congruent figures.

9.

O W

M N U V

  a. $\triangle MNO \cong$ ___?___
  b. $\angle N \cong$ _?_
  c. $\overline{MO} \cong$ _?_

10.

M L D C

H K A B

  a. Quadrilateral $HKLM \cong$ ___?___
  b. $\angle B \cong$ _?_
  c. $\overline{HM} \cong$ _?_

State which of the rigid motions is needed to match the vertices of the triangles in each pair and give a reason why the triangles are congruent.

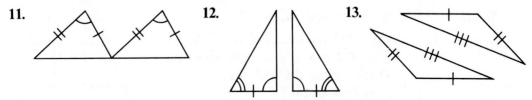

11.   12.   13.

Written Exercises

Which statement is correct?

A **1.**

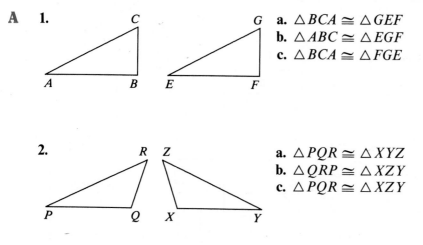

a. $\triangle BCA \cong \triangle GEF$
b. $\triangle ABC \cong \triangle EGF$
c. $\triangle BCA \cong \triangle FGE$

2.

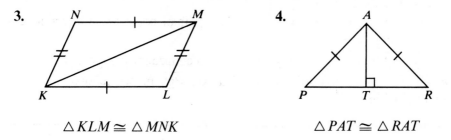

a. $\triangle PQR \cong \triangle XYZ$
b. $\triangle QRP \cong \triangle XZY$
c. $\triangle PQR \cong \triangle XZY$

Explain why the triangles in each pair are congruent.

3.

$\triangle KLM \cong \triangle MNK$

4.

$\triangle PAT \cong \triangle RAT$

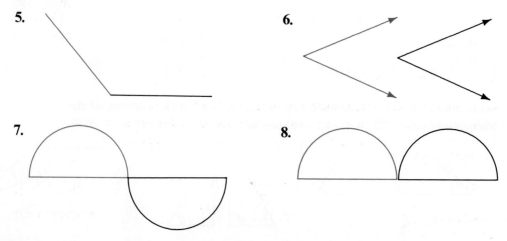

What type of rigid motion would make the red figure coincide with the black one?

5.

6.

7.

8.

Name a pair of congruent triangles and explain why they are congruent.

B 9. 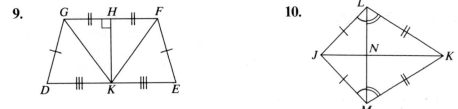 10.

Complete each statement.

11. $\triangle XRL \cong \triangle NYS$
    a. $\angle X \cong$ ____?____
    b. $\angle R \cong$ ____?____
    c. $\overline{XL} \cong$ ____?____
    d. $\overline{YS} \cong$ ____?____

12. $PQTV \cong HJKM$
    a. $\angle Q \cong$ ____?____
    b. $\angle M \cong$ ____?____
    c. $\overline{VP} \cong$ ____?____
    d. $\overline{JK} \cong$ ____?____

13. $ABCD \cong EFGH$
    a. $\overline{BC} \cong$ ____?____
    b. $\overline{AD} \cong$ ____?____
    c. $\angle ABC \cong$ ____?____
    d. $\overline{GH} \cong$ ____?____

C 14. $ABCDEF$ is a regular hexagon. If all the diagonals from F are drawn, name the following.
    a. all pairs of congruent triangles
    b. a pair of congruent quadrilaterals
    c. a pair of congruent pentagons

15. Let $\overline{AB}$ and $\overline{PQ}$ be corresponding sides of two congruent polygons. If one polygon is moved so that $\overline{AB}$ falls on $\overline{PQ}$, must the two polygons coincide?

Review Exercises

Solve.

1. $6x = 42$
2. $5x = 50$
3. $y \times 4 = 44$
4. $y \times 7 = 56$

5. $x \div 9 = 8$
6. $x \div 11 = 6$
7. $84 \div y = 21$
8. $65 \div y = 13$

 Calculator Key-In

Many ancient civilizations used approximations for π. Use a calculator to determine the following approximations for π as decimals. Which approximation is closest to the modern approximation of 3.14159265358?

1. Egyptian: $\frac{256}{81}$

2. Greek: $\frac{223}{71}$

3. Roman: $\frac{377}{120}$

4. Chinese: $\frac{355}{113}$

5. Hindu: $\frac{3927}{1250}$

6. Babylonian: $\frac{25}{8}$

5-8 Geometric Constructions

There is a difference between making a drawing and a **geometric construction.** For drawings, we may measure segments and angles; that is, we may use a ruler and a protractor to draw the figures. For geometric constructions, however, we may use only a compass and a straightedge. (We may use a ruler, but we must ignore the markings.)

Here are some important constructions. Construction I and Construction II involve dividing a segment or angle into two congruent parts. This process is called **bisecting** the segment or the angle.

Construction I: To bisect a segment $\overline{AB}$.

Use the compass to draw an arc (part of a circle) with center A and radius greater than $\frac{1}{2}AB$. Using the same radius but with center B, draw another arc. Call the points of intersection X and Y. $\overleftrightarrow{XY}$ is the **perpendicular bisector** of $\overline{AB}$ because it is perpendicular to $\overline{AB}$ and divides $\overline{AB}$ into two congruent segments.

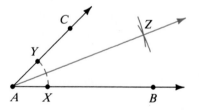

Construction II: To bisect an angle BAC.

Draw an arc with center A. Let X and Y be the points where the arc intersects the sides of the angle. Draw arcs of equal radii with centers X and Y. Call the point of intersection Z. $\overrightarrow{AZ}$ is the **angle bisector** of $\angle BAC$, and $\angle CAZ \cong \angle ZAB$.

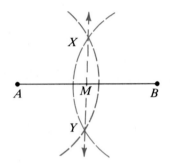

Construction III: To construct an angle congruent to a given angle Y.

Draw $\overrightarrow{MN}$. Draw an arc on $\angle Y$ with center Y. Let X and Z be the points where the arc intersects the sides of the angle. Draw an arc with center M and the same radius as arc XZ. Let S be the point where this arc intersects $\overrightarrow{MN}$. Call the other end of the arc R. With S as center draw an arc with radius equal to XZ. Let Q be the point where this arc intersects arc RS. Draw $\overrightarrow{MQ}$. $\angle NMQ \cong \angle Y$.

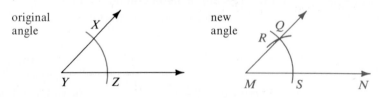

EXAMPLE 1 Construct a line that is perpendicular to $\overleftrightarrow{AB}$ and contains A.

Solution

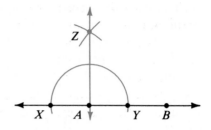

1. Place the compass at point A and draw an arc intersecting $\overleftrightarrow{AB}$ at two points. Call these two points X and Y, respectively. A is now the midpoint of $\overline{XY}$.

2. Place the compass at X and, as in Construction I, draw an arc with radius greater than $\overline{YA}$. Keeping the same radius, place the compass at Y and draw a second arc that intersects the first arc. Call the point of intersection of the two arcs Z.

3. Draw $\overleftrightarrow{AZ}$. Since $\overleftrightarrow{AZ}$ is the perpendicular bisector of $\overline{XY}$, and thus perpendicular to $\overleftrightarrow{AB}$, it is the required line.

EXAMPLE 2 Construct a 60° angle.

Solution

1. Draw a ray with endpoint A.

2. Draw an arc, with center A and any radius, intersecting the ray at B.

3. Draw an arc, with center B and the same radius as in step 2, intersecting the first arc at C.

4. Draw $\overrightarrow{AC}$. Since $\triangle ABC$ is equilateral, $m\angle BAC = 60°$.

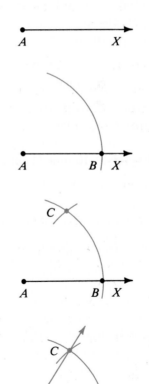

Written Exercises

In this exercise set use a compass and straightedge as your only construction tools.

A 1. Construct a 45° angle. (Method: Construct a right angle as in Example 1 and then bisect it.)

2. Construct a 30° angle. (Method: Construct a 60° angle as in Example 2 and then bisect it.)

3. Construct a 22.5° angle. (Use Exercise 1.)

4. Construct a 15° angle. (Use Exercise 2.)

5. Use a protractor to draw an angle with measure 75°. Construct an angle congruent to this angle.

6. Use a protractor to draw an angle with measure 130°. Construct an angle congruent to this angle.

7. Draw a large isosceles triangle. Using this triangle, construct the perpendicular bisector of the base. Through what point does the perpendicular bisector appear to pass?

8. Draw a large scalene triangle. Bisect its three angles. Are the angle bisectors **concurrent;** that is, do all three have a point in common?

9. Draw a large scalene triangle. Construct the perpendicular bisectors of its sides. Are these bisectors concurrent?

In Exercises 10 and 11, draw $\overleftrightarrow{ST}$ and a point P not on $\overleftrightarrow{ST}$.

B 10. Construct a line through P perpendicular to $\overleftrightarrow{ST}$. (Method: Draw an arc with center P to intersect $\overleftrightarrow{ST}$ in two points, A and B. Construct the perpendicular bisector of $\overline{AB}$.)

11. Construct a line through P parallel to $\overleftrightarrow{ST}$. (Method: 1. Construct $\overleftrightarrow{PQ}$ perpendicular to $\overleftrightarrow{ST}$ as in Exercise 10. 2. Construct $\overleftrightarrow{PR}$ perpendicular to $\overleftrightarrow{PQ}$ as in Example 1.)

12. Draw a large scalene triangle. A line through a vertex that is perpendicular to the opposite side is called an **altitude** of the triangle. Construct the three altitudes of the triangle (see Exercise 10). Are they concurrent?

13. Draw a large scalene triangle. A line through a vertex and the midpoint of the side opposite the vertex is called a **median** of the triangle. Construct the three medians (see Construction I). Are they concurrent?

C 14. Draw three noncollinear points, *A*, *B*, and *C*. Construct the circle that passes through these points. (*Hint:* The perpendicular bisectors of $\overline{AB}$ and $\overline{BC}$ both pass through the center of the circle.)

15. Use a compass to construct a regular hexagon. (*Hint:* The length of each side of a regular hexagon inscribed in a circle equals the radius of the circle.)

Self-Test B

Complete each statement.

1. A triangle with three congruent sides is __?__ .   [5–4]

2. The sum of the measures of the angles of a triangle is __?__ °.

3. An acute triangle has __?__ acute angle(s).

4. A(n) __?__ has eight sides.   [5–5]

5. A __?__ has its opposite sides parallel and congruent.

6. A trapezoid has sides of 7 cm, 5 cm, 7 cm, and 14 cm. Find its perimeter.

7. The radius of a circle is 16 cm. Find its circumference. Use   [5–6]
   $\pi \approx 3.14$ and round to three digits.

True or false?

8. A diameter cuts a circle into two semicircles.

9. A radius is a chord.

10. Pentagon *ABCDE* ≅ Pentagon *FGHIJ*. Complete each statement.   [5–7]
    a. $\overline{AB} \cong$ __?__   **b.** $\angle E \cong \angle$ __?__   **c.** $\angle DEA \cong \angle$ __?__

11. Construct an isosceles right triangle.   [5–8]

12. Construct an equilateral triangle.

Self-Test answers and Extra Practice are at the back of the book.

■■■ **Challenge**

You have your choice of your height in nickels that are stacked or in quarters that are laid side by side. Which would you choose?

More Programming in BASIC

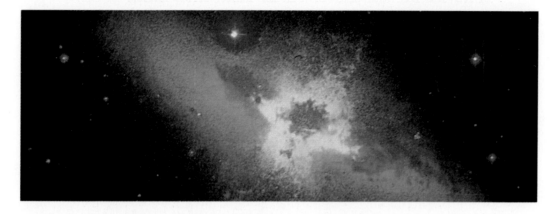

In Chapter 3 we learned that to enter different values of a variable in BASIC we can use the INPUT statement.

To assign a value to a variable that will be repeated over and over again, we use the **LET** statement. For example, the statement

$$20 \quad \text{LET K} = 4037$$

assigns the value 4037 to the variable K. This statement tells the computer to store 4037 in its memory at location K. The value of a variable can be changed by assigning a new value. When we write

$$20 \quad \text{LET K} = 0.025$$

the original value, 4037, is replaced by the new value, 0.025.

The program below converts miles to kilometers by using the fact that 1 mi = 1.61 km.

```
10   PRINT "FROM MILES TO KILOMETERS"
20   PRINT "DISTANCE IN MILES";
30   INPUT X
40   LET A = 1.61
50   PRINT X;" MI = ";A*X;" KM"
60   END
```

Let us use the program to convert the approximate distance in miles from the planet Saturn to the Sun. That is, convert 887,000,000 mi to kilometers.

```
RUN
FROM MILES TO KILOMETERS
DISTANCE IN MILES? 887000000          do not use commas
887000000 MI = 1428070000 KM          to enter the distance
```

Use the program on the previous page to complete the table.

	Planet	Distance (in mi) from the Sun	Distance (in km) from the Sun
1.	Mercury	36,000,000	?
2.	Venus	67,000,000	?
3.	Earth	93,000,000	?

Instead of running the program three times, we can modify it to repeat lines 20 through 50 so that all three distances are converted in one RUN. To do this, we use the **FOR** and **NEXT** statements to create a *loop*. The loop starts with the FOR statement, and ends with the NEXT statement. These two statements tell the computer how many times to repeat a group of statements located between them. The program below is now modified to repeat the loop three times. The output for Exercises 1–3 is shown at the right.

```
10   PRINT "FROM MILES TO KILOMETERS"
15   FOR I = 1 TO 3
20   PRINT "DISTANCE IN MILES";
30   INPUT X
40   LET A = 1.61
50   PRINT X;" MI = ";A*X;" KM"
55   NEXT I
60   END
```

```
RUN
FROM MILES TO KILOMETERS
DISTANCE IN MILES? 36000000
36000000 MI = 57960000 KM
DISTANCE IN MILES? 67000000
67000000 MI = 107870000 KM
DISTANCE IN MILES? 93000000
93000000 MI = 149730000 KM
```

Depending on the computer you are using, the output displayed for the conversions above may be expressed in *scientific notation*. That is, a number such as 376770000 may be expressed as

$$3.7677E+08.$$

The code E+08 means "times 10 raised to the power of 8." Therefore

$$3.7677E+08 \text{ means } 3.7677 \times 10^8, \text{ or } 376770000.$$

Complete.

4. $37{,}492{,}000{,}000 = 3.7492E+\underline{\ ?\ }$

5. $5{,}491{,}000{,}000{,}000 = 5.491E+\underline{\ ?\ }$

6. $9.4678E+07 = \underline{\ ?\ }$

7. $3.2186E+10 = \underline{\ ?\ }$

8. Write a program to print out the multiples of 2 from one to ten.

9. Write a program to print out the distance traveled at a constant rate of 760 mi/h for 15, 27, 31, 40, and 55 hours. Use the formula $d = rt$.

Chapter Review

Complete.

1. Points on the same line are called ___?___. [5–1]

2. A ___?___ has one endpoint.

3. Z divides $\overline{XY}$ into two congruent segments. Z is called the ___?___ of $\overline{XY}$. [5–2]

4. 927 mm = ___?___ cm = ___?___ m

True or false?

5. A right angle is obtuse. [5–3]

6. In $\angle ABC$, A is the vertex.

7. The supplement of a 40° angle has measure 140°.

8. A triangle that has three sides of different lengths is called scalene. [5–4]

9. In a triangle, the longest side is opposite the smallest angle.

10. All quadrilaterals are parallelograms. [5–5]

Write the letter of the correct answer.

11. A hexagon is regular. One side has length 8 cm. What is the perimeter?
   a. 40 cm   **b.** 64 cm   **c.** 80 cm   **d.** 48 cm

12. Name the segment joining the center of a circle to a point on the circle. [5–6]
   a. diameter   **b.** chord   **c.** radius   **d.** circumference

13. A circle has diameter 16 cm. Use $\pi \approx 3.14$ to find the circumference and round to three digits.
   a. 50.24 cm   **b.** 50.3 cm   **c.** 50.2 cm   **d.** 50 cm

14. Which is the symbol for congruence? [5–7]
   a. $\cong$ **b.** $\perp$ **c.** $\angle$ **d.** $\triangle$

15. Construct a 120° angle. [5–8]

16. Construct a right triangle.

Chapter Test

Exercises 1–3 refer to the diagram at the right.

1. Name a pair of perpendicular lines.   [5-1]

2. Name two rays that are not parallel, but do not intersect.

3. Name three collinear points.

Complete.

4. 27 m = _?_ cm   5. 3.6 km = _?_ m   [5-2]

6. 5000 cm = _?_ km   7. 4 mm = _?_ m

8. Give the measures of the complement and the supplement of $\angle A$ if   [5-3]
   $m \angle A = 27°$.

9. If $\angle X \cong \angle Y$, then $m \angle X = $ _?_ .

10. True or false? The sides of a right angle are perpendicular.

11. One angle of an isosceles triangle has measure 98°. Find the meas-   [5-4]
    ures of the two congruent angles.

12. An obtuse triangle has how many obtuse angles?

13. True or false? A square is a rhombus.   [5-5]

14. A quadrilateral has sides of length 8 cm, 13 cm, 9 cm, and 16 cm.
    Find the perimeter.

15. A regular hexagon has perimeter 84 mm. Find the length of each
    side.

16. The diameter of a circle is 18 cm. Find the radius.   [5-6]

17. A circle has radius 50 mm. Find the circumference. Use $\pi \approx 3.14$.

18. True or false? Every triangle can be inscribed in a circle.

19. If quadrilateral $ABCD \cong$ quadrilateral $WXYZ$, then $\overline{AD} \cong$ _?_ .   [5-7]

20. Draw a segment. Construct the perpendicular bisector. Then con-   [5-8]
    struct the bisector of one of the right angles.

Cumulative Review (Chapters 1–5)

Exercises

Evaluate the expression if $x = 3$ and $y = 5$.

1. $x + y$ **2.** $2x + y$ **3.** $2y - x$ **4.** $x + 6y$

5. $y + x + 4$ **6.** $-x - y$ **7.** $-3x - 2y$ **8.** $5x + (-y) - 7$

9. x^2 **10.** xy^2 **11.** $(-x)^2 y$ **12.** $-(xy)^2$

Solve using transformations.

13. $x + 36 = 50$ **14.** $x - 11 = -4$ **15.** $-4x = 75$

16. $-7x = -105$ **17.** $\frac{x}{8} = 9$ **18.** $\frac{x}{7} = -8$

19. $\frac{2}{3}x = 16$ **20.** $-\frac{5}{6}x = 25$ **21.** $0.45x = 13.5$

22. $\frac{x}{1.8} = 2.7$ **23.** $\frac{4}{5}x + 8 = 20$ **24.** $\frac{15}{4}x + 6 = -4$

Write in lowest terms.

25. $\frac{32}{40}$ **26.** $\frac{56}{80}$ **27.** $-\frac{12}{108}$

28. $-\frac{13}{182}$ **29.** $\frac{98}{147}$ **30.** $\frac{72}{96}$

Write as a terminating or repeating decimal. Use a bar to indicate repeating digits.

31. $\frac{2}{5}$ **32.** $\frac{3}{4}$ **33.** $\frac{7}{16}$

34. $\frac{3}{10}$ **35.** $-\frac{5}{18}$ **36.** $-\frac{2}{3}$

Write as a proper fraction in lowest terms or as a mixed number in simple form.

37. 0.07 **38.** 0.007 **39.** $1.\overline{9}$

40. $4.\overline{20}$ **41.** $-1.\overline{24}$ **42.** $-4.\overline{862}$

True or false?

43. An equilateral triangle is acute.   **44.** A diameter is a chord.

Problems

Solve.

1. Susan purchased the following items for the school dance: streamers, $2.89; tape, $4.59; bunting, $8.88; paper decorations, $14.75. How much did Susan spend?

2. Fred's Fish Farm started the week with 2078 fish. On Monday Fred sold 473 fish, on Tuesday he sold 509 fish, and on Wednesday 617 fish were sold. Fred bought 675 fish on Thursday and sold 349 on Friday. How many fish did Fred have at the end of the week?

3. Mr. Chou was putting a certain amount into his savings account each month. Last month he increased the amount by $38. If Mr. Chou deposited $162 into his savings account last month, how much was he putting in before the increase?

4. Yonora bought 7 gallons of paint at $16.95 a gallon, 3 brushes at $6.99 each, 4 rollers at $2.95 each, and a dropcloth for $7.88. How much did Yonora spend on painting supplies?

5. A side of a square is 13 m long. Find the perimeter.

6. If a number is multiplied by 3, the result is 51. Find the number.

7. The seventh grade sold greeting cards to raise money for a trip. There were 12 cards and 12 envelopes in each box. If the class sold 1524 cards with envelopes, how many boxes did they sell?

8. Elgin had $150 in his checking account. He wrote checks for $17.95, $23.98, $45.17, and $31.26. How much does Elgin have left in his account?

9. Becky bought a round pool that is 7 m in diameter. What is the circumference of the pool to the nearest meter?

10. Juanita is 7 years older than her brother Carlos, who is 3 years older than their sister Maria. If Carlos is 6 years old, how old are Juanita and Maria?

6

Ratio, Proportion, and Percent

Before the invention of the microscope, objects appeared to consist only of those materials seen with the unaided eye. Today the ability to magnify objects, such as the salt crystals shown at the right, has enabled scientists to understand the structures of various compounds in detail. The most advanced microscopes in use at the present time are electron microscopes. Electron microscopes can magnify objects hundreds of thousands of times by using beams of focused electrons.

The visibility of fine detail in a magnification depends on several factors, including the light and the magnifying power of the microscope. For a simple microscope, the magnifying power can be expressed as this ratio:

$$\frac{\text{size of the image on the viewer's eye}}{\text{size of the object seen without a microscope}}.$$

In this chapter, you will learn how scales and ratios are used.

Career Note

When you think of photography, you probably think of it as a means of portraying people and places. When used in conjunction with a microscope (photomicrography), or with infrared or ultraviolet light, photography can become an important research tool. Scientific photographers must have a knowledge of film, filters, lenses, illuminators, and all other types of camera equipment. They must also have a thorough understanding of scale and proportion in order to find the best composition for a particular photograph.

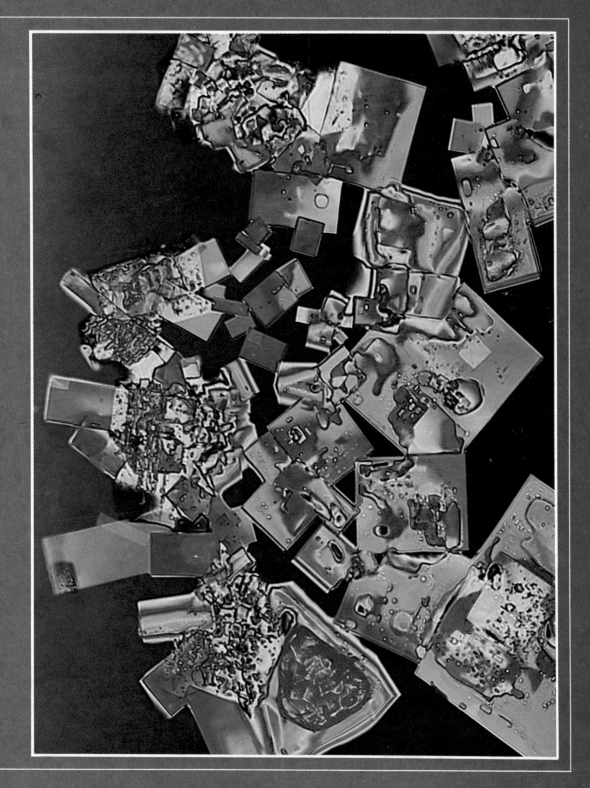

6-1 Ratios

At Fair Oaks Junior High School there are 35 teachers and 525 students. We can compare the number of teachers to the number of students by writing a quotient.

$$\frac{\text{number of teachers}}{\text{number of students}} = \frac{35}{525}, \text{ or } \frac{1}{15}$$

The indicated quotient of one number divided by a second number is called the **ratio** of the first number to the second number. We can write the ratio above in the following ways.

$$\frac{1}{15} \qquad 1:15 \qquad 1 \text{ to } 15$$

All of these expressions are read *one to fifteen*. If the colon notation is used, the first number is divided by the second. A ratio is said to be in **lowest terms** if the two numbers are relatively prime. You do not change an improper fraction to a mixed number if the improper fraction represents a ratio.

EXAMPLE 1 There are 9 players on a baseball team. Four of these are infielders and 3 are outfielders. Find each ratio in lowest terms.

        a. infielders to outfielders

        b. outfielders to total players

Solution   **a.** $\dfrac{\text{infielders}}{\text{outfielders}} = \dfrac{4}{3}$,   or $4:3$,   or   4 to 3

            b. $\dfrac{\text{outfielders}}{\text{total players}} = \dfrac{3}{9} = \dfrac{1}{3}$,   or $1:3$,   or   1 to 3

Some ratios compare measurements. In these cases, we must be sure that the measurements are expressed in the same unit.

EXAMPLE 2 It takes Herb 4 min to mix some paint. Herb can paint a room in 3 h. What is the ratio of the time it takes Herb to mix the paint to the time it takes Herb to paint the room?

Solution Use minutes as a common unit for measuring time.

$$3\,\text{h} = 3 \times 60\,\text{min} = 180\,\text{min}$$

The ratio is $\dfrac{\text{min to mix}}{\text{min to paint}} = \dfrac{4}{180} = \dfrac{1}{45}$, or $1:45$.

Problem Solving Reminder

There is *not enough information* given in some problems. To solve such problems, you must recall facts that are part of your general knowledge. In Example 2, you must recall that 1 h = 60 min.

Class Exercises

Express each ratio as a fraction in lowest terms.

1. 5 to 7   **2.** 11 to 6   **3.** 10:30   **4.** 12:24

5. 8 to 2   **6.** 32 to 4   **7.** 68:17   **8.** 45:18

Rewrite each ratio so that the numerator and denominator are expressed in the same unit of measure.

9. $\dfrac{2 \text{ dollars}}{50 \text{ cents}}$ **10.** $\dfrac{5 \text{ months}}{2 \text{ years}}$ **11.** $\dfrac{35 \text{ cm}}{1 \text{ m}}$ **12.** $\dfrac{12 \text{ min}}{2 \text{ h}}$

Written Exercises

For each diagram below, name each ratio as a fraction in lowest terms.
a. The number of shaded squares to the number of unshaded squares
b. The number of shaded squares to the total number of squares
c. The total number of squares to the number of unshaded squares

A **1.** 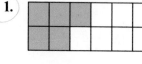   **2.**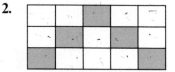

3. 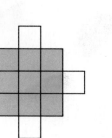   **4.**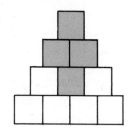

Express each ratio as a fraction in lowest terms.

5. 18 hours to 2 days   **6.** 25 cm to 3 m   **7.** 4 days:2 weeks

8. 48 s:5 min   **9.** 3 kg:800 g   **10.** 6 lb:24 oz

Find each ratio as a fraction in lowest terms.

B **11. a.** The number of vowels to the number of consonants in the alphabet (consider y a consonant)
    b. The number of consonants to the total number of letters
    c. The total number of letters to the number of vowels

12. a. The number of weekdays to the number of weekend days (Saturdays and Sundays) in the month of February (not in a leap year)
    b. The number of weekdays in the month of February (not a leap year) to the number of days in February
    c. The number of days to the number of Sundays in the month of February (not a leap year)

13. a. The number of diagonals drawn in the figure at the right to the total number of segments
    b. The number of sides of the figure to the number of diagonals
    c. The total number of segments to the number of sides

14. a. The number of prime numbers between 10 and 25 to the number of whole numbers between 10 and 25
    b. The number of prime numbers between 10 and 25 to the number of composite numbers between 10 and 25
    c. The number of whole numbers between 10 and 25 to the number of composite numbers between 10 and 25

In Exercises 15–18, $AB = 7\frac{1}{5}$, $CD = 10\frac{1}{2}$, $EF = 12$, and $GH = 6\frac{3}{4}$. Express each ratio in lowest terms.

C **15.** $\dfrac{AB}{EF}$ **16.** $\dfrac{EF}{GH}$ **17.** $\dfrac{CD}{GH}$ **18.** $\dfrac{GH}{AB}$

Problems

Solve.

A **1.** The *mechanical advantage* of a simple machine is the ratio of the weight lifted by the machine to the force necessary to lift it. What is the mechanical advantage of a jack that lifts a 3200-lb car with a force of 120 lb?

2. The *C*-string of a cello vibrates 654 times in 5 seconds. How many vibrations per second is this?

3. At sea level, 4 ft³ of water weighs 250 lb. What is the density of water in pounds per cubic foot?

4. The *index of refraction* of a transparent substance is the ratio of the speed of light in space to the speed of light in the substance. Using the table, find the index of refraction of
a. glass.   **b.** water.

Substance	Speed of Light (in km/s)
space	300,000
glass	200,000
water	225,000

5. A share of stock that cost $88 earned $16 last year. What was the price-to-earnings ratio of this stock?

In Exercises 6 and 7, find the ratio in lowest terms.

B   **6. a.** $\dfrac{AB}{DE}$

  b. $\dfrac{\text{Perimeter of } \triangle ABC}{\text{Perimeter of } \triangle DEF}$

7. a. $PQ:TU$
  b. $QR:UV$
  c. $\dfrac{\text{Perimeter of } PQRS}{\text{Perimeter of } TUVW}$

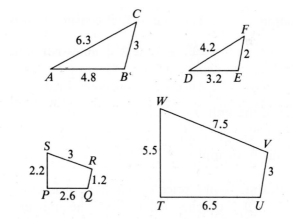

For Exercises 8–11, refer to the table to find the ratios in lowest terms.

8. The population of Centerville in 1980 to its population in 1970

9. The growth in the population of Easton to its 1980 population

Population (in thousands)		
Town	**1970**	**1980**
Centerville	36	44
Easton	16	28

10. The total population of both towns in 1970 to their total population in 1980

11. The total growth in the population of both towns to their total 1980 population

---

Review Exercises

Solve.

1. $6x = 54$ **2.** $11x = 99$ **3.** $5x = 45$ **4.** $3x = 39$

5. $20x = 100$ **6.** $10x = 80$ **7.** $12x = 144$ **8.** $9x = 72$

6-2 Rates

Some ratios are of the form

40 miles per hour   or   5 for a dollar.

These ratios involve quantities of different kinds and are called **rates.** Rates may be expressed as decimals or mixed numbers. Rates should be simplified to a *per unit* form.

EXAMPLE 1   Alice's car went 258 mi on 12 gal of gasoline. Express the rate of fuel consumption in miles per gallon.

Solution   The rate of fuel consumption is

$$\frac{258}{12} = \frac{43}{2} = 21\frac{1}{2} \text{ miles per gallon.}$$

Alice's car consumes 1 gal of gasoline every $21\frac{1}{2}$ mi.

Some of the units in which rates are given are:

mi/gal (or mpg)	miles per gallon	km/L	kilometers per liter
mi/h (or mph)	miles per hour	km/h	kilometers per hour

If a rate is the price of one item, it is called the **unit price.** For example, if 2 peaches sell for 78¢, the unit price is $\frac{78}{2}$, or 39, cents per peach.

EXAMPLE 2   If 5 oranges sell for 95¢, what is the cost of 12 oranges?

Solution   You can plan to find the price of one orange and then multiply by 12 to answer the question in the problem.

$$\text{unit price} = \frac{95}{5} = 19 \text{ (cents per orange)}$$

$$\text{cost of 12 oranges} = 12 \times 19 = 228 \text{ (cents)}$$

The cost of 12 oranges is 228¢, or $2.28.

Class Exercises

Express each rate in per unit form.

1. 120 km in 3 h

2. 70 mi on 5 gal of gasoline

3. $1000 in 4 months

4. 30 km on 3 L of gasoline

5. Three melons for $1.59

6. Two cans of tennis balls for $5.88

7. Six cans of water per 2 cans of juice

8. 28 bicycles sold in 7 days

9. 192.5 km in 3.5 h

10. A dozen eggs for $1.08

11. Ten oranges for $1.65

12. 225 m in 25 s

13. 28 teachers per 56 students

14. 18°F in 2 hours

15. 11 tickets for $30.80

16. Seven days for $399

Problems

Give the unit price of each item.

A 1. 7 oz of crackers for $1.19

2. 14 oz of cottage cheese for $1.19

3. 5 yd of upholstery fabric for $80

4. 16 boxes of raisins for $5.60

Solve.

5. A certain kind of lumber costs $3.00 for 8 ft. At this rate, how much does a piece that is 14 ft long cost?

6. A package of 3 lb of ground beef costs $5.10. How much ground beef could you buy for $3.40 at this rate?

7. A car travels for 3 h at an average speed of 65 km/h. How far does the car travel?

8. A boat covers 48 km in 2 h. What is the boat's average speed?

9. A homing pigeon flies 180 km in 3 h. At this average speed, how far could the pigeon travel in 4 h?

10. A bicyclist travels for 2 h at an average speed of 12 km/h. How far does the bicyclist travel? At this speed, how long will it take the bicyclist to travel 54 km?

Determine the better buy based on unit price alone.

B 11. A can of 35 oz of Best Brand Pear Tomatoes is on sale for 69¢. A can of 4 lb of Sun Ripe Pear Tomatoes costs $1.88. Which brand is the better buy?

12. A can of Favorite Beef Dog Food holds $14\frac{1}{2}$ oz. Four cans cost $1.00. Three cans of Delight Beef Dog Food, each containing 12 oz, cost $.58. Which is the better buy?

13. Three bottles of Bright Shine Window Cleaner, each containing 15 oz, cost $2.75. Two bottles of Sparkle Window Cleaner, each containing 18.75 oz, can be purchased for $1.98. Which is the better buy?

14. A bottle of Harvest Time Apple Juice contains 64 oz and costs 99¢. Farm Fresh Juice is available in bottles that contain 1 gal for $1.88 each. Which is the better buy?

Solve.

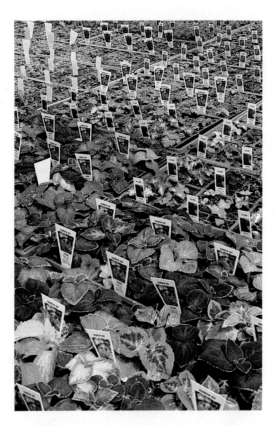

15. A car uses 3 gal of gasoline every 117 mi. During the first part of a trip, the car traveled 130 mi in 4 h. If the car continues to travel at the same average speed and the trip takes a total of 6 h, how many gallons of gasoline will be consumed?

16. Emily Depietro purchased 3 trays of strawberry plants for $16.47. Emily also purchased 10 trays of ivy plants. If the ratio of the price per tray of strawberry plants to the price per tray of ivy plants is 3 to 2, what is the total cost of the plants?

C 17. In the time that it takes one car to travel 93 km, a second car travels 111 km. If the average speed of the second car is 12 km/h faster than the speed of the first car, what is the speed of each car?

Review Exercises

Find the perimeter of a regular polygon whose sides have the given length.

1. pentagon, 4 cm

2. square, 6.2 m

3. octagon, 10.5 cm

4. triangle, 8.9 m

5. rhombus, 35.6 m

6. hexagon, 21.75 cm

7. quadrilateral, 14.35 m

8. decagon, 64.87 cm

9. rhombus, 12.36 cm

6-3 Proportions

The seventh grade at Madison Junior High School has 160 students and 10 teachers. The seventh grade at Jefferson Junior High School has 144 students and 9 teachers. Let us compare the two teacher-student ratios.

$$\frac{10}{160} = \frac{1}{16} \qquad \frac{9}{144} = \frac{1}{16}$$

Thus, the two ratios are equal.

$$\frac{10}{160} = \frac{9}{144}$$

An equation that states that two ratios are equal is called a **proportion.** The proportion above may be read as

10 is to 160 as 9 is to 144.

The numbers 10, 160, 9, and 144 are called the **terms** of the proportion.

Sometimes one of the terms of a proportion is a variable. If, for example, 192 students will be in the seventh grade at Madison Junior High next year, how many teachers will be needed if the teacher-student ratio is to remain the same?

Let n be the number of teachers needed next year. Then, if the teacher-student ratio is to be the same, we must have

$$\frac{n}{192} = \frac{10}{160}.$$

To **solve** this proportion, we find the value of the variable that makes the equation true. This can be done by finding equivalent fractions with a common denominator. For example:

$$\frac{160 \times n}{160 \times 192} = \frac{10 \times 192}{160 \times 192}$$

Since the denominators are equal, the numerators also must be equal.

$$160 \times n = 10 \times 192$$

Notice that this result could also be obtained by **cross-multiplying** in the original proportion.

$$\frac{n}{192} \diagup \frac{10}{160}$$

$$160 \times n = 10 \times 192$$
$$160n = 1920$$
$$n = 1920 \div 160 = 12$$

Therefore, the seventh grade will need 12 teachers next year.

The example on the previous page illustrates the following property of proportions.

> ## *Property*
>
> If $\frac{a}{b} = \frac{c}{d}$, with $b \neq 0$ and $d \neq 0$, then $ad = bc$.

In the proportion $\qquad \frac{a}{b} = \frac{c}{d}$

the terms a and d are called the **extremes,** and the terms b and c are called the **means.** The property above can therefore be stated:

The product of the means equals the product of the extremes.

EXAMPLE   Solve $\frac{3}{8} = \frac{12}{n}$.

Solution $\qquad\qquad \frac{3}{8} = \frac{12}{n}$

$$3 \times n = 8 \times 12$$
$$3n = 96$$
$$n = 96 \div 3 = 32$$

It is a simple matter to check your answer when solving a proportion. You merely substitute your answer for the variable and cross-multiply. For instance, in the example above:

$$\frac{3}{8} \overset{?}{=} \frac{12}{32}$$
$$3 \times 32 \overset{?}{=} 8 \times 12$$
$$96 = 96$$

Class Exercises

Cross-multiply and state an equation that does not involve fractions.

1. $\frac{n}{9} = \frac{2}{3}$ **2.** $\frac{3}{5} = \frac{n}{20}$ **3.** $\frac{2}{7} = \frac{6}{n}$ **4.** $\frac{3}{n} = \frac{6}{10}$

5. $\frac{12}{15} = \frac{n}{5}$ **6.** $\frac{2}{n} = \frac{3}{9}$ **7.** $\frac{n}{16} = \frac{3}{4}$ **8.** $\frac{8}{3} = \frac{24}{n}$

Written Exercises

Solve and check.

A 1. $\dfrac{n}{3} = \dfrac{12}{9}$ 2. $\dfrac{7}{2} = \dfrac{x}{10}$ 3. $\dfrac{21}{r} = \dfrac{3}{8}$ 4. $\dfrac{3}{75} = \dfrac{2}{m}$

5. $\dfrac{8}{5} = \dfrac{56}{u}$ 6. $\dfrac{14}{n} = \dfrac{7}{9}$ 7. $\dfrac{80}{c} = \dfrac{4}{3}$ 8. $\dfrac{b}{24} = \dfrac{15}{9}$

9. $\dfrac{8}{7} = \dfrac{x}{63}$ 10. $\dfrac{d}{20} = \dfrac{14}{8}$ 11. $\dfrac{15}{11} = \dfrac{n}{33}$ 12. $\dfrac{13}{11} = \dfrac{26}{m}$

13. $\dfrac{5}{r} = \dfrac{2}{3}$ 14. $\dfrac{4}{3} = \dfrac{n}{7}$ 15. $\dfrac{17}{20} = \dfrac{v}{10}$ 16. $\dfrac{c}{2} = \dfrac{6}{18}$

B 17. $\dfrac{x}{5} = \dfrac{20}{10}$ 18. $\dfrac{3}{m} = \dfrac{9}{27}$ 19. $\dfrac{4}{n} = \dfrac{12}{36}$ 20. $\dfrac{a}{16} = \dfrac{4}{8}$

21. $\dfrac{20}{25} = \dfrac{16}{y}$ 22. $\dfrac{v}{50} = \dfrac{18}{30}$ 23. $\dfrac{25}{x} = \dfrac{15}{9}$ 24. $\dfrac{49}{16} = \dfrac{n}{4}$

25. $\dfrac{n}{8} = \dfrac{7}{10}$ 26. $\dfrac{15}{4} = \dfrac{9}{r}$ 27. $\dfrac{9}{10} = \dfrac{b}{5}$ 28. $\dfrac{9}{n} = \dfrac{15}{7}$

29. If $\dfrac{x}{7} = \dfrac{3}{21}$, what is the ratio of x to 3?

30. If $\dfrac{27}{m} = \dfrac{9}{2}$, what is the ratio of m to 27?

31. If $\dfrac{3}{5} = \dfrac{12}{n}$, what is the ratio of n to 5?

C 32. Choose nonzero whole numbers a, b, c, d, x, and y such that $\dfrac{a}{b} = \dfrac{x}{y}$ and $\dfrac{c}{d} = \dfrac{x}{y}$. Use these numbers to check whether $\dfrac{a+c}{b+d} = \dfrac{x}{y}$.

33. Find nonzero whole numbers a, b, c, and d to show that if $\dfrac{a+c}{b+d} = \dfrac{x}{y}$, it may not be true that $\dfrac{a}{b} = \dfrac{x}{y}$ and $\dfrac{c}{d} = \dfrac{x}{y}$.

Review Exercises

Multiply.

1. $2\dfrac{2}{3} \times 5$ 2. $3\dfrac{5}{8} \times 6$ 3. $5 \times 4\dfrac{5}{9}$

4. $7 \times 6\dfrac{3}{4}$ 5. $3\dfrac{4}{9} \times 2\dfrac{1}{2}$ 6. $4\dfrac{1}{3} \times 5\dfrac{1}{4}$

7. $6 \times 7\dfrac{1}{4}$ 8. $5 \times 8\dfrac{3}{5}$ 9. $9 \times 6\dfrac{7}{10}$

6-4 Solving Problems with Proportions

Proportions can be used to solve problems. The following steps are helpful in solving problems using proportions.

1. Decide which quantity is to be found and represent it by a variable.
2. Determine whether the quantities involved can be compared using ratios (rates).
3. Equate the ratios in a proportion.
4. Solve the proportion.

EXAMPLE   Linda Chu bought 4 tires for her car at a total cost of $264. How much would 5 tires cost at the same rate?

Solution   Let c = the cost of 5 tires. Set up a proportion.

$$\frac{4}{264} = \frac{5}{c} \quad \longleftarrow \text{ number of tires}$$
$$\phantom{\frac{4}{264} = \frac{5}{c}} \quad \longleftarrow \text{ cost}$$

Solve the proportion.

$$\frac{4}{264} = \frac{5}{c}$$
$$4c = 5 \times 264$$
$$4c = 1320$$
$$c = 330$$

Therefore, 5 tires would cost $330.

Notice that the proportion in the Example could also be written as:

$$\frac{264}{4} = \frac{c}{5} \quad \longleftarrow \text{ cost}$$
$$\phantom{\frac{264}{4} = \frac{c}{5}} \quad \longleftarrow \text{ number of tires}$$

Class Exercises

State a proportion you could use to solve each problem.

1. If 4 bars of soap cost $1.50, how much would 8 bars cost?

2. If you can buy 4 containers of cottage cheese for $4.20, how many could you buy for $9.45?

3. If a satellite travels 19,500 km in 3 h, how far does it travel in 7 h?

4. If a car uses 5 gal of gasoline to travel 160 mi, how many gallons would the car use in traveling 96 mi?

5. A recipe for 20 rolls calls for 5 tablespoons of butter. How many tablespoons are needed for 30 rolls?

6. If 9 kg of fertilizer will feed 300 m² of grass, how much fertilizer would be required to feed 500 m²?

7. If 2 cans of paint will cover a wall measuring 900 ft², what area will 3 cans cover?

Problems

Solve.

A 1. A train traveled 720 km in 9 h.
   a. How far would it travel in 11 h?
   b. How long would it take to go 1120 km?

2. Five pounds of apples cost $3.70.
   a. How many pounds could you buy for $5.92?
   b. How much would 9 lb cost? 6.66

3. Eight oranges cost $1.50.
   a. How much would 20 oranges cost?
   b. How many oranges could you buy for $5.25? 28

4. Due to Earth's rotation, a point on the equator travels about 40,000 km every 24 h.
   a. How far does a point on the equator travel in 33 h?
   b. How long does it take a point on the equator to travel 95,000 km?

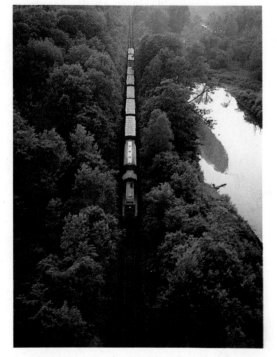

5. Seventy-five cubic centimeters of maple sap can be boiled down to make 2 cm³ of maple syrup.
   a. How much maple syrup would 200 cm³ of sap make?
   b. How much sap would be needed to make 9 cm³ of syrup?

6. A long-playing record revolves 100 times every 3 min.
   a. How many revolutions does it make in 2.25 min? 75
   b. How long does it take for 275 revolutions? 8.25 min.

7. Three and a half pounds of peaches cost $1.68. How much would 2½ lb of peaches cost? $1.20

Ratio, Proportion, and Percent **221**

Solve.

8. A type of steel used for bicycle frames contains 5 g of manganese in every 400 g of steel. How much manganese would a 2200 g bicycle frame contain?

9. Five cans of paint will cover 130 m² of wall space. How many cans will be needed to cover 208 m²?

10. To obtain the correct strength of a medicine, 5 cm³ of distilled water is added to 12 cm³ of an antibiotic. How much water should be added to 30 cm³ of the antibiotic? 12.5

11. A receipe that serves 8 calls for 15 oz of cooked tomatoes. How many ounces of tomatoes will be needed if the recipe is reduced to serve 6 people? How many servings can be made with 20 oz of cooked tomatoes?

12. A geologist found that silt was deposited on a river bed at the rate of 4 cm every 170 years. How long would it take for 5 cm of silt to be deposited? How much silt would be deposited in 225 years?
    212.5 , 5,294

13. A printing press can print 350 sheets in 4 min. How long would it take to print 525 sheets?

14. A pharmacist combines 5 g of a powder with 45 cm³ of water to make a prescription medicine. How much powder should she mix with 81 cm³ of water to make a larger amount of the same medicine?
    9

B 15. A baseball team has won 8 games and lost 6. If the team continues to have the same ratio of wins to losses, how many wins will the team have after playing 21 games?

16. The ratio of cars to trucks passing a certain intersection is found to be 7:2. If 63 vehicles (cars and trucks) pass the intersection, how many might be trucks?

17. Five vests can be made from 2½ yd of fabric. How many vests can be made from 6 yd of fabric?

18. A fruit punch recipe calls for 3 parts of apple juice to 4 parts of cranberry juice. How many liters of cranberry juice should be added to 4.5 L of apple juice?

19. A 3 lb bag of Fairlawn's Number 25 grass seed covers a 4000 ft² area. How great an area will 16 oz of the Number 25 grass seed cover?

20. A wall hanging requires 54 cm of braided trim. How many wall hangings can be completed if 3 m of braided trim is available?

C 21. In a recent election, the ratio of votes *for* a particular proposal to votes *against* the proposal was 5 to 2. There were 4173 more votes for the proposal than against the proposal. How many votes were for and how many votes were against the proposal?

22. A certain soil mixture calls for 8 parts of potting soil to 3 parts of sand. To make the correct mixture, Vern used 0.672 kg of sand and 2 bags of potting soil. How much potting soil was in each bag?

23. In the third century B.C., the Greek mathematician Eratosthenes calculated that an angle of $7\frac{1}{2}°$ at Earth's center cuts off an arc of about 1600 km on Earth's surface. From this information compute the circumference of Earth.

24. In the diagram $\overline{PQ}$ is perpendicular to $\overline{MN}$. It can be shown that $\frac{a}{x} = \frac{x}{b}$. If $a = 50$ and $b = 2$, find x.

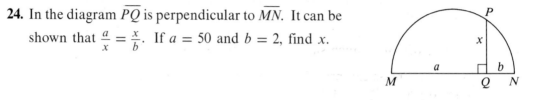

Review Exercises

Rewrite each ratio so that the numerator and denominator are expressed in the same unit of measure.

1. $\dfrac{2 \text{ m}}{15 \text{ cm}}$ 2. $\dfrac{20 \text{ mm}}{7 \text{ cm}}$ 3. $\dfrac{10 \text{ yd}}{5 \text{ ft}}$ 4. $\dfrac{8 \text{ in.}}{3 \text{ ft}}$

5. $\dfrac{2 \text{ km}}{450 \text{ m}}$ 6. $\dfrac{85 \text{ cm}}{4 \text{ m}}$ 7. $\dfrac{1 \text{ yd}}{20 \text{ in.}}$ 8. $\dfrac{310 \text{ m}}{3 \text{ km}}$

▮▮▮ Calculator Key-In

It is fairly simple to find the reciprocal of a fraction or a whole number. It is harder to find the reciprocal of a decimal. However, many calculators have a reciprocal key to carry out this procedure.

Use a calculator with a reciprocal key to find each reciprocal.

1. 0.67   **2.** 0.579   **3.** 0.2539   **4.** 1.564   **5.** 4.7851

6-5 Scale Drawing

In the drawing of the house the actual height of 9 m is represented by a length of 3 cm, and the actual length of 21 m is represented by a length of 7 cm. This means that 1 cm in the drawing represents 3 m in the actual building. Such a drawing in which all lengths are in the same ratio to actual lengths is called a **scale drawing.** The relationship of length in the drawing to actual length is called the **scale.** In the drawing of the house the scale is 1 cm : 3 m.

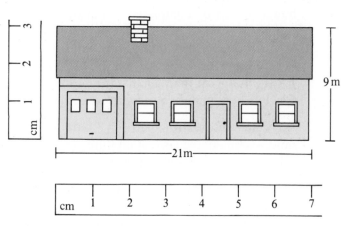

We can express the scale as a ratio, called the scale ratio, if a common unit of measure is used. Since 3 m equals 300 cm, the scale ratio above is $\frac{1}{300}$.

EXAMPLE Find the length and width of the room shown if the scale of the drawing is 1 cm : 1.5 m.

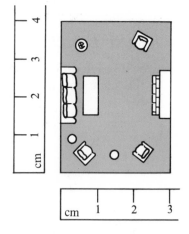

Solution Measuring the drawing, we find that it has length 4 cm and width 3 cm.

Method 1 Write a proportion for the length.

$$\frac{1}{1.5} = \frac{4}{l} \quad\begin{matrix}\leftarrow \text{ unit lengths in the drawing}\\ \leftarrow \text{ actual length}\end{matrix}$$

$l = 1.5 \times 4 = 6$
The room is 6 m long.

Write a proportion for the width. $\frac{1}{1.5} = \frac{3}{w}$

$w = 1.5 \times 3 = 4.5$ The room is 4.5 m wide.

Method 2 Use the scale ratio: $\frac{1 \text{ cm}}{1.5 \text{ m}} = \frac{1 \text{ cm}}{150 \text{ cm}} = \frac{1}{150}$

The actual length is 150 times the length in the drawing.

$l = 150 \times 4 = 600 \text{ cm} = 6 \text{ m}$ $w = 150 \times 3 = 450 \text{ cm} = 4.5 \text{ m}$

Class Exercises

A drawing of a bureau is to be made with a scale of 1 cm to 10 cm. Find the dimension on the drawing if the actual dimension is given.

1. Height of bureau (70 cm)   **2.** Width of bureau (80 cm)

3. Height of legs (17.5 cm)   **4.** Width of top (75 cm)

5. Height of top drawer (10 cm)   **6.** Height of second drawer (12.5 cm)

7. Height of third drawer (15 cm)   **8.** Width of drawer (72.5 cm)

Written Exercises

An O-gauge model railroad has a scale of 1 in.:48 in. Find the actual length of each railroad car, given the scale dimension.

A   **1.** Flat car: 23 in.   **2.** Freight car: 11 in.   **3.** Tank car: 12 in.

     4. Caboose: 9 in.   **5.** Passenger car: 20 in.   **6.** Refrigerator car: 15 in.

Exercises 7–14, on the next page, refer to the map below.
a. Measure each distance in the map shown to the nearest 0.5 cm.
b. Compute the actual distance to the nearest 100 km.

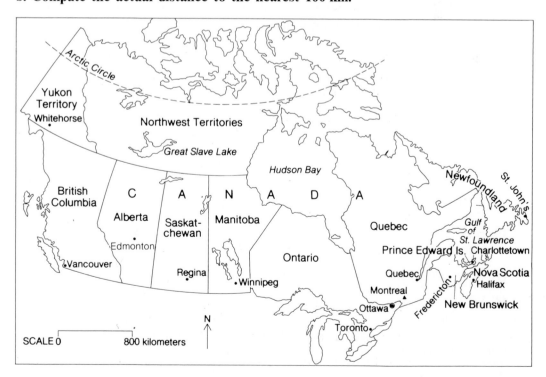

7. Vancouver to Edmonton

8. Toronto to Winnipeg

9. Whitehorse to Montreal

10. Ottawa to Charlottetown

11. Toronto to Halifax

12. Fredericton to St. John's

B 13. By how many kilometers would an airplane route from Winnipeg to Montreal be extended if the plane went by way of Toronto?

14. How much farther is it by air from Vancouver to Edmonton to Whitehorse than it is from Vancouver directly to Whitehorse?

If Earth had the diameter of a peppercorn (5 mm), the sun would have the diameter of a large beach ball (54.5 cm) and it would be about the length of two basketball courts (58.75 m) away. Assuming that the diameter of Earth is about 12,700 km, compute each measurement.

15. The actual diameter of the sun

16. The distance from Earth to the sun

17. In the scale described above, the diameter of the planet Jupiter would be 55 mm. What is the actual diameter of Jupiter?

Self-Test A

Express each ratio as a fraction in lowest terms.

1. $12:8$

2. 51 to 27

3. $\dfrac{18}{99}$

[6–1]

Give the unit price of each item.

4. 8 gal of gasoline for $9.20

5. 11 cans of pet food for $6.72

[6–2]

Solve.

6. $\dfrac{x}{3} = \dfrac{8}{12}$

7. $\dfrac{12}{9} = \dfrac{n}{3}$

8. $\dfrac{180}{n} = \dfrac{4}{3}$

[6–3]

9. Find the price per gram of a metal that costs $154.10 for 230 g.

[6–4]

10. A company paid a dividend of $30 on 12 shares of stock. How much will it pay on 44 shares?

11. On a map, 3 in. represents 16 ft. What length represents $5\frac{1}{3}$ ft?

[6–5]

12. What is the scale in a drawing in which a vase 28 cm tall is drawn 1.75 cm high?

Self-Test answers and Extra Practice are at the back of the book.

6-6 Percents and Fractions

During basketball season, Alice made 17 out of 25 free throws, while Nina made 7 out of 10. To see who did better, we compare the fractions representing each girl's successful free throws:

$$\frac{17}{25} \quad \text{and} \quad \frac{7}{10}$$

In comparing fractions it is often convenient to use the common denominator 100, even if 100 is not the LCD of the fractions.

$$\frac{17}{25} = \frac{17 \times 4}{25 \times 4} = \frac{68}{100} \qquad \frac{7}{10} = \frac{7 \times 10}{10 \times 10} = \frac{70}{100}$$

Since Alice makes 68 free throws per hundred and Nina makes 70 per hundred, Nina is the better free-throw shooter.

The ratio of a number to 100 is called a **percent.** We write percents by using the symbol %. For example,

$$\frac{17}{25} = \frac{68}{100} = 68\% \qquad \text{and} \qquad \frac{7}{10} = \frac{70}{100} = 70\%.$$

Rule

To express the fraction $\frac{a}{b}$ as a percent, solve the equation

$\frac{n}{100} = \frac{a}{b}$ for the variable n and write $n\%$.

EXAMPLE 1 Express $\frac{17}{40}$ as a percent.

Solution $\frac{n}{100} = \frac{17}{40}$

Cross-multiply.

$40 \times n = 17 \times 100$

$$n = \frac{17}{40} \times 100 = \frac{17}{\underset{2}{40}} \times \overset{5}{100} = \frac{85}{2} = 42\frac{1}{2}$$

Therefore, $\frac{17}{40} = 42\frac{1}{2}\%$, or 42.5%.

> ## Rule
>
> To express $n\%$ as a fraction, write the fraction
>
> $$\frac{n}{100}$$
>
> in lowest terms.

EXAMPLE 2 Express $7\frac{1}{2}\%$ as a fraction in lowest terms.

Solution $7\frac{1}{2}\% = 7.5\% = \frac{7.5}{100} = \frac{7.5 \times 10}{100 \times 10} = \frac{75}{1000} = \frac{3}{40}$

Since a percent is the ratio of a number to 100, we can have percents that are greater than or equal to 100%. For example,

$$\frac{100}{100} = 100\% \qquad \text{and} \qquad \frac{165}{100} = 165\%.$$

EXAMPLE 3 Write 250% as a mixed number in simple form.

Solution $250\% = \frac{250}{100}$

$$= 2\frac{50}{100} = 2\frac{1}{2}$$

EXAMPLE 4 A certain town spends 42% of its budget on education. What percent is used for other purposes?

Solution The whole budget is represented by 100%. Therefore, the part used for other purposes is

$$100 - 42, \text{ or } 58\%.$$

Class Exercises

Express as a fraction in lowest terms or as a mixed number in simple form.

1. 17%	**2.** 90%	**3.** 50%	**4.** 25%
5. 20%	**6.** 100%	**7.** 4%	**8.** 150%
9. 300%	**10.** 30%	**11.** 35%	**12.** 210%

Express as a percent.

13. $\frac{1}{50}$ 14. $\frac{1}{10}$ 15. $\frac{7}{10}$ 16. 1

17. 2   18. $\frac{1}{20}$ 19. $3\frac{1}{2}$ 20. $\frac{9}{10}$

21. $\frac{3}{4}$ 22. $4\frac{1}{2}$ 23. $\frac{2}{25}$ 24. $\frac{3}{20}$

Written Exercises

Express as a fraction in lowest terms or as a mixed number in simple form.

A   1. 75%   2. 60%   3. 45%   4. 95%

5. 12%   6. 76%   7. 125%   8. 220%

9. $15\frac{1}{2}\%$ 10. $8\frac{4}{5}\%$ 11. $10\frac{3}{4}\%$ 12. $5\frac{3}{8}\%$

Express as a percent.

13. $\frac{4}{5}$ 14. $\frac{1}{4}$ 15. $\frac{3}{10}$ 16. $\frac{1}{25}$

17. $\frac{12}{25}$ 18. $\frac{17}{20}$ 19. $\frac{31}{50}$ 20. $1\frac{3}{4}$

21. $2\frac{1}{5}$ 22. $3\frac{11}{25}$ 23. $\frac{51}{50}$ 24. $\frac{31}{25}$

B   25. $\frac{7}{8}$ 26. $\frac{7}{40}$ 27. $\frac{1}{200}$ 28. $\frac{12}{125}$

29. $\frac{3}{400}$ 30. $\frac{9}{250}$ 31. $\frac{121}{40}$ 32. $\frac{25}{8}$

EXAMPLE   Express $33\frac{1}{3}\%$ as a fraction in lowest terms.

Solution $33\frac{1}{3}\% = \dfrac{33\frac{1}{3}}{100} = 33\frac{1}{3} \div 100$

$$= \frac{100}{3} \times \frac{1}{100} = \frac{1}{3}$$

Express each percent as a fraction in lowest terms.

C   33. $16\frac{2}{3}\%$ 34. $66\frac{2}{3}\%$ 35. $41\frac{2}{3}\%$ 36. $83\frac{1}{3}\%$

Problems

A   1. In a public opinion poll 62% of the questionnaires sent out were returned. What percent were not returned?

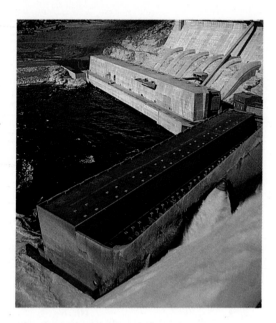

2. The efficiency of a machine is the percent of energy going into the machine that does useful work. A turbine in a hydroelectric plant is 92% efficient. What percent of the energy is wasted?

3. Of the 300 acres on Swanson's farm, 180 acres are used to grow wheat. What percent of the land is used to grow wheat?

4. Of the selling price of a pair of gloves, 42% pays the wholesale cost of the gloves, 33% pays store expenses, and the rest is profit. What percent is profit?

B   5. In a 500 kg metal bar, 475 kg is iron and the remainder is impurities. What percent of the bar is impurities?

6. A baseball team won 42 games out of its first 80. What percent of the games did the team win?

7. One year the Caterpillars lost 5 games out of 16. If the Caterpillars also tied 1 game, what percent of their games did they win?

C   8. The Bears won 40 games and lost 24, while the Bulls won 32 games and lost 18. Which team had the higher percent of wins?

9. At a company sales conference there were 4 executives, 28 salespeople, and 8 marketing consultants. What percent of the people were executives? Salespeople? Not marketing consultants?

Review Exercises

Change each fraction to a decimal.

1. $\frac{9}{20}$ 2. $\frac{19}{25}$ 3. $\frac{11}{40}$ 4. $\frac{17}{80}$ 5. $\frac{1}{25}$

6. $\frac{13}{30}$ 7. $\frac{8}{11}$ 8. $\frac{19}{22}$ 9. $\frac{43}{75}$ 10. $\frac{83}{90}$

6-7 Percents and Decimals

By looking at the following examples, you may be able to see a general relationship between decimals and percents.

$$57\% = \frac{57}{100} = 0.57 \qquad\qquad 0.79 = \frac{79}{100} = 79\%$$

$$113\% = \frac{113}{100} = 1\frac{13}{100} = 1.13 \qquad 0.06 = \frac{6}{100} = 6\%$$

These examples suggest the following rules.

> ## *Rules*
>
> 1. To express a percent as a decimal, move the decimal point two places to the left and remove the percent sign.
>
> $$57\% = 0.57 \qquad 113\% = 1.13$$
>
> 2. To express a decimal as a percent, move the decimal point two places to the right and add a percent sign.
>
> $$0.79 = 79\% \qquad 0.06 = 6\%$$

EXAMPLE 1 Express each percent as a decimal.
   a. 83.5%   **b.** 450%   **c.** 0.25%

Solution   **a.** $83.5\% = 0.835$

b. $450\% = 4.50 = 4.5$

c. $0.25\% = 0.0025$

EXAMPLE 2 Express each decimal as a percent.
   a. 10.5   **b.** 0.0062   **c.** 0.574

Solution   **a.** $10.5 = 1050\%$

b. $0.0062 = 00.62\%$

c. $0.574 = 57.4\%$

In the previous lesson you learned one method of changing a fraction to a percent. The ease of changing a decimal to a percent suggests the alternative method shown on the following page.

> ## Rule
>
> To express a fraction as a percent, first express the fraction as a decimal and then as a percent.

EXAMPLE 3   Express $\frac{7}{8}$ as a percent.

Solution   Divide 7 by 8.

$$\begin{array}{r} 0.875 \\ 8\overline{)7.000} \\ \underline{6\,4} \\ 60 \\ \underline{56} \\ 40 \\ \underline{40} \\ 0 \end{array}$$

$\frac{7}{8} = 0.875 = 87.5\%$

EXAMPLE 4   Express $\frac{1}{3}$ as a percent. Round to the nearest tenth of a percent.

Solution   Divide 1 by 3 to the ten-thousandths' place.

Round the quotient to the nearest thousandth.

$$0.3333 \approx 0.333$$

Express the decimal as a percent.

$$0.333 = 33.3\%$$

To the nearest tenth of a percent, $\frac{1}{3} = 33.3\%$.

$$\begin{array}{r} 0.3333 \\ 3\overline{)1.0000} \\ \underline{9} \\ 10 \\ \underline{9} \\ 10 \\ \underline{9} \\ 10 \\ \underline{9} \\ 1 \end{array}$$

Class Exercises

Express each percent as a decimal.

1. 39%   **2.** 4%   **3.** 150%   **4.** 0.8%   **5.** 1080%   **6.** 1%

Express each decimal as a percent.

7. 0.56   **8.** 0.005   **9.** 0.07   **10.** 1.6   **11.** 5.3   **12.** 0.0001

Express each of the following first as a decimal and then as a percent.

13. $\frac{1}{2}$ **14.** $\frac{1}{4}$ **15.** $\frac{3}{5}$ **16.** $2\frac{1}{2}$ **17.** $\frac{1}{1000}$ **18.** $\frac{23}{1000}$

Written Exercises

Express each percent as a decimal.

A
1. 93%
2. 46%
3. 114%
4. 175%

5. 260%
6. 1150%
7. 49.5%
8. 78.2%

9. 0.6%
10. 99.44%
11. 0.05%
12. 0.032%

Express each decimal as a percent.

13. 0.59
14. 0.87
15. 0.09
16. 0.075

17. 2.6
18. 10.6
19. 12.83
20. 5.01

21. 0.007
22. 0.033
23. 0.0867
24. 0.0026

Express each fraction as a decimal and then as a percent. Round to the nearest tenth of a percent if necessary.

B
25. $\frac{3}{8}$
26. $\frac{9}{125}$
27. $\frac{3}{500}$
28. $\frac{27}{40}$

29. $1\frac{5}{8}$
30. $2\frac{37}{40}$
31. $\frac{47}{80}$
32. $\frac{7}{11}$

33. $\frac{17}{24}$
34. $\frac{19}{12}$
35. $\frac{2}{7}$
36. $\frac{16}{9}$

Express each fraction as an exact percent.

EXAMPLE $\frac{1}{3}$

Solution Divide 1 by 3 to the hundredths' place: $1 \div 3 = 0.33$ R 1, or $0.33\frac{1}{3}$

Express the quotient as a percent: $0.33\frac{1}{3} = 33\frac{1}{3}\%$

Thus, as a percent, $\frac{1}{3} = 33\frac{1}{3}\%$.

C
37. $\frac{1}{6}$
38. $\frac{2}{3}$
39. $\frac{8}{9}$
40. $\frac{1}{15}$
41. $\frac{5}{6}$

Review Exercises

Solve.

1. $x + 2.47 = 5.42$
2. $x - 3.43 = 1.91$
3. $x \div 3.72 = 4.15$

4. $2.48x = 8.1096$
5. $x \div 4.03 = 5.92$
6. $1.37x = 11.4806$

6-8 Computing with Percents

The statement 20% of 300 is 60 can be translated into the equations

$$\frac{20}{100} \times 300 = 60 \quad \text{and} \quad 0.20 \times 300 = 60.$$

Notice the following relationship between the words and the symbols.

$$
\begin{array}{ccccc}
\underline{20\%} & \underline{of} & 300 & \underline{is} & 60 \\
\downarrow & \downarrow & & \downarrow & \\
\left.\begin{array}{c} \frac{20}{100} \\ \\ 0.20 \end{array}\right\} & \times & 300 & = & 60
\end{array}
$$

A similar relationship occurs whenever a statement or a question involves a number that is a percent of another number.

EXAMPLE 1   What number is 8% of 75?

Solution   Let n represent the number asked for.

$$
\begin{array}{ccc}
\underline{\text{What number}} & \text{is} & 8\% \text{ of } 75? \\
\downarrow & \downarrow & \downarrow \\
n & = & 0.08 \times 75
\end{array}
$$

6 is 8% of 75.

EXAMPLE 2   What percent of 40 is 6?

Solution   Let $n\%$ represent the percent asked for. We can translate the question into an equation as follows.

$$
\begin{array}{ccccc}
\underline{\text{What percent}} & \text{of} & 40 & \text{is} & 6? \\
\downarrow & \downarrow & & \downarrow & \\
n\% & \times & 40 & = & 6
\end{array}
$$

$$n\% \times 40 = 6$$

$$n\% = \frac{6}{40}$$

$$\frac{n}{100} = \frac{3}{20}$$

$$n = \frac{3}{20} \times 100 = 15$$

15% of 40 is 6.

EXAMPLE 3   140 is 35% of what number?

Solution   Let n represent the number asked for.

$$140 \quad\quad \text{is} \quad 35\% \quad \text{of} \quad \text{what number?}$$

$$140 \quad\quad = 0.35 \quad\quad \times \quad\quad n$$

$$140 = 0.35n$$

$$140 \div 0.35 = 0.35n \div 0.35$$

$$140 \div 0.35 = n$$

$$400 = n$$

140 is 35% of 400

Class Exercises

State an equation involving a variable that expresses the conditions of the question.

1. What number is 10% of 920?

2. What percent of 650 is 130?

3. 28 is 80% of what number?

4. 120 is what percent of 150?

5. 40% of 25 is what number?

6. What percent of 80 is 100?

7. 60 is 75% of what number?

8. What number is 125% of 160?

Written Exercises

Answer each question by writing an equation and solving it. Round your answer to the nearest tenth of a percent if necessary.

A **1.** What percent of 225 is 90?

2. What number is 76% of 350?

3. 45% of 600 is what number?

4. What percent of 150 is 48?

5. 52 is 4% of what number?

6. 56 is 4% of what number?

7. What number is 36% of 15?

8. 96% of 85 is what number?

9. What percent of 36 is 30?

10. 48 is what percent of 72?

B **11.** What is 110% of 95?

12. 0.5% of what number is 15?

13. 116% of 75 is what number?

14. What percent of 40 is 86?

15. What is 0.35% of 256?

16. 12 is 150% of what number?

Answer each question by writing an equation and solving it. Round your answer to the nearest tenth of a percent if necessary.

17. What percent of 21 is 24?

18. What is 81% of 60?

19. 12.5% of what number is 28?

20. What percent of 45 is 600?

C   21. 18 is $33\frac{1}{3}$% of what number?

(*Hint:* Write the percent as a fraction in lowest terms.)

22. What is $41\frac{2}{3}$% of 300?

23. 231 is $91\frac{2}{3}$% of what number?

Problems

Solve.

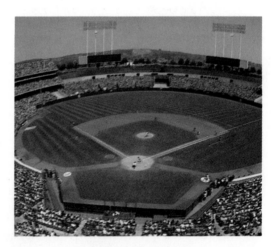

A   1. Lisa earns $250 a week and lives in a state that taxes income at 5%. How much does Lisa pay in state tax each week?

2. A baseball park has 40,000 seats of which 13,040 are box seats and 18,200 are reserved seats. What percent of the seats are box seats? Reserved seats?

3. A basketball player made 62 out of 80 free-throw shots. What percent of the free throws did she make?

4. A sweater is 65% wool by weight. If the sweater weighs 12.4 ounces, how much wool is in the sweater?

B   5. In a class of 40 students, 36 received passing grades on a geography test. What percent of the students in the class did not receive passing grades?

6. A service contract offered by a washing machine manufacturer can be purchased for 9% of the price of a washing machine. If a certain washer costs $580, what is the price of the service contract?

7. Of the 427 people responding to a public opinion poll, 224 answered *Yes* to a certain question and 154 answered *No*. What percent of those corresponding were undecided? Give your answer to the nearest tenth of a percent.

8. In 1979 the United States produced 3112 million barrels of oil. This was 13.7% of the world oil output. What was the world oil output to the nearest million barrels?

9. It is estimated that 60% of the people of the world live in Asia. If there are 2.4 billion people living in Asia, what is the population of the world?

C **10.** In a recent election, 45% of the eligible voters actually voted. Of these, 55% voted for the winner.
   a. What percent of eligible voters voted for the winning candidate?
   b. Suppose 495 people voted for the winner. How many eligible voters were there?

11. Of a city's 180,000 workers, 25% use the subway system. Of these, 18,000 use the subway between 7 A.M. and 9:30 A.M.
   a. What percent of the city's total number of workers ride the subway between 7 A.M. and 9:30 A.M.?
   b. What percent of the total number of subway riders use the subway between 7 A.M. and 9:30 A.M.?

Self-Test B

Express as a fraction in lowest terms or as a mixed number in simple form.

1. 27%	**2.** 83%	**3.** 164%	**4.** 290%	[6-6]

Express as a percent.

5. $\frac{1}{20}$	**6.** $\frac{3}{8}$	**7.** 4	**8.** $3\frac{1}{4}$

Express as a decimal.

9. 45%	**10.** 78%	**11.** 348%	**12.** 0.8%	[6-7]

Express as a percent.

13. 0.64   **14.** 0.81   **15.** 7.85   **16.** 0.068

17. What percent of 56 is 14?   **18.** 82 is what percent of 40?   [6-8]

19. What is 44% of 25?   **20.** 70% of what number is 84?

Self-Test answers and Extra Practice are at the back of the book.

Fibonacci Numbers

In the thirteenth century, an Italian mathematician named Leonardo of Pisa, nicknamed Fibonacci, discovered a sequence of numbers that has many interesting mathematical properties, as well as applications to biology, art, and architecture. Fibonacci defined the sequence as the number of pairs of rabbits you would have, starting with one pair, if each pair produced a new pair after two months and another new pair every month thereafter.

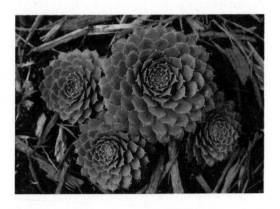

The diagram below illustrates the process that Fibonacci described for the first six months:

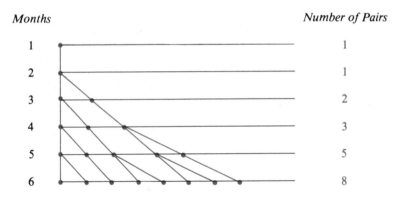

The sequence formed by the numbers of pairs is called the **Fibonacci sequence.** Note that any number in the sequence is the sum of the two numbers that precede it (for example, $2 + 3 = 5, 3 + 5 = 8$). Thus the sequence would continue:

1, 1, 2, 3, 5, 8, 13, 21, 34, 55, 89, 144, 233, 377, 610, . . .

To see one of the many mathematical properties of this sequence, study the sums of the squares of some pairs of consecutive Fibonacci numbers:

$$2^2 + 3^2 = 4 + 9 = 13$$
$$5^2 + 8^2 = 25 + 64 = 89$$
$$13^2 + 21^2 = 169 + 441 = 610$$

Note that in each case the sum is another number in the sequence.

The Fibonacci sequence also relates to a historically important number called the **Golden Ratio,** or the **Golden Mean.** The Golden Ratio is the ratio of the length to the width of a "perfect" rectangle. A rectangle was considered to be "perfect" if the ratio of its length to its width was the same as the ratio of their sum to its length, as written in the proportion at the right. If we let the width of the rectangle be 1, the length is the nonterminating, nonrepeating decimal 1.61803 . . . . Thus, the Golden Ratio is the ratio 1.61803 . . . to 1.

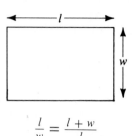

$$\frac{l}{w} = \frac{l + w}{l}$$

It is remarkable that the ratios of successive terms of the Fibonacci sequence get closer and closer to this number. For example,

$\frac{8}{5} = 1.6$ $\frac{13}{8} = 1.625$ $\frac{21}{13} = 1.615384\ldots$

$\frac{34}{21} = 1.61904\ldots$ $\frac{55}{34} = 1.61764\ldots$ $\frac{89}{55} = 1.61818\ldots$

1. Examine the fourth, eighth, twelfth, and sixteenth terms of the Fibonacci sequence. What do these numbers have in common? Try the fifth, tenth, and fifteenth terms.

Find some other numerical patterns by performing these calculations with the numbers in the Fibonacci sequence listed on the previous page. Tell what you notice about each new pattern.

2. Find the difference of two numbers that are two places apart in the sequence (the first and the third terms, the second and the fourth terms, the third and the fifth terms, and so on).

3. Subtract the squares of two numbers that are two places apart (as in Exercise 2).

4. Multiply two consecutive numbers (the first and second terms), multiply the next two consecutive numbers (the second and third terms), and then add the products.

5. Multiply two numbers that are two places apart (begin with the second and fourth terms), multiply two other numbers that "straddle" one of these (the first and third terms), and then add the products.

Career Activity Botanists have discovered that Fibonacci numbers occur naturally in many plant forms. For example, a pine cone is made up of 8 spirals swirling upward in one direction and 13 spirals swirling upward in the opposite direction. Find some other instances of Fibonacci numbers that botanists have found in nature.

Chapter Review

Match.

1. 2 min to 90 sec   2. 1 lb : 8 oz   **a.** 4 : 3   **b.** 22 mi/gal   [6–1]

3. 682 mi on 31 gal   **4.** 40 km in 30 min   **c.** 2 : 1   **d.** $1\frac{1}{3}$ km/min   [6–2]

Write the letter of the correct answer.

5. Solve $\frac{6}{x} = \frac{9}{75}$.   [6–3]

   a. 450   **b.** 54   **c.** 50   **d.** 37.5

6. A bicyclist went 7 mi in 30 min. How far would the cyclist go in   [6–4]
   45 min?

   a. 4.2 mi   **b.** 14 mi   **c.** $10\frac{1}{2}$ mi   **d.** $\frac{14}{3}$ mi

7. Three cans of paint will cover 80 m² of wall. What area will 5 cans
   cover?

   a. $133\frac{1}{3}$ m²   **b.** 48 m²   **c.** 1200 m²   **d.** 400 m²

8. A model truck has a scale of 1 cm : 25 cm. The model is 14 cm high.   [6–5]
   How high is the actual truck?

   a. 60 cm   **b.** 160 cm   **c.** 24 cm   **d.** 350 cm

9. On an engineering diagram the scale is 5 mm : 1 mm. A circuit
   measures 4 mm across. What is the length of the circuit in the
   drawing?

   a. 0.8 mm   **b.** 20 mm   **c.** 1.25 mm   **d.** 4 cm

Match.

10. 75%   **11.** $\frac{13}{20}$ **a.** 600%   **b.** 7.5%   [6–6]

12. 6   **13.** 0.6%   **c.** 65%   **d.** 60%

14. $\frac{3}{5}$ **15.** 0.075   **e.** 0.006   **f.** $\frac{3}{4}$ [6–7]

Write the letter of the correct answer.

16. What is 65% of 140?   [6–8]

    a. 215   **b.** 9100   **c.** 0.46   **d.** 91

17. 18 is what percent of 40?

    a. 222%   **b.** 0.45   **c.** 45%   **d.** 7.2%

Chapter Test

Express each ratio as a fraction in lowest terms.

1. 35 min : 3 h

2. 2 m to 85 cm

[6–1]

Give the unit price of each item.

3. 5 basketballs for $59.75

4. 12 oz of cereal for $1.32

[6–2]

Solve.

5. $\frac{n}{40} = \frac{3}{8}$

6. $\frac{24}{5} = \frac{x}{10}$

7. $\frac{5}{11} = \frac{20}{a}$

[6–3]

8. A car traveled 162 mi in 3 h. How many hours would it take to travel 351 mi?

[6–4]

9. On a map, 2 in. represents 300 mi. If two points are separated by 5 in. on the map, what is the actual distance between them?

[6–5]

Express as a fraction in lowest terms or as a mixed number in simple form.

10. 48%

11. 6%

12. 215%

13. 190%

[6–6]

Express as a percent.

14. $\frac{11}{20}$

15. $\frac{5}{8}$

16. 3

17. $2\frac{1}{8}$

Express as a decimal.

18. 93%

19. 42%

20. 259%

21. 0.86%

[6–7]

Express as a percent.

22. 0.81

23. 0.07

24. 2.91

25. 1.01

Solve.

26. What percent of 85 is 51?

[6–8]

27. 27 is what percent of 60?

28. What is 30% of 80?

29. 20% of what number is 25?

Cumulative Review (Chapters 1–6)

Exercises

Evaluate the expression when $x = 2$, $y = 3$, and $z = -2$.

1. $5y - 10$
2. $6x + 3y$
3. $2z + 6$
4. $8 - z$
5. $4xy \div (-2z)$
6. $3x + 3y \div z$
7. $5y \div (2 + y)$
8. $10x - (3y + 1)$
9. x^z
10. $2y^2$
11. $(2y)^2$
12. $(3x)^{-2}$

True or false?

13. $2.1(3 \times 4.7) = (2.1 \times 3)(2.1 \times 4.7)$
14. $9.51 + (-6.21) = (-6.21) + 9.51$
15. $1(-10.3) = 10.3$
16. $7.4 \times 0 = 0$

Write as equivalent fractions using the LCD.

17. $\frac{2}{3}, \frac{1}{5}$
18. $\frac{3}{4}, \frac{6}{7}$
19. $-\frac{1}{8}, \frac{1}{3}$
20. $\frac{7}{10}, -\frac{4}{9}$
21. $\frac{2}{5}, \frac{1}{6}, \frac{1}{4}$
22. $\frac{3}{11}, \frac{1}{2}, \frac{3}{4}$

Use transformations to solve each equation.

23. $x + 7 = 12$
24. $x - 3 = -6$
25. $6x = 18$
26. $-9x = 27$
27. $\frac{3}{4}x = 12$
28. $2x + 9 = 27$

Solve.

29. $\frac{x}{4} = \frac{2}{8}$
30. $\frac{x}{7} = \frac{9}{21}$
31. $\frac{3}{8} = \frac{24}{x}$
32. $\frac{48}{176} = \frac{8}{x}$
33. $\frac{13}{11} = \frac{3}{x}$
34. $\frac{148}{4} = \frac{x}{5}$

Complete.

35. A __?__ is a parallelogram with four equal sides.

36. If two lines are __?__ , they form four right angles.

37. A __?__ is a chord of a circle which is twice as long as the radius.

38. To the nearest hundredth, the ratio of the circumference of a circle to its diameter is __?__ .

242 Chapter 6

Problems

Problem Solving Reminders

Here are some reminders that may help you solve some of the problems on this page.

• Consider whether a chart will help to organize information.
• Supply additional information if needed.
• Reread the problem to be sure that your answer is complete.

Solve.

1. Donald bought a pair of hiking boots for $35.83, a sweater for $24.65, and a backpack for $18. The tax on his purchase was $.90. How much did Donald spend?

2. This week, Marisa worked $1\frac{1}{2}$ h on Monday, $2\frac{1}{4}$ h on Tuesday, $1\frac{1}{3}$ h on Wednesday, and $7\frac{1}{2}$ h on Saturday. How many hours did she work this week?

3. An airplane flying at an altitude of 25,000 ft dropped 4000 ft in the first 25 s and rose 2500 ft in the next 15 s. What was the altitude of the airplane after 40 s?

4. Carolyn Cramer spent 3 h 15 min mowing and raking her lawn. She spent twice as long raking as she did mowing. How long did she spend on each task?

5. At a milk processing plant 100 lb of farm milk are needed to make 8.13 lb of nonfat dry milk. To the nearest pound, how many pounds of farm milk are needed to produce 100 lb of nonfat dry milk?

6. A highway noise barrier that is 120 m long is constructed in two pieces. One piece is 45 m longer than the other. Find the length of each piece.

7. The perimeter of a rectangle is 40 m. The length of the rectangle is 10 m greater than the width. Find the length and the width.

8. Oak Hill School, Longview School, and Peabody School participated in a clean-up campaign to collect scrap aluminum. Oak Hill School collected 40% more scrap aluminum than Longview School. Longview School collected 25% more than Peabody School. If the total collected by the 3 schools was 560 kg, how much did Oak Hill School collect?

9. Eladio invested $200 at 6% annual interest and $350 at 5.75% annual interest, both compounded annually. If he makes no deposits or withdrawals, how much will he have after two years?

7

Percents and Problem Solving

The photograph shows a strand of DNA, or deoxyribonucleic acid, as seen through the center of the strand. In 1953 James Watson and Francis Crick developed a model for the DNA. They called it the double helix. In 1962 Watson and Crick were awarded the Nobel Prize in Medicine for their work with the double helix model.

According to the model, a strand of DNA is built much like a spiral staircase with phosphates and sugars forming the frame of the staircase. The four bases, adenine, guanine, thymine, and cytosine, form the steps. In analysis of DNA obtained from different organisms, it can be shown that the percentages of the four bases vary considerably. Thus, the sequence of the four bases are thought to determine individual heredity.

In this chapter, you will learn some interesting applications of percents to business, consumer, and financial situations.

Career Note

Chemists analyze the structure, composition, and nature of matter. They can specialize in a variety of fields from developing new products to organic analysis of moon rocks. Their work involves quantitative and qualitative analyses, as well as practical applications of basic research. A strong background in science and mathematics and an inquisitive mind are essential for this career.

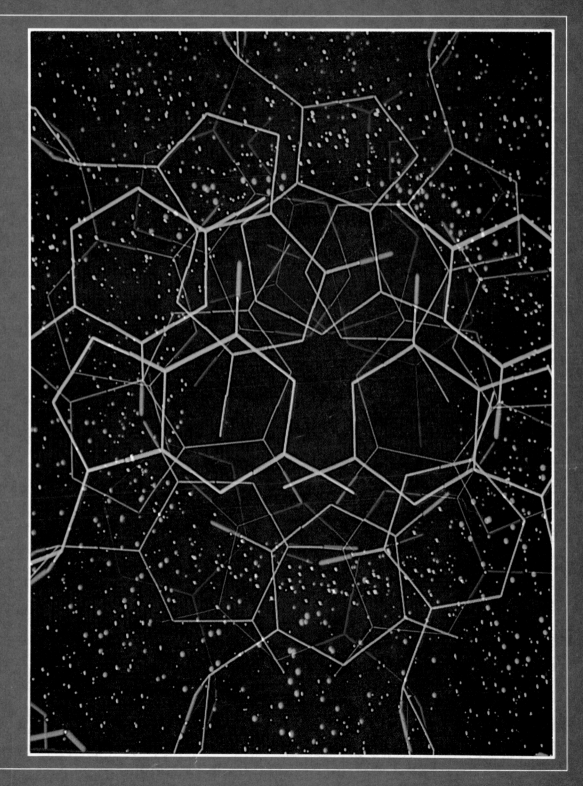

7-1 Percent of Increase or Decrease

A department store has a sale on audio equipment. An amplifier that originally sold for $260 is selling for $208. To find the **amount of change** in the price, we subtract the sale price from the original price.

$$\$260 - \$208 = \$52$$

To find the **percent of change** in the price we divide the amount of change by the original price and express the result as a percent.

$$\frac{52}{260} = 0.20 = 20\%$$

Formula

$$\text{percent of change} = \frac{\text{amount of change}}{\text{original amount}}$$

The denominator in the formula above is always the *original* amount, whether smaller or larger than the new amount.

EXAMPLE 1   Find the percent of increase from 20 to 24.

Solution   amount of change $= 24 - 20 = 4$

percent of change $= \dfrac{\text{amount of change}}{\text{original amount}} = \dfrac{4}{20} = 0.2 = 20\%$

The formula above can be rewritten to find the amount of change when the original amount and the percent of change are known.

Formula

amount of change = percent of change × original amount

EXAMPLE 2   Find the new number when 75 is decreased by 26%.

Solution   First find the amount of change.

amount of change = percent of change × original amount
$$= \quad 26\% \quad \times \quad 75$$
$$= 0.26 \times 75 = 19.5$$

Since the original number is being decreased, we subtract to find the new number. $75 - 19.5 = 55.5$

EXAMPLE 3 The population of Eastown grew from 25,000 to 28,000 in 3 years. What was the percent of increase for this period?

Solution The problem asks for the percent of increase.

amount of change $= 28{,}000 - 25{,}000 = 3000$

$$\text{percent of change} = \frac{\text{amount of change}}{\text{original amount}}$$

$$= \frac{3000}{25{,}000} = \frac{3}{25} = 0.12 = 12\%$$

The percent of increase was 12%.

Problem Solving Reminder

Sometimes *extra information* is given in a problem. The time period, 3 years, is not needed for the solution of the problem in Example 3.

Class Exercises

a. State the amount of change from the first number to the second.
b. State the percent of increase or decrease from the first number to the second.

1. 10 to 12	**2.** 4 to 3	**3.** 12 to 6	**4.** 6 to 12
5. 2 to 5	**6.** 5 to 7	**7.** 25 to 4	**8.** 1 to 4
9. 4 to 7	**10.** 100 to 55	**11.** 100 to 160	**12.** 125 to 100

Find the new number produced when the given number is increased or decreased by the given percent.

13. 120; 20% decrease	**14.** 30; 10% decrease
15. 48; 50% increase	**16.** 24; 25% increase

Written Exercises

Find the percent of increase or decrease from the first number to the second. Round to the nearest tenth of a percent if necessary.

A	**1.** 20 to 17	**2.** 25 to 12	**3.** 70 to 98	**4.** 16 to 10
	5. 40 to 73	**6.** 63 to 79	**7.** 32 to 17	**8.** 8 to 19
	9. 125 to 124	**10.** 160 to 380	**11.** 12 to 8.7	**12.** 240 to 245.5

Find the new number produced when the given number is increased or decreased by the given percent.

13. 165; 20% decrease   **14.** 76; 25% increase

15. 65; 12% decrease   **16.** 250; 63% decrease

17. 84; 145% increase   **18.** 260; 105% increase

19. 125; 0.4% decrease   **20.** 1950; 0.8% increase

Find the new number produced when the given number is changed by the first percent, and then the resulting number is changed by the second percent.

B **21.** 80; increase by 50%; decrease by 50%

  22. 128; decrease by 25% increase by 25%

  23. 150; increase by 40%; increase by 60%

  24. 480; decrease by 35%; decrease by 65%

  25. 350; increase by 76%; decrease by 45%

  26. 136; decrease by 85%; increase by 175%

Find the original number if the given number is the result of increasing or decreasing the original number by the given percent.

C **27.** 80; original number increased by 25%

  28. 63; original number increased by 75%

  29. 78; original number decreased by 35%

  30. 30; original number decreased by 85%

Problems

Solve. Round to the nearest tenth of a percent if necessary.

A **1.** The number of employees at a factory was increased by 5% from its original total of 1080 workers. What was the new number of employees?

  2. The cost of a basket of groceries at the Shopfast Supermarket was $62.50 in April. In May the cost of the same groceries had risen by 0.8%. What was the cost in May?

3. The attendance at a baseball stadium went from 1,440,000 one year to 1,800,000 the next year. What was the percent of increase?

4. The number of registered motor vehicles in Smalltown dropped from 350 in 1978 to 329 in 1979. What percent of decrease is this?

5. The new Maple City Library budget will enable the library to increase its collection of books by 3.6%. If the library now has 7250 books, how many will it have after the increase?

B 6. The number of students at Center State University is 22,540. Ten years ago there were only 7000 students. What is the percent of increase?

7. The annual budget of Brictown was $9,000,000 last year. Currently, the budget is only $7,500,000. Find the percent of decrease.

8. Last year the population of Spoon Forks grew from 1250 to 1300. If the population of the town grows by the same percent this year, what will the population be?

9. This year, Village Realty sold 289 homes. Last year the realty sold 340 homes. If sales decrease by the same percent next year, how many homes can Village Realty expect to sell?

C 10. Contributions to the annual Grayson School fund raising campaign were 10% greater in 1984 than they were in 1983. In 1983, contributions were 15% greater than they were in 1982. If contributions for 1984 total $8855, what was the total in 1982?

11. In July the price of a gallon of gasoline at Quick Sale Service Station rose 12%. In August it fell 15% of its final July price, ending the month at $1.19. What was its price at the beginning of July?

Review Exercises

Solve.

1. $p = 0.36 \times 27$

2. $1.89 = r \times 7$

3. $144.5 = 8.5n$

4. $21.65 \times 0.7 = m$

5. $156 = 0.3q$

6. $a \times 0.15 = 4.125$

7. $\frac{x}{21} = 10.5$

8. $91.53 \times 0.4 = t$

9. $\frac{324}{y} = 8100$

7-2 Discount and Markup

A **discount** is a decrease in the price of an item. A **markup** is an increase in the price of an item. Both of these changes can be expressed as an amount of money or as a percent of the original price of the item. For example, a store may announce a discount of $3 off the original price of a $30 basketball, or a discount of 10%.

EXAMPLE 1   A warm-up suit that sold for $42.50 is on sale at a 12% discount. What is the sale price?

Solution   *Method 1* Use the formula:

amount of change = percent of change × original amount
                 =   12%   ×   42.50
Therefore, the discount is 0.12 × 42.50, or $5.10.

The amount of the discount is $5.10.
The sale price is 42.50 − 5.10, or $37.40.

Method 2 Since the discount is 12%, the sale price is 100% − 12%, or 88%, of the original price. The sale price is 0.88 × 42.50, or $37.40.

As shown in the solutions to Example 1, when you know the amount of discount you subtract to find the new price. When dealing with a markup, you add to find the new price.

EXAMPLE 2   The price of a new car model was marked up 6% over the previous year's model. If the previous year's model sold for $7800, what is the cost of the new car?

Solution   *Method 1* Use the formula:

amount of change = percent of change × original amount
                 =   6%   ×   7800
Therefore, the markup is 0.06 × 7800, or $468.

The amount of the markup is $468.
The new price is 7800 + 468, or $8268.

Method 2 Since the markup is 6%, the new price is 100% + 6%, or 106%, of the original price. The new price is 1.06 × 7800, or $8268.

A method similar to the second method of the previous examples can be used to solve problems like the one in the next example.

EXAMPLE 3   This year a pair of ice skates sells for $46 after a 15% markup over last year's price. What was last year's price?

Solution   This year's price is 100 + 15, or 115%, of last year's price. Let n represent last year's price.

$$46 = \frac{115}{100} \times n$$

$$46 = 1.15 \times n$$

$$\frac{46}{1.15} = n$$

$$40 = n$$

The price of the skates last year was $40.

Example 4 illustrates how to find the original price if you know the discounted price.

EXAMPLE 4   A department store advertised electric shavers at a sale price of $36. If this is a 20% discount, what was the original price?

Solution   The sale price is 100 − 20, or 80%, of the original price. Let n represent the original price.

$$36 = \frac{80}{100} \times n$$

$$36 = 0.8 \times n$$

$$36 \div 0.8 = n$$

$$45 = n$$

The original price was $45.

Problem Solving Reminder

Be sure that your *answers are reasonable.* In Example 3, last year's price should be less than this year's marked-up price. In Example 4, the original price should be greater than the sale price.

We can use the following formula to find the percent of discount or the percent of markup.

$$\text{percent of change} = \frac{\text{amount of change}}{\text{original amount}}$$

For example, if the original price of an item was $25 and the new price is $20, the amount of discount is $5 and the percent of discount is $5 \div 25 = 0.2$, or 20%.

Class Exercises

Copy and complete the following table.

	Old price	Percent of change	Amount of change	New price
1.	$12	25% discount	?	?
2.	$60	10% markup	?	?
3.	$50	?	?	$60
4.	$120	?	?	$240
5.	$200	?	$30 markup	?
6.	$250	?	$100 discount	?
7.	?	12% discount	$48 discount	?
8.	?	5% markup	$2.50 markup	?
9.	?	20% discount	?	$160
10.	?	150% markup	?	$50

Problems

Solve.

A 1. A basketball backboard set that sold for $79 is discounted 15%. What is the new price?

2. A parka that sold for $65 is marked up to $70.20. What is the percent of markup?

3. A stereo tape deck that sold for $235 was on sale for $202.10. What was the percent of discount?

4. At the end-of-summer sale, an air conditioner that sold for $310 was discounted 21%. What was the sale price?

5. Because of an increase of 8% in wholesale prices, a shoe store had to mark up its new stock by the same percent. What was the new price of a pair of shoes that had sold for $24.50?

6. A department store has a sale on gloves. The sale price is 18% less than the original price, resulting in a saving of $2.97. What was the original price of the gloves? What is the sale price?

7. A coat that originally cost $40 was marked up 50%. During a sale the coat was discounted 50%. What was the sale price?

8. A 7% sales tax added $3.15 to the selling price of a pair of ski boots. What was the selling price of the boots? What was the total price including the tax?

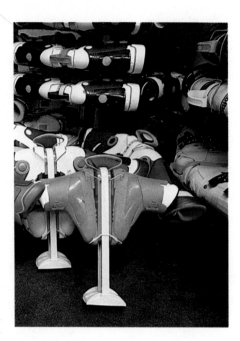

B **9.** A tape recorder that cost $50 was discounted 20% for a sale. It was then returned to its original price. What percent of markup was the original price over the sale price?

10. At an end-of-season sale a power lawnmower was on sale for $168. A sign advertised that this was 20% off the original price. What was the original price?

11. At a paint sale a gallon can of latex was discounted 24%. If the sale price of a gallon is $9.50, what was the original price?

12. The cost of a record album was $10.53, including an 8% sales tax. What was the price of the album without the tax?

C **13.** An item is discounted 20%. Then another 10% discount is given on the new price. What percent of the original price is the final price?

14. An item is marked up 20% and then discounted 15% based on the new price. What percent of the original price is the final price?

15. Which of the following situations will produce a lower final price on a given item?
  a. The item is marked up 30% and then discounted 30% of the new price.
  b. The item is discounted 30% and then marked up 30% of the new price.

Review Exercises

Complete.

1. circumference = $2\pi \times$ __?__

2. amount of change = __?__ $\times$ original amount

3. circumference = $\pi \times$ __?__

4. percent of change = $\dfrac{?}{\text{original amount}}$

7-3 Commission and Profit

In addition to a salary, many salespeople are paid a percent of the price of the products they sell. This payment is called a **commission.** Like a discount, a commission can be expressed as a percent or as an amount of money. The following formula applies to commissions.

> ### Formula
> amount of commission = percent of commission × total sales

EXAMPLE 1 Maria Bertram sold $42,000 worth of insurance in January. If her commission is 3% of the total sales, what was the amount of her commission in January?

Solution
amount of commission = percent × total sales
$$= 0.03 \times 42{,}000 = 1260$$

Her commission was $1260.

Profit is the difference between total income and total operating costs.

> ### Formula
> profit = total income − total costs

The **percent of profit** is the percent of total income that is profit.

> ### Formula
> $$\text{percent of profit} = \frac{\text{profit}}{\text{total income}}$$

EXAMPLE 2 In April, a shoe store had an income of $8600 and operating costs of $7310. What percent of the store's income was profit?

Solution
profit = total income − total costs = 8600 − 7310 = 1290

$$\text{percent of profit} = \frac{\text{profit}}{\text{total income}} = \frac{1290}{8600} = 0.15$$

The percent of profit was 15%.

Class Exercises

Copy and complete the following table.

	Total sales	Percent of commission	Amount of commission
1.	$3250	10%	?
2.	$680	20%	?
3.	$900	?	$225
4.	$2500	?	$125
5.	?	15%	$300
6.	?	10%	$14.50

a. State the amount of profit.
b. Give an equation that could be used to find the percent of profit.
c. Find the percent of profit.

7. Income $12,000; costs $9000

8. Income $10,000; costs $8700

9. Income $14,000; costs $12,600

10. Income $3000; costs $2850

11. Income $5000; costs $4950

12. Income $24,000; costs $16,800

13. Income $12,300; costs $9840

14. Income $105,360; costs $63,216

Problems

Solve.

A 1. Esther Simpson receives a 15% commission on magazine subscriptions. One week her sales totaled $860. What was her commission for the week?

2. The Greenwood Lumber Company had an income of $7680 for one week in May. If the company's profit for this period was 15% of its income, what were its costs for the week?

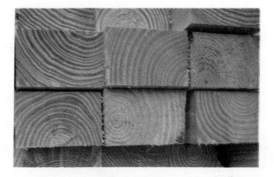

3. Margaret DeRosa's day-care service makes a profit of $222 per week. What are her costs if this profit is 18.5% of her total income?

4. Harvey Williams sold new insurance policies worth $5120 in August. If he receives a 4.5% commission on new policies, how much did he earn in commissions in August?

B 5. Sole Mates Shoes has expenses of $9592 per month. What must the store's total income be if it is to make a 12% profit?

6. The Top Drawer Furniture Company made a profit of $4360 in one month. What were its operating costs if this profit was 16% of its total income?

Nina Perez is a real estate agent who receives a commission of 6% of the selling price of each house she sells. The seller of the house pays Nina's commission out of the selling price and keeps the remainder. What should be the selling price of each house if the seller wants to keep the amount indicated below?

7. $61,000   8. $66,000   9. $55,000   10. $70,500

C 11. In May Sal's Bakery had operating costs of $6630 and made a profit of $1170. In June the operating costs are expected to be $6273. What must the bakery's income be if its profit is to remain the same percent of its income?

12. Each month Fran Parks receives a 6% commission on all her sales of barber supplies up to $15,000. She receives 8% commission on the portion of her sales that are above $15,000. Her commission for March was $1260. What were her sales?

13. Mildred Hofstadter receives a 5% commission on her sales of exercise equipment and a 6% commission on her sales of weight-training equipment. One month she sold $7900 worth of exercise equipment and made a total of $650 in commissions. How much were her sales of weight-training equipment that month?

14. Norman's Natural Foods has weekly expenses of $1075 and makes a profit of 14% of sales. If his weekly expenses increase to $1225 and he wants to make the same dollar profit as before, what percent of sales will this profit represent?

Review Exercises

Evaluate if $w = 8$, $x = 0.25$, $y = 0.8$, and $z = 5$.

1. wxz 2. xyz 3. $wx + yz$ 4. $wy - xz$

5. $(wyz) \div x$ 6. $(wy) \div (xz)$ 7. $0.2wx$ 8. $1.3wyz$

7-4 Percents and Proportions

In Chapter 6, you learned how to use a proportion to write a fraction as a percent. You can also use proportions to solve problems involving percents. The following discussion shows how we may write a proportion that relates percentage, rate, and base.

The statement *9 is 15% of 60* can be written as $9 = 15\% \times 60$. Because a percent is an amount *per hundred*, we can think of 15% as 15 per hundred, or the ratio of 15 to 100, $\frac{15}{100}$. Substituting, we can write the original statement as

$$9 = \frac{15}{100} \times 60.$$

Dividing both sides of the equation by 60, we obtain the proportion

$$\frac{9}{60} = \frac{15}{100},$$

or 9 is to 60 as 15 is to 100.

Note that $\frac{9}{60}$ is the ratio of the percentage (p) to the base (b).

Percentage, base, and rate are related as shown in the following proportion:

$$\frac{p}{b} = \frac{n}{100},$$

where $\frac{n}{100}$ is the rate expressed as an amount per hundred.

EXAMPLE 1   143 is 65% of what number?

Solution   The rate, 65%, expressed in the form $\frac{n}{100}$, is $\frac{65}{100}$.

The percentage, p, is 143. Write a proportion to find the base, b.

$$\frac{p}{b} = \frac{n}{100}$$

$$\frac{143}{b} = \frac{65}{100}$$

$$65b = 100 \times 143$$

$$b = \frac{14{,}300}{65} = 220$$

EXAMPLE 2   In a recent survey, 38 of 120 people preferred the Bright Light
disposable flashlight to other flashlights. What percent of the people surveyed preferred Bright Light?

Solution   The question asks what percent, or how many people per hundred,
prefer Bright Light.

Let n equal the number per hundred.
You know that p is 38 and b is 120.
Set up a proportion and then solve for n.

$$\frac{p}{b} = \frac{n}{100}$$

$$\frac{38}{120} = \frac{n}{100}$$

$$38 \times 100 = 120n$$

$$\frac{3800}{120} = n$$

$$n = 31\frac{2}{3}$$

In the survey, $31\frac{2}{3}\%$ of the people preferred Bright Light.

EXAMPLE 3   The price of a pocket cassette player has been discounted 25%. The
original price was $59. What is the sale price?

Solution   The question asks you to find the sale price.

First find the amount of the discount.
p is to be found, b is 59, and n is 25.
Set up a proportion and then solve for p.

$$\frac{p}{b} = \frac{n}{100}$$

$$\frac{p}{59} = \frac{25}{100}$$

$$100p = 59 \times 25$$

$$p = \frac{1475}{100} = 14.75$$

The amount of the discount is $14.75.

Next find the sale price.

$$59 - 14.75 = 44.25$$

The sale price is $44.25.

Class Exercises

For each exercise, set up a proportion to find the number or percent. Do not solve the proportion.

1. What percent of 32 is 20?

2. 14 is 25% of what number?

3. What is 58% of 24?

4. A digital clock is selling at a discount of 15%. The original price was $8.98. How much money will you save by buying the clock at the sale price?

5. Catherine answered 95% of the test questions correctly. If she answered 38 questions correctly, how many questions were on the test?

6. This year, 360 people ran in the town marathon. Only 315 people finished the race. What percent of the people finished the race?

Written Exercises

Use a proportion to solve.

A 1. What is 16% of 32?

     2. 306 is 51% of what number?

     3. What percent of 20 is 16?

     4. What is 104% of 85?

     5. 15 is 37.5% of what number?

     6. What percent of 72 is 18?

Problems

Use a proportion to solve.

A 1. The Plantery received a shipment of 40 plants on Wednesday. By Friday, 33 of the plants had been sold. What percent of the plants were sold?

2. The Eagles have won 6 of the 8 games they have played this season. What percent of this season's games have the Eagles won?

3. The library ordered 56 new books. 87.5% of the books are nonfiction. How many books are nonfiction?

4. This year 18.75% more students have joined the Long Hill High School Drama Club. The records show that 6 new students have joined. How many students were members last year?

5. A water purifier is discounted 20% of the original price for a saving of $6.96. What is the original price of the water purifier? What is the sale price?

6. The original price of a Sportsmaster 300 fishing pole was $37.80. The price has now been discounted 15%. What is the amount of the discount? What is the sale price?

B 7. Steve recently received a raise of 6% of his salary at his part-time job. He now earns $38.69 per week. How much did he earn per week before his raise?

8. Since the beginning of the year, the number of subscriptions to *New Tech Magazine* has increased by 180%. The number of subscriptions is now 140,000. What was the number of subscriptions at the beginning of the year?

EXAMPLE This **pie chart,** or **circle graph,** shows the distribution of the Valley Springs annual budget. Use a proportion to find the measure of the angle for the wedge for education.

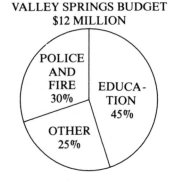

VALLEY SPRINGS BUDGET
$12 MILLION

Solution The number of degrees in a circle is 360°. The circle represents the total budget. 45% of the total budget is for education. Therefore,

$$\frac{45}{100} = \frac{n}{360}$$

$$100n = 45 \times 360$$

$$n = \frac{16,200}{100}$$

$$n = 162$$

There are 162° in the wedge for education.

Use proportions to answer these questions about the pie chart above.

9. a. What is the measure of the angle for the wedge for police and fire expenses?
   b. How much money is budgeted for police and fire expenses?

10. a. What is the measure of the angle for the wedge for other expenses?
   b. How much money is budgeted for other expenses?

For Exercises 11–13, (a) use a compass and protractor to draw a pie chart to represent the budget, and (b) use proportions to find the dollar value of each expense.

C 11. The monthly budget of the Miller family allows for spending 25% on food, 15% on clothing, 30% on housing expenses, 10% on medical expenses, and 20% on other expenses. Their total budget is $1800 per month.

12. The total weekly expenses of Daisy's Diner average $8400. Of this total, 20% is spent for employee's salaries, 60% is spent on food, 5% is spent on advertising, 10% is spent on rent, and 5% is used for other expenses.

13. The Chimney Hill school budget allows 72% for salaries, 8% for maintenance and repair, and 5% for books and supplies. The remainder is divided equally among recreation, after-school programs, and teacher training. The budget totals $680,000.

Self-Test A

Find the percent of increase or decrease.

  1. 12 to 15   2. 20 to 13   3. 200 to 246   [7–1]

  4. A sleeping bag that cost $85 is marked up 22%. What is the new price?   [7–2]

  5. A toy that had sold for $16.50 was on sale for $11.55. What was the percent of discount?

  6. A real estate agency charges a commission of 6% on sales. How much is the commission on a house that sells for $106,000?   [7–3]

  7. In August, Middle Mountain Mines had an income of $82,600. If profit for August was 12% of income, what were the company's costs that month?

Use a proportion to solve.

  8. What is 81% of 540?   9. 64 is what percent of 80?   [7–4]

  10. Of the traffic violations cited by Officer Huang, 64% were for speeding. If Officer Huang cited 48 motorists for speeding, how many violations were there altogether?

Self-Test answers and Extra Practice are at the end of the book.

7-5 Simple Interest

When you lease a car or an apartment, you pay the owner rent for the use of the car or the apartment. When you borrow money, you pay the lender **interest** for the use of the money. The amount of interest you pay is usually a percent of the amount borrowed figured on a yearly basis. This percent is called the **annual rate.** For example, if you borrow $150 at an annual rate of 12%, you pay:

$$\$150 \times 0.12 = \$18 \text{ interest for one year}$$
$$\$150 \times 0.12 \times 2 = \$36 \text{ interest for two years}$$
$$\$150 \times 0.12 \times 3 = \$54 \text{ interest for three years}$$

When interest is computed year by year in this manner we call it **simple interest.** The example above illustrates the following formula.

Formula

Let I = simple interest charged
   P = amount borrowed, or **principal**
   r = annual rate
   t = time in years for which the amount is borrowed

Then, interest = principal $\times$ rate $\times$ time, or $I = Prt$.

EXAMPLE 1   How much simple interest do you pay if you borrow $640 for 3 years at an annual rate of 15%?

Solution   Use the formula: $I = Prt$
$$I = 640 \times 0.15 \times 3 = 288$$

The interest is $288.

EXAMPLE 2   Sarah Sachs borrowed $3650 for 4 years at an annual rate of 16%. How much money must she repay in all?

Solution   Use the formula: $I = Prt$
$$I = 3650 \times 0.16 \times 4 = 2336$$

The interest is $2336.
The total to be repaid is the principal plus the interest: 3650 + 2336, or $5986.

Problem Solving Reminder

When solving a problem, be certain to *answer the question asked.* In Example 2, you are asked to find the total amount to be repaid, not just the interest. To get the total amount to be repaid, you must add the interest to the amount borrowed.

EXAMPLE 3 Renny Soloman paid $375 simple interest on a loan of $1500 at 12.5%. What was the length of time for the loan?

Solution Let t = time.

Use the formula: $I = Prt$
$$375 = 1500 \times 0.125 \times t$$
$$375 = 187.5t$$
$$\frac{375}{187.5} = t$$
$$t = 2$$

The loan was for 2 years.

EXAMPLE 4 George Landon paid $585 simple interest on a loan of $6500 for 6 months. What was the annual rate?

Solution Let r = annual rate.

Use the formula: $I = Prt$
$$585 = 6500 \times r \times \frac{1}{2}$$
$$585 = 3250r$$
$$r = \frac{585}{3250} = 0.18$$

The annual rate was 18%.

In Example 4 notice that the time, 6 months, is expressed as $\frac{1}{2}$ year, since the rate of interest in the formula is the *annual or yearly rate.*

Class Exercises

Give the simple interest on each loan at the given annual rate for 1 year, 3 years, and 6 months.

1. $100 at 8%

2. $200 at 12%

3. $5000 at 10%

4. $400 at 5%

5. $1500 at 6%

6. $100 at 8.4%

Find the annual rate of interest for each loan.

7. principal: $1100, time: 2 years, simple interest: $220

8. principal: $1600, time: $1\frac{1}{2}$ years, simple interest: $120

Find the length of time for each loan.

9. principal: $1200, interest rate: 6%, simple interest: $144

10. principal: $500, interest rate: 8%, simple interest: $30

Find the total amount that must be repaid on each loan.

11. principal: $200, interest rate: 15%, time: 2 years

12. principal: $600, interest rate: 9%, time: 3 years

Written Exercises

Find the simple interest on each loan and the total amount to be repaid.

A   1. $1280 at 15% for 2 years   2. $4250 at 12% for 3 years

3. $2760 at 18% for 1 year, 6 months   4. $3500 at 16% for 9 months

5. $5640 at 7.5% for 4 years   6. $7250 at 12.8% for $2\frac{1}{2}$ years

7. $6380 at 14.5% for 6 years   8. $14,650 at 16.4% for $3\frac{1}{2}$ years

Find the annual rate of interest for each loan.

9. $4360 for 2 years, 6 months; simple interest: $1526

10. $1240 for 3 years, 6 months; simple interest: $651

11. $2600 for 4 years; total to be repaid: $3484

12. $5760 for 2 years, 9 months; total to be repaid: $8532

13. $6520 for 3 years, 3 months; simple interest: $3390.40

14. $3980 for $4\frac{1}{2}$ years; total to be repaid: $7024.70

Find the length of time for each loan.

15. $3775 at 12%; simple interest: $226.50

16. $7850 at 6.5%; simple interest: $510.25

Find the original amount (principal) of the given loan.

EXAMPLE   9% for 4 years; total to be repaid: $7140

Solution   Let P = the original amount of the loan.

$$
\begin{aligned}
\text{amount to be repaid} &= P + Prt \\
&= P + P \times 0.09 \times 4 \\
&= P + 0.36P \\
&= P(1 + 0.36) \\
7140 &= 1.36P \\
P &= \frac{7140}{1.36} = 5250
\end{aligned}
$$

The original amount of the loan was $5250.

B **17.** 8% for $4\frac{1}{2}$ years; total to be repaid: $6052

18. 13.5% for 5 years; total to be repaid: $3417

19. 16% for 2 years, 3 months; total to be repaid: $9139.20

20. 12.4% for 3 years, 6 months; total to be repaid: $2222.70

21. 9.6% for 4 years; total to be repaid: $2560.40

22. 10.8% for 2 years, 9 months; total to be repaid: $4734.05

Solve.

C **23.** If the simple interest on $250 for 1 year, 8 months is $30, how much is the interest on $425.50 for 3 years, 4 months?

24. If $150 earns $28.75 simple interest in 1 year and 8 months, what principal is required to earn $747.50 interest in 2 years, 6 months?

Problems

Solve.

A **1.** Lois Pocket owns bonds worth $10,500 that pay 11% annual interest. The interest is paid semiannually in two equal amounts. How much is each payment?

2. A car loan of $4650 at an annual rate of 16% for 2 years is to be repaid in 24 equal monthly payments, including principal and interest. How much is each of these payments?

3. Gilbert White wants to borrow $2250 for 3 years to remodel his garage. The annual rate is 18%. If the principal and interest are repaid in equal monthly installments, how much will each installment be?

4. Fernando Lopez can borrow $5640 at 12.5% for 4 years, or he can borrow the same amount for 3 years at 15%. Find the total amount to be repaid on each loan. Which amount is smaller?

B 5. An education loan of $8400 for ten years is to be repaid in monthly installments of $122.50. What is the annual rate of this loan, computed as simple interest?

6. Will Darcy's three-year home improvement loan is to be repaid in monthly installments of $375.90 each. If the annual rate (as simple interest) is 14.4%, what is the principal of the loan?

C 7. In how many years would the amount to be repaid on a loan at 12.5% simple interest be double the principal of the loan?

8. At what rate of simple interest would the amount to be repaid on a loan be triple the principal of the loan after 25 years?

Review Exercises

Multiply. Round to the nearest thousandth if necessary.

1. $\frac{1}{2} \times 0.75$ 2. $\frac{1}{4} \times 0.3$ 3. $\frac{1}{5} \times 0.25$

4. $\frac{3}{4} \times 0.61$ 5. $\frac{4}{5} \times 1.87$ 6. $\frac{3}{10} \times 2.03$

7. $\frac{2}{3} \times 1.25$ 8. $\frac{7}{9} \times 2.375$ 9. $\frac{5}{6} \times 2.875$

▮▮▮ Calculator Key-In

Some calculators have a percent key. Use a calculator with a percent key to do the following exercises.

1. What is 8% of 200?   2. 35 is 20% of what number?

3. What percent of 75 is 36?   4. Express $\frac{17}{20}$ as a percent.

5. Express $\frac{13}{15}$ as a percent.   6. Express $\frac{7}{11}$ as a percent.

7-6 Compound Interest

If you deposited $100 in an account that paid 10% interest, you would have $10 interest after one year for a total of $110. You could then withdraw the $10 interest or leave it in the account. By withdrawing the interest, your principal would remain $100, and you would again receive simple interest. If, however, you left the $10 interest in the account, your principal would become $110, and you would accumulate **compound interest,** that is, interest on principal plus interest. The following chart illustrates these alternatives.

	Simple Interest		Compound Interest	
After	Interest	Principal	Interest	Principal
0 years	0	$100	0	$100
1 year	10% of $100 = $10	$100	10% of $100 = $10	$100 + $10 = $110
2 years	10% of $100 = $10	$100	10% of $110 = $11	$110 + $11 = $121
3 years	10% of $100 = $10	$100	10% of $121 = $12.10	$121 + $12.10 = $133.10
	Total interest: $30		Total interest: $33.10	

Notice that because the principal increases as interest is compounded, the total amount of interest paid on $100 after 3 years is greater than what is paid at the same rate of simple interest.

Interest is often compounded in one of the following manners.

monthly: 12 times a year
quarterly: 4 times a year
semiannually: 2 times a year

EXAMPLE If $500 is deposited in an account paying 8% interest compounded quarterly, how much will the principal amount to after 1 year?

Solution Use the formula $I = Prt$.

After 1 quarter:
$I = 500 \times 0.08 \times \frac{1}{4} = \$10$ $\qquad P = 500 + 10 = \$510$

After 2 quarters:
$I = 510 \times 0.08 \times \frac{1}{4} = \$10.20$ $\qquad P = 510 + 10.20 = \$520.20$

After 3 quarters:
$I = 520.20 \times 0.08 \times \frac{1}{4} \approx \$10.40$ $\qquad P = 520.20 + 10.40 = \$530.60$

After 4 quarters:
$I = 530.60 \times 0.08 \times \frac{1}{4} \approx \$10.61$ $\qquad P = 530.60 + 10.61 = \$541.21$

After you read an interest problem, ask yourself the following questions:
What is asked for, simple interest or compound interest?
What is the time period? For example, is it 3 months or 3 years?
Is the answer to be the interest, the new principal, or the total amount to be repaid?

Class Exercises

$8000 is deposited in a bank that compounds interest annually at 5%. Find the following.

1. The interest paid at the end of the first year

2. The new principal at the beginning of the second year

3. The interest paid at the end of the second year

4. The new principal at the beginning of the third year

5. The interest paid at the end of the third year

$1000 is invested at 12%, compounded quarterly. Find the following.

6. The interest paid after 3 months

7. The new principal after 3 months

8. The interest paid after 6 months

9. The new principal after 6 months

Written Exercises

How much will each principal amount to if it is deposited for the given time at the given rate? (If you do not have a calculator, round to the nearest penny at each step.)

A   1. $6400 for 2 years at 5%, compounded annually

2. $500 for 1 year at 8%, compounded semiannually

3. $1500 for 6 months at 8%, compounded quarterly

4. $8000 for 2 months at 6%, compounded monthly

5. $2500 for 18 months at 16%, compounded semiannually

6. $1280 for 9 months at 10%, compounded quarterly

7. $1800 for 1 year, 3 months at 14%, compounded quarterly

8. $3475 for $2\frac{1}{2}$ years at 6%, compounded semiannually

How much will each principal amount to if it is deposited for the given time at the given rate? (If you do not have a calculator, round to the nearest penny at each step.)

B **9.** $3200 for 3 years at 7.5%, compounded annually

10. $3125 for 3 months at 9.6%, compounded monthly

11. $8000 for 2 years at 10%, compounded semiannually

12. $6250 for 1 year at 16%, compounded quarterly

13. What is the difference between the simple and compound (compounded semiannually) interest on $250 in 2 years at 14% per year?

14. What is the difference between the interest on $800 in 1 year at 8% per year compounded semiannually and compounded quarterly?

C **15.** How long would it take $2560 to grow to $2756.84 at 10% compounded quarterly?

16. What principal will grow to $1367.10 after 1 year at 10% compounded semiannually?

Problems

Solve. (If you do not have a calculator, round to the nearest penny at each step.)

A **1.** The River Bank and Trust Company pays 10%, compounded semiannually, on their 18-month certificates. How much would a certificate for $1600 be worth at maturity?

2. Mike Estrada invested $1250 at 9.6%, compounded monthly. How much was his investment worth at the end of 3 months?

B **3.** Jennifer Thornton can invest $3200 at 12% simple interest or at 10% interest compounded quarterly. Which investment will earn more in 9 months?

4. Which is a better way to invest $6400 for $1\frac{1}{2}$ years: 16% simple interest or 15% compounded semiannually?

C **5.** A money market fund pays 12.8% per year, compounded semiannually. For a deposit of $5000, this compound interest rate is equivalent to what simple interest rate for 1 year? Give your answer to the nearest tenth of a percent.

7-7 Percents and Problem Solving

Percents are used frequently to express facts about situations we encounter. The skills acquired earlier for working with percents can be used to solve problems that are involved in these situations.

EXAMPLE 1 Eve Malik has a yearly salary of $27,600. She is paid in equal amounts twice a month. She and her employer each pay 6.7% of her salary to her social security account. What is the combined amount paid to social security for Eve each pay period?

Solution The problem asks for the combined amount paid to social security.
Given facts: yearly salary $27,600
                2 paychecks a month
                6.7% each for social security

2 payments a month for 12 months: $2 \times 12 = 24$ payments
$27,600 \div 24 = \$1150$, salary per payment
social security paid by each is 6.7% of $1150

$$0.067 \times 1150 = \$77.05$$

Combined amount paid to social security is $2 \times \$77.05$, or $154.10.

EXAMPLE 2 Property taxes in Jackson County are $1.42 per $100 of assessed value of the property. Assessed value is 60% of the actual market value. If taxes on a home are $681.60, what is the market value of the property?

Solution The problem asks for the market value.
Given facts: Taxes are $681.60
                Tax rate is $1.42 per $100 of assessed value.
                Assessed value is 60% of market value.

Divide $681.60 by $1.42 to find how many $100's are in the assessed value: $681.60 \div 1.42 = 480$
Assessed value is $480 \times 100 = 48,000$
Assessed value is 60% ($= 0.6$) of market value.

$$48,000 = 0.6 \times m$$

$$\frac{48,000}{0.6} = m$$

$$80,000 = m$$

The market value is $80,000.

EXAMPLE 3 Central Electric Co. charges $.055 per kW·h for the first 500 kW·h and $.05 per kW·h for the next 2000 kW·h. There is a discount of 2% for paying bills promptly. In March the Gronskis used 1450 kW·h. How much did they pay if they paid in time to receive the discount for prompt payment?

Solution The problem asks how much the Gronskis paid.

Given facts: Cost is $.55 per kW·h for the first 500 kW·h,
$.05 per kW·h for the next 2000 kW·h.
1450 kW·h were used.
Discount is 2%.

First find the total charge.
500 kW·h at $.055 each: $500 \times 0.055 = \$27.50$
$1450 - 500 = 950$
950 kW·h at $.05 each: $950 \times 0.05 = \$47.50$
Total charge: $\$27.50 + \$47.50 = \$75.00$

Since the discount is 2%, they only paid 100% − 2%, or 98%, of the actual charge.

$$75 \times 0.98 = 73.50$$

The Gronskis paid $73.50.

Problem Solving Reminder

In some problems, it is necessary to use several operations. Notice that Example 3 above required that the charge for the first 500 kW·h and the charge for the next 950 kW·h be found separately and then added to find the total charge. Finally, the discounted price was calculated.

Problems

Solve.

A **1.** Jim Damato charged $86.50 on his FasterCharge card and got a cash advance of $120. There is a finance charge of 1.5% on purchases and 1% on cash advances. How much was his total finance charge?

2. Esther Upperman invested $1250 in 50 shares of BU + U stock, which pays an annual dividend of $1.90 per share. Which investment gives a greater yield, the BU + U shares or a certificate of deposit that pays 7% interest?

3. A guitarist is to be paid a royalty of 6% of the selling price of a new album. If 46,000 copies of the album were sold at $7.95 each, how much should the guitarist be paid?

4. The publisher of *Lost in the Jungle* receives $12.60 from each copy sold. The remaining portion of the $15 selling price goes to the author. What royalty rate does the author earn?

5. At a clearance sale, a gas-powered lawn mower was discounted 32%. The lawn mower was sold for $117.81, including a sales tax of 5% of the sale price. What was the original price of the mower?

6. The Ransoms intend to reduce their electricity use by 15% in September. In August they used 2200 kW·h. Their electric company charges $0.062 per kW·h for the first 1000 kW·h, $0.055 per kW·h for the next 1000 kW·h, and $0.05 per kW·h for any additional use. How much can the Ransoms expect to save?

B 7. Anita Ramirez owns two bonds, one paying 8.5% interest and the other paying 9% interest. Every six months Anita receives a total of $485 in interest from both bonds. If the 8.5% bond is worth $4000, how much is the 9% bond worth?

8. Mike Robarts owns two bonds, one worth $3000, the other worth $5000. The $3000 bond pays 12% interest. Every 6 months, Mike receives a total of $530 interest from both bonds. What is the annual rate of the $5000 bond?

C 9. The property tax rate in Glendale is $2.15 per $100 of assessed value. Assessed value is 60% of market value. This year the Prestons' tax bill was $129 more than last year, when the market value of their house was $84,000. What is the present assessed value of their house?

10. In the primary election, 56% of eligible voters voted. Smith received 65% of the votes, Jones got 30%, and 5% of the voters chose other candidates. Smith won by a margin of 5488 votes over Jones. How many eligible voters are there?

11. David Cho deposited $10,000 in a six-month savings certificate that paid simple interest at an annual rate of 12%. After 6 months, David deposited the total value of his investment in another six-month savings certificate. David made no other deposits or withdrawals. After 6 months, David's investment was worth $11,130. What was the annual simple interest rate of the second certificate?

12. A savings account pays 5% interest, compounded annually. Show that if $1000 is deposited in the account, the account will contain

1000×1.05 dollars after 1 year.

$1000 \times (1.05)^2$ dollars after 2 years.

$1000 \times (1.05)^3$ dollars after 3 years, and so on.

Self-Test B

Solve.

1. A loan of $6400 at 12.5% simple interest is to be repaid in $4\frac{1}{2}$ years. What is the total amount to be repaid? [7-5]

2. A $6500 automobile loan is to be repaid in 3 years. The total amount to be repaid is $9230. If the interest were simple interest, what would be the annual rate?

3. You borrow $2500 at 16% interest, compounded semiannually. No interest is due until you repay the loan. If you repay the loan at the end of 18 months, how much will you pay? [7-6]

4. Julian Dolby invested $5000 in a special savings account that pays 8% interest, compounded quarterly. How long must Julian keep his money in the account to earn at least $250 in interest?

5. Mary Barnes earns $9.00 an hour. In 1984 she worked an average of 38 h a week. She pays 5% of her wages to a pension plan, and her employer pays an additional 7.2% of her wages to the same plan. How much was paid to the plan for Mary in 1984? [7-7]

Self-Test answers and Extra Practice are at the back of the book.

Credit Balances

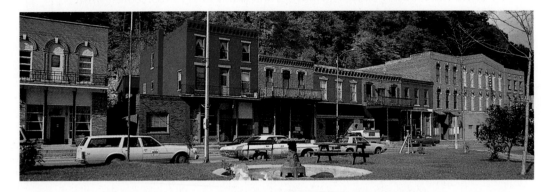

Before stores or banks issue credit cards, they do a complete credit check of the prospective charge customer. Why? Because issuing credit is actually lending money. When customers use credit cards they are getting instant loans. For credit loans, interest, in the form of a *finance charge,* is paid for the favor of the loan.

To keep track of charge account activity, monthly statements are prepared. The sample statement below is a typical summary of activity.

Customer's Statement Account Number 35–0119–4G			Billing Cycle Closing Date 9/22 Payment Due Date 10/17	
Date	**Dept. No.**	**Description**	**Purchases & Charges**	**Payments & Credits**
9/3 9/14 9/17	753 212	TOYS HOUSEWARES PAYMENT	30.00 12.50	 20.00

Previous Balance	**Payments & Credits**	**Unpaid Balance**	**Finance Charge**	**Purchases & Charges**	**New Balance**	**Minimum Payment**
40.99	20.00	20.99	.61	42.50	64.10	20.00

Statements usually show any finance charges and a complete list of transactions completed during the billing cycle. Finance charges are determined in a variety of ways. One common method is to compute the amount of the unpaid balance and make a charge based on that amount. Then new purchases are added to compute the new balance on which a minimum payment is due.

To manage the masses of data generated by a credit system, many merchants use computerized cash registers. The cash registers work in the following way. When a customer asks to have a purchase charged, the salesperson enters the amount of the purchase and the customer's credit card number into the computer. The computer then retrieves the account balance from memory, adds in the new purchase, and compares the total to the limit allowed for the account. If the account limit has not been reached, the transaction is completed and the amount of the new purchase is stored in memory. At the end of the billing cycle, the computer totals the costs of the new purchases, deducts payments or credits, adds any applicable finance charges, and prints out a detailed statement.

Copy and complete. Use the chart below to find the minimum payment.

	Previous Balance	Payments and Credits	Unpaid Balance	Finance Charge	Purchases and Charges	New Balance	Minimum Payment
1.	175.86	50.00	?	1.89	35.00	?	?
2.	20.00	20.00	?	0	30.00	?	?
3.	289.75	40.00	?	5.25	68.80	?	?
4.	580.00	52.00	?	8.00	189.65	?	?
5.	775.61	110.00	?	10.48	0	?	?

Solve.

6. Debra Dinardo is comparing her sales receipts to her charge account statement for the month. The billing cycle closing date for the statement is 4/18. Debra has sales receipts for the following dates and amounts.
3/30 $17.60   4/8 $21.54
4/16 $33.12   4/26 $9.75
On April 14, Debra paid the balance on her last statement with a check for $139.80. Her statement shows the information below. Is the statement correct? Explain.

New Balance	Minimum Payment
Up to $20.00	New Balance
$ 20.01 to $200.00	$20.00
$200.01 to $250.00	$25.00
$250.01 to $300.00	$30.00
$300.01 to $350.00	$35.00
$350.01 to $400.00	$40.00
$400.01 to $450.00	$45.00
$450.01 to $500.00	$50.00
Over $500.00	$50.00 plus $10.00 for each $50.00 (or fraction thereof) of New Balance over $500

Previous Balance	Payments & Credits	Unpaid Balance	Finance Charge	Purchases & Charges	New Balance	Minimum Payment
139.80	139.80	0	0	72.26	72.26	20.00

Research Activity Find out why stores and banks are willing to extend credit. How are the expenses of running the credit department paid for? Why do some stores offer discounts to customers who pay cash?

Chapter Review

Complete each statement.

1. The percent of increase from 24 to 30 is __?__. [7-1]

2. The percent of decrease from 50 to 37 is __?__.

3. The percent of increase from 76 to __?__ is 25%.

Write the letter of the correct answer.

4. A pair of shoes that regularly sells for $32 is on sale for $24. What is [7-2]
the percent of discount?

   a. $33\frac{1}{3}\%$ **b.** 25%   **c.** 8%   **d.** 125%

5. The Vico Manufacturing Company makes a 12% profit. If the com- [7-3]
pany sold $15,250 worth of goods in April, what was its profit?
   a. $13,420   **b.** $15,250   **c.** $1830   **d.** $18,300

6. The Ski Club has 50 members. If 36 members attend the ski trip, [7-4]
what percent attends the ski trip? Which of the following proportions could be used to solve this problem?

   a. $\dfrac{36}{100} = \dfrac{n}{50}$ **b.** $\dfrac{n}{100} = \dfrac{36}{50}$

True or false?

7. If George's aunt gives him a loan of $650 for one year at 12% simple [7-5]
interest, George will owe $728 at the end of the year.

8. An investment of $500 for 2 years at 12% simple interest will pay
more than one of $500 at $8\frac{1}{2}\%$ for 30 months.

Write the letter of the correct answer.

9. Lorraine Eldar invested $6000 at 8% interest compounded semian- [7-6]
nually. How long will it take her investment to exceed $7000?

   a. 1 year   **b.** $1\frac{1}{2}$ years   **c.** 2 years   **d.** $2\frac{1}{2}$ years

10. Anita Ramirez owns two bonds, one paying 8.5% interest and the [7-7]
other paying 9% interest. Every six months Anita receives a total of
$485 in interest from both bonds. If the 8.5% bond is worth $4000,
how much is the 9% bond worth?
   a. $7000   **b.** $4000   **c.** $1611.11   **d.** $10,777.78

Chapter Test

Solve.

1. Sam Golden's salary increased $30 a week. If his salary was $400 a week before the raise, by what percent did his salary increase? [7–1]

2. A clock ratio that sells for $30 is on sale at a 20% discount. What is the sale price? [7–2]

3. Edna's Autos sold $24,000 worth of cars last week. If Edna's costs were $16,800, how much profit did Edna make and what was the percent of profit? [7–3]

4. Computer Village had sales of $16,000 for December. The store's profits were $2880. What was the percent of profit?

Use proportions to solve Exercises 5 and 6.

5. The Pro Shop sold 6 of 20 tennis rackets in May. What percent of the tennis rackets were sold? [7–4]

6. This term, 36% of the students in one class are on the honor roll. If 9 students are on the honor roll, how many students are in the class?

Solve.

7. John Anthony borrowed $1200 for $1\frac{1}{2}$ years at 13% simple interest. How much must he repay when the loan is due? [7–5]

8. Joan Wu invested $5000 in an account that pays 13% simple interest. If the interest is paid 4 times a year, how much is each payment?

9. Billtown Bank pays 8% interest compounded quarterly. To the nearest penny, how much will $2500 earn in one year? [7–6]

10. You deposit money in a savings account and make no other deposits or withdrawals. How much is in the account at the end of three months if you deposit $350 at 6% interest, compounded monthly?

11. A major credit card charges a 1.5% interest rate each month on unpaid balances. If you were charged $8.50 in interest in June, what was your balance? [7–7]

Cumulative Review (Chapters 1–7)

Exercises

Evaluate the expression if $x = 3$ and $y = 5$.

1. $x + y$ **2.** $2x + y$ **3.** $2y - x$ **4.** $x + 6y$

5. $y + x + 4$ **6.** $-x - y$ **7.** $-3x - 2y$ **8.** $5x + (-y) - 7$

9. x^2 **10.** xy^2 **11.** $(-x)^2 y$ **12.** $-(xy)^2$

Write the numbers in order from least to greatest.

13. $3, -2.5, 0, -7, 6.4, -2.2$ **14.** $4, -6.2, -7.3, 0, 3.5, 2.5$

15. $-1.6, -8.4, -3, -1.0, 0.5$ **16.** $-4.7, -11.9, 1, 3.8, 0.7, -0.6$

Tell whether the statement is true or false for the given value of the variable.

17. $t - 3 \leq -6; \ -4$ **18.** $-m - 3 > 0; \ -3$ **19.** $2b < 3; \ 1$

20. $3 - x = 2; \ 5$ **21.** $n + 1 \geq -7; \ -6$ **22.** $r < -2r - 4; \ -2$

Write the fractions as equivalent fractions having the least common denominator (LCD).

23. $\frac{2}{3}, \frac{5}{9}$ **24.** $-\frac{3}{5}, \frac{7}{20}$ **25.** $-\frac{8}{3}, \frac{9}{11}$ **26.** $-\frac{5}{7}, -\frac{12}{17}$

27. $\frac{7}{3}, \frac{3}{4}$ **28.** $\frac{8}{45}, \frac{11}{75}$ **29.** $\frac{17}{32}, -\frac{3}{128}$ **30.** $\frac{3}{34}, \frac{5}{39}$

Solve.

31. $\frac{n}{4} = \frac{36}{12}$ **32.** $\frac{5}{n} = \frac{60}{12}$ **33.** $\frac{90}{n} = \frac{4}{8}$

34. $\frac{4}{6} = \frac{n}{30}$ **35.** $\frac{21}{28} = \frac{n}{84}$ **36.** $\frac{20}{10} = \frac{10}{n}$

State which of the rigid motions are needed to match the vertices of the triangles and explain why the triangles are congruent.

37.   **38.**   **39.**

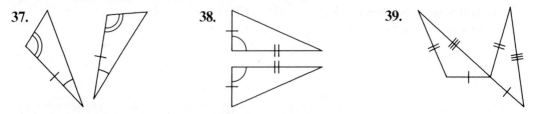

Problems

Solve.

1. The perimeter of an equilateral triangle is 45 cm. What is the length of each side?

2. A photographer works 35 h a week and earns $295. What is the hourly rate to the nearest cent?

3. Elena commutes to work. She travels 2.6 km by subway and 1.8 km by bus. How far is that in all?

4. The temperature at 11:30 P.M. was 7° below zero. By the next morning, the temperature had fallen 6°. What was the temperature then?

5. During one week, the stock of DataTech Corporation had the following daily changes in price: Monday, up $1\frac{1}{2}$ points; Tuesday, down 2 points; Wednesday, down $\frac{3}{4}$ of a point; Thursday, up $3\frac{1}{8}$ points; Friday, up $2\frac{3}{4}$ points. What was the change in the price of the stock for the week?

6. A rope 25 m long is cut into 2 pieces so that one piece is 9 m shorter than the other. Find the length of each piece.

7. A water purification device can purify 15.5 L of water in one hour. How many liters can it purify in $3\frac{3}{4}$ hours?

8. The Onagas have a wall at the back of their property. They want to fence off a rectangular garden using 7 m of the existing wall for the back part of the fence. If they have 15 m of fencing, what will be the length of each of the shorter sides?

9. Maria Sanchez gave 8% of her mathematics students a grade of A. If she had 125 students in her 4 classes, how many of these students received an A?

8

Equations and Inequalities

The trains pictured at the right were introduced in France. They can travel at speeds of up to 160 km/h on conventional tracks and nearly triple that on their own continuously welded tracks. The speed of a train on an actual trip depends, of course, on the number of curves and the type of track. A trip of 425 km from Paris to Lyon that takes about 4 h in a conventional train, for instance, can be completed in about 2.5 h in one of these trains.

The time it takes a train to complete a trip depends on the speed of the train and the distance traveled. Some relationships, such as the relationship between time, rate, and distance, can be expressed as equations. Other relationships can be expressed as inequalities. You will learn more about equations and inequalities and methods to solve both in this chapter. You will also learn how to use equations to help solve problems.

Career Note

Reporters representing newspapers, magazines, and radio and television stations often attend newsworthy events such as the introduction of new trains. Reporters need a wide educational background. They must report facts, not their own opinions. They must be willing to meet deadlines and often to work at irregular hours.

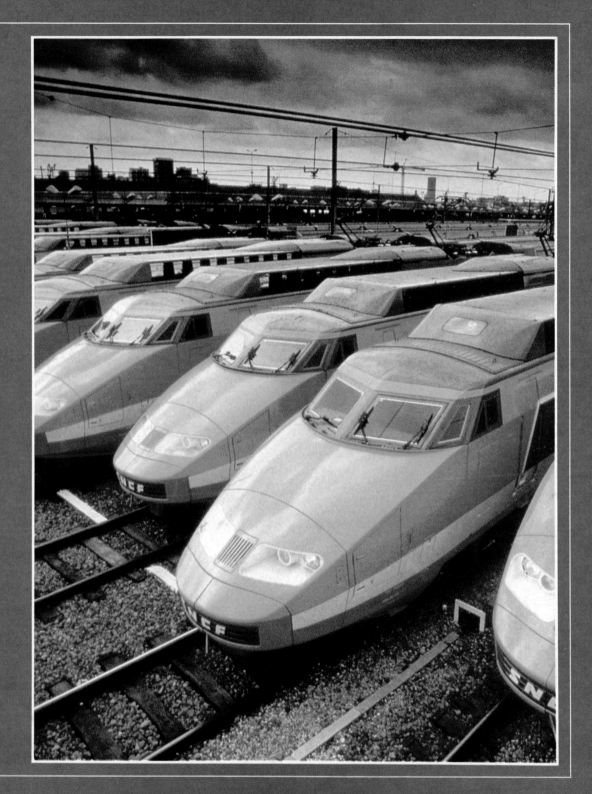

8-1 Equations: Variable on One Side

In Chapter 4, you learned the transformations that are used in solving equations. In this chapter, you will learn how these transformations can be used to solve more difficult equations.

Two terms are called **like terms** if their variable parts are the same. For example, x and $11x$ are like terms, as are $-4y$ and $7y$. Because their variable parts are different, $4x$, $3x^2$, and $6xy$ are not like terms.

We can use the properties of addition and multiplication to simplify expressions with like terms. To simplify $3a + 11 + 4a$, we use the commutative and distributive properties.

$$3a + 11 + 4a = (3a + 4a) + 11$$
$$= (3 + 4)a + 11$$
$$= 7a + 11$$

The terms $7a$ and 11 cannot be combined because they are not like terms. When an expression is in *simplest form,* it contains no like terms.

We can use the distributive property $a(b + c) = ab + ac$ to simplify certain variable expressions that involve parentheses.

EXAMPLE 1   Simplify $-2(x - 6) + 8x$.

Solution
$$-2(x - 6) + 8x = -2x + 12 + 8x$$
$$= -2x + 8x + 12$$
$$= 6x + 12$$

These procedures may be used when solving an equation.

EXAMPLE 2   Solve $2x + 15 + 8x = 20$.

Solution
$$2x + 15 + 8x = 20$$
$$2x + 8x + 15 = 20$$
$$10x + 15 = 20$$
$$10x + 15 - 15 = 20 - 15$$
$$10x = 5$$
$$\frac{10x}{10} = \frac{5}{10}$$
$$x = \frac{1}{2}$$

The solution is $\frac{1}{2}$.

EXAMPLE 3 Solve $3(x + 3) + 6x = 12$.

Solution

$$3(x + 3) + 6x = 12$$
$$3x + 9 + 6x = 12$$
$$3x + 6x + 9 = 12$$
$$9x + 9 = 12$$
$$9x + 9 - 9 = 12 - 9$$
$$9x = 3$$
$$\frac{9x}{9} = \frac{3}{9}$$
$$x = \frac{1}{3}$$

The solution is $\frac{1}{3}$.

Class Exercises

Which pairs of terms are like terms?

1. $7a, 12a$
2. $4x, -6x$
3. $3r, 4rs$
4. $6a, 6b$
5. $-8y, y$
6. $-11, -11x$
7. $a^2, 7a$
8. $3a^2, 3a$

Simplify.

9. $4c + 7c$
10. $13y - 8y$
11. $z - 7z$
12. $2t + t + 4t$
13. $-5x + 6x - x$
14. $4p - p + 5p$
15. $2(b + 5)$
16. $-3(x + 7)$
17. $9(c - 4)$
18. $4(n + 4) + 3$
19. $-5(x - 1) - 6$
20. $3(y + 4) + 2y$
21. $12(d - 4) - 10d$
22. $-10(p - 3) + 6p$
23. $15(y + 1) + 10(y - 2)$

Written Exercises

Simplify.

A

1. $10m - 8m$
2. $-3a + 11a$
3. $-8c + c$
4. $-3n + 8 + 8n$
5. $-5 + 6c - 5c$
6. $12 + 10z - 12z$
7. $-7(y - 11)$
8. $6(n + 3) + 2n$
9. $-10(a + 3) + 6a$
10. $8(p + 4) + 6(p - 3)$
11. $4(x - 3) + 2(x - 1)$
12. $-5(n - 5) + 7(n + 1)$

Solve.

13. $4x + 8x = 6$ **14.** $5z - 7z = -4$ **15.** $-2y + 6y = 36$

16. $p - 10p = -27$ **17.** $-7c - 9c = 20$ **18.** $-z - 10z = -3$

19. $3n + 2n - 8 = 17$ **20.** $-6a + 7a - 3 = 8$ **21.** $-x + 9 - 5x = 12$

22. $4t - 8 + 8t = 32$ **23.** $5 - 4y - 7y = 16$ **24.** $-7 + 3n + 9n = 29$

25. $12 = 8y + 16y$ **26.** $-9 = 3y - 9y$ **27.** $15 = x + 6 - 10x$

28. $-4 = 3z - 10 + 4z$ **29.** $-14 = 6 + z - 9z$ **30.** $3 = t - 4t + 15$

B **31.** $2(x + 1) = 4$ **32.** $-3(y + 4) = -6$ **33.** $8(t - 1) = -16$

34. $-7(c - 3) = 35$ **35.** $3(7 - p) = 3$ **36.** $-6(4 - z) = 20$

37. $2(n + 4) + 6n = 2$ **38.** $6(c - 2) + 4c = 8$ **39.** $-5(d + 3) - 7d = 5$

40. $-4(x - 5) - 16x = 10$ **41.** $2(3 - y) + 6y = 12$ **42.** $-3(2 - z) - 8z = 15$

C **43.** $3(a + 2) - (a - 1) = 17$ **44.** $5(c - 3) - (5 - c) = 0$

45. $4(p + 2) - 2(1 - p) - 4p = 0$ **46.** $5(v - 2) - 2(v + 4) = 6$

47. $2(y - 5) + 7 = 4(y + 7) - 3$ **48.** $-3(x + 2) + 3 = 5(x - 1) + 10$

Review Exercises

Solve.

1. $\dfrac{n}{4} = \dfrac{8}{32}$ **2.** $\dfrac{n}{48} = \dfrac{5}{6}$ **3.** $\dfrac{6}{n} = \dfrac{24}{60}$

4. $\dfrac{50}{n} = \dfrac{5}{15}$ **5.** $\dfrac{2}{11} = \dfrac{n}{66}$ **6.** $\dfrac{1}{6} = \dfrac{n}{18}$

7. $\dfrac{2}{3} = \dfrac{7}{n}$ **8.** $\dfrac{12}{84} = \dfrac{1}{n}$ **9.** $\dfrac{36}{n} = \dfrac{72}{8}$

■■■ **Challenge**

Fill in the blanks.

1. 6, 10, 15, 21, __?__, 36, 45   **2.** 103, __?__, 305, 406, 507

3. 5, 3, 4, 2, __?__, 1, 2   **4.** 132, 243, 354, 465, __?__

5. 17, 16, 18, __?__, 19, 14, 20, 13   **6.** 6, 11, 21, 41, __?__

8-2 Equations: Variable on Both Sides

Some equations have variables on each side. To solve such an equation, add a variable expression to each side, or subtract a variable expression from each side.

EXAMPLE 1 Solve $8c = c + 14$.

Solution Subtract c from both sides.

$$8c = c + 14$$
$$8c - c = c + 14 - c$$
$$7c = 14$$
$$\frac{7c}{7} = \frac{14}{7}$$
$$c = 2$$

The solution is 2.

EXAMPLE 2 Solve $7c = 3 - 2c$.

Solution Add $2c$ to both sides.

$$7c = 3 - 2c$$
$$7c + 2c = 3 - 2c + 2c$$
$$9c = 3$$
$$\frac{9c}{9} = \frac{3}{9}$$
$$c = \frac{1}{3}$$

The solution is $\frac{1}{3}$.

EXAMPLE 3 Solve $2(a - 3) = 5(a + 3)$.

Solution

$$2(a - 3) = 5(a + 3)$$
$$2a - 6 = 5a + 15$$
$$2a - 6 + 6 = 5a + 15 + 6$$
$$2a = 5a + 21$$
$$2a - 5a = 5a + 21 - 5a$$
$$-3a = 21$$
$$\frac{-3a}{-3} = \frac{21}{-3}$$
$$a = -7$$

The solution is -7.

Class Exercises

Solve.

1. $2y = y + 1$ **2.** $t + 3 = 2t$ **3.** $4a + 2 = 5a$ **4.** $3n + 5 = 4n$

5. $a - 1 = 2a$ **6.** $6p = 5p - 4$ **7.** $2a - 7 = 3a$ **8.** $6t + 1 = 7t$

Written Exercises

Solve.

A   **1.** $6c = 4c + 10$ **2.** $13z = 15 + 8z$ **3.** $49 + a = 8a$

     4. $8x + 16 = 4x$ **5.** $7y = 5y - 12$ **6.** $17t = 8t - 36$

     7. $32y = 24y - 4$ **8.** $17z = 15z - 3$ **9.** $3s = -6s - 36$

     10. $-14p = 6p + 10$ **11.** $11n + 9 = -4n$ **12.** $-4x + 6 = -2x$

     13. $2c + 6 = 5c - 6$ **14.** $6y + 3 = 8y + 2$ **15.** $-3d - 8 = 7d + 17$

     16. $10a - 1 = 2a - (-5)$ **17.** $15 - 7x = 8x - 30$ **18.** $y - 11 = 24 - 9y$

B   **19.** $2(x + 1) = 4x$ **20.** $-3(y + 4) = -6y$ **21.** $8(t - 1) = -16t$

     22. $-5(d + 3) = 7d + 5$ **23.** $6(c - 2) + 4c = 8c$ **24.** $-4(x - 5) = 16x + 10$

     25. $6(d + 1) = 4(d + 2)$ **26.** $8(p + 4) = 6(p - 2)$

     27. $-2(c - 3) = 4(c + 6)$ **28.** $-2(x - 4) = 5(x - 2)$

     29. $10(y + 2) + 4 = 6(y - 3) + 8$ **30.** $-12(x + 3) + 2 = 6(x - 1) + 8$

C   **31.** $\frac{1}{2}(x + 4) = \frac{1}{4}(x - 8)$ **32.** $\frac{1}{3}(y - 6) = \frac{2}{9}(y + 18)$

     33. $\frac{2}{5}(a + 10) = \frac{1}{4}(a + 20)$ **34.** $\frac{5}{8}(t - 24) = \frac{1}{4}(t + 12)$

     35. $\frac{9}{10}(n - 30) = \frac{1}{2}(n + 10)$ **36.** $\frac{1}{3}(p + 21) = \frac{1}{6}(p - 9)$

Review Exercises

Use inverse operations to solve.

1. $x + 8 = 12$ **2.** $x + (-5) = -3$ **3.** $x - 5 = 1$ **4.** $x - (-3) = 4$

5. $6x = 72$ **6.** $-9x = 81$ **7.** $\frac{x}{4} = 6$ **8.** $-\frac{x}{7} = 11$

8-3 Equations in Problem Solving

The five-step method that was shown in Chapter 4 may be applied with the procedures shown in this chapter.

Solving a Word Problem Using an Equation

Step 1   Read the problem carefully. Make sure that you understand what it says. You may need to read it more than once.

Step 2   Decide what numbers are asked for. Choose a variable and use it to represent the number(s) asked for.

Step 3   Write an equation based on the given conditions.

Step 4   Solve the equation and find the required number(s).

Step 5   Check your results with the words of the problem. Give the answer.

EXAMPLE 1   An electrician has a length of wire that is 120 m long. The wire is cut into two pieces, one 30 m longer than the other. Find the lengths of the two pieces of wire.

Solution

- The problem says: length of wire is 120 m, one piece is 30 m longer than the other

- The problem asks for: the lengths of the two pieces of wire
  Let l = the length of shorter piece of wire.
  The length of the other piece of wire = $l + 30$.

- We set the sum of the lengths $(l + l + 30)$ equal to 120.

$$l + l + 30 = 120$$

- Solve.

$$l + l + 30 = 120$$
$$2l + 30 = 120$$
$$2l + 30 - 30 = 120 - 30$$
$$2l = 90$$
$$\frac{2l}{2} = \frac{90}{2}$$
$$l = 45, \; l + 30 = 75$$

- Check: $45 + 75 = 120$, and $75 - 45 = 30$. The result checks.

The lengths are 45 m and 75 m.

EXAMPLE 2   The sum of two consecutive integers is 137. Name the larger integer.

Solution

- The problem says: the sum of two consecutive integers is 137

- The problem asks for: the larger of the two integers

    Let n = the smaller integer.
    Then the larger integer = $n + 1$.
    The sum of the two integers is $n + n + 1$.
    The sum of the two integers is 137.

- We set the expression for the sum of the two integers $(n + n + 1)$ equal to 137.

$$n + n + 1 = 137$$

- Solve.
$$n + n + 1 = 137$$
$$2n + 1 = 137$$
$$2n + 1 - 1 = 137 - 1$$
$$2n = 136$$
$$\frac{2n}{2} = \frac{136}{2}$$
$$n = 68$$
$$n + 1 = 69$$

- Check: $68 + 69 = 137$.

    The larger integer is 69.

Reading Mathematics: Study Skills

When you find a reference in the text to material you learned earlier, reread the material in the earlier lesson to help you understand the new lesson. For example, page 287 includes a reference to the five-step method learned in Chapter 4. Turn back to Chapter 4 to review how the five-step method was used.

Problems

Solve.

A   1. A 40 ft board is cut into two pieces so that one piece is 8 ft longer than the other piece. Find the lengths of the two pieces.

2. The sum of two numbers is 60. One number is 16 less than the other number. What is the larger number?

3. Marisa Gonzalez is training for a cross-country race. Yesterday, it took her 80 minutes to jog to the reservoir and back. The return trip took 10 minutes longer than the trip to the reservoir. How long did it take her each way?

4. Mark Johnson's weight is 18 kg greater than his sister's. If they weigh a total of 110 kg, what are their weights?

5. The perimeter of an isosceles triangle is 50 cm. If the congruent sides of the triangle are each twice as long as the remaining side, what is the length of each side of the triangle?

6. Find two consecutive integers whose sum is 115.

7. West High School defeated Central High by eleven points in the city championship basketball game. If a total of 159 points were scored in the game, how many points did Central High score?

8. Together, a table and a set of four chairs cost $499. If the table costs $35 more than the set of chairs, what is the cost of the table?

B 9. A 50 ft rope is cut into two pieces. One piece is 2 ft longer than twice the length of the other. Find the length of the longer piece.

10. Twice the sum of two consecutive integers is 42. What are the two integers?

11. A collection of jewelry includes two rings, one 18 years old and the other 46 years old. In how many years will the older ring be twice as old as the newer ring?

12. Neil is 4 years older than Andrea. If Neil was twice as old as Andrea four years ago, how old was Andrea?

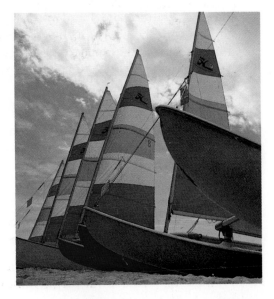

C 13. A sailing race takes place on a 3000 m course. The second leg of the course is 100 m longer than the first, and the third leg is 100 m longer than the second. How long is the second leg?

14. A teller's supply of dimes and nickels totals $3.60. If the teller's supply of dimes numbers one more than three times the number of nickels, how many dimes are there?

Self-Test A

Solve.

1. $3x + 9x = 48$

2. $2a - 4a = 1$ [8-1]

3. $-y + 6 - 5y = 18$

4. $6 - z - 4z = -4$

5. $5(y - 6) = -60$

6. $-4(x - 3) - 6x = 10$

7. $2(z - 4) - z = 8$

8. $-4(n + 3) + 2n = 6$

9. $3c = c + 10$

10. $9t = 4t - 20$ [8-2]

11. $3p - 1 = 8p + 9$

12. $3(a + 1) = 19 - 5a$

13. $2(p - 1) = 5(p + 2)$

14. $-4(t + 2) = 5(t - 3)$

15. $3(c + 4) + c = 2(c - 5)$

16. $5(x - 3) = 3(x + 5) - 2x$

17. A 60 ft long piece of chain link fence is cut into two pieces, one   [8-3] twice as long as the other. What is the length of the shorter piece?

18. The sum of two consecutive integers is 211. What is the larger integer?

Self-Test answers and Extra Practice are at the back of the book.

▮▮▮ Challenge

Flanders, Fulton, and Farnsworth teach two subjects each in a small junior high school. The courses are mathematics, science, carpentry, music, social studies, and English.

1. The carpentry and music teachers are next-door neighbors.

2. The science teacher is older than the mathematics teacher.

3. The teachers ride together going to school and coming home. Farnsworth, the science teacher, and the music teacher each drive one week out of three.

4. Flanders is the youngest.

5. When they can find another player, the English teacher, the mathematics teacher, and Flanders spend their lunch period playing bridge.

What subjects does each teach?

8-4 Writing Inequalities

In previous chapters, you have learned how to use the *inequality symbols* < (less than) and > (greater than). Sentences written using these symbols are called **inequalities.**

EXAMPLE   Write an inequality for each word sentence.

> **a.** Two is less than ten.
> **b.** A number $2 + x$ is greater than a number t.
> **c.** A number n is between 6 and 12.

Solution   **a.** $2 < 10$
b. $2 + x > t$
c. $6 < n < 12$, or $12 > n > 6$

Class Exercises

Suppose the numbers given in Exercises 1–6 have been graphed on a number line. Replace the first __?__ with "left" or "right." Replace the second __?__ with < or >.

1. The graph of 9 is to the __?__ of the graph of 2.   9 __?__ 2

2. The graph of 4 is to the __?__ of the graph of 7.   4 __?__ 7

3. The graph of 3 is to the __?__ of the graph of 8.   3 __?__ 8

4. The graph of 10 is to the __?__ of the graph of 0.   10 __?__ 0

5. The graph of 0 is to the __?__ of the graph of 5.   0 __?__ 5

6. The graph of 6 is to the __?__ of the graph of 1.   6 __?__ 1

Written Exercises

Write an inequality for each word sentence.

A   1. Twelve is less than twenty-two.   2. Nineteen is greater than nine.

3. Six is greater than zero.   4. Twenty-two is less than thirty-three.

5. On a number line eight is between zero and ten.

B   6. On a number line twenty-five is between fifty-two and five.

Pictured below is a portion of a number line showing the graph of a whole number *m*. Copy this number line and graph each of the following numbers.

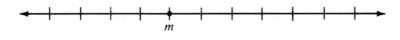

7. $m + 1$ **8.** $m - 2$ **9.** $m + 2 - 3$ **10.** $m - 2 + 3$

Write an inequality for each word sentence.

11. Six is greater than a number *t*.

12. Twenty-seven is less than a number $3m$.

13. A number *p* is greater than a number *q*.

14. A number *a* is less than a number *b*.

15. The value in cents of *d* dimes is less than the value in cents of *n* nickels.

16. The value in cents of *m* pennies is greater than the value in cents of *y* quarters.

17. On a number line a number $2n$ is between 6 and 8.

18. On a number line a number $r + 1$ is between 10 and 4.

19. On a number line a number *a* is between a number *x* and a number *y*, where $x < y$.

20. On a number line a number $4x$ is between a number *m* and a number *n*, where $m > n$.

C **21.** On a number line 6 is between 2 and 10, and 20 is between 10 and 50.

22. On a number line a number *x* is between 0 and 10, and a number *y* is between 10 and 14.

23. On a number line 5 is between a number *a* and a number *b*, where $a < b$, and 8 is also between *a* and *b*.

Review Exercises

Solve using transformations.

1. $x + 4 = 9$ **2.** $x + 11 = 14$ **3.** $x - 3 = 2$ **4.** $x - 6 = -4$

5. $4x = 36$ **6.** $-5x = 70$ **7.** $\frac{x}{7} = 11$ **8.** $-\frac{x}{5} = 6$

8-5 Equivalent Inequalities

To solve an inequality, we transform the inequality into an **equivalent inequality.** The transformations that we use are similar to those we use to solve equations.

> Simplify numerical expressions and variable expressions.
>
> Add the same number to, or subtract the same number from, both sides of the inequality.
>
> Multiply or divide both sides of the inequality by the same *positive* number.
>
> Multiply or divide both sides of the inequality by the same *negative number and reverse the inequality sign.*

Notice that we do not multiply the sides of an inequality by 0.

It is easy to see that when the inequality $-6 < 5$ is multiplied by 2, the inequality sign does not change. The following shows why we must reverse the inequality sign when multiplying or dividing by a negative number.

$$-6 < 5$$
$$-2(-6) \ ? \ -2(5)$$
$$12 > -10$$

EXAMPLE 1 Solve each inequality.
  a. $x + 7 \leq -18$ **b.** $y - 4.5 > 32$

Solution **a.** Subtract 7 from both sides of the inequality.

$$x + 7 \leq -18$$
$$x + 7 - 7 \leq -18 - 7$$
$$x \leq -25$$

The solutions are all the numbers less than or equal to -25.

b. Add 4.5 to both sides of the inequality.

$$y - 4.5 > 32$$
$$y - 4.5 + 4.5 > 32 + 4.5$$
$$y > 36.5$$

The solutions are all the numbers greater than 36.5.

EXAMPLE 2 Solve $2\frac{1}{4} - \frac{1}{2} \geq n$.

Solution We may exchange the sides of the inequality and *reverse the inequality sign* before we simplify the numerical expression.

$$2\frac{1}{4} - \frac{1}{2} \geq n$$

$$n \leq 2\frac{1}{4} - \frac{1}{2}$$

$$n \leq \frac{7}{4}, \text{ or } 1\frac{3}{4}$$

The solutions are all the numbers less than or equal to $\frac{7}{4}$.

EXAMPLE 3 Solve each inequality.

a. $7a < 91$ **b.** $-3x \geq 18$ **c.** $26 \leq \frac{y}{4}$ **d.** $\frac{d}{-9} > -108$

Solution **a.** Divide both sides by 7.

$$7a < 91$$

$$\frac{7a}{7} < \frac{91}{7}$$

$$a < 13$$

The solutions are all the numbers less than 13.

b. Divide both sides by -3 and *reverse the inequality sign.*

$$-3x \geq 18$$

$$\frac{-3x}{-3} \leq \frac{18}{-3}$$

$$x \leq -6$$

The solutions are all the numbers less than or equal to -6.

c. Multiply both sides by 4.

$$26 \leq \frac{y}{4}$$

$$4 \times 26 \leq 4 \times \frac{y}{4}$$

$$104 \leq y$$

The solutions are all the numbers greater than or equal to 104.

d. Multiply both sides by -9 and *reverse the inequality sign.*

$$\frac{d}{-9} > -108$$

$$-9 \times \frac{d}{-9} < -9 \times (-108)$$

$$d < 972$$

The solutions are all the numbers less than 972.

Class Exercises

Identify the transformation used to transform the first inequality into the second.

1. $e + 5 > 8$
   $e + 5 - 5 > 8 - 5$

2. $q - 3 < 7$
   $q - 3 + 3 < 7 + 3$

3. $\frac{1}{2}k < 4$
   $2 \times \frac{1}{2}k < 2 \times 4$

4. $6a > 12$
   $\frac{6a}{6} > \frac{12}{6}$

5. $-\frac{1}{4}u > 3$
   $-4 \times -\frac{1}{4}u < -4 \times 3$

6. $-9m < 27$
   $\frac{-9m}{-9} > \frac{27}{-9}$

Identify each transformation and complete the equivalent inequality.

7. $n - 6 > 9$
   $n - 6 + 6 \underline{\ ?\ } 9 + 6$

8. $d + 4 < -3$
   $d + 4 - 4 \underline{\ ?\ } -3 - 4$

9. $3r < 15$
   $\frac{3r}{3} \underline{\ ?\ } \frac{15}{3}$

10. $\frac{1}{5}v > 6$
    $5 \times \frac{1}{5}v \underline{\ ?\ } 5 \times 6$

11. $-4z > 32.8$
    $\frac{-4z}{-4} \underline{\ ?\ } \frac{32.8}{-4}$

12. $-\frac{1}{3}s < 2\frac{1}{3}$
    $-3 \times -\frac{1}{3}s \underline{\ ?\ } -3 \times \frac{7}{3}$

Written Exercises

Use transformations to solve the inequality. Write down all the steps.

A

1. $-4 + 16 > k$
2. $g < -18 - 9$
3. $(17 + 4)2 < j$
4. $f \geq 7(23 - 9)$
5. $a + 7 < 10$
6. $c + 8 > 13$
7. $e - 11 \geq 9$
8. $m - 5 \leq 15$
9. $-16 > n + 2$
10. $-13 < q - 6$
11. $8w < 56$
12. $7y > 42$
13. $-5t > 35$
14. $-6a < 18$
15. $-48 \leq -4b$
16. $-49 \geq -7m$
17. $\frac{u}{3} \leq 5$
18. $\frac{w}{4} \geq 9$

Use transformations to solve the inequality. Write down all the steps.

19. $\frac{f}{-2} > 13$

20. $\frac{n}{-5} < 12$

21. $-10 \le \frac{y}{-6}$

22. $-9 \ge \frac{d}{4}$

23. $\frac{4h - 2h}{2} \le -6 - 5$

24. $\frac{16}{4} > \frac{7n - 2n}{5}$

B **25.** $-8(13.4 + 7.6) > a$

26. $12 \le p - 4.27$

27. $3r > 63.9$

28. $10\left(3\frac{1}{2} + 4\frac{2}{5}\right) \ge g$

29. $j + 3\frac{4}{7} < 9$

30. $d + 5\frac{1}{4} > -8$

31. $-10 \ge n - 6.13$

32. $c < (18.7 - 7.6)4$

33. $e \le \left(5\frac{1}{3} + 2\frac{1}{2}\right)6$

34. $42.4 < 4t$

35. $\frac{d}{0.6} \le -18$

36. $\frac{1}{5}w \ge \frac{2}{5}$

37. $\frac{3}{4} \le \frac{1}{4}n$

38. $\frac{m}{3.1} \ge 12$

39. $-7 > -\frac{1}{3}d$

40. $-\frac{1}{2}f \le -13$

41. $-6y < 24.6$

42. $42.5 > -5b$

43. $\frac{a}{-13.2} \ge 7$

44. $\frac{x}{-0.3} < -9$

45. $h - 10\frac{2}{3} > 12\frac{1}{5}$

46. $-8.27 \le k + 17.41$

47. $22.5 \ge -2.5m$

48. $3.2u \ge 25.6$

C **49.** $\frac{3}{4}n + \frac{1}{2}n > \frac{2}{3} \times \frac{3}{8}$

50. $\frac{-5}{8}p - \frac{1}{8}p > \frac{1}{4} \div 7$

51. $3.4(21.2 - 18.9) < 4.6(-3b + 2b)$

52. $\frac{5(-1.6t)}{2} < -14.3 - 9.7$

Review Exercises

Write the numbers in order from least to greatest.

1. $-1.4,\ 1.2,\ -2.6,\ 3.2$

2. $3.7,\ 4.02,\ -3.07,\ -4.1,\ 3$

3. $12,\ -12.2,\ -12.09,\ 112,\ -11.2$

4. $9.8,\ -8.09,\ 0.89,\ -0.98,\ -9$

5. $-5.03,\ 3.05,\ -30.05,\ 0.35,\ -5.3$

6. $-0.2,\ -0.02,\ -2,\ -20,\ 200$

7. $2.89,\ 2.089,\ -2.8,\ 28.9,\ -2.89$

8. $-7.6,\ -0.76,\ -7.06,\ -0.076,\ -76.0$

8-6 Solving Inequalities by Several Transformations

We may need to use more than one transformation to solve some inequalities. It is helpful to follow the same steps that we use for solving equations.

> **1.** Simplify each side of the inequality.
>
> **2.** Use the inverse operations to undo any indicated additions or subtractions.
>
> **3.** Use the inverse operations to undo any indicated multiplications or divisions.

EXAMPLE 1 Solve $-4r + 6 + 2r - 18 < -8$.

Solution Simplify the left side.
$$-4r + 6 + 2r - 18 < -8$$
$$-2r - 12 < -8$$

Add 12 to both sides.
$$-2r - 12 + 12 < -8 + 12$$
$$-2r < 4$$

Divide both sides by -2 and reverse the inequality sign.
$$\frac{-2r}{-2} > \frac{4}{-2}$$
$$r > -2$$

The solutions are all the numbers greater than -2.

The solutions to the inequality in Example 1 include all numbers greater than -2. We show the graph of the solutions on the number line in the following way.

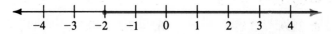

The open dot at -2 indicates that -2 is not on the graph of the solutions of the inequality.

We use a solid dot to show that a number is on the graph of the solutions. We graph the solutions of $r \geq -2$ in the following way.

EXAMPLE 2   Solve $3(5 + x) \leq -3$ and graph the solutions.

Solution   Simplify the left side.

$$3(5 + x) \leq -3$$
$$3(5) + 3x \leq -3$$
$$15 + 3x \leq -3$$

Subtract 15 from both sides.

$$15 + 3x - 15 \leq -3 - 15$$
$$3x \leq -18$$

Divide both sides by 3.

$$\frac{3x}{3} \leq \frac{-18}{3}$$
$$x \leq -6$$

The solutions are all the numbers less than or equal to -6.

Because -6 is on the graph, we used a solid dot to graph the solutions of the inequality.

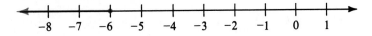

Like equations, inequalities may have variables on both sides. We may add a variable expression to both sides or subtract a variable expression from both sides to obtain an equivalent inequality.

EXAMPLE 3   Solve $-z + 7 \leq 3z - 18$.

Solution   Add z to both sides.

$$-z + 7 \leq 3z - 18$$
$$z + (-z) + 7 \leq z + 3z - 18$$
$$7 \leq 4z - 18$$

Add 18 to both sides.

$$7 + 18 \leq 4z - 18 + 18$$
$$25 \leq 4z$$

Divide both sides by 4.

$$\frac{25}{4} \leq \frac{4z}{4}$$
$$6.25 \leq z$$

The solutions are all the numbers greater than or equal to 6.25.

Class Exercises

State which transformations you would use to solve the inequality. State them in the order in which you would use them.

1. $8x + 7 - 5x + 2 \leq 30$

2. $-29 > 5 - 2y - 10 - 4y$

3. $7 \geq \frac{-4}{5}m + 6 + \frac{3}{5}m - 4$

4. $\frac{6}{7}k - 8 - \frac{5}{7}k + 3 < -3$

5. $4(h - 3) > 16$

6. $-4 \geq \frac{1}{2}(w + 12)$

7. $2 < (k + 45)\frac{-1}{5}$

8. $(3 - s)7 \leq 42$

9. $-u + 8 \geq 4u - 10$

10. $a - 6 < -5a - 18$

Written Exercises

Solve and graph the solutions.

A   **1.** $3q + 5 < -13$

2. $-7 + 5m > 28$

3. $30 \geq -4b - 6$

4. $-57 \leq -8z - 9$

5. $-\frac{w}{2} + 8 > 23$

6. $-\frac{c}{3} + 7 < -18$

7. $-12 \leq -5 + \frac{r}{6}$

8. $13 \geq 6 + \frac{e}{4}$

Solve.

9. $3v + 11 - 8v - 5 < -21$

10. $9 - 12u + 4 + 6u > -5$

11. $12 \geq \frac{3}{5}f + 6 - \frac{4}{5}f + 4$

12. $19 \leq 7 + \frac{1}{3}k + 2 - \frac{2}{3}k$

13. $h > -5h + 18 - 6$

14. $t < 17 - 4t - 2$

15. $38 - 8 - 7n \leq 3n$

16. $-9q + 18 - 3 \geq 6q$

17. $\frac{1}{4}(20 - x) < 6$

18. $\frac{1}{6}(42 - p) > 12$

19. $21 \geq 7(m - 2)$

20. $-25 \leq 5(w + 3)$

21. $j + 8 > 4j - 16$

22. $-6f + 7 < 2f - 9$

23. $10 + \frac{3}{4}a \leq \frac{-7}{8}a + 5$

24. $\frac{5}{6}g - 4 \geq \frac{2}{3}g + 6$

B   **25.** $-12.8c + 8 + 7.8c - 6 \geq 17$

26. $4 + 7.5y - 9 + 2.5y > 25$

Solve.

27. $1\frac{4}{5} < 8m + 4\frac{1}{5} - 3m - 7\frac{2}{5}$

28. $-2\frac{2}{3} \leq 5\frac{2}{3} - 9u + 4\frac{2}{3} + 3u$

29. $0.2(40k + 62.5) \leq -3.5$

30. $-0.5(12v - 18.6) < 21.3$

31. $-2\frac{7}{8} > \left(\frac{5}{8} - t\right)\frac{1}{5}$

32. $5\frac{3}{4} \leq \frac{1}{3}\left(x - \frac{3}{4}\right)$

33. $2.7e + 8.2 < -9.3e + 32.2$

34. $5.4 - 10.9w \geq 9.1w - 14.6$

35. $\frac{5}{6}f - 2\frac{4}{5} > 1\frac{1}{5} + \frac{2}{3}f$

36. $-2\frac{1}{9}d + \frac{3}{5} \leq -3\frac{2}{9}d - 4\frac{2}{5}$

C 37. $0.11(360 + 25n) < (1.86n \div 6) - 3.06n$

38. $\frac{1}{5}\left(w - 5\frac{5}{9}\right) + \frac{2}{9} + \frac{3}{4}w \geq \frac{1}{8}w - 1 + \frac{5}{8}w$

39. $[(250.25x - 10.5) \div -5] - 14.6 \leq -0.05x + 502.5$

40. $9\frac{4}{5} + \frac{2}{7}k - 7\frac{3}{5} > -\frac{11}{12} + \left[\left(\frac{4}{7}k + 2\frac{1}{3}\right) \div \frac{4}{5}\right]$

Review Exercises

Use *n* to write a variable expression for the word phrase.

1. A number increased by nine

2. Twice a number

3. Sixteen less than a number

4. Half of a number

5. The sum of a number and three

6. Six more than a number

7. A number divided by five

8. Eight times a number

Challenge

Each letter in each exercise stands for a digit from 0 through 9. Find the value of each letter to make the computation correct. (There may be more than one correct answer.)

1.
```
  H O W
+ A R E
-------
  Y O U
```

2.
```
  T I M E
+ S U R E
---------
  F L I E S
```

3.
```
  M A T H
-      I S
---------
  F U N
```

8-7 Inequalities in Problem Solving

The five-step method is also helpful in solving problems that require inequalities.

EXAMPLE   The sum of two consecutive integers is less than 40. What pair of integers with this property has the greatest sum?

Solution
- The problem says:
  the sum of two consecutive integers is less than 40

- The problem asks for:
  the greatest pair of integers whose sum is less than 40
  Let $n =$ the smaller of the two integers.
  Then the other integer $= n + 1$.
  The sum of the two integers is $n + n + 1$.
  The sum of the two integers is less than 40.

- We now have enough information to write an inequality.

$$n + n + 1 < 40$$

- Solve.
$$n + n + 1 < 40$$
$$2n + 1 < 40$$
$$2n + 1 - 1 < 40 - 1$$
$$2n < 39$$
$$\frac{2n}{2} < \frac{39}{2}$$
$$n < 19.5$$
$$n = 19$$
$$n + 1 = 20$$

- Check: $19 + 20 = 39$, $39 < 40$. The result checks.

  The two integers are 19 and 20.

Class Exercises

Using x as the variable, write an inequality based on the given information. Do not solve.

1. A used-car dealer has sold 30 of his compact cars and now has fewer than 70 left.

2. Alejandro Mendoza, who had more than 60 base hits during his school team's baseball season, had 25 more hits than his teammate Peter Evans.

3. Deborah's bowling score was 8 less than half of Lydia's score. Deborah's score was less than 95.

4. A house and lot together cost more than $120,000. The cost of the house was $2000 more than six times the cost of the lot.

5. The number of students at Ivytown High School who study computer science is twice the number who study home economics. The total number of students enrolled in these courses exceeds 600.

6. The sum of two consecutive integers is greater than 30.

Problems

Solve.

A 1. The sum of two consecutive integers is less than 75. Find the pair of integers with the greatest sum.

2. Of all pairs of consecutive integers whose sum is greater than 100, find the pair whose sum is the least.

3. Two trucks start from the same point traveling in different directions. One truck travels at a speed of 54 mi/h, the other at 48 mi/h. How long must they travel to be at least 408 mi apart?

4. A purse contains 30 coins, all either quarters or dimes. The total value of the coins is greater than $5.20. At least how many of the coins are quarters? At most how many are dimes?

5. A home and adjoining lot cost more than $160,000 together. The cost of the house was $1000 more than six times the cost of the lot. What is the smallest possible cost of the lot?

6. Paul is two fifths as old as Janet. Five years from now, he will be at least half as old as Janet. At most how old is Paul now?

B 7. The sum of three consecutive integers, decreased by five, is greater than twice the smallest of the integers. What are the three least positive integers with this property?

8. A pair of consecutive integers has the property that five times the smaller is less than four times the greater. Find the greatest pair of integers with this property.

9. The number of Software Services employees who use public transportation to commute to work is 200 more than twice the number who drive their own cars. If there are 1400 employees, how many drive their own cars?

C **10.** Bonanza Rent-A-Car rents cars for $40 per day and 10¢ for every mile driven. Autos Unlimited rents cars for $50 per day with no extra charge for mileage. How many miles per day can you drive a Bonanza car if it is to cost you less than an Auto Unlimited car?

11. A bank offers two types of checking accounts. Account A has a $4 maintenance fee each month and charges 10¢ for each check cashed. Account B has a $6 maintenance fee and charges 6¢ for each check. What is the least number of checks that can be written each month for the "A" account to be more expensive?

Self-Test B

Write an inequality for each word sentence.

1. A number a is less than a number b. [8–4]

2. Thirty-five is greater than a number $4z$.

Use transformations to solve the inequality.

3. $m - 8 \leq 20$ **4.** $t + 3 > 6$ **5.** $c + 7 \geq 14$ [8–5]

6. $9p > 42$ **7.** $-4b < 56$ **8.** $-7x < -35$

Solve.

9. $2x + 4 + 6x - 2 < 18$ **10.** $12 - 6u + 4 + 8u > 20$ [8–6]

11. $\frac{1}{2}(30 - 6y) \geq 15$ **12.** $-30 \leq 6(t + 1)$

13. The sum of two consecutive integers is less than 150. Find the greatest pair of integers with this property. [8–7]

▮▮▮ Challenge

Using each of the digits 1, 3, 5, 7, and 9 exactly once, create a three-digit integer and a two-digit integer. The integers may be either positive or negative.

1. What is the greatest possible sum of the two integers? the least possible sum?

2. What is the greatest possible difference between the two integers? the least possible difference?

3. What is the greatest possible product of the two integers? the least possible product?

People in Mathematics

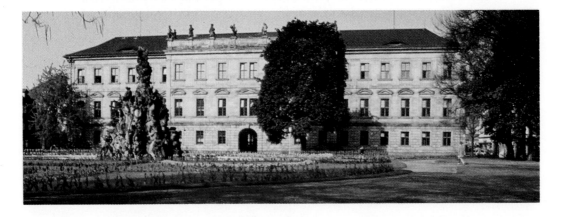

Archimedes (287–212 B.C.)

Archimedes is considered to be one of the greatest mathematicians of all time. He was a native of the Greek city of Syracuse, although he did spend some time at the University of Alexandria in Egypt.

Archimedes is the subject of many stories and legends. The most famous story about Archimedes is that of King Hieron's crown. The crown was supposedly all gold, but the king suspected that it contained silver and he asked Archimedes to determine whether it was pure gold. Archimedes hit upon the solution, while bathing, by discovering the first law of hydrostatics. The story relates that he jumped from the bath and ran through the streets shouting "Eureka."

Archimedes discovered many important mathematical facts. He found formulas for the volumes and surface areas of many geometric solids. He invented a method for approximating π and studied spirals, one of which bears his name. His work, as shown by a paper not found until 1906, even contained the beginning of calculus, a branch of mathematics not developed until the seventeenth century.

Sonya Kovaleski (1850–1891)

Sonya Kovaleski was one of the great mathematicians of the nineteenth century. Her work includes papers on such diverse topics as partial differential equations (a theorem is named in her honor), Abelian integrals, and the rings of Saturn. Her other work included research in the topics of analysis and physics. In 1888 her research paper entitled *On the Rotation of a Solid Body about a Fixed Point* was awarded the Prix Bordin of the French Academy of Sciences. It was considered so outstanding that the prize of 3000 francs was doubled.

Kovaleski's rise to prominence was far from easy. In order to leave Russia to study at a foreign university, she had to arrange a marriage, at age eighteen, to Vladimir Kovaleski. In 1868 they went to Heidelberg where she studied with Kirchhoff and Helmholtz, two famous physicists. In 1871 she went to Berlin to study with Karl Weierstrass. Since women were not admitted to university lectures, all her studying was done privately. Finally, in 1874, the University of Gottingen awarded her a doctorate *in absentia*. However, she was unable to find an academic position for ten years despite strong letters of recommendation from Weierstrass. Finally, in 1884, she was appointed as a lecturer at the University of Stockholm where she was made a full professor five years later.

Emmy Noether (1882–1935)

Emmy Noether is considered one of the brilliant mathematicians of the twentieth century. Her most important work was done in the field of advanced algebra, a branch of mathematics that deals with structures called "groups" and "rings." An important theorem in advanced algebra is called the Noether-Lasker Decomposition Theorem. Noether is also known for work she did on Einstein's theory of relativity.

Although her father was a mathematician, Noether faced many of the same obstacles as Sonya Kovaleski. She sat in on courses at the University of Erlangen (shown in the photograph) and the University of Gottingen from 1900 to 1903, but was not allowed to officially enroll until 1904 when Erlangen changed its policy toward women. She received her doctorate in 1907.

In 1915 Noether was invited to Gottingen by David Hilbert. There, she worked with Hilbert and Felix Klein, two prominent mathematicians, although she was not appointed to the faculty until 1922. She left Gottingen in 1933 and took a professorship at Bryn Mawr College in Pennsylvania.

Research Activities

1. Look up the statement of the law of physics known as Archimedes' principle. Using a measuring cup, devise a simple experiment to verify this law.

2. Archimedes discovered a way to calculate the number π very accurately. Look up the history of π in an encyclopedia. Find what values ancient civilizations thought it had.

3. Two other people considered important in the history of mathematics are Hypatia and Maria Agnesi. Find out about the lives and work of these mathematicians.

Chapter Review

True or false?

1. If $2y + 8y = -20$, $y = 2$.

2. If $p + 6 - 6p = -8$, $p = -3$.

3. If $4(n - 3) = 6$, $n = 4\frac{1}{2}$.

4. If $-4(a + 3) = 15$, $a = \frac{3}{4}$.

5. If $5z + 4 = 3z + 6$, $z = 1$.   **6.** If $6x - 11 = 12x - 7$, $x = 4$.   [8-2]

7. If $2(x - 4) = 5(x + 3)$, $x = 20$.   **8.** If $4(y + 7) = 3(y - 6)$, $y = -2$.

Write the letter of the correct answer.

9. The perimeter of an isosceles triangle is 63 cm. If the congruent   [8-3]
sides of the triangle are each three times as long as the remaining
side, how long are the congruent sides?
    a. 7 cm   **b.** 27 cm   **c.** 9 cm   **d.** 18 cm

10. A 60 ft board with a thickness of 1 in. is to be cut into two pieces,
one three times as long as the other. Find the lengths of the two
pieces.
    a. 30 ft, 30 ft   **b.** 40 ft, 20 ft   **c.** 45 ft, 15 ft   **d.** 48 ft, 12 ft

11. Which inequality represents the word sentence? Thirty is greater   [8-4]
than a number x.
    a. $30 < x$ **b.** $30 \le x$ **c.** $30 > x$ **d.** $30 \ge x$

Match the equivalent inequalities.

12. $-8 + 12 < x$ **13.** $6x > 54$ **A.** $x \le 8$ **B.** $x > 8$ [8-5]

14. $-64 \le -8x$ **15.** $2x < 8$ **C.** $x > 4$ **D.** $x > 9$

16. $\frac{1}{2}x + 6 < 26$ **17.** $\frac{x}{-5} + 5 \ge 10$ **E.** $x \le -25$ **F.** $x < 40$ [8-6]

18. $-17 \le -5 + \frac{x}{3}$ **19.** $-\frac{x}{6} + 5 > -3$ **G.** $x < 48$ **H.** $x \ge -36$

Write the letter of the correct answer.

20. The sum of two consecutive integers is greater than 60. Find the   [8-7]
least pair of integers having this property.
    a. 29, 30   **b.** 20, 21   **c.** 30, 31   **d.** 31, 32

21. NewBank offers two checking accounts. Account A has a monthly
fee of $2 and charges 15¢ for each check cashed. Account B has a
monthly fee of $5 and charges 10¢ for each check cashed. What is
the greatest number of checks that can be cashed for Account A to
be less expensive than Account B?
    a. 60   **b.** 59   **c.** 61   **d.** 20

Chapter Test

Solve.

1. $9a + 6a = 120$ 2. $-6z - (-4z) = -5$ [8-1]

3. $4 + (-4a) + 20 = 16$ 4. $-7n - 6 + 8n = -6$

5. $4(x - 5) = 10$ 6. $8(y + 5) = -20$

7. $5y + 4 = 6y - 3$ 8. $6(x + 4) = -2x$ [8-2]

9. $-3(a + 1) = 6a + 12$ 10. $6(p + 1) = 4(p + 2)$

11. $-3(n - 3) = 2n + 5$ 12. $4(y + 2) = -6y + 8$

Use an equation to solve.

13. The sum of two numbers is 100. One number is 24 less than the other number. What is the larger number?   [8-3]

Write an inequality for each word sentence.

14. Sixty-eight is less than eighty.   [8-4]

15. Nineteen is between fourteen and thirty.

16. Zero is less than a number y.

17. A number z is greater than a number r.

Solve.

18. $a + 12 < 19$ 19. $\frac{m}{4} > -8$ 20. $-3y \le 42$ [8-5]

21. $\frac{w}{-6} \ge 9$ 22. $75 < 5p$ 23. $27 \ge n - 16$

Solve and graph the solutions.

24. $\frac{1}{4}d - 2 \le 18$ 25. $-35 \le -5(r + 8)$ [8-6]

26. $\frac{a}{9} + 17 \ge 20$ 27. $8x - 4 < 5x + 23$

Solve.

28. Two trucks start from the same point traveling in opposite directions. One truck travels at a speed of 50 mi/h, the other travels at a speed of 45 mi/h. How long must they travel to be 380 mi apart?   [8-7]

Cumulative Review (Chapters 1–8)

Exercises

Evaluate the expression when $a = 2$, $b = -4$, and $c = 3$.

1. $a + b - c$
2. $c - b + a$
3. $3ac$
4. $-2b$
5. $4c - 5a$
6. $10a - 3b$
7. $8c \div (-3b)$
8. $50 \div (a + c)$
9. a^2
10. b^2
11. $(-b)^3$
12. $(ab)^2$

Solve.

13. $x + 9 = 12$
14. $x - 4 = -11$
15. $2x = 14$
16. $-5x = 35$
17. $3x + 7 = 22$
18. $-7x + 3 = -32$
19. $2x + 3x = 20$
20. $10x - 18x = 4$
21. $-7x - 9x + 7 = 11$
22. $5x = 30 - 10x$
23. $7x - 3 = 3x + 9$
24. $x - 14 = 26 - 9x$

Write as equivalent fractions using the LCD.

25. $\frac{1}{2}, \frac{7}{8}$
26. $\frac{3}{5}, \frac{9}{20}$
27. $\frac{1}{5}, \frac{3}{4}$
28. $\frac{2}{7}, \frac{5}{9}$
29. $\frac{2}{3}, \frac{1}{4}, \frac{5}{12}$
30. $\frac{21}{24}, \frac{5}{8}, \frac{7}{9}$

Complete.

31. Two nonparallel lines that do not intersect are called ___?___ lines.
32. In a ___?___ triangle, no two sides are congruent.
33. The number π is the ratio of the circumference of a circle to its ___?___.
34. The ___?___ of a figure is the distance around it.
35. The common endpoint of the two rays of an angle is called the ___?___.
36. A ___?___ of a polygon is a segment joining two nonconsecutive vertices.

Solve.

37. What percent of 60 is 55?
38. What is 81% of 120?
39. 30 is 15% of what number?
40. What percent of 100 is 49?

Problems

Solve.

1. Donald bought a pair of hiking boots for $35.83, a sweater for $24.65, and a backpack for $18. The tax on his purchase was $.90. How much did Donald spend?

2. This week, Marisa worked $1\frac{1}{2}$ h on Monday, $2\frac{1}{4}$ h on Tuesday, $1\frac{1}{3}$ h on Wednesday, and $7\frac{1}{2}$ h on Saturday. How many hours did she work this week?

3. An airplane flying at an altitude of 25,000 ft dropped 4000 ft in the first 25 s and rose 2500 ft in the next 15 s. What was the altitude of the airplane after 40 s?

4. The difference between twice a number and 50 is 10. What is the number?

5. At a milk processing plant 100 lb of farm milk are needed to make 8.13 lb of nonfat dry milk. To the nearest pound, how many pounds of farm milk are needed to produce 100 lb of nonfat dry milk?

6. A highway noise barrier that is 120 m long is constructed in two pieces. One piece is 45 m longer than the other. Find the length of each piece.

7. A side of a square is 13 cm long. What is the perimeter of the square?

8. Oak Hill School, Longview School, and Peabody School participated in a clean-up campaign to collect scrap aluminum. Oak Hill School collected 40% more scrap aluminum than Longview School. Longview School collected 25% more than Peabody School. If the total collected by the 3 schools was 560 kg, how much did Oak Hill School collect?

9. Eladio invested $200 at 6% annual interest and $350 at 5.75% annual interest, both compounded annually. If he makes no deposits or withdrawals, how much will he have after two years?

9

The Coordinate Plane

One of the most fascinating aspects of computer science is the field of computer-aided design (C.A.D.). Computers are used to design a wide variety of goods ranging from televisions and cars to skyscrapers, airplanes, and spacecraft. Computers are also used to generate designs for decorative purposes, such as the rug pattern shown at the right. A particular advantage of using the computer is the ease with which the design can be prepared and modified. The designer may use a light pen to create the design on the computer screen and may type in commands to tell the computer to enlarge, reduce, or rotate the design. Although the actual programs for computer graphics are often complicated, the underlying idea is based on establishing a grid with labeled reference points. The grid is actually an application of the coordinate plane that is presented in this chapter.

Career Note

If you enjoy working with fabrics and drawing your own patterns, you might consider a career as a textile designer. Textile designers create the graphic designs printed or woven on all kinds of fabrics. In addition to having a good understanding of graphics, textile designers must possess a knowledge of textile production. Another important part of textile design is the ability to appeal to current tastes.

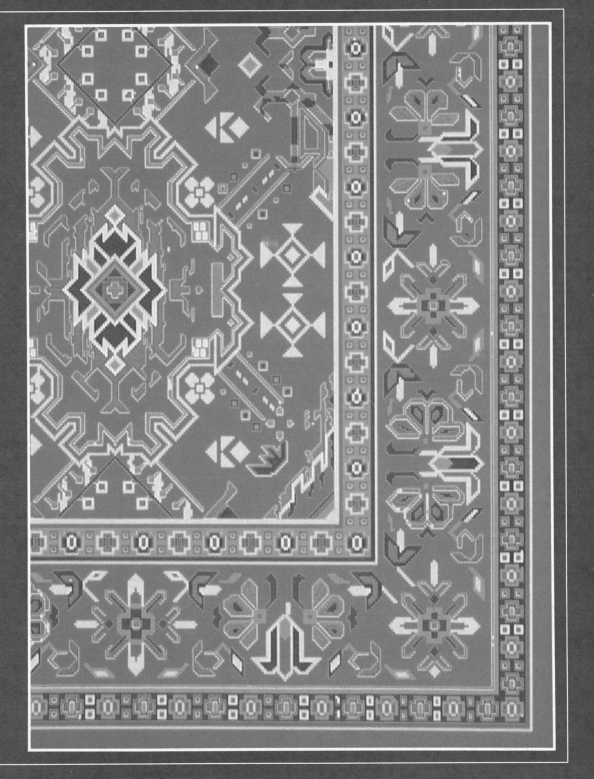

9-1 The Coordinate Plane

We describe the position of a point on a number line by stating its coordinate. Similarly, we can describe the position of a point in a plane by stating a pair of coordinates that locate it in a **rectangular coordinate system.** This system consists of two number lines perpendicular to each other at point *O*, called the **origin.** The horizontal line is called the *x*-**axis,** and the vertical line is called the *y*-**axis.** The positive direction is to the right of the origin on the *x*-axis and upward on the *y*-axis. The negative direction is to the left of the origin and downward.

Reading Mathematics: *Diagrams*

As you read text that is next to a diagram, stop after each sentence and relate what you have read to what you see in the diagram. For example, as you read the first paragraph next to the diagram below, locate point *M* on the graph, and find the vertical line from *M* to the *x*-axis.

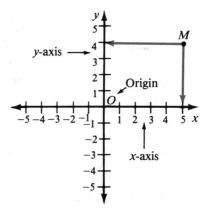

To assign a pair of coordinates to point *M* located in the **coordinate plane,** first draw a vertical line from *M* to the *x*-axis. The point of intersection on the *x*-axis is called the *x*-**coordinate,** or **abscissa.** The abscissa of *M* is 5.

Next draw a horizontal line from *M* to the *y*-axis. The point of intersection on the *y*-axis is called the *y*-**coordinate,** or **ordinate.** The ordinate of *M* is 4.

Together, the abscissa and ordinate form an **ordered pair of numbers** that are the coordinates of a point. The coordinates of *M* are (5, 4).

EXAMPLE 1   Give the coordinates of each point.

      a. *F*   **b.** *S*   **c.** *P*   **d.** *T*

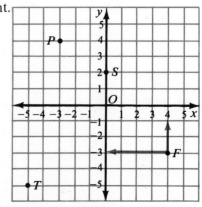

Solution   **a.** Point *F* has *x*-coordinate 4 and *y*-coordinate -3.
          F has coordinates (4, -3).

         Similarly,

      b. *S* has coordinates (0, 2).

      c. *P* has coordinates (-3, 4).

      d. *T* has coordinates (-5, -5).

Notice that $(4, -3)$ and $(-3, 4)$ are coordinates of different points. In an ordered pair of numbers the x-coordinate is listed first, followed by the y-coordinate, in the form **(x, y).**

Just as each point in the plane is associated with exactly one ordered pair, each ordered pair of numbers determines exactly one point in the plane.

EXAMPLE 2   Graph these ordered pairs:
$(-6, 5)$, $(5, -4)$, $(0, 3)$,
$(-3, -2)$, and $\left(2\frac{1}{2}, 1\right)$.

Solution   First locate the x-coordinate on the x-axis. Then move up or down to locate the y-coordinate.

The x- and y-axes divide the coordinate plane into **Quadrants I, II, III,** and **IV.** The ranges of values for the x-coordinate and y-coordinate of any point in each quadrant are shown at the right.

Class Exercises

Give the coordinates of the point.

1. A 2. K 3. E

4. J 5. L 6. F

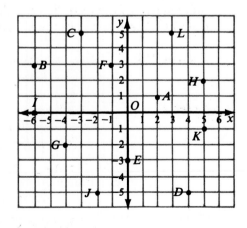

Name the point for the ordered pair.

7. $(5, 2)$ H   8. $(-6, 0)$ I

9. $(4, -5)$ D   10. $(-4, -2)$ G

11. $(-3, 5)$ C   12. $(-6, 3)$ B

Name the quadrant containing the point.

13. F 14. D 15. H 16. J 17. K

Written Exercises

For Exercises 1-18, use the graph at the right.

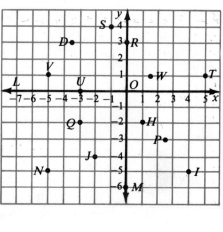

Give the coordinates of the point.

A   **1.** N   **2.** P   **3.** T   **4.** R

     5. Q   **6.** M   **7.** S   **8.** V

Name the point for the ordered pair.

9. $(4, -5)$ **10.** $(-3, -2)$

11. $(-5, 1)$ **12.** $\left(\frac{5}{2}, -3\right)$

13. $\left(-\frac{7}{2}, 3\right)$ **14.** $(1, -2)$ **15.** $\left(\frac{3}{2}, 1\right)$

16. $(-1, 4)$ **17.** $(0, -6)$ **18.** $(0, 3)$

a. Graph the given ordered pairs on a coordinate plane.

b. Draw line segments to connect the points in the order listed and to connect the first and last points.

c. Name the closed figure as specifically as you can.

EXAMPLE $(-3, -2), (-1, 2), (4, 2), (2, -2)$

Solution   **a.**

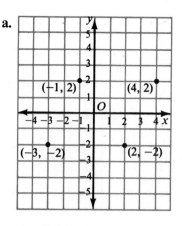

            b.

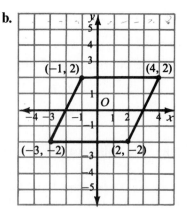

         c. parallelogram

B   **19.** $(1, -2), (3, -2), (3, 4), (1, 4)$ **20.** $(0, 1), (3, -2), (6, 1), (3, 4)$

    21. $(0, -5), (0, 2), (-3, 6), (-3, -1)$ **22.** $(-5, 0), (-1, 2), (1, 6), (-3, 4)$

We can translate a figure on a coordinate plane by changing the ordered pairs. We can reflect a figure on a coordinate plane by changing the signs of the ordered pairs.

   a. **Graph the given ordered pairs on a coordinate plane, connect the points in the order listed, and connect the first and last points.**
   b. **Change the values of the coordinates as directed.**
   c. **Graph and connect all the new points to form a second figure.**
   d. **Identify the change as translation or reflection.**

C 23. $(-5, 4)$, $(-2, 1)$, $(2, 1)$, $(2, 4)$
   Decrease all y-coordinates by 3.
   (*Hint:* $(-5, 4)$ becomes $(-5, 1)$)

24. $(1, 5)$, $(1, 1)$, $(5, 3)$
   Decrease all x-coordinates by 2.

25. $(-2, -2)$, $(2, -2)$, $(4, -4)$, $(4, -6)$, $(1, -4)$, $(-1, -4)$, $(-4, -6)$, $(-4, -4)$
   Increase all y-coordinates by 5.

26. $(-8, 4)$, $(-4, 4)$, $(-4, 5)$, $(-1, 3)$, $(-4, 1)$, $(-4, 2)$, $(-8, 2)$
   Increase all x-coordinates by 9.

27. $(6, 5)$, $(2, 1)$, $(9, 3)$
   Multiply all x-coordinates by -1.

28. $(1, 7)$, $(4, 2)$, $(7, 3)$, $(4, 8)$
   Multiply all y-coordinates by -1.

Review Exercises

Complete.

1. If $x + 5 = 13$, then $x = \underline{\ ?\ }$.

2. If $8 + x = -1$, then $x = \underline{\ ?\ }$.

3. If $9x = 243$, then $x = \underline{\ ?\ }$.

4. If $-4x = 52$, then $x = \underline{\ ?\ }$.

5. If $2x + 11 = 1$, then $x = \underline{\ ?\ }$.

6. If $99 - 9x = 18$, then $x = \underline{\ ?\ }$.

7. If $-\frac{4}{5}x = 12$, then $x = \underline{\ ?\ }$.

8. If $9 + \frac{2}{3}x = 15$, then $x = \underline{\ ?\ }$.

■■■ | **Challenge**

Set up a pair of coordinate axes on graph paper. Connect the following points in the order given:

$$(-9, 3), (-4, 3), (-1.5, 1), (2, -1),$$
$$(2, -4), (8.5, -5), (9.5, -1), (2, -1)$$

Do you recognize the figure? (*Hint:* It is a well-known group of stars that is part of the constellation *Ursa Major*.)

9-2 Equations in Two Variables

The equation

$$x + y = 5$$

has two variables, x and y. A solution to this equation consists of two numbers, one for each variable. The solution can be expressed as an ordered pair of numbers, (x, y). There are many ordered pairs that satisfy this equation. Some solutions are

$$(-3, 8), (5, 0), (4, 1), (0, 5), (11, -6).$$

In fact, there are *infinitely* many ordered pairs that satisfy this equation.

EXAMPLE 1   Tell whether each ordered pair is a solution of the equation $2x + y = 7$.

   a. $(4, -1)$ **b.** $(-4, 1)$

Solution   Substitute the given values of x and y in the equation.

a.
$$2x + y = 7$$
$$2(4) + (-1) \overset{?}{=} 7$$
$$8 - 1 \overset{?}{=} 7$$
$$7 = 7$$

$(4, -1)$ is a solution.

b.
$$2x + y = 7$$
$$2(-4) + 1 \overset{?}{=} 7$$
$$-8 + 1 \overset{?}{=} 7$$
$$-7 \neq 7$$

$(-4, 1)$ is not a solution.

An equation in the two variables x and y establishes a correspondence between values of x and values of y. To find a solution of a given equation in x and y, we can choose any value for x, substitute it in the equation, and solve for the corresponding value for y.

EXAMPLE 2   Give one solution of the equation $x - 3y = 2$.

Solution   Choose any value for x. For example, if $x = 14$:

$$x - 3y = 2$$
$$14 - 3y = 2$$
$$-3y = 2 - 14$$
$$y = \frac{-12}{-3} = 4$$

The values $x = 14$ and $y = 4$ correspond.

$(14, 4)$ is one solution of the equation.

To find the value of y corresponding to any given value of x, we could substitute the value of x into a given equation and solve for y, as in Example 2. An easier method is to solve for y in terms of x first, and then substitute, as in Example 3.

EXAMPLE 3 Find the solutions for $2x + 3y = 6$ for the following values of x: -9, -3, 0, 3, 6.

Solution First solve for y in terms of x by writing an equation with y on one side and x on the other.

$$2x + 3y = 6$$
$$3y = 6 - 2x$$
$$y = 2 - \frac{2}{3}x$$

Then substitute the values of x in the new equation and solve for the corresponding values of y.

x	$y = 2 - \frac{2}{3}x$	(x, y)
-9	$2 - \frac{2}{3}(-9) = 8$	$(-9, 8)$
-3	$2 - \frac{2}{3}(-3) = 4$	$(-3, 4)$
0	$2 - \frac{2}{3}(0) = 2$	$(0, 2)$
3	$2 - \frac{2}{3}(3) = 0$	$(3, 0)$
6	$2 - \frac{2}{3}(6) = -2$	$(6, -2)$

Thus $(-9, 8)$, $(-3, 4)$, $(0, 2)$, $(3, 0)$, and $(6, -2)$ are solutions of the equation for the given values of x.

Notice in the table above that each given value of x corresponds to exactly one value of y. In general, any set of ordered pairs such that no two different ordered pairs have the same x-coordinate is called a **function.** An equation, as the one above, that produces such a set of ordered pairs defines a function.

Class Exercises

Tell whether the ordered pair is a solution of the given equation.

$2x + y = 7$
  1. $(2, 3)$ **2.** $(1, 5)$ **3.** $(7, 0)$ **4.** $(0, 7)$

$x - 3y = 1$
  5. $(2, 1)$ **6.** $(4, 1)$ **7.** $(7, 2)$ **8.** $(-2, 1)$

Solve the equation for y in terms of x.

  9. $x - y = 5$ **10.** $x - y = 9$ **11.** $-3x + y = 7$

If $y = x - 12$, give the value of y such that the ordered pair is a solution of the equation.

12. $(9, ?)$ **13.** $(-4, ?)$ **14.** $(0, ?)$ **15.** $(-6, ?)$

Written Exercises

Tell whether the ordered pair is a solution of the given equation.

A $-x + 3y = 15$
  1. $(0, 5)$ **2.** $(6, -7)$ **3.** $(6, 7)$ **4.** $(-3, 6)$

$x - 4y = 12$
  5. $(4, 2)$ **6.** $(-6, -12)$ **7.** $(0, 3)$ **8.** $\left(13, \frac{1}{4}\right)$

$3x - 2y = 8$
  9. $(1, 6)$ **10.** $(0, 4)$ **11.** $(4, 0)$ **12.** $\left(3, \frac{1}{2}\right)$

$-5x - 2y = 18$
13. $(-2, -4)$ **14.** $(-4, 1)$ **15.** $\left(1, -\frac{23}{2}\right)$ **16.** $(0, 0)$

Solve the equation for y in terms of x.

17. $2x + y = 7$ **18.** $-8x + 5y = 10$ **19.** $-12x + 3y = 48$

20. $4x - 9y = 36$ **21.** $x - \frac{3}{2}y = 3$ **22.** $5x - 4y = 20$

a. Solve the equation for y in terms of x.
b. Find the solutions of the equation for the given values of x.

23. $y - x = 7$
    values of x: $2, -5, 7$

24. $x + y = -1$
    values of x: $3, 1, -2$

25. $-x + 2y = 10$
values of x: 4, 0, 6

26. $x - 3y = 12$
values of x: -3, 6, 12

27. $x + 4y = 20$
values of x: 4, -8, 0

28. $-x - 2y = 8$
values of x: -6, -2, 10

B **29.** $3x - 2y = 6$
values of x: 4, -2, -8

30. $-2x + 3y = 12$
values of x: 3, -3, -12

31. $2y - x = 5$
values of x: 3, 5, -1

32. $-3y + x = 7$
values of x: 1, 7, -5

33. $2y - 5x = 6$
values of x: 2, 1, -3

34. $4y - 3x = 1$
values of x: 9, -1, -5

Give any three ordered pairs that are solutions of the equation.

35. $y + x = -1$

36. $x - y = 6$

37. $x + y = 0$

38. $4y - x = 7$

39. $5x - y = -5$

40. $-3x - 2y = 0$

41. $2x - 3y = 12$

42. $-\frac{1}{4}y - x = 0$

43. $-x + \frac{1}{2}y = 3$

Write an equation that expresses a relationship between the coordinates of each ordered pair.

EXAMPLE $(1, 4), (2, 3), (5, 0), (-1, 6)$

Solution   Notice that all the coordinates share a common property: the sum of the coordinates in each pair is 5. You can express this relationship by the equation $x + y = 5$.

C **44.** $(7, 6), (11, 10), (4, 3)$

45. $(3, -3), (6, -6), (-4, 4)$

46. $(-2, -4), (-3, -5), (4, 2)$

47. $(3, -6), (-3, 0), (6, -9)$

Review Exercises

Solve.

1. $8a = 24$

2. $6 - 5m = 11$

3. $6t - 31 = 137$

4. $-7x + 4 = -10$

5. $9c = 18 + 3c$

6. $\frac{4}{5}y = 16$

7. $2 + \frac{7}{8}d = -47$

8. $-10 - \frac{2}{3}f = 12$

9. $5(8 + 2h) = 0$

9-3 Graphing Equations in the Coordinate Plane

The equation in two variables

$$x + 2y = 6$$

has infinitely many solutions. The **table of values** below lists some of the solutions. When we graph the solutions on a coordinate plane, we find that they all lie on a straight line.

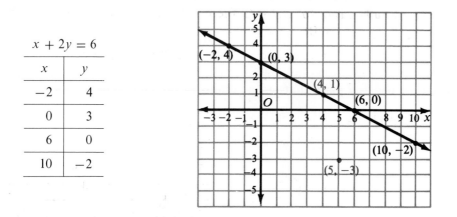

$$x + 2y = 6$$

x	y
-2	4
0	3
6	0
10	-2

If we choose any other point on this line, we will find that the coordinates also satisfy the equation. For example, the ordered pair (4, 1) is a solution:

$$x + 2y = 6$$
$$4 + 2(1) = 6$$

If we choose a point *not* on this line, such as the graph of (5, −3), we find that its coordinates *do not* satisfy the equation:

$$x + 2y = 6$$
$$5 + 2(-3) \neq 6$$

The graph of an ordered pair is on the line if and only if it is a solution of the equation. The set of all points that are the graphs of solutions of a given equation is called the **graph of the equation.**

Note that the graph of $x + 2y = 6$ crosses the y-axis at (0, 3). The y-coordinate of a point where a graph crosses the y-axis is called the **y-intercept** of the graph. In this case, the y-intercept is 3. Since the graph also crosses the x-axis at (6, 0), the **x-intercept** of the graph is 6.

In general, any equation that can be written in the form

$$ax + by = c$$

where x and y are variables and a, b, and c are numbers (with a and b

not both zero), is called a **linear equation in two variables** because its graph is always a straight line in the plane.

In order to graph a linear equation, we need to graph only two points whose coordinates satisfy the equation and then join them by means of a line. It is wise, however, to graph a third point as a check.

EXAMPLE   Graph the equation $x + 3y = 6$.

Solution   First find three points whose coordinates satisfy the equation. It is usually easier to start with the y-intercept and the x-intercept, that is, $(0, y)$ and $(x, 0)$.

If $x = 0$: $0 + 3y = 6$ If $y = 0$: $x + 3(0) = 6$
$3y = 6$ $x = 6$
$y = 2$

As a check, if $x = 3$: $3 + 3y = 6$
$3y = 3$
$y = 1$

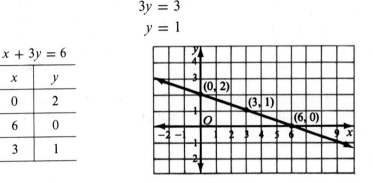

$x + 3y = 6$	
x	y
0	2
6	0
3	1

Class Exercises

Find three solutions of the linear equation. Include those that are in the form $(0, y)$ and $(x, 0)$.

1. $x - y = 7$ **2.** $y + x = -4$ **3.** $-x - 2y = 8$

4. $3y - x = 9$ **5.** $2x + y = 10$ **6.** $3x - 2y = 3$

7. $y = x$ **8.** $y = 3x$ **9.** $y = \frac{1}{2}x$

Written Exercises

A 1–9. Graph each equation in Class Exercises 1–9. Use a separate set of coordinate axes for each equation.

Graph the equation on a coordinate plane. Use a separate set of axes for each equation.

10. $x + y = 5$

11. $x - 6 = y$

12. $y - x = 4$

13. $y + x = -3$

14. $2x - y = 10$

15. $8x + 2y = 8$

16. $3y + x = 0$

17. $3x - y = -6$

18. $-2x + 3y = 12$

19. $2y - \frac{1}{2}x = 4$

20. $\frac{1}{3}y + 2x = 3$

21. $4y - 3x = 12$

22. $4x - 3y = 6$

23. $-2x + 5y = 5$

24. $\frac{1}{2}y + 2x = 3$

B 25. $\frac{x + y}{3} = 2$

26. $\frac{x - y}{4} = -1$

27. $\frac{3x - y}{2} = 3$

28. $\frac{2x + y}{3} = 1$

29. $\frac{x - 2y}{3} = -4$

30. $\frac{x + 3}{4} = y$

31. $\frac{3x - 1}{2} = y$

32. $\frac{-3y + 2x}{4} = -2$

33. $\frac{-4x + 3y}{6} = -4$

Graph the equation. Use a separate set of axes for each equation.

EXAMPLE $y = 6$

Solution   Rewrite the equation in the form

$$y = 0x + 6.$$

Find three solutions.

If $x = -1$: $y = 0(-1) + 6 = 6$

If $x = 2$: $y = 0(2) + 6 = 6$

If $x = 3$: $y = 0(3) + 6 = 6$

Three solutions are $(-1, 6)$, $(2, 6)$, and $(3, 6)$. Graph these points and draw the line.

The graph of $y = 6$ is a horizontal line.

34. $y = 2$

35. $x = -4$

36. $y = 0$

37. $y = -3$

38. $x = 6$

39. $y = \frac{3}{2}$

C 40. Graph the equation $y = x^2$ by graphing the points with x-coordinates -3, -2, -1, 0, 1, 2, and 3. Join the points by means of a curved line. (This curve is called a **parabola.**)

41. Graph the equation $xy = 12$ by graphing the points with x-coordinates 1, 3, 6, and 12. Join the points by means of a curved line. On the same set of axes, graph the points with x-coordinates -1, -3, -6, and -12. Join the points by means of a curved line. (This two-branched curve is called a **hyperbola**.)

Graph the equation using the following values of x: -5, -2, 0, 2, 5. Join the points by means of a straight line.

42. $y = |x|$ **43.** $y = -|x|$ **44.** $y = |x - 2|$ **45.** $y - 4 = |x|$

For what value of k is the graph of the given ordered pair in the graph of the given equation?

46. $(3, -2)$; $2y + kx = 14$ **47.** $(-5, 4)$; $3x - ky = -12$

Self-Test A

Exercises 1–6 refer to the diagram. Give the coordinates of each point.

1. M **2.** Z **3.** L

Name the point for the given ordered pair.

4. $(-6, -3)$ **5.** $(2, 2)$ **6.** $(-5, 3)$

[9-1]

Graph the given ordered pairs on one set of axes.

7. $(-3, 5)$ **8.** $(9, 7)$ **9.** $(-4, -8)$

10. $(11, -10)$ **11.** $(0, -2)$ **12.** $(-4, 2)$

Find the solutions of the equation for the given values of x.

13. $4y - x = 2$
values of x: 0, -4, 9

14. $y + 2x = 6$
values of x: -3, $\frac{1}{2}$, 11

[9-2]

Graph each equation on a coordinate plane. Use a separate set of axes for each equation.

15. $y = x - 1$ **16.** $y = 2x$ **17.** $4x - y = 9$ **18.** $x = 7$ [9-3]

Self-Test answers and Extra Practice are at the back of the book.

9-4 Graphing a System of Equations

Two equations in the same variables are called a **system of equations.** If the graphs of two linear equations in a system have a point in common, the coordinates of that point must be a solution of both equations. We can find a solution of a system of equations such as

$$x - y = 2$$
$$x + 2y = 5$$

by finding the *point of intersection* of the graphs of the two equations.

The graphs of the two equations above are shown on the same set of axes. The point with coordinates (3, 1) appears to be the point of intersection of the graphs. To check whether (3, 1) satisfies the given system, we substitute its coordinates in both equations:

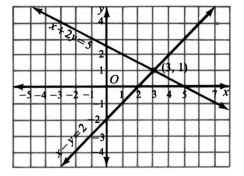

$$x - y = 2 \qquad x + 2y = 5$$
$$3 - 1 = 2 \qquad 3 + 2(1) = 5$$

Since the coordinates satisfy both equations, (3, 1) is the solution of the given system of equations.

EXAMPLE 1 Use a graph to solve the system of equations:

$$y - x = 4$$
$$3y + x = 8$$

Solution First make a table of values for each equation, then graph both equations on one set of axes.

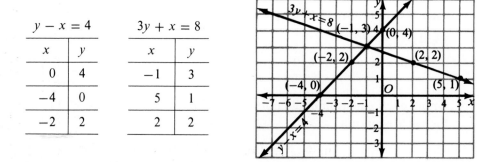

$y - x = 4$		$3y + x = 8$	
x	y	x	y
0	4	−1	3
−4	0	5	1
−2	2	2	2

The point of intersection appears to be (−1, 3).

To check, substitute the coordinates $(-1, 3)$ in both equations:

$$y - x = 4 \qquad\qquad 3y + x = 8$$
$$3 - (-1) \overset{?}{=} 4 \qquad\qquad 3(3) + (-1) \overset{?}{=} 8$$
$$3 + 1 = 4 \checkmark \qquad\qquad 9 - 1 = 8 \checkmark$$

The solution for the given system is $(-1, 3)$.

EXAMPLE 2 Use a graph to solve the system of equations: $2y - x = 2$
$2y - x = -4$

Solution Make a table of values for each equation and graph both equations on one set of axes.

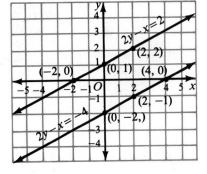

$2y - x = 2$

x	y
0	1
-2	0
2	2

$2y - x = -4$

x	y
0	-2
4	0
2	-1

The graphs do not intersect; they are **parallel lines.** Thus, the system has *no solution.*

A system may have infinitely many solutions, as the following example illustrates.

EXAMPLE 3 Use a graph to solve the system of equations: $6x + 3y = 18$
$2x + y = 6$

Solution Make a table of values for each equation and graph both equations on one set of axes.

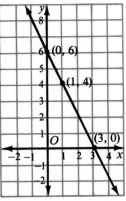

$6x + 3y = 18$

x	y
0	6
3	0
1	4

$2x + y = 6$

x	y
0	6
3	0
1	4

The graphs *coincide.* The coordinates of all points on the line satisfy both equations. This system has *infinitely many solutions.*

To solve a system of equations, first graph the equations on one set of axes. Then consider:

If the graphs intersect, the system has one solution. The coordinates of the point of intersection form the solution.

If the graphs are parallel, the system has no solution.

If the graphs coincide, the system has infinitely many solutions.

Class Exercises

Is the ordered pair a solution of the system of equations?

1. $(4, -1)$ $x + y = 3$
                 $x - y = 5$

2. $(5, -1)$ $x + y = -6$
                 $x - y = 4$

3. $(3, 1)$ $x + 2y = 5$
                 $x - y = 2$

4. $(-4, -4)$ $2x + y = -12$
                 $x - y = 0$

5. A system of two linear equations has no solution. What does the graph of this system look like?

6. The coordinates $(-3, -1)$, $(0, 0)$, and $(3, 1)$ are solutions of a system of two linear equations. What does the graph of this system look like?

7. The graphs of two equations appear to intersect at $(-4, 5)$. How can you check to see whether $(-4, 5)$ satisfies the system?

Written Exercises

Use a graph to solve the system. Do the lines intersect or coincide, or are they parallel?

A

1. $x + y = 6$
   $x - y = 0$

2. $x + y = 5$
   $3y + 3x = 15$

3. $x - y = -3$
   $x - y = 2$

4. $x - y = 4$
   $x + y = 0$

5. $-2y - 2x = -6$
   $x + y = 3$

6. $2x - y = 4$
   $y + 2x = 2$

7. $x - 2y = 8$
   $2y - x = 4$

8. $6y + 4x = 24$
   $2x + 3y = 12$

9. $3x - y = -6$
   $y - x = 6$

10. $x - 2y = -8$
    $2y - 3x = 12$

11. $7x - 14y = 70$
    $x - 2y = 10$

12. $3x + 2y = 6$
    $3x + 2y = 12$

B 13. $2x + \frac{3}{2}y = 2$
       $x + 2y = 6$

14. $x + 3y = 2$
    $2x + 5y = 3$

15. $\frac{2}{3}x - y = 2$
    $6y - 4x = 18$

16. $3x - 5y = 9$
    $\frac{1}{2}x - 2y = 5$

17. $\frac{3}{2}x + 2y = 4$
    $2x + 5y = 3$

18. $-7x - 2y = 7$
    $-\frac{7}{2}x - y = 1$

C 19. Find the value of k in the equations

$$6x - 4y = 12$$
$$3x - ky = 6$$

such that the system has infinitely many solutions.

20. Find the value of k in the equations

$$5x - 3y = 15$$
$$kx - 9y = 30$$

such that the system has no solution.

Review Exercises

Write in lowest terms.

1. $\frac{18}{16}$

2. $\frac{12}{27}$

3. $\frac{49}{56}$

4. $\frac{18}{81}$

5. $\frac{24}{30}$

6. $\frac{48}{144}$

7. $\frac{13}{169}$

8. $\frac{17}{101}$

▮▮▮ **Calculator Key-In**

On Roger's first birthday he received a dime from his parents. For each birthday after that, they doubled the money. How much will Roger receive for his eighteenth birthday?

9-5 Using Graphs to Solve Problems

In the drawing at the left below, the slope of the hill changes. It becomes steeper partway up, and then flattens out near the top.

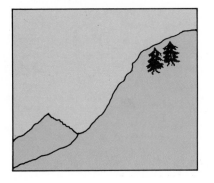
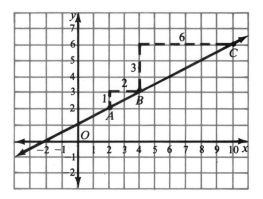

On the other hand, the slope of the straight line shown in the graph above does not change. It remains constant. The **slope of a line** is the ratio of the change in the *y*-coordinate to the change in the *x*-coordinate when moving from one point on the line to another.

Moving from *A* to *B*: slope $= \dfrac{\text{change in } y}{\text{change in } x} = \dfrac{1}{2}$

Moving from *B* to *C*: slope $= \dfrac{\text{change in } y}{\text{change in } x} = \dfrac{3}{6} = \dfrac{1}{2}$

A basic property of a straight line is that its slope is constant.

A straight-line graph sometimes expresses the relationship between two physical quantities. For example, such a graph can represent the conditions of temperature falling at a constant rate or of a hiker walking at a steady pace. If we can locate two points of a graph that is known to be a straight line, then we can extend the graph and get more information about the relationship.

EXAMPLE 1　The temperature at 8 A.M. was 3°C. At 10 A.M. it was 7°C. If the temperature climbed at a constant rate from 6 A.M. to 12 noon, what was it at 6 A.M.? What was it at 12 noon?

Solution　Set up a pair of axes.

Let the coordinates on the horizontal axis represent the hours after 6 A.M.

Let the vertical axis represent the temperature.

Use the information given to plot the points.

At 8 A.M., or 2 h after 6 A.M., the temperature was 3°C. This gives us the point (2, 3).

At 10 A.M., or 4 h after 6 A.M., the temperature was 7°C. This gives us the point (4, 7).

Since we know that the temperature climbed at a constant rate, we can first graph the two points and then draw a straight line through them.

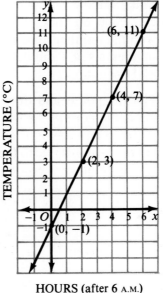

HOURS (after 6 A.M.)

We can see that the line crosses the vertical axis at −1. Therefore, at 6 A.M., or 0 h after 6 A.M., the temperature was −1°C. At 12 noon, or 6 h after 6 A.M., the temperature was 11°C.

Sometimes we are given information about the relationship between two quantities. We can use the information to write and graph an equation. We can then read additional information from the graph.

EXAMPLE 2   Maryanne uses 15 Cal of energy in stretching before she runs and 10 Cal for every minute of running time. Write an equation that relates the total number of Calories (*y*) that she uses when she stretches and goes for a run to the number of minutes (*x*) that she spends running. Graph this equation. From your graph, determine how long Maryanne must run after stretching to use a total of 55 Cal.

(The solution is on the next page.)

The Coordinate Plane   **329**

Solution

Consider the facts given:

15 Cal used in stretching

10 Cal/min used in running

Use the variables suggested.

If x = running time in minutes, then $10x$ = Cal used in running for x min.

If y = Cal used in stretching *and* running for x min, then $y = 15 + 10x$.

Make a table of values to locate two points. Because the number of Calories is large compared with the number of minutes, mark the vertical axis in intervals of 5 and the horizontal axis in intervals of 1.

$y = 15 + 10x$

x	y
0	15
2	35

Plot the points and draw the graph.

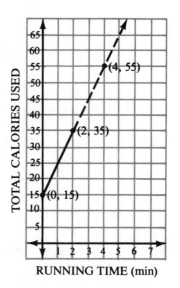

From the graph, you can see that Maryanne must run 4 min after stretching to use a total of 55 Cal.

Problem Solving Reminder

To help identify the conditions of a problem, it may be useful strategy to *rewrite the facts in simpler form.* In Example 2, we list the given facts before writing an equation based on the conditions of the problem.

Class Exercises

Complete for each graph.

1. change in $y =$ ___?___
change in $x =$ ___?___
slope $=$ ___?___

2. change in $y =$ ___?___
change in $x =$ ___?___
slope $=$ ___?___

3. change in $y =$ ___?___
change in $x =$ ___?___
slope $=$ ___?___

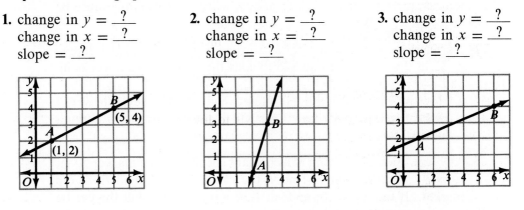

Use a straight-line graph to complete the ordered pairs, then find the slope.

4. $A(1, 3)$, $B(5, 5)$, $C(9, ?)$, $D(?, -1)$

5. $A(0, -3)$, $B(2, 2)$, $C(4, ?)$, $D(?, -8)$

6. $A(8, 4)$, $B(-1, -8)$, $C(5, ?)$, $D(?, -4)$

7. $A(0, 1)$, $B(2, 3)$, $C(-2, ?)$, $D(?, 0)$

8. $A(-1, 6)$, $B(0, 4)$, $C(2, ?)$, $D(?, -4)$

Problems

Solve. Use the same intervals for both axes.

A

1. A pack of greeting cards costs $1.50. Five packs will cost $7.50. Draw a straight-line graph to show the relationship between the number of packs and the cost. Let the x-axis represent the number of packs and the y-axis represent the cost in dollars. What is the slope of the line?

2. An object of 2 g suspended from a spring stretches the spring to a length of 6 cm. An object of 5 g stretches the spring to a length of 11 cm. Draw a straight-line graph to show the relationship between the number of grams of the object and the length of the stretched spring. Let the x-axis represent grams, and the y-axis represent centimeters. What is the slope of the line?

Use a graph to solve the problem.

B **3.** At 1 A.M. the temperature was −6°C. At 5 A.M. it was −1°C. If the temperature continues to rise steadily, what will the temperature be at 9 A.M.?

4. Hernando is saving money for a camping trip. Each week he deposits $5 in the bank. He had $25 to start the account. In 3 weeks he had $40 in the account.
a. How much money will Hernando have by the seventh week?
b. If the trip costs $85, how long will it take him to save enough money?

5. At 9 A.M. a test car driving at a constant speed passes a marker 50 mi from its starting point. At noon the car is about 130 mi from the marker. If the test drive ends at 1:30 P.M., how far will the car be from its starting point?

6. Between 1970 and 1980, the Rockfort Corporation used a 10-year expansion plan to increase its annual earnings steadily. The corporation had earnings of $3.6 million in 1975 and $6 million in 1977.
a. About how much were the corporation's annual earnings in 1972?
b. About how much did it earn by the end of the 10-year plan?

a. Write an equation relating the quantity labeled *y* to the quantity labeled *x*.
b. Graph the equation.
c. Use the graph to answer the question.

C **7.** A butcher charges $4.50 a pound for the best cut of beef. For an additional $2.00, any order will be delivered. Relate the total cost (*y*) to the amount of beef (*x*) ordered and delivered. How many pounds of beef can be ordered and delivered for $33.50?

8. It takes a work crew 15 min to set up its equipment, and 3 min to paint each square meter of a wall. Relate the number of minutes (*y*) it takes to complete a job to the number of square meters (*x*) to be painted. If it took the crew 33 hours to complete the job, about how many square meters was the wall?

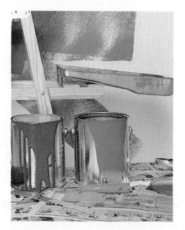

9. A word processor can store documents in its memory. It takes about 10 s to get the information, and about 35 s to print each page of it. Therefore, in about 360 s, or 6 min, the processor can complete a 10-page document. Relate the time (y) in minutes it takes to complete a document to the number of pages (x) to be typed. How many minutes will it take to complete an 18-page document?

10. Shaoli Hyatt earns a salary of $215 a week, plus a $15 commission for each encyclopedia she sells. Relate her total pay for one week (y) to the number of encyclopedias she sells during the week (x). How many encyclopedias must she sell to receive $350 for one week?

Use a graph to solve.

11. The velocity of a model rocket is 3 km/min at 1 s after takeoff. The velocity decreases to 2 km/min at 2.5 s after takeoff. When the rocket reaches its maximum height, the velocity will be 0. Assume that the decrease in velocity is constant. How long will it take the rocket to reach its maximum height?

Review Exercises

Solve.

1. $3x + 4 > 8$

2. $5y - 10 < 0$

3. $7 + 3y \geq -4y$

4. $2(8x + 3) < -2$

5. $6(2y + 7) \leq 42$

6. $-3\left(9x - \frac{2}{3}\right) > -7$

7. $4(9x + 10) \geq 4$

8. $5(4y + 9) \leq 15$

9. $12\left(\frac{x}{6} - \frac{5}{6}\right) > 72$

■■■ | **Calculator Key-In**

Use a calculator to find the product.

$$1^2 = \underline{\ ?\ }$$
$$11^2 = \underline{\ ?\ }$$
$$111^2 = \underline{\ ?\ }$$
$$1111^2 = \underline{\ ?\ }$$

Use the pattern to predict the products $11,111^2$, $111,111^2$, $1,111,111^2$, $11,111,111^2$, and $111,111,111^2$.

9-6 Graphing Inequalities

When we graph a linear equation such as

$$y = x + 1$$

we see that the graph separates the coordinate plane into three sets of points:

(1) those above the line, such as $(-4, 5)$,

(2) those below the line, such as $(3, 1)$, and

(3) those on the line, such as $(2, 3)$.

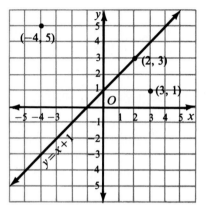

The region *above* the line is the graph of the set of solutions of the inequality

$$y > x + 1.$$

The region *below* the line is the graph of the set of solutions of the inequality

$$y < x + 1.$$

The line $y = x + 1$ forms the **boundary line** of the graphs of the inequalities $y > x + 1$ and $y < x + 1$. For any inequality we can get the boundary line by replacing the inequality symbol with the "equals" symbol.

Since the graph of an inequality consists of all the points above or below a boundary line, we use shading to indicate the region. If the boundary line is part of the graph, it is drawn with a solid line. If the boundary line is not part of the graph, use a dashed line.

$y > x + 1$ $y \geq x + 1$ $y < x + 1$ $y \leq x + 1$

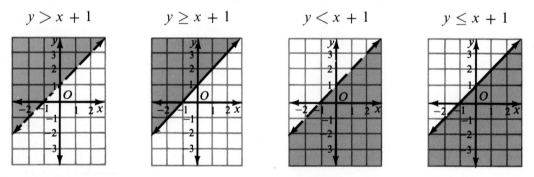

To check whether the shading is correct, choose a point in the shaded region. Then substitute its coordinates for x and y in the inequality. If the coordinates satisfy the inequality, then the shading is correct.

Any set of ordered pairs is a **relation.** Each of the open sentences

$y = x + 1, y > x + 1, y \geq x + 1, y < x + 1$, and $y \leq x + 1$ defines a relation. The equation $y = x + 1$ is a special kind of relation because it defines a function. Not all relations are functions. Recall that for a function, every value of x has only one corresponding value of y. Notice in the shaded region of each graph above, more than one value of y may be associated with each value of x. For example, the following ordered pairs all satisfy the inequalities $y > x + 1$ and $y \geq x + 1$:

$$(-2, 0), (-2, 1), (-2, 2), (-2, 3)$$

Therefore, the relation defined by the inequalities $y > x + 1$ and $y \geq x + 1$ is not a function.

EXAMPLE 1   Graph $y - x < 4$.

Solution   First transform $y - x < 4$ into an equivalent inequality with y alone on one side.

$$y < 4 + x$$

Then locate the boundary line by graphing

$$y = 4 + x.$$

Use a dashed line to draw the boundary line, and shade the region below.

Check: Use $(4, -2)$.
$$y - x \underset{?}{<} 4$$
$$-2 - 4 \overset{?}{<} 4$$
$$-6 < 4 \quad \checkmark$$

EXAMPLE 2   Graph $x \geq -7$.

Solution   Locate the boundary line by graphing

$$x = -7.$$

Use a solid line to draw the boundary. Shade the region to the right since all values of x greater than -7 lie to the right of the boundary line.

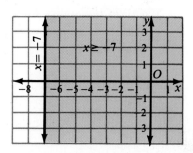

Class Exercises

Transform the inequality into an equivalent inequality with y alone on one side. State the equation of the boundary line.

1. $4x + y < 8$

2. $y - 9x < 2$

3. $4y + 2x > 10$

4. $6x - y > 0$

5. $3 \leq 5x + y$

6. $9y \geq 18$

State whether each point belongs to the graph of the given inequality.

7. $y \leq x + 2$ $(0, 1), (3, 6)$

8. $-x + 2y \geq 0$ $(4, 4), (-2, 1)$

9. $x \leq -7$ $(-4, -10), (-8, 0)$

10. $5 \leq -x + y$ $(-6, -5), (2, 7)$

11. $0 \geq x + y - 5$ $(2, 1), (4, 1)$

12. $y \geq 3$ $(9, 4), (0, 8)$

Written Exercises

State the equation of the boundary line.

A

1. $3x + y > -6$

2. $x + y \geq 2$

3. $x - y \leq 2$

4. $2y - 4 > 0$

5. $-x \geq y - 3$

6. $2y - 6x < 0$

Graph the inequality.

7. $x + y \geq 9$

8. $y > -3x + 3$

9. $-2x + y \geq 2$

10. $x + 6y \leq -5$

11. $4x + 2y \geq 8$

12. $3y - x < -3$

13. $y \geq 2x + 5$

14. $x + 2y \leq 6$

15. $3y - 4 > 2x - 5$

B

16. $3(x - y) > 6$

17. $y \leq 8$

18. $6x + 2y + 3 < 2x - 1$

19. $4x + 3y \leq x - 3$

20. $3y - 6 > 0$

21. $x \leq -3$

22. $y > 0$

23. $2(x + y) < 6x + 10$

24. $3y - 6 \geq 3(x + 2y)$

Write an inequality for the graph shown.

25.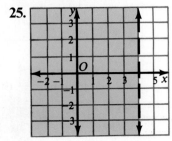

26.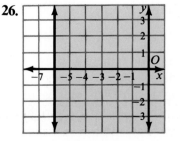

27.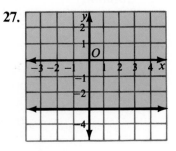

Graph the solutions of each system of inequalities.

EXAMPLE $y \geq -3 + x$
$\quad\quad\quad\quad\quad y \leq 2 - x$

Solution   First graph $y \geq -3 + x$. Use blue to shade the region. Then graph
$y \leq 2 - x$. Use gray to shade the region.

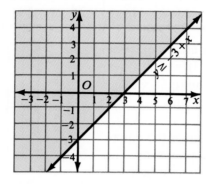 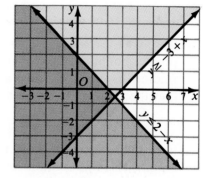

The graph of the solutions of the system is the region where the blue and gray shading overlap.

C   **28.** $y \geq -4$
$\quad\quad x \leq 2$

29. $y > 5 - x$
$\quad\quad y \geq x + 5$

30. $x \leq 9 - y$
$\quad\quad y < x + 3$

31. $x \geq -6$
$\quad\quad x < 3$

Self-Test B

Use a graph to solve the system. Do the lines intersect or coincide, or are they parallel?

1. $x + y = 6$
$\quad\quad y - x = -2$

2. $x + 2y = 6$
$\quad\quad 6y + 3x = 18$

3. $2x + y = 3$
$\quad\quad -2x - y = 2$

[9-4]

Use a graph to solve.

4. When Fritz enrolled in a speed-reading class, he read about 250 words per minute. Two weeks later, his reading speed was about 750 words per minute. If his reading speed increases steadily, how many weeks after enrollment will it take Fritz to read about 1250 words per minute?

[9-5]

Graph each inequality.

5. $x + y \leq 10$

6. $3y - x > 9$

7. $x - 5y \geq 5$

[9-6]

Self-Test answers and Extra Practice are at the back of the book.

The Computer and Linear Equations

For a science project, Nina watered 6 identical lima bean gardens by different amounts. The crop yields were as recorded below.

Water applied daily in cm (x)	0.5	1.0	1.5	2.0	2.5	3.0
Yield of lima beans in kg (y)	1.6	1.8	2.0	2.4	2.6	2.8

Can Nina use these data to predict crop yields for other amounts of daily watering? If we plot her findings as shown on the graph at the right, we see that the points are very nearly on a line.

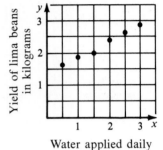

Water applied daily
in centimeters

The computer program below gives the equation of the line that best fits the points on the graph. This line is often called the **line of best fit.** The instruction in line 40 provides the program with all the coordinates of the points. Compare the numbers in line 40 to the numbers in the chart.

```
10    DIM L(50)
20    PRINT "NUMBER OF POINTS ON GRAPH IS";
30    INPUT N
40    DATA .5,1.6,1,1.8,1.5,2,2,2.4,2.5,2.6,3,2.8
50    FOR I = 1 TO N
60    READ X,Y
70    LET A = A + X
80    LET B = B + Y
90    LET C = C + X * X
100   LET D = D + X * Y
110   NEXT I
120   LET Q = N * C - A * A
130   LET R =  INT (100 * (N * D - A * B) / Q + .5) / 100
140   LET S =  INT (100 * (B * C - A * D) / Q + .5) / 100
145   PRINT
150   PRINT "EQUATION OF BEST FITTING LINE IS"
155   PRINT " Y = ";R;"X";
160   IF S >  = 0 THEN 190
170   PRINT S
180   STOP
190   PRINT " ";"+ ";S
200   END
```

1. RUN the program to find the equation of the best fitting line for Nina's data.

2. Draw the graph of the equation.

3. Use the graph to predict the yield (y) if Nina applied 3.3 cm of water daily (x).

Use the computer program to find the equation of the line of best fit for the data given in each chart. Graph each equation and use the equation to answer each question.

4. The chart below shows the distance a spring stretches when different masses are hung from it.

Mass in kg	0.3	0.6	0.9	1.2	1.5	1.8
Stretch in cm	2.1	4.9	6.0	7.1	8.9	10.8

About how much stretch would a 1 kg mass produce?

5. The chart below shows temperature changes as a cold front approached.

Time in hours from 1st reading	0	1	2	3	4
Temperature in °C	21	17	14	12	7

a. Estimate the temperature 1.5 hours from the first reading.

b. If the temperature continues to decrease steadily, about how many hours will it take to reach 0°C?

6. The chart below shows the profit earned by a bookstore on the sale of a bestseller.

No. sold	3	4	7	9	11
Profit	$13.50	$18.00	$31.50	$40.50	$49.50

How many sales will it take to earn a profit of at least $80?

7. The chart below shows the cost of college education for the past 5 years.

Year	1	2	3	4	5
Cost (in thousands)	$7.8	$8.6	$9.4	$9.9	$10.1

Predict the cost of college education for the next two years.

Chapter Review

True or false?

1. The coordinates of point G are $(3, 2)$.

2. The abscissa of point W is 2.

3. The ordinate of point T is 1.

4. Point B is associated with the ordered pair $(2, -3)$.

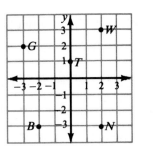

[9-1]

Match each equation with an ordered pair that satisfies the equation.

5. $2y - 7x = 4$ **A.** $(-18, 1)$ [9-2]

6. $10x + \frac{5}{9}y = 0$ **B.** $(9, 2)$

7. $-2x + 9y = 0$ **C.** $(2, 9)$

8. $y - \frac{1}{3}x = 7$ **D.** $(1, -18)$

Graph the equation on a coordinate plane. Use a separate set of axes for each equation.

9. $x + y = 0$ 10. $2y - 3x = -6$ 11. $y - 2x = 2$ [9-3]

Use a graph to solve the system of equations. Match the system with the word that describes its graphs.

12. $y + x = -3$ 13. $y - 3x = -6$ 14. $5y - 2x = 4$ [9-4]
    $2y - 3x = 4$ $y - 3x = 3$ $15y - 6x = 12$

A. intersect   **B.** coincide   **C.** parallel

Complete.

15. A basic property of a straight line is that its slope remains __?__.   [9-5]

16. The slope of a line is the ratio of the change in the __?__-coordinate to the change in the __?__-coordinate when moving from one point on the line to another.

17. The boundary line for the graph of $y > x + 6$ is a __?__ line.   [9-6]

18. If the boundary line is part of the graph of an inequality, it is drawn with a __?__ line.

Chapter Test

Give the coordinates of the point.

1. I **2.** M **3.** E **4.** R

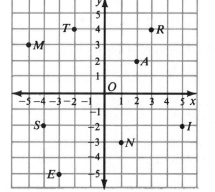

[9–1]

Name the point for the ordered pair.

5. $(-2, 4)$ **6.** $(1, -3)$

7. $(-4, -2)$ **8.** $(5, -2)$

a. Solve the equation for y in terms of x.
b. Find solutions of the equation for the given values of x: -3, 0, 4.

9. $y + 7x = 23$ **10.** $2y - 4x = 1$ **11.** $3y - 6x = 0$ [9–2]

Graph the equation on a coordinate plane. Use a separate set of axes for each equation.

12. $y - 3x = 7$ **13.** $4y - x = 8$ **14.** $2y + x = -10$ [9–3]

Use a graph to solve the system. Do the lines intersect or coincide, or are they parallel?

15. $x - 2y = 0$ **16.** $3x - y = -4$ **17.** $5x + y = 2$ [9–4]
$\quad\;\; 2x + y = 5$ $\quad\;\; 3x - y = 3$ $\quad\;\; 10x + 2y = 4$

Use a graph to solve the problem.

18. One hour after the start of an experiment, the temperature of a solution was $-15°C$. Three hours later it was $-6°C$. If the temperature continues to rise steadily, about how many hours will it take for the temperature to reach $0°C$? [9–5]

19. It takes the window washers 24 min to get ready and 4 min to wash a 6 m by 6 m window.
   a. Write an equation relating the total time (y) required on the job to the number of windows (x) to be washed.
   b. Graph the equation.
   c. About how many 6 m by 6 m windows can they wash in 2 h?

a. State the equation of the boundary line.
b. Graph the inequality.

20. $y \geq 2x + 1$ **21.** $x + y > -4$ **22.** $y - 3x < 0$ [9–6]

Cumulative Review (Chapters 1–9)

Exercises

Write a variable expression for the word phrase.

1. The product of b and five

2. Eight times a number x

3. Twelve less than the sum of y and z

4. A number q divided by seven

5. The sum of three times a number p and seven

Round to the nearest hundredth.

6. 46.871   **7.** 288.005   **8.** 0.7826   **9.** 100.758   **10.** 33.663

Perform the indicated operation.

11. $-8.709 + 13.6001$

12. $7615.7 - 333.61$

13. $606.08 + (-51.99)$

14. $272.65 - (-0.88)$

15. 37.61×0.08

16. $1.5798 \div 0.03$

17. -11.56×36.77

18. $72.5 \div 5$

19. $6.7 \times (-1.22)$

20. $-\frac{1}{3} + \frac{4}{5}$

21. $\frac{4}{7} \times \left(-\frac{3}{8}\right)$

22. $6\frac{1}{2} \div \left(-2\frac{1}{2}\right)$

23. $\frac{7}{8} - \left(-\frac{1}{4}\right)$

24. $3\frac{1}{2} - 1\frac{7}{8}$

25. $-3\frac{4}{5} \times 1\frac{3}{10}$

Write an equation or inequality for the word sentence and solve.

26. The sum of x and three is seven.

27. A number t is the product of negative three fourths and one fifth.

28. The quotient of negative eight divided by w is seven.

29. The sum of x and twelve is greater than the product of x and 2.

Find the circumference of the circle described. Use $\pi \approx 3.14$.

30. diameter $= 28$ cm

31. radius $= 3.3$ m

32. diameter $= 88.5$ km

Solve the proportion.

33. $\frac{n}{4.8} = \frac{0.4}{1.2}$

34. $\frac{1.5}{n} = \frac{1}{4}$

35. $\frac{13}{14} = \frac{39}{n}$

36. $\frac{1.2}{2.0} = \frac{n}{3.0}$

Tell whether the ordered pair is a solution of the given equation.

$2x + y = 15$ **37.** $(0, 12)$ **38.** $(-5, 25)$ **39.** $(5, 5)$ **40.** $(4, 13)$

Problems

Solve.

1. Bill Murphy earns $4.85 an hour working in a day care center. Last week he worked from 1:00 P.M. to 4:30 P.M. on Monday through Friday. How much did he earn?

2. "I feel like I ran a mile," gasped Marge. If Marge ran 5 times around a circular track with a diameter of 210 ft, did she really run a mile? (*Hint:* 5280 ft = 1 mi)

3. Light travels at a speed of 297,600 km/s. If the circumference of Earth is about 39,800 km, about how many times could light travel around Earth in 1 s?

4. Michael Woolsey bought $5671 worth of stock. The commission rate was $28 plus 0.6% of the dollar amount. How much was the commission?

5. A car dealer is expecting a price increase of between $2\frac{1}{2}\%$ and 5% over the price of last year's models. If a certain car sold for $9560 last year, what is the least it can be expected to sell for this year? the most?

6. Myra Daley was given an advance of $18,000 on royalties expected from a book she wrote. If the selling price of the book is $15.95 and her royalty rate is 5%, how many books must be sold before her royalties exceed her advance?

7. A baby that weighed 7 lb 6 oz at birth weighed 10 lb 10 oz at 6 weeks of age. To the nearest tenth of a percent, what was the percent of increase?

8. It took Thomas 25 min longer to do his math homework than to do his French homework. He spent a total of 2.25 h on both subjects. How much time did he spend on math?

9. If a microwave oven uses 1.5 kilowatt hours (kW·h) of electricity in 15 min, how much electricity does it use in 5 min?

10

Areas and Volumes

Pyramids are one type of space figure in geometry. The bottom, or base, of a pyramid is in the shape of a polygon and the sides are always triangular. When your study of measurement is extended to include area, volume, and capacity, you can then describe the pyramid shown in the photograph in more mathematical terms.

The pyramid in the photograph is one of the pyramids built by the Egyptian kings, or Pharaohs, as a monumental tomb. The largest is the Great Pyramid, built by Pharaoh Khufu around 2600 B.C. The Great Pyramid has a square base measuring about 230 m on a side and originally rose to an approximate height of 150 m. When built, it contained about 2,300,000 stone blocks, each having a mass of nearly 2.5 t.

Career Note

Architects are responsible for the design and visual appearance of buildings. Good architectural designs are appealing, safe, and functional. Architects must combine technical skills with a strong sense of style. Course work in mathematics, engineering, and art provide the necessary background for this profession.

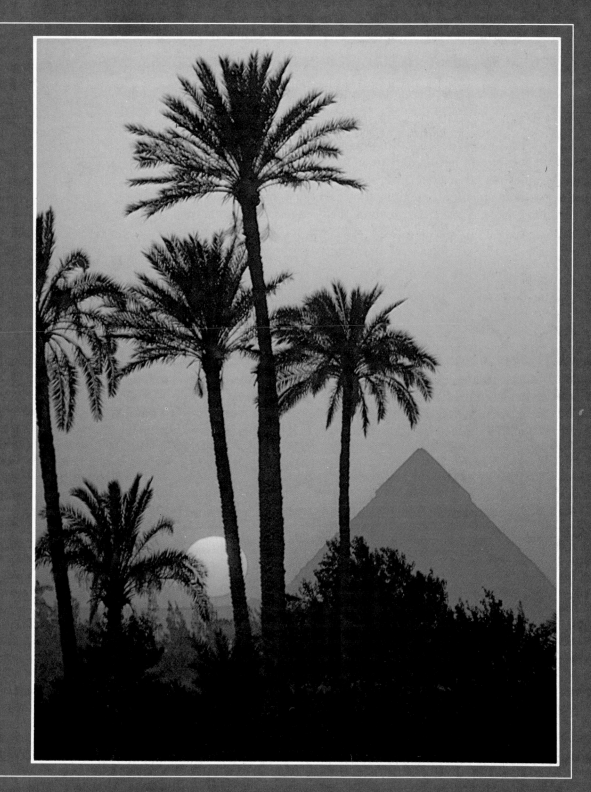

10-1 Areas of Rectangles and Parallelograms

Earlier we measured lengths of segments and found perimeters of polygons. Now we will measure the part of the plane enclosed by a polygon. We call this measure the **area** of the polygon.

Just as we needed a unit length to measure segments, we now need a unit area. In the metric system a unit area often used is the **square centimeter (cm²).**

The rectangular regions shown in the diagrams have been divided into square centimeters to show the areas of the rectangles.

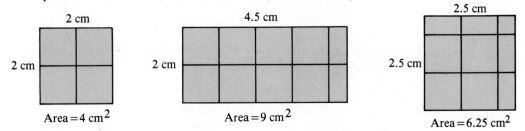

Notice that the area of each rectangle is the product of the lengths of two consecutive sides. These sides are called the **length** and the **width** of the rectangle. The length names the longer side and the width names the shorter side. We have the following formula for any rectangle.

Formula

Area of rectangle = length × width

$$A = lw$$

The length and width of a rectangle are called its **dimensions.**

In the case of a parallelogram, we may consider either pair of parallel sides to be the **bases.** (The word *base* is also used to denote the length of the base.) The **height** is the perpendicular distance between the bases.

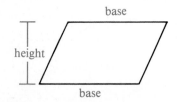

The colored region in the figure at the top of the next page can be moved to the right, as shown in the second figure, to form a rectangle having dimensions b and h. Thus, the area of the parallelogram is the same as the area of the rectangle, bh.

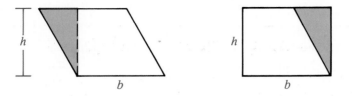

The area of any parallelogram can be found by using the following formula.

> ## Formula
>
> Area of parallelogram = base × height
>
> $$A = bh$$

EXAMPLE 1 Find the area of each parallelogram.

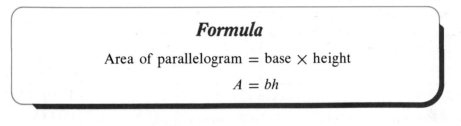

a. 30 m 25 m

b. 15 mm 20 mm

Solution

a. $A = bh$
$= 25 \times 30 = 750$
The area is 750 m².

b. $A = bh$
$= 15 \times 20 = 300$
The area is 300 mm².

EXAMPLE 2 A parallelogram has an area of 375 cm² and a height of 15 cm. Find the length of the base.

Solution

$A = bh$

$375 = b \times 15$

$\dfrac{375}{15} = b$

$25 = b$

The length of the base is 25 cm.

The unit areas used in the examples are **square meters (m²)**, **square millimeters (mm²)**, and **square centimeters (cm²)**. For very large regions, such as states or countries, we could use **square kilometers (km²)**.

Sometimes we may work with an unspecified unit of length. Then the unit of area is simply called a **square unit.** Thus, the area of the rectangle shown at the right is 250 square units.

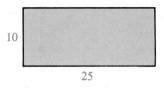

10

25

Class Exercises

Find the area of each shaded region.

1. 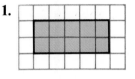   **2.** 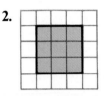   **3.**    **4.**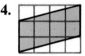

5. Find the perimeters of the regions in Exercises 1 and 2.

6. Find the area of a square with sides 4 cm long.

Complete.

7. $1 \text{ cm} = \underline{\ ?\ } \text{ mm}$

    $1 \text{ cm}^2 = \underline{\ ?\ } \text{ mm}^2$

8. $1 \text{ m} = \underline{\ ?\ } \text{ cm}$

    $1 \text{ m}^2 = \underline{\ ?\ } \text{ cm}^2$

9. $1 \text{ km} = \underline{\ ?\ } \text{ m}$

    $1 \text{ km}^2 = \underline{\ ?\ } \text{ m}^2$

10. Explain why the blue parallelogram and the gray one have equal areas.

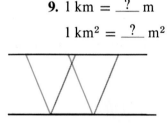

Written Exercises

Find the area and the perimeter of each rectangle or parallelogram.

A   **1.**   30 cm   35 cm

2.   11 m   4 m   5 m

3.   65 km   41 km

4.   5.6   1.3   1.2

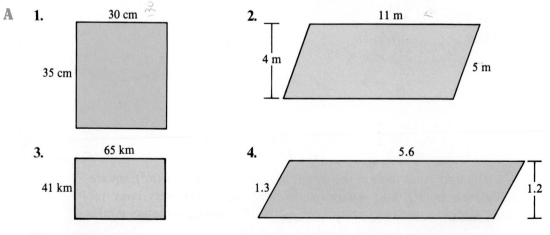

Find the area and the perimeter of a rectangle having the given dimensions.

5. 48 mm by 92 mm

6. 55 cm by 32 cm

7. 63.7 km by 39.1 km

8. 206.3 m by 33.15 m

Copy and complete the tables.

Rectangle	9.	10.	11.	12.	13.	14.
length	12.5	12	? *80*	? *6*	8.6	?
width	7.5	*5* ?	45	2.5	? *.4*	?
perimeter	?	? *34*	? *250*	17.0	18.0	4
area	?	60	3600	? *15*	? *3*	1

Parallelogram	15.	16.	17.	18.	19.	20.
base	18.5	2.7	? *.5*	14.3	2.9	?
height	4.0	? *3*	1.6	3.2	?	0.4
area	? *74*	8.1	0.8	? *45.76*	11.6	3.6

Find the area of each region. (*Hint:* Subdivide each region into simpler ones if necessary.)

B

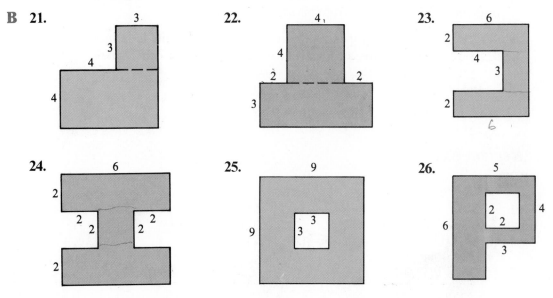

21.

22.

23.

24.

25.

26.

Problems

Solve.

A **1.** How many square meters of wallpaper are needed to cover a wall 8 m long and 3 m high?

2. a. How many square yards of carpeting are needed to cover a floor that measures 8 yd by 5 yd?
   b. How much will the carpeting cost at $24 per square yard?

3. a. How many square feet of vinyl floor covering are needed to cover a floor measuring 60 ft by 12 ft?
   b. How much will the floor covering cost at $1.50 per square foot?

4. Jose wishes to line the open box shown at the right using five sheets of plastic. How many square centimeters will he need?

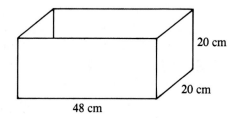

48 cm
20 cm
20 cm

B **5.** Yoneko wishes to obtain 6 m² of plastic from a roll 40 cm wide. How many meters should she unroll?

6. A square pool 5 m on each side is surrounded by a brick walk 2 m wide. What is the area of the walk?

7. A construction site in the shape of a square is surrounded by a wooden wall 2 m high. If the length of one side of the wall is 45 m, find the area of the construction site.

8. A rectangular cow pasture has an area of 1925 m². If the length of one side of the pasture is 55 m, find the lengths of the other sides.

Review Exercises

Multiply.

1. $\frac{1}{2} \times 8 \times 7$
2. $\frac{1}{3} \times 11 \times 9$
3. $\frac{1}{2} \times 1.3 \times 1.6$

4. $\frac{1}{2}(8 + 9)11$
5. $\frac{1}{4}(20 + 12)5$
6. $\frac{1}{2}(0.11 + 0.17)0.6$

7. $\frac{1}{3}(0.26 + 0.52)0.3$
8. $\frac{1}{4}(1.76 + 2.69)1.94$

10-2 Areas of Triangles and Trapezoids

Any side of a triangle can be considered to be the **base.** The **height** is then the perpendicular distance from the opposite vertex to the base line.

Let us find the area of a triangle having base b and height h. The triangle and a congruent copy of it can be put together to form a parallelogram as shown in the diagrams.

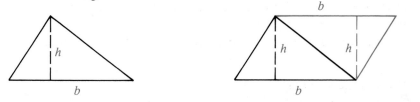

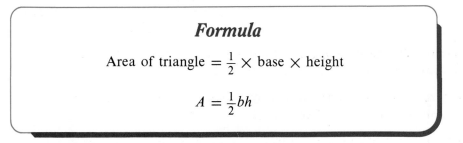

Since the area of the parallelogram is bh and the area of the triangle is half the parallelogram, we have the following formula.

> ## Formula
>
> Area of triangle $= \frac{1}{2} \times$ base $\times$ height
>
> $$A = \frac{1}{2}bh$$

EXAMPLE   Find the area of each triangle.

a.

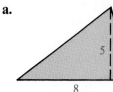

b.

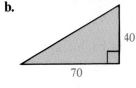

c.

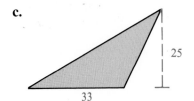

Solution

a. $A = \frac{1}{2}bh$

$\quad = \frac{1}{2} \times 8 \times 5$

$\quad = 20$

$\quad A = 20$ square units

b. $A = \frac{1}{2}bh$

$\quad = \frac{1}{2} \times 70 \times 40$

$\quad = 1400$

$\quad A = 1400$ square units

c. $A = \frac{1}{2}bh$

$\quad = \frac{1}{2} \times 33 \times 25$

$\quad = 4125$

$\quad A = 412.5$ square units

Note in part (b) of Example 1 that the lengths of the sides of the *right angle* of the triangle were used as the base and the height. This can be done for any *right* triangle, even if the triangle is positioned so that it is "standing" on the side opposite the right angle.

The **height** of a trapezoid is the perpendicular distance between the parallel sides. These parallel sides are called the **bases** of the trapezoid. The method used to find the formula for the area of a triangle can be used to find the formula for the area of a trapezoid having bases b_1 and b_2 and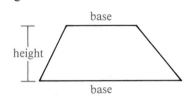
height h. The trapezoid and a congruent copy of it can be put together to form a parallelogram. The area of the parallelogram is $(b_1 + b_2)h$ and the area of the original trapezoid is half of the area of the parallelogram.

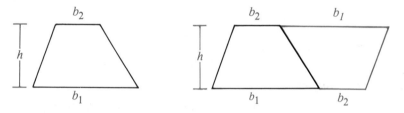

We, therefore, have the following formula.

Formula

Area of trapezoid $= \frac{1}{2} \times$ (sum of bases) $\times$ height

$$A = \frac{1}{2}(b_1 + b_2)h$$

EXAMPLE 2 Find the area of each trapezoid.

a.

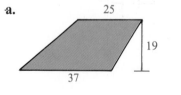

b.

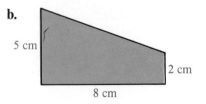

Solution

a. $A = \frac{1}{2}(b_1 + b_2)h$

$= \frac{1}{2} \times (37 + 25) \times 19 = 589$

$A = 589$ square units

b. $A = \frac{1}{2}(b_1 + b_2)h$

$= \frac{1}{2} \times (5 + 2) \times 8 = 28$

$A = 28$ m^2

EXAMPLE 3   A trapezoid has an area of 200 cm² and bases of 15 cm and 25 cm.
            Find the height.

Solution $A = \frac{1}{2}(b_1 + b_2)h$

            $200 = \frac{1}{2} \times (15 + 25) \times h$

            $200 = \frac{1}{2} \times 40 \times h$

            $200 = 20h$
            $\ \ 10 = h$

            The height is 10 cm.

Class Exercises

Find the area of each polygon.

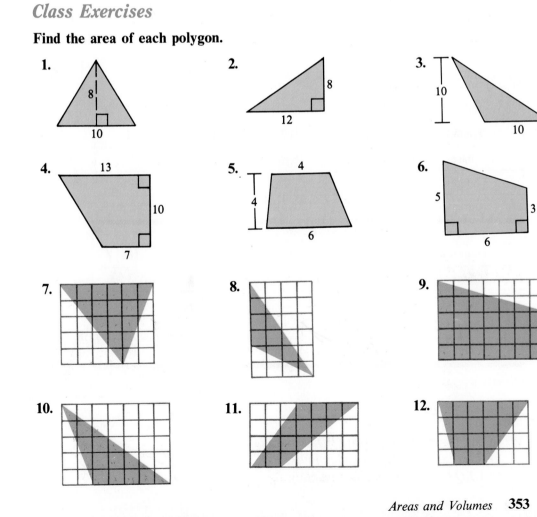

1.

8
10

2.

8
12

3.

10
10

4.

13
10
7

5.

4
4
6

6.

5
3
6

7.

8.

9.

10.

11.

12.

Written Exercises

Find the area of each polygon.

A

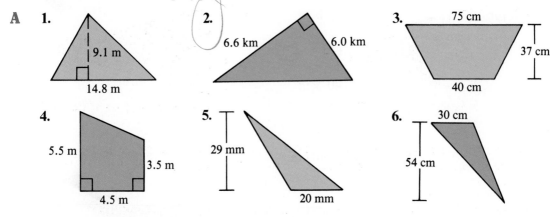

1.

9.1 m

14.8 m

2.

6.6 km   6.0 km

3.   75 cm

37 cm

40 cm

4.

5.5 m

3.5 m

4.5 m

5.

29 mm

20 mm

6.   30 cm

54 cm

7. Triangle: base 122 km, height 30 km

8. Triangle: base 480 m, height 480 m

9. Trapezoid: bases 12.3 cm and 6.2 cm, height 4.8 cm

10. Trapezoid: bases 14.6 km and 22.4 km, height 14.0 km

Copy and complete the tables.

Triangle	11.	12.	13.	14.
base	6 cm	16 mm	?	?
height	?	?	2.4 m	1.4 m
area	72 cm²	80 mm²	4.8 m²	0.42 m²

B

Trapezoid	15.	16.	17.	18.
base	0.7 mm	0.8 m	3	2
base	1.7 mm	1.2 m	?	?
height	?	?	2	3
area	9.6 mm²	1.0 m²	18	18

R ‒ ‒ ‒ S ‒ ‒ ‒ ‒ ‒ T

19. In the figure at the right, $\overline{PQ}$ is parallel to $\overline{RT}$. Explain why triangles PQR, PQS, and PQT all have the same area.

P   Q

In Exercises 20 and 21 find the area of (a) the blue part and (b) the red part of the pennant.

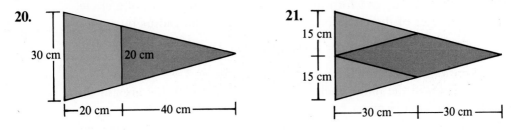

20. 30 cm / 20 cm / 20 cm / 40 cm

21. 15 cm / 15 cm / 30 cm / 30 cm

C **22.** One triangle has a base and a height that are twice as large as the base and the height of another triangle. What is the ratio of their areas?

23. One rectangle has a base and a height that are 3 times the base and the height of another rectangle. What is the ratio of their areas? their perimeters?

Review Exercises

Simplify.

1. 3×5^2

2. 1.2×9^2

3. 4×1.3^2

4. $3 \times 7^2 - 2 \times 4^2$

5. $4 \times 5^2 + 3 \times 8^2$

6. $11^2 \times 3 - 6^2 \times 4$

7. $5 \times 1.4^2 - 7 \times 1.1^2$

8. $2.5^2 \times 4 + 3.2^2 \times 7$

9. $17 \times 14^2 + 6 \times 16^2$

▊▊▊ **Challenge**

The ancient Egyptians worked primarily with fractions with a numerator of 1. They expressed fractions such as $\frac{2}{5}$ as the sum of these fractions: $\frac{2}{5} = \frac{1}{3} + \frac{1}{15}$. These sums were listed in a table. Find the following sums selected from the Egyptian fraction table.

1. $\frac{1}{8} + \frac{1}{52} + \frac{1}{104}$

2. $\frac{1}{12} + \frac{1}{51} + \frac{1}{68}$

3. $\frac{1}{12} + \frac{1}{76} + \frac{1}{114}$

4. $\frac{1}{24} + \frac{1}{58} + \frac{1}{174} + \frac{1}{232}$

5. $\frac{1}{20} + \frac{1}{124} + \frac{1}{155}$

6. $\frac{1}{24} + \frac{1}{111} + \frac{1}{296}$

10-3 Areas of Circles

Recall that there are two formulas for the circumference, C, of a circle. If the diameter of the circle is denoted by d and the radius by r, then

$$C = \pi d \quad \text{and} \quad C = 2\pi r.$$

Two approximations for the number π are 3.14 and $\frac{22}{7}$.

The part of the plane enclosed by a circle is called the **area of the circle.** This area is given by the following formula.

Formula

Area of circle $= \pi \times (\text{radius})^2$

$$A = \pi r^2$$

EXAMPLE 1 Find the areas of the shaded regions. Use $\pi \approx 3.14$.

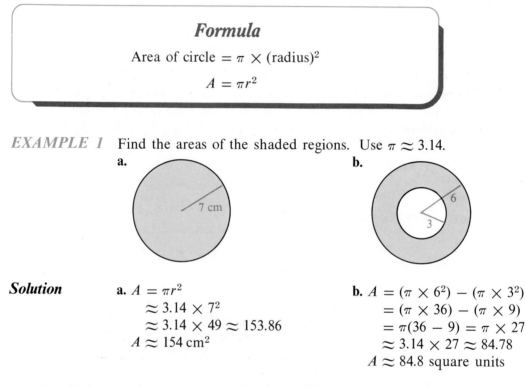

a.

7 cm

b.

6

3

Solution

a. $A = \pi r^2$
$\approx 3.14 \times 7^2$
$\approx 3.14 \times 49 \approx 153.86$
$A \approx 154 \text{ cm}^2$

b. $A = (\pi \times 6^2) - (\pi \times 3^2)$
$= (\pi \times 36) - (\pi \times 9)$
$= \pi(36 - 9) = \pi \times 27$
$\approx 3.14 \times 27 \approx 84.78$
$A \approx 84.8$ square units

Recall that we give answers to only three digits when we use the approximation $\pi \approx 3.14$. Sometimes, to avoid approximations, we give an answer in terms of π.

EXAMPLE 2 Find the area of the shaded region. Leave your answer in terms of π.

2 m

O

Solution Area of shaded region
$= (\text{Area of large circle}) -$
$\qquad\qquad (\text{Area of small circle})$
We first find the area of the small circle.

$$A = \pi r^2 = \pi \times 2^2 = 4\pi$$

We then find the area of the large circle.
Since the radius of the large circle is the same as the diameter of the small circle, we know that the radius of the large circle is 4 m.

$$A = \pi r^2 = \pi \times 4^2 = 16\pi$$

Thus, area of shaded region is equal to $16\pi - 4\pi = 12\pi$
The area of the shaded region is 12π m².

To make the formula $A = \pi r^2$ seem reasonable to you, think of the circular region below cut like a pie.

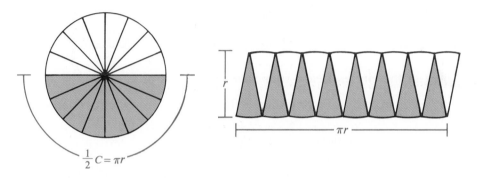

The pieces can be arranged to form a figure rather like a parallelogram with base πr and height r. This suggests that the area is given by

$$\pi r \times r = \pi r^2.$$

Reading Mathematics: *Diagrams*
To read and understand an explanation that is illustrated by a diagram, ask yourself questions about the diagram as you read. In the explanation above, for example, ask yourself, why is the figure "rather like" a parallelogram. How is it different? Why is the measure of the base πr?

Class Exercises

Solve.

1. A circle has radius 10 cm. What is its area? Use $\pi \approx 3.14$.

2. A circle has diameter 14 units. What is its area? Use $\pi \approx \frac{22}{7}$.

3. A circle has diameter 6. What is its area? Give your answer in terms of π.

4. A circle has radius 5. What is its area? Give your answer in terms of π.

5. A circle has area 4π cm². What is its radius?

6. A circle has area 9π. What is its diameter?

Written Exercises

Find the area of the circle. Use $\pi \approx 3.14$ and round the answer to three digits.

A **1.** radius = 5 km   **2.** radius = 8 cm   **3.** diameter = 0.6 m

Find the area of the circle. Use $\pi \approx \frac{22}{7}$.

4. radius = 14 cm   **5.** diameter = $3\frac{1}{2}$ **6.** diameter = 28 cm

Find the area of the circle. Leave your answer in terms of π.

7. diameter = 20 m   **8.** radius = 15 cm   **9.** circumference = 4π

Find the radius of a circle having the given area. Use $\pi \approx 3.14$.

10. $A = 78.5$ cm²   **11.** $A = 314$ m²

Find the diameter of a circle having the given area. Use $\pi \approx \frac{22}{7}$.

12. $A = 154$ km²   **13.** $A = 3\frac{1}{7}$ cm²

Find the circumference of a circle with the given area in terms of π.

B **14.** $A = 16\pi$ **15.** $A = 4\pi$

Find the area of the shaded region. Leave your answer in terms of π.

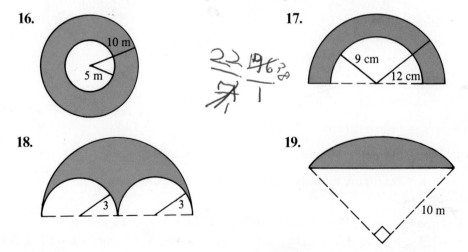

16.   10 m   5 m

17.   9 cm   12 cm

18.   3   3

19.   10 m

C 20. Find a formula giving the area of a circle in terms of the diameter.

21. Find the formula giving the area of a circle in terms of the circumference.

Problems

Solve. Draw a sketch illustrating the problem if necessary. Use $\pi \approx 3.14$ and round the answer to three digits.

A 1. A circular lawn 10 m in diameter is to be resodded at a cost of $14 per m². Find the total cost.

2. The Connaught Centre building in Hong Kong has 1748 circular plate glass windows, each 2.4 m in diameter. If glass costs $12 per m², what is the cost of the glass in a single window?

3. The circumference of a circular pond is 62.8 m. If its diameter is 20 m, find the area.

B 4. A circular pond 20 m in diameter is surrounded by a gravel path 5 m wide. The path is to be replaced by a brick walk costing $30 per square meter. How much will the walk cost?

5. The inner and outer radii of the grooved part of a phonograph record are 7 cm and 14 cm. What is the area of the grooved part?

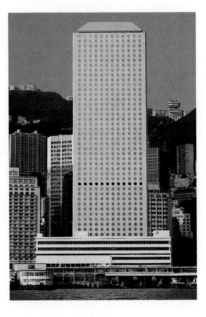

Hint for Problems 6 and 7: Let the radius of the circle be 1 unit.

C 6. A circle is inscribed in a square. What fraction of the area of the square is taken up by the circle?

7. A square is inscribed in a circle. What fraction of the area of the circle is taken up by the square?

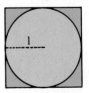

Review Exercises

Estimate to the nearest whole number.

1. $(3.9)^2$	**2.** $(5.3)^2$	**3.** $(2.72)^2$	**4.** $(6.18)^2$
5. 2.7×6	**6.** 3.1×4.9	**7.** 3.14×5.3	**8.** 4.92×5.13

10-4 Using Symmetry to Find Areas

We say that the figure at the right is **symmetric with respect to a line,** $\overleftrightarrow{AB}$, because if it were folded along $\overrightarrow{AB}$, the lower half would fall exactly on the upper half. $\overleftrightarrow{AB}$ is called a **line of symmetry.**

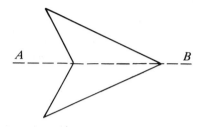

The diagrams below show that figures may have more than one line of symmetry.

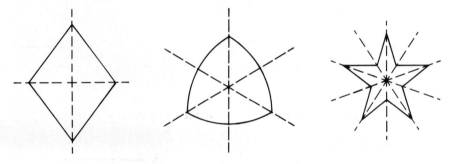

Symmetry can be helpful in finding areas.

EXAMPLE 1 Find the area of the symmetric figure.

Solution The symmetry of this figure is such that the four triangles are congruent. Therefore,

$$A = 4 \times \frac{1}{2}bh$$

$$= 4 \times \left(\frac{1}{2} \times 7 \times 6\right) = 84$$

Thus, the area is 84 square units.

Figures can also be **symmetric with respect to a point.** Although the figure at the right has no line of symmetry, it is symmetric with respect to point O. A figure is symmetric with respect to a point, O, if for every point P on the figure there corresponds an opposite point Q on the figure such that O is the midpoint of the segment $\overline{PQ}$. Every line through the point of symmetry divides the figure into two congruent figures.

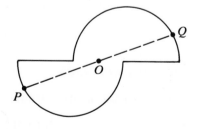

EXAMPLE 2 Find the area of the symmetric figure.

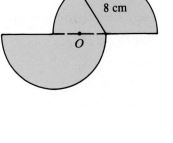

Solution The dashed line divides the region into two semicircles of radius 8 cm.

$$A = 2 \times \left(\frac{1}{2}\pi r^2\right)$$

$$= 2 \times \left(\frac{1}{2}\pi \times 8^2\right)$$

$$\approx 3.14 \times 64 = 200.96$$

The area is approximately 201 cm².

Class Exercises

Copy each figure and show on your drawing any lines or points of symmetry.

1.

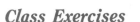

Equilateral
Triangle

2.

Semicircle

3.

Square

4.

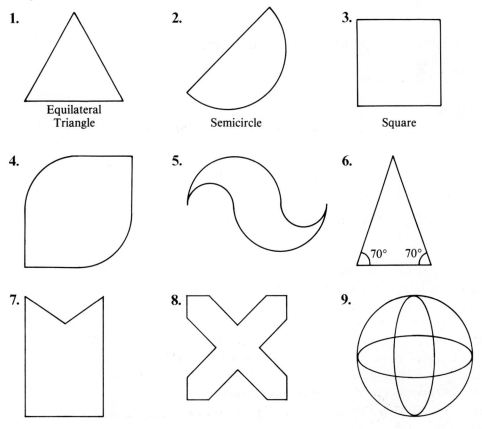

5.

6.

70°   70°

7.

8.

9.

Written Exercises

Copy each figure and show on your drawing any lines or points of symmetry.

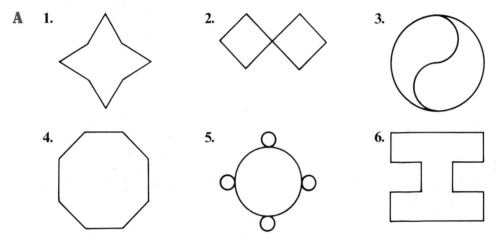

A 1.

2.

3.

4.

5.

6.

Find the areas of the following symmetric figures. Give your answers in terms of π if necessary.

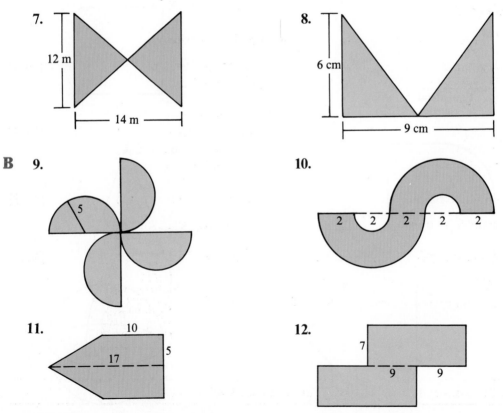

7.

12 m

14 m

8.

6 cm

9 cm

B 9.

5

10.

2 2 2 2 2

11.

10

17

5

12.

7

9 9

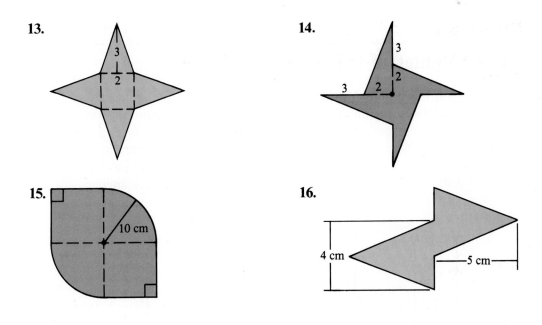

13. 3 ┬ 2

14. 3 2 3 2

15. 10 cm

16. 4 cm 5 cm

Self-Test A

Find the area. Round the answer to three digits if necessary.

1. rectangle
length: 21 cm
width: 13 cm

2. parallelogram
base: 7 m
height: 12 m   [10–1]

3. triangle
base: 18 cm
height: 8 cm

4. trapezoid
bases: 11 m and 7 m
height: 4 m   [10–2]

5. circle: Use $\pi \approx 3.14$.

radius: 15 mm

6. circle: Use $\pi \approx \frac{22}{7}$.

diameter: 28 cm   [10–3]

7. Copy the figure and show any lines or points of
symmetry.

8. Find the area of the symmetric figure.   [10–4]

2   2

2   6

6

Self-Test answers and Extra Practice are at the back of the book.

10-5 Volumes of Prisms and Cylinders

A **polyhedron** is a figure formed of polygonal parts of planes, called **faces,** that enclose a region of space. A **prism** is a polyhedron that has two congruent faces, called **bases,** that are parallel. The other faces are regions bounded by parallelograms. The bases may also be parallelograms. Prisms are named according to their bases. Unless otherwise stated, we will only consider prisms whose other faces are rectangles.

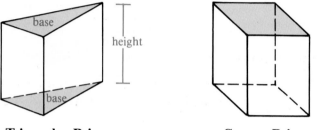

Triangular Prism   **Square Prism**

In each figure above, the bases are shaded. The perpendicular distance between the bases is the **height** of the prism.

A polyhedron together with the region inside it is called a **solid.** The measure of the space occupied by a solid is called the **volume** of the solid. The prism at the right, filled with 3 layers of 8 unit cubes, has 24 unit cubes. In this case, each unit cube is a cubic centimeter (cm³). Thus the volume of the cube is 24 cm³.

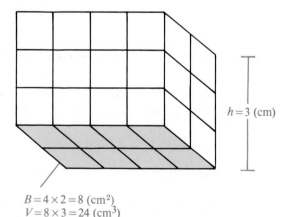

$h = 3$ (cm)

This example suggests a formula for finding the volume of any prism.

$B = 4 \times 2 = 8$ (cm²)
$V = 8 \times 3 = 24$ (cm³)

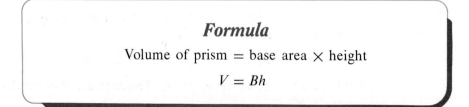

Formula

Volume of prism = base area × height

$$V = Bh$$

EXAMPLE 1   A watering trough is in the form of a trapezoidal prism. Its ends have the dimensions shown. How long is the trough if it holds 12 m³?

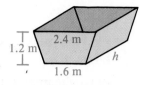

Solution   Examine the diagram carefully to determine which regions are the bases. In this diagram, one of the bases is at the front. You know that the volume is 12 m³. Find the area of the base.

$$B = \frac{1}{2}(1.6 + 2.4) \times 1.2 = 2.4 \,(\text{m}^2)$$

Then, use the formula.
$$V = Bh$$
$$12 = 2.4h$$
$$5 = h$$

The length of the trough is 5 m.

A **cylinder** is like a prism except that its bases are circles instead of polygons. We will only consider cylinders with congruent bases. The area of the base, B, is πr^2. Thus:

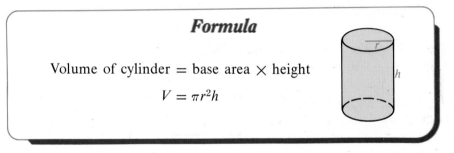

Formula

Volume of cylinder = base area × height

$$V = \pi r^2 h$$

The volume of a container is often called its **capacity.** The capacity of containers of fluids is usually measured in **liters** (L) or **milliliters** (mL).

$$1 \text{ L} = 1000 \text{ cm}^3 \qquad 1 \text{ mL} = 1 \text{ cm}^3$$

It is easy to show that 1 m³ = 1000 L.

EXAMPLE 2   A cylindrical storage tank 1 m in diameter is 1.2 m high. Find its capacity in liters. Use $\pi \approx 3.14$.

Solution   Use the formula $V = \pi r^2 h$. The height is 1.2 m and, because the diameter is 1 m, the radius is 0.5 m.

$$V \approx 3.14 \times (0.5)^2 \times 1.2 = 0.942 \,(\text{m}^3)$$

Since 1 m³ = 1000 L, 0.942 m³ = 942 L. The capacity of the tank is approximately 942 L.

Class Exercises

Find the volume of the solid. In Exercises 5 and 6, leave your answer in terms of π.

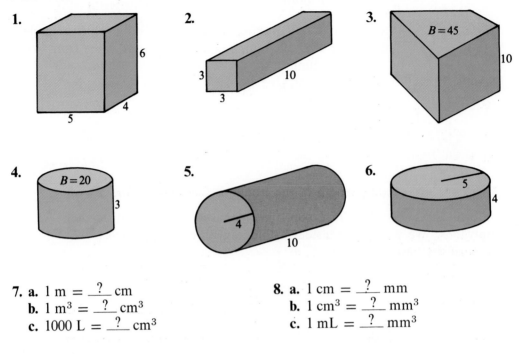

1.

6
4
5

2.

3
3
10

3.

B=45
10

4.

B=20
3

5.

4
10

6.

5
4

7. a. 1 m = _?_ cm
  b. 1 m³ = _?_ cm³
  c. 1000 L = _?_ cm³

8. a. 1 cm = _?_ mm
  b. 1 cm³ = _?_ mm³
  c. 1 mL = _?_ mm³

Written Exercises

In this exercise set, use π ≈ 3.14 and round the answer to three digits.

Find the volume of the solid.

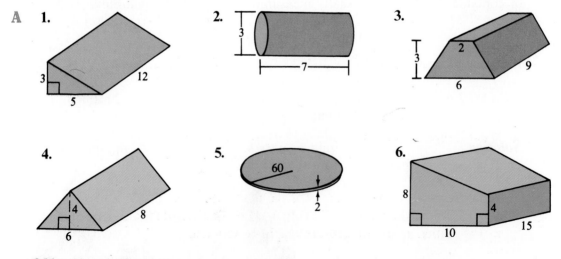

A 1.

3
5
12

2.

3
7

3.

2
3
6
9

4.

4
6
8

5.

60
2

6.

8
10
4
15

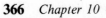

7.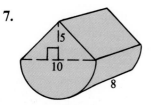

8.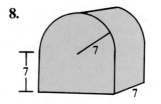

Find the capacity in liters of the prism or cylinder.

9. Square prism: 25 cm by 25 cm by 80 cm

10. Prism: base area = 1.2 m², height = 2.3 m

11. Cylinder: base radius = 1.2 m, height = 1.4 m

12. Cylinder: base diameter = 1 m, height = 75 cm

The table below refers to cylinders. Copy and complete it. Leave your answers in terms of π.

B

	13.	**14.**	**15.**	**16.**	**17.**	**18.**
volume	12π	150π	100π	20π	18π	100π
base radius	2	5	?	?	?	?
base area	?	?	25π	4π	?	?
height	?	?	?	?	2	25

Find the volume of the prism if the pattern were folded.

19.   **20.**

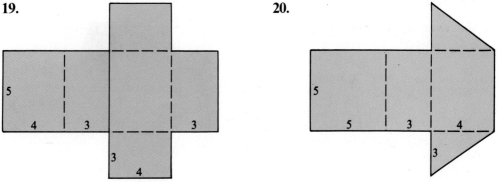

C **21.** What happens to the volume of a cylinder if this change is made?
    a. The radius is doubled.   **b.** The height is halved.
    c. The radius is doubled and the height is halved.

22. What happens to the volume of a cylinder if this change is made?
    a. The radius is halved.   **b.** The height is doubled.
    c. The radius is halved and the height is doubled.

In an *oblique prism,* the bases are *not* perpendicular to the other faces. The volume formula $V = Bh$ still applies, where h is the perpendicular distance between the bases. **Find the volume of each figure shown in red.**

23.

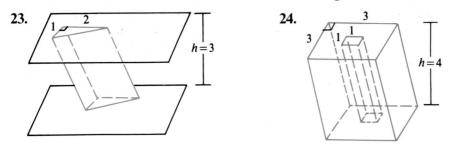

24.

Problems

Solve. Use $\pi \approx 3.14$ and round the answer to three digits.

A **1.** Find the capacity in liters of the V-shaped trough shown below.

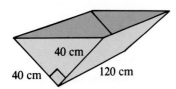

2. Find the capacity in liters of the half-cylinder trough shown below.

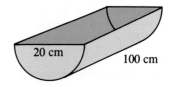

B **3.** Find the volume of metal in the copper pipe shown below.

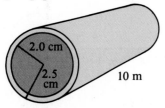

4. Find the volume of concrete in the construction block shown below.

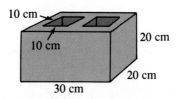

C **5.** A cylindrical water bottle is 28 cm in diameter. How many centimeters does the water level drop when one liter is drawn off?

Review Exercises

Solve for x.

1. $x = \frac{1}{3} \times 6.4 \times 15$ **2.** $x = \frac{1}{2}(7.2) \times 3$ **3.** $3.38 = 4x$ **4.** $\frac{1}{3}x = 11$

5. $3.14 \times 20^2 = x$ **6.** $(0.8)^2 x = 5.12$ **7.** $314 = 3.14x^2$ **8.** $x^2 = 169$

10-6 Volumes of Pyramids and Cones

If we shrink one base of a prism to a point, we obtain a **pyramid** with that point as its **vertex.** A **cone** is obtained in the same way from a cylinder. In each case, the **height** of the solid is the perpendicular distance from its vertex to its base. As for a prism, the shape of the base of a pyramid determines its name. All other faces of a pyramid are triangles. A cone is like a pyramid except that its base is a circle instead of a polygon.

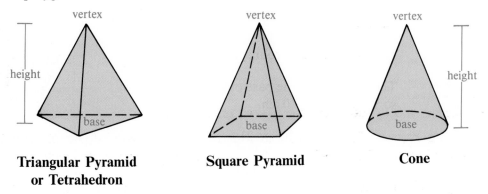

**Triangular Pyramid
or Tetrahedron**   **Square Pyramid**   **Cone**

The volume of a pyramid can be found using this formula:

Formula

Volume of pyramid $= \frac{1}{3} \times$ base area $\times$ height

$$V = \frac{1}{3}Bh$$

EXAMPLE 1   Find the volume of the square pyramid shown at the right.

Solution   First find the base area. Since the base is a square,

$$B = 12^2 = 144 \text{ (cm}^2).$$

Then use the volume formula.

$$V = \frac{1}{3}Bh$$

$$= \frac{1}{3} \times 144 \times 25 = 1200 \text{ (cm}^3)$$

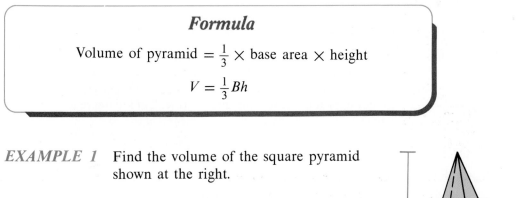

For a cone, the base area is given by the formula $B = \pi r^2$.

Formula

Volume of cone $= \frac{1}{3} \times$ base area $\times$ height

$$V = \frac{1}{3}\pi r^2 h$$

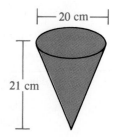

EXAMPLE 2   A conical container is 20 cm across the top and 21 cm deep. Find its capacity in liters. Use $\pi \approx 3.14$ and round to three digits.

Solution   The diameter of the base of the cone is 20 cm, so the radius is 10 cm.

$$V = \frac{1}{3}\pi \times 10^2 \times 21$$

$$\approx \frac{1}{3} \times 3.14 \times 100 \times 21 = 2198$$

Rounding the product to three digits, the volume is approximately 2200 cm³. Because 1000 cm³ equals 1 L, the capacity of the conical container is approximately 2.2 L.

Reading Mathematics: *Vocabulary*
Words that we use in everyday speech may have different meanings in mathematics. For example, the everyday word *base* often refers to the part of an object that it is resting on. The geometrical term *base* refers to a particular face of a figure that may appear at the top, the side, or the end of the figure in a drawing. In Example 2, above, the base appears at the top of the container.

Class Exercises

Find the volume of the solid. In Exercise 3, the base is a square. In Exercise 4, leave your answer in terms of π.

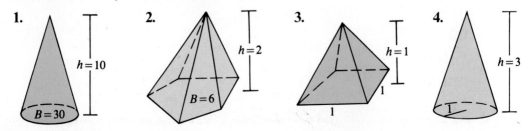

1. $h = 10$, $B = 30$

2. $h = 2$, $B = 6$

3. $h = 1$, 1, 1

4. $h = 3$

Complete.

5. Except for the base, the shapes of all the faces of a pyramid are __?__ .

6. The shapes of all the faces of a tetrahedron are __?__ .

7. A cone has base radius 3 and height 6. The volume of the cone is __?__ π.

Written Exercises

For Exercises 1–10, use $\pi \approx 3.14$ and round the answer to three digits if necessary.

Find the volume of the solid pictured.

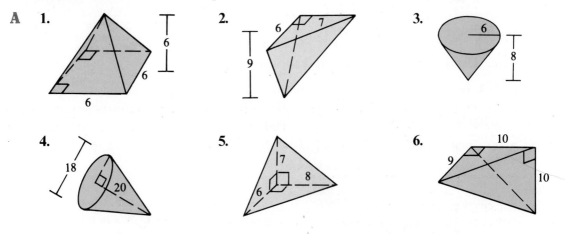

A 1.

6
6
6

2.

6 7
9

3.

6
8

4.

18
20

5.

7
8
6

6.

10
9
10
10

Find the capacity in liters of the cone or pyramid described.

7. A pyramid of height 12 cm having a 5 cm by 8 cm rectangle as base

8. A pyramid having height 10 m and a square base 15 m on a side

9. A cone having base radius 0.8 m and height 1.5 m

10. A cone of height 24 cm and base diameter 11 cm

Copy and complete the table for pyramids.

	11.	12.	13.	14.	15.	16.
base area, *B*	5	33	4	13	?	?
height, *h*	6	12	?	?	10	15
volume, *V*	?	?	8	13	10	20

Copy and complete the table for cones.

B

	17.	18.	19.	20.
radius, r	1	2	?	?
height, h	?	?	4	15
volume, V	5π	12π	12π	5π

Complete.

C **21.** A cone has volume 6 cm³. The volume of a cylinder having the same base and same height is __?__ cm³.

22. A cylinder of height 2 m has the same base and same volume as a cone. The cone's height is __?__ m.

Problems

Solve. Use $\pi \approx 3.14$ and round the answer to three digits.

A **1.** The Great Pyramid in Egypt has a square base approximately 230 m on a side. Its original height was approximately 147 m. What was its approximate volume originally?

2. A volcano is in the form of a cone approximately 1.8 km high and 12 km in diameter. Find its volume.

B **3.** Find the volume of this buoy.

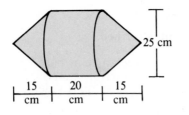

4. Find the volume of this tent. The floor of the tent is square.

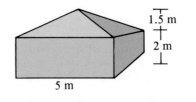

Review Exercises

Find the perimeter of the figure whose sides have the given lengths.

1. rhombus: 9 m per side

2. trapezoid: 4 cm, 4 cm, 5 cm, 7 cm

3. triangle: 35 cm per side

4. parallelogram: 15 m, 7 m, 15 m, 7 m

5. square: 12.8 km per side

6. rectangle: 24.63 km by 37.40 km

7. square: 145.2 km per side

8. triangle: 3.70 m, 12.90 m, 14.85 m

10-7 Surface Areas of Prisms and Cylinders

The **surface area** of every prism and cylinder is made up of its two **bases** and its **lateral surface** as illustrated in the figures below. The lateral surface of a prism is made up of its **lateral faces.** Each lateral face is a rectangle.

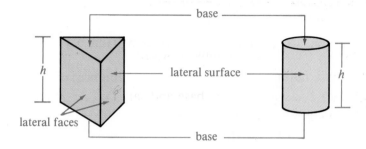

If we were to cut open and flatten out the prism and cylinder shown above, the bases and the lateral surfaces of the figures would look like this:

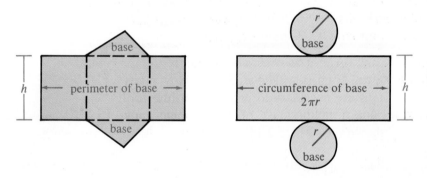

In each of the figures above, the area of the lateral surface, called the **lateral area,** is the product of the perimeter of the base and the height of the figure. To find the **total surface area** of a prism or cylinder, we simply add the area of the two bases to the lateral area of the figure.

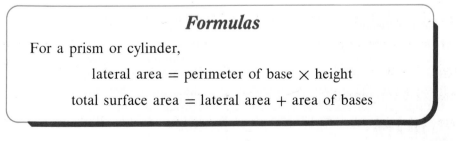

Formulas

For a prism or cylinder,

lateral area = perimeter of base × height

total surface area = lateral area + area of bases

EXAMPLE 1 Find (a) the lateral area, (b) the area of the bases, and (c) the total surface area of the prism shown.

Solution

a. perimeter of base $= 5 + 12 + 13 = 30$ (cm)
height $= 15$ cm
lateral area $= 30 \times 15 = 450$ (cm^2)

b. area of bases $= 2 \times \left(\frac{1}{2} \times 12 \times 5\right) = 60$ (cm^2)

c. total surface area $= 450 + 60 = 510$ (cm^2)

In a cylinder of base radius r, the perimeter (circumference) of the base is $2\pi r$. Thus:

Formulas

For a cylinder,

lateral area $= 2\pi rh$

area of bases $= 2\pi r^2$

total surface area $= 2\pi rh + 2\pi r^2$

EXAMPLE 2 A can of paint will cover 50 m^2. How many cans are necessary to paint the inside (top, bottom, and sides) of the storage tank shown? Use $\pi \approx 3.14$.

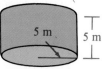

Solution

Since $r = 5$ and $h = 5$,
total surface area $= (2\pi \times 5 \times 5) + (2\pi \times 5^2)$
$\approx (3.14 \times 50) + (3.14 \times 50) = 314$

The total surface area is approximately 314 m^2.

The number of cans of paint is $314 \div 50$, or 6.28. Rounding *up* to the nearest whole number, the answer is 7 cans.

Problem Solving Reminder

For problems whose answers are the result of division, take time to consider whether it is reasonable *to round up or round down*. In Example 2, the answer to the division was 6.28 cans of paint. Because paint cannot be purchased in hundredths of a can, the answer was rounded up to the nearest whole number. If the answer had been rounded down, there would not have been enough paint to cover the interior of the tank.

Class Exercises

1. If a prism has hexagonal bases, how many lateral faces does it have? How many faces does it have in all?

Find the lateral area and the total surface area. Use $\pi \approx 3.14$ and round the answer to three digits.

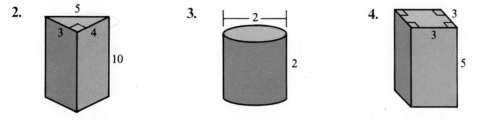

2.

3.

4.

5. If each edge of a cube is one unit long, what is the total surface area in square units?

Written Exercises

Find the total surface area of a rectangular prism having the given dimensions.

A 1. 45 cm by 30 cm by 20 cm

2. 5 cm by 18 cm by 25 cm

3. 2.5 m by 1.6 m by 0.8 m

4. 1.8 m by 0.6 m by 2.0 m

Find (a) the lateral area and (b) the total surface area of the cylinder or prism. Use $\pi \approx 3.14$ and round the answer to three digits.

5. A cylinder having base radius 12 cm and height 22 cm

6. A cylinder having base diameter 6 m and height 4.5 m

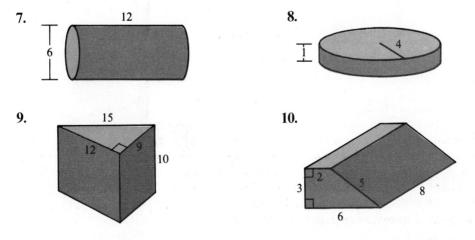

7.

8.

9.

10.

If the patterns below were drawn on cardboard, they could be folded along the dotted lines to form prisms. Find (a) the volume and (b) the total surface area of each.

B 11.

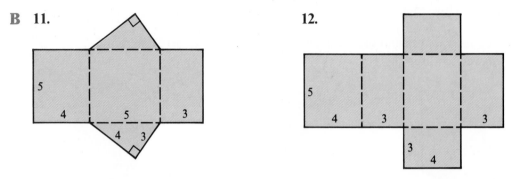

12.

13. Find the length of the edge of a cube whose total area is 150 cm².

14. Three faces of a box have a common vertex and their combined area is 20 cm². What is the total surface area of the box?

15. One can of varnish will cover 64 m² of wood. If you want to put one coat of varnish on each of 24 wooden cubes with the dimensions shown at the right, how many cans of varnish should you buy?

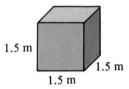

16. You have two cans of red paint, each of which will cover 100 m². Which of the two cylinders pictured below can you paint completely using just the paint that you have?

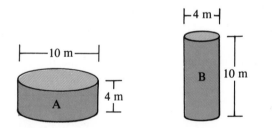

17. A prism of height 3 m has bases that are right triangles with sides 6 m, 8 m, and 10 m. Find the lateral area and the total surface area. (Be sure to draw and label a sketch.)

18. A prism of height 10 cm has bases that are right triangles with sides 5 cm, 12 cm, and 13 cm. Find the lateral area and the surface area. (Be sure to draw and label a sketch.)

19. If the number of faces of a prism is represented by *n*, write an algebraic expression to represent the number of lateral faces.

C **20.** The lateral surface of a cone is made up of many small wedges like the one shown in color. Thinking of the wedge as a triangle of base b and height s, we see that its area is $\frac{1}{2}bs$. When we add all these areas together, we obtain $\frac{1}{2}(2\pi r)s$, or πrs, because the sum of all the b's is $2\pi r$, the circumference of the base. Thus, for a cone:

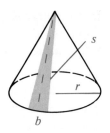

$$\text{lateral area} = \pi rs$$

$$\text{area of base} = \pi r^2$$

$$\text{total surface area} = \pi rs + \pi r^2$$

The length s is called the **slant height** of the cone.

Find the total surface area of each figure.

a.   **b.**   **c.**

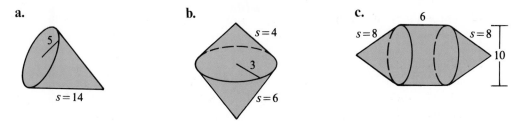

Review Exercises

Find the radius of the circle with the given circumference C or diameter d. Use $\pi \approx 3.14$ and round the answer to three digits.

1. $d = 12$ **2.** $C = 62.8$ **3.** $d = 210$ **4.** $C = 83.6$

5. $C = 220$ **6.** $d = 25$ **7.** $d = 76$ **8.** $C = 2.42$

▌▌▌ Challenge

1. Copy the square at the right and cut it into four pieces along the dashed lines. Re-form the four pieces into a larger square with a "hollow" square at the center.

2. Repeat step 1 several times, assigning different values to a and b each time. In each case, what is the area of the "hollow" square?

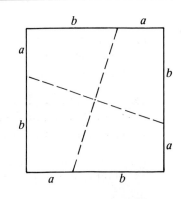

10-8 Volumes and Surface Areas of Spheres

The **sphere** with **radius** r and **center** at C consists of all points at the distance r from point C. The word *radius* also is used for any segment having C as one endpoint and a point of the sphere as another (for example, $\overline{CP}$ in the figure). The word **diameter** is also used in two ways: for a *segment* through C having its endpoints on the sphere (for example, $\overline{AB}$), and for the *length* of such a segment.

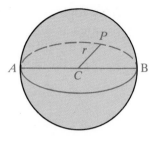

The following formulas for the surface area and volume of a sphere can be proved using higher mathematics.

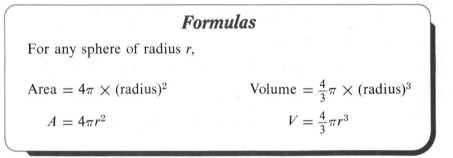

Formulas

For any sphere of radius r,

Area $= 4\pi \times$ (radius)^2 Volume $= \frac{4}{3}\pi \times$ (radius)^3

$A = 4\pi r^2$ $V = \frac{4}{3}\pi r^3$

The surface area of a sphere is usually referred to simply as the *area* of the sphere.

Reading Mathematics: *Diagrams*
Reading diagrams correctly is an important reading skill in mathematics. When three-dimensional objects are pictured on a two-dimensional page, the lines used to draw congruent segments may be of different lengths. For example, in the drawing above, you understand that all radii of a sphere are congruent and that $CP = CB$. Yet these radii cannot be drawn to be of equal length if the picture is to look realistic.

EXAMPLE 1   Find (a) the surface area and (b) the volume of a sphere having diameter 18. Leave your answer in terms of π.

Solution   The radius equals $\frac{1}{2}$ the diameter, so $r = 9$.
   a. $A = 4\pi r^2 = 4\pi \times 9^2 = 4\pi \times 81 = 324\pi$

   b. $V = \frac{4}{3}\pi r^3 = \frac{4}{3}\pi \times 9^3 = \frac{4}{3}\pi \times 729 = 972\pi$

EXAMPLE 2 The area of a sphere is 1600π cm². What is the radius?

Solution Substitute 1600π for A in the formula $A = 4\pi r^2$.

$$1600\pi = 4\pi r^2$$
$$\frac{1600\pi}{4\pi} = \frac{4\pi r^2}{4\pi}$$
$$400 = r^2$$

Since $20^2 = 400$, $r = 20$ cm.

Class Exercises

Complete. In Exercises 1 and 2, give your answers in terms of π.

1. The area of a sphere of radius 1 is __?__, and the volume is __?__.

2. The area of a sphere of radius 2 is __?__, and the volume is __?__.

3. If the radius of a sphere is doubled, the area is multiplied by __?__.

4. If the radius of a sphere is doubled, the volume is multiplied by __?__.

5. If $\overline{AB}$ is a diameter of a sphere having center C, then $\overline{AC}$ and $\overline{BC}$ are __?__ of the sphere.

Complete the following analogies with choice a, b, c, or d.

6. Sphere: Circle = Cube: __?__
   a. Pyramid   **b.** Prism   **c.** Square   **d.** Cylinder

7. Cone: Pyramid = Cylinder: __?__
   a. Sphere   **b.** Prism   **c.** Circle   **d.** Triangle

Written Exercises

Copy and complete the table below. Leave your answers in terms of π.

A

	1.	2.	3.	4.	5.	6.
radius of sphere	3	5	6	9	10	12
surface area	?	?	?	?	?	?
volume	?	?	?	?	?	?

Half of a sphere is called a *hemisphere*. Solve. Leave your answers in terms of π.

7. Find the volume of a hemisphere of radius 2.

8. Find the area of the curved surface of a hemisphere of radius 8.

9. Find the area of the curved surface of a hemisphere of radius 2.2.

10. Find the volume of a hemisphere of radius 3.3.

Copy and complete the table below. Leave your answers in terms of π.

B

	11.	12.	13.	14.	15.	16.
radius of sphere	3.6	?	?	4.5	?	?
surface area	?	64π	?	?	256π	?
volume	?	?	972π	?	?	288π

Solve. Leave your answers in terms of π.

17. The observatory building shown at the right consists of a cylinder surmounted by a hemisphere. Find its volume.

18. The water tank at the right consists of a cone surmounted by a cylinder surmounted by a hemisphere. Find its volume.

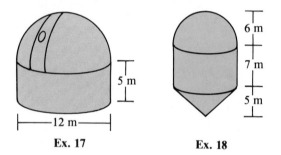

Ex. 17   Ex. 18

19. Earth's diameter is about $3\frac{2}{3}$ times that of the moon. How do their volumes compare?

20. The sun's diameter is about 110 times that of Earth. How do their volumes compare?

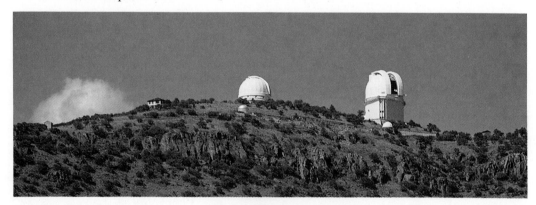

If a sphere fits snugly inside a cylinder it is said to be *inscribed* in the cylinder. Use the diagram at the right for Exercises 21 and 22.

C **21. a.** A sphere of radius 4 is inscribed in a cylinder of height 8. What is the ratio of the volume of the sphere to the volume of the cylinder?
  b. A sphere of radius 5 is inscribed in a cylinder of height 10. What is the ratio of the volume of the sphere to the volume of the cylinder?
  c. A sphere of radius r is inscribed in a cylinder. What is the ratio of the volume of the sphere to the volume of the cylinder?

22. a. A sphere of radius 6 is inscribed in a cylinder of height 12. What is the ratio of the surface area of the sphere to the lateral area of the cylinder?
  b. A sphere of radius 7 is inscribed in a cylinder of height 14. What is the ratio of the surface area of the sphere to the lateral area of the cylinder?
  c. A sphere of radius r is inscribed in a cylinder. What is the ratio of the surface area of the sphere to the lateral area of the cylinder?

Review Exercises

Simplify these in your head if you can. Write down the answers.

1. 7×0.3 **2.** 4×5.1 **3.** 0.8×0.8 **4.** 23.3×100

5. $3500 \div 1000$ **6.** $10.75 \div 100$ **7.** 300×2.7 **8.** 0.0004×0.2

▌▌▌▌ **Calculator Key-In**

The surface area of Earth is approximately 510,070,000 km². The surface area of Jupiter is approximately 64,017,000,000 km². About how many times greater than the surface area of Earth is the surface area of Jupiter?

If you try to enter the numbers as they are shown above on your calculator, you may find it will not accept more than eight digits. Many calculators have a key marked *EXP* that allows you to use scientific notation to express very large (or very small) numbers. For example, you can enter 510,070,000 by thinking of the number as 5.1007×10^8 and entering 5.1007 ⎡EXP⎤ 8. Your calculator may show 5.1007   08.

Try to find a calculator that will accept scientific notation and solve the problem above.

10-9 Mass and Density

The **mass** of an object is a measure of the amount of matter it contains. In the metric system, units of mass are the **gram (g),** the **kilogram (kg),** and the **metric ton (t).**

> 1 g = mass of 1 cm³ of water under standard conditions. (Standard conditions are 4°C at sea-level pressure.)
>
> $$1 \text{ kg} = 1000 \text{ g}$$
>
> $$1 \text{ t} = 1000 \text{ kg}$$

The *weight* of an object is the force of gravity acting on it. While the mass of an object remains constant, its weight would be less on a mountaintop or on the moon than at sea level. In a given region, mass and weight are proportional (so that mass can be found by weighing).

The tables below give the masses of unit volumes (1 cm³) of several substances.

TABLE 1				TABLE 2		
Substance	Mass of 1 cm³	Mass of 1 m³		Substance	Mass of 1 cm³	Mass of 1 L
Pine	0.56 g	0.56 t		Helium	0.00018 g	0.00018 kg
Ice	0.92 g	0.92 t		Air	0.0012 g	0.0012 kg
Water	1.00 g	1.00 t		Gasoline	0.66 g	0.66 kg
Aluminum	2.70 g	2.70 t		Water	1.00 g	1.00 kg
Steel	7.82 g	7.82 t		Milk	1.03 g	1.03 kg
Gold	19.3 g	19.3 t		Mercury	13.6 g	13.6 kg

The mass per unit volume of a substance is its **density.** In describing densities we use a slash (/) for the word *per.* For example, the density of gasoline is 0.66 kg/L.

EXAMPLE   Find the mass of a block 3 cm by 5 cm by 10 cm made of wood having density 0.8 g/cm³.

Solution   The volume of the block is 3 × 5 × 10, or 150, cm³.

Since 1 cm³ of the wood has mass 0.8 g, 150 cm³ has mass 0.8 × 150, or 120, g.

The example illustrates the following formula.

> ## Formula
> Mass = Density × Volume

In Table 2, the number of grams per cubic centimeter is the same as the number of kilograms per liter. This is because there are 1000 g in a kilogram and 1000 cm³ in a liter. Similarly in Table 1, the number of grams per cubic centimeter is the same as the number of metric tons per cubic meter.

Class Exercises

Complete.

1. $1 \, t = \underline{\;?\;} \, kg$

2. $1 \, kg = \underline{\;?\;} \, g$

3. $1 \, t = \underline{\;?\;} \, g$

4. $2400 \, kg = \underline{\;?\;} \, t$

5. $0.62 \, kg = \underline{\;?\;} \, g$

6. $400 \, g = \underline{\;?\;} \, kg$

Use the tables in this lesson to give the mass of the following.

7. 2 L of water

8. 10 cm³ of gasoline

9. 100 cm³ of milk

10. 4 L of gasoline

11. helium filling a 1000 L tank

12. a cube of ice 2 cm on each edge

13. the block of steel shown

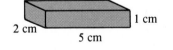
2 cm   1 cm   5 cm

Written Exercises

Complete.

A 1. $6.3 \, kg = \underline{\;?\;} \, g$

2. $2500 \, kg = \underline{\;?\;} \, t$

3. $4.3 \, t = \underline{\;?\;} \, kg$

Use the tables in this lesson to find the mass of the following.

4. 50 cm³ of gold

5. 300 cm³ of aluminum

6. 25 L of gasoline

7. 2.5 L of mercury

8. 500 m³ of water

9. 500 m³ of ice

10. 1 m³ of air

11. 1 m³ of helium

12. 4 L of milk

In Exercises 13–18, use $\pi \approx 3.14$ and round the answer to three digits.
In Exercises 13–15, the solid pictured is made of the specified material.
Use the tables in this lesson to find the mass of the solid.

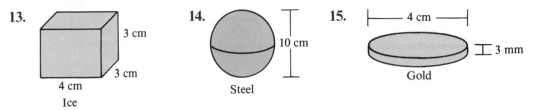

13.

3 cm

3 cm

4 cm

Ice

14.

10 cm

Steel

15.

4 cm

3 mm

Gold

In Exercises 16–18, use the tables in this lesson to find the mass of the
named content of the container pictured.

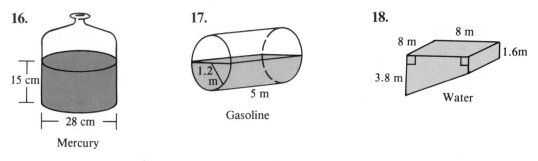

16.

15 cm

28 cm

Mercury

17.

1.2 m

5 m

Gasoline

18.

8 m

8 m

1.6 m

3.8 m

Water

Problems

Solve. Use the tables in this lesson if no density is given. Use $\pi \approx 3.14$
and round the answer to three digits.

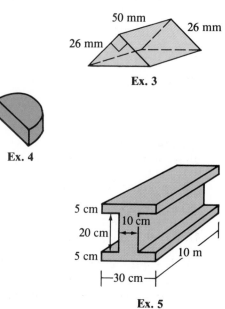

A 1. A solid gold bar has dimensions of
approximately 17 cm by 9 cm by
4.5 cm. Find its mass in kilograms.

2. A solid pine board has dimensions of
approximately 100 cm by 30 cm by
1.5 cm. Find its mass in grams.

3. The optical prism shown at the right
is made of glass having density
4.8 g/cm³. Find its mass.

4. A piece of ice is in the form of a
half-cylinder 5 cm in radius and
3 cm high. What is its mass?

B 5. What is the mass in metric tons of the
steel I-beam shown at the right?

50 mm

26 mm

26 mm

Ex. 3

Ex. 4

5 cm

10 cm

20 cm

5 cm

10 m

30 cm

Ex. 5

6. The drawing at the right shows the cross section of a two-kilometer-long tunnel that is to be dug through a mountain. How many metric tons of earth must be removed if its density is 2.8 t/m³?

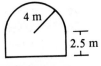

Ex. 6

Self-Test B

Use $\pi \approx 3.14$ and round answers involving π to three digits.

Complete.

1. Triangular prism: base area = 7.6 m², height = 5.5 m, volume = __?__ m³   [10–5]

2. Cylinder: base diameter = 38 cm, height = 24 cm, volume = __?__ cm³

3. Square prism: 17 cm by 17 cm by 32 cm, volume = __?__ cm³, capacity = __?__ L

Find the volume of the solid.

4. A cone with base radius 0.5 m and height 1.2 m   [10–6]

5. A pyramid with base of 180 m² and height 20 m

6. A square pyramid with base 26 cm on a side and height 48 cm

Find (a) the lateral area and (b) the total surface area of the solid.

7. A rectangular prism with base 4 by 3 and height 7   [10–7]

8. A cylinder with base diameter 10 and height 3

9. A square prism with height 42 and base 18 per side

Find (a) the surface area and (b) the volume of a sphere with the given dimensions. Leave your answers in terms of π.

10. radius = 18 cm   11. diameter = 12 m   [10–8]

Find the mass of the solid.

12. A sphere of aluminum with diameter 18 cm, density 2.70 g/cm³   [10–9]

13. A 4 cm by 4 cm by 20 cm block of pine, density of 0.568 g/cm³

Self-Test answers and Extra Practice are at the back of the book.

Locating Points on Earth

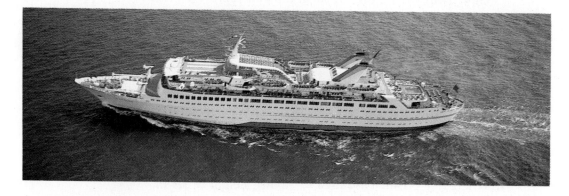

We can think of Earth as a sphere rotating on an axis that is a diameter with endpoints at the North Pole (N) and South Pole (S). A **great circle** on a sphere is the intersection of the sphere with a plane that contains the center of the sphere. The great circle whose plane is perpendicular to Earth's axis is called the **equator.** The equator divides Earth into the Northern and Southern Hemispheres.

Semicircles with endpoints at the North and South Poles are called **meridians.** The meridian that passes through Greenwich, England, is called the **prime meridian.** The great circle on which the prime meridian lies divides Earth into the Eastern and Western Hemispheres.

The prime meridian and the equator are important parts of a degree-coordinate system that we use to describe the location of points on Earth. A series of circles whose planes are parallel to the equator, called **parallels of latitude,** identify the **latitude** of a point as a number of degrees between 0° and 90° *north* or *south of the equator.* The meridians identify the **longitude** of a point as the number of degrees between 0° and 180° *east* or *west of the prime meridian.*

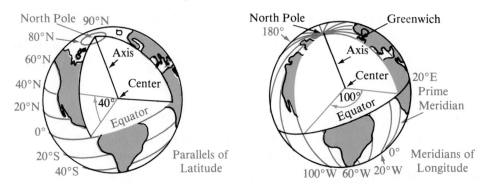

Thus, each point on the surface of Earth can be assigned an ordered pair of degree-coordinates: (latitude, longitude).

The flat map below, called a **Mercator projection,** shows the meridians and parallels of latitude marked off in 10° intervals as perpendicular lines. Notice that the city of Paris, France, is located at about 48°N, 2°E.

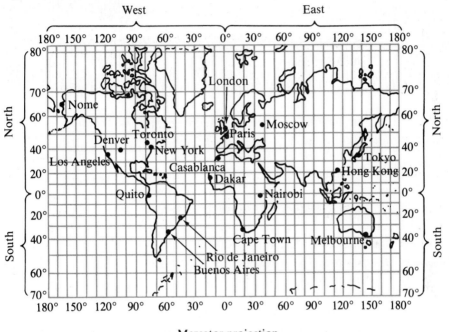

Mercator projection

Use the map above to name the major city at the location specified.

1. 40°N, 74°W   **2.** 34°S, 58°W   **3.** 23°S, 43°W   **4.** 34°S, 18°E

5. 55°N, 37°E   **6.** 37°S, 145°E   **7.** 33°N, 7°W   **8.** 34°N, 118°W

Give the latitude and longitude of the following cities to the nearest 5°.

9. Denver   **10.** Nairobi   **11.** London   **12.** Quito

13. Dakar   **14.** Toronto   **15.** Nome   **16.** Hong Kong

Career Activity

Ancient navigators determined their position by observing the sun and the stars. Modern navigators use much more sophisticated methods. If you were a navigator today what are some of the instruments and methods you might use?

Chapter Review

Write the letter of the correct answer.

1. Find the area of a rectangle 17 cm long and 5 cm wide. [10–1]
   a. 44 cm²   **b.** 85 cm²   **c.** 42.5 cm²   **d.** 22 cm²

2. A parallelogram has a base of 16 m and a height of 4 m. Find the area.
   a. 32 m²   **b.** 40 m²   **c.** 20 m²   **d.** 64 m²

3. A triangle has a base of 14 m and a height of 10 m. Find the area. [10–2]
   a. 140 m²   **b.** 34 m²   **c.** 70 m²   **d.** 35 m²

4. A trapezoid has bases of 9 cm and 15 cm and a height of 6 cm. Find the area.
   a. 72 cm²   **b.** 144 cm²   **c.** 810 cm²   **d.** 189 cm²

5. A circle has a diameter of 18 cm. Find the area. Use $\pi \approx 3.14$ and round to three digits. [10–3]
   a. 28.3 cm²   **b.** 1020 cm²   **c.** 56.5 cm²   **d.** 254 cm²

Complete. Use $\pi \approx 3.14$ and round answers involving π to three digits.

6. Figures may be symmetric with respect to a __?__ or a __?__. [10–4]

7. A rectangular prism has a base 12 cm by 14 cm and height 23 cm. Its volume is __?__. [10–5]

8. A cylinder has base radius 4 cm and height 15 cm. Its capacity is __?__ liters.

9. A cone with base diameter 6 and height 4.8 has volume __?__. [10–6]

10. A pyramid with base area 160 cm² and height 24 cm has volume __?__.

11. A cylinder with base radius 7 and height 12 has lateral area __?__ π and surface area __?__ π. [10–7]

12. A prism has height 16. Its bases are triangles with base 15, height 12, and remaining side 18. Its total surface area is __?__.

13. A sphere with radius 24 has surface area __?__ π and volume __?__ π. [10–8]

14. A sphere with radius 32 has surface area __?__ π and volume __?__ π.

15. A rectangular storage tank has dimensions 14 m by 6 m by 4 m. It is filled with helium of density 0.00018 kg/L. The mass of the helium is __?__. [10–9]

Chapter Test

Find the area. Use $\pi \approx 3.14$ and round the answer to three digits.

1. rectangle:
length = 14 cm
width = 9 m

2. parallelogram:
base = 23 cm
height = 11 cm

[10-1]

3. triangle:
base = 9 mm
height = 16 mm

4. trapezoid:
bases = 8 m and 14 m
height = 7 m

[10-2]

5. circle:
radius = 17 mm

6. circle:
diameter = 42 cm

[10-3]

7. Copy the figure at the right and show any lines or points of symmetry.

8. Find the area of the symmetric figure at the right.

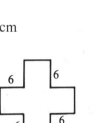

[10-4]

Find the volume. Use $\pi \approx 3.14$ and round the answer to three digits.

9. Cylinder: base radius = 7.2 m, height = 5.8 m

[10-5]

10. Prism: base area = 45 cm², height = 33 cm

11. Cone: base diameter = 6 cm, height = 14 cm

[10-6]

12. Pyramid: square base 17 cm on a side, height = 21 cm

Find (a) the lateral area and (b) the total surface area of each. Use $\pi \approx 3.14$ and round the answer to three digits.

13.

14.

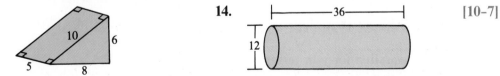

[10-7]

Find (a) the surface area and (b) the volume of a sphere with the given dimensions. Leave your answer in terms of π.

15. diameter = 18 cm

16. radius = 45 m

[10-8]

17. Find the mass of a sphere with diameter 20 cm and density 8.9 g/cm³. Use $\pi \approx 3.14$ and round the answer to three digits.

[10-9]

18. Find the mass of a cube 9 cm on each edge with density 0.56 g/cm³.

Cumulative Review (Chapters 1–10)

Exercises

Evaluate the expression if $a = 0.5$, $b = 5$, and $c = 2$.

1. abc

2. $a + b + c$

3. $b \div a$

4. $3a - 3b$

5. ab^2

6. $c^2 + b^3$

7. $6(a^2 - c^2)$

8. $10a - \dfrac{b}{c}$

Evaluate the expression if $x = \dfrac{1}{3}$, $y = 2\dfrac{3}{4}$, and $z = -\dfrac{3}{5}$.

9. $x + y$

10. xz

11. $3x + z$

12. $5z - x$

13. $x + 4y - 10z$

14. $6x + 8y + z$

15. $20z - (-y)$

16. $12x \div z$

Solve.

17. $15n + 7 > 52$

18. $6 - 2x < 21$

19. $38 \geq x - 2$

20. $\dfrac{n}{8} > 3$

21. $27 \leq 3x$

22. $3b + 5 < 56$

23. $4x + 7 = 35$

24. $-y + 10 = 26$

25. $\dfrac{3w}{7} = 9$

26. Find the measure of each angle of an equilateral triangle.

27. The measure of one angle in an isosceles triangle is 90°. Find the measures of the other angles.

28. An equilateral triangle has perimeter 37.5 cm. Find the length of each side.

29. What is 18% of 45?

30. 8 is what percent of 4000?

31. 6.48 is what percent of 27?

32. 105 is 42% of what number?

33. 316 is 0.5% of what number?

34. What is $34\frac{1}{2}\%$ of 1100?

Solve the equation for y in terms of x.

35. $4x + y = 18$

36. $x + 2y = 15$

37. $6x - 6y = 50$

38. $\dfrac{x}{2} + y = 17$

39. $xy = 20$

40. $x^2 + y = 100$

Find the area of the circle described. Leave your answer in terms of π.

41. radius 14 cm

42. diameter 46 mm

43. radius 125 km

44. diameter 286 m

45. radius 1805 cm

46. diameter 305.6 m

Find the surface area and volume for the sphere described. Leave your answer in terms of π.

47. radius 8   **48.** radius 15   **49.** radius 36

Problems

Problem Solving Reminders
Here are some reminders that may help you solve some of the problems on this page.
- Determine what information is necessary to solve the problem.
- Consider whether drawing a sketch will help.
- If more than one method can be used to solve a problem, use one method to solve and one to check.

Solve.

1. The Aleutian Trench in the Pacific Ocean is 8100 m deep. Each story of an average skyscraper is about 4.2 m high. How many stories would a skyscraper as tall as the Aleutian Trench have? Round your answer to the nearest whole number.

2. These announcements were heard at a rocket launch: "Minus 45 seconds and counting," and "We have second-stage ignition at plus 110 seconds." How much time elapsed between the announcements?

3. A rancher bought 15 fence sections at $58 each to complete one side of a corral. If the length of the side is 375 m and each section is the same length, what is the length of a section?

4. George had 15 flat tires last year. The cost of repairing each tire was $6.35 plus 5% tax. How much did he spend on repairs for the year?

5. Fred bought a bag of nuts. He gave $\frac{1}{4}$ of it to one brother, $\frac{1}{6}$ to another, $\frac{1}{3}$ to his sister, and kept the rest. How much did he keep?

6. Gus is canning tomato sauce. He has 20 jars that have a diameter of 9 cm and height of 9 cm. If he must leave one centimeter of air space at the top of each jar, what volume of sauce can a jar hold? Use $\pi \approx 3.14$ and round the answer to three digits.

7. The cost of an average basket of groceries rose from $78.80 in April to $82.74 in June. What was the percent of increase?

8. A roll of 36-exposure film costs $5.85. Processing for color prints costs $.42 per print. What is the total cost for film and processing of 36 prints?

11

Applying Algebra to Right Triangles

One of the basic shapes used in building hang-gliders such as the one shown at the right is the triangle. Triangles are especially well-suited for use in building because they are the simplest rigid forms. A rigid form is a figure that preserves its shape under pressure. Because of their rigidity, triangles are used in the construction of many large-scale projects, such as bridges, towers, and statues.

One important type of triangle is the right triangle. The ratios of the lengths of the sides of a right triangle are called trigonometric ratios. In this chapter, you will extend your knowledge of triangles and learn about trigonometric ratios. You will also study some methods for finding angles and lengths where triangles are involved.

Career Note

The job of surveyor is a career in which knowledge of right triangles and trigonometry plays an important role. Surveyors are responsible for establishing legal land boundaries. About half of their time is spent on location measuring sites and collecting data for maps and charts. The remaining part of their time is spent preparing reports, drawing maps, and planning future surveys.

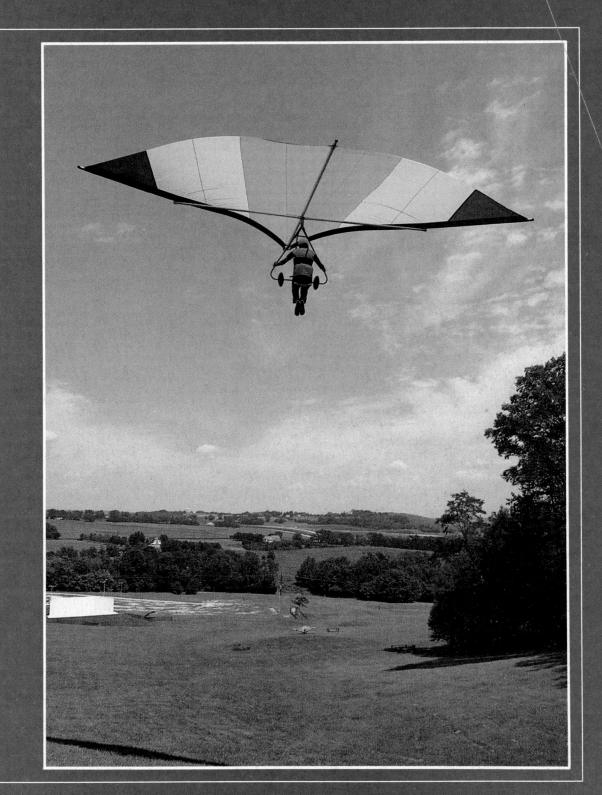

11-1 Square Roots

Recall that we can write $b \times b$ as b^2 and call it the *square* of b. The factor b is a **square root** of b^2. A given number a has b as a square root if

$$b^2 = a.$$

Thus 9 has 3 as a square root because $3^2 = 9$.

Every positive number has two square roots, and these are opposites of each other. For example, the square roots of 25 are 5 and -5 because

$$5^2 = 5 \times 5 = 25 \quad \text{and} \quad (-5)^2 = (-5) \times (-5) = 25.$$

The only square root of 0 is 0 because $b \times b = 0$ only when $b = 0$.

In this chapter we will work mostly with positive square roots. We use $\sqrt{a}$ to denote the *positive* square root of a. Thus $\sqrt{25} = 5$, not -5. A symbol such as $2\sqrt{25}$ means *2 times the positive square root of 25*. The negative square root of 25 is $-\sqrt{25}$, or -5.

Negative numbers have no real-number square roots because no real number has a square that is negative.

If $\sqrt{a}$ is an integer, we call a a **perfect square.** For example, 36 is a perfect square because $\sqrt{36}$ is the integer 6. Also, 144 is a perfect square because $\sqrt{144} = 12$.

If a is not a perfect square, we can estimate $\sqrt{a}$ by finding the two consecutive integers between which the square root lies. In the process, we use the fact that the smaller of two positive numbers has the smaller positive square root.

EXAMPLE   Between which two consecutive integers does $\sqrt{40}$ lie?

Solution   40 lies between the consecutive perfect squares 36 and 49.

$$36 < 40 < 49$$
$$\sqrt{36} < \sqrt{40} < \sqrt{49}$$
$$\text{Thus} \quad 6 < \sqrt{40} < 7.$$

Class Exercises

Read each symbol.

1. $\sqrt{7}$ **2.** $3\sqrt{10}$ **3.** $-\sqrt{81}$ **4.** $\sqrt{64}$ **5.** $2\sqrt{14}$

If the given symbol names an integer, state the integer. If not, name
two consecutive integers between which the number lies.

6. $\sqrt{16}$ **7.** $-\sqrt{36}$ **8.** $\sqrt{21}$ **9.** $\sqrt{70}$

11. $-\sqrt{49}$ **12.** $\sqrt{81}$ **13.** $\sqrt{69}$ **14.** $-\sqrt{144}$

Written Exercises

If the given symbol names an integer, state the integer. If not, name the
two consecutive integers between which the number lies.

A   **1.** $\sqrt{43}$ **2.** $\sqrt{64}$ **3.** $-\sqrt{16}$ **4.** $\sqrt{24}$ **5.** $\sqrt{1}$

    6. $\sqrt{0}$ **7.** $-\sqrt{6^2}$ **8.** $\sqrt{13}$ **9.** $\sqrt{54}$ **10.** $\sqrt{9}$

    11. $\sqrt{30}$ **12.** $\sqrt{48}$ **13.** $\sqrt{15}$ **14.** $\sqrt{8^2}$ **15.** $\sqrt{2}$

    16. $\sqrt{25} + \sqrt{16}$ **17.** $\sqrt{100} - \sqrt{49}$ **18.** $\sqrt{144} + \sqrt{25}$

    19. $\sqrt{79 - 61}$ **20.** $-\sqrt{66 - 2}$ **21.** $\sqrt{100 - 19}$

Replace the __?__ with <, >, or = to make a true statement.

EXAMPLE $\sqrt{9} + \sqrt{25}$ __?__ $\sqrt{9 + 25}$

Solution $\sqrt{9} + \sqrt{25} = 3 + 5 = 8$; $\sqrt{9 + 25} = \sqrt{34} < 8$.
Thus $\sqrt{9} + \sqrt{25} > \sqrt{9 + 25}$.

B   **22.** $\sqrt{9} + \sqrt{16}$ __?__ $\sqrt{9 + 16}$ **23.** $\sqrt{16} + \sqrt{4}$ __?__ $\sqrt{16 + 4}$

    24. $\sqrt{16} - \sqrt{9}$ __?__ $\sqrt{16 - 9}$ **25.** $\sqrt{25} - \sqrt{9}$ __?__ $\sqrt{25 - 9}$

    26. $\sqrt{4} \times \sqrt{9}$ __?__ $\sqrt{4 \times 9}$ **27.** $\sqrt{25} \times \sqrt{4}$ __?__ $\sqrt{25 \times 4}$

    28. $2\sqrt{2}$ __?__ $\sqrt{2 \times 2}$ **29.** $3\sqrt{12}$ __?__ $\sqrt{3 \times 12}$

Evaluate the expression.

C   **30.** $\left(\sqrt{25}\right)^2$ **31.** $\left(\sqrt{81}\right)^2$ **32.** $\left(\sqrt{49}\right)^2$ **33.** $\left(\sqrt{11}\right)^2$ **34.** $\left(\sqrt{2}\right)^2$

Review Exercises

Divide. Round the answer to the nearest hundredth.

    1. $44 \div 6.7$ **2.** $35 \div 5.9$ **3.** $72 \div 8.3$ **4.** $96 \div 9.5$

    5. $147 \div 12.3$ **6.** $230 \div 14.7$ **7.** $0.0165 \div 0.13$ **8.** $0.68 \div 0.81$

11-2 Approximating Square Roots

To get a close approximation of a square root, we can use the *divide-and-average* method. This method is based on the fact that

$$\text{if } \sqrt{a} = b, \text{ then } a = b \times b \text{ and } \frac{a}{b} = b.$$

In other words, when we divide a number a by its square root b, the quotient is b. When we use an estimate for b that is *less* than b for a divisor, the quotient is then *greater* than b. The average of the divisor and quotient can be used as a new estimate for b.

EXAMPLE 1 Approximate $\sqrt{55}$ to the tenths' place.

Solution   Step 1   To estimate $\sqrt{55}$, first find the two integers between which $\sqrt{55}$ lies.

$$49 < \quad 55 < \quad 64$$
$$\sqrt{49} < \sqrt{55} < \sqrt{64}$$
$$7 < \sqrt{55} < \quad 8$$

Since 55 is closer to 49 than to 64, you might try 7.3 as an estimate of $\sqrt{55}$.

Step 2   Divide 55 by the estimate, 7.3. Compute to one more place than you want in the final answer.

```
      7.53
7.3)55.000
    51 1
    3 90
    3 65
      250
      219
       31
```

Step 3   Average the divisor and quotient.

$$\frac{7.3 + 7.53}{2} \approx 7.42$$

Use the average as the next estimate and repeat Steps 2 and 3 until your divisor and quotient agree in the tenths' place.

In this case, use 7.42 as your next estimate and divide.

```
       7.41
7.42)55.0000
     51 94
     3 060
     2 968
       920
       742
       178
```

As you can see, $\sqrt{55} \approx 7.4$ to the tenths' place.

We can approximate $\sqrt{55}$ to whatever decimal place we wish by repeating the steps shown in Example 1 on the previous page. Because $\sqrt{55}$ is a nonterminating, nonrepeating decimal, we say that $\sqrt{55}$ is an **irrational number.** Together, irrational and rational numbers form the set of **real numbers.** Other irrational numbers are discussed on page 119.

To find the square root of a number that is not an integer by the divide-and-average method, we use the same steps as in Example 1. The first step, finding the two integers between which a square root lies, is shown below.

EXAMPLE 2   Complete the first step in estimating each square root.

  a. $\sqrt{12.3}$ **b.** $\sqrt{0.7}$

Solution   The first step in estimating a square root is to find the two integers between which it lies.

  a. $9 < 12.3 < 16$ **b.** $0 < 0.7 < 1$
  $\sqrt{9} < \sqrt{12.3} < \sqrt{16}$ $\sqrt{0} < \sqrt{0.7} < \sqrt{1}$
  $3 < \sqrt{12.3} < 4$ $0 < \sqrt{0.7} < 1$

Class Exercises

Give the first digit of the square root.

1. $\sqrt{7}$ **2.** $\sqrt{11}$ **3.** $\sqrt{30}$ **4.** $\sqrt{50}$ **5.** $\sqrt{94}$

Give the next estimate for the square root of the dividend.

EXAMPLE $3.8\overline{)15.000}$ (quotient 3.95)

Solution $\dfrac{3.8 + 3.95}{2} \approx 3.88$

Thus 3.88 is the next estimate.

6. $2\overline{)4.8}$ (2.4)   **7.** $3\overline{)11}$ (3.7)   **8.** $5\overline{)28.5}$ (5.7)   **9.** $4.3\overline{)21.000}$ (4.88)

10. $14\overline{)225}$ (16)   **11.** $0.7\overline{)0.53}$ (0.76)   **12.** $0.6\overline{)0.3}$ (0.5)   **13.** $0.9\overline{)0.83}$ (0.92)

Written Exercises

Approximate to the tenths' place.

A
1. $\sqrt{11}$ 2. $\sqrt{13}$ 3. $\sqrt{33}$ 4. $\sqrt{23}$

5. $\sqrt{8}$ 6. $\sqrt{5}$ 7. $\sqrt{26}$ 8. $\sqrt{42}$

9. $\sqrt{57}$ 10. $\sqrt{75}$ 11. $\sqrt{91}$ 12. $\sqrt{69}$

13. $\sqrt{5.7}$ 14. $\sqrt{7.5}$ 15. $\sqrt{9.1}$ 16. $\sqrt{6.9}$

17. $\sqrt{8.2}$ 18. $\sqrt{4.6}$ 19. $\sqrt{3.5}$ 20. $\sqrt{1.6}$

B
21. $\sqrt{152}$ 22. $\sqrt{285}$ 23. $\sqrt{705}$ 24. $\sqrt{328}$

25. $\sqrt{15.2}$ 26. $\sqrt{28.5}$ 27. $\sqrt{70.5}$ 28. $\sqrt{32.4}$

29. $\sqrt{0.4}$ 30. $\sqrt{0.6}$ 31. $\sqrt{0.05}$ 32. $\sqrt{0.21}$

Approximate to the hundredths' place.

33. $\sqrt{2}$ 34. $\sqrt{3}$ 35. $\sqrt{5}$ 36. $\sqrt{10}$

Review Exercises

Simplify.

1. $4(11 - 2) + 3(2) + 2(5 + 3)$

2. $5(81 \div 9) - 36 + 11$

3. $7.3 + (9.14 - 6.91) - 2.81$

4. $11.32 - 67(8.01 - 7.92)$

5. $3.617 + 0.7(5.301 - 4.911)$

6. $14.95 + 5(3.2 + 14) - 90.84$

7. $(72 - 65) + 11(8.76 - 0.89)$

8. $5.143 + 0.3(8.914 - 7.126)$

Calculator Key-In

On many calculators there is a square-root key. If you have access to such a calculator, use it to find the square roots below.

1. a. $\sqrt{1}$ b. $\sqrt{100}$ c. $\sqrt{10,000}$

2. a. $\sqrt{7}$ b. $\sqrt{700}$ c. $\sqrt{70,000}$

3. a. $\sqrt{70}$ b. $\sqrt{7000}$ c. $\sqrt{700,000}$

4. a. $\sqrt{0.08}$ b. $\sqrt{8}$ c. $\sqrt{800}$

5. a. $\sqrt{0.54}$ b. $\sqrt{54}$ c. $\sqrt{5400}$

11-3 Using a Square-Root Table

Part of the Table of Square Roots on page 508 is shown below. Square roots of integers are given to the nearest thousandth.

Number	Positive Square Root	Number	Positive Square Root	Number	Positive Square Root	Number	Positive Square Root
N	$\sqrt{N}$	N	$\sqrt{N}$	N	$\sqrt{N}$	N	$\sqrt{N}$
1	1	26	5.099	51	7.141	76	8.718
2	1.414	27	5.196	52	7.211	77	8.775
3	1.732	28	5.292	53	7.280	78	8.832
4	2	29	5.385	54	7.348	79	8.888

We can use the table to approximate the square roots of integers from 1 to 100. For example, to find $\sqrt{78}$, first locate 78 under a column headed "Number." Then read off the value beside 78 in the "Square Root" column.

$$\sqrt{78} \approx 8.832$$

Reading Mathematics: *Tables*
Some tables may have many columns of information. When you are reading a table, use a ruler to help guide your eyes across the page or down a column. This way you can be sure to find the correct entry.

To find an approximate square root of a number that lies between two entries in the column headed "Number," we can use a process called **interpolation.** The interpolation process may cause an error in the last digit of the approximation.

EXAMPLE 1 Approximate $\sqrt{3.8}$ to the nearest thousandth by interpolation.

Solution On a number line $\sqrt{3.8}$ lies between $\sqrt{3}$ and $\sqrt{4}$. We can assume that $\sqrt{3.8}$ is about 0.8 of the distance between $\sqrt{3}$ and $\sqrt{4}$.

$$\sqrt{3.8} \approx \sqrt{3} + 0.8(\sqrt{4} - \sqrt{3})$$
$$\approx 1.732 + 0.8(2.000 - 1.732)$$
$$\approx 1.732 + 0.2144 = 1.9464$$

Thus, rounded to the thousandths' place, $\sqrt{3.8} = 1.946$.

EXAMPLE 2 The area of a square display room is 71 m². Find the length of a side to the nearest hundredth of a meter.

Solution Recall that the formula for the area of a square is $A = s^2$.

$$s^2 = 71$$
$$s = \sqrt{71}$$

Using the table on page 508, we see that $\sqrt{71} = 8.426$.
To the nearest hundredth of a meter, the length of a side is 8.43 m.

Class Exercises

Use the table on page 508 to find the approximate square root.

1. $\sqrt{39}$ 2. $\sqrt{83}$ 3. $\sqrt{20}$ 4. $\sqrt{95}$ 5. $\sqrt{34}$

6. $\sqrt{49}$ 7. $\sqrt{11}$ 8. $\sqrt{52}$ 9. $10\sqrt{87}$ 10. $\frac{1}{10}\sqrt{22}$

Find two decimals in the table on page 508 between which the square root lies.

11. $\sqrt{54.3}$ 12. $\sqrt{1.7}$ 13. $\sqrt{60.7}$ 14. $\sqrt{4.5}$ 15. $\sqrt{28.6}$

Written Exercises

For Exercises 1–37, refer to the table on page 508.

Approximate to the nearest hundredth.

A 1. $\sqrt{65}$ 2. $\sqrt{31}$ 3. $\sqrt{56}$ 4. $\sqrt{13}$ 5. $\sqrt{97}$

6. $10\sqrt{37}$ 7. $10\sqrt{41}$ 8. $\frac{1}{10}\sqrt{83}$ 9. $\frac{1}{10}\sqrt{75}$ 10. $\frac{1}{10}\sqrt{24}$

11. $3\sqrt{55}$ 12. $2\sqrt{30}$ 13. $6\sqrt{19}$ 14. $4\sqrt{18}$ 15. $7\sqrt{72}$

B 16. $\sqrt{39} + \sqrt{16}$ 17. $\sqrt{28} + \sqrt{53}$ 18. $\sqrt{71} - \sqrt{25}$

19. $\sqrt{91} - \sqrt{84}$ 20. $2\sqrt{56} - \sqrt{4}$ 21. $\sqrt{37} - 2\sqrt{8}$

Approximate to the nearest hundredth by interpolation.

22. $\sqrt{13.2}$ 23. $\sqrt{5.9}$ 24. $\sqrt{14.7}$ 25. $\sqrt{81.6}$ 26. $\sqrt{24.3}$

27. $\sqrt{8.7}$ 28. $\sqrt{69.2}$ 29. $\sqrt{50.9}$ 30. $5\sqrt{84.4}$ 31. $3\sqrt{81.9}$

Approximate to the nearest hundredth.

C **32.** $\sqrt{700}$ (*Hint:* $\sqrt{100 \times 7} = \sqrt{100} \times \sqrt{7} = 10\sqrt{7}$)   **33.** $\sqrt{500}$ **34.** $\sqrt{1100}$

   35. $\sqrt{380}$ (*Hint:* $\sqrt{100 \times 3.8} = \sqrt{100} \times \sqrt{3.8} = 10\sqrt{3.8}$)   **36.** $\sqrt{420}$ **37.** $\sqrt{3470}$

Problems

Solve.

A **1.** The area of a square is 85 m². Find the length of a side to the nearest hundredth of a meter.

   2. A square floor has an area of 32 m². Find the length of a side to the nearest tenth of a meter.

   3. The area of a square room measures 225 ft². How much will it cost to put molding around the ceiling at $.35 per foot?

B **4.** An isosceles right triangle has an area of 13.5 cm². Find the length of the equal sides to the nearest tenth of a centimeter.

   5. A circle has an area of 47.1 cm². Find its radius to the nearest hundredth of a centimeter. (Use $\pi \approx 3.14$.)

   6. The height of a parallelogram is half the length of its base. The parallelogram has an area of 67 cm². Find the height to the nearest tenth of a centimeter.

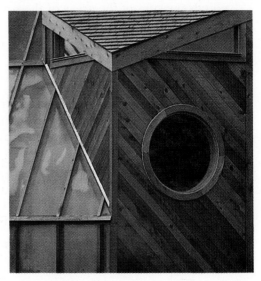

C **7.** The total surface area of a cube is 210 m². Find the length of an edge to the nearest hundredth of a meter.

   8. One base of a trapezoid is three times as long as the other base. The height of the trapezoid is the same as the shorter base. The trapezoid has an area of 83 cm². Find the height to the nearest tenth of a centimeter.

Review Exercises

Write the value of the product.

  1. 0.9^2 **2.** 0.05^2 **3.** 0.06^2 **4.** 0.7^2 **5.** 3.7^2 **6.** 1.9^2 **7.** 24.3^2 **8.** 5.03^2

11-4 The Pythagorean Theorem

The longest side of a right triangle is opposite the right angle and is called the **hypotenuse.** The two shorter sides are called **legs.**

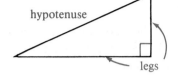

About 2500 years ago, the Greek mathematician Pythagoras proved the following useful fact about right triangles.

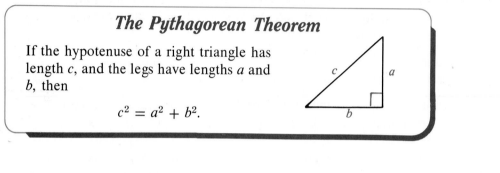

The Pythagorean Theorem

If the hypotenuse of a right triangle has length c, and the legs have lengths a and b, then

$$c^2 = a^2 + b^2.$$

The figure at the right illustrates the Pythagorean theorem. We see that the area of the square on the hypotenuse equals the sum of the areas of the squares on the legs:

$$25 = 9 + 16,$$

$$\text{or } 5^2 = 3^2 + 4^2.$$

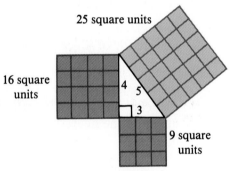

25 square units

16 square units

9 square units

The converse of the Pythagorean theorem is also true. It can be used to test whether a triangle is a right triangle.

Converse of the Pythagorean Theorem

If the sides of a triangle have lengths a, b, and c, such that $c^2 = a^2 + b^2$, then the triangle is a right triangle.

EXAMPLE 1 Is the triangle with sides of the given lengths a right triangle?
  a. 4, 5, 7   **b.** 5, 12, 13

Solution   **a.** $4^2 = 16$, $5^2 = 25$, $7^2 = 49$
            No, since $16 + 25 \neq 49$. The triangle with sides of lengths 4, 5, and 7 *cannot* be a right triangle.

b. $5^2 = 25$, $12^2 = 144$, $13^2 = 169$

Yes, since $25 + 144 = 169$. The triangle with sides of lengths 5, 12, and 13 is a right triangle.

Sometimes it may be necessary to solve for the length of a missing side of a right triangle. The example below illustrates the steps involved.

EXAMPLE 2   For right triangle ABC, find the length of the missing side to the nearest hundredth. Use the table on page 508.

a. $a = 3$, $b = 7$ **b.** $a = 4$, $c = 9$

Solution   Using the equation $c^2 = a^2 + b^2$:

a. $c^2 = 3^2 + 7^2$
    $= 9 + 49 = 58$
    $c = \sqrt{58}$
    $c \approx 7.62$

b. $9^2 = 4^2 + b^2$
    $9^2 - 4^2 = b^2$
    $81 - 16 = b^2$
    $65 = b^2$
    $\sqrt{65} = b$
    $b \approx 8.06$

Class Exercises

Without actually counting them, tell how many unit squares there are in the shaded square.

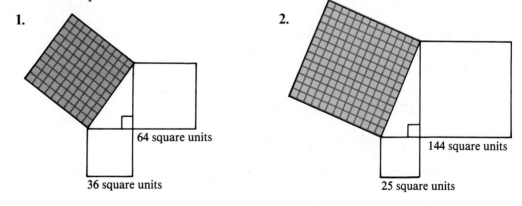

1. 64 square units / 36 square units

2. 144 square units / 25 square units

Replace _?_ **with = or ≠ to make a true statement.**

3. 6^2 _?_ $4^2 + 5^2$ **4.** 5^2 _?_ $3^2 + 4^2$ **5.** 10^2 _?_ $6^2 + 8^2$

The lengths of the sides of a triangle are given. Is it a right triangle?

6. 3, 4, 5   **7.** 7, 24, 25   **8.** 5, 10, 12   **9.** 10, 24, 26

Written Exercises

Find the area of the square.

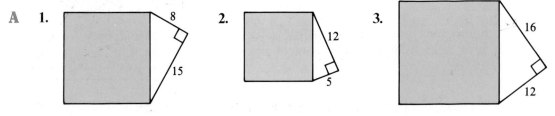

A 1.   8   15

2.   12   5

3.   16   12

Is the triangle with sides of the given lengths a right triangle?

4. 6, 8, 10

5. 8, 15, 17

6. 16 cm, 30 cm, 34 cm

7. 9 m, 12 m, 15 m

8. 1.5 mm, 2.0 mm, 2.5 mm

9. 0.6 km, 0.8 km, 1.0 km

10. 9 m, 21 m, 23 m

11. 20 cm, 21 cm, 29 cm

12. 9 km, 40 km, 41 km

13. 8 m, 37 m, 39 m

A right triangle has sides of lengths a, b, and c, with c the length of the hypotenuse. Find the length of the missing side. If necessary, use the table on page 508 for the square-root values and round answers to the nearest hundredth.

B 14. $a = 2$, $b = 1$ 15. $a = 8$, $b = 6$ 16. $a = 4$, $c = 9$ 17. $b = 5$, $c = 6$

18. $a = 5$, $b = 12$ 19. $a = 9$, $b = 7$ 20. $b = 11$, $c = 19$ 21. $a = 24$, $c = 74$

A **Pythagorean triple** consists of three positive integers a, b, and c that satisfy the equation $a^2 + b^2 = c^2$. You can find as many Pythagorean triples as you wish by substituting positive integers for m and n (such that $m > n$) in the following expressions for a, b, and c.

$$a = m^2 - n^2 \qquad b = 2mn \qquad c = m^2 + n^2$$

Find Pythagorean triples using the given values of m and n.

C 22. $m = 5$, $n = 1$ 23. $m = 6$, $n = 3$ 24. $m = 4$, $n = 2$

Problems

Solve. Round your answer to the nearest tenth.

A 1. A plane flies 90 km due east and then 60 km due north. How far is it then from its starting point?

2. The foot of a 6 m ladder is 2.5 m from the base of a wall. How high up the wall does the ladder reach?

3. The figure shows two cables bracing a television tower. What is the distance between the points where the cables touch the ground?

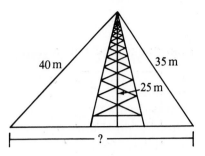

40 m 35 m 25 m ?

4. Find the length of a diagonal of a 10 cm by 10 cm square.

B **5.** A square has diagonals 10 cm long. Find the length of a side.

6. The diagonals of a rhombus are perpendicular and bisect each other. Find the length of a side of a rhombus whose diagonals have lengths 12 m and 18 m.

C **7.** Find the length of a diagonal of a 10 by 10 by 10 cube. (*Hint:* First find AQ using right triangle PQA. Then find the required length AB using right triangle AQB.)

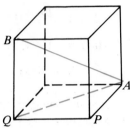

8. Find the length of a diagonal of a box having dimensions 2 by 3 by 6. (See the *Hint* for Problem 7.)

Self-Test A

If the given symbol names an integer, state the integer. If not, name the two consecutive integers between which the number lies.

1. $\sqrt{56}$ **2.** $-\sqrt{81}$ **3.** $\sqrt{9} + \sqrt{25}$ **4.** $\sqrt{106 - 57}$ [11-1]

5. Use the divide-and-average method to approximate $\sqrt{86.4}$ to the nearest tenth.   [11-2]

Use the table on page 508 and interpolation to approximate each square root to the nearest tenth.

6. $\sqrt{18}$ **7.** $\sqrt{50}$ **8.** $\sqrt{9.8}$ **9.** $\sqrt{5.6}$ [11-3]

A right triangle has sides of lengths *a*, *b*, and *c*, with *c* the length of the hypotenuse. Find the length of the missing side.

10. $a = 3, b = 4$ **11.** $b = 96, c = 100$ **12.** $c = 20, a = 12$ [11-4]

Self-Test answers and Extra Practice are at the back of the book.

11-5 Similar Triangles

As you know, we say that two figures are congruent when they are identical in both shape and size. When two figures have the same shape, but do not necessarily have the same size, we say that the figures are **similar.**

For two *triangles* to be similar it is enough that the measures of their corresponding angles are equal.

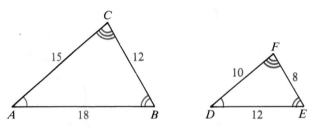

To indicate that the triangles shown above are similar, we can write the following:

$$\triangle ABC \sim \triangle DEF$$

The symbol $\sim$ means *is similar to*. Note that when we write expressions such as the one above, we list corresponding vertices in the same order.

In triangles *ABC* and *DEF*, we see that the lengths of the corresponding sides have the same ratio:

$$\frac{AB}{DE} = \frac{18}{12} = \frac{3}{2} \qquad \frac{BC}{EF} = \frac{12}{8} = \frac{3}{2} \qquad \frac{CA}{FD} = \frac{15}{10} = \frac{3}{2}$$

Therefore,

$$\frac{AB}{DE} = \frac{BC}{EF} = \frac{CA}{FD}.$$

Because the ratios are equal, we say that the lengths of the corresponding sides are *proportional.*

In general, we can say the following:

> For two similar triangles,
>
> corresponding angles are congruent
>
> and
>
> lengths of corresponding sides are proportional.

If $\triangle RUN \sim \triangle JOG$, find the lengths marked x and y.

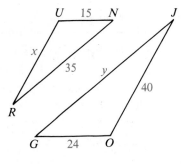

Solution

Since the corresponding vertices are listed in the same order, we know the following.

$$\angle R \cong \angle J$$

$$\angle U \cong \angle O$$

$$\angle N \cong \angle G$$

$$\frac{RU}{JO} = \frac{UN}{OG} = \frac{NR}{GJ}$$

Substituting the values that are given in the diagram, we obtain

$$\frac{x}{40} = \frac{15}{24} = \frac{35}{y}.$$

Therefore, we can set up one proportion involving x and another involving y.

$$\frac{x}{40} = \frac{15}{24} \qquad\qquad \frac{15}{24} = \frac{35}{y}$$

$$24x = 15 \times 40 \qquad\qquad 15y = 35 \times 24$$

$$x = \frac{15 \times 40}{24} \qquad\qquad y = \frac{35 \times 24}{15}$$

$$x = \frac{600}{24} = 25 \qquad\qquad y = \frac{840}{15} = 56$$

The length marked x is 25 and the length marked y is 56.

In the two *right triangles* shown at the right, the measures of two acute angles are equal. Since all right angles have equal measure, 90°, the two remaining acute angles must also have equal measure. (Recall that the sum of the angle measures of any triangle is 180°.) Thus the two right triangles are similar.

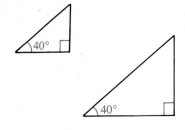

> If an acute angle of one *right* triangle is congruent to an angle of a second *right* triangle, then the triangles are similar.

EXAMPLE 2 At the same time a tree on level ground casts a shadow 48 m long, a 2 m pole casts a shadow 5 m long. Find the height, h, of the tree.

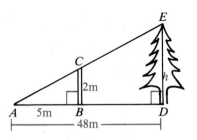

Solution In the diagram, right triangles ABC and ADE share acute $\angle A$ and thus are similar. Since $\frac{AD}{AB} = \frac{DE}{BC} = \frac{EA}{CA}$, we can set up a proportion to solve for h.

$$\frac{h}{2} = \frac{48}{5}$$

$$5h = 48 \times 2$$

$$h = \frac{48 \times 2}{5} = 19.2$$

The height of the tree is 19.2 m.

Reading Mathematics: *Diagrams*

To help you read a diagram that has overlapping triangles, you can redraw the diagram, pulling apart the individual triangles. For example, $\triangle ADE$ above can be separated as shown below.

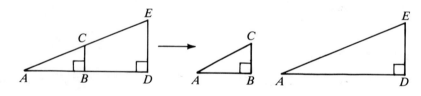

Class Exercises

In Exercises 1–4, $\triangle LOG \sim \triangle RIT$.

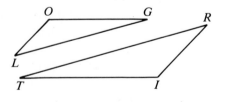

1. Name all pairs of corresponding angles.

2. Name all pairs of corresponding sides.

3. $\frac{OL}{IR} = \frac{OG}{?}$

4. $\frac{LG}{?} = \frac{GO}{TI}$

True or false?

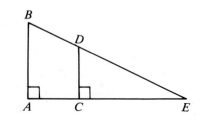

5. $\triangle BAE$ and $\triangle DCE$ are right triangles.

6. $m \angle ABE = m \angle CDE$

7. $\triangle BAE \sim \triangle DCE$

8. $\frac{CE}{AE} = \frac{BA}{DE}$

9. $\frac{BA}{DC} = \frac{BE}{DE}$

Written Exercises

Exercises 1–5 refer to the diagram at the right. $\triangle ABC \sim \triangle PQR$.

A   **1.** $\dfrac{PR}{AC} = \dfrac{?}{CB}$

2. $\dfrac{BA}{?} = \dfrac{CB}{RQ}$

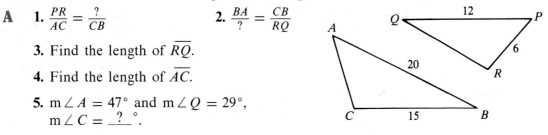

3. Find the length of $\overline{RQ}$.

4. Find the length of $\overline{AC}$.

5. m $\angle A = 47°$ and m $\angle Q = 29°$,
m $\angle C = \underline{\ ?\ }°$.

Exercises 6–10 refer to the diagram at the right. $\triangle AED \sim \triangle ACB$.

6. The length of $\overline{AE} = \underline{\ ?\ }$.

7. The length of $\overline{AB} = \underline{\ ?\ }$.

8. The length of $\overline{AD} = \underline{\ ?\ }$.

9. If m $\angle A = 25°$, then m $\angle ABC = \underline{\ ?\ }°$
and m $\angle ADE = \underline{\ ?\ }°$.

10. If $\dfrac{BC}{DE} = \dfrac{1}{2}$, then $\dfrac{AB}{AD} = \underline{\ ?\ }$.

Find the lengths marked x and y.

11. $\triangle MAB \sim \triangle SRO$

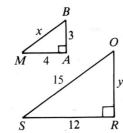

12. $\triangle DIP \sim \triangle MON$

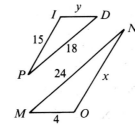

13. $\triangle RST \sim \triangle RUV$

B   **14.** $\triangle GEM \sim \triangle TIM$

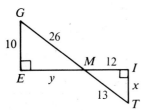

15. $\triangle PAR \sim \triangle PBT$

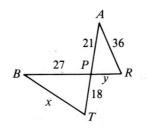

16. $\triangle ART \sim \triangle ABC$

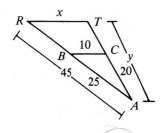

17. One day Jessica, who is 150 cm tall, cast a shadow that was 200 cm long while her father's shadow was 240 cm long. How tall is her father?

18. A person 1.8 m tall standing 7 m from a streetlight casts a shadow 3 m long. How high is the light?

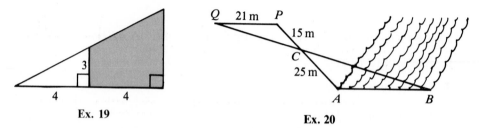

1.8m

3 m   7 m

Ex. 18

19. Find (a) the perimeter and (b) the area of the shaded trapezoid in the figure at the left below.

3

4   4

Ex. 19

Q   21 m   *P*

15 m

C

25 m

A   *B*

Ex. 20

20. To find the distance *AB* across a river, surveyors laid off $\overline{PQ}$ parallel to $\overline{AB}$ and created 2 similar triangles. They made the measurements shown in the figure at the right above. Find the length of $\overline{AB}$.

Exercises 21–22 refer to the diagram at the right.

C **21.** Explain why $\triangle ADC \sim \triangle ACB$.

22. Explain why $\triangle ADC \sim \triangle CDB$.

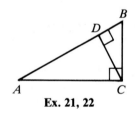

B

D

A   *C*

Ex. 21, 22

23. If $\triangle MNO \sim \triangle PQR$ and $\triangle PQR \sim \triangle STU$, is $\triangle MNO \sim \triangle STU$? Explain your answer.

24. If $\triangle MNO \cong \triangle PQR$, is $\triangle MNO \sim \triangle PQR$? Explain your answer.

25. If $\triangle MNO \sim \triangle PQR$, is $\triangle MNO \cong \triangle PQR$? Explain your answer.

Review Exercises

Multiply.

1. 300×1.73 **2.** 500×3.9 **3.** 7.81×200

4. 16.34×120 **5.** 2.18×1.03 **6.** 3.17×6.01

7. 54.2×0.09 **8.** 683×2.48 **9.** 71.4×52.4

11-6 Special Right Triangles

In an *isosceles right triangle* the two acute angles are congruent. Since the sum of the measures of these two angles is 90°, each angle measures 45°. For this reason, an isosceles right triangle is often called a **45° right triangle.**

In the diagram each leg is 1 unit long. If the hypotenuse is c units long, by the Pythagorean theorem we know that $c^2 = 1^2 + 1^2 = 2$ and thus

$$c = \sqrt{2}.$$

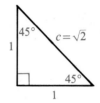

Every 45° right triangle is similar to the one shown. Since corresponding sides of similar triangles are proportional, we have the following property.

> If each leg of a 45° right triangle is a units long, then the hypotenuse is $a\sqrt{2}$ units long.

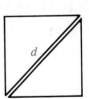

EXAMPLE 1 A square park measures 200 m on each edge. Find the length, d, of a path extending diagonally from one corner to the opposite corner. Use $\sqrt{2} \approx 1.414$.

Solution Since the park is square, we can apply the property of 45° right triangles to solve for d. We use the fact that d is the hypotenuse of the right triangle and that each side measures 200 m.

$$d = 200\sqrt{2} \approx 200 \times 1.414 = 282.8$$

Thus the path measures approximately 282.8 m.

A **30°-60° right triangle,** such as $\triangle ACB$, may be thought of as half an equilateral triangle. If hypotenuse $\overline{AB}$ is 2 units long, then the shorter leg $\overline{AC}$ (half of $\overline{AD}$) is 1 unit long. To find BC, we use the Pythagorean theorem:

$$(AC)^2 + (BC)^2 = (AB)^2$$
$$1^2 + (BC)^2 = 2^2$$
$$(BC)^2 = 2^2 - 1^2 = 3$$
$$BC = \sqrt{3}$$

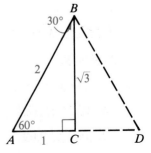

Every 30°–60° right triangle is similar to the one shown on the preceding page, and since corresponding sides of similar triangles are proportional, we have the following property.

If the shorter leg of a 30°–60° right triangle is a units long, then the longer leg is $a\sqrt{3}$ units long, and the hypotenuse is $2a$ units long.

EXAMPLE 2   The hypotenuse of a 30°–60° right triangle is 8 cm long. Find the lengths of the legs.

Solution   Using the 30°–60° right triangle property, we know that
$$2a = 8, \ a = 4, \text{ and } a\sqrt{3} = 4\sqrt{3}.$$
Thus the lengths of the legs are 4 cm and $4\sqrt{3}$ cm.

The symbol $\sqrt{\ }$ is called the **radical sign.** An expression such as $\sqrt{3}$ or $\sqrt{x}$ is called a **radical.** We often leave answers *in terms of radicals* with the radical in the numerator. To rewrite expressions such as $\dfrac{6}{\sqrt{3}}$ so that the radical appears in the numerator, we may use the fact that $\sqrt{x} \times \sqrt{x} = x$.

EXAMPLE 3   Rewrite $\dfrac{6}{\sqrt{3}}$ in lowest terms with the radical in the numerator.

Solution   If we multiply the numerator and denominator by $\sqrt{3}$, we will find an equivalent fraction with the radical in the numerator.

$$\frac{6}{\sqrt{3}} = \frac{6 \times \sqrt{3}}{\sqrt{3} \times \sqrt{3}}$$

$$= \frac{6\sqrt{3}}{3}$$

$$= 2\sqrt{3}$$

Thus, $2\sqrt{3}$ is equivalent to $\dfrac{6}{\sqrt{3}}$ in lowest terms with the radical in the numerator.

Class Exercises

Rewrite the expression in lowest terms with the radical in the numerator.

1. $\dfrac{1}{\sqrt{3}}$ **2.** $\dfrac{2}{\sqrt{3}}$ **3.** $\dfrac{2}{\sqrt{2}}$ **4.** $\dfrac{6}{\sqrt{2}}$ **5.** $\dfrac{1}{\sqrt{x}}$ **6.** $\dfrac{x}{\sqrt{x}}$

Find the lengths marked x and y in the triangle. Give your answer in terms of radicals when radicals occur.

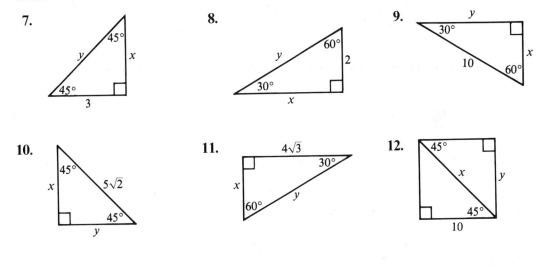

7.   **8.**   **9.**

10.   **11.**   **12.**

Written Exercises

Rewrite the expression in lowest terms with the radical in the numerator.

A   **1.** $\dfrac{6}{\sqrt{10}}$ **2.** $\dfrac{12}{\sqrt{13}}$ **3.** $\dfrac{3}{\sqrt{3}}$ **4.** $\dfrac{1}{\sqrt{2}}$ **5.** $\dfrac{2}{\sqrt{x}}$ **6.** $\dfrac{3x}{\sqrt{x}}$

Approximate the lengths marked x and y to the nearest tenth. Use $\sqrt{2} \approx 1.414$ and $\sqrt{3} \approx 1.732$.

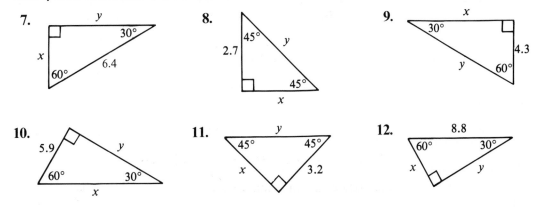

7.   **8.**   **9.**

10.   **11.**   **12.**

In Exercises 13–16, give answers in terms of radicals with the radical in the numerator.

B **13.** The hypotenuse of an isosceles right triangle has length 4. How long is each leg?

14. The hypotenuse of a 45° right triangle has length 10. How long is each leg?

15. The longer leg of a 30°–60° right triangle has length 15. How long are the other sides?

16. The side opposite the 60° angle of a right triangle has length 3. How long are the other sides?

In Exercises 17–22, $\angle C$ is a right angle in $\triangle ABC$. Find the length of the missing side to the nearest tenth.

17. $AC = 2$, $BC = 5$ **18.** $AB = 18$, $AC = 9$

19. $AB = 6\sqrt{2}$, $AC = 6$ **20.** $AC = CB = x$

C **21.** $\frac{1}{2}BA = CA = y$ **22.** $2BC = BA = z$

Approximate the lengths marked x and y to the nearest tenth.

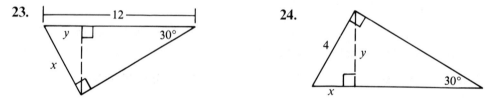

23.

24.

Problems

Solve. Round answers to the nearest tenth.

A **1.** A ladder 10 m long resting against a wall makes a 60° angle with the ground. How far up the wall does it reach?

2. A baseball diamond is a square 90 ft on each side. How far is it diagonally from home plate to second base?

3. A hillside is inclined at an angle of 30° with the horizontal. How much altitude has Mary gained after hiking 40 m up the hill?

4. The diagram on the right shows the roof of a house. Find the dimensions marked x and y.

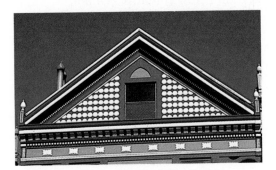

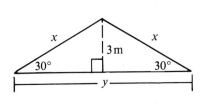

B **5.** A checkerboard has 8 squares on each side. If one side of a square is 5 cm long, how far is it from one corner of the board to the opposite corner?

6. Find the height of an equilateral triangle with sides 12 cm long.

7. Find the perimeters of the two squares shown in the diagram.

8. An equilateral triangle has sides 10 units long. Find (a) the height and (b) the area.

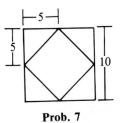

Prob. 7

C **9.** An equilateral triangle has sides r units long. Find both (a) the height and (b) the area in terms of r.

10. The area of a square pan is 900 cm². What is the length of a diagonal of the pan?

11. A 10 m pole is supported in a vertical position by three 6 m guy wires. If one end of each wire is fastened to the ground at a 60° angle, how high on the pole is the other end fastened?

12. A rhombus has angles of 60° and 120°. Each side of the rhombus is 8 cm long. What are the lengths of the diagonals? (*Hint:* The diagonals bisect the angles of the rhombus.)

Review Exercises

Write the fraction as a decimal. Use a bar to show a repeating decimal.

1. $\frac{5}{4}$ **2.** $\frac{3}{5}$ **3.** $\frac{2}{9}$ **4.** $\frac{7}{12}$ **5.** $\frac{11}{10}$ **6.** $\frac{3}{16}$ **7.** $\frac{1}{6}$ **8.** $\frac{4}{11}$

11-7 Trigonometric Ratios

Since each of the three triangles in the diagram below contains $\angle A$ and a right angle, the triangles are *similar* and the lengths of their sides are *proportional.* Thus, the ratios written below for the smallest triangle apply to all three triangles.

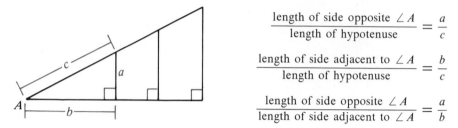

$$\frac{\text{length of side opposite } \angle A}{\text{length of hypotenuse}} = \frac{a}{c}$$

$$\frac{\text{length of side adjacent to } \angle A}{\text{length of hypotenuse}} = \frac{b}{c}$$

$$\frac{\text{length of side opposite } \angle A}{\text{length of side adjacent to } \angle A} = \frac{a}{b}$$

These ratios, called the **trigonometric ratios,** are so useful that each has been given a special name.

$\dfrac{a}{c}$ is called the **sine** of $\angle A$, or **sin A.**

$\dfrac{b}{c}$ is called the **cosine** of $\angle A$, or **cos A.**

$\dfrac{a}{b}$ is called the **tangent** of $\angle A$, or **tan A.**

It is important to understand that each trigonometric ratio depends only on the measure of $\angle A$ and *not* on the size of the right triangle.

The following shortened forms of the definitions may help you remember the trigonometric ratios.

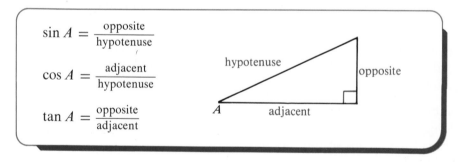

$$\sin A = \frac{\text{opposite}}{\text{hypotenuse}}$$

$$\cos A = \frac{\text{adjacent}}{\text{hypotenuse}}$$

$$\tan A = \frac{\text{opposite}}{\text{adjacent}}$$

EXAMPLE 1   For $\angle A$ find the value of each trigonometric ratio in lowest terms.

a. sin A **b.** cos A **c.** tan A

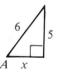

Solution To find the value of the trigonometric ratios for $\angle A$, first find the value of x. By the Pythagorean theorem:

$$x^2 + 5^2 = 6^2$$
$$x^2 + 25 = 36$$
$$x^2 = 36 - 25$$
$$x^2 = 11$$
$$x = \sqrt{11}$$

a. $\sin A = \dfrac{\text{opposite}}{\text{hypotenuse}} = \dfrac{5}{6}$

b. $\cos A = \dfrac{\text{adjacent}}{\text{hypotenuse}} = \dfrac{\sqrt{11}}{6}$

c. $\tan A = \dfrac{\text{opposite}}{\text{adjacent}} = \dfrac{5}{\sqrt{11}} = \dfrac{5 \times \sqrt{11}}{\sqrt{11} \times \sqrt{11}} = \dfrac{5\sqrt{11}}{11}$

EXAMPLE 2 Find the sine, cosine, and tangent of a 30° angle to the nearest thousandth.

Solution To find the values of these trigonometric ratios, first draw a 30°–60° right triangle. Let the shorter leg be 1 unit long and write in the lengths of the other sides according to the property of 30°–60° triangles that you learned in the previous lesson.

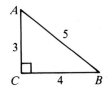

$$\sin 30° = \frac{1}{2} = 0.500$$

$$\cos 30° = \frac{\sqrt{3}}{2} \approx 0.866$$

$$\tan 30° = \frac{1}{\sqrt{3}} = \frac{\sqrt{3}}{3} \approx 0.577$$

Class Exercises

Find the value of the trigonometric ratio.

1. $\sin A$

2. $\cos A$

3. $\tan A$

4. $\sin B$

5. $\cos B$

6. $\tan B$

Find the value of the trigonometric ratio.

7. $\sin P$ 8. $\cos P$

9. $\tan P$ 10. $\sin R$

11. $\cos R$ 12. $\tan R$

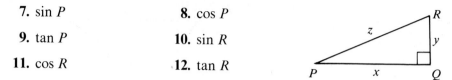

Written Exercises

Give the value of the sine, cosine, and tangent of $\angle A$ and $\angle B$. Give all ratios in lowest terms.

A

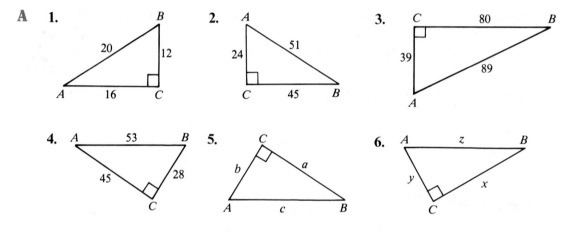

1.

2.

3.

4.

5.

6.

B   In Exercises 7–12, give all ratios in lowest terms and with the radical in the numerator.

Find the value of x. Then find $\tan A$.

7.

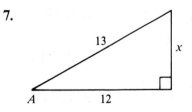

8.

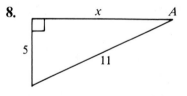

Find the value of x. Then find $\sin A$.

9.

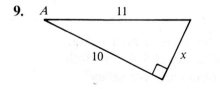

10.

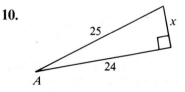

Find the value of *x*. Then find cos *A*.

11.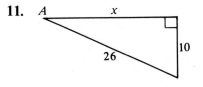

12.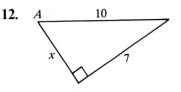

Find the sine, cosine, and tangent. Write the answer both as a fraction and as a decimal to the nearest thousandth. (*Hint:* See Example 2.)

13. **a.** sin 60°   **b.** cos 60°   **c.** tan 60°   14. **a.** sin 45°   **b.** cos 45°   **c.** tan 45°

Give answers to the nearest tenth.

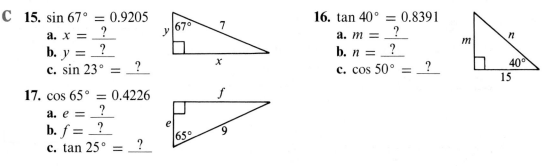

C 15. sin 67° = 0.9205
   a. x = ___?___
   b. y = ___?___
   c. sin 23° = ___?___

16. tan 40° = 0.8391
   a. m = ___?___
   b. n = ___?___
   c. cos 50° = ___?___

17. cos 65° = 0.4226
   a. e = ___?___
   b. f = ___?___
   c. tan 25° = ___?___

Review Exercises

Select the number that is closest to the one given.

1. 0.3765
   a. 0.3774   **b.** 0.3759

2. 8.1443
   a. 8.1430   **b.** 8.1451

3. 0.9004
   a. 0.9019   **b.** 0.8954

4. 1.8040
   a. 1.829   **b.** 1.788

5. 0.2126
   a. 0.2666   **b.** 0.1986

6. 11.4301
   a. 12.0801   **b.** 10.6801

7. 0.1758
   a. 0.1744   **b.** 0.1764

8. 3.2709
   a. 3.2712   **b.** 3.2705

▮▮▮ Challenge

Leslie is considering two job offers. Alloid Metals pays an hourly wage of $7.30. Acme Steel Company pays an annual salary of $14,040. Both jobs have a 40-hour work week. Which job offers a better salary?

11-8 Solving Right Triangles

The table on page 509 gives approximate values of the sine, the cosine, and the tangent of angles with measure 1°, 2°, 3°, . . . , 90°. To find sin 45°, look down the column headed "Angle" to 45°. To the right of it in the column headed "Sine," you see that sin 45° ≈ 0.7071.

The values in the table on page 509 are, in general, accurate to only four decimal places. However, in computational work with sine, cosine, and tangent, it is customary to use = instead of ≈. In this lesson, we will write *sin 45° = 0.7071* instead of *sin 45° ≈ 0.7071*.

We can use the values in the table to **solve right triangles,** that is, to find approximate measures of all the sides and all the angles of any right triangle.

EXAMPLE 1 Solve $\triangle ABC$ by finding each measure.
  a. c to the nearest tenth
  b. m $\angle A$
  c. m $\angle B$

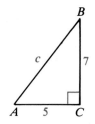

Solution **a.** The diagram indicates that $\angle C$ is a right triangle, therefore by the Pythagorean theorem:

$$c^2 = 7^2 + 5^2 = 74$$
$$c = \sqrt{74} = 8.6$$

To the nearest tenth, $c = 8.6$.

b. $\tan A = \frac{7}{5} = 1.4$

In the tangent column in the table, the closest entry to 1.4 is 1.3764, for angle measure 54°. Thus, to the nearest degree, m $\angle A = 54°$.

c. m $\angle A$ + m $\angle B$ + m $\angle C = 180°$
    $54°$ + m $\angle B$ + $90° = 180°$
          m $\angle B = 180° - 90° - 54°$
          m $\angle B = 36°$

Problem Solving Reminder

To solve some problems, you might need to *use previously obtained solutions* in order to complete the answer. In Example 1, it was convenient to use the m $\angle A$ found in part *b* to solve for the m $\angle B$.

EXAMPLE 2 Solve △ABC by finding each measure.

        a. m ∠ B
        b. *a* to the nearest tenth
        c. *b* to the nearest tenth

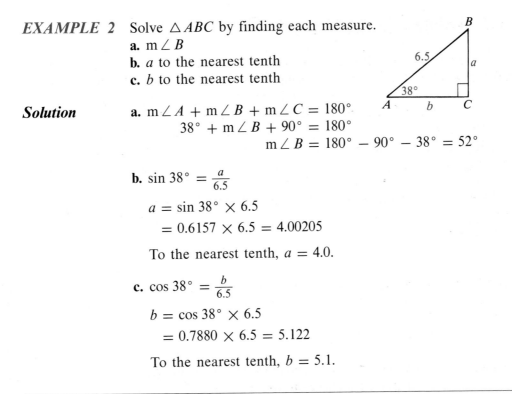

Solution

a. m ∠ A + m ∠ B + m ∠ C = 180°
    38° + m ∠ B + 90° = 180°
            m ∠ B = 180° − 90° − 38° = 52°

b. $\sin 38° = \dfrac{a}{6.5}$

    $a = \sin 38° \times 6.5$
      $= 0.6157 \times 6.5 = 4.00205$

    To the nearest tenth, $a = 4.0$.

c. $\cos 38° = \dfrac{b}{6.5}$

    $b = \cos 38° \times 6.5$
      $= 0.7880 \times 6.5 = 5.122$

    To the nearest tenth, $b = 5.1$.

Class Exercises

State whether you would use the sine, cosine, or tangent ratio to find x in each diagram.

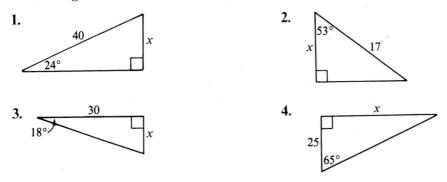

For Exercises 5–18, use the table on page 509.

Find a value for the trigonometric ratio.

5. cos 8°   **6.** sin 67°   **7.** tan 36°   **8.** tan 82°

9. sin 15°   **10.** cos 75°   **11.** cos 20°   **12.** sin 70°

Find the measure of $\angle A$ to the nearest degree.

13. $\sin A = 0.4$ **14.** $\tan A = 1.6$ **15.** $\cos A = 0.85$

16. $\cos A = 0.19$ **17.** $\tan A = 0.819$ **18.** $\sin A = 0.208$

Written Exercises

For Exercises 1–40, use the tables on page 508 and page 509.

Find $\sin A$, $\cos A$, and $\tan A$ for the given measure of $\angle A$.

A   **1.** $25°$ **2.** $76°$ **3.** $88°$ **4.** $11°$ **5.** $39°$ **6.** $42°$

      7. $74°$ **8.** $13°$ **9.** $40°$ **10.** $52°$ **11.** $65°$ **12.** $81°$

Find the measure of $\angle A$ to the nearest degree.

13. $\sin A = 0.9877$ **14.** $\cos A = 0.9205$ **15.** $\tan A = 0.0175$

16. $\cos A = 0.8572$ **17.** $\tan A = 4.0108$ **18.** $\sin A = 0.2250$

Find the measure of the angle to the nearest degree or the length of the side to the nearest whole number.

19. $m \angle A$

21. $m \angle B$

23. t

20. x

22. $m \angle L$

24. u

Find the measure of $\angle A$ to the nearest degree.

B   **25.** $\sin A = 0.8483$ **26.** $\cos A = 0.2758$ **27.** $\tan A = 0.4560$

      28. $\sin A = 0.6559$ **29.** $\tan A = 2.7500$ **30.** $\cos A = 0.5148$

Solve $\triangle ABC$. Round angle measures to the nearest degree and lengths to the nearest tenth.

31. $a = 5, b = 8$ **32.** $a = 4, b = 7$

33. $m \angle A = 72°, c = 10$ **34.** $m \angle B = 26°, c = 8$

35. $b = 4, c = 9$ **36.** $a = 5, c = 7$

37. $m \angle B = 20°, b = 15$ **38.** $m \angle A = 80°, a = 9$

39. $m \angle A = 58°, b = 12$ **40.** $m \angle B = 39°, a = 20$

Problems

Give angle measures to the nearest degree and lengths to the nearest tenth.

A

1. How tall is the tree in the diagram below?

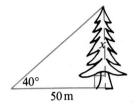
40°
50 m

2. How tall is the flagpole in the diagram below?

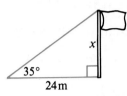
35°
24 m
x

3. In the diagram below, the road rises 20 m for every 100 m traveled horizontally. What angle does it make with the horizontal?

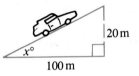
20 m
x°
100 m

4. What angle does the rope make with the horizontal in the diagram below?

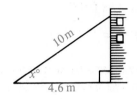
10 m
x°
4.6 m

B

5. a. How tall is the building in the diagram below?
b. How tall is the antenna?

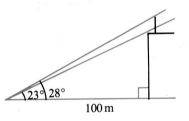
23° 28°
100 m

6. What is the height of the child in the diagram below?

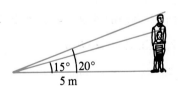
15° 20°
5 m

7. In △ABC, $\overline{AC}$ is 8 cm long. The length of the altitude to $\overline{AB}$ is 5 cm. Find the measure of ∠A.

8. Triangle MNO is an isosceles triangle with $\overline{MO}$ congruent to $\overline{NO}$. The third side of the triangle, $\overline{MN}$, is 36 cm long. The perimeter of the triangle is 96 cm.
a. Find the lengths of $\overline{MO}$ and $\overline{NO}$.
b. The altitude from O to $\overline{MN}$ bisects $\overline{MN}$. Find the measure of ∠OMN.

Give angle measures to the nearest degree and lengths to the nearest tenth.

9. A surveyor is determining the direction in which tunnel $\overline{AB}$ is to be dug through a mountain. She locates point C so that $\angle C$ is a right angle, the length of $\overline{AC}$ is 1.5 km, and the length of $\overline{BC}$ is 3.5 km. Find the measure of $\angle A$.

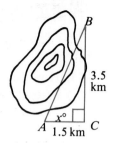

C 10. In $\triangle RST$, the measure of $\angle S$ is 142°. The length of $\overline{RS}$ is 10. Find the length of the altitude from vertex R.

Self-Test B

Exercises 1–4 refer to the diagram below. Complete.

1. $\triangle TOY \underline{\ ?\ } \triangle TIN$ [11-5]

2. $\dfrac{TI}{TO} = \dfrac{IN}{OY} = \dfrac{?}{?}$

3. $TY = \underline{\ ?\ }$

4. $m \angle TIN \underline{\ ?\ } m \angle TOY$

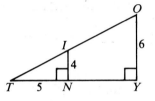

In Exercises 5 and 6, give answers in terms of radicals with the radical in the numerator.

5. The hypotenuse of a 45° right triangle is $6\sqrt{2}$ cm long. What is the length of each leg?   [11-6]

6. The longer leg of a 30°–60° right triangle has length 12. What are the lengths of the shorter leg and the hypotenuse?

Exercises 7–13 refer to the diagram at the right.

Complete in terms of p, q, and r.

7. $\sin P = \underline{\ ?\ }$ 8. $\cos P = \underline{\ ?\ }$ [11-7]

9. $\tan P = \underline{\ ?\ }$

Find the measure of the angles to the nearest degree and the lengths to the nearest tenth. Use the tables on page 508 and page 509.

10. $r = 3$, $q = 6$ 11. $m \angle P = 78°$, $r = 5$ [11-8]

12. $m \angle R = 23°$, $p = 8$ 13. $m \angle R = 57°$, $q = 24$

Self-Test answers and Extra Practice are at the back of the book.

The following program produces a Pythagorean triple using any counting number greater than 2.

```
10   PRINT "INPUT THE DESIRED NUMBER";
20   INPUT N
30   IF N * (N − 1) * (N − 2) < > 0 THEN 60
40   PRINT "THERE IS NO SUCH TRIPLE."
50   GOTO 150
60   IF INT (N / 2) < > N / 2 THEN 120
70   IF N = 4 THEN 110
80   LET N = N / 2
90   LET C = C + 1
100  GOTO 60
110  LET N = 3
120  PRINT "A PYTHAGOREAN TRIPLE IS:"
130  LET B = INT (N ↑ 2 / 2)
140  PRINT 2 ↑ C * N,2 ↑ C * B,2 ↑ C * (B + 1)
150  END
```

1. Use the program to find a triple with the number 3. Does it give you the triple you had expected?

2. Use the program to find a triple with the number 4. Does it give you the triple you had expected?

3. Now try 5. Is the output what you had expected?

4. Input each of these numbers to produce Pythagorean triples:

$$6, 7, 8, 11, 17, 24, 101$$

Check three of your answers by multiplying.

5. Try 1 or 2 in the program. Can you explain why this output is true?

Trace the two squares as they are shown at the right. Can you draw one line that will divide each of the squares into two parts of equal area?

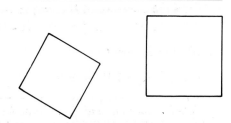

Other Roots and Fractions as Exponents

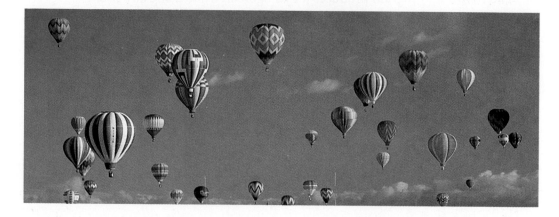

As you learned earlier, $\sqrt{49} = 7$ because $7^2 = 49$. Recall that we chose 7 and not -7 since 7 is the positive square root of 49.

We can extend the idea of square roots to other roots. The fourth root of 16, denoted $\sqrt[4]{16}$, is 2 since $2^4 = 16$. In general,

> For any positive *even* integer n, and positive integer c,
>
> $$\sqrt[n]{a} = c, \text{ if } c^n = a.$$

The third root, or cube root, of a number may be positive or negative depending on the sign of the number. For example,

$$\sqrt[3]{64} = 4 \text{ because } 4^3 = 64$$

and $$\sqrt[3]{-27} = -3 \text{ because } (-3)^3 = -27.$$

In general,

> For any positive *odd* integer n, and any integers a and c,
>
> $$\sqrt[n]{a} = c, \text{ if } c^n = a.$$

The following cases will complete our discussion of roots.

If $a = 0$, then $\sqrt[n]{a} = 0$ because $a^n = 0^n = 0$.

If a is a negative number and n is *even,* there is no real nth root of a.

Recall that you add exponents when multiplying powers of the same base.

$$9^1 \times 9^2 = 9^{1+2} = 9^3$$

When this rule is applied to fractional exponents, we have

$$9^{\frac{1}{2}} \times 9^{\frac{1}{2}} = 9^{\frac{1}{2}+\frac{1}{2}} = 9^1 = 9.$$

This example suggests that we define $9^{\frac{1}{2}}$ as $\sqrt{9}$, since $(\sqrt{9})^2 = 9$.
   In general,

$$a^{\frac{1}{n}} = \sqrt[n]{a}.$$

Find the root. If the root does not exist, explain why.

1. $\sqrt[3]{27}$ 2. $\sqrt[6]{0}$ 3. $\sqrt[4]{16}$ 4. $\sqrt[3]{1000}$

5. $\sqrt[3]{64}$ 6. $\sqrt[3]{-27}$ 7. $\sqrt{-49}$ 8. $\sqrt[4]{-16}$

9. $\sqrt[3]{-1000}$ 10. $\sqrt[5]{-32}$ 11. $\sqrt[3]{125}$ 12. $\sqrt[7]{-1}$

Write the expression without exponents.

13. $36^{\frac{1}{2}}$ 14. $27^{\frac{1}{3}}$ 15. $64^{\frac{1}{3}}$ 16. $64^{\frac{1}{6}}$ 17. $16^{\frac{1}{4}}$ 18. $1000^{\frac{1}{3}}$ 19. $81^{\frac{1}{4}}$

Calculator Activity

Most scientific calculators have a $\boxed{\sqrt[x]{y}}$ key that can be used to approximate roots that are not integers. For example, to obtain $\sqrt[4]{7}$, enter $\boxed{7}$ $\boxed{\sqrt[x]{y}}$ $\boxed{4}$ $\boxed{=}$ to get 1.6265766. On some calculators, the $\boxed{\sqrt[x]{y}}$ key may be a second function. In this case, push the $\boxed{2\text{nd F}}$ key to activate the root function.

   Other calculators have a $\boxed{y^x}$ and a $\boxed{1/x}$ key. In this case, we can obtain $\sqrt[4]{7}$ by calculating $7^{\frac{1}{4}}$ in the following way.

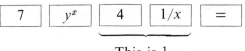

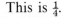

This is $\frac{1}{4}$.

Use a calculator to approximate the following.

1. $\sqrt[3]{10}$ 2. $\sqrt[3]{4}$ 3. $\sqrt[5]{50}$ 4. $\sqrt[4]{44}$ 5. $5^{\frac{1}{4}}$ 6. $11^{\frac{1}{3}}$

7. The volume of a sphere is related to its radius by the formula $V = \frac{4}{3}\pi r^3$. Use the formula to find the radius of a balloon that has a volume of 3500 ft³. Use $\pi \approx 3.14$.

Chapter Review

Complete.

1. A positive number has exactly __?__ different square root(s).   [11–1]

2. $\sqrt{169}$ is 13, therefore 169 is a __?__ square.

3. If 5.2 is used as an estimate for $\sqrt{28.6}$ in the divide-and-average   [11–2]
   method, the next estimate will be __?__.

4. Using the divide-and-average method, $\sqrt{53} =$ __?__ to the tenths'
   place.

5. In the table on page 508, $\sqrt{24.6}$ lies between __?__ and __?__.   [11–3]

6. Using interpolation and the table on page 498, $\sqrt{5.7} =$ __?__ to the
   nearest hundredth.

True or false?

7. The Pythagorean theorem applies to all triangles.   [11–4]

8. The hypotenuse is the longest side of a right triangle and is opposite
   the right angle.

9. The measure of the diagonal of a 5 cm by 5 cm square is 50 cm.

Exercises 10–12 refer to the diagram below.
$\triangle ABC \sim \triangle DEF$. **Complete.**

10. $\frac{BA}{?} = \frac{AC}{DF}$ 11. $\angle C \cong \angle$ __?__   [11–5]

12. $\overline{BC}$ corresponds to __?__.

13. An isosceles right triangle is also called a __?__° right triangle.   [11–6]

14. An equilateral triangle with sides 16 cm long has an altitude of
    __?__ cm.

15. The legs of an isosceles right triangle are 7 cm long. The length of
    the hypotenuse is __?__ cm.

Exercises 16–21 refer to the diagram at the right. Match.

16. sin F 17. cos F **A.** $\frac{x}{7}$ **B.** cos 42° × 7   [11–7]

18. tan N 19. y **C.** $\frac{y}{7}$ **D.** sin 42° × 7   [11–8]

20. x 21. m $\angle N$ **E.** $\frac{x}{y}$ **F.** 48°

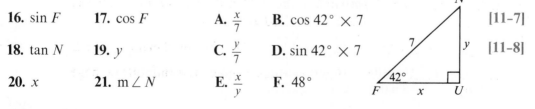

Chapter Test

If the given symbol names an integer, state the integer. If not, name the
two consecutive integers between which the number lies.

1. $\sqrt{16}$ 2. $-\sqrt{144}$ 3. $\sqrt{169} - \sqrt{121}$ 4. $\sqrt{38 + 43}$ [11–1]

Solve. Round your answer to the nearest tenth.

5. Use the divide-and-average method to approximate $\sqrt{13.7}$. [11–2]

6. Using interpolation and the table on page 508, $\sqrt{12.6} \approx$ __?__. [11–3]

7. The area of a square deck is 65.6 m². Find the length of the side.

Is the triangle with sides of the given lengths a right triangle?

8. 6, 8, 10 9. 7, 11, 19 10. 8, 15, 17 [11–4]

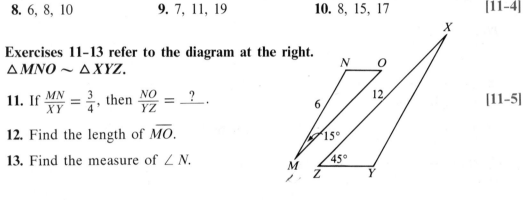

Exercises 11–13 refer to the diagram at the right.
$\triangle MNO \sim \triangle XYZ$.

11. If $\frac{MN}{XY} = \frac{3}{4}$, then $\frac{NO}{YZ} =$ __?__. [11–5]

12. Find the length of $\overline{MO}$.

13. Find the measure of $\angle N$.

Give answers in terms of radicals with the radical in the numerator.

14. In a 30°–60° right triangle, the shorter leg has length 5. How long is [11–6]
    (a) the longer leg and (b) the hypotenuse?

15. The hypotenuse of a 45° right triangle has a
    length of 36. How long is each leg?

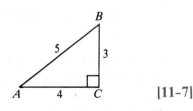

Exercises 16–19 refer to the diagram at the right.
Find a value for the trigonometric ratio.

16. $\cos A$ 17. $\tan A$ 18. $\cos B$ 19. $\sin B$ [11–7]

$\triangle KLM$ is an isosceles triangle with $\overline{KL} \cong \overline{LM}$. The third side, $\overline{KM}$, is
42 cm long. The perimeter of $\triangle KLM$ is 112 cm.

20. Find the lengths of $\overline{KL}$ and $\overline{LM}$. 21. Find the height of $\triangle KLM$. [11–8]

22. Find m $\angle K$ and m $\angle M$ to the nearest degree. Use the table on page
    509.

Cumulative Review (Chapters 1–11)

Exercises

Simplify the expression.

1. $(8 + 2) \div (3 \times 9)$

2. $15 \div 8 + 7 \div 9$

3. $[48(2 + 5) - 6] \times 10$

4. $-26 - 7 + 9 \times 3$

5. $2(10 + 5) \div (-3 - 6)$

6. $[(7 - 5)(3 \times 5)] - 5$

Evaluate the expression when $a = 10$, $b = -10$, and $c = 0.5$.

7. ab

8. ac

9. $a + b$

10. $a - b$

11. $2ab$

12. b^2

13. ac^2

14. a^2c

15. $\dfrac{b}{a}$

16. $\dfrac{ab}{c}$

Replace $\underline{\ ?\ }$ with $<$, $>$, or $=$ to make a true statement.

17. $\dfrac{1}{2} \underline{\ ?\ } \dfrac{3}{8}$

18. $\dfrac{1}{5} \underline{\ ?\ } \dfrac{2}{8}$

19. $-\dfrac{4}{5} \underline{\ ?\ } \dfrac{3}{4}$

20. $-\dfrac{1}{3} \underline{\ ?\ } -\dfrac{7}{9}$

Solve the equation.

21. $12 + a = 50$

22. $x - 27 = 56$

23. $43m = 107.5$

24. $\dfrac{n}{38.6} = 15$

25. $a + \dfrac{2}{3} = 8$

26. $w - \dfrac{1}{5} = 12$

27. $2x + 4x = 48$

28. $5c - 12c = 35$

29. $3(t - 4) = 24$

30. $6z = 32 + z$

31. $2 + 5a = 30$

32. $7(x - 6) = 3x$

Find the perimeter of the given polygon.

33. square: sides of 2.9 ft

34. triangle: 7.11 in., 8.11 in., 12.45 in.

Solve the proportion.

35. $\dfrac{n}{15} = \dfrac{12}{45}$

36. $\dfrac{6}{7} = \dfrac{n}{35}$

37. $\dfrac{8}{n} = \dfrac{32}{40}$

38. $\dfrac{3}{5} = \dfrac{24}{n}$

Graph each equation on a separate coordinate plane.

39. $x + 2y = 7$

40. $2x + 2y = 9$

41. $x + \dfrac{1}{5}y = 1$

Find the volume of a cylinder with the given dimensions. Leave your answer in terms of π.

42. radius: 7   height: 12

43. radius: 2.3   height: 10.5

Rewrite the expression in lowest terms with the radical in the numerator.

44. $\dfrac{4}{\sqrt{10}}$ **45.** $\dfrac{5}{\sqrt{2}}$ **46.** $\dfrac{18}{\sqrt{37}}$ **47.** $\dfrac{2n}{\sqrt{n}}$ **48.** $\dfrac{6m}{\sqrt{m}}$

Problems

> **Problem Solving Reminders**
> Here are some problem solving reminders that may help you solve some of the problems on this page.
> • Sometimes more than one method can be used to solve.
> • Supply additional information if necessary.
> • Check your results with the facts given in the problem.

Solve.

1. Evan is a parking lot attendant at the Lonestar Garage. When counting his tips from Monday he discovered he had 12 more quarters than dimes and 3 fewer nickels than quarters. If Evan earned a total of $19.45 in tips, how many of each type of coin did he have?

2. A regular pentagon has a perimeter of 378.5 m. Find the length of each side.

3. A discount store has an automatic markdown policy. Every 7 days, the price of an item is marked down 25% until the item is sold or 4 weeks have elapsed. If the first price of an item is $40 on September 17, what will the price be on October 1?

4. A window washer uses a vinegar and water solution in the ratio of one-half cup of vinegar to three cups of water. How much vinegar will be in two gallons of solution?

5. Lavender soap is sold in boxes of 3 bars for $6.50. To the nearest cent, what is the cost of one bar?

6. Bertha Magnuson had purchased 2500 shares of ABC stock for $3.50 per share. When she sold the stock, its value had gone down to $\frac{5}{8}$ of the total purchase price. How much did Bertha lose?

7. The area of a square table is 1936 in.^{2}. What will be the dimensions of a square tablecloth that drops 4 in. over each side of the table?

8. Mary has $300 to spend on new boots and a winter coat. She expects to spend $\frac{2}{5}$ as much for boots as for a coat. What is the most she can spend on boots?

12
Statistics and Probability

For ecological and other reasons, it is sometimes important to determine the size and geographical location of a group of migrating birds such as those shown in the photograph. A total count of a particular kind of bird obviously poses a difficult problem. By using a sample count, however, only a small part of the bird population needs to be counted. The total number of birds in the entire area can then be estimated from the number in the sampled area.

The simplest method of counting birds and studying migration is direct observation. Because of the disadvantages of this method, more sophisticated methods are being developed and used. These include banding, radio tracking, and radar observation. With the help of computers, this data can be quickly collected and examined.

In this chapter, you will learn some methods for gathering and analyzing data.

Career Note

Statisticians collect, analyze, and interpret numerical results of surveys and experiments. They may use the information that is gathered to determine suitable choices, evaluate a report, or redesign an existing program. Statisticians are usually employed in manufacturing, finance, or government positions. A thorough knowledge of mathematics and a background in economics or natural science is needed.

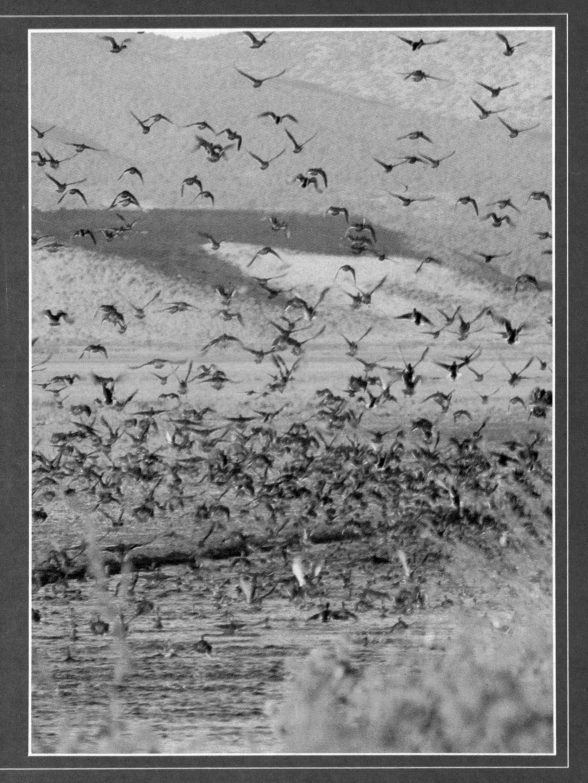

12-1 Picturing Numerical Data

Many scientific, social, and economic studies produce numerical facts. Such numerical information is called **data.** At the right are some data about the number of automobiles sold in the United States.

These data can be pictured by using a **bar graph** (below left) or a **broken-line graph** (below right). On the bar graph the height of each bar is drawn to the scale marked at the left and so is proportional to the data it represents. All bars have the same width. The broken-line graph can be made by joining the midpoints of the tops of the bars.

We can see from either graph that the most rapid 10-year increase in auto sales occurred between 1940 and 1950.

Car Sales	
Year	**Number Sold (nearest 100,000)**
1920	2,200,000
1930	3,400,000
1940	4,500,000
1950	8,000,000
1960	7,900,000
1970	8,200,000
1980	8,000,000

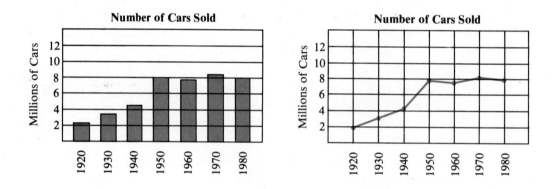

To draw a graph we must choose a **data unit** to mark off one of the axes. If the data are small numbers, the data unit can be a small number, such as 1 or 5. If the data are large numbers, a larger data unit should be chosen so that the graph will be a reasonable size. For example, the data unit in the graphs above is 2,000,000 automobiles.

EXAMPLE The following table gives the average monthly temperatures in Minneapolis, Minnesota. Construct a bar graph to illustrate the data.

Month	J	F	M	A	M	J	J	A	S	O	N	D
°C	−11.1	−8.3	−2.2	7.2	13.9	19.4	22.2	21.1	15.6	10.0	0	−7.2

Solution   Label the horizontal axis with symbols for the months.   Label the vertical axis using a data unit of 5°. Then draw bars of equal widths and proper lengths. Draw the bars downward for negative data. Finally, give the graph a title.

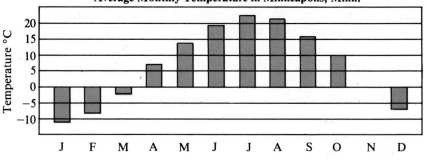

Average Monthly Temperature in Minneapolis, Minn.

Sometimes it is more convenient to arrange the bars in a graph horizontally. In the graph at the right, the data unit for the horizontal axis is 10,000 km² and the vertical axis is labeled with the names of the lakes.

We can estimate data from graphs. For example, we see from the graph that the area of Lake Erie is approximately 25,000 km².

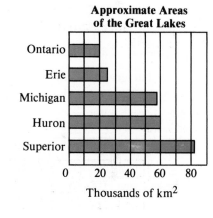

Approximate Areas of the Great Lakes

Thousands of km²

Class Exercises

Exercises 1-5 refer to the bar graph at the right.

1. What data unit is used on the vertical axis?

2. Which mountain has the lowest elevation? What is its elevation?

3. Which mountain has the highest elevation? What is its elevation?

4. Which two mountains have nearly the same elevation?

5. Find the ratio of the elevation of Mount Vinson to the elevation of Mount McKinley.

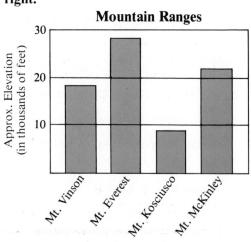

Mountain Ranges

Exercises 6–10 refer to the broken-line graph at the right.

6. What data unit is used on the vertical axis?

7. What was the approximate population in 1900? In 1950?

8. In approximately what year did the population pass 100 million? 150 million? 200 million?

9. In which 20-year period did the population increase the most?

10. Find the approximate total increase in population during the twentieth century.

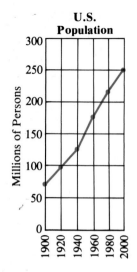

U.S.
Population

Written Exercises

The bar graph below shows the seven nations having populations over 100 million. Use the graph for Exercises 1–6.

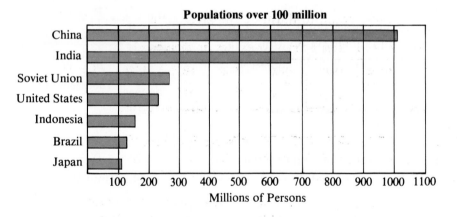

Populations over 100 million

A
1. What data unit is used on the horizontal axis?

2. Estimate the total population of the three largest nations.

3. Estimate the total population of the three smallest nations.

4. Estimate the total population of the seven nations.

5. To the nearest percent, what percent of the world's 4.5 billion people live in China?

6. To the nearest percent, what percent of the world's 4.5 billion people live in the seven nations shown on the graph?

In Exercises 7–9, make a bar graph to illustrate the given data.

7. The six longest highway tunnels are: Saint Gotthard, 16.2 km; Arlberg, 14 km; Frejus, 12.8 km; Mont Blanc, 11.7 km; Enasson, 8.5 km; and San Bernadino, 6.6 km.

8. The areas of the world's five largest islands in thousands of square kilometers are: Greenland, 2175; New Guinea, 792; Borneo, 725; Madagascar, 587; and Baffin, 507.

9. The table below gives the length of each continent's longest river.

Continent	River	Length (km)
Africa	Nile	6632
Asia	Yangtze	6342
Australia	Murray-Darling	3693
Europe	Volga	3510
North America	Mississippi-Missouri	5936
South America	Amazon	6400

10. Make a broken-line graph to illustrate the given data.

Number of U.S. High School Graduates (in thousands)

1920	1930	1940	1950	1960	1970	1980
311	667	1221	1200	1864	2896	3078

B 11. Make a bar graph to illustrate the data. Net profits of the XYZ Company in thousands of dollars were: 30 in 1981; −20 (loss) in 1982; −5 (loss) in 1983; 45 in 1984; and 60 in 1985.

12. Make a broken-line graph to illustrate the average monthly temperatures in Minneapolis. (Use the table in the example in this lesson.)

Review Exercises

Perform the indicated operation.

1. $\frac{47}{60} \times 360$ 2. $\frac{74}{83} \times 249$ 3. $\frac{118}{37} \times 111$ 4. $\frac{85}{156} \times 312$

5. 25% of 540   6. 47% of 360   7. 73% of 180   8. 81% of 360

12-2 Pictographs and Circle Graphs

Nontechnical magazines often present data using pictures. These **pictographs** take the form of bar graphs with the bars replaced by rows or columns of symbols. Each symbol represents an assigned quantity. This amount must be clearly indicated on the pictograph. For example, the pictograph below illustrates the data on automobile sales given in the previous lesson.

Number of Cars Sold

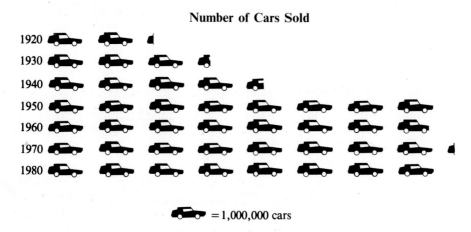

= 1,000,000 cars

EXAMPLE 1   The approximate numbers of different book titles published in the United States in selected years are: 11,000 in 1950; 15,000 in 1960; 36,000 in 1970; and 42,000 in 1980. Illustrate the data with a pictograph.

Solution   Stacks of books are appropriate symbols. We let one thick book represent 5000 titles and one thin book represent 1000 titles.

Books Published in the U.S.

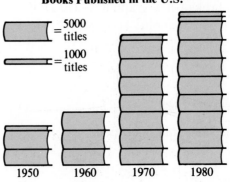

The **circle graph** at the right shows how the world's water is distributed. Circle graphs are often more effective than other graphs in picturing how a total amount is divided into parts.

The following example illustrates how to make a circle graph.

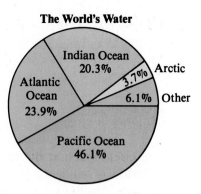

The World's Water

EXAMPLE 2 The seventh-grade class voted to decide where to have their year-end picnic. The results were as follows: Mountain Park, 62 votes; State Beach, 96 votes; City Zoo, 82 votes. Draw a circle graph to illustrate this distribution.

Solution The whole circle represents the total number of votes. We plan to divide the circle into wedges to represent the distribution of the votes. Since the sum of all the adjacent angles around a point is 360°, the sum of the angle measures of all the wedges is 360°.

First find the total of all votes cast.

$$62 + 96 + 82 = 240$$

Then find the fraction of the vote cast for each place and the corresponding angle measure.

For Mountain Park:

$$\frac{62}{240} \times 360° = 93°$$

For State Beach:

$$\frac{96}{240} \times 360° = 144°$$

For City Zoo:

$$\frac{82}{240} \times 360° = 123°$$

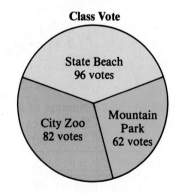

Class Vote

Now use a compass to draw a circle and a protractor to draw three radii forming the angles found above. Finally, label the wedges and give the graph a title.

Class Exercises

1. Draw a circle and divide it into 4 equal parts.

2. Draw a circle and divide it into 6 equal parts.

3. Draw a circle and divide it into 9 equal parts.

4. Draw a circle and divide it into 12 equal parts.

The circle graph at the right pictures the distribution of students playing the various instruments in the school orchestra.

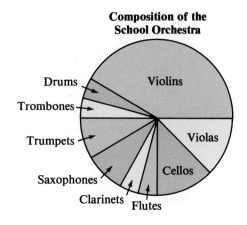

Composition of the School Orchestra

5. Which instrument is played by the greatest number of students in the orchestra?

6. How does the number of students playing stringed instruments (violins, violas, and cellos) compare with the number of students playing all the other instruments?

7. Which four instruments are played by the fewest students?

8. How does the number of saxophone players compare with the number of trumpet players?

Written Exercises

Complete the following tables and construct a circle graph for each.

A **1.** The Junior Athletic Association decided to raise money by selling greeting cards. Orders were obtained for the following kinds of cards.

Kind of Card	Number of Boxes	Fraction of the Whole	Number of Degrees in the Angle
birthday	60	?	?
get well	72	?	?
friendship	48	?	?
thank you	60	?	?
Total	?	?	?

2. The winter issue of the school magazine contained the following kinds of material.

Kind of Material	Number of Pages	Fraction of the Whole	Number of Degrees in the Angle
fiction	32	?	?
essays	8	?	?
sports	16	?	?
advertisements	8	?	?
Total	?	?	?

Illustrate, using a circle graph.

3. The surface of Earth is 30% land and 70% water.

4. Earth's atmosphere is 78% nitrogen, 21% oxygen, and 1% other gases.

Illustrate, using a pictograph. The parentheses contain a suggestion as to what symbol to use.

5. The XYZ Car Rental Company rented 520 cars in July, 350 cars in August, 350 cars in September, 400 cars in October, and 110 cars in November. (cars)

6. The Meadowbrook School ordered 200 cartons of milk the first week, 220 the second week, 240 the third week, and 180 the fourth week. (milk cartons)

7. The number of fish caught in Clear Lake: 4500 in 1970; 3500 in 1975; 4200 in 1980; 4800 in 1985. (fish)

8. The cost of higher education in the United States in billions of dollars: 1965 — $13; 1970 — $23; 1975 — $39; 1980 — $55. (dollars)

Illustrate, using (a) a circle graph and (b) a pictograph. The parentheses contain a suggestion as to what symbol to use in the pictograph.

B **9.** In the United States about 167 million people live in cities and about 59 million live in rural areas. (people)

10. A fund-raising event made $420 from the sale of antiques, $280 from crafts items, and $240 from food. (dollars)

Illustrate, using (a) a circle graph and (b) a pictograph. The parentheses contain a suggestion as to what symbol to use in the pictograph.

11. The average seasonal rainfall in Honolulu is 26 cm in winter, 7 cm in spring, 5 cm in summer, and 21 cm in autumn. (raindrops)

12. Of each dollar the United States government takes in, 47¢ comes from individual income taxes, 27¢ from Social Security, 12¢ from corporation taxes, and 14¢ from other sources. (piles of coins)

13. A family spends $440.75 of the monthly budget on food, $530.00 on rent, $617.00 total on clothes, medicine, and other items, and $175.25 on transportation. (dollars)

14. A total of 387 people were polled on Proposition Q, 46% favored it, 33% opposed it, and 21% had no opinion. (people)

15. The library received a $1300 grant. The librarian plans to spend 10% of the grant to extend magazine subscriptions, 35% to buy new books, 15% to repair damaged books, 30% to buy new furniture, and 10% to locate missing books. (books)

C 16. Which pictograph correctly shows that the production of a certain oil field doubled between 1975 and 1985? Explain your answer.

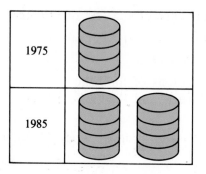
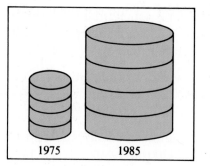

Review Exercises

Arrange in order from least to greatest.

1. 4, 2.6, 7, 0.84, 3

2. 4, -8, -3, 1, 10, -5

3. 7, $3\frac{1}{2}$, -5, $4\frac{1}{4}$, -6

4. $\frac{7}{8}$, $\frac{5}{6}$, $\frac{11}{9}$, $\frac{7}{12}$, $\frac{12}{7}$

5. -6, -10, -2, -12, -9

6. $3\frac{7}{8}$, $2\frac{9}{10}$, $2\frac{8}{9}$, $3\frac{11}{16}$

7. 1.09, 1.1, 0.9, 0.09

8. $\frac{17}{4}$, $\frac{11}{2}$, $\frac{15}{8}$, $\frac{9}{4}$, $\frac{7}{5}$

12-3 Mean, Median, and Range

The daytime high temperatures in °C for five days in May were

$$23°, \ 14°, \ 18°, \ 28°, \ \text{and} \ 25°.$$

Here are two ways to summarize this information.

(1) The **mean** of the temperatures is their sum divided by the number of temperatures.

$$\frac{23° + 14° + 18° + 28° + 25°}{5} = \frac{108°}{5} = 21.6°$$

(2) The **median** of the temperatures is the middle temperature when they are arranged in order of size.

$$14°, \ 18°, \ 23°, \ 25°, \ 28° \qquad \text{Median} = 23°$$

For an even number of data items the median is midway between the two middle numbers.

The **range** of a set of data is the difference between the greatest and least numbers in the set. For example, the range of the above temperatures is $28° - 14°$, or $14°$.

EXAMPLE Find the mean, median, and range of each set of numbers. Round to the nearest tenth.

    a. 11, 19, 7, 45, 22, 38   **b.** 0, 1, 3, −4, 4, −6, 7

Solution   **a.** Mean $= \dfrac{11 + 19 + 7 + 45 + 22 + 38}{6} = \dfrac{142}{6} \approx 23.7$

            Arrange the numbers in order of size: 7, 11, 19, 22, 38, 45

            Median $= \dfrac{19 + 22}{2} = 20.5$ Range $= 45 - 7 = 38$

    b. Mean $= \dfrac{0 + 1 + 3 + (-4) + 4 + (-6) + 7}{7} = \dfrac{5}{7} \approx 0.7$

            Arrange the numbers in order of size: −6, −4, 0, 1, 3, 4, 7

            Median $= 1$ Range $= 7 - (-6) = 13$

In everyday conversation the word *average* is usually used for mean.

Analyzing data as we have been doing is part of the branch of mathematics called **statistics**.

Class Exercises

Find the mean, median, and range of each set of data.

1. 1, 2, 3, 4, 5
2. 5, 3, 1
3. 10, 10, 6, 2
4. 3, 4, 5, 6, 8, 10
5. −4, −2, 0, 2, 4
6. 3, 2, 1, 0, −1, −2, −3
7. −3, −1, 0, 4, 5
8. 6, 5, 5, 0, −1
9. −15, −11, −7, −7, −7, 0, 2, 5, 9, 15, 18, 22
10. −37, −28, −15, −15, −6, 1, 13, 26, 34
11. 11, 17, 31, 43, 58, 61, 58, 89, 94, 58, 94, 107, 215

1-14, 17-20 &22

Written Exercises

Find the mean, median, and range of each set of data. If necessary, round to the nearest tenth.

A
1. 30, 18, 21, 28, 23
2. 42, 58, 55, 61, 39
3. 7, 16, 20, 13, 26, 14
4. 85, 70, 93, 101, 116, 111
5. 47, 61, 53, 69, 45, 58
6. 17, 11, 9, 13, 7, 21, 8, 18
7. 3.6, 2.7, 2.9, 3.4, 3.4
8. 8.1, 9.2, 6.8, 7.3, 7.9, 6.9

B
9. −3, 2, −2, −5, 3
10. 8, −8, −12, 16, −8, 7
11. 1.3, −0.8, −0.1, 0.2, 0.9
12. 4.1, −3.2, −0.8, −1.5, 2.7, −0.1

13. Low Temperatures in February (°C)
  −13° −8° −10° −4° 1° 0° −2°
  −5° −7° −12° −8° −7° −5° 0°
  −2° −3° −5° 1° 2° 3° 1°
  2° 4° 2° 4° 4° 5° 6°

14. Elevations Along the Salton Sea Railway (meters)

6.82	2.55	1.60	−0.21	−1.35
−2.68	−1.95	−2.06	−0.88	−0.02
0.41	1.15	3.15	6.51	5.86

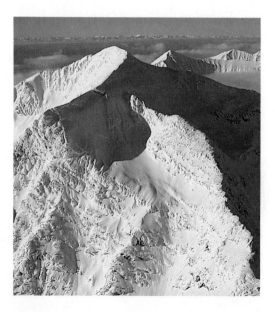

15. Insert another number in the list 15, 23, 11, 17 in such a way that the median is not changed.

16. Replace one of the numbers in the list 15, 23, 11, 17 so that the median becomes 17.

Find the value of x such that the mean of the given list is the specified number.

17. 6, 9, 13, x; mean = 11

18. 8, 14, 16, 12, x; mean = 15

19. Janet's scores on her first four mathematics tests were 98, 78, 84, and 96. What score must she make on the fifth test to have the mean of the five tests equal 90?

20. The heights of the starting guards and forwards on the basketball team are 178 cm, 185 cm, 165 cm, and 188 cm. How tall is the center if the mean height of the starting five is 182 cm?

C 21. If each number in a list is increased by 5, how is the median affected?

22. If each number in a list is increased by 5, how is the mean affected?

Review Exercises

Perform the indicated operations. Round to the nearest tenth if necessary.

1. $(4 \times 2 + 7 \times 5 + 6 \times 8) \div 15$

2. $(9 \times 4 + 6 \times 7 + 11 \times 5) \div 16$

3. $(14 \times 6 + 3 \times 0 + 16 \times 4) \div 10$

4. $(12 \times 1 + 8 \times 11 + 5 \times 6) \div 18$

5. $(18 \times 3 + 20 \times 5 + 7 \times 6) \div 14$

6. $(7 \times 15 + 4 \times 9 + 7 \times 2) \div 26$

7. $(11 \times 3 \times 2 + 8 \times 3 + 9) \div 33$

8. $(12 \times 2 \times 8 + 9 \times 3 \times 4) \div 15$

		Challenge

Cellini and Valdez were each appointed to a new job. Cellini is paid a starting salary of $16,500 a year with a $1000 raise at the end of each year. Valdez is paid a starting salary of $8000 for the first 6 months with a raise of $500 at the end of every 6 months. How much does each make at the end of the first year? The third year? Who has the better pay plan?

12-4 Frequency Distributions

Forty students took a quiz and received the following scores.

8	7	10	6	8	7	9	7	8	5
9	7	8	8	7	9	3	8	8	6
7	5	6	8	10	10	7	10	8	9
7	7	9	7	8	7	9	10	10	7

Score	Frequency
3	1
4	0
5	2
6	3
7	12
8	10
9	6
10	6

In order to analyze these data, we can arrange them in a **frequency table** as shown at the right. The number of times a score occurs is its **frequency.** Since a score of 9 was received by 6 students, we can say that the frequency of 9 is 6. The pairing of the scores with their frequencies is called a **frequency distribution.**

EXAMPLE Find the range, mean, and median for the data above.

Solution Since the lowest score is 3 and the highest is 10, the range is $10 - 3$, or 7.

To find the *mean* of the data, first multiply each possible score by its frequency. Enter the product in a third column as shown. The sum of the numbers in this column equals the sum of the 40 scores. Therefore:

$$\text{mean} = \frac{309}{40} = 7.725$$

Score x	Frequency f	$x \times f$
3	1	3
4	0	0
5	2	10
6	3	18
7	12	84
8	10	80
9	6	54
10	6	60
Total	40	309

To find the median, first rearrange the data in order from least to greatest. Since there are 40 scores, the median is the average of the twentieth and twenty-first scores, both of which are 8.

$$\text{median} = \frac{8 + 8}{2} = 8$$

Reading Mathematics: *Tables*

As you use a table, reread the headings to remind yourself what each number represents. For example, the frequency table above shows that the *score* of 8 had a *frequency* of 10; that is, there are 10 scores of 8, not 8 scores of 10.

The **mode** of a set of data is the item that occurs with the greatest frequency. In the example on the preceding page, the mode is 7 since it has the greatest frequency, 12. Sometimes there is more than one mode. The mode usually is used with nonnumerical data, such as to determine the popularity of car colors.

Class Exercises

Find the range, the mean, the median, and the mode(s) of each student's test score, *x*.

1. Evelyn

x	f
70	1
80	4
90	3
100	2

2. Bruce

x	f
75	2
85	3
90	1
100	4

3. Shana

x	f
70	4
85	3
95	2
100	1

4. Elroy

x	f
75	1
80	2
95	3
100	4

Written Exercises

In Exercises 1–6, find the range, the mean, the median, and the mode(s) of the data in each frequency table.

A

1.

x	f
5	2
6	4
7	8
8	5
9	1

2.

x	f
0	3
1	2
2	7
3	8
4	5

3.

x	f
25	1
20	0
15	3
10	5
5	6

4.

x	f
18	1
15	0
12	3
9	6
6	7
3	1
0	2

5.

x	f
14	2
15	5
16	11
17	11
18	8
19	0
20	3

6.

x	f
28	2
27	4
26	11
25	11
24	4
23	2
22	1

In Exercises 7–12, make a frequency table for the given data, and then find the range, the mean, the median, and the mode(s) of the data. Round the mean to the nearest tenth if necessary.

B 7. The number of runs scored by Jan's team in recent softball games:
5, 1, 4, 4, 8, 6, 4, 1, 5, 0, 1, 5, 3, 8, 4, 5, 3, 4

8. Jim's 200 m dash practice times: 28 s, 29 s, 27 s, 27 s, 28 s, 29 s, 28 s, 26 s, 27 s, 26 s, 28 s, 27 s, 27 s, 25 s, 26 s

9.

April in Pleasantville
Average Temperatures (°C)

		16	15	14	16	17
17	18	18	18	19	19	18
17	18	17	18	19	20	20
19	19	18	17	18	19	20
20	20	19	20			

10.

Class Test Scores

16	14	20	15	15	17
15	17	17	16	14	18
17	15	14	14	20	15
14	16	15	18	17	16
15	16	18	14	18	17

11.

Samples of Steel Rods (diameters in millimeters)

101	102	100	97	101	103	100	100	101	100	99	100
99	100	101	103	102	100	101	99	100	100	101	

12.

Ages of Members of the Moose Hill Hiking Club

15	14	15	13	16	14	18	16	15	14	14	15	18	15
13	13	14	15	14	16	16	17	14	15	13	12	14	16
14	16	15	13	16	14	15	17	12	13	16	15		

Exercises 13 and 14 refer to a class of 24 boys and 16 girls. (*Hint:* If you know the number of scores and their mean, you can find the sum of the scores.)

C 13. On test A, the mean of the boys' scores was 70 and the mean of the girls' scores was 75. What was the class mean?

14. On test B, the class mean was 75 and the mean of the girls' scores was 72. What was the mean of the boys' scores?

Review Exercises

Explain the meaning of each term.

1. mean   2. median   3. mode   4. range

5. odd number   6. even number   7. prime number   8. multiple of 7

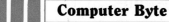

The following computer program will find the average, or mean, of several numbers. The program finds the sum of the numbers and then divides this sum by the number of numbers. For example, if you input 2, 4, 7, 8, and 11, the computer would find their sum, 32, and divide it by 5, the number of items, resulting in an answer of 6.4.

```
10   PRINT "TO FIND THE AVERAGE,"
20   PRINT "INPUT THE NUMBERS ONE AT A TIME."
30   PRINT "TYPE -1 AT END OF LIST."
40   PRINT
50   LET N = 0
60   LET S = 0
70   INPUT A
80   IF A = - 1 THEN 120
90   LET N = N + 1
100  LET S = S + A
110  GOTO 70
120  PRINT
130  PRINT "N = ";N
140  PRINT "SUM = ";S
150  PRINT "AVERAGE = ";S/N
160  END
```

Use the program to find the average of the following. Be sure to type −1 at the end of each list.

1. 12, 19, 23, 8, 17, 31

2. 57, 3, 86, 79, 101, 9

3. 542, 863, 921, 254, 378, 511

4. 1649, 15,241, 8463, 11,684

5. 887, 3105, 6324, 7048, 2103, 1298, 5541, 7201, 4961, 1114, 2260, 1954, 7322, 5665, 5321, 3742, 4457, 8916, 9923, 4309, 2385, 3342, 4187

6.

21,542	11,372	63,982	14,320
78,864	24,953	21,419	17,160
47,922	72,315	18,560	21,000
91,254	94,456	41,215	35,743
20,964	34,290	38,730	44,287

7.

502,784	339,065	764,290	274,415
114,902	765,329	314,675	441,823
345,245	465,367	468,901	687,390
113,823	589,001	892,030	389,210
992,084	314,675	440,871	572,903

12-5 Histograms and Frequency Polygons

When a bar graph is used to picture a frequency distribution, it is called a **histogram.**
No spaces are left between the bars. The histogram for the quiz-score data of the table is
shown at the left below.

Score x	Frequency f
3	1
4	0
5	2
6	3
7	12
8	10
9	6
10	6

The broken-line graph shown at the right
below is the **frequency polygon** for the same
distribution. The broken-line graph of the frequencies is connected to the horizontal axis at
each end to form a polygon.

We can find the range, the mode, the
mean, and the median from a histogram and
from a frequency polygon.

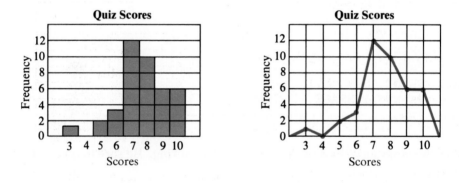

EXAMPLE   Find the range, the mode, the mean, and the median for the data
represented in the graphs above.

Solution   The range is the difference between the least number representing
data on the horizontal axis and the greatest number.

The range is 10 − 3, or 7.

The tallest bar or highest point represents the mode.

The mode is 7.

To find the mean, we first multiply each data item by its frequency.

$3 \times 1 = 3$ $4 \times 0 = 0$ $5 \times 2 = 10$ $6 \times 3 = 18$
$7 \times 12 = 84$ $8 \times 10 = 80$ $9 \times 6 = 54$ $10 \times 6 = 60$

We then add the products.

$3 + 0 + 10 + 18 + 84 + 80 + 54 + 60 = 309$

We then add the frequencies.

$$1 + 0 + 2 + 9 + 12 + 8 + 5 + 3 = 40$$

We then divide the sum of the products by the sum of the frequencies.

$$309 \div 40 = 7.725$$

The mean is 7.725.

Since there are 40 data items, the median is the average of the middle two items, both of which are 8. Thus, their average is 8.

The median is 8.

Class Exercises

Refer to the histogram at the right.

1. What is the mode of the scores?

2. What is the range of the scores?

3. How many students received scores of 90? 60? 50? 40?

4. How many students took the test?

5. What is the median score?

6. What is the mean of the scores? Round to the nearest tenth.

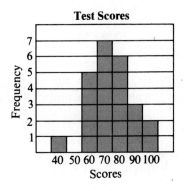

Test Scores

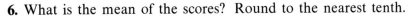

Written Exercises

Exercises 1–10 refer to the frequency polygon below.

A   1. What is the range of the data?   2. What is the mode of the data?

How many students did the following numbers of pushups?

3. 25   4. 30   5. 35   6. 40

7. How many students are in the class?

8. What is the median of the data?

9. What is the mean of the data?

10. Draw a histogram for the data.

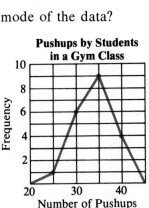

Draw a histogram and a frequency polygon for the data in the following exercises of Lesson 12-4.

B **11.** Exercise 7   **12.** Exercise 8   **13.** Exercise 9

14. Exercise 10   **15.** Exercise 11   **16.** Exercise 12

C **17.** Arrange the data listed below into the following intervals.

10–15, 15–20, 20–25, 25–30, 30–35, 35–40, 40–45

Then draw a histogram for the seven intervals.

23, 43, 27, 41, 12, 13, 19, 32, 43, 22, 36, 28, 44, 29, 31, 24, 34, 44, 37, 23, 17, 14, 23, 32, 36, 33, 43, 28, 39, 19

Self-Test A

The number of people employed in farming in the United States was: 11,100,000 in 1900; 10,400,000 in 1920; 9,500,000 in 1940; 5,400,000 in 1960; and 3,400,000 in 1980.

1. Draw a bar graph.   [12–1]

2. Draw a broken-line graph.

3. Draw a pictograph. Use people as symbols.   [12–2]

4. The sign-up records at the school's computer room showed the following usage: students, 40%; teachers, 30%; administration, 25%; other, 5%. Draw a circle graph for the given data.

5. Find the mean, median, and range of 13, 6, 20, 20, 9, 15, 11, 10.   [12–3]

6. Make a frequency table for 12, 18, 15, 12, 9, 15, 15, 16, 9, 12, 18, 12. [12–4]

Exercises 7–10 refer to the histogram.

7. How many runners had a time of 16 s?   [12–5]

8. How many runners were there in all?

9. Draw a frequency polygon for the data.

10. What are the range, the mode, the mean, and the median of the data?

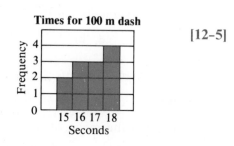

Self-Test answers and Extra Practice are at the back of the book.

12-6 Permutations

After school, Vilma plans to go to the music store and then to the pool. She can take any one of 3 routes from school to the music store and then take either of 2 routes from the store to the pool. In how many different ways can Vilma go from school to the pool?

School

Music Store

Pool

To answer, consider that for each route Vilma can take from school to the music store, she has a choice of either of 2 routes to continue from there. Thus, she has a choice of 3 × 2, or 6, possible different ways to go from school to the pool.

This example illustrates a general counting principle:

> If there are *m* ways to do one thing and *n* ways to do another, then there are *m* × *n* ways to do both things.

In mathematics, an arrangement of a group of things in a particular order is called a **permutation.** The counting principle can help you count the number of different permutations of any group of items.

EXAMPLE 1 In how many different ways can you arrange the three cards shown at the right if you arrange them side by side in a row?

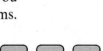
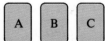

Solution Notice that there are 3 possibilities for the first card: A, B, or C. After the first card is selected, there are 2 possibilities for the second card. After the first and second cards have been selected, there is just 1 possibility for the third card.

Applying the counting principle, there are 3 × 2 × 1, or 6, possible ways to arrange the three cards.

To check, list the permutations: A B C   B A C   C A B
                                   A C B   B C A   C B A

Notice that the number of permutations of 3 things is 3 × 2 × 1. We can write 3! (read *3 factorial*) to represent the expression 3 × 2 × 1. In general, the number of permutations of *n* things is

$$n \times (n - 1) \times (n - 2) \times \cdots \times 3 \times 2 \times 1.$$

We can write this expression as *n*!.

If we let $_nP_n$ represent the number of permutations of a group of n things when using all n things, we can write the following formula.

Formula

For the number of permutations of n things taken n at a time,

$$_nP_n = n \times (n - 1) \times (n - 2) \times \cdots \times 3 \times 2 \times 1 = n!$$

EXAMPLE 2 How many four-digit whole numbers can you write using the digits 1, 2, 3, and 4 if no digit appears more than once in each number?

Solution You need to find the number of permutations of 4 things taken 4 at a time.
Using the formula,

$$_4P_4 = 4! = 4 \times 3 \times 2 \times 1 = 24.$$

Therefore, 24 four-digit whole numbers can be written using the given digits.

Sometimes we work with arrangements that involve just a portion of the group at one time.

EXAMPLE 3 This year, 7 dogs are entered in the collie competition at the annual Ridgedale Kennel Club show. In how many different ways can first, second, and third prizes be awarded in the competition?

Solution You want to find the number of permutations of 7 things taken 3 at a time. There are 7 choices for first prize, 6 for second, and 5 for third. Thus,

$$7 \times 6 \times 5 = 210.$$

There are 210 possible ways to award the prizes.

If we let $_nP_r$ represent the number of permutations of n objects taken r at a time, we can write the following formula.

Formula

For the number of permutations of n things taken r at a time, we use the following formula carried out to r factors:

$$_nP_r = n \times (n - 1) \times (n - 2) \times \cdots$$

Using the formula in Example 3 above, we find $_7P_3 = 7 \times 6 \times 5 = 210.$

Class Exercises

Find the value of each.

1. 4! **2.** 3! **3.** 2! **4.** 1!

5. $_5P_5$ **6.** $_3P_3$ **7.** $_5P_4$ **8.** $_6P_3$

Solve.

9. In wrapping a gift, you have a choice of 3 different boxes and 4 different wrapping papers. In how many different ways can you wrap the gift?

10. There are 3 roads from Craig to Hartsdale, 2 roads from Hartsdale to Lee, and 4 roads from Lee to Trumbull. In how many different ways can you travel from Craig to Trumbull by way of Hartsdale and Lee?

Use the formula to answer. Then list all of the permutations to check.

11. In how many different ways can you arrange the letters in the word CAR?

12. In how many different ways can you arrange the 4 cards shown at the right if you take 3 at a time and arrange them side by side?

R Y G B

Written Exercises

Find the value of each.

A **1.** 5! **2.** 6! **3.** 7! **4.** 8!

5. $_6P_6$ **6.** $_7P_7$ **7.** $_8P_8$ **8.** $_5P_5$

9. $_6P_4$ **10.** $_8P_4$ **11.** $_{43}P_3$ **12.** $_{23}P_2$

Problems

Exercises 1–4 refer to the map at the right. Tell how many different ways you can travel from one city to the other.

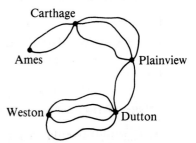

A **1.** Ames to Plainview **2.** Carthage to Dutton

3. Carthage to Weston **4.** Ames to Dutton

5. A furniture store sells couches that are available in 3 different styles, 7 different colors, and 2 different sizes. How many different couches are available?

6. How many different sandwiches can you make using one kind of bread, one kind of meat, and one kind of cheese with these choices?

Bread: white, rye, whole wheat
Cheese: Swiss, cheddar
Meat: turkey, chicken, roast beef

Use a formula to solve. List the permutations to check your answer.

7. In how many different ways can you arrange the 4 books shown side by side on a shelf?

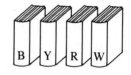

8. In how many different ways can Carla, Dean, and Ellen be seated in a row of 3 chairs?

9. How many different two-digit whole numbers can you make with the digits 1, 3, 5, and 7 if no digit appears more than once in each number?

10. In how many different ways can you arrange the letters in the word RING if you take the letters 3 at a time?

Solve.

B **11.** In how many different ways can 7 books be arranged side by side on a shelf?

12. In how many different ways can 6 students stand in a row of 6?

13. In how many different ways can you arrange the letters in the word ANSWER if you take the letters 5 at a time?

14. How many different four-digit numbers can you make using the digits 1, 2, 3, 5, 7, 8, and 9 if no digit appears more than once in a number?

Using the digits 1, 2, 4, 5, 7, and 8, how many different three-digit numbers can you form according to each of the following rules?

C **15.** Each digit may be repeated any number of times in a number.

16. The numbers are even numbers and no digit appears more than once in a number.

17. There is a 5 in the ones' place and no digit appears more than once in a number.

18. In how many different ways can you arrange the letters in the word ROOT? (*Hint:* Notice that two of the letters are indistinguishable.)

19. In how many different ways can you arrange the letters in the word NOON?

The diagram at the right, called a **Venn diagram,** illustrates the following statement.

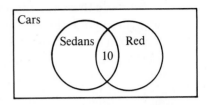

> Of 100 cars, 35 are sedans, 25 are red, and 10 are red sedans.

The rectangular region represents the number of cars. One circular region represents the number of sedans; the other represents the number of red cars. The overlapping portion of the two circular regions represents the number of cars that are red and sedans. The number of red cars that are not sedans is 25 − 10, or 15.

Draw a Venn diagram to illustrate the statement. Then answer the questions.

20. Of 240 knit caps, 110 are striped, 65 are blue, and 45 are striped and blue.
  a. How many are striped but not blue?
  b. How many are blue but not striped?
  c. How many are striped or blue (striped, or blue, or both)?
  d. How many are neither striped nor blue?

Review Exercises

Simplify.

1. $\dfrac{70}{5} \times \dfrac{1}{2}$

2. $\dfrac{15}{12} \times \dfrac{36}{60}$

3. $\dfrac{21}{5} \times \dfrac{10}{14}$

4. $\dfrac{27}{51} \times \dfrac{17}{3}$

5. $\dfrac{9 \times 8}{3 \times 2}$

6. $\dfrac{7 \times 6}{4 \times 3}$

7. $\dfrac{11 \times 10 \times 9}{3 \times 2 \times 1}$

8. $\dfrac{23 \times 22 \times 21 \times 20}{4 \times 3 \times 2 \times 1}$

▮▮▮ Challenge

You and a friend have decided to jog through Peachtree Park. The park has five entrance gates and several paths as shown in the diagram at the right. To jog along all of the paths without covering any path more than once, through which gate would you enter?

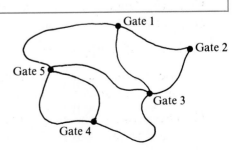

12-7 Combinations

Sometimes we select groups of objects from a larger group without regard to the order of the objects selected. Such groups in which the order is not considered are called **combinations.**

Suppose there is a group of 4 students—Jon, Lin, Meg, and Ray—who wish to go to the computer center today. If only 3 of them may go today, what are the possible combinations of these students who may be selected to go? To find any one combination, just leave out 1 student from the group of 4. The possible combinations are listed below.

Jon, Lin, Meg   Jon, Lin, Ray   Jon, Meg, Ray   Lin, Meg, Ray

The number of groups of 3 students that can be selected from a group of 4 students is 4.

Here is another way to approach the problem.

$$
\begin{bmatrix} \text{number of groups} \\ \text{of 3 students you} \\ \text{can select from 4} \end{bmatrix} \times \begin{bmatrix} \text{number of ways of} \\ \text{arranging 3 stu-} \\ \text{dents in a group} \end{bmatrix} = \begin{bmatrix} \text{number of ways of} \\ \text{arranging 3 out} \\ \text{of 4 students} \end{bmatrix}
$$

$$
N \qquad \times \qquad {}_3P_3 \qquad = \qquad {}_4P_3
$$

Solving for N, we find that

$$
N = \frac{{}_4P_3}{{}_3P_3} = \frac{4 \times 3 \times 2}{3 \times 2 \times 1} = 4.
$$

This formula gives us the same answer that we found by showing and counting the number of combinations of 3 students that may be selected from a group of 4 students.

EXAMPLE 1 How many combinations of 4 cards can be chosen from the cards shown at the right?

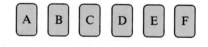

Solution Use the formula to find the number of combinations of 6 cards taken 4 at a time.

$$
N = \frac{{}_6P_4}{{}_4P_4} = \frac{\overset{3}{\cancel{6}} \times 5 \times \overset{1}{\cancel{4}} \times \overset{1}{\cancel{3}}}{\underset{1}{\cancel{4}} \times \underset{1}{\cancel{3}} \times \underset{1}{\cancel{2}} \times 1} = \frac{15}{1} = 15
$$

List the combinations to check.

A B C D	A B D E	A C D E	A D E F	B C E F
A B C E	A B D F	A C D F	B C D E	B D E F
A B C F	A B E F	A C E F	B C D F	C D E F

In general, if we let $_nC_r$ represent the number of combinations of n things taken r at a time, we can use the following formula.

Formula

For the number of combinations of n things taken r at a time,

$$_nC_r = \frac{_nP_r}{_rP_r} = \frac{n \times (n-1) \times \cdots \text{(to } r \text{ factors)}}{r!}$$

EXAMPLE 2   Four of 7 students who have volunteered will be chosen to hand out programs at the drama club performance. How many combinations of these students can be selected?

Solution   We wish to find the number of combinations of 7 students taken 4 at a time.
Using the formula, we find

$$_7C_4 = \frac{_7P_4}{_4P_4} = \frac{7 \times 6 \times 5 \times 4}{4 \times 3 \times 2 \times 1} = \frac{35}{1} = 35.$$

Class Exercises

Find the value of each.

1. $_5C_3$ **2.** $_5C_4$ **3.** $_6C_2$ **4.** $_7C_2$ **5.** $_8C_4$ **6.** $_8C_6$ **7.** $_{12}C_3$ **8.** $_{20}C_2$

Use the formula to solve. List the combinations to check your answer.

9. How many combinations of 2 cards can be chosen from the cards shown at the right?

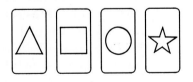

10. How many combinations of 3 letters can be chosen from the letters A, B, C, D, and E?

Problems

A   **1.** How many combinations of 4 books can you choose from 6 books?

2. How many groups of 3 types of plants can be selected from 6 types?

3. How many straight lines can be formed by connecting any 2 of 6 points, no 3 of which are on a straight line?

4. How many groups of 4 fabrics can be selected from 7 fabrics?

B **5.** How many ways can a class of 21 students select 2 of its members as class representatives for student government?

6. The school photographer wants to photograph 3 students from a club with 14 members. How many combinations can be made?

7. Kristen must answer 5 of 10 questions on her quiz. How many combinations of questions are possible?

8. Philip wishes to check 2 books out of his school library. If the library contains 800 books, in how many ways might Philip make his choice of books?

9. You have a total of 4 coins: a penny, a nickel, a dime, and a quarter. How many different amounts of money can you form using the given number of these coins?
  a. 1 coin **b.** 2 coins **c.** 3 coins **d.** 4 coins **e.** one or more coins

10. There are three books left in the sale rack: a book about sailing, a cookbook, and a book about baseball. How many combinations can be formed using the given number of these books?
  a. 1 book **b.** 2 books **c.** 3 books **d.** one or more books

C **11.** In how many ways can a five-member committee of 3 seniors and 2 juniors be selected from a group of 14 seniors and 8 juniors? (*Hint:* Find the number of combinations of each type and determine their product.)

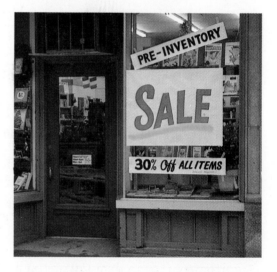

12. A basketball squad has 17 members. The coach has designated 3 members to play center, 6 to play guard, and 8 to play forward. How many ways can the coach select a starting team of 1 center, 2 guards, and 2 forwards? (*Hint:* See the hint in Exercise 11.)

Review Exercises

Explain the meaning of each term.

1. factor   **2.** multiple   **3.** even number   **4.** odd number

5. cube   **6.** at least one   **7.** at most one   **8.** exactly one

12-8 The Probability of an Event

In a simple game, the five cards shown are turned face down and mixed so that all choices are *equally likely.*

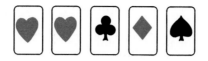

You then draw a card. If the card is a heart, you win a prize. To find your chance of winning, notice that there are 5 possible **outcomes.** Notice, too, that 2 of the outcomes are hearts. We say that 2 of the outcomes **favor** the event of drawing a heart. The **probability,** or chance, of drawing a heart is $\frac{2}{5}$. If we let H stand for the event of drawing a heart, we may write $P(H) = \frac{2}{5}$. This statement is read as *the probability of event H is $\frac{2}{5}$.*

In general we have the following:

Formula

The probability of an event E is

$$P(E) = \frac{\text{number of outcomes favoring event } E}{\text{number of possible outcomes}}$$

for equally likely outcomes.

When all outcomes are equally likely, as in drawing one of the cards in the game described above, we say that the outcomes occur *at random,* or *randomly.*

In this chapter, we shall often refer to *experiments* such as drawing cards, drawing marbles from a bag, or rolling game cubes. We shall always assume that the outcomes of these experiments occur at random. When we refer to spinners like the one shown at the right, we shall always assume that the pointer stops at random but not on a division line.

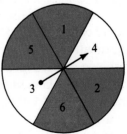

Often it is helpful to list all possible outcomes of an experiment. We could show the possible outcomes for the spinner shown above by using letters to represent the colors and by writing the following:

R1	B2	W3
R6	B5	W4

EXAMPLE 1   Find the probability that the pointer of the spinner shown on the preceding page stops on a wedge of the type described.

a. even-numbered   **b.** odd-numbered

c. red   **d.** not red

e. even-numbered *and* red   **f.** green

g. not green

Solution   The number of possible outcomes is 6.

a. $P(\text{even-numbered}) = \frac{3}{6} = \frac{1}{2}$

b. $P(\text{odd-numbered}) = \frac{3}{6} = \frac{1}{2}$

c. $P(\text{red}) = \frac{2}{6} = \frac{1}{3}$

d. $P(\text{not red}) = \frac{4}{6} = \frac{2}{3}$

e. $P(\text{even-numbered and red}) = \frac{1}{6}$

f. $P(\text{green}) = \frac{0}{6} = 0$

g. $P(\text{not green}) = \frac{6}{6} = 1$

The events in parts (f) and (g) of the example illustrate these facts:

> The probability of an impossible event is 0.
> The probability of a certain event is 1.

Sometimes it is useful to picture the possible outcomes of an experiment. Consider the experiment of rolling the two game cubes that are shown at the right. One cube is blue, one cube is red. The numbers 1 through 6 are printed on each cube, one number per face. An outcome can be represented by an ordered pair of numbers. The array at the right shows the 36 possible outcomes when the two cubes are rolled. The encircled dot stands for the outcome of a 5 on the top face of the red cube and a 3 on the top face of the blue cube, or the ordered pair (5, 3).

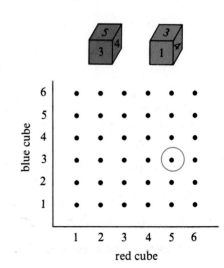

EXAMPLE 2 Two game cubes are rolled.

    a. Find the probability that one cube *or* the other cube shows a 5 (that is, that the number 5 is on the top face of either or both cubes).

    b. Find the probability that the sum of the top faces is 5.

Solution   First, make a sketch to show the possible outcomes. Then circle the event.

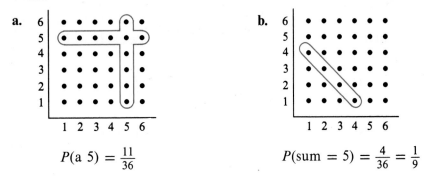

$$P(\text{a } 5) = \frac{11}{36} \qquad\qquad P(\text{sum} = 5) = \frac{4}{36} = \frac{1}{9}$$

Problem Solving Reminder

Sometimes *making a sketch* can help you solve a problem. In Example 2, above, picturing an outcome as the graph of an ordered pair simplifies the problem.

Class Exercises

Two red, one white, and three blue marbles are put into a bag. Find each probability for a marble chosen at random.

1. $P(\text{red})$ **2.** $P(\text{white})$ **3.** $P(\text{blue})$ **4.** $P(\text{green})$

5. $P(\text{not green})$ **6.** $P(\text{red or white})$

7. $P(\text{white or blue})$ **8.** $P(\text{red or blue})$

Exercises 9–12 refer to the spinner at the right. Find the probability that the pointer stops on a wedge of the type described.

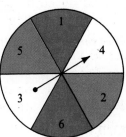

9. numbered with a factor of 6

10. numbered with a multiple of 3

11. even-numbered or blue

12. even-numbered and blue

Written Exercises

Find the probability of each roll if you use a single game cube.

A **1.** a 5

2. an odd number

3. a number less than 5

4. a number greater than 3

5. a 7

6. a number less than 7

Each of the 20 cards shown at the right has a letter, a number, and a color. Each card is equally likely to be drawn. Find each probability.

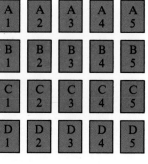

7. $P(C)$

8. $P(A)$

9. $P(1)$

10. $P(2)$

11. $P(red)$

12. $P(blue)$

13. $P(not\ A)$

14. $P(not\ D)$

15. $P(1\ or\ 2)$

16. $P(1, 2, 3, or\ 4)$

17. $P(neither\ 1\ nor\ 2)$

18. $P(not\ 1, or\ 2, or\ 3, or\ 4)$

Exercises 19–28 refer to the spinner below. Find the probability that the pointer stops on a wedge of the type described.

19. red

20. white or blue

21. numbered with a factor of 12

22. even-numbered

23. numbered with a multiple of 3

24. numbered with a multiple of 4

25. odd-numbered or red

26. odd-numbered and red

27. red and a factor of 6

28. blue and a multiple of 5

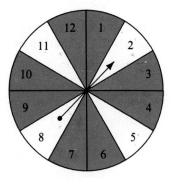

Two game cubes are rolled. Find the probability that this sum shows.

B **29.** 7 **30.** 12 **31.** 3 **32.** 9

33. 7 or 11 **34.** 2 or 12 **35.** less than 7 **36.** 6, 7, or 8

For Exercises 37 and 38, use a *tree diagram* to picture the possible outcomes of the random experiment.

EXAMPLE   Two coins are tossed. Find the probability of obtaining at least one head.

Solution   Let H stand for heads and T stand for tails.

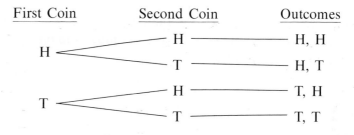

First Coin   Second Coin   Outcomes

H ── H ──────── H, H
H
T ── T ──────── H, T

H ── H ──────── T, H
T
T ── T ──────── T, T

There are 4 possible outcomes. Three of the outcomes have one or more heads.

$$P(\text{at least one H}) = \frac{3}{4}$$

37. You have two bags of marbles, each of which holds one blue marble, one red marble, and one green marble. You choose one marble at random from each bag. Find the probability of obtaining the following.
   a. two red marbles   **b.** at least one blue marble   **c.** no green marbles
   d. at most one green marble   **e.** exactly one red marble

38. Three coins are tossed. Find the probability of obtaining the following.
   a. at least two heads   **b.** three heads   **c.** no heads
   d. at most two tails   **e.** exactly one head

C   39. You have one penny, one nickel, one dime, and one quarter in your pocket. You select two coins at random. What is the probability that you have taken at least 25¢ from your pocket?

Review Exercises

Evaluate each expression using the given values of the variable.

$1 - x$

1. $x = 1$ **2.** $x = \frac{1}{2}$ **3.** $x = \frac{2}{3}$ **4.** $x = -1$

$\dfrac{x}{1 - x}$

5. $x = \frac{1}{3}$ **6.** $x = \frac{2}{3}$ **7.** $x = \frac{3}{7}$ **8.** $x = \frac{4}{7}$

12-9 Odds in Favor and Odds Against

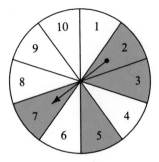

EXAMPLE 1   A game is played with the spinner shown at the right. To win the game, the pointer must stop on a wedge that shows a prime number. Find each probability.
a. You win.   **b.** You do not win.

Solution   There are 10 possible outcomes.
For you to win, the pointer must stop on 2, 3, 5, or 7. Therefore:

a. $P(\text{win}) = \frac{4}{10} = \frac{2}{5}$

b. $P(\text{not win}) = \frac{6}{10} = \frac{3}{5}$

Example 1 illustrates this general fact:

> If the probability that an event occurs is p, then the probability that the event does not occur is $1 - p$.

In Example 1 there are 4 ways of winning and 6 ways of not winning. We therefore say:

a. The *odds in favor* of winning are 4 to 6, or 2 to 3.

b. The *odds against* winning are 6 to 4, or 3 to 2.

> ### *Formula*
> If the probability that an event occurs is p (where $p \neq 0$ and $p \neq 1$), then:
>
> $$\text{Odds in favor of the event} = \frac{p}{1 - p}$$
>
> $$\text{Odds against the event} = \frac{1 - p}{p}$$

Odds are usually expressed in the form "x to y," where x and y are integers having no common factor.

EXAMPLE 2 Find the odds (a) in favor of and (b) against rolling a sum of 6 with two game cubes.

Solution From the array of possible outcomes, we see that:

$$P(\text{sum} = 6) = \frac{5}{36} = p$$

$$P(\text{sum} \neq 6) = 1 - p = 1 - \frac{5}{36} = \frac{31}{36}$$

a. Odds in favor $= \dfrac{p}{1-p}$

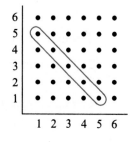

$$\frac{\frac{5}{36}}{\frac{31}{36}} = \frac{5}{36} \div \frac{31}{36} = \frac{5}{36} \times \frac{36}{31} = \frac{5}{31}$$

Odds in favor are 5 to 31.

b. Odds against are 31 to 5.

EXAMPLE 3 The chance of rain tomorrow is 40%. What are the odds against its raining?

Solution The probability of rain is $p = 40\% = 0.4$.

Odds against rain $= \dfrac{1-p}{p} = \dfrac{1-0.4}{0.4} = \dfrac{0.6}{0.4} = \dfrac{3}{2}$

Odds against rain are 3 to 2.

Class Exercises

1. The chance of rain tomorrow is 20%. Find the odds against rain.

2. Find the odds against rolling a 4 with one game cube.

Exercises 3–6 refer to the spinner at the right. Find the odds (a) in favor of and (b) against the pointer stopping on a wedge of the type described.

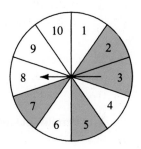

3. an odd number

4. a multiple of 3

5. a factor of 10

6. a number less than 7

7. The odds are 1 to 1 that an event will occur. What is the probability that the event will occur?

8. The probability that an event will occur is $\frac{1}{2}$. What are the odds against the event?

Written Exercises

Exercises 1–6 refer to a bag containing 6 red, 2 white, and 4 blue marbles. Find the odds in favor of drawing a marble of the type described.

A **1.** red   **2.** white   **3.** blue

       4. white or blue   **5.** blue or red   **6.** red or white

       7. The chance of rain tomorrow is 60%. What are the odds against rain?

       8. The probability that the Lions football team will win the next game is 0.6. What are the odds that it will win?

       9. The Student Union Party has a 30% chance of winning in the next school election. What are the odds against its winning?

In Exercises 10–15 a card has been drawn at random from the 20 cards that are shown. Find the odds against drawing a card of the type described.

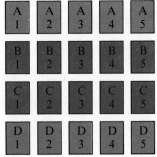

10. an A

11. a blue card

12. a red card

13. a C

14. a 1, 2, or 3

15. B2, B3, B4, or B5

Two game cubes are rolled. Find the odds against obtaining the sum described.

16. 7   **17.** 11   **18.** 7 or 11

19. 2 or 12   **20.** greater than 7   **21.** less than 6

B **22. a.** even   **b.** odd

       23. a. divisible by 3   **b.** not divisible by 3

The two game cubes are rolled again. Find the odds in favor of the event described.

24. Exactly one 5 shows.   **25.** At least one 5 shows.

26. Two even numbers show.   **27.** At least one odd number shows.

C **28.** The odds in favor of the Melodies winning the music competition are 5 to 3. What is the probability that the Melodies will win?

29. The odds in favor of drawing a red marble at random from a bag of marbles are 1 to 8. What is the probability of drawing a red marble?

Review Exercises

Perform the indicated operations. Simplify.

1. $\dfrac{5}{6} + \dfrac{7}{12} - \dfrac{11}{24}$ **2.** $\dfrac{7}{8} + \dfrac{15}{16} - \dfrac{7}{24}$ **3.** $\dfrac{11}{20} + \dfrac{9}{10} - \dfrac{8}{15}$ **4.** $\dfrac{5}{9} + \dfrac{25}{27} - \dfrac{71}{81}$

5. $\dfrac{17}{18} - \dfrac{2}{3} + \dfrac{5}{12}$ **6.** $\dfrac{37}{40} - \dfrac{41}{60} + \dfrac{11}{12}$ **7.** $\dfrac{11}{14} - \dfrac{17}{28} + \dfrac{9}{49}$ **8.** $\dfrac{7}{9} - \dfrac{5}{12} + \dfrac{13}{18}$

███ **Computer Byte**

If we toss a coin, there are two possible outcomes—a head or a tail. If these two outcomes are equally likely, then the probability of each is $\frac{1}{2}$. Does this mean that if we toss a coin 10 times, we will get 5 heads and 5 tails? (Not necessarily.)

The following program will simulate tossing a coin. The program is based on a list of "random numbers" that are decimals between 0 and 1. (Usage of the RND function varies. Check this program with the manual for the computer that you are using, and make any necessary changes.)

```
10   PRINT "HOW MANY TOSSES";
20   INPUT N
30   LET H = 0
40   FOR I = 1 to N
50   LET A = RND (1)
60   IF A < .5 THEN 90
70   PRINT TAB( 6);"TAIL"
80   GOTO 110
90   LET H = H + 1
100   PRINT "HEAD"
110   NEXT I
120   PRINT
130   PRINT "H = ";H; TAB( 10);"T = ";N - H;
140   PRINT  TAB( 20);"H/N = ";H/N
150   END
```

1. Run the program 10 times for N = 25.
   a. For how many runs was 0.45 < H/N < 0.55?
   b. What percent was this?

12-10 Mutually Exclusive Events

The pointer shown at the right stops at random but not on a division line. Consider the following events.

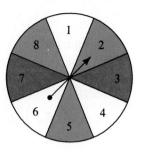

R: The pointer stops on a red wedge.

B: The pointer stops on a blue wedge.

O: The pointer stops on an odd-numbered wedge.

E: The pointer stops on an even-numbered wedge.

Events *R* and *B* cannot both occur at once. Such events are said to be **mutually exclusive.** Notice that events *B* and *E* are *not* mutually exclusive because they both occur when the pointer stops on a blue wedge that is even-numbered.

In the spinner above, five of the eight wedges are colored red or blue. Therefore,

$$P(R \text{ or } B) = \frac{5}{8}.$$

Notice that

$$P(R) = \frac{1}{4}, \ P(B) = \frac{3}{8}, \text{ and } P(R) + P(B) = \frac{1}{4} + \frac{3}{8} = \frac{5}{8}.$$

Thus, $P(R \text{ or } B) = P(R) + P(B)$.

If *A* and *B* are mutually exclusive events, then

$$P(A \text{ or } B) = P(A) + P(B)$$

EXAMPLE The probability that a randomly chosen car is green is 0.15 and that it is red is 0.25.
   a. Find the probability that the next car you see will be red or green.
   b. Find the odds against its being red or green.

Solution   **a.** The events described are mutually exclusive. Thus,

$$P(\text{red or green}) = P(\text{red}) + P(\text{green})$$
$$= 0.25 + 0.15 = 0.40$$

The probability that the next car will be red or green is 40%.

   b. Odds against red or green $= \dfrac{1 - 0.40}{0.40} = \dfrac{0.6}{0.4} = \dfrac{3}{2}$

The odds against the next car's being red or green are 3 to 2.

Class Exercises

Are events *A* and *B* mutually exclusive?

1. You take a test.
 A: You pass it.
 B: You fail it.

2. You take a test.
 A: You score less than 9.
 B: You score more than 6.

3. Two coins are tossed.
 A: Two heads result.
 B: Two tails result.

4. Two game cubes are rolled.
 A: The sum is 5.
 B: A 5 shows on one cube.

5. Two game cubes are rolled.
 A: Cubes show the same number.
 B: The sum is 7.

6. Two game cubes are rolled.
 A: Cubes show the same number.
 B: The sum is 8.

***A* and *B* are mutually exclusive events. Find *P*(*A* or *B*).**

7. $P(A) = \frac{1}{4}$, $P(B) = \frac{3}{8}$

8. $P(A) = 0.2$, $P(B) = 0.5$

9. $P(A) = \frac{1}{2}$ and $P(B) = \frac{2}{3}$. Are *A* and *B* mutually exclusive events?

Written Exercises

Solve. *A* and *B* are mutually exclusive events.

A **1.** $P(A) = \frac{1}{5}$, $P(B) = \frac{2}{3}$. Find *P*(*A* or *B*).

2. $P(A) = 0.32$, $P(B) = 0.45$. Find *P*(*A* or *B*).

3. $P(A) = 0.4$, $P(A \text{ or } B) = 0.7$. Find *P*(*B*).

4. $P(B) = \frac{1}{3}$, $P(A \text{ or } B) = \frac{3}{4}$. Find *P*(*A*).

In Exercises 5–10, find the probability that the pointer stops on a wedge of the type described.

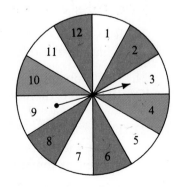

5. a. red   **b.** white   **c.** red or white

6. a. blue   **b.** red   **c.** blue or red

7. a. blue   **b.** not blue

8. a. white   **b.** not white

9. a. odd-numbered   **b.** red   **c.** odd-numbered or red

10. a. odd-numbered   **b.** blue   **c.** odd-numbered or blue

Exercises 11–15 refer to the cards at the right. Find the probability that a card drawn at random is of the type described.

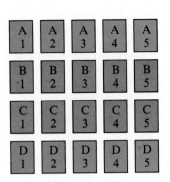

11. a. a 5   **b.** less than 3
     c. a 5 or less than 3

12. a. a 2   **b.** greater than 3
     c. a 2 or greater than 3

13. a. a D   **b.** a red card greater than 2
     c. a D or a red card greater than 2

14. a. a B   **b.** a blue card greater than 3
     c. a B or a blue card greater than 3

15. a. a C   **b.** a red card less than 4
     c. a C or a red card less than 4

Two game cubes are rolled. Find the probability of the event described.

B **16. a.** The sum is 5.
     b. A 5 shows.
     c. Neither is the sum 5 nor does a 5 show.

17. a. The sum is 4.
     b. A 6 shows.
     c. Neither is the sum 4 nor does a 6 show.

18. a. The sum is 9.
     b. The roll is a double (for example, $\boxed{3}$ $\boxed{3}$).
     c. The sum is 9 or a double is rolled.

19. a. The sum is 7.
     b. The roll is a double.
     c. The sum is 7 or a double is rolled.

20. Joe's batting average (the probability of his getting a hit) is 0.350. What are the odds against his getting a hit?

21. The probability of Jan's team winning the next softball game is 55%. Find the odds that the team will lose.

C **22.** The probability that the next soup ordered will be chicken is 0.45; that it will be tomato is 0.35. What are the odds against its being chicken or tomato?

23. At West High School the probability that a randomly chosen student is a senior is 0.20. The probability that the student is a junior is 0.25. Find the odds against the student's being a junior or senior.

A sightseer at Breathless Gorge dropped his sandwich from a gondola. The object fell at the rate of 9.8 meters per second (m/s) after the first second, 19.6 m/s after the second second, and 29.4 m/s after the third second. How fast will the sandwich be falling at 4 s?

Self-Test B

1. In how many different ways can you arrange 4 boxes side by side on a shelf?   [12-6]

2. How many different three-digit numbers can you make with the digits 1, 2, 3, 4, and 5 if no digit appears more than once in each number?

3. How many combinations of 3 letters can be chosen from the letters A, B, C, D, and E?   [12-7]

4. In how many ways can a committee of 2 people be selected from a group of 15 people?

Find the probability that the pointer on the spinner shown at the right stops on a wedge of the type described.

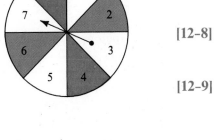

5. 3   6. odd-numbered   [12-8]

7. red   8. a number less than 9

9. What are the odds in favor of the pointer on the spinner shown stopping on a wedge with a number greater than 6?   [12-9]

10. What are the odds against the pointer on the spinner shown stopping on a blue wedge?

11. The probability of snow next week is 75%. What are the odds in favor of snow?

12. Events A and B are mutually exclusive. $P(A) = \frac{5}{12}$. $P(B) = \frac{1}{6}$. Find $P(A \text{ or } B)$.   [12-10]

13. Events A and B are mutually exclusive. $P(A) = 0.5$. $P(A \text{ or } B) = 0.7$. Find $P(B)$.

Self-Test answers and Extra Practice are at the back of the book.

Standard Deviation

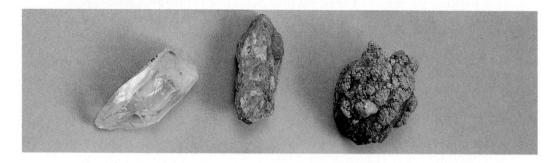

For many purposes the *range* of a set of data is a poor measure of its spread. Consider, for example, the frequency distributions and histograms below for the mass in kilograms of various rocks found by three groups of rock collectors.

Group A	
Mass (kg)	Frequency
1	4
3	1
7	1
9	4

Group B	
Mass (kg)	Frequency
1	1
3	3
5	2
7	3
9	1

Group C	
Mass (kg)	Frequency
1	1
3	2
5	4
7	2
9	1

Group A

Group B

Group C

Each distribution has a range of 8. But a glance at each histogram reveals that distribution A is more spread out around its center, or mean, than are distributions B and C.

A more useful measure of the spread of a distribution is the **deviation** from the mean. Suppose a bowler has scores of 198, 210, and 156. The mean score is 188. The table at the right shows how much each score varies, or *deviates*, from the mean.

Score	Deviation
198	+10
210	+22
156	−32

The **variance** and **standard deviation** are two commonly used measures of how data are scattered around the mean. The variance is computed by squaring each deviation from the mean, adding these squares, and dividing the sum by the number of entries in the distribution. The standard deviation is found by computing the positive square root of the variance. The standard deviation is a more useful statistic than the variance because comparisons are being made of common units. For example, when data are given in meters, the variance will be in square meters, but the standard deviation will be in meters.

The table below shows the calculation of the variance and standard deviation for each frequency distribution on the preceding page. In each case, x is the mass and m is the mean, which is 5. Notice that the more a distribution is spread out from its mean, the larger its standard deviation.

Group A			Group B			Group C		
x	deviation $(x-m)$	$(x-m)^2$	x	deviation $(x-m)$	$(x-m)^2$	x	deviation $(x-m)$	$(x-m)^2$
1	−4	16	1	−4	16	1	−4	16
1	−4	16	3	−2	4	3	−2	4
1	−4	16	3	−2	4	3	−2	4
1	−4	16	3	−2	4	5	0	0
3	−2	4	5	0	0	5	0	0
7	2	4	5	0	0	5	0	0
9	4	16	7	2	4	5	0	0
9	4	16	7	2	4	7	2	4
9	4	16	7	2	4	7	2	4
9	4	16	9	4	16	9	4	16
		136 kg²			56 kg²			48 kg²

variance $= \frac{136}{10} = 13.6$ kg²   variance $= \frac{56}{10} = 5.6$ kg²   variance $= \frac{48}{10} = 4.8$ kg²

standard deviation $= \sqrt{13.6}$ ≈ 3.7 kg

standard deviation $= \sqrt{5.6}$ ≈ 2.4 kg

standard deviation $= \sqrt{4.8}$ ≈ 2.2 kg

Find (a) the mean, (b) the deviation, (c) the variance, and (d) the standard deviation of the given data. Use the table on page 508, or approximate the square root to the nearest hundredth by interpolation.

1. From a sample of four dairy cows, a farmer recorded the following yields for one day: 11 gal, 13 gal, 9 gal, and 15 gal.

2. In a survey of local stores, the following prices were quoted for a World watch: $34, $27, $41, and $38.

3. The fuel efficiency ratings of five new cars were 20, 19, 20, 22, and 33 mi/gal.

Chapter Review

Complete.
Refer to the bar graph for Exercises 1–3.

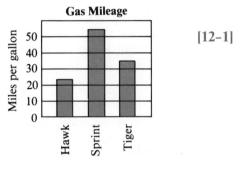

Gas Mileage

1. The car with the best gas mileage is the ___?___. [12–1]

2. The Tiger gets approximately __?__ miles per gallon.

3. If we join the midpoints of the tops of the bars in the bar graph, we obtain a ___?___ graph.

4. To show on a circle graph that 25% of a team is in the seventh grade, you would use a wedge of a circle that has an angle measure of __?__ degrees. [12–2]

Use the data 65, 67, 67, 69, 70, 73 for Exercises 5–9.

5. The range is __?__.   6. The median is __?__. [12–3]

7. The mean is __?__.   8. The mode is __?__. [12–4]

9. The frequency of 67 is __?__.

Refer to the frequency table for Exercises 10 and 11.

10. If you drew a histogram for the data, the tallest bar would represent __?__. [12–5]

11. The range of the data is ___?___.

Cost of a Quart of Milk				
Price	59¢	60¢	61¢	62¢
Frequency	4	5	2	1

True or false?

12. You can arrange the letters in the word DRAW in 4 different ways if you take the letters 3 at a time. [12–6]

13. A group of 3 people can be selected from 8 people in 56 ways. [12–7]

14. When a single game cube is rolled, the probability that the roll shows a number greater than 3 is $\frac{1}{2}$. [12–8]

15. The odds in favor of rolling a 2 with a single game cube are 1 to 5. [12–9]

16. The probability of rolling a 3 or a 6 with a single game cube is $\frac{1}{3}$. [12–10]

Chapter Test

Refer to the bar graph for Exercises 1 and 2.

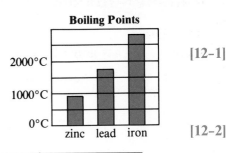

Boiling Points

1. Give the approximate boiling points of the three elements.   [12–1]

2. Draw a broken-line graph for the data.

3. Draw a pictograph for the data below.   [12–2]

Number of Shares of Stock Sold			
1980	1,546,000	**1981**	2,341,000
1982	3,995,000	**1983**	4,784,000

4. Find the mean, the median, and the range of 28, 14, 19, 24, 30.   [12–3]

Refer to the frequency table for Exercises 5–7.

5. Give the mean, the median, the range, and the mode of the data. Round the mean to the nearest tenth.   [12–4]

6. Draw a histogram for the data.   [12–5]

7. Draw a frequency polygon for the data.

Number of Minutes	Frequency
155	2
158	3
159	1
162	1
163	1
166	2
167	3
168	5

Solve.

8. In how many different ways can 3 people sit in a row of 5 seats?   [12–6]

9. How many combinations of 3 colors can you choose from 7 colors?   [12–7]

Exercises 10–13 refer to the spinner shown below at the right. Find the probability that the pointer will stop on a wedge of the type described.

10. blue   11. green   [12–8]

12. odd-numbered and red

13. What are the odds in favor of the pointer stopping on a red wedge?   [12–9]

14. Events A and B are mutually exclusive. $P(A) = \frac{1}{3}$. $P(B) = \frac{5}{12}$. Find $P(A \text{ or } B)$.   [12–10]

Cumulative Review (Chapters 1–12)

Exercises

Simplify.

1. $5.4 + (7 \times 6.3)$

2. $\frac{16 + 9}{32 + 8}$

3. $13(9.2 \div 16)$

4. $4x - y + xy + 3y$

5. $2m + 2n - m + n$

6. $3p^2(p + 5)$

Perform the indicated operation. Write the answer as a proper fraction in lowest terms or as a mixed number in simple form.

7. $\frac{3}{5} + \frac{4}{7}$

8. $\frac{8}{11} - \frac{1}{3}$

9. $\frac{3}{4} \times \frac{7}{8}$

10. $-1\frac{1}{2} \div -2\frac{1}{2}$

Solve.

11. $6x = -4 + (-18)$

12. $-3 - 7 = x + 1$

13. $x(4 - 2) = 40$

14. $x + (-9) > -2$

15. $4 + (-12) \le x - 6$

16. $11 - x > 0$

Find the radius of a circle with the given circumference. Use $\pi \approx \frac{22}{7}$.

17. $C = 264$

18. $C = 343.2$

19. $C = 83.6$

20. $C = 897.6$

Solve.

21. What is 39% of 120?

22. What is 125% of 89?

23. What percent of 60 is 12?

24. What percent of 75 is 35?

25. 18 is 50% of what number?

26. 35 is 8% of what number?

Use a straight-line graph to complete the ordered pairs, then find the slope.

27. $A(7, 0)$, $B(5, 1)$, $C(-1, ?)$, $D(?, 7)$

28. $A(0, 0)$, $B(2, 1)$, $C(4, ?)$, $D(?, 3)$

Find the perimeter and the area of the polygon described.

29. A rectangle with sides 136.5 m and 97.5 m

30. A parallelogram with base 15 cm, one side 7 cm, and height 6 cm

31. A triangle with base 63 m, sides 51 m and 30 m, and height 24 m

Is the triangle with sides of the given lengths a right triangle?

32. 12, 16, 20

33. 4, 6, 9

34. 9, 12, 15

Problems

> **Problem Solving Reminders**
> Here are some problem solving reminders that may help you solve some of the problems on this page.
> - Some steps in your plan may not involve operations.
> - Consider whether a chart will help to organize information.
> - Check by using rounding to find an estimated answer.

Solve.

1. Rosalie has 2 ten-dollar bills. She would like to buy a book for $6.95, some puzzles for a total cost of $12.50, and birthday cards for a total cost of $3.60. Does she have enough money?

2. A faucet leaks at the rate of $\frac{1}{4}$ cup of water per hour. How much water will leak in 24 hours?

3. A Rosebud rocking chair can be purchased for $245.70 in a furniture store or for $189 at a factory store. What is the percent of markup for the furniture store?

4. In order for two elements to combine, the sum of their valence numbers must be equal to 0. One atom of carbon has a valence number of 4, and one atom of fluorine has a valence number of -1. How many atoms of fluorine are needed to combine with 1 atom of carbon?

5. Find the length of a diagonal of a square if each side of the square has a length of 7 cm. Round to the nearest tenth.

6. Two cyclists depart at the same time from the same point, traveling in opposite directions. One cyclist travels at a speed of 14 mi/h, while the other cyclist travels at a speed of 16 mi/h. How long must the cyclists travel to be at least 135 mi apart?

7. Find the area of a rectangular yard that has one side of length 12 m and perimeter 54 m.

8. You can buy whole chickens at Sal's Market for $1.09/lb. For an additional $.25/lb, the butcher will cut up the chicken and remove the bones. If chicken is sold in tenths of a pound, how much boneless chicken can be purchased for $7.50?

9. A rectangular painting is 5 ft wide and has an area of 15 ft^2. The frame around the painting is 3 in. wide. What are the dimensions of the framed painting?

Skill Review

Addition

```
  236
    4
  108
+  57
  405


   14.71
    3.009
+ 291.681
  309.400
```

Add.

1. 84
  + 15

2. 46
  + 32

3. 25
  + 18

4. 59
  + 16

5. 26
  + 95

6. 79
  + 56

7. 653
  + 88

8. 296
  + 35

9. 8.7
  + 0.5

10. 0.36
  + 2.44

11. 299.1
  + 68.33

12. 933.068
  + 724.3997

13. 5.4
  12.137
  1.25
  + 306.49

14. 1.6256
  6.006
  9.36
  + 1.49

15. 24.603
  18.4
  2.9
  + 0.216

16. 911.34
  0.52
  26.1
  + 83.192

17. $257 + 631$

18. $463 + 451$

19. $358 + 164$

20. $10.4 + 3.25$

21. $19.6 + 0.462$

22. $4.78 + 31.1$

23. $5.176 + 2.98$

24. $67.4 + 45.93$

25. $19.71 + 2.388$

26. $27.0564 + 281.4$

27. $3.51032 + 14.99$

28. $6.8 + 37.51 + 108.2$

29. $89.71 + 5.5 + 0.62$

30. $5326 + 703 + 9427 + 8$

31. $1027 + 349 + 8 + 12$

32. $16.24 + 5.6 + 18.09 + 6.7$

33. $2.55 + 0.34 + 0.42 + 3.57$

34. $61.476 + 14.1 + 0.59 + 366$

35. $90.072 + 32.4 + 24 + 8.6$

36. $115 + 20 + 9 + 7603$

37. $70 + 1328 + 94 + 5$

38. $193.7 + 4.08 + 11.5 + 1.9026$

39. $0.428 + 83.7 + 6.999 + 7.06$

40. $29 + 72 + 604 + 396$

41. $785 + 120 + 7 + 653$

42. $356 + 9 + 12 + 2301$

43. $6 + 24 + 315 + 1409$

44. $37.7 + 0.6 + 6.834 + 16$

45. $1165 + 0.08 + 17.1 + 94.028$

46. $570.2 + 74.4 + 6.553 + 9.2$

47. $7.8118 + 27.6 + 5.302 + 14$

Skill Review

Subtraction

```
  630
- 249
  381


  300.710
-  46.008
  254.702
```

Subtract.

1. 64
    − 51

2. 98
    − 37

3. 56
    − 30

4. 79
    − 42

5. 896
    − 241

6. 613
    − 402

7. 978
    − 365

8. 784
    − 463

9. 18.636
    − 13.435

10. 67.86
    − 54.22

11. 27.954
    − 16.21

12. 46.5822
    − 24.001

13. 8.434
    − 6.297

14. 35.061
    − 9.875

15. 6.952
    − 5.06

16. 583.86
    − 279.9

17. 453
    − 17.46

18. 55.7
    − 3.9

19. 0.081
    − 0.007

20. 2.0056
    − 0.918

21. 57 − 32

22. 86 − 45

23. 98 − 36

24. 49 − 26

25. 78 − 34

26. 76 − 65

27. 85 − 37

28. 42 − 29

29. 90 − 57

30. 94.7 − 39

31. 48.08 − 7.95

32. 279.5 − 33.7

33. 64.08 − 7.05

34. 605.01 − 31.23

35. 0.072 − 0.009

36. 1314 − 197

37. 6240 − 3078

38. 8521 − 2364

39. 7017 − 3468

40. 4320 − 2006

41. 9481 − 2556

42. 22.916 − 17.4

43. 25.006 − 3.98

44. 518.2 − 327.41

45. 2.7736 − 0.1531

46. 800.6 − 315

47. 0.9001 − 0.035

48. 207.001 − 44.62

49. 91.003 − 17.6

50. 23,025 − 18,769

51. 55,317 − 40,769

Skill Review

Multiplication

```
  476
 ×15
 2380
  476
 7140
```

```
 341.6    1 place
×0.27    2 places
23912
 6832
92.232   3 places
```

Multiply.

1. $\begin{array}{r} 13 \\ \times 2 \\ \hline \end{array}$ **2.** $\begin{array}{r} 21 \\ \times 4 \\ \hline \end{array}$ **3.** $\begin{array}{r} 53 \\ \times 3 \\ \hline \end{array}$ **4.** $\begin{array}{r} 64 \\ \times 2 \\ \hline \end{array}$

5. $\begin{array}{r} 47 \\ \times 3 \\ \hline \end{array}$ **6.** $\begin{array}{r} 16 \\ \times 5 \\ \hline \end{array}$ **7.** $\begin{array}{r} 90 \\ \times 4 \\ \hline \end{array}$ **8.** $\begin{array}{r} 34 \\ \times 6 \\ \hline \end{array}$

9. $\begin{array}{r} 84 \\ \times 12 \\ \hline \end{array}$ **10.** $\begin{array}{r} 63 \\ \times 23 \\ \hline \end{array}$ **11.** $\begin{array}{r} 71 \\ \times 65 \\ \hline \end{array}$ **12.** $\begin{array}{r} 40 \\ \times 31 \\ \hline \end{array}$

13. $\begin{array}{r} 785 \\ \times 1.2 \\ \hline \end{array}$ **14.** $\begin{array}{r} 6.61 \\ \times 3 \\ \hline \end{array}$ **15.** $\begin{array}{r} 808 \\ \times 17.2 \\ \hline \end{array}$ **16.** $\begin{array}{r} 22.5 \\ \times 8.9 \\ \hline \end{array}$

17. $\begin{array}{r} 89.06 \\ \times 0.5 \\ \hline \end{array}$ **18.** $\begin{array}{r} 37.5 \\ \times 0.28 \\ \hline \end{array}$ **19.** $\begin{array}{r} 212.8 \\ \times 0.67 \\ \hline \end{array}$ **20.** $\begin{array}{r} 93.65 \\ \times 4.11 \\ \hline \end{array}$

21. 20×30 **22.** 60×50 **23.** 10×90

24. 50×700 **25.** 900×80 **26.** 600×80

27. 3400×200 **28.** 400×1500 **29.** 300×470

30. 18×345 **31.** 563×27

32. 99×198 **33.** 314×16

34. 408×70 **35.** 923×60

36. 11.6×38.51 **37.** 47.3×6.05

38. 86.9×121.75 **39.** 36.91×0.51

40. 8.05×0.003 **41.** 20.35×3.7

42. 854.6×2.19 **43.** 41.6×212.5

44. 5129.36×0.008 **45.** 85.004×93.11

46. 9.8413×16.55 **47.** 3.7509×0.031

48. 83.751×98.230 **49.** 251×0.0074

50. 326.11×7.001 **51.** 0.8612×0.0101

Skill Review

Division

$$\begin{array}{r} 12.51 \\ 6.8\overline{)85.068} \\ \underline{68} \\ 170 \\ \underline{136} \\ 346 \\ \underline{340} \\ 68 \\ \underline{68} \\ 0 \end{array}$$

Divide.

1. $5\overline{)85}$ **2.** $8\overline{)96}$ **3.** $2\overline{)92}$

4. $13\overline{)273}$ **5.** $32\overline{)512}$ **6.** $17\overline{)714}$

7. $4\overline{)140.8}$ **8.** $7\overline{)160.3}$ **9.** $18\overline{)13.68}$

10. $5.06\overline{)480.7}$ **11.** $3.8\overline{)59.66}$ **12.** $8.1\overline{)423.63}$

Divide. Round to the nearest tenth if necessary.

13. $8\overline{)86}$ **14.** $6\overline{)50}$ **15.** $4\overline{)63}$

16. $49\overline{)172}$ **17.** $32\overline{)424}$ **18.** $26\overline{)817}$

19. $7.3\overline{)4001}$ **20.** $6.9\overline{)117}$ **21.** $0.56\overline{)27.8}$

To round a quotient to a particular place, divide to one place beyond the place specified and then round.

$$\begin{array}{r} 22.988 \\ 2.71\overline{)62.30000} \\ 54\,2 \\ 8\,10 \\ 5\,42 \\ 2\,680 \\ 2\,439 \\ 2410 \\ 2168 \\ 2420 \\ 2168 \\ 252 \end{array}$$

Rounded to the nearest hundredth the quotient is 22.99.

Divide. Round to the nearest hundredth if necessary.

22. $315 \div 9$ **23.** $513 \div 7$ **24.** $536 \div 8$

25. $405 \div 5$ **26.** $341 \div 6$ **27.** $11 \div 4$

28. $3775 \div 15.6$ **29.** $6.3 \div 2.4$ **30.** $11.9 \div 4.6$

31. $276 \div 37.5$ **32.** $88.01 \div 0.6$ **33.** $764 \div 0.4$

34. $21.6 \div 28$ **35.** $12.75 \div 51$ **36.** $1066 \div 27$

37. $17,063 \div 33$ **38.** $24,474 \div 60$ **39.** $19,412 \div 0.15$

40. $1.0472 \div 0.66$ **41.** $565.28 \div 11.8$ **42.** $47.611 \div 0.4$

43. $29,919 \div 56$ **44.** $15,960 \div 38$ **45.** $23,674 \div 77$

46. $11,500 \div 25$ **47.** $21,984 \div 36$ **48.** $87,048 \div 403$

49. $186.22 \div 0.038$ **50.** $28,400 \div 75$ **51.** $1234.5 \div 67$

52. $8.7553 \div 0.47$ **53.** $96.14 \div 0.026$ **54.** $0.054 \div 1.86$

55. $0.0269 \div 4.001$ **56.** $365.4 \div 74.1$ **57.** $11.99 \div 0.121$

Extra Practice: Chapter 1

Simplify the numerical expression.

1. $44.23 - 1.6$ **2.** 83×6 **3.** $4.80 \div 30$ **4.** $74 + 116$

Evaluate the expression when $d = 6$ and $y = 4$.

5. $y - 3$ **6.** $d + d$ **7.** $2y \times 3$ **8.** $y + d + 2$

Simplify the numerical expression.

9. $18 \div (2 \times 3) + 6$ **10.** $5 \times (5 - 2) \div 3$ **11.** $\dfrac{8 - 2 \times 3}{(6 - 4)(5 + 1)}$

Evaluate the expression when $x = 4.2$ and $y = 9$.

12. $4(x + y)$ **13.** $5y - x$ **14.** $(y - x)(x + y)$

Evaluate the expression when $a = 5$ and $b = 10$.

15. $3a - \dfrac{a}{5}$ **16.** $a(b - 2) \div 3$ **17.** $\dfrac{ab - 20}{a + b}$

Evaluate.

18. 3^4 **19.** 13^2 **20.** 25^3 **21.** 34^2

22. 17^3 **23.** 7^5 **24.** 30^3 **25.** 9^4

Multiply.

26. $9^2 \times 3^4$ **27.** $10^3 \times 2^4$ **28.** $7^3 \times 13^2$ **29.** $15^3 \times 4^5$

30. $6^3 \times 100^2$ **31.** $4^3 \times 1^5$ **32.** $2^5 \times 11^3$ **33.** $3^3 \times 2^6$

Write the decimal in expanded form.

34. 734   **35.** 516.21   **36.** 0.024   **37.** 25.2

38. 2138   **39.** 91.9   **40.** 0.38   **41.** 307.009

Write as a decimal.

42. 18 and 21 hundredths   **43.** 5 and 4 thousandths   **44.** 242 and 6 tenths

45. 9 and 9 ten-thousandths   **46.** 85 thousandths   **47.** 6 ten-thousandths

Round to the place specified.

48. hundreds; 871.21   **49.** tenths; 113.93   **50.** thousandths; 1.00414

51. hundredths; 0.0577   **52.** tens; 382.45   **53.** hundredths; 45.552

54. thousandths; 3.4279   **55.** hundreds; 84   **56.** tenths; 74.991

What value of the variable makes the statement true?

57. $7.4 \times n = 1.84 \times 7.4$ **58.** $6.81 = r + 6.81$

59. $8.726z = z$ **60.** $3.4(5.12 + 9.4) = (5.12 + 9.4)p$

61. $(79 \times k) + (79 \times 4) = 79 \times 12$ **62.** $a \times 24.5 = 24.5$

Solve for the given replacement set.

63. $q + 9 = 17$; $\{8, 9, 10\}$ **64.** $b - 12 = 35$; $\{45, 46, 47\}$

65. $x \div 14 = 8$; $\{110, 112, 114\}$ **66.** $53 + m = 66$; $\{13, 15, 17\}$

67. $8f = 56$; $\{5, 6, 7\}$ **68.** $17t = 102$; $\{7, 8, 9\}$

69. $2g - 8 = 14$; $\{10, 11, 12\}$ **70.** $4(a + 6) = 36$; $\{1, 2, 3\}$

Use inverse operations to solve.

71. $k + 16 = 28$ **72.** $n \div 6 = 122$ **73.** $7p = 217$ **74.** $p - 11 = 41$

75. $m \div 12 = 204$ **76.** $17 + z = 53$ **77.** $6m = 240$ **78.** $a - 35 = 41$

Solve, using the five-step plan.

79. Recently, Ken ran a 400 m race in 52.3 s. This was 0.2 s slower than the school record. What is the school record?

80. On July 1, Kay had $542.07 in her savings account. On September 1, she had $671.82 in her account. How much did she save between July 1 and September 1?

81. A machine produces 3 plastic parts each minute that it runs. If the machine runs for 7 h, how many parts will it produce?

82. Exercise World is buying 4 new exercise bicycles for $129.95 each and 6 exercise mats for $47.85 each. What is the total cost?

Solve and check.

83. John owes Tom $18. John earns $5 an hour and already has $3. How long must John work to earn enough to pay Tom back?

84. Rosa sells newspapers at the bus stop. If each paper costs $.25, how many must Rosa sell to take in $10?

Extra Practice: Chapter 2

Express as an integer.

1. $|^-3|$ **2.** $|5|$ **3.** $|1|$ **4.** $|0|$ **5.** $|^-6|$

6. $|4|$ **7.** $|^-2|$ **8.** $|^-7|$ **9.** $|9|$ **10.** $|^-8|$

Graph the number and its opposite on the same number line.

11. 6 **12.** $^-9$ **13.** 8 **14.** 5 **15.** $^-1$

Write the integers in order from least to greatest.

16. 0, 4, $^-4$, 3, $^-3$ **17.** 5, 0, $^-2$, $^-8$, 6 **18.** 7, $^-3$, $^-2$, 1, 9

19. $^-1$, 3, $^-7$, 5, $^-4$ **20.** $^-6$, $^-7$, 0, $^-5$, $^-2$ **21.** $^-4$, 5, 4, $^-5$, 0

Replace __?__ with =, >, or < to make a true statement.

22. 31 __?__ 61 **23.** 18 × 4 __?__ 82 **24.** 47 __?__ 49 − 9

List the integers that can replace x to make the statement true.

25. $|x| = 5$ **26.** $|x| = 2$ **27.** $|x| = 0$

28. $|x| = 4$ **29.** $|x| \le 6$ **30.** $|x| \le 3$

Graph the numbers in each exercise on the same number line.

31. 1, $^-1.5$, 0, $^-2$ **32.** $^-2$, $^-4$, 2.5, $^-3.5$ **33.** 3, 1.2, $^-2.4$, $^-5$

34. 7.6, $^-6.7$, 6, $^-7$ **35.** 1, 1.5, $^-2$, 2.5 **36.** 2, $^-1.8$, $^-2.1$, 0

Draw an arrow to represent the decimal number described.

37. The number 5, with starting point $^-4$

38. The number $^-8$, with starting point 6

39. The number 6, with starting point $^-5$

40. The number $^-6$, with starting point 3

Find the sum.

41. 2.7 + 7.2 **42.** $^-4.9 + {}^-7.6$ **43.** $^-2.25 + 2.25$

44. $^-3.8 + {}^-3.8$ **45.** $^-148 + {}^-256$ **46.** 6.1 + $^-2.3$

47. $^-0.6 + {}^-2.3$ **48.** 18.12 + 1.66 **49.** $^-5.2 + 2.9$

50. $^-2.8 + {}^-3.9$ **51.** 1.9 + 19 **52.** $^-14.75 + 9.94$

Find the difference.

53. $30.5 - 18$

54. $16 - 24.3$

55. $10.6 - 11.2$

56. $16.2 - (-7)$

57. $5 - (-15.3)$

58. $18 - (-9.7)$

59. $-8.3 - 5.2$

60. $-7 - 14.6$

61. $-12.3 - 8$

62. $43.4 - (-136)$

63. $-3 - (-8.2)$

64. $-12.9 - (-4.5)$

Evaluate when $x = -3.2$ and $y = -5.7$.

65. $-y$

66. $-x$

67. $-|x|$

68. $-|y|$

69. $y - x$

70. $-x - y$

71. $x - (-y)$

72. $-x - (-y)$

73. $-y - (-x)$

Find the quotient.

74. $-15.5 \div 0.5$

75. $-16.4 \div 4$

76. $-150 \div 7.5$

77. $36.6 \div -0.06$

78. $38 \div -0.4$

79. $8.19 \div (-9)$

80. $-3.038 \div (-7)$

81. $-63.7 \div (-0.007)$

82. $-246 \div (-0.6)$

83. $-0.003 \div (1)$

84. $0 \div (-0.85)$

85. $-0.9 \div (-1.8)$

Find the product.

86. $2.4(-1.2)$

87. $-1.4(3.4)$

88. $4.5(-1.7)$

89. $-8.2(-6.1)$

90. $-4.3(-3.4)$

91. $-6.2(-5.3)$

92. $-2.15(1.15)$

93. $3.14(-8.1)$

94. $-5.22(8.11)$

95. $4.25(-3.14)$

96. $1.11(-1.11)$

97. $-6.75(2.32)$

Evaluate the expression if $a = 4$, $b = 2$, and $c = 6$.

98. $5c^3$

99. $(4b)^3$

100. $2ab^4$

101. $2a^3$

102. $3(ab)^2$

103. $(3c)^b$

104. $a^2 - b^4$

105. c^2a

Write the expression without exponents.

106. 7^{-3}

107. $(-4)^{-2}$

108. 2^{-5}

109. $(-6)^{-4}$

110. 8^{-1}

111. $(-9)^{-2}$

112. 5^{-4}

113. $(-1)^{-7}$

114. 3^{-6}

115. $(-5)^{-3}$

116. $8^5 \times 8^{-7}$

117. $10^4 \times 10^{-3}$

118. $5^9 \times 5^{-9}$

119. $4^{-2} \times 4^0$

120. $9^{17} \times 9^{-17}$

121. $3^{-6} \times 3^4$

122. $6^{-2} \times 6^5$

123. $2^{10} \times 2^{-8}$

Extra Practice: Chapter 3

List all the factors of each number.

1. 6   **2.** 7   **3.** 10   **4.** 13   **5.** 15   **6.** 18

7. 41   **8.** 42   **9.** 52   **10.** 56   **11.** 59   **12.** 64

Which of the numbers 2, 3, 4, 5, 9, and 10 are factors of the given number?

13. 155   **14.** 168   **15.** 189   **16.** 210   **17.** 272   **18.** 305

19. 1080   **20.** 1100   **21.** 1260   **22.** 1362   **23.** 1423   **24.** 1485

Determine whether each number is prime or composite. If the number is composite, give the prime factorization.

25. 10   **26.** 34   **27.** 54   **28.** 41   **29.** 30   **30.** 18

Write as a proper fraction in lowest terms or as a mixed number in simple form.

31. $\frac{15}{45}$ **32.** $-\frac{22}{64}$ **33.** $\frac{7}{5}$ **34.** $\frac{180}{240}$

35. $-\frac{144}{96}$ **36.** $-\frac{58}{12}$ **37.** $\frac{75}{125}$ **38.** $\frac{-145}{95}$

39. $\frac{14}{-8}$ **40.** $\frac{32}{28}$ **41.** $\frac{-63}{81}$ **42.** $-\frac{48}{54}$

Complete.

43. $\frac{1}{4} + \frac{1}{4} + \frac{1}{4} + \frac{1}{4} = \underline{\ ?\ }$ **44.** $\underline{\ ?\ } \times \frac{1}{3} = -\frac{2}{3}$

45. $5 \times \underline{\ ?\ } = -1$ **46.** $\frac{3}{10} = 3 \div \underline{\ ?\ }$

47. $\left(-\frac{1}{7}\right) + \left(-\frac{1}{7}\right) = \underline{\ ?\ }$ **48.** $4 \times \underline{\ ?\ } = \frac{4}{9}$

49. $\frac{2}{5} = \frac{?}{20}$ **50.** $\frac{-8}{9} = \frac{?}{27}$ **51.** $-\frac{12}{30} = -\frac{2}{?}$

52. $\frac{20}{-36} = \frac{?}{-9}$ **53.** $3 = \frac{12}{?}$ **54.** $-4 = \frac{-28}{?}$

Write as an improper fraction.

55. $5\frac{2}{3}$ **56.** $3\frac{4}{5}$ **57.** $-4\frac{3}{10}$ **58.** $-15\frac{1}{6}$

59. $-7\frac{1}{8}$ **60.** $9\frac{3}{25}$ **61.** $6\frac{1}{4}$ **62.** $-5\frac{11}{12}$

Write the set of fractions as equivalent fractions with the least common denominator (LCD).

63. $\frac{5}{6}, \frac{3}{8}$

64. $\frac{4}{5}, -\frac{3}{10}$

65. $\frac{4}{8}, \frac{5}{12}$

66. $-\frac{8}{15}, -\frac{7}{20}$

67. $-\frac{11}{28}, \frac{17}{42}$

68. $\frac{7}{30}, \frac{19}{70}$

Add or subtract. Write the answer as a proper fraction in lowest terms or as a mixed number in simple form.

69. $\frac{5}{13} + \frac{4}{13}$

70. $-\frac{7}{8} - \frac{5}{8}$

71. $\frac{5}{12} - \frac{1}{12}$

72. $\frac{5}{9} + \left(-\frac{1}{4}\right)$

73. $-\frac{9}{14} - \frac{5}{32}$

74. $\frac{3}{7} - \left(-\frac{4}{5}\right)$

75. $-4\frac{1}{12} + 2\frac{4}{5}$

76. $5\frac{2}{3} - 2\frac{5}{8}$

77. $-3\frac{7}{12} + 7\frac{5}{16}$

78. $2\frac{3}{7} - \left(-4\frac{5}{6}\right)$

79. $-1\frac{3}{28} + \left(-4\frac{10}{21}\right)$

80. $-15\frac{1}{2} - \left(-8\frac{3}{4}\right)$

Multiply or divide. Write the answer as a proper fraction in lowest terms or as a mixed number in simple form.

81. $-\frac{3}{4} \times \frac{4}{5}$

82. $\frac{21}{56} \times \frac{20}{25}$

83. $\frac{7}{8} \times \left(-\frac{4}{7}\right)$

84. $6\frac{3}{4} \times \left(-1\frac{1}{3}\right)$

85. $-2\frac{5}{8} \times \left(-\frac{16}{19}\right)$

86. $-4\frac{2}{7} \times 2\frac{1}{4}$

87. $\frac{4}{9} \div \frac{2}{9}$

88. $-\frac{3}{8} \div \left(-\frac{5}{16}\right)$

89. $-\frac{8}{15} \div \left(-2\frac{2}{7}\right)$

90. $-3\frac{3}{5} \div \left(2\frac{4}{15}\right)$

91. $-\frac{5}{6} \div 4\frac{1}{2}$

92. $3\frac{5}{9} \div (-32)$

Write as a terminating or repeating decimal. Use a bar to show a repeating decimal.

93. $\frac{3}{8}$

94. $\frac{3}{5}$

95. $\frac{21}{22}$

96. $-\frac{5}{16}$

97. $\frac{1}{6}$

98. $-\frac{5}{9}$

99. $-\frac{8}{15}$

100. $-\frac{161}{189}$

101. $\frac{287}{385}$

102. $3\frac{5}{12}$

103. $-2\frac{3}{11}$

104. $4\frac{1}{18}$

Write as a proper fraction in lowest terms or as a mixed number in simple form.

105. 0.6

106. -0.04

107. 1.34

108. -4.22

109. -3.025

110. $0.\overline{6}$

111. $-2.\overline{09}$

112. $1.\overline{7}$

113. $8.2121\ldots$

114. $-2.1666\ldots$

Extra Practice: Chapter 4

Use transformations to solve each equation. Write down all the steps.

1. $r + 30 = 80$

2. $31 + d = 47$

3. $\frac{1}{4}b = \frac{3}{4}$

4. $x - 21 = 19$

5. $79 - a = 17$

6. $14 + 12 = 17 + a$

7. $1.23 = 1.50 - a$

8. $\frac{7}{8} + a = 4$

9. $13t = 52$

10. $84 = 14k$

11. $\frac{n}{6} = 12$

12. $15 = \frac{x}{3}$

13. $28 = 7v$

14. $3 = \frac{p}{3}$

15. $\frac{t}{7} = 5(3 + 4)$

16. $9 = \frac{x}{10}$

17. $\frac{1}{7} = \frac{3}{7}k$

18. $\frac{12}{5}c = \frac{3}{10}$

19. $0.25a = 1.0$

20. $1.7 = 1.7x$

21. $\frac{5}{9} = \frac{12}{5}k$

22. $1.25 = 0.6f$

23. $6.25n = 1.25$

24. $\frac{11}{15} = \frac{3}{5}y$

25. $\frac{p}{6} - 12 = 3$

26. $72 = \frac{p}{3} + 3$

27. $3.6x - 2.5 = 15.5$

28. $1.24 - 1.2m = 1.0$

29. $17 = 5y - 3$

30. $\frac{8}{3} = \frac{2}{5}v - \frac{1}{3}$

31. $\frac{m}{3} = \frac{1}{3}(6 + 12)$

32. $2x - 3 = 15 - 6$

Write a variable expression for the word phrase.

33. The difference when a number t is subtracted from eighteen

34. Five added to the product of a number x and nine

35. Forty divided by a number m, decreased by sixteen

36. The remainder when a number q is subtracted from two hundred

37. Eleven more than three times a number y

38. The sum of a number r and six, divided by twelve

Write an equation for each word sentence.

39. The product of six and a number n is fifty-four.

40. Twelve less than two times a number n is seventy.

41. The sum of a number n and nineteen is sixty-one.

Choose a variable and write an equation for each problem.

42. The altitude of the Dead Sea is 1296 ft below sea level. How much greater is the altitude of Death Valley, California, at 282 ft below sea level?

43. An astronaut enters a space capsule 1 hr 40 min before launch time. How long has the astronaut been in the capsule 2 h 32 min after the launch?

44. The Torrance baseball team scored 10 runs in the first 3 innings. Gardena scored 2 in the first and 5 in the fourth. If Torrence does not score again, how many more runs does Gardena need to win?

Write an equation for each problem. Solve the equation using the five-step method. Check your answer.

45. Mercury melts at 38.87° below 0°C and boils at 356.9°C. What is the difference between these temperatures?

46. Yolanda rode the bus from a point 53 blocks south of Carroll Avenue to a point 41 blocks north of Carroll Avenue. How many blocks did she travel?

47. John sailed for 7 hours on Swan Lake. If he sailed for two more hours than he fished, how long did he fish?

48. In a local election 1584 people voted. The winner received 122 votes more than the loser. How many votes did each candidate receive?

49. It takes Fritz 55 min to commute to and from work. The ride home takes 7 min less than the ride to work. How long does it take each way?

50. Ann swam a total of 78 laps on Monday and Tuesday. She swam 12 more laps on Tuesday than on Monday. How far did she swim each day?

Extra Practice: Chapter 5

Draw a sketch to illustrate each of the following.

1. Three points on a line
2. Two intersecting lines
3. Three noncollinear points
4. Two intersecting planes
5. Two rays with a common endpoint, A
6. Two segments with a common endpoint, B

Complete.

7. $10 \text{ km} = \underline{\ ?\ } \text{ m}$ 8. $0.27 \text{ km} = \underline{\ ?\ } \text{ m}$ 9. $9 \text{ m} = \underline{\ ?\ } \text{ cm}$

10. $0.5 \text{ km} = \underline{\ ?\ } \text{ m}$ 11. $77 \text{ m} = \underline{\ ?\ } \text{ cm}$ 12. $175 \text{ mm} = \underline{\ ?\ } \text{ m}$

13. $1500 \text{ m} = \underline{\ ?\ } \text{ km}$ 14. $81 \text{ cm} = \underline{\ ?\ } \text{ mm}$ 15. $0.1575 \text{ km} = \underline{\ ?\ } \text{ m}$

16. $900 \text{ mm} = \underline{\ ?\ } \text{ m} = \underline{\ ?\ } \text{ cm}$ 17. $2 \text{ m} = \underline{\ ?\ } \text{ cm} = \underline{\ ?\ } \text{ mm}$

18. If the sum of the measures of two angles is $180°$, the angles are $\underline{\ ?\ }$.

19. A small square is often used to indicate a(n) $\underline{\ ?\ }$ angle.

20. Perpendicular lines form $\underline{\ ?\ }°$ angles.

21. The $\underline{\ ?\ }$ is the common endpoint of two rays that form an angle.

22. If $m\angle A = 40°$, the complement of $\angle A$ measures $\underline{\ ?\ }°$.

23. A(n) $\underline{\ ?\ }$ angle has a measure between $90°$ and $180°$.

24. A triangle with at least two sides congruent is called a(n) $\underline{\ ?\ }$ triangle.

25. Triangles can be classified by their $\underline{\ ?\ }$ or their $\underline{\ ?\ }$.

26. The sum of the measures of the angles of a triangle is $\underline{\ ?\ }°$.

27. A(n) $\underline{\ ?\ }$ triangle has two perpendicular sides.

28. The sum of the lengths of any two sides of a triangle is $\underline{\ ?\ }$ than the length of the third side.

29. A triangle with three congruent sides is called a(n) $\underline{\ ?\ }$ triangle.

30. A triangle with all its angles less than $90°$ is called a(n) $\underline{\ ?\ }$ triangle.

True or false?

31. A regular polygon has all the sides equal.

32. All the angles of a rectangle have a measure of $90°$.

33. A trapezoid always has one pair of congruent sides.

34. The opposite sides of a parallelogram are congruent.

35. Only two sides of a rhombus are congruent.

36. A square with a perimeter of 24 cm has 4 sides that measure 6 cm.

37. A regular decagon, 5 cm on a side, has a perimeter of 50 cm.

Solve. Use $\pi \approx 3.14$ and round answers to three digits.

38. The radius of a circle is 30 cm. Find the diameter.

39. The radius of a circle is 56 mm. Find the circumference.

40. The diameter of a circle is 3 m. Find the circumference.

41. The diameter of a circle is 16 mm. Find the circumference.

42. The circumference of a circle is 20 m. Find the diameter.

43. The circumference of a circle is 25.8 m. Find the radius.

Complete the statements about the pair of congruent figures.

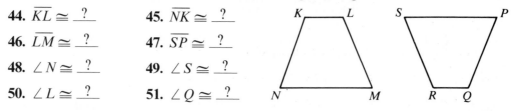

44. $\overline{KL} \cong$? **45.** $\overline{NK} \cong$?

46. $\overline{LM} \cong$? **47.** $\overline{SP} \cong$?

48. $\angle N \cong$? **49.** $\angle S \cong$?

50. $\angle L \cong$? **51.** $\angle Q \cong$?

Are the triangles in each pair congruent? If so, name the triangles that are congruent and explain why they are congruent.

52.

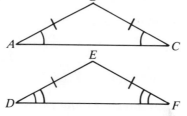

53.

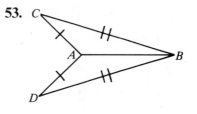

Use a compass and a straightedge to make each construction.

54. Draw a segment AB. Construct the perpendicular bisector.

55. Draw an acute angle ABC. Construct $\overrightarrow{BX}$ so that it bisects $\angle ABC$.

56. Construct an angle congruent to $\angle ABC$ of Exercise 55.

Extra Practice: Chapter 6

Express each ratio as a fraction in lowest terms.

1. $\dfrac{10 \text{ min}}{1 \text{ h}}$

2. $\dfrac{6 \text{ cm}}{2 \text{ m}}$

3. $\dfrac{250 \text{ mL}}{2 \text{ L}}$

4. $\dfrac{6 \text{ kg}}{600 \text{ g}}$

5. $\dfrac{7 \text{ days}}{4 \text{ weeks}}$

6. $\dfrac{3 \text{ h}}{45 \text{ min}}$

7. $\dfrac{15 \text{ mm}}{5 \text{ cm}}$

8. $\dfrac{60 \text{ cm}}{150 \text{ mm}}$

Solve. Express each ratio in lowest terms.

9. A student walked 25 km in 4 h. What was the average speed in kilometers per hour?

10. A special typewriter has 46 keys. Of these 46 keys, 26 are used for letters of the alphabet. What is the ratio of the number of keys not used for letters to the total number of keys?

Solve.

11. In order to make 4 servings, a recipe calls for 3 eggs to be used. How many eggs will be needed to make 32 servings?

12. Charlie runs 5 mi in 37 min. If he could maintain the same speed, how long would it take him to run 15 mi?

13. A dozen apples cost $1.80. What is the unit price?

14. A car travels 234 km in 4.5 h. What is the car's average speed?

15. $\dfrac{19}{20} = \dfrac{n}{10}$

16. $\dfrac{8}{48} = \dfrac{n}{4}$

17. $\dfrac{4}{13} = \dfrac{12}{n}$

18. $\dfrac{n}{27} = \dfrac{12}{81}$

19. $\dfrac{40}{n} = \dfrac{5}{9}$

20. $\dfrac{n}{64} = \dfrac{12}{8}$

21. $\dfrac{100}{40} = \dfrac{20}{n}$

22. $\dfrac{7}{3} = \dfrac{n}{18}$

23. Joe bought 4 shock absorbers for the price of 3 at a clearance sale. He paid a total of $39. How much would the 4 shock absorbers cost at their regular price?

24. Billie runs 4 km in 25 min. How long will it take to run 10,000 m?

25. A supermarket sells 12 oranges for $1.30. How much would 18 oranges cost at the same rate?

A map has a scale of 1 cm : 8 km. What actual distance does each map length represent?

26. 8 cm

27. 5.5 cm

28. 3 cm

29. 7.9 cm

30. 3.75 cm

31. 10.2 cm

32. 6.25 cm

33. 15.25 cm

Express as a fraction in lowest terms or as a mixed number in simple form.

34. 5% **35.** 10% **36.** 72% **37.** 39% **38.** 2%

39. 27% **40.** 25% **41.** 200% **42.** 163% **43.** 215%

Express as a percent.

44. $\frac{3}{4}$ **45.** $\frac{1}{10}$ **46.** $\frac{3}{5}$ **47.** $\frac{1}{8}$ **48.** 7

49. $\frac{7}{16}$ **50.** $\frac{43}{20}$ **51.** $\frac{36}{25}$ **52.** $\frac{23}{4}$ **53.** $\frac{22}{5}$

Express each percent as a decimal.

54. 15% **55.** 71% **56.** 5% **57.** 15.2% **58.** 98%

59. 2.4% **60.** 7.5% **61.** 625% **62.** 0.42% **63.** 200%

Express each decimal as a percent.

64. 0.45 **65.** 0.23 **66.** 1.33 **67.** 0.05 **68.** 12.5

69. 0.0025 **70.** 10.2 **71.** 0.53 **72.** 0.008 **73.** 0.125

Express each fraction as a decimal, then as a percent.

74. $\frac{2}{5}$ **75.** $\frac{1}{4}$ **76.** $\frac{7}{10}$ **77.** $\frac{5}{8}$ **78.** $\frac{1}{16}$

79. $1\frac{3}{8}$ **80.** $\frac{5}{16}$ **81.** $8\frac{3}{4}$ **82.** $\frac{13}{16}$ **83.** $5\frac{1}{5}$

Answer each question by writing an equation and solving it. Round to the nearest tenth of a percent if necessary.

84. 12% of 50 is what number? **85.** 110% of 99 is what number?

86. What percent of 81 is 27? **87.** 85% of what number is 425?

88. 15% of $30 is how much? **89.** What percent of 250 is 75?

90. What percent of 256 is 32? **91.** 60% of what number is 144?

92. 5% of 1000 is what number? **93.** 140% of what number is 35?

94. 18% of $85 is how much? **95.** What percent of 825 is 25?

96. 30% of what number is 23.7? **97.** 6% of what number is 3.48?

98. What percent of 325 is 65? **99.** 12% of 408 is what number?

Extra Practice: *Chapter 7*

Find the percent increase or decrease from the first number to the second. Round to the nearest tenth of a percent if necessary.

1. 45 to 66   **2.** 50 to 60   **3.** 140 to 84   **4.** 256 to 500

5. 15 to 75   **6.** 144 to 96   **7.** 360 to 234   **8.** 196 to 49

Find the new number produced when the given number is increased or decreased by the given percent.

9. 64; 25% increase   **10.** 80; 65% decrease

11. 78; 150% increase   **12.** 480; 35% increase

Solve.

13. Mervyn's is having a sale on batteries. The regular price of $2.40 is decreased by 20%. What is the sale price?

14. A bicycle that usually sells for $120 is on sale for $96. What is the percent of discount?

15. Great Hikes purchases backpacks from the manufacturer at $10 each. Then the backpacks are sold at the store for $25 each. What is the percent of markup?

16. If there is a sales tax of 5%, how much will it cost to buy a $57 handbag?

17. A wheelbarrow sells for $36. Next month the price will be marked up 6%. How much will the wheelbarrow cost next month?

18. A furniture store has a total income of $3600 per week and total operating costs of $3096 per week. To the nearest tenth, what percent of the income is profit?

19. The Thort Company made a profit of $32,175 on sales of $371,250. To the nearest tenth, what percent of the sales was profit?

20. Dora's commission last month was $621. Her total sales were $8280. What is her rate of commission?

21. Foster Realty Co. charges a 6% commission for the sale of property. If a homeowner wishes to clear $130,000 after paying the commission, for how much must the home be sold?

22. Ivan works for salary plus commission. He earns $500 per month plus 4% commission on all sales. What sales level is needed for Ivan to earn $675 in a given month?

23. Last Friday, 720 people at Data Tech drove cars to work. Of these, 585 bought gas on the way home. What percent of the drivers bought gas on the way home? Use a proportion to solve.

24. How much does a $53.00 iron cost if it is taxed at 5%? Use a proportion to solve.

25. Jill has $525 in a savings account that pays 6% simple interest. How much will she have in the account after 1 year, if she makes no deposits or withdrawals?

26. Holly has a savings account that pays 6.5% interest, compounded monthly. If she started the account with $750 and makes no deposits or withdrawals, how much will be in the account after 3 months?

27. Phil borrowed $5000 for one year. The interest on the loan came to $689.44. To the nearest tenth, what was the interest rate?

28. Victor had a two-year loan with a simple interest rate of 13% annually. At the end of the two years he had paid $1454.44 in interest. What was the original of Victor's loan?

29. Consider a principal of $2750 earning an interest rate of 10.5%. If compounded semiannually for one year, what is the total interest earned on $2750? (If you do not have a calculator, round to the nearest penny at every step.)

30. A $600 deposit is left in an account for 9 months. If the account earns an 8% interest compounded quarterly, what is the total interest earned at the end of the 9 months? (If you do not have a calculator, round to the nearest penny at every step.)

31. Carol has 60 boxes of light bulbs. If she sells 15% of the boxes today, how many will be left?

32. At a pet store, fish that usually cost $1.25 each are on sale for $.75 each. What is the percent of decrease?

33. A restaurant raises its price for the salad bar 20% to $1.50. What did the salad bar cost before?

34. The band concert drew an audience of 270 on Thursday. On Friday, attendance increased 30%. How many people attended on Friday?

35. The discount rate at an appliance store sale is 15%. What is the sale price of a dishwasher if the original price was $600?

36. Nancy Allen earns a 12% commission on her sales. Last month she earned $4800. What was the total value of her sales?

Extra Practice: Chapter 8

Solve.

1. $2a + 7a = 36$
2. $12x - 8x = 4$
3. $-10y + 12y = 1$
4. $d - 7d = -72$
5. $-5t + 12t = 3$
6. $-3p - 9p = 6$
7. $x + 3x + 6 = 8$
8. $4c + 8c - 3 = 9$
9. $-n - 3 + 10n = 9$
10. $5z + 10 - 12z = -4$
11. $8 + y - 9y = -4$
12. $d + 12 - 7d = 48$
13. $4a = a + 3$
14. $16p = 12 + 8p$
15. $32 - 6x = 2x$
16. $50 + t = 6t$
17. $3x = -6x + 36$
18. $y = 12y - 44$
19. $3c + 4 = 5c + 5$
20. $2n - 5 = 7n + 20$
21. $d - 9 = 24 - 10d$
22. $-x + 7 = 6x + 21$
23. $3 - 4y = 13 + 2y$
24. $-3a + 6 = 5 - 2a$

Solve.

25. At Moor's Deli, a ham sandwich and a glass of milk cost a total of $3.25. If the sandwich costs four times as much as the milk, what is the cost of each?

26. The sum of two consecutive integers is 135. What are the two integers?

27. A 60 ft piece of rope is cut into two pieces, one three times as long as the other. What is the length of each piece?

28. The perimeter of an isosceles triangle is 75 cm. If the congruent sides of the triangle are each twice as long as the remaining side, what is the length of each side?

Replace __?__ with < or >.

29. 15 __?__ 23
30. 57 __?__ 49
31. 35 __?__ 18
32. $7 + 11$ __?__ 31
33. 17 __?__ $12 + 4$
34. $29 - 15$ __?__ 17

Write an inequality for each word sentence.

35. Seventeen is greater than twelve.

36. A number plus twelve is less than twenty-two.

37. Twice a number is greater than sixty-nine.

38. Seven is smaller than two times five.

39. Eighty minus twenty-six is greater than two times twenty-one.

40. Thirty-three is less than six times a number.

Use transformations to solve the inequality. Write down all the steps.

41. $y + 5 \le -17$

42. $q - 8 > 24$

43. $5\frac{1}{6} - \frac{1}{3} < k$

44. $7.8 + 4.3 \ge m$

45. $f < (17 - 3)0.5$

46. $z \le \frac{1}{2}(25 - 7)$

47. $6e > 42$

48. $-5a \le 45$

49. $28 < -7u$

50. $52 \ge 4x$

51. $\frac{w}{-3} > 21$

52. $\frac{c}{4} \ge 17$

53. $-11 \le \frac{a}{5}$

54. $\frac{e}{-2} < -23$

55. $10 > \frac{v}{7}$

56. $-5x + 7 + 2x - 13 < 9$

57. $-22 \ge 10d - 4 - 3d + 12$

58. $2 > \frac{4}{5}n + 3 - \frac{1}{5}n + 6$

59. $5 + \frac{3}{7}u - 8 + \frac{2}{7}u \le 5$

60. $-w + 8 \le 4w - 17$

61. $-6s - 4 < s + 31$

62. $10 + \frac{2}{3}h > -\frac{5}{3}h + 6$

63. $8 - \frac{1}{6}p \ge 4 - \frac{1}{3}p$

64. $4(m + 3) \ge 48$

65. $35 < -5(x + 2)$

66. $34 < (18t - 6)\frac{1}{3}$

67. $\frac{-1}{7}(14 + 21u) \ge 7$

Solve.

68. Of all pairs of consecutive integers whose sum is greater than 250, find the pair whose sum is least.

69. Two cars start from the same point traveling in different directions. One car travels at a speed of 52 mi/h, and the other car travels at a speed of 48 mi/h. How long must they travel to be 300 mi apart?

70. A purse contains 20 coins, all either quarters or dimes. If the total value of the coins is greater than $3.50, at least how many are quarters?

Extra Practice: Chapter 9

For Exercises 1–6, give the coordinates of the point.

1. A 2. B 3. C

4. D 5. E 6. F

Name the point for the ordered pair.

7. $(2, -2)$ 8. $(-3, -4)$

9. $(4, 2)$ 10. $(-6, -3)$

11. $(1, -4)$ 12. $(-3, 1)$

a. Graph the given ordered pairs on a coordinate plane.
b. Connect all the points in the order listed by means of line segments to produce a closed figure.
c. Name the figure as specifically as you can.

13. $(3, 3), (3, 0), (-2, 0), (-5, 0), (-5, 3), (3, 3)$

14. $(2, -2), (2, -6), (-2, -6), (-2, -2), (0, -2), (2, -2)$

15. $(1, 5), (-2, 2), (-5, -1), (0, -1), (6, -1), (1, 5)$

16. $(0, 7), (3, 5), (2, 2), (-2, 2), (-3, 5), (0, 7)$

17. $(7, -4), (4, -1), (2, 1), (1, 2), (1, -4), (7, -4)$

Tell whether the ordered pair is a solution of the given equation.

$-x + 2y = 4$
18. $(4, 0)$ 19. $(-4, 0)$ 20. $(2, 3)$ 21. $(-2, 3)$

$x + 3y = 6$
22. $(0, 2)$ 23. $(6, 0)$ 24. $(2, 1)$ 25. $(3, 1)$

$2x + y = 5$
26. $(3, 1)$ 27. $(2, 1)$ 28. $(1, 3)$ 29. $(0, 5)$

a. Solve the equation for y in terms of x.
b. Find the solutions of the equation for the given values of x.

30. $2x + y = 8$
    values of x: $-1, 0, 1$

31. $y - 3x = 4$
    values of x: $-5, 0, 5$

32. $-x + y = 1$
    values of x: $-1, \frac{1}{2}, 2$

33. $3x - 2y = -6$
    values of x: $-2, 0, 2$

34. $2x + y = 6$
   values of x: 0, 3, 1

35. $x - y = 3$
   values of x: 6, -1, -3

Graph the equation on a coordinate plane. Use a separate set of axes for each equation.

36. $2x + y = 4$

37. $x - 3y = -3$

38. $x + 2y = -4$

39. $3x + 4y = 12$

40. $2x + 5y = 10$

41. $-x + y = -1$

42. $x + y = 2$

43. $3x - y = 3$

44. $4x - 2y = 3$

45. $2x = y - 2$

46. $y = x - 3$

47. $-3x + 4y = 12$

Use a graph to solve the system. Do the lines intersect, coincide, or are they parallel?

48. $x - y = -2$
   $2x + y = 5$

49. $x - y = 6$
   $2x + y = 0$

50. $2x + y = -2$
   $x - y = -4$

51. $2x + y = 2$
   $2x + y = -3$

52. $6x + 3y = 6$
   $2x + y = 2$

53. $3x + y = -6$
   $2x - y = 1$

54. A parking lot attendant charges $3 for the first hour and $1 for each extra hour after that. Write an equation that relates the total cost of parking (y) to the number of extra hours a car is parked (x). Graph the equation. What is the slope of the graph? From your graph determine how much it would cost to park a car for 5 h after the initial hour.

55. The initial charge for a phone call to Jonesboro is 25¢ for the first 3 min. After that the charge is 5¢ for every additional minute. Write an equation that relates the total cost of a phone call (y) to the number of additional minutes on the phone (x). Graph the equation. What is the slope of the graph? From the graph determine the cost of a call requiring 7 min beyond the initial 3.

56. The temperature in a town rose at a constant rate from 5 A.M. to 12 noon. At 9 A.M. the temperature was 17°C. At 11 A.M. the temperature was 21°C. Use this information to draw a graph and determine what the temperature was at 5 A.M. and at 12 noon.

Graph the inequality.

57. $x + 2y < 4$

58. $2x - y < 1$

59. $6x + y \geq 7$

60. $-x + 3y < 0$

61. $2x + y \geq 1$

62. $3x + y \leq -2$

Extra Practice: Chapter 10

Find the area and perimeter of a rectangle with the given dimensions.

1. 100 m by 50 m   **2.** 27 mm by 13 mm   **3.** 125 cm by 61 cm

4. If a rectangle has a width of 57 km and an area of 3648 km², what is
   (a) the length and (b) the perimeter?

Find the area of a parallelogram with the given dimensions.

5. $b = 12$ cm, $h = 11$ cm   **6.** $b = 105$ m, $h = 28$ m   **7.** $b = 17$ km, $h = 7$ km

8. If a parallelogram has a height of 13 cm and an area of 201.5 cm²,
   what is the base?

Find the area of each polygon.

9. Triangle: base 23 cm, height 7 cm   **10.** Triangle: base 35 m, height 41 m

11. Trapezoid: bases 11.5 m and 6.5 m, height 15 m

12. If a triangle has a height of 113 cm and an area of 4576.5 cm², what
   is the base?

13. If a trapezoid has an area of 531 mm² and bases of 32.1 mm and
   21 mm, what is the height?

Solve. Use $\pi \approx 3.14$ and round the answer to three digits.

14. A circle has a radius of 42 cm. What is the area?

15. A circle has a diameter of 22 m. What is the area?

16. A circle has an area of $12\frac{4}{7}$ ft². What is the diameter?

17. A circle has a radius of 56 m. What is the area?

Copy each figure and show on your drawing any lines or points of symmetry.

18.   **19.**   **20.**

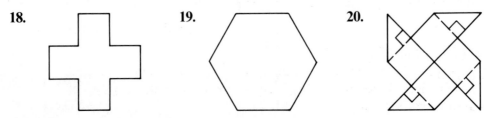

21. A prism with height 5 m has base area 173 m². Find the volume.

22. Find the volume of a cylinder with height 82 cm and base area 50 cm².

23. A right triangle with legs 15 mm and 7 mm is the base of a prism with height 24 mm. Find the volume of the prism.

24. Find the volume of a cylinder with height 300 cm and diameter 15 cm.

25. The volume of a triangular prism is 2340 cm³. Find the height of the prism if the base area is 78 cm².

26. A cone with base area 234 mm² is 82 mm high. Find its volume and its capacity in liters.

27. A pyramid with height 52 cm has a rectangular base measuring 12 cm by 17 cm. Find the volume.

28. The base of a cone has diameter 70 cm. If the height of the cone is 120 cm, what is the volume?

For Exercises 29–32, find (a) the lateral surface area and (b) the total surface area of the figure described.

29. A prism of height 15 cm whose bases are right triangles with sides 15 cm, 36 cm, and 39 cm

30. A cylinder with radius 4 cm and height 11 cm

31. A cube with edges that are 15 cm

32. A rectangular prism of height 27 cm and base 15 cm by 12 cm

For Exercises 33–36, leave your answers in terms of π.

33. Find the surface area of a sphere with radius 18 cm.

34. Find the volume of a sphere with diameter 30 cm.

35. Find the radius of a sphere whose surface area is 576π m².

36. Find the volume of a sphere whose radius is 16 cm.

37. If the mass of 1 L of gasoline is 0.66 kg, what is the mass of 4 L?

38. Each edge of a cube of steel measures 12 cm. Find the mass of the cube if the mass of 1 cm³ of steel is 7.82 g.

39. A rectangular prism of aluminum is 15 cm long, 7 cm wide, and 30 cm high. Find the mass of the prism if the mass of 1 cm³ of aluminum is 2.708 g.

Extra Practice: *Chapter 11*

If the given symbol names an integer, state the integer. If not, name the two consecutive integers between which the number lies.

1. $\sqrt{9}$ 2. $\sqrt{39}$ 3. $-\sqrt{27}$ 4. $\sqrt{10}$

5. $\sqrt{17}$ 6. $\sqrt{5}$ 7. $\sqrt{81}$ 8. $-\sqrt{12}$

9. $\sqrt{60}$ 10. $-\sqrt{78}$ 11. $\sqrt{25}$ 12. $\sqrt{19}$

13. $\sqrt{16}$ 14. $\sqrt{43}$ 15. $\sqrt{84}$ 16. $\sqrt{64}$

Approximate to the tenths' place, using the divide-and-average method.

17. $\sqrt{24}$ 18. $\sqrt{30}$ 19. $\sqrt{92}$ 20. $\sqrt{74}$

21. $\sqrt{51}$ 22. $\sqrt{29}$ 23. $\sqrt{10}$ 24. $\sqrt{86}$

25. $\sqrt{37}$ 26. $\sqrt{80}$ 27. $\sqrt{5.6}$ 28. $\sqrt{9.8}$

For Exercises 29–53, refer to the table on page 508.
Approximate the square root to the nearest hundredth.

29. $\sqrt{8}$ 30. $\sqrt{19}$ 31. $\sqrt{5}$ 32. $\sqrt{11}$

33. $\sqrt{24}$ 34. $\sqrt{52}$ 35. $\sqrt{39}$ 36. $\sqrt{2}$

37. $\sqrt{31}$ 38. $2\sqrt{18}$ 39. $\sqrt{58}$ 40. $5\sqrt{45}$

Approximate the square root to the nearest hundredth by interpolation.

41. $\sqrt{15.8}$ 42. $\sqrt{6.3}$ 43. $\sqrt{21.4}$ 44. $\sqrt{83.6}$

State whether or not a triangle with sides of the given lengths is a right triangle.

45. 2, 3, 4   46. 3, 4, 5   47. 10, 20, 24

48. 8, 15, 17   49. 10, 12, 15   50. 6, 8, 10

51. 30, 40, 50   52. 7, 9, 12   53. 12, 16, 20

A right triangle has sides of lengths *a*, *b*, and *c*, with *c* the length of the hypotenuse. Find the length of the missing side. If necessary, use the table on page 508 for the square root values and round answers to the nearest hundredth.

54. $a = 5, b = 8$ 55. $a = 4, b = 5$ 56. $a = 3, c = 5$

57. $b = 12, c = 15$ 58. $b = 15, c = 17$ 59. $a = 7, b = 7$

60. $a = 6, c = 10$ **61.** $b = 8, c = 17$ **62.** $a = 13, c = 14$

Find the lengths marked x and y. In each exercise, the triangles are similar.

63.
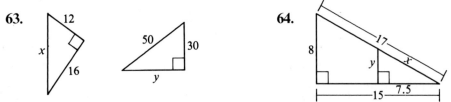
64.

Find the lengths marked x and y in the triangle. Give your answer in terms of radicals when radicals occur.

65.   **66.**   **67.**   **68.**
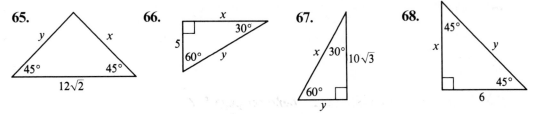

Rewrite the expression in lowest terms with the radical in the numerator.

69. $\dfrac{2}{\sqrt{3}}$ **70.** $\dfrac{5}{\sqrt{x}}$ **71.** $\dfrac{x}{\sqrt{2a}}$ **72.** $\dfrac{7}{\sqrt{4}}$

Use the diagram to name each ratio.

73. $\tan A$ **74.** $\sin A$

75. $\cos A$ **76.** $\tan B$

77. $\cos B$ **78.** $\sin B$

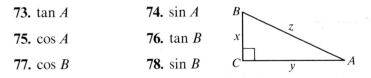

For Exercises 79–88, use the tables on pages 508 and 509. Find $\sin A$, $\cos A$, and $\tan A$ for the given measure of $\angle A$.

79. $27°$ **80.** $68°$ **81.** $89°$ **82.** $5°$

Find the measure of $\angle A$ to the nearest degree.

83. $\sin A = 0.436$ **84.** $\cos A = 0.224$ **85.** $\tan A = 1.35$

Refer to the diagram at the right.

86. Find the value of x.

87. Find $\angle D$ to the nearest degree.

88. Find $\angle E$ to the nearest degree.

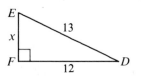

Extra Practice: *Chapter 12*

Illustrate.

1. Make a broken-line graph and a bar graph to illustrate the given data.

Class Typing Speed

Words per minute	20	19	18	17	16	15	14
Number of students	1	5	1	12	6	4	1

2. During the baseball season, Tom hit 16 home runs, Fred hit 12, Jamie hit 10, Dale hit 6, and Corey hit 6. Illustrate the data using both a pictograph and a circle graph.

Find the mean, the median, and the range of each set of data.

3. 2, 4, 5, 8, 8, 10, 12

4. 6, 7, 7, 9, 11, 12, 12, 16

5. 1, 2, 3, 3, 3, 4, 4, 7, 8, 9

6. 310, 220, 300, 300, 240, 220, 300

7. 210, 250, 190, 180, 155

8. 1.4, 1.7, 2.7, 1.9, 2.1, 2.2

9. 8000, 6000, 3000, 8000, 7000, 1000

10. 1.9, 2.1, 2.1, 1.7, 1.5, 2.1, 1.5, 1.9

Make a frequency table for the given data. Then find the mean, the median, the range, and the mode.

11. 8, 9, 10, 11, 9, 12, 12, 16, 12, 14, 11, 10, 10, 11, 10

12. 9, 7, 9, 12, 10, 11, 5, 8, 8, 7, 12, 7, 11, 10

13. 4, 2, 1, 2, 4, 2, 5, 1, 3, 3, 4, 3, 5, 2, 1, 2, 5, 5

14. 16, 17, 15, 16, 17, 18, 18, 16, 15, 17

Make a table, and arrange the data listed below into the following intervals: 4.5–34.5, 34.5–64.5, 64.5–94.5. Then use the table to make a histogram and a frequency polygon.

15. 64 91 86 23 67
    16 42 63 25 46
    44 88 48 67 86
    68 25 46 86 67
    52 25 67 32 86

16. 61 84 88 8 17
    23 27 46 10 23
    65 42 65 46 65
    23 35 46 27 46
     5 42 27 46 84

Find the value of each.

17. 6!   **18.** 3!   **19.** 10!   **20.** 2!   **21.** 5!

22. In how many different ways can you arrange the letters in the word DIRECT if you take the letters 3 at a time?

23. $_4C_2$ **24.** $_{10}C_3$ **25.** $_6C_3$ **26.** $_{12}C_2$ **27.** $_{10}C_5$

28. How many combinations of 3 fish can you choose from 7 fish?

29. There are 52 basketball teams entered in a tournament. How many combinations can make it to the final game?

A bag contains 3 green, 2 blue, 1 red, and 1 white marble. Find the probability for a marble chosen at random.

30. P(green)   **31.** P(not green)   **32.** P(yellow)

33. P(not yellow)   **34.** P(green or red)   **35.** P(red, white, or green)

Kate has 24 albums: 4 by the Deltas, 6 by the Squares, 6 by the Tuscon Band, 3 by Eliot Smith, 3 by the Marks, and 2 by the Deep River Quartet. She selects one at random.

36. Find the odds in favor of selecting a record by the following.
     a. the Marks   **b.** the Deep River Quartet   **c.** the Squares

37. Find the odds against selecting a record by the following.
     a. Eliot Smith   **b.** the Tuscon Band   **c.** the Squares

Two game cubes are rolled. Find the probability of each.

38. a. The cubes show the same number.   **39. a.** The difference is 1.
     b. The sum is 3.   **b.** The sum is 12.
     c. The cubes show the same number   **c.** The difference is 1 or the sum is
        or the sum is 3.   12.

40. $P(A) = 0.40$, $P(B) = 0.60$, $P(A \text{ and } B) = 0.24$. Find $P(A \text{ or } B)$.

41. Find the probability that a month, chosen at random, begins with the letter J or has 30 days.

42. $P(A) = 0.25$, $P(B) = 0.20$, $P(A \text{ and } B) = 0.05$. Find $P(A \text{ or } B)$.

43. Two game cubes are rolled. Find the probability of each event.
     a. The cubes show the same number.
     b. The sum is 8.
     c. The cubes show the same number and the sum is 8.
     d. The cubes show the same number or the sum is 8.

Table of Square Roots of Integers from 1 to 100

Number	Positive Square Root	Number	Positive Square Root	Number	Positive Square Root	Number	Positive Square Root
N	$\sqrt{N}$	N	$\sqrt{N}$	N	$\sqrt{N}$	N	$\sqrt{N}$
1	1	26	5.099	51	7.141	76	8.718
2	1.414	27	5.196	52	7.211	77	8.775
3	1.732	28	5.292	53	7.280	78	8.832
4	2	29	5.385	54	7.348	79	8.888
5	2.236	30	5.477	55	7.416	80	8.944
6	2.449	31	5.568	56	7.483	81	9
7	2.646	32	5.657	57	7.550	82	9.055
8	2.828	33	5.745	58	7.616	83	9.110
9	3	34	5.831	59	7.681	84	9.165
10	3.162	35	5.916	60	7.746	85	9.220
11	3.317	36	6	61	7.810	86	9.274
12	3.464	37	6.083	62	7.874	87	9.327
13	3.606	38	6.164	63	7.937	88	9.381
14	3.742	39	6.245	64	8	89	9.434
15	3.873	40	6.325	65	8.062	90	9.487
16	4	41	6.403	66	8.124	91	9.539
17	4.123	42	6.481	67	8.185	92	9.592
18	4.243	43	6.557	68	8.246	93	9.644
19	4.359	44	6.633	69	8.307	94	9.695
20	4.472	45	6.708	70	8.367	95	9.747
21	4.583	46	6.782	71	8.426	96	9.798
22	4.690	47	6.856	72	8.485	97	9.849
23	4.796	48	6.928	73	8.544	98	9.899
24	4.899	49	7	74	8.602	99	9.950
25	5	50	7.071	75	8.660	100	10

Exact square roots are shown in red. For the others, rational approximations are given correct to three decimal places.

Table of Trigonometric Ratios

Angle	Sine	Cosine	Tangent	Angle	Sine	Cosine	Tangent
1°	.0175	.9998	.0175	46°	.7193	.6947	1.0355
2°	.0349	.9994	.0349	47°	.7314	.6820	1.0724
3°	.0523	.9986	.0524	48°	.7431	.6691	1.1106
4°	.0698	.9976	.0699	49°	.7547	.6561	1.1504
5°	.0872	.9962	.0875	50°	.7660	.6428	1.1918
6°	.1045	.9945	.1051	51°	.7771	.6293	1.2349
7°	.1219	.9925	.1228	52°	.7880	.6157	1.2799
8°	.1392	.9903	.1405	53°	.7986	.6018	1.3270
9°	.1564	.9877	.1584	54°	.8090	.5878	1.3764
10°	.1736	.9848	.1763	55°	.8192	.5736	1.4281
11°	.1908	.9816	.1944	56°	.8290	.5592	1.4826
12°	.2079	.9781	.2126	57°	.8387	.5446	1.5399
13°	.2250	.9744	.2309	58°	.8480	.5299	1.6003
14°	.2419	.9703	.2493	59°	.8572	.5150	1.6643
15°	.2588	.9659	.2679	60°	.8660	.5000	1.7321
16°	.2756	.9613	.2867	61°	.8746	.4848	1.8040
17°	.2924	.9563	.3057	62°	.8829	.4695	1.8807
18°	.3090	.9511	.3249	63°	.8910	.4540	1.9626
19°	.3256	.9455	.3443	64°	.8988	.4384	2.0503
20°	.3420	.9397	.3640	65°	.9063	.4226	2.1445
21°	.3584	.9336	.3839	66°	.9135	.4067	2.2460
22°	.3746	.9272	.4040	67°	.9205	.3907	2.3559
23°	.3907	.9205	.4245	68°	.9272	.3746	2.4751
24°	.4067	.9135	.4452	69°	.9336	.3584	2.6051
25°	.4226	.9063	.4663	70°	.9397	.3420	2.7475
26°	.4384	.8988	.4877	71°	.9455	.3256	2.9042
27°	.4540	.8910	.5095	72°	.9511	.3090	3.0777
28°	.4695	.8829	.5317	73°	.9563	.2924	3.2709
29°	.4848	.8746	.5543	74°	.9613	.2756	3.4874
30°	.5000	.8660	.5774	75°	.9659	.2588	3.7321
31°	.5150	.8572	.6009	76°	.9703	.2419	4.0108
32°	.5299	.8480	.6249	77°	.9744	.2250	4.3315
33°	.5446	.8387	.6494	78°	.9781	.2079	4.7046
34°	.5592	.8290	.6745	79°	.9816	.1908	5.1446
35°	.5736	.8192	.7002	80°	.9848	.1736	5.6713
36°	.5878	.8090	.7265	81°	.9877	.1564	6.3138
37°	.6018	.7986	.7536	82°	.9903	.1392	7.1154
38°	.6157	.7880	.7813	83°	.9925	.1219	8.1443
39°	.6293	.7771	.8098	84°	.9945	.1045	9.5144
40°	.6428	.7660	.8391	85°	.9962	.0872	11.4301
41°	.6561	.7547	.8693	86°	.9976	.0698	14.3007
42°	.6691	.7431	.9004	87°	.9986	.0523	19.0811
43°	.6820	.7314	.9325	88°	.9994	.0349	28.6363
44°	.6947	.7193	.9657	89°	.9998	.0175	57.2900
45°	.7071	.7071	1.0000	90°	1.0000	.0000	Undefined

Summary of Formulas

Circumference

$C = \pi d$

$C = 2\pi r$

Area

Rectangle: $A = lw$

Triangle: $A = \frac{1}{2}bh$

Parallelogram: $A = bh$

Trapezoid: $A = \frac{1}{2}(b_1 + b_2)h$

Circle: $A = \pi r^2$

Volume

Prism: $V = Bh$

Cylinder: $V = \pi r^2 h$

Pyramid: $V = \frac{1}{3}Bh$

Cone: $V = \frac{1}{3}\pi r^2 h$

Sphere: $V = \frac{4}{3}\pi r^3$

Lateral Area

Prism: lateral area = perimeter of base $\times$ height

Cylinder: lateral area = $2\pi rh$

Surface Area

Prism: total surface area = lateral area + area of bases

Cylinder: total surface area = $2\pi rh + 2\pi r^2$

Sphere: $A = 4\pi r^2$

Mass

Mass = Density $\times$ Volume

Distance

distance = rate $\times$ time

Percentage

percentage = rate $\times$ base

Interest

Interest = Principal $\times$ rate $\times$ time

APPENDIX A: *Estimation*

Sometimes solving a problem involves long and repetitive calculations. To avoid doing these, it is often possible to use **estimation.** We *estimate* when we need to find only an approximate answer to a problem or to test the reasonableness of the calculated answer. For example, suppose that we want to find the total number of rainy days this summer, and it rained 7 days in June, 12 days in July, and 9 days in August. To find the sum we approximate each number. Notice that the numbers all *cluster* around, or are close to, 10. Thus the sum is about 10 + 10 + 10, or 30. There were approximately 30 rainy days this summer.

Estimation strategies that are frequently used include *rounding, clustering, front-end estimation,* and choosing *compatible numbers.* The example above illustrates the use of *clustering* in estimation. The **clustering** method is appropriate to use when finding a sum in which the addends are all close to the same number.

EXAMPLE 1   Estimate the total grocery bill for the following items.
$2.19, $1.88, $1.79, $2.31, $1.74, $1.98, $2.08, $2.26

Solution   Each item costs about $2.00.
The total grocery bill will be close to 8 × $2.00, or $16.00.

Front-end estimation helps us to add or subtract numbers quickly. Determine the highest place value shown for the given numbers. Add or subtract all the digits in that place value. Then adjust the answer by calculating with the digits in the next highest place value.

EXAMPLE 2   Fabric remnants are on sale for $.50 per yard. One bundle has 3 pieces of fabric, all having the same width but with lengths $1\frac{2}{3}$ yd, $1\frac{5}{8}$ yd, and 1 yd. About how much does the bundle cost?

Solution   When working with fractions, first add the whole numbers.

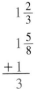

Then compensate for the fractions. Both $\frac{2}{3}$ and $\frac{5}{8}$ are close to $\frac{1}{2}$ so that the sum $\frac{2}{3} + \frac{5}{8}$ is about equal to the sum $\frac{1}{2} + \frac{1}{2}$, or 1. Thus the bundle contains around 3 + 1, or 4, yards. Since each yard costs $.50, the bundle costs about 4 × $.50, or $2.00.

Rounding is a common way of estimating. Refer to pages 14–15 for a detailed explanation of rounding. When rounding more than one number in order to estimate an answer, round each number to its highest place value to allow for fast computation.

EXAMPLE 3 Denise Crosby earns a salary of $214.33 each week. Deductions of $20.28 for federal income tax, $7.94 for state income tax, and $14.61 for Social Security are taken from her pay. About how much money does Denise take home each week?

Solution Round each deduction and then add the deductions.
Round $20.28 to $20, $7.94 to $8, and $14.61 to $10.

$$20 + 8 + 10 = 38$$

The total deductions are close to $38.

Subtract the total from the salary.
Round $214.33 to $200 and $38 to $40.

$$200 - 40 = 160$$

Denise takes home about $160 each week.

Choosing **compatible numbers** makes solving multiplication and division problems simpler. Select numbers that are easy to multiply or divide and that are close to the actual numbers.

EXAMPLE 4 A recent survey shows that about 23% of a class will vote for Bill Donnway for class treasurer. If 768 students vote, about how many can be expected to vote for Bill?

Solution Find an estimate for 23% of 768. First change the percent to one that is close to 23% and that can be converted easily to a fraction. 23% is about 25%, or $\frac{1}{4}$. Then choose a number close to 768 that has 4 as a factor. Pick 800.

$$23\% \text{ of } 768 \longrightarrow \tfrac{1}{4} \times 800 = 200$$

About 200 students will vote for Bill Donnway.

Exercises

Select the best estimate.

A **1.** $0.16 + 2.34 + 9.5$
    a. 0.12   **b.** 1.2   **c.** 12   **d.** 120

2. 4.01×8.2
    a. 0.32   **b.** 3.2   **c.** 12   **d.** 32

Select the best estimate.

3. $72{,}197 - 38{,}846$
   a. 300   b. 3000   c. 30,000   d. 300,000

4. $4213 \div 6.7$
   a. 0.6   b. 6.0   c. 60   d. 600

B 5. $489.233 + 256.1 + 133.26$
   a. 90   b. 900   c. 9000   d. 90,000

6. $\dfrac{7}{16} \times 6104$
   a. 30   b. 300   c. 3000   d. 30,000

7. 18% of 3477
   a. 0.7   b. 7   c. 70   d. 700

8. $\dfrac{7}{12} + \dfrac{4}{10}$
   a. 1   b. 2   c. 11   d. 22

C 9. $\$32.14 \div 0.78$
   a. $.04   b. $4   c. $40   d. $400

10. $0.04 + 0.0006 + 1.009$
   a. 0.019   b. 0.05   c. 0.1   d. 1

Problems

Estimate each answer.

A 1. Garth takes $1\frac{7}{12}$ hours to ride his bicycle to the lake. He rides around the lake in $2\frac{2}{3}$ hours. About how much more time does he take to ride around the lake than to the lake?

2. What is the greatest number of cassette tapes costing $6.45 each that Carolyn can buy with $20.00?

B 3. The digits in the product of 3.008×2.79 are 839232. Where should the decimal point be placed?

4. At Parts Inc. 0.023 of the parts built are defective. About how many of the 4140 parts built in an average day are defective?

C 5. A $489.66 VCR is on sale for 18% off. Approximately what is the sale price?

6. To get the most for his money, should Adam buy 60 vitamins for $6.82 or 90 of the same vitamins for $8.85?

APPENDIX B: *Stem-and-Leaf Plots*

Like a frequency distribution, a **stem-and-leaf plot** is a method of displaying data. Consider the following centimeter heights of plants in a laboratory experiment:

25 16 32 28 25 11 29 17 43 24 37 33 30

In order to create a stem-and-leaf plot, you first draw a vertical line and list the tens' digits from least to greatest to the left of the line. These are the "stems."

```
1 |
2 |
3 |
4 |
```

Next, list the units' digit for each item of data to the right of its corresponding stem. These are the "leaves."

```
1 | 6, 1, 7
2 | 5, 8, 5, 9, 4
3 | 2, 7, 3, 0
4 | 3
```

Finally, rewrite your diagram with the leaves listed from least to greatest, reading from left to right. This is the finished stem-and-leaf plot.

```
1 | 1, 6, 7
2 | 4, 5, 5, 8, 9
3 | 0, 2, 3, 7
4 | 3
```

EXAMPLE Construct a stem-and-leaf plot for the following test scores:

75 83 72 56 92 74 87 88 91 76 74 80

Solution

```
5 | 6
6 |
7 | 2, 4, 4, 5, 6
8 | 0, 3, 7, 8
9 | 1, 2
```

Note that the stem 6 is included for completeness, even though no scores require that stem.

Class Exercises

1. List the data items from which the stem-and-leaf plot shown at the right was constructed.

```
0 | 4
1 | 2, 3, 3, 7
2 | 2, 5, 6
3 | 4, 7
4 | 5, 9, 9
```

Use the following data for Exercises 2 and 3:

| 54 | 65 | 76 | 83 | 47 | 62 | 76 | 89 | 77 | 88 | 71 | 80 |

2. List the stems for this set of data.

3. List the leaves for the stems 7 and 8.

4. What are the advantages of a stem-and-leaf plot over a frequency distribution? What are the disadvantages?

Written Exercises

Construct a stem-and-leaf plot for each set of data.

A
1. 22, 14, 14, 25, 27, 31, 35, 29, 18

2. 54, 40, 41, 32, 55, 57, 58, 58, 36, 43

3. 62, 65, 43, 44, 44, 44, 50, 53, 72, 67

4. 81, 85, 70, 76, 92, 65, 97, 85, 87, 53, 66

5. 7, 23, 27, 24, 9, 5, 13, 16, 5, 30, 2, 12, 10

6. 45, 37, 28, 22, 45, 56, 25, 28, 37, 40, 42, 48

7. 92, 90, 58, 87, 56, 77, 91, 53, 53, 91, 95, 84

8. 11, 19, 5, 33, 9, 7, 5, 35, 16, 44, 5, 46, 41

B
9. Numbers of customers at a car wash on different days:
   46, 42, 45, 36, 57, 72, 54, 32, 30, 44, 73, 31, 45, 53

10. Numbers of seeds out of samples of 50 that germinated:
   42, 35, 31, 30, 9, 28, 27, 37, 35, 30, 41, 22, 25, 8, 33

11. Point totals for a basketball team in successive games:
   87, 94, 82, 78, 95, 91, 87, 83, 101, 83, 82, 77, 80, 102, 75

12. Daily patient counts at a health clinic:
   47, 39, 32, 32, 58, 63, 55, 67, 52, 44, 37, 50, 40, 71, 50

C
13. Consider the following standardized test scores:
   570, 650, 780, 460, 550, 530, 580, 610, 720, 640, 490, 520, 480

   How would you alter the rule for constructing a stem-and-leaf plot so that these data could be best displayed? Construct a stem-and-leaf plot according to your rule.

APPENDIX C: *Box-and-Whisker Plots*

A **box-and-whisker plot** is a method of displaying data that gives a quick picture of the distribution of the data items. Consider the data below, which are scores on a job aptitude test whose maximum score is 100.

56 48 66 72 37 62 49 37 29 83 74 55 46 48 52 57 44

To make a box-and-whisker plot, first put the data items in increasing order, reading from left to right.

29 37 37 44 46 48 48 49 52 55 56 57 62 66 72 74 83

Next, find the three numbers that split the data into four equal-sized parts. The second of these numbers will be the median. In this example, the median is 52. The other two numbers, called the **first quartile** and the **third quartile,** are, respectively, the medians of the lower and upper halves of the data, not including the median.

lower half	upper half

29 37 37 44 46 48 48 49 52 55 56 57 62 66 72 74 83

first quartile: median: third quartile:

$$\frac{44 + 46}{2} = 45 \qquad 52 \qquad \frac{62 + 66}{2} = 64$$

Draw a number line that includes all the *possible* data values. Underneath the line, mark with dots the boundaries of the range, the median, and the two quartiles.

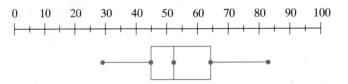

Finally, using the dots as a guide, draw a "box" around the middle half of the range, a vertical line through the median, and "whiskers" out to the two ends of the range.

Class Exercises

Exercises 1–4 refer to the box-and-whisker plot below.

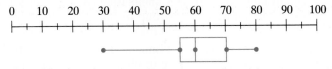

1. What is the range of the data? What is the median of the data?

2. What are the first and third quartiles?

3. Name the interval into which the middle half of the data falls.

4. Name the interval that contains the quarter of the data in which the data items are *most concentrated*.

Written Exercises

Construct a box-and-whisker plot for each set of data.

A **1.** 18, 32, 35, 37, 45, 50, 53, 55, 60, 75, 80

   2. 36, 38, 40, 45, 46, 55, 57, 60, 70, 77, 82

   3. 6.6, 5.4, 8.3, 9.2, 9.0, 7.4, 8.2, 5.8, 6.3, 6.5

   4. 114, 128, 105, 122, 130, 136, 118, 110, 129, 140

For each pair of sets of data construct two box-and-whisker plots using a common number line.

B **5.** Monthly rainfall (in inches):

   Antrim: 2.5, 2.0, 4.9, 3.4, 2.1, 1.6, 1.3, 0.7, 1.4, 3.6, 3.5, 3.5

   Brewster: 3.2, 4.1, 5.5, 7.2, 3.6, 2.1, 1.5, 1.4, 2.5, 3.8, 5.0, 4.4

   6. Scores on a math test (out of 100):

   Class 1: 92, 86, 74, 56, 82, 85, 78, 94, 95, 98, 80, 72, 63, 77

   Class 2: 82, 84, 83, 48, 56, 64, 72, 90, 88, 86, 80, 79, 68, 92

Construct a set of data that would give rise to each box-and-whisker plot.

C **7.**  **8.**

Glossary

Absolute value (p. 46) The distance from 0 to the graph of a number on the number line.

Acute angle (p. 174) An angle with measure between 0° and 90°.

Acute triangle (p. 179) A triangle with three acute angles.

Angle (p. 173) A figure formed by two rays with a common endpoint.

Annual rate of interest (p. 262) A percent of the principal figured on a yearly basis.

Arc (p. 198) A part of a circle.

Area (p. 346) Amount of surface, measured in square units.

Bar graph (p. 434) A graph in which the length of each bar is proportional to the number it represents.

Base of a geometric figure (pp. 346, 351, 352, 364) A selected side or face.

Base, numerical (p. 9) A number that is raised to some power. In 5^2, 5 is the base.

Bisector (p. 198) The line dividing a geometric figure into two congruent parts.

Broken-line graph (p. 434) A graph made by joining successive plotted points.

Capacity (p. 365) A measure of the volume of a container.

Center (pp. 188, 378) The point that is equidistant from all points on a circle or a sphere.

Chord (p. 188) A segment joining two points on a circle.

Circle (p. 188) A plane figure composed of all points measuring the same distance from a given point in the plane.

Circle graph (p. 260) A graph that uses the area of a circle to represent a sum of data. The area is divided into segments proportional to the data.

Circumference (p. 188) The perimeter of a circle.

Collinear points (p. 164) Two or more points that lie on the same line.

Combination (p. 458) An arrangement of a group of things in which order does not matter.

Common denominator (p. 100) A common multiple used as the denominator of two or more fractions that are equivalent to the given fractions.

Common factor (p. 97) A number that is a factor of two or more numbers.

Common multiple (p. 100) A number that is a multiple of two or more numbers.

Compass (p. 188) A tool used to draw a circle.

Complementary angles (p. 174) Two angles whose measures have a sum of 90°.

Cone (p. 369) A closed figure formed by a circular region and a curved surface that come to a point.

Congruent figures (pp. 192, 360) Figures that have the same size and shape.

Coordinate (p. 14) The number paired with a point on the number line.

Coordinate plane (p. 310) A plane marked with two perpendicular number lines, used to graph ordered pairs of numbers.

Corresponding angles (p. 192) The angles at matching vertices of congruent figures.

Cosine of an angle (p. 416) If $\angle A$ is one of the acute angles in a right triangle, the cosine of $\angle A$ is the ratio of the length of the side adjacent to $\angle A$ to the length of the hypotenuse.

Counting numbers (p. 89) The set of numbers 1, 2, 3, 4 . . . .

Cross-multiplying (p. 217) A method for solving and checking proportions.

Cube (p. 364) A rectangular prism having square faces.

Cube root of a number (p. 426) One of the three equal factors of a number.

Cylinder (p. 365) A geometric solid having two parallel bases that are congruent and one curved surface joining the bases.

Data (p. 434) Numerical information.

Decimal system (p. 13) The place-value numeration system that uses 10 as a base.

Degree (p. 173) Unit of angle measure.

Density (p. 382) The mass per unit volume of a substance.

Diameter (pp. 188, 378) A chord that contains the center of a circle or a sphere. Also, the length of such a chord.

Dimensions (p. 346) Length, width and height of a space figure.

Endpoint (p. 164) The point at the end of a line segment or ray.

Equation (p. 23) A mathematical sentence with an equals sign to indicate that two expressions name the same number.

Equilateral triangle (p. 179) A triangle in which all sides are congruent.

Equivalent equations (p. 130) Equations that have the same solution.

Equivalent fractions (p. 96) Fractions that name the same number.

Equivalent inequalities (p. 293) Inequalities that have the same solutions.

Evaluate an expression (p. 3) To replace variables in an expression with specified values and then complete the indicated arithmetic.

Expanded form (p. 13) The method of representing a number as the sum of products of each digit and powers of 10.

Even number (p. 84) Any multiple of 2.

Exponent (p. 9) A number indicating how many times the base is used as a factor.

Extremes of a proportion (p. 218) The first and last terms of a proportion.

Factor (p. 9) Any of two or more whole numbers that are multiplied to form a product.

Fraction (p. 97) An indicated quotient, for example $\frac{2}{5}$. The denominator, 5 in the example, tells the number of equal parts into which the whole has been divided. The numerator, 2, tells how many of these parts are being considered.

Frequency distribution (p. 446) A table that pairs each item in a set of data with its frequency.

Frequency polygon (p. 450) A line graph of frequencies connected to the horizontal axis at each end to form a polygon.

Function (p. 317) A set of ordered pairs in which no two different ordered pairs have the same x-coordinate.

Geometric construction (p. 198) A geometric drawing for which only a compass and a straightedge may be used.

Graph of an equation (p. 320) The line consisting of all points whose coordinates satisfy the equation.

Graph of a number (p. 14) The point on the number line paired with the number.

Graphs *See* Bar graph, Broken-line graph, Circle graph, Histogram, Pictograph.

Greatest common factor (GCF) (p. 97) The greatest whole number that is a factor of two or more given whole numbers.

Grouping symbols (p. 5) Symbols such as parentheses, ( ), and brackets, [ ], that are used to group expressions.

Height (p. 346) The perpendicular distance between the bases of a geometric figure. In triangles, cones, and pyramids, the perpendicular distance from the base to the opposite vertex.

Histogram (p. 450) A bar graph that shows a frequency distribution.

Hypotenuse (p. 402) The side opposite the right angle in a right triangle.

Identity elements (p. 19) 0 is the identity element for addition, because it can be added to any number without changing the value of the number. 1 is the identity element for multiplication, because it may be multiplied by any number without changing the value of the number.

Improper fraction (p. 98) A positive fraction whose numerator is greater than or equal to its denominator, or the opposite of such a fraction.

Inequality (p. 47) A mathematical sentence formed by placing an inequality sign between two expressions.

Inscribed polygon (p. 189) A polygon that has all of its vertices on the circle.

Integers (p. 46) The whole numbers and their opposites: . . . , $-2, -1, 0, 1, 2, ...$

Interest (p. 262) The amount of money paid for the use of money.

Interpolation (p. 399) A method of approximation.

Inverse operations (p. 26) Operations that undo each other. Addition and subtraction are inverse operations, as are multiplication and division.

Irrational number (p. 119) All real numbers that are not rational.

Isosceles triangle (p. 179) A triangle with at least two sides congruent.

Lateral area (p. 373) The surface area of a solid, not including the bases.

Least common denominator (LCD) (p. 100) The least common multiple of two or more denominators.

Least common multiple (LCM) (p. 100) The least number that is a multiple of two or more nonzero numbers.

Legs of a right triangle (p. 402) The two sides forming the right angle.

Like terms (p. 282) Terms in which the variable parts are the same.

Line (p. 164) A figure determined by two points and extending in both directions without end.

Line segment (p. 164) Two points on a line and all the points between them.

Linear equation in two variables (p. 321) An equation with two variables that can be written in the form $ax + by = c$, where a and b are both not 0.

Lowest terms (p. 97) A fraction is in lowest terms when the numerator and the denominator have no common factor but 1.

Mass (p. 382) The measure of the amount of matter an object contains.

Mean (p. 443) The value found by dividing the sum of a group of numbers by the number of numbers in the group. Also called *average*.

Means of a proportion (p. 218) The second and third terms of a proportion.

Median (p. 443) The number that falls in the middle when data are listed from least to greatest. If the number of data is even, the median is the mean of the two middle items.

Midpoint (p. 169) The point of a segment that divides it into two congruent segments.

Mixed number (p. 98) A whole number plus a proper fraction.

Mode (p. 447) The number that occurs most often in a set of data.

Multiple (p. 84) A product of a given number and any whole number.

Mutually exclusive events (p. 470) Events that cannot both occur at the same time.

Noncollinear points (p. 164) Points not on the same line.

Number line (p. 14) A line on which consecutive integers are assigned to equally spaced points on the line in increasing order from left to right.

Number sentence (p. 23) An equation or inequality indicating the relationship between two mathematical expressions.

Numerical coefficient (p. 3) In an expression such as $3ab$, the number 3 is the numerical coefficient of ab.

Numerical expression (p. 2) An expression that names a number, such as $2 + 3$.

Obtuse angle (p. 174) An angle with measure between 90° and 180°.

Obtuse triangle (p. 179) A triangle that has one obtuse angle.

Odd number (p. 84) A whole number that is not a multiple of 2.

Odds of an event (p. 466) A ratio that compares the probability of an event occurring and the probability of the event not occurring.

Open sentence (p. 23) A mathematical sentence that contains one or more variables.

Opposites (p. 46) A pair of numbers such as −4 and 4.

Ordered pair of numbers (p. 312) A pair of numbers whose order is important.

Origin (pp. 14, 312) The graph of zero on a number line, or $(0, 0)$ in a rectangular coordinate plane.

Outcome (p. 461) The result of an event.

Parallel lines (p. 165) Lines in the same plane that do not intersect.

Parallel planes (p. 165) Planes that do not intersect.

Parallelogram (p. 183) A quadrilateral with both pairs of opposite sides parallel.

Percent (p. 227) A ratio of a number to 100, shown by the symbol %.

Percent of change (p. 246) The amount of change divided by the original amount.

Perfect square (p. 394) A number whose square root is an integer.

Perimeter (p. 184) The distance around a plane figure.

Permutation (p. 453) An arrangement of a group of things in a particular order.

Perpendicular bisector (p. 198) The line that is perpendicular to a segment at its midpoint.

Perpendicular lines (p. 173) Two lines that intersect to form 90° angles.

Pi (p. 188) The ratio of the circumference of a circle to its diameter.

Pictograph (p. 438) A form of bar graph with the bars replaced by rows or columns of symbols.

Plane (p. 165) A flat surface extending infinitely in all directions.

Point (p. 164) The simplest figure in geometry representing an exact location.

Polygon (p. 183) A closed plane figure made up of line segments.

Polyhedron (p. 364) A three-dimensional figure formed of polygonal parts of planes.

Power of a number (pp. 9, 70) A product in which all the factors, except 1, are the same. For example, $2^3 = 2 \times 2 \times 2 = 8$, so 8 is the third power of 2.

Prime factorization (p. 90) An expression showing a positive integer as the product of prime factors.

Prime number (p. 89) A whole number greater than 1 that has only two whole number factors, itself and 1.

Principal (p. 262) An amount of money on which interest is paid.

Prism (p. 364) A polyhedron that has two parallel, congruent faces called bases. The other faces are parallelograms.

Probability (p. 461) The ratio of the number of outcomes favoring an event to the total number of possible outcomes.

Proper fraction (p. 98) A positive fraction whose numerator is less than its denominator, or the opposite of such a fraction.

Proportion (p. 217) An equation stating that two ratios are equal.

Protractor (p. 173) A device used to measure angles.

Pyramid (p. 369) A polyhedron that has a polygonal base and three or more triangular faces.

Quadrilateral (p. 183) A polygon with four sides.

Radical (p. 412) An expression such as $\sqrt{5}$ or $\sqrt{a}$; the radical sign symbol used to denote the square root of a number.

Radius (pp. 188, 356) A line segment joining any point on a circle or sphere to the center. Also, the length of that segment.

Random variable (p. 461) A variable whose value is determined by the outcome of a random experiment.

Range (p. 443) The difference between the greatest and the least numbers in a set of data.

Rate (p. 214) A ratio that compares quantities of different kinds of units.

Ratio (p. 210) An indicated quotient of two numbers.

Ray (p. 164) A part of a line with one endpoint.

Real number (p. 119) Any number that is either a rational number or an irrational number.

Reciprocals (p. 113) Two numbers whose product is 1.

Rectangle (p. 184) A quadrilateral with four right angles.

Regular polygon (p. 183) A polygon in which all sides are congruent and all angles are congruent.

Relatively prime numbers (p. 97) Two or more numbers that have no common factor but 1.

Replacement set (p. 23) The given set of numbers that a variable may represent.

Rhombus (p. 184) A parallelogram in which all sides are congruent.

Right angle (p. 174) An angle with measure 90°.

Right triangle (p. 179) A triangle with a right angle.

Rigid motions (p. 193) Motions such as rotation, translation, and reflection, used to move a figure to a new position without changing its shape or size.

Rounding (p. 14) A method of approximating a number.

Scalene triangle (p. 179) A triangle with no two sides congruent.

Scientific notation (p. 76) A method of expressing a number as the product of a power of 10 and a number between 1 and 10.

Segment (p. 164) *See* line segment.

Semicircle (p. 188) Half of a circle.

Sides of an equation (p. 23) The mathematical expressions to the right and to the left of the equals sign.

Sides of a figure (pp. 178, 183, 212) The rays that form an angle or the segments that form a polygon.

Similar figures (p. 196) Figures that have the same shape but not necessarily the same size.

Simple form (p. 106) A mixed number is in simple form if its fractional part is expressed in lowest terms.

Simplify an expression (p. 2) To replace an expression with its simplest name.

Sine of an angle (p. 416) If $\angle A$ is an acute angle of a right triangle, the sine of $\angle A$ is the ratio of the length of the side opposite $\angle A$ to the length of the hypotenuse.

Skew lines (p. 166) Two nonparallel lines that do not intersect.

Slope of a line (p. 328) The steepness of a line; that is, the ratio of the change in the y-coordinate to the change in the x-coordinate when moving from one point on a line to another point.

Solid (p. 364) An enclosed region of space bounded by planes.

Solution (pp. 23, 130) A value of a variable that makes an equation or inequality a true sentence.

Solving a right triangle (p. 420) The process of finding the measures of the sides and angles of a right triangle.

Sphere (p. 378) A figure in space made up of all points equidistant from a given point.

Square (p. 184) A rectangle with all four sides congruent.

Square root of a number (p. 394) One of the two equal factors of the number.

Statistical measures (p. 443) Measures including the range, mean, median, and mode used to analyze numerical data.

Supplementary angles (p. 174) Two angles whose measures have a sum of 180°.

Surface area (p. 373) The total area of a solid.

Symmetric (p. 360) A figure is symmetric with respect to a line if it can be folded on that line so that every point on one side coincides exactly with a point on the other side. A figure is symmetric with respect to a point O if for each point A on the figure there is a point B on the figure for which O is the midpoint of AB.

System of equations (p. 324) A set of two or more equations in the same variables.

Tangent of an angle (p. 416) If $\angle A$ is an acute angle of a right triangle, the tangent of $\angle A$ is the ratio of the length of the side opposite $\angle A$ to the length of the side adjacent to $\angle A$.

Terms of an expression (p. 3) The parts of a mathematical expression that are separated by a $+$ sign.

Terms of a proportion (p. 217) The numbers in a proportion.

Transformation (pp. 130, 282) Rewriting an equation or inequality as an equivalent equation or inequality.

Trapezoid (p. 183) A quadrilateral with exactly one pair of parallel sides.

Triangle (p. 178) A polygon with three sides.

Trigonometric ratios (p. 416) Any of the sine, cosine, or tangent ratios.

Value of a variable (p. 2) Any number that a variable represents.

Variable (p. 2) A symbol used to represent one or more numbers.

Variable expression (p. 2) A mathematical expression that contains a variable.

Vertex of an angle (p. 173) The common endpoint of two intersecting rays.

Vertex of a polygon or polyhedron (p. 178) The point at which two sides of a polygon or three or more edges of a polyhedron intersect.

Volume (p. 364) A measure of the space occupied by a solid.

x-axis (p. 312) The horizontal number line on a coordinate plane.

x-coordinate (p. 312) The first number in an ordered pair of numbers that designates the location of a point on the coordinate plane. Also called the *abscissa*.

y-axis (p. 312) The vertical number line on a coordinate plane.

y-coordinate (p. 312) The second number in an ordered pair of numbers that designates the location of a point on the coordinate plane. Also called the *ordinate*.

Index

in dividing fractions, 113
in solving equations, 134, 139
in solving inequalities, 293, 297
Inverted short division, 89
Irrational numbers, 119, 397
Irrigation, center-pivot, 162

Keyboard, computer, 39
Kilobyte (K), 38
Kilogram, 382
Kilometers, 170, 202, 214
KOVALESKI, SONYA, 304, 305

Languages, computer, 39
Lateral surface, 373
    area, 373
    faces, 373
Latitude, 386
Least common denominator (LCD), 100
Least common multiple (LCM), 100, 121
Legs, of triangle, 402, 411
    See also Sides
Length
    golden ratio of, 239
    measures of, 169, 224, 346, 402–403
    radius and diameter, 188, 378
    scale drawings and, 224
Less than, 13, 47
Less than or equal to, 13, 47
LET statement, 202
Lightning, 44
Like terms, 282
Line segments, 50, 164
Linear equation(s)
    the computer and, 338
    in two variables, 321
Line(s), 164
    boundary, 334
    intersecting, 165, 173, 312
    parallel, 165, 325
    perpendicular, 173, 387
    skew, 166
    slope of, 328
    of symmetry, 360
LIST command, 123
Liter, 365
LOGO, 39
Longitude, 386

Loop, programming, 203
Lowest terms
    of fractions, 97, 118
    of ratios, 210

Magnifying power, 208
Mainframes, 38
Markup, price, 250
Mass, 382
Mathematical expressions, 2
    compared using inequality symbols, 47
    in equations, 23
    in scientific notation, 76
Mathematicians, 304–305
Mean, 443, 474
Means, of a proportion, 218
Measurement(s), 169
    of angles, 173
    in ratios, 210
    of volume, 364
    in right triangles, 411
    of a distribution, 474
    using scientific notation, 76–77
    statistical, 432, 443
    units of, 224, 364, 365, 382
Mechanical advantage, 212
Median, 443
Memory, computer
    ROM and RAM, 38
Mercator projection, 387
Meridian(s), 386
    prime, 386
Meter, 169
Metric system, 169, 382
    rates, 214
Metric ton, 382
Microchip, facing page 1
Microcomputers, 38, 122
Microprocessor, 38
Microscope, electron, 208
Midpoint, 169
Mile, 202, 214
Milliliters, 365
Millimeters, 169
Minicomputers, 38
Minimum payment, 274–275
Mixed numbers, 98
    adding and subtracting, 106
    converting to fractions, 106
    from percentages, 228
    multiplying, 111
Mode, 447
Modem, computer, 39

Molecules, 156
Multiple, 84–85
    least common (LCM), 100
Multiplication
    cross-, 217, 218
    to find percentages, 234
    of fractions, 96, 109
    and identity elements, 19
    and inverse operations, 26, 139
    of mixed numbers, 111
    to obtain multiples, 84
    in order of operations, 5
    of positive and negative numbers, 63
    properties of, 18–19, 282
    symbols, 5
    transformation by, 134
Multiplication property of one, 19
    in multiplying fractions, 109
Multiplication property of zero, 19
    in multiplying positive and negative numbers, 63
    in dividing positive and negative numbers, 67
Multiplier, 20
Mutually exclusive, 470

National Aeronautics and Space Administration (NASA), 128
Negative numbers, 46
    adding, 54
    as decimals, 50
    dividing, 67, 293
    as exponents, 73
    expressed in scientific notation, 76
    as integers, 46–47, 73
    multiplying, 63, 293
    subtracting, 59
NEXT statement, 203
Nobel prize, 244
NOETHER, EMMY, 305
Noncollinear points, 164
North pole, 386
Not equal to, 47
Number line, 14, 119, 312
    addends and sums on, 54
    decimals on, 50, 119
    fractions on, 92, 96

Credits

Mechanical art: ANCO/Boston. Cover concept: Kirchoff/Wohlberg, Inc., cover photograph: Balthazar Korab. Page 1, Gregory Heisler/Gamma-Liaison; 32, Milt & Joan Mann/The Marilyn Gartman Agency; 45, Ralph Wetmore/Photo Researchers, Inc.; 58, Clyde H. Smith/Peter Arnold, Inc.; 62, Gary Milburn/Tom Stack & Associates; 76, NASA; 83, © Paulo Bonino 1982/Photo Researchers, Inc.; 88, © Dan McCoy/Rainbow; 116, Greig Cranna; 129, NASA; 151, VANSCAN™ Thermogram by Daedalus Enterprises; 156, © Julie Houck 1983; 163, Grant Heilman Photography; 186, © S.L.O.T.S./Taurus Photos; 190, NASA; 200, Rainbow; 202, Dr. J. Lorre/Photo Researchers, Inc.; 209, Peter Arnold, Inc.; 216, Benn Mitchell © 1981/The Image Bank; 221, Greig Cranna; 230, Brian Parker/Tom Stack & Associates; 236, © Peter Menzel/Stock, Boston; 238, Greig Cranna; 245, Langridge/McCoy/Rainbow; 255, © Dick Luria 1982/The Stock Shop; 272, © John Lee/The Image Bank; 274, Thomas Hovland/Grant Heilman Photography; 281, Courtesy of French National Railroads; 289, Hank Morgan/Rainbow; 304, German Information Center; 311, Photo Courtesy of LEXIDATA; 333, © Lou Jones 1981/The Image Bank; 345; Owen Franken/Stock, Boston; 359, © Rick Smolan/Stock, Boston; 380, © Van Bucher 1982/Photo Researchers, Inc.; 386, © Dick Davis 1972/Photo Researchers, Inc.; 393, © Jerry Wachter Photography/Focus on Sports; 401, Milt & Joan Mann/The Marilyn Gartman Agency; 415, © 1979 Stuart Cohen/Stock, Boston; 426, © C. B. Jones 1982/Taurus Photos; 433, Robert C. Fields/Animals Animals; 444, Frederic Lewis Inc.; 460, Mike Mazzaschi/Stock, Boston; 474, Russ Kinne/Photo Researchers, Inc.

Answers to Selected Exercises

1 Introduction to Algebra

PAGE 4 WRITTEN EXERCISES **1.** 48
3. 105 **5.** 14.15 **7.** 4.5 **9.** 25 **11.** 4 **13.** 12
15. 27 **17.** 2 **19.** 47 **21.** 26 **23.** 512 **25.** 9
27. 24 **29.** 2.5 **31.** 112.5 **33.** 680.805
35. 3.15 **37.** 2

PAGE 4 REVIEW EXERCISES **1.** 51.87
3. 45.93 **5.** 0.27 **7.** 6.3

PAGES 7–8 WRITTEN EXERCISES **1.** 92
3. 51 **5.** 2 **7.** 126 **9.** 7 **11.** 36 **13.** 10
15. 70 **17.** 36 **19.** 196 **21.** 3 **23.** 1512
25. 91 **27.** 84 **29.** 0.5 **31.** 4.1 **33.** 5827.248
35. 14.6 **37.** $2x \times (y - 4) + 2x$
or $2x \times y - (4 + 2)x$
39. $x \times [y + (z \div 3 + 1)] - z$

PAGE 8 REVIEW EXERCISES **1.** 5 **3.** 6
5. 3 **7.** 168

PAGE 8 CALCULATOR KEY-IN **1.** 288
3. 16.5 **5.** 6048

PAGES 11–12 WRITTEN EXERCISES **1.** 5^6
3. 8^9 **5.** 7^7 **7.** 4^6 **9.** 10^1 **11.** 10^6
13. 1,000,000 **15.** 10,000 **17.** 16 **19.** 256
21. 400 **23.** 3375 **25.** 6400 **27.** 256 **29.** 1296
31. 4096 **33.** 125 **35.** 169 **37.** 400
39. 1,680,700 **41.** 0 **43.** 961 **45.** 256
47. 6912 **49.** 72,000 **51.** 0 **53.** 27 **55.** 90,000
57. 27 **59.** 218 **61.** 25 **63.** 225 **65.** 3375
67. 16

PAGE 12 REVIEW EXERCISES **1.** 60 **3.** 57
5. 30 **7.** 24

PAGES 16–17 WRITTEN EXERCISES
1. $(3 \times 10) + 8$ **3.** $(8 \times 1000) + (9 \times 10) + 1$
5. $(4 \times 0.1) + (7 \times 0.01)$
7. $(6 \times 0.01) + (3 \times 0.001)$
9. $(1 \times 0.1) + (8 \times 0.01) + (7 \times 0.001)$
11. 54.57 **13.** 9002.146 **15.** 7.43 **17.** 19.005
19. 0.0048 **21.** 6.025 **23.** 30 **25.** 290 **27.** 650
29. 160 **31.** 72.46 **33.** 0.06 **35.** 0.01 **37.** 18.17
39. 0.001 **41.** 401.090 **43.** 250.341
45. 8.100 **47.** $(5 \times 10^3) + (2 \times 10^2) + (8 \times 10^1)$
49. $(1 \times 10^2) + (8 \times 10^1) +$
$$(3 \times 10^0) + \left(8 \times \frac{1}{10^2}\right)$$
51. $\left(9 \times \frac{1}{10^2}\right) + \left(1 \times \frac{1}{10^3}\right)$

53. $(7 \times 10^0) + \left(4 \times \frac{1}{10^1}\right) + \left(8 \times \frac{1}{10^2}\right) +$
$$\left(2 \times \frac{1}{10^3}\right)$$
55. $(2 \times 10^2) + (4 \times 10^0) + \left(5 \times \frac{1}{10^1}\right)$
57. $(3 \times 10^1) + (8 \times 10^0) + \left(3 \times \frac{1}{10^3}\right)$ **59.** b
61. a **63.** b **65.** c

PAGE 17 REVIEW EXERCISES **1.** 9.4
3. 960 **5.** 60 **7.** 14.8

PAGES 21–22 WRITTEN EXERCISES
1. 14.6; associative **3.** 14.24; distributive
5. 18.97; commutative and associative
7. 0.21; commutative and associative
9. False **11.** True **13.** $n = 0$ **15.** $t = 3.2$
17. $w = 0$ **19.** $g = 15.9$ **21.** $n = 3$
23. $d = 1565$ **25.** $t = 0$ **27.** 3.88 **29.** 400
31. 900 **33.** 32 For exercises 35 and 37,
answers will vary. An example is given.
35. $a = 2, b = 3, c = 4$
37. $a = 2, b = 4, c = 6$

PAGE 22 SELF-TEST A **1.** 46 **2.** 15 **3.** 168
4. 9 **5.** 4 **6.** 6 **7.** 16 **8.** 512 **9.** 9
10. 100,000 **11.** 100,000 **12.** 80 **13.** 3.18
14. 300 **15.** 102 **16.** 93 **17.** 21 **18.** 67.96

PAGES 24–25 WRITTEN EXERCISES
1. True **3.** False **5.** False **7.** True **9.** True
11. True **13.** 29 **15.** 8 **17.** No solution
19. No solution **21.** 1518 **23.** 1.26 **25.** 11
27. 12 **29.** 9 **31.** 2 **33.** No solution **35.** 4
For exercises 37 and 39, answers will vary. An
example is given. **37.** $3x + 5 = 35$
39. $(x + 20) \div 6 - 10 = 10$ **41.** $+, -$
43. $+, \div$ **45.** $\div, -, \times$ **47.** $-, +, \div$

PAGE 25 REVIEW EXERCISES **1.** 11.67
3. 27.14 **5.** 7.337 **7.** 2.84

PAGE 28 WRITTEN EXERCISES
1. $x = 15 - 8; 7$ **3.** $f = 74 - 38; 36$
5. $y = 14 + 9; 23$ **7.** $b = 32 + 25; 57$
9. $c = 27 \div 3; 9$ **11.** $m = 108 \div 9; 12$
13. $n = 9 \times 6; 54$ **15.** $g = 7 \times 16; 112$
17. $a = 17 - 17; 0$ **19.** $n = 42 \div 14; 3$
21. $h = 297 \times 11; 3267$ **23.** $d = 110 + 87; 197$
25. $q = 465 \div 31; 15$ **27.** $p = 358 - 208; 150$
29. $c = 536 - 511; 25$ **31.** $g = 401 + 19; 420$
33. $x = 31.9 - 1.6; 30.3$ **35.** $c = 2.56 \div 1.6;$
1.6 **37.** 6 **39.** 7 **41.** 13 **43.** 17 **45.** 24

47. 120 **49.** 0.54 **51.** 3.3 **53.** 12.84
55. ×, + **57.** ×, − **59.** ÷, +

PAGE 28 REVIEW EXERCISES **1.** 2 **3.** 52
5. 60 **7.** 31

PAGES 31–32 PROBLEMS **1.** 11.65 m
3. $41,520 **5.** $7.20 **7.** 936 people **9.** $1596
11. $4.25

PAGE 32 REVIEW EXERCISES **1.** 340
3. 175 **5.** 500 **7.** 400

PAGES 35–37 PROBLEMS **1.** $113.70
3. $24.79 **5.** 22 bonus points **7.** smaller:
4265 square ft; larger: 16,620 square ft
9. 41 points **11.** $488.25 **13.** 12,948 shares
15. $3.90

PAGE 37 SELF-TEST B **1.** 29 **2.** 8 **3.** No
solution **4.** 3 **5.** 44 **6.** 16 **7.** 9 **8.** $114.15
9. 49 passengers **10.** $182.24

PAGE 40 CHAPTER REVIEW **1.** F **3.** A
5. D **7.** False **9.** True **11.** True **13.** False
15. False **17.** False **19.** False **21.** d

PAGE 42 CUMULATIVE REVIEW
EXERCISES **1.** 809 **3.** 3.1 **5.** 351.9 **7.** 27
9. 25 **11.** 2 **13.** 43 **15.** 16.5 **17.** 6 **19.** 27
21. 64 **23.** 15,625 **25.** a **27.** a **29.** False
31. False **33.** 7 **35.** 3 **37.** 19 **39.** 2 **41.** 13
43. 2

PAGE 43 CUMULATIVE REVIEW
PROBLEMS **1.** $3010 **3.** $42.95 **5.** $20
7. $17

2 Positive and Negative Numbers
PAGES 48–49 WRITTEN EXERCISES

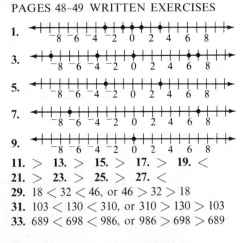

11. > **13.** > **15.** > **17.** > **19.** <
21. > **23.** > **25.** > **27.** <
29. 18 < 32 < 46, or 46 > 32 > 18
31. 103 < 130 < 310, or 310 > 130 > 103
33. 689 < 698 < 986, or 986 > 698 > 689

35. 3 **37.** 0 **39.** 9 **41.** 8 **43.** ⁻15, ⁻2, 0, 6
45. ⁻12, ⁻8, ⁻1, 1, 7 **47.** ⁻14, ⁻10, 4, 8, 14
49. ⁻6.4, ⁻2.7, 0.6, 3.1
51. 6, ⁻6

53. 4, ⁻4

55. 0

57. ⁻1, 0, 1

59. ⁻4, ⁻3, ⁻2, ⁻1, 0, 1, 2, 3, 4

61. ⁻7, ⁻6, ⁻5, ⁻4, ⁻3, 3, 4, 5, 6, 7

63. positive **65.** No number has a negative
absolute value.

PAGE 49 REVIEW EXERCISES

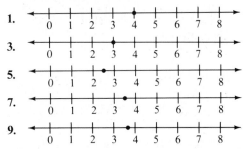

PAGES 52–53 WRITTEN EXERCISES

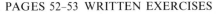

11.

$-0.3\ 0.3$

(number line from $^-6$ to 4)

13. 2.36 **15.** 16 **17.** 3.03 **19.** $<$ **21.** $<$
23. $<$ **25.** $>$ **27.** $<$ **29.** $^-8,\ ^-7.6,\ ^-1.75,$
6.03, 6.3 **31.** $^-100.5,\ ^-46.8,\ ^-2.1,\ ^-2,\ 3.11$
33. $^-3.3,\ ^-0.33,\ ^-0.3,\ 30.3,\ 33$
35.

2.5 ; $^-0.5$

(number line from $^-6$ to 4)

37.

$^-3$; $^-3.5\ ^-0.5$

(number line from $^-6$ to 4)

39.

$^-4$

(number line from $^-6$ to 4)

41. 4.1, $^-4.1$ **43.** 26.3, $^-26.3$ **45.** 1.19, $^-1.19$
47. $^-4.5$ **49.** $^-12$ **50.** 8.25 **51. a.** 4, 3, 2, 1, 0,
$^-1,\ ^-2,\ ^-3,\ ^-4$
b.

(number line from $^-6$ to 4)

53. a. $^-5,\ ^-4,\ ^-3,\ ^-2,\ ^-1,\ 0,\ 1,\ 2,\ 3,\ 4,\ 5$
b.

(number line from $^-6$ to 4)

PAGE 53 REVIEW EXERCISES **1.** 11.14;
distributive **3.** 27.18; multiplicative property
of one **5.** 132.3; distributive **7.** 1075;
commutative and associative **9.** 0;
multiplicative property of zero

PAGE 57 WRITTEN EXERCISES
1.

$^-11$; $^-8$; $^-3$

(number line from $^-12$ to 10)

3.

22 ; 9.5 ; $^-12.5$

(number line from $^-12$ to 10)

5. $^-19$ **7.** $^-13$ **9.** $^-0.3$ **11.** 0 **13.** 16.2
15. 4.17 **17.** 0 **19.** $^-0.12$ **21.** 6.3 **23.** $^-10.8$
25. $^-7.25$ **27.** 12 **29.** $^-12$ **31.** $^-18.5$
33. $^-2.4$ **35.** $^-19.8$ **37.** $^-25.9$ **39.** $<$ **41.** $>$
43. a. $=$ **b.** $<$ **c.** $<$ **d.** $<$ **e.** $=$ **f.** $<$
g. $|x + y| \leq |x| + |y|$

PAGE 58 PROBLEMS **1.** $^-7 + 13 + ^-3$;
$3°C$ **3.** $3.5 + ^-11 + 2$; lost; 5.5 yd lost
5. $^-4.30 + 2.50 + 2.60$; gain

PAGE 58 REVIEW EXERCISES **1.** 156.1
3. 64.9 **5.** 44.89 **7.** 4.2 **9.** 285

PAGES 60–61 WRITTEN EXERCISES
1. $7 + (-19)$ **3.** $6.2 + 8.3$ **5.** -12 **7.** 14.5
9. -6 **11.** -27 **13.** 42 **15.** 15 **17.** -43
19. 20 **21.** 44 **23.** -1.1 **25.** 2.2 **27.** -24.6
29. -24.6 **31.** 3.37 **33.** 24.8 **35.** -41.3
37. 1.8 **39.** 4.5 **41.** -6.2 **43.** 1.7 **45.** 10.7
47. -10.7 **49.** 1.7 **51.** 8 **53.** 8 **55.** -19
57. -18 **59.** 7 **61.** -8 **63. a.** $=$ **b.** $>$
c. $>$ **d.** $>$ **e.** $|x - y| \geq |x| - |y|$

PAGES 61–62 PROBLEMS **1.** $-3 - (-11)$;
$8°C$ change **3.** $1266 - 1455$; 229 m
5. $18.75 - 1.00 - 1.75 - 1.50$; \$14.50
7. $78 - 5.8 - 7.5 - 12$; 52.7 cm **9.** \$44.22

PAGE 62 SELF-TEST A **1.** $<$ **2.** $>$ **3.** $<$
4. $=$ **5.** $=$ **6.** $^-54,\ ^-4.52,\ ^-0.25,\ 0,\ 5.4$
7. $^-7.3,\ ^-3.79,\ ^-0.37,\ ^-0.09,\ 37$ **8.** 33 **9.** 0
10. $^-1.44$ **11.** 35 **12.** 0 **13.** -36 **14.** 11.6
15. -11.6 **16.** -11.6

PAGES 65–66 WRITTEN EXERCISES
1. 27 **3.** -56 **5.** 96 **7.** 0 **9.** -12
11. 5.1 **13.** -2.9 **15.** 15.4 **17.** -5 **19.** 459
21. -66.69 **23.** 0 **25.** 3.42 **27.** -111.24
29. 37.875 **31.** 61.38 **33.** -1.054 **35.** 0
37. 361.9 **39.** -40.81 **41.** -8.2 **43.** -100
45. -2 **47.** -2 **49.** 0 **51.** 2 **53.** -30
55. 0

PAGE 66 REVIEW EXERCISES **1.** 56
3. 154 **5.** 13 **7.** 26

PAGE 66 CALCULATOR KEY-IN 8192

PAGES 68–69 WRITTEN EXERCISES
1. -6 **3.** 3 **5.** 0 **7.** -12 **9.** -7.5 **11.** 3.6
13. -35 **15.** -5.3 **17.** 8 **19.** 0 **21.** -0.5
23. -9.5 **25.** -2.2 **27.** 13.8 **29.** 0.1545
31. -6.3 **33.** 4.7 **35.** -1.85 **37.** -3.2
39. 0.625 **41.** -4.2 **43.** -1.2 **45.** -2
47. -72 **49.** -8

PAGE 69 REVIEW EXERCISES **1.** 49
3. 784 **5.** 112 **7.** 1 **9.** 37

PAGE 69 CALCULATOR KEY-IN **1.** 1.1
3. -28.201 **5.** 5101.015

PAGES 71–72 WRITTEN EXERCISES
1. 64 **3.** 100 **5.** 14 **7.** 225 **9.** 1 **11.** 3^2
13. 9^2 **15.** $(16 \times 4)^2$ **17.** 2^7 **19.** 10^5 **21.** n^{11}
23. 100 **25.** 81 **27.** 576 **29.** 1 **31.** 1875

33. 225 **35.** 1 **37.** 1000 **39.** 96 **41.** 52
43. 4 **45.** $\frac{1}{8}$ **47.** 1

PAGE 72 REVIEW EXERCISES **1.** -2
3. 2 **5.** 12 **7.** 1

PAGE 72 CALCULATOR KEY-IN **1.** 56,
56 **3.** 3243, 3243 $\qquad a^2 - b^2, (a + b)(a - b)$

PAGE 74 WRITTEN EXERCISES **1.** $-\frac{1}{32}$
3. $\frac{1}{1000}$ **5.** 1 **7.** $\frac{1}{25}$ **9.** $\frac{1}{64}$ **11.** $\frac{1}{49}$ **13.** 1
15. $\frac{1}{27}$ **17.** $\frac{1}{256}$ **19.** $-\frac{1}{8}$ **21.** 1 **23.** -3
25. 5 **27.** -2 **29.** -2 **31.** 8 **33.** 0 **35.** 1
37. -4 **39.** -3 **41.** $\frac{1}{x^5}$ **43.** $\frac{1}{a^5}$ **45.** $\frac{1}{w^8}$

PAGE 75 SELF-TEST B **1.** -47.46
2. -136.68 **3.** 378 **4.** -11 **5.** -31 **6.** 8
7. 8 **8.** 225 **9.** 1296 **10.** $\frac{1}{16}$ **11.** $-\frac{1}{216}$
12. $\frac{1}{343}$ **13.** $\frac{1}{81}$

PAGES 76–77 ENRICHMENT
1. 5.798×10^3 **3.** 8.915673×10^6 **5.** 1.75
7. 5.01×10^{-2} **9.** 3790 **11.** 301,000
13. 0.056 **15.** 0.0000000399 **17.** 7.4×10^{-4}
19. 1.5×10^{11}

PAGE 78 CHAPTER REVIEW **1.** $<$ **3.** $>$
5. $=$ **7.** $<$ **9.** $>$ **11.** $>$ **13.** False
15. True **17.** True **19.** False **21.** True
23. False **25.** False **27.** True **29.** True
31. True **33.** True **35.** True **37.** c **39.** d
41. d

PAGES 80–81 CUMULATIVE REVIEW
EXERCISES **1.** 6 **3.** 180 **5.** 3 **7.** 17
9. True **11.** True **13.** False **15.** False
17. True **19.** $^-6.18$ **21.** -8 **23.** 4.3
25. -0.12 **27.** -9 **29.** -1.6 **31.** 4.009
33. 7700 **35.** 909.1 **37.** 103.6 **39.** 10^{10} or
10,000,000,000 **41.** 64 **43.** 6 **45.** 100
47. $-20, -7, 0, 6, 12, 15$ **49.** $-5, -3, 0, 1, 7,$
9

PAGE 81 CUMULATIVE REVIEW
PROBLEMS **1.** \$59.46 **3.** 4 times **5.** Deli
Delights

3 Rational Numbers

PAGES 87–88 WRITTEN EXERCISES **1.** 1,
2, 3, 6, 7, 14, 21, 42 **3.** 1, 2, 4, 8, 16, 32 **5.** 1,
2, 4, 7, 8, 14, 28, 56 **7.** 1, 2, 3, 4, 6, 7, 12, 14,
21, 28, 42, 84 **9.** 1, 41 **11.** 2, 3, 4 **13.** 3, 5
15. 3, 9 **17.** 2, 3, 4, 5, 10 **19.** none

21. a. yes **b.** no **c.** no **23. a.** yes **b.** yes
c. yes **25. a.** yes **b.** yes **c.** yes **27.** 4
29. 5 **31.** 9 **33.** if number represented by last
three digits is a multiple of 8 **35.** if last two
digits are 00, 25, 50, or 75

PAGE 88 REVIEW EXERCISES **1.** $<$
3. $>$ **5.** $<$ **7.** $>$

PAGE 91 WRITTEN EXERCISES
1. composite **3.** composite **5.** composite
7. prime **9.** composite **11.** composite
13. $2^2 \cdot 3$ **15.** $2^3 \cdot 3$ **17.** $3 \cdot 13$ **19.** $2 \cdot 3 \cdot 11$
21. $2 \cdot 3^3$ **23.** $2^2 \cdot 3 \cdot 7$ **25.** $2^2 \cdot 7^2$
27. $2^2 \cdot 7 \cdot 11$ **29.** $2 \cdot 3 \cdot 19$ **31.** All other even
numbers are divisible by 2. **33.** All prime
numbers greater than 2 are odd numbers. The
sum of two odd numbers is an even number.
35. 1, 3, 7, 9 **37.** 1001; the three digit number

PAGE 91 REVIEW EXERCISES **1.** 2
3. -1 **5.** 240 **7.** 2

PAGE 94–95 WRITTEN EXERCISES
1.
3.
5.
7. $\frac{-1}{2}, \frac{1}{-2}$ **9.** $\frac{1}{-11}, -\frac{1}{11}$ **11.** $\frac{-2}{9}, -\frac{2}{9}$
13. $\frac{-13}{6}, \frac{13}{-6}$ **15.** $\frac{-3}{4}, \frac{3}{-4}$ **17.** 6 **19.** $\frac{1}{4}$
21. 3 **23.** -3 **25.** $-\frac{7}{8}$ **27.** -1 **29.** $-\frac{1}{3}$
31. -3 **33.** -9 **35.** $\frac{7}{6}$ **37.** $\frac{3}{7}$ **39.** $-\frac{1}{9}$
41. $-\frac{2}{7}$ **43.** $-\frac{3}{8}$

PAGE 95 REVIEW EXERCISES **1.** 3, 4, 8,
18, 36 **3.** 1, 5, 6, 10, 15, 30, 45 **5.** 6, x

PAGE 99 WRITTEN EXERCISES **1.** 4
3. 5 **5.** 7 **7.** 3 **9.** 125 **11.** $\frac{3}{5}$ **13.** $2\frac{3}{4}$
15. $-\frac{1}{9}$ **17.** $-5\frac{2}{3}$ **19.** $-\frac{2}{5}$ **21.** $10\frac{5}{12}$
23. $-6\frac{1}{13}$ **25.** $-42\frac{6}{7}$ **27.** $\frac{17}{8}$ **29.** $\frac{99}{16}$
31. $-\frac{35}{8}$ **33.** $-\frac{49}{3}$ **35.** $-\frac{83}{10}$ **37.** 3 **39.** -1
41. 0 **43.** 24 **45.** $\frac{b}{5}$ **47.** $\frac{d}{e}$ **49.** $\frac{n}{3}$ **51.** $\frac{v}{3u}$

PAGE 99 REVIEW EXERCISES 1. 49
3. 1296 5. 1 7. 5184 9. 243

PAGES 101–102 WRITTEN EXERCISES
1. $\frac{4}{12}, \frac{1}{12}$ 3. $\frac{6}{8}, \frac{5}{8}$ 5. $\frac{6}{27}, -\frac{1}{27}$ 7. $\frac{70}{147}, \frac{6}{147}$
9. $-\frac{20}{30}, \frac{7}{30}$ 11. $\frac{16}{300}, \frac{21}{300}$ 13. $-\frac{48}{112}, -\frac{7}{112}$
15. $\frac{35}{294}, \frac{30}{294}$ 17. $\frac{70}{80}, \frac{25}{80}, \frac{42}{80}$ 19. $\frac{108}{252}, \frac{441}{252},$
$\frac{112}{252}$ 21. $\frac{2}{130}, \frac{78}{130}, \frac{45}{130}$ 23. $-\frac{60}{72}, \frac{16}{72}, -\frac{63}{72}$
25. $\frac{2a}{6}, \frac{b}{6}$ 27. $\frac{20h}{500}, \frac{5h}{500}, \frac{4h}{500}$ 29. $\frac{3}{3c}, \frac{2}{3c}$
31. $\frac{3yz}{xyz}, \frac{xz}{xyz}, \frac{5xy}{xyz}$ 33. $<$ 35. $<$ 37. $>$

PAGE 102 SELF-TEST A 1. 2, 3, 4, 9 2. 3,
9 3. 2, 3, 4, 5, 9, 10 4. none 5. composite;
$2^2 \cdot 3^3$ 6. prime 7. composite; $3 \cdot 29$
8. prime 9. $-\frac{1}{3}$ 10. $\frac{7}{9}$ 11. $\frac{2}{-3}$ 12. $\frac{1}{4}$
13. $-2\frac{2}{5}$ 14. $\frac{16}{21}$ 15. $-1\frac{23}{48}$ 16. $4\frac{1}{4}$ 17. $\frac{11}{5}$
18. $-\frac{11}{3}$ 19. $\frac{94}{15}$ 20. $\frac{19}{12}$ 21. $-\frac{69}{8}$ 22. $\frac{28}{40},$
$\frac{35}{40}$ 23. $-\frac{30}{147}, \frac{14}{147}$ 24. $\frac{27}{450}, \frac{12}{450}$ 25. $-\frac{16}{30},$
$-\frac{1}{30}$

PAGES 104–105 WRITTEN EXERCISES
1. $\frac{2}{3}$ 3. $-\frac{4}{17}$ 5. 0 7. $-\frac{11}{5}$ 9. $\frac{16}{21}$ 11. $\frac{7}{2}$
13. $-\frac{3}{8}$ 15. $-\frac{51}{10}$ 17. $\frac{287}{156}$ 19. $-\frac{41}{72}$
21. $\frac{7}{12}$ 23. $\frac{3}{5}$ 25. $-\frac{17}{18}$ 27. $\frac{19}{12}$ 29. $\frac{1}{10}$

PAGE 105 REVIEW EXERCISES 1. $1\frac{3}{8}$
3. $3\frac{2}{7}$ 5. $5\frac{11}{12}$ 7. $9\frac{4}{13}$

PAGES 107–108 WRITTEN EXERCISES
1. $8\frac{4}{5}$ 3. $\frac{10}{11}$ 5. $6\frac{2}{3}$ 7. $-20\frac{1}{7}$ 9. $3\frac{5}{6}$
11. $2\frac{1}{2}$ 13. $-2\frac{5}{24}$ 15. $-3\frac{17}{30}$ 17. $5\frac{3}{4}$
19. $-3\frac{7}{8}$ 21. $11\frac{2}{3}$ 23. $-19\frac{1}{5}$ 25. $9\frac{11}{12}$
27. $-8\frac{1}{4}$ 29. $-8\frac{2}{7}$ 31. 4 33. $\frac{2}{15}$ 35. $\frac{1}{4}$

PAGE 108 PROBLEMS 1. $14\frac{11}{16}$ yd 3. $\frac{5}{6}$ mi

5. $1\frac{5}{8}$ in. 7. right : $1\frac{5}{16}$ in.; bottom : $\frac{11}{16}$ in.

PAGE 108 REVIEW EXERCISES 1. $\frac{2}{-7}$
3. $\frac{5}{-9}$ 5. $-\frac{1}{7}$ 7. 4 9. 3

PAGES 111–112 WRITTEN EXERCISES
1. 7 3. -2 5. $\frac{1}{28}$ 7. $-\frac{1}{60}$ 9. $\frac{10}{27}$ 11. $-\frac{1}{4}$
13. $-\frac{2}{27}$ 15. $\frac{5}{8}$ 17. 0 19. $\frac{15}{64}$ 21. 1
23. $43\frac{11}{12}$ 25. $-22\frac{1}{7}$ 27. $3\frac{10}{27}$ 29. $\frac{1}{24}$
31. $\frac{1}{72}$ 33. $-4\frac{1}{2}$ 35. $6n$ 37. $-\frac{y}{2}$ 39. $\frac{2}{5}$
41. 3

PAGE 112 REVIEW EXERCISES 1. 60
3. -36 5. 8 7. $-3\frac{1}{9}$

PAGE 115 WRITTEN EXERCISES 1. $\frac{2}{3}$
3. 25 5. $\frac{25}{72}$ 7. $3\frac{8}{9}$ 9. 6 11. $5\frac{1}{5}$ 13. $-\frac{9}{16}$
15. 7 17. $5\frac{23}{64}$ 19. -2 21. -9 23. $\frac{1}{3}$
25. $-\frac{1}{2}$

PAGES 115–116 PROBLEMS 1. $\frac{1}{19}$
3. $7,500 5. $4 per hour 7. $6.50 9. $\frac{1}{6}$ of
the class 11. $\frac{3}{20}$ of the workers

PAGE 116 REVIEW EXERCISES
1. $n = 240 - 135$; 105 3. $y = 156 \div 4$; 39
5. $x = 432 \div 12$; 36 7. $m = 418 \div 38$; 11

PAGE 120 WRITTEN EXERCISES 1. 0.25
3. $0.\overline{2}$ 5. 0.9 7. $-0.\overline{6}$ 9. -0.375
11. -0.12 13. 1.1 15. $0.58\overline{3}$ 17. $0.2\overline{6}$
19. $-1.3\overline{8}$ 21. 0.15 23. $3.\overline{285714}$ 25. $\frac{1}{20}$
27. $-\frac{3}{5}$ 29. $2\frac{7}{100}$ 31. $5\frac{1}{8}$ 33. $-1\frac{3}{8}$
35. $12\frac{5}{8}$ 37. $\frac{9}{40}$ 39. $-1\frac{413}{500}$ 41. $-\frac{5}{9}$
43. $-1\frac{1}{90}$ 45. $\frac{5}{33}$ 47. $\frac{35}{99}$ 49. $-1\frac{4}{33}$
51. $2\frac{121}{900}$ 53. $\frac{41}{333}$ 55. rational 57. rational
59. 3.0, 3.00$\overline{9}$, 3.0$\overline{9}$, 3.1 61. a. 1 b. $=$
63. a. $-1\frac{1}{4}$ b. $=$

PAGE 121 SELF-TEST B 1. $\frac{7}{12}$ 2. $-\frac{21}{30}$

3. $-\frac{2}{15}$ 4. $22\frac{4}{9}$ 5. $-10\frac{1}{24}$ 6. $17\frac{3}{8}$ 7. $3\frac{3}{4}$

8. $-\frac{1}{24}$ 9. $-8\frac{1}{7}$ 10. $1\frac{1}{2}$ 11. $-\frac{1}{8}$

12. $-4\frac{1}{2}$ 13. 0.625 14. $0.\overline{18}$ 15. -0.0125

16. $1.1\overline{6}$ 17. $\frac{7}{8}$ 18. $1\frac{2}{3}$ 19. $-2\frac{213}{1000}$ 20. $\frac{7}{30}$

PAGE 121 COMPUTER BYTE 1. 300
3. 510 5. 2640

PAGE 123 ENRICHMENT 1. Answers will vary.

PAGE 124 CHAPTER REVIEW 1. 4, 6, 8, 12, 24 3. c 5. False 7. True 9. False
11. False 13. F 15. G 17. K 19. L 21. I
23. J

PAGE 126 CUMULATIVE REVIEW EXERCISES 1. 58 3. 7 5. 5 7. 12
9. 225 11. 8 13. 25 15. 250
17. $75.70 > 75.40 > 75.06$
19. $0.33 > 0.30 > 0.03$ 21. $-7, 7$ 23. $-5,$
$-6, -7$ and so on; also 5, 6, 7, and so on
25. $-5, 5$ 27. $-32, -33, -34, -35, -36,$
$-37, -38, -39, 32, 33, 34, 35, 36, 37, 38, 39$
29. 18 31. 12 33. -4 35. $-\frac{4}{5}$ 37. $\frac{2}{5}$

39. $-\frac{10}{7}$ 41. $-\frac{2}{7}$ 43. $\frac{2}{5}$ 45. $-5\frac{5}{8}$

47. $8\frac{23}{136}$

PAGE 127 CUMULATIVE REVIEW PROBLEMS 1. $196.88 3. No 5. $787.50
7. $444.75

Chapter 4 Solving Equations

PAGE 133 WRITTEN EXERCISES 1. 12
3. -1 5. -4 7. 23 9. 17 11. 7 13. 12
15. 6 17. 8 19. $-\frac{2}{5}$ 21. $3\frac{2}{3}$ 23. 1.1
25. 0.253 27. 1.196 29. $9\frac{3}{4}$ 31. $2\frac{7}{12}$
33. 0.358 35. $3\frac{4}{5}$ 37. 1.73

PAGE 133 REVIEW EXERCISES 1. 5 3. 3
5. 9

PAGE 135 WRITTEN EXERCISES 1. 15
3. 18 5. 6 7. 54 9. -84 11. 28 13. 5
15. -10 17. 91 19. 11 21. $7\frac{1}{2}$ 23. -221

25. -252 27. $-\frac{5}{6}$ 29. $9\frac{2}{3}$ 31. 364 33. 247
35. $\frac{2}{19}$ 37. $10\frac{1}{2}$

PAGE 135 REVIEW EXERCISES 1. $\frac{3}{14}$
3. $\frac{2}{15}$ 5. $3\frac{1}{19}$

PAGE 138 WRITTEN EXERCISES 1. 88
3. 20 5. -1.5 7. -24 9. 60 11. 19.5
13. 18 15. 20 17. -30 19. -49.5 21. $13\frac{1}{2}$
23. $10\frac{1}{2}$ 25. 6.5 27. -0.8 29. $-\frac{1}{9}$ 31. $-\frac{5}{6}$
33. 7.595 35. 0.02148 37. 5.7 39. 15.6
41. 3.3

PAGE 138 REVIEW EXERCISES 1. 30
3. 55 5. 103 7. 17 9. 19

PAGE 138 CALCULATOR KEY-IN 1. 0.3
3. 2.7203791 5. 3.3807

PAGES 141–142 WRITTEN EXERCISES
1. 11 3. 7 5. 11 7. 10 9. 3 11. 80
13. 30 15. 55 17. 24 19. $4\frac{1}{3}$ 21. $22\frac{1}{2}$
23. $7\frac{1}{2}$ 25. $3\frac{1}{3}$ 27. $1\frac{7}{9}$ 29. $1\frac{17}{21}$ 31. $4\frac{3}{7}$ 33. $\frac{1}{4}$
35. $\frac{25}{66}$ 37. $\frac{5}{11}$ 39. $\frac{2}{15}$ 41. 27

PAGE 142 SELF-TEST A 1. -24 2. 10
3. 9 4. 56 5. -13 6. -68 7. 17 8. -33
9. 150 10. $-2\frac{4}{13}$ 11. -80 12. -1.74
13. $27\frac{1}{2}$ 14. 120 15. 6 16. -3

PAGE 142 CALCULATOR KEY-IN 852

PAGES 145–146 WRITTEN EXERCISES
1. $8b$ 3. $53 - d$ 5. $30 + t$ 7. $g + 9$
9. $78 - m$ 11. $n + 19$ 13. $d \div 11$
15. $12 - z$ 17. $11t + 15$ 19. $91(m + n)$
21. $r \div (83 - 10)$ 23. $c[(12 + 9) + 3]$
25. $(60 + 40 + 10) \div d$ 27. $b + 3$ 29. $x + 6$
31. $25q$ 33. $x \div 60$ 35. $x - 10$

PAGE 146 REVIEW EXERCISES 1. 27
3. 576 5. -15 7. 19

PAGE 148 WRITTEN EXERCISES
1. $5d = 20$ 3. $3w - 7 = 8$ 5. $5 \div r = 42$
7. $n - 1 = 5$ 9. $2n \div 3 = 15$
11. $(4 + x) \div 2 = 34$ 13. $59 - x = 3 + 2x$
15. $(x - 5) \div 3 = 2$

PAGE 148 REVIEW EXERCISES 1. $n - 4$
3. $n \div 7$ 5. $40 - n$ 7. $2n$

PAGES 150–151 PROBLEMS 1. $9n = 1170$
3. $18n = 13.50$ 5. $144 - n = 116$
7. $n = (12 + 18) - 19$ 9. $2000 + n = 2650$

11. $\frac{4}{5}n = 180$ **13.** $2n - 30 = 20$ **15.** $\frac{1}{9}n = 5$

PAGE 151 REVIEW EXERCISES
1. $n - 8 = 43$ **3.** $n + 14 = 70$
5. $n - 17 = 34$

PAGES 154–155 PROBLEMS **1.** 250 lb
3. 480 books **5.** 24 shirts **7.** 25 people
9. 150 lb **11.** 24 gal

PAGE 155 SELF-TEST B **1.** $12x$ **2.** $60 - d$
3. d **4.** c **5.** a **6.** $21n = 189$
7. $n - 450 = 1845$ **8.** 412 tennis balls

PAGE 157 ENRICHMENT **1.** 3 **3.** 3
5. 2; 7

PAGE 158 CHAPTER REVIEW **1.** 20
3. divide **5.** a **7.** c **9.** b **11.** b

PAGE 160 CUMULATIVE REVIEW
EXERCISES **1.** 5 **3.** 5 **5.** -1 **7.** 32
9. 16 **11.** $<$ **13.** $<$ **15.** $<$ **17.** $>$
19. $x = 8$ **21.** $x = -20$ **23.** $x = -18.5$
25. $x = 5$ **27.** $x = -12$ **29.** $-3\frac{7}{12}$ **31.** $-1\frac{3}{8}$
33. $1\frac{3}{20}$ **35.** -21 **37.** $-\frac{1}{9}$ **39.** $3\frac{11}{48}$ **41.** 20
43. 24 **45.** -14 **47.** 0.75 **49.** 11 **51.** -6

PAGE 161 CUMULATIVE REVIEW
PROBLEMS **1.** $2.97 **3.** 220,000 readers
5. $418.50 **7.** $656.38 **9.** 100 inquiries

5 Geometric Figures

PAGES 167–168 WRITTEN EXERCISES
1. $\overline{YX}$ **3.** $\overrightarrow{PQ}$ **5.** $\overleftrightarrow{XY}, \overleftrightarrow{XZ}, \overleftrightarrow{XY}, \overleftrightarrow{YX}$ **7.** S, P,
O or T, Q, O **9.** $\overrightarrow{PS}, \overrightarrow{PO}, \overrightarrow{PQ}$ **11.** $\overline{ST}$ and
$\overrightarrow{PQ}$ **13.** Answers may vary; for example, $\overrightarrow{PS}$
and $\overrightarrow{OT}$ **15.** Answers may vary; for example,
$\overrightarrow{OS}$ and $\overrightarrow{OT}$ **17.** $\overrightarrow{OS}$ **19.** $\overrightarrow{OP}, \overrightarrow{OQ}, \overrightarrow{OS}, \overrightarrow{OT}$
21. Answers may vary; for example, $\overleftrightarrow{AX}$ and
$\overleftrightarrow{XY}$; X **23.** Answers may vary; for example,
$\overleftrightarrow{XW}$ and $\overleftrightarrow{AD}$, plane XWD **25.** true **27.** false
29. false **31.** true **33.** one **35.** Two
nonparallel lines in a plane must intersect, and
their intersection is a point.

PAGE 168 REVIEW EXERCISES **1.** 2.9
3. 4.6 **5.** 3.0 **7.** 9.3

PAGES 171–172 WRITTEN EXERCISES
1. a. 8 cm **b.** 80 mm **3. a.** 9 cm **b.** 92 mm
5. a. 8 cm **b.** 82 mm **7.** $\overline{AE}$ and $\overline{PT}$; $\overline{VZ}$ and
$\overline{GJ}$ **9.** 450; 4500 **11.** 2.5, 2500 **13.** 60; 6000

15. 2 **17.** 0.625 **19.** 4500 **21.** 3.74 m by
5.2 m **23.** 4.675 m by 7.05 m **25.** 27 mm
27. 65 cm **29.** 2.1875 **31.** 35

PAGE 172 REVIEW EXERCISES **1.** 90
3. 40 **5.** 140 **7.** 105 **9.** 65

PAGES 175–177 WRITTEN EXERCISES

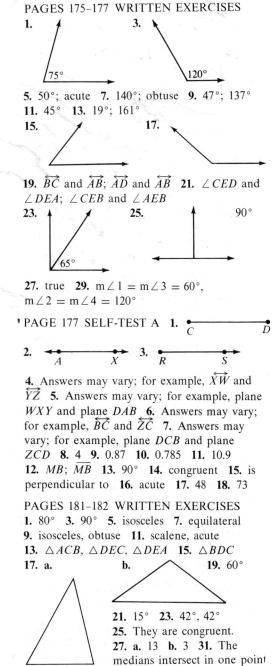

1. **3.**
75° 120°

5. 50°; acute **7.** 140°; obtuse **9.** 47°; 137°
11. 45° **13.** 19°; 161°
15. **17.**

19. $\overrightarrow{BC}$ and $\overleftrightarrow{AB}$; $\overleftrightarrow{AD}$ and $\overleftrightarrow{AB}$ **21.** $\angle CED$ and
$\angle DEA$; $\angle CEB$ and $\angle AEB$
23. **25.** 90°
65°

27. true **29.** $m\angle 1 = m\angle 3 = 60°$,
$m\angle 2 = m\angle 4 = 120°$

' PAGE 177 SELF-TEST A **1.**
C D

2. **3.**
A X R S

4. Answers may vary; for example, $\overleftrightarrow{XW}$ and
$\overleftrightarrow{YZ}$ **5.** Answers may vary; for example, plane
WXY and plane DAB **6.** Answers may vary;
for example, $\overleftrightarrow{BC}$ and $\overleftrightarrow{ZC}$ **7.** Answers may
vary; for example, plane DCB and plane
ZCD **8.** 4 **9.** 0.87 **10.** 0.785 **11.** 10.9
12. MB; $\overline{MB}$ **13.** 90° **14.** congruent **15.** is
perpendicular to **16.** acute **17.** 48 **18.** 73

PAGES 181–182 WRITTEN EXERCISES
1. 80° **3.** 90° **5.** isosceles **7.** equilateral
9. isosceles, obtuse **11.** scalene, acute
13. $\triangle ACB$, $\triangle DEC$, $\triangle DEA$ **15.** $\triangle BDC$
17. a. **b.** **19.** 60°

21. 15° **23.** 42°, 42°
25. They are congruent.
27. a. 13 **b.** 3 **31.** The
medians intersect in one point

PAGE 182 REVIEW EXERCISES 1. 15.08
3. 15.52 **5.** 20.33 **7.** 21.873 **9.** 24.768

PAGES 185–187 WRITTEN EXERCISES
1. pentagon **3.** hexagon **5.** triangle **7.** square
9. 14.1 **11.** 312 cm **13.** 72.6 mm **15.** 1356 m
17. 108° **19.** 2.56 m **21.** 12 m **23.** 3
25.   **27.** 22

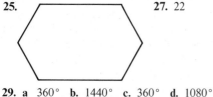

29. a 360° **b.** 1440° **c.** 360° **d.** 1080°
31. 5

PAGE 187 REVIEW EXERCISES 1. 22.4
3. 49 **5.** 10.9 **7.** 44.8

PAGES 190–191 WRITTEN EXERCISES
1. 25.1 cm **3.** 2830 mm **5.** 134 m **7.** 90.1 m
9. 143 km **11.** 199 m **13.** 1.59 mm
15. 3 74 km **17.** 2.79 cm **19.** 40,074 km
21. 47.1 km **23.** 94.2 m **25.** 35.7 **27.** 41.4

29. 22.7 **31.** $S = \frac{\pi d}{2}$ **33.** Draw a circle and
label three points A, B, C on the circle. Let
point D be a point not on the circle.
Quadrilateral $ABCD$ cannot be inscribed in the
circle **35.** An angle inscribed in a semicircle is
a right angle.

PAGE 191 REVIEW EXERCISES 1. 18
3. 27 **5.** 8 **7.** 14

PAGES 196–197 WRITTEN EXERCISES
1. c **3.** SSS **5.** rotation or reflection **7.** a
rotation, two reflections, or a translation and a
reflection **9.** $\triangle GHK \cong \triangle FHK$; SAS
11. a. $\angle N$ **b.** $\angle Y$ **c.** $\overline{NS}$ **d.** $\overline{RL}$ **13. a.** $\overline{FG}$
b. $\overline{EH}$ **c.** $\angle EFG$ **d.** $\overline{CD}$ **15.** no

PAGE 197 REVIEW EXERCISES 1. 7
3. 11 **5.** 72 **7.** 4

PAGE 197 CALCULATOR KEY-IN
1. 3.1604938 **3.** 3.141$\overline{6}$ **5.** 3.1416 The closest
approximation is $\frac{355}{113}$.

PAGES 200–201 WRITTEN EXERCISES
1.   **5.**

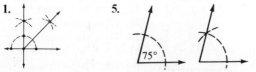

7. The perpendicular bisector appears to
pass through the vertex of the angle
formed by the two congruent sides. **9.** yes
11.   **13.** yes

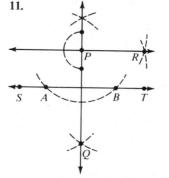

PAGE 201 SELF-TEST B 1. equilateral
2. 180 **3.** 3 **4.** octagon **5.** parallelogram
6. 33 cm **7.** 100 cm **8.** true **9.** false
10. $\overline{FG}$, J, IJF
11.   **12.**

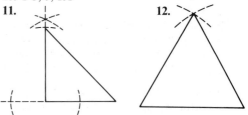

PAGE 203 ENRICHMENT 1. 57,960,000
3. 149,730,000 **5.** 12 **7.** 32,186,000,000
9.

```
10  FOR I=1 TO 5
20  PRINT "HOW MANY HOURS";
30  INPUT T
40  LET R=760
50  PRINT "DISTANCE TRAVELED"
60  PRINT "IS ";R*T;" MILES."
70  NEXT I
80  END
```

PAGE 204 CHAPTER REVIEW 1. collinear
points **3.** midpoint **5.** false **7.** true
9. false **11.** d **13.** c
15.

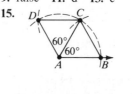

$\triangle ABC$ is
equilateral, thus
$\angle CAB = 60°$.
$\triangle ABC \cong DAC$,
thus $\angle DAC = 60°$,
$\angle DAB = 120°$.

**PAGE 206 CUMULATIVE REVIEW
EXERCISES 1.** 8 **3.** 7 **5.** 12 **7.** −19

9. 9 **11.** 45 **13.** 14 **15.** $-18\frac{3}{4}$ **17.** 72
19. 24 **21.** 30 **23.** 15 **25.** $\frac{4}{5}$ **27.** $-\frac{1}{9}$ **29.** $\frac{2}{3}$
31. 0.4 **33.** 0.4375 **35.** $-0.2\overline{7}$ **37.** $\frac{7}{100}$ **39.** 2
41. $-1\frac{8}{33}$ **43.** true

PAGE 207 CUMULATIVE REVIEW
PROBLEMS **1.** $31.11 **3.** $124 **5.** 52 m
7. 127 boxes **9.** 22 m

6 Ratio, Proportion, and Percent

PAGES 211–212 WRITTEN EXERCISES
1. a. $\frac{5}{7}$ **b.** $\frac{5}{12}$ **c.** $\frac{12}{7}$ **3. a.** $\frac{9}{4}$ **b.** $\frac{9}{13}$ **c.** $\frac{13}{4}$
5. $\frac{3}{8}$ **7.** $\frac{2}{7}$ **9.** $\frac{15}{4}$ **11. a.** $\frac{5}{21}$ **b.** $\frac{21}{26}$ **c.** $\frac{26}{5}$
13. a. $\frac{1}{3}$ **b.** $\frac{2}{1}$ **c.** $\frac{3}{2}$ **15.** $\frac{3}{5}$ **17.** $\frac{14}{9}$

PAGES 212–213 PROBLEMS **1.** $\frac{80}{3}$
3. $62\frac{1}{2}$ lb/ft^3 **5.** $\frac{11}{2}$ **7. a.** 2:5 **b.** 2:5 **c.** $\frac{2}{5}$
9. $\frac{3}{7}$ **11.** $\frac{5}{18}$

PAGE 213 REVIEW EXERCISES **1.** 9 **3.** 9
5. 5 **7.** 12

PAGES 215–216 PROBLEMS **1.** 17¢ **3.** $16
5. $5.25 **7.** 195 km **9.** 240 km **11.** Best
Brand Pear Tomatoes **13.** Sparkle Window
Cleaner **15.** 5 gal **17.** 62 km/h; 74 km/h

PAGE 216 REVIEW EXERCISES **1.** 20 cm
3. 84 cm **5.** 142.4 m **7.** 57.4 m **9.** 49.44 cm

PAGE 219 WRITTEN EXERCISES **1.** 4
3. 56 **5.** 35 **7.** 60 **9.** 72 **11.** 45 **13.** $7\frac{1}{2}$
15. $8\frac{1}{2}$ **17.** 10 **19.** 12 **21.** 20 **23.** 15
25. $5\frac{2}{5}$ **27.** $4\frac{1}{2}$ **29.** $\frac{1}{3}$ **31.** $\frac{4}{1}$

PAGE 219 REVIEW EXERCISES **1.** $13\frac{1}{3}$
3. $22\frac{7}{9}$ **5.** $8\frac{11}{18}$ **7.** $43\frac{1}{2}$ **9.** $60\frac{3}{10}$

PAGES 221–223 PROBLEMS **1. a.** 880 km
b. 14 h **3. a.** $3.75 **b.** 28 oranges
5. a. 5.3 cm^3 **b.** 337.5 cm^3 **7.** $1.20 **9.** 8 cans
11. $11\frac{1}{4}$ oz; $10\frac{2}{3}$ servings **13.** 6 min
15. 12 wins **17.** 12 vests **19.** $1333\frac{1}{3}$ ft^2
21. 6955 votes for; 2782 votes against
23. 76,800 km

PAGE 223 REVIEW EXERCISES **1.** $\frac{200 \text{ cm}}{15 \text{ cm}}$

3. $\frac{30 \text{ ft}}{5 \text{ ft}}$ **5.** $\frac{2000 \text{ m}}{450 \text{ m}}$ **7.** $\frac{36 \text{ in.}}{20 \text{ in.}}$

PAGE 223 CALCULATOR KEY-IN
1. 1.4925373 **3.** 3.9385584 **5.** 0.208982

PAGES 225–226 WRITTEN EXERCISES
1. 1104 in. **3.** 576 in. **5.** 960 in. **7. a.** 2 cm

b. 800 km **9. a.** 10.5 cm **b.** 4200 km
11. a. 3 cm **b.** 1200 km **13.** 400 km
15. 1,384,300 km **17.** 139,700 km

PAGE 226 SELF-TEST A **1.** $\frac{3}{2}$ **2.** $\frac{17}{9}$ **3.** $\frac{2}{11}$
4. $1.15 **5.** $.61 **6.** 2 **7.** 4 **8.** 135 **9.** $.67
10. $110 **11.** 1 in. **12.** 1 cm : 16 cm

PAGE 229 WRITTEN EXERCISES **1.** $\frac{3}{4}$
3. $\frac{9}{20}$ **5.** $\frac{3}{25}$ **7.** $1\frac{1}{4}$ **9.** $\frac{31}{200}$ **11.** $\frac{43}{400}$ **13.** 80%
15. 30% **17.** 48% **19.** 62% **21.** 220%
23. 102% **25.** $87\frac{1}{2}$% **27.** $\frac{1}{2}$% **29.** $\frac{3}{4}$%
31. $302\frac{1}{2}$% **33.** $\frac{1}{6}$ **35.** $\frac{5}{12}$

PAGE 230 PROBLEMS **1.** 38% **3.** 60%
5. 5% **7.** $62\frac{1}{2}$ **9.** 10%; 70%; 80%

PAGE 230 REVIEW EXERCISES **1.** 0.45
3. 0.275 **5.** 0.04 **7.** $0.\overline{72}$ **9.** $0.57\overline{3}$

PAGE 233 WRITTEN EXERCISES **1.** 0.93
3. 1.14 **5.** 2.6 **7.** 0.495 **9.** 0.006 **11.** 0.0005
13. 59% **15.** 9% **17.** 260% **19.** 1283%
21. 0.7% **23.** 8.67% **25.** 0.375; 37.5%
27. 0.006; 0.6% **29.** 1.625; 162.5% **31.** 0.5875;
58.8% **33.** $0.70\overline{83}$; 70.8% **35.** 0.2857143;
28.6% **37.** $16\frac{2}{3}$% **39.** $88\frac{8}{9}$% **41.** $83\frac{1}{3}$%

PAGE 233 REVIEW EXERCISES **1.** 2.95
3. 15.438 **5.** 23.8576

PAGES 235–236 WRITTEN EXERCISES
1. 40% **3.** 270 **5.** 1300 **7.** 5.4 **9.** 83.3%
11. 104.5 **13.** 87 **15.** 0.896 **17.** 114.3%
19. 224 **21.** 54 **23.** 252

PAGES 236–237 PROBLEMS **1.** $12.50
3. $77.5% **5.** 10% **7.** 11.5% **9.** 4 billion
11. a. 10% **b.** 40%

PAGE 237 SELF-TEST B **1.** $\frac{27}{100}$ **2.** $\frac{83}{100}$
3. $1\frac{16}{25}$ **4.** $2\frac{9}{10}$ **5.** 5% **6.** 37.5% **7.** 400%
8. 325% **9.** 0.45 **10.** 0.78 **11.** 3.48
12. 0.008 **13.** 64% **14.** 81% **15.** 785%
16. 6.8% **17.** 25% **18.** 205% **19.** 11 **20.** 120

PAGE 239 ENRICHMENT **1.** 3, 21, 144, and
987 are divisible by 3; 5, 55, and 610 are
divisible by 5. **3.** The new pattern consists of
every other Fibonacci number, starting with 3.
5. The new pattern consists of every other
Fibonacci number, starting with 5.

PAGE 240 CHAPTER REVIEW **1.** a **3.** b
5. c **7.** a **9.** b **11.** c **13.** e **15.** b **17.** c

PAGE 242 CUMULATIVE REVIEW
EXERCISES **1.** 5 **3.** 2 **5.** 6 **7.** 3 **9.** 4
11. 36 **13.** false **15.** false **17.** $\frac{10}{15}, \frac{3}{15}$
19. $-\frac{3}{24}, \frac{8}{24}$ **21.** $\frac{24}{60}, \frac{10}{60}, \frac{15}{60}$ **23.** 5 **25.** 3
27. 16 **29.** 1 **31.** 64 **33.** $2\frac{7}{13}$ **35.** rhombus
37. diameter

PAGE 243 CUMULATIVE REVIEW
PROBLEMS **1.** $79.38 **3.** 23,500 ft
5. 1230 lb **7.** l: 15 m; w: 5 m **9.** $616.13

7 Percents and Problem Solving

PAGES 247–248 WRITTEN EXERCISES
1. 15% **3.** 40% **5.** 82.5% **7.** 46.9% **9.** 0.8%
11. 27.5% **13.** 132 **15.** 57.2 **17.** 205.8
19. 124.5 **21.** 60 **23.** 336 **25.** 338.8 **27.** 64
29. 120

PAGES 248–249 PROBLEMS **1.** 1,134
employees **3.** 25% **5.** 7511 books **7.** 16.7%
9. 246 homes **11.** $1.25

PAGE 249 REVIEW EXERCISES **1.** 9.72
3. 17 **5.** 520 **7.** 220.5 **9.** 0.04

PAGES 252–253 PROBLEMS **1.** $67.15
3. 14% discount **5.** $26.46 **7.** $30 **9.** 25%
markup **11.** $12.50 **13.** 72% of the original
price **15.** The final prices will be equal.

PAGE 253 REVIEW EXERCISES **1.** radius
3. diameter

PAGES 255–256 PROBLEMS **1.** $129
3. $978 **5.** $10,900 **7.** $64,893.62
9. $58,510.64 **11.** $7,380 **13.** $4,250

PAGE 256 REVIEW EXERCISES **1.** 10
3. 6 **5.** 128 **7.** 0.4

PAGE 259 WRITTEN EXERCISES **1.** 5.12
3. 80% **5.** 40

PAGES 259–261 PROBLEMS **1.** 82.5%
3. 49 books **5.** $34.80; $27.84 **7.** $36.50
9. a. 108° **b.** $3.6 million
11. b. food $450; clothing $270; housing $540;
medical $180; other $360
13. b. salaries $489,600;
maintenance/repair $54,400; books/supplies
$34,000; recreation $34,000; after-school
programs $34,000; teacher training $34,000

PAGE 261 SELF-TEST A **1.** 25% **2.** 35%
3. 23% **4.** $103.70 **5.** 30% discount

6. $6,360 **7.** $72,688 **8.** 437.4 **9.** 80% **10.** 75
violations

PAGES 264–265 WRITTEN EXERCISES
1. $384; $1664 **3.** $745.20; $3505.20 **5.** $1692;
$7332 **7.** $5550.60; $11,930.60 **9.** 14%
11. 8.5% **13.** 16% **15.** $\frac{1}{2}$ yr **17.** $4450
19. $6720 **21.** $1850 **23.** $102.12

PAGES 265–266 PROBLEMS **1.** $577.50
3. $96.25 **5.** 7.5% **7.** 8 yr

PAGE 266 REVIEW EXERCISES **1.** 0.375
3. 0.05 **5.** 1.496 **7.** 0.833 **9.** 2.396

PAGE 266 CALCULATOR KEY-IN **1.** 16
3. 48% **5.** 86.$\overline{6}$%

PAGES 268–269 WRITTEN EXERCISES
1. $7056 **3.** $1560.60 **5.** $3149.28
7. $2137.84 **9.** $3975.35 **11.** $9724.05
13. $7.70 **15.** 9 mo

PAGE 269 PROBLEMS **1.** $1852.20 **3.** 12%
simple interest will earn more. **5.** 13.2%

PAGES 271–273 PROBLEMS **1.** $2.50
3. $21,942 **5.** $165 **7.** $7000 **9.** $56,400
11. 10%

PAGE 273 SELF-TEST B **1.** $10,000
2. 14% **3.** $3,149.28 **4.** 9 mo **5.** $2,169.65

PAGE 275 ENRICHMENT **1.** 125.86; 162.75;
20.00 **3.** 249.75; 323.80; 35.00 **5.** 665.61;
676.09; 90.00

PAGE 276 CHAPTER REVIEW **1.** 25%
3. 95 **5.** c **7.** true **9.** c

PAGE 278 CUMULATIVE REVIEW
EXERCISES **1.** 8 **3.** 7 **5.** 12 **7.** −19
9. 9 **11.** 45 **13.** −7, −2.5, −2.2, 0, 3, 6.4
15. −8.4, −3, −1.6, −1.0, 0.5 **17.** True
19. True **21.** True **23.** $\frac{6}{9}, \frac{5}{9}$ **25.** $-\frac{88}{33}, \frac{27}{33}$
27. $\frac{28}{12}, \frac{9}{12}$ **29.** $\frac{68}{128}, -\frac{3}{128}$ **31.** 12 **33.** 180
35. 63 **37.** rotation and translation; ASA
39. rotation and translation; SSS

PAGE 279 CUMULATIVE REVIEW
PROBLEMS **1.** 15 cm **3.** 4.4 km **5.** up $4\frac{5}{8}$
points **7.** 58.125 L **9.** 10 students

8 Equations and Inequalities

PAGES 283–284 WRITTEN EXERCISES
1. $2m$ **3.** $-7c$ **5.** $c - 5$ **7.** $-7y + 77$

9. $-4a - 30$ 11. $6x - 14$ 13. $\frac{1}{2}$ 15. 9
17. $-1\frac{1}{4}$ 19. 5 21. $-\frac{1}{2}$ 23. -1 25. $\frac{1}{2}$
27. -1 29. $2\frac{1}{2}$ 31. 1 33. -1 35. 6
37. $-\frac{3}{4}$ 39. $-1\frac{2}{3}$ 41. $1\frac{1}{2}$ 43. 5 45. -3
47. -14

PAGE 284 REVIEW EXERCISES 1. 1
3. 15 5. 12 7. $10\frac{1}{2}$ 9. 4

PAGE 286 WRITTEN EXERCISES 1. 5
3. 7 5. -6 7. $-\frac{1}{2}$ 9. -4 11. $-\frac{3}{5}$ 13. 4
15. $-2\frac{1}{2}$ 17. 3 19. 1 21. $\frac{1}{3}$ 23. 6 25. 1
27. -3 29. $-8\frac{1}{2}$ 31. -16 33. $6\frac{2}{3}$ 35. 80

PAGE 286 REVIEW EXERCISES 1. 4 3. 6
5. 12 7. 24

PAGES 288–289 PROBLEMS 1. 16 ft, 24 ft
3. 35 min, 45 min 5. 10 cm, 20 cm, 20 cm
7. 74 points 9. 34 ft 11. 10 yr 13. 1000 m

PAGE 290 SELF-TEST A 1. 4 2. $-\frac{1}{2}$
3. -2 4. 2 5. -6 6. $\frac{1}{5}$ 7. 16 8. -9
9. 5 10. -4 11. -2 12. 2 13. -4 14. $\frac{7}{9}$
15. -11 16. $7\frac{1}{2}$ 17. 20 ft 18. 106

PAGE 291–292 WRITTEN EXERCISES
1. $12 < 22$ 3. $6 > 0$ 5. $0 < 8 < 10$
7.
11. $6 > t$ 13. $p > q$ 15. $10d < 5n$
17. $6 < 2n < 8$ 19. $x < a < y$
21. $2 < 6 < 10 < 20 < 50$ 23. $a < 5 < 8 < b$

PAGE 292 REVIEW EXERCISES 1. 5 3. 5
5. 9 7. 77

PAGES 295–296 WRITTEN EXERCISES All
the numbers: 1. less than 12 3. greater than
42 5. less than 3 7. greater than or equal
to 20 9. less than -18 11. less than 7
13. less than -7 15. less than or equal to 12
17. less than or equal to 15 19. less than
-26 21. less than or equal to 60 23. less
than or equal to -11 25. less than -168
27. greater than 21.3 29. less than $5\frac{3}{7}$
31. less than or equal to -3.87 33. less than
or equal to 47 35. less than or equal to -10.8
37. greater than or equal to 3 39. greater
than 21 41. greater than -4.1 43. less than
or equal to -92.4 45. greater than $22\frac{13}{15}$
47. greater than or equal to -9 49. greater
than $\frac{1}{5}$ 51. less than -1.7

PAGE 296 REVIEW EXERCISES 1. -2.6,
-1.4, 1.2, 3.2 3. -12.2, -12.09, -11.2, 12,
112 5. -30.05, -5.3, -5.03, 0.35, 3.05
7. -2.89, -2.8, 2.089, 2.89, 28.9

PAGES 299–300 WRITTEN EXERCISES All
the numbers: 1. less than -6
3. greater than or equal to -9
5. less than -30
7. greater than or equal to -42
9. greater than $5\frac{2}{5}$ 11. greater than or equal to
-10 13. greater than 2 15. greater than or
equal to 3 17. greater than -4 19. less than
or equal to 5 21. less than 8 23. less than or
equal to $-3\frac{1}{13}$ 25. less than or equal to -3
27. greater than 1 29. less than or equal
to -2 31. greater than 15 33. less than 2
35. greater than 24 37. less than -7.2
39. greater than or equal to -10.3

PAGE 300 REVIEW EXERCISES 1. $n + 9$
3. $n - 16$ 5. $n + 3$ 7. $\frac{n}{5}$

PAGES 302–303 PROBLEMS 1. 36, 37
3. 4 hr 5. $22,714.29 7. 3, 4, 5 9. 400
employees 11. 51 checks

PAGE 303 SELF-TEST B 1. $a < b$
2. $35 > 4z$ All the numbers: 3. less than or
equal to 28 4. greater than 3 5. greater than
or equal to 7 6. greater than $4\frac{2}{3}$ 7. greater
than -14 8. greater than 5 9. less than 2
10. greater than 2 11. less than or equal to 0
12. greater than or equal to -6 13. 74, 75

PAGE 306 CHAPTER REVIEW 1. False
3. True 5. True 7. False 9. b 11. c
13. D 15. B 17. E 19. G 21. b

PAGE 308 CUMULATIVE REVIEW
EXERCISES 1. -5 3. 18 5. 2 7. 2 9. 4
11. 64 13. 3 15. 7 17. 5 19. 4 21. $-\frac{1}{4}$
23. 3 25. $\frac{4}{8}, \frac{7}{8}$ 27. $\frac{4}{20}, \frac{15}{20}$ 29. $\frac{8}{12}, \frac{3}{12}, \frac{5}{12}$
31. skew 33. diameter 35. vertex 37. $91\frac{2}{3}\%$
39. 200

PAGE 309 CUMULATIVE REVIEW
PROBLEMS **1.** $79.38 **3.** 23,500 ft
5. 1230 lb **7.** 52 cm **9.** $616.13

9 The Coordinate Plane

PAGES 314–315 WRITTEN EXERCISES
1. $(-5, -5)$ **3.** $(5, 1)$ **5.** $(-3, -2)$
7. $(-1, 4)$ **9.** I **11.** V **13.** D **15.** W **17.** M
19. c. rectangle **21. c.** parallelogram
23. b. $(-5, 1), (-2, -2), (2, -2), (2, 1)$
d. Translation **25. b.** $(-2, 3), (2, 3), (4, 1),$
$(4, -1), (1, 1), (-1, 1), (-4, -1), (-4, 1)$
d. Translation **27. b.** $(-6, 5), (-2, 1), (-9, 3)$
d. Reflection

PAGE 315 REVIEW EXERCISES **1.** 8
3. 27 **5.** -5 **7.** -15

PAGES 318–319 WRITTEN EXERCISES
1. Yes **3.** Yes **5.** No **7.** No **9.** No **11.** No
13. Yes **15.** Yes **17.** $y = -2x + 7$
19. $y = 4x + 16$ **21.** $y = \frac{2}{3}x - 2$
23. a. $y = x + 7$ **b.** $(2, 9), (-5, 2), (7, 14)$
25. a. $y = \frac{1}{2}x + 5$ **b.** $(4, 7), (0, 5), (6, 8)$
27. a. $y = -\frac{1}{4}x + 5$ **b.** $(4, 4), (-8, 7), (0, 5)$
29. a. $y = \frac{3}{2}x - 3$ **b.** $(4, 3), (-2, -6),$
$(-8, -15)$ **31. a.** $y = \frac{1}{2}x + \frac{5}{2}$ **b.** $(3, 4), (5, 5),$
$(-1, 2)$ **33. a.** $y = \frac{5}{2}x + 3$ **b.** $(2, 8), (1, 5\frac{1}{2}),$
$(-3, -4\frac{1}{2})$ In Exercises 35–43, answers will
vary. Examples are given. **35.** $(-1, 0), (0, -1),$
$(1, -2)$ **37.** $(-1, 1), (0, 0), (1, -1)$
39. $(-1, 0), (0, 5), (1, 10)$ **41.** $(-3, -6),$
$(0, -4), (3, -2)$ **43.** $(-1, 4), (0, 6), (1, 8)$
45. $x + y = 0$ **47.** $x + y = -3$

PAGE 319 REVIEW EXERCISES **1.** 3
3. 28 **5.** 3 **7.** -56 **9.** -4

PAGES 321–323 WRITTEN EXERCISES
1.

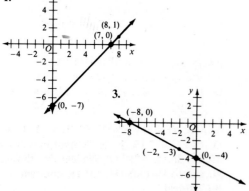

5.–33. Each graph is a straight line through the
points listed: **5.** $(0, 10), (1, 8), (5, 0)$ **7.** $(0, 0),$
$(1, 1), (2, 2)$ **9.** $(-2, -1), (0, 0)$ **11.** $(0, -6),$
$(6, 0)$ **13.** $(-3, 0), (0, -3)$ **15.** $(0, 4), (1, 0)$
17. $(-2, 0), (0, 6)$ **19.** $(-8, 0), (0, 2)$
21. $(-4, 0), (0, 3)$ **23.** $(-\frac{5}{2}, 0), (0, 1)$
25. $(0, 6), (6, 0)$ **27.** $(0, -6), (2, 0)$ **29.** $(-12, 0), (0, 6)$
31. $(0, -\frac{1}{2}), (\frac{1}{3}, 0)$ **33.** $(0, -8), (6, 0)$
35.   **37.**

39.   **47.** $-\frac{3}{4}$

PAGE 323 SELF-TEST A **1.** $(-3, 6)$
2. $(4, -4)$
3. $(6, 6)$
4. C
5. T
6. P **7.–12.**

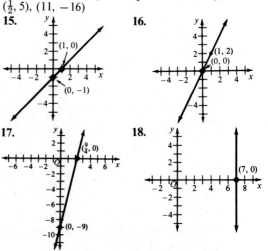

13. $(0, \frac{1}{2}), (-4, -\frac{1}{2}), (9, 2\frac{3}{4})$ **14.** $(-3, 12),$
$(\frac{1}{2}, 5), (11, -16)$
15.   **16.**

17.   **18.**

544 *Answers*

PAGES 326–327 WRITTEN EXERCISES
1. Intersect **3.** Parallel **5.** Coincide
7. Parallel **9.** Intersect **11.** Coincide
13. Intersect **15.** Parallel **17.** Intersect **19.** 2

PAGE 327 REVIEW EXERCISES **1.** $1\frac{1}{8}$
3. $\frac{7}{8}$ **5.** $\frac{4}{5}$ **7.** $\frac{1}{13}$

PAGE 327 CALCULATOR KEY-IN
$13,107.20

PAGES 331–333 PROBLEMS **1.** $\frac{3}{2}$ **3.** 4°C
5. 245 mi **7. a.** $y = 4.5x + 2$ **c.** 7 lb
9. a. $y = \frac{7}{12}x + \frac{1}{6}$ **c.** $10\frac{2}{3}$ min **11.** 5.5 s

PAGE 333 REVIEW EXERCISES All the
numbers: **1.** greater than $1\frac{1}{3}$ **3.** greater than or
equal to -1 **5.** less than or equal to 0
7. greater than or equal to -1 **9.** greater
than 41

PAGE 333 CALCULATOR KEY-IN 1; 121;
12,321; 1,234,321; 123,454,321; and so on.

PAGES 336–337 WRITTEN EXERCISES
1. $y = -3x - 6$ **3.** $y = x - 2$
5. $y = -x + 3$
7.

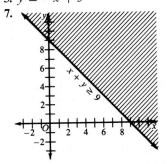

9. Solid line through $(-1, 0)$ and $(0, 2)$, shaded
region at left above line **11.** Solid line
through $(0, 4)$ and $(2, 0)$, shaded region at right
above line **13.** Solid line through $(-\frac{5}{2}, 0)$ and
$(0, 5)$, shaded region at left above line
15. Dashed line through $(0, -\frac{1}{3})$ and $(\frac{1}{2}, 0)$,
shaded region at left above line **17.** Solid line
through $(0, 8)$ parallel to x-axis, shaded region
below line **19.** Solid line through $(-1, 0)$ and
$(0, -1)$, shaded region at left below line.
21. Solid line through $(-3, 0)$ parallel to y-
axis, shaded region to left of line. **23.** Dashed
line through $(-\frac{5}{2}, 0)$ and $(0, 5)$, shaded region
at right below line **25.** $x < 4$ **27.** $y \geq -3$

PAGE 337 SELF-TEST B **1.** intersect
2. coincide **3.** parallel **4.** 4 wk

5.

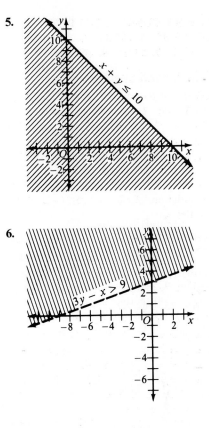

6.

7.

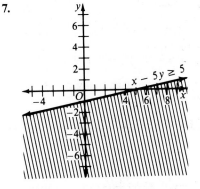

PAGES 338–339 ENRICHMENT
1. $y = 0.5x + 1.32$ **3.** 2.9 kg
5. $y = -3.3x + 20.8$ **a.** 15.85°C **b.** 6.3 h
7. $y = 0.59x + 7.39$; $10,930; $11,520

PAGE 340 CHAPTER REVIEW **1.** False
3. True **5.** C **7.** B **9.** Straight line through
$(0, 0)$ and $(1, -1)$ **11.** Straight line through
$(0, 2)$ and $(-1, 0)$ **13.** C **15.** constant
17. dashed

PAGE 342 CUMULATIVE REVIEW
EXERCISES **1.** $5b$ **3.** $y + z - 12$
5. $3p + 7$ **7.** 288.01 **9.** 100.76 **11.** 4.8911
13. 554.09 **15.** 3.0088 **17.** -425.0612
19. -8.174 **21.** $-\frac{3}{14}$ **23.** $1\frac{1}{8}$ **25.** $-4\frac{47}{50}$
27. $t = -\frac{3}{4}(\frac{1}{5})$; $-\frac{3}{20}$ **29.** $x + 12 > 2x$; the
solutions are all the numbers less than 12
31. 20.7 m **33.** 1.6 **35.** 42 **37.** no **39.** yes

PAGE 343 CUMULATIVE REVIEW
PROBLEMS **1.** $84.88 **3.** 7.5 times
5. $9799; $10,038 **7.** 44.1% **9.** 0.5 kW·h

10 Areas and Volumes

PAGES 348–349 WRITTEN EXERCISES
1. 1050 cm²; 130 cm **3.** 2665 km²; 212 km
5. 4416 mm²; 280 mm **7.** 2490.67 km²;
205.6 km **9.** perimeter: 40; area: 93.75
11. length: 80; perimeter: 250 **13.** width: 0.4;
area: 3.44 **15.** 74 **17.** 0.5 **19.** 4 **21.** 37
square units **23.** 30 square units **25.** 72
square units

PAGE 350 PROBLEMS **1.** 24 m²
3. a. 720 ft² **b.** $1080 **5.** 15 m **7.** 2025 m²

PAGE 350 REVIEW EXERCISES **1.** 28
3. 1.04 **5.** 40 **7.** 0.078

PAGES 354–355 WRITTEN EXERCISES
1. 67.34 m² **3.** 2127.5 cm² **5.** 290 mm²
7. 1830 km² **9.** 44.4 cm² **11.** 24 cm **13.** 4 m
15. 8 mm **17.** 15 **19.** The base and the height
are the same for each triangle. **21.** 450 cm²;
450 cm² **23.** 9 : 1; 3 : 1

PAGE 355 REVIEW EXERCISES **1.** 75
3. 6.76 **5.** 292 **7.** 1.33 **9.** 4868

PAGES 358–359 WRITTEN EXERCISES
1. 78.5 km² **3.** 0.283 m² **5.** $9\frac{5}{8}$ square units
7. 100π m² **9.** 4π square units **11.** 10 m
13. 2 cm **15.** 4π **17.** $31\frac{1}{2}\pi$ cm²
19. $(25\pi - 50)$m² **21.** $A = \dfrac{C^2}{4\pi}$

PAGE 359 PROBLEMS **1.** $1100 **3.** 314 m²
5. 462 cm² **7.** $\frac{100}{157}$

PAGE 359 REVIEW EXERCISES **1.** 16
3. 9 **5.** 18 **7.** 15

PAGES 362–363 WRITTEN EXERCISES
1.

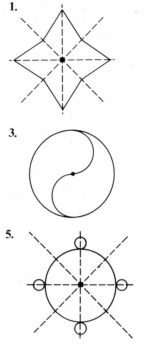

3.

5.

7. 84 m² **9.** 50π square units **11.** 135
square units **13.** 16 square units
15. $(200 + 50\pi)$cm²

PAGE 363 SELF-TEST A **1.** 273 cm²
2. 84 m² **3.** 72 cm² **4.** 36 m² **5.** 707 mm²
6. 616 cm² **7.** **8.** 28 square
units

PAGES 366–368 WRITTEN EXERCISES
1. 90 cubic units **3.** 108 cubic units **5.** 22,608
cubic units **7.** 514 cubic units **9.** 50 L
11. 6330 L **13.** 4π; 3 **15.** 5; 4 **17.** 3; 9π
19. 60 cubic units **21. a.** quadrupled
b. halved **c.** doubled **23.** 3

PAGE 368 PROBLEMS **1.** 96 L
3. 7070 cm³ **5.** 1.62 cm

PAGE 368 REVIEW EXERCISES **1.** 32
3. 0.845 **5.** 1256 **7.** 10; -10

PAGES 371–372 WRITTEN EXERCISES
1. 72 cubic units **3.** 301 cubic units **5.** 56
cubic units **7.** 0.16 L **9.** 1000 L **11.** 10
13. 6 **15.** 3 **17.** 15 **19.** 3 **21.** 18

PAGE 372 PROBLEMS **1.** 2,590,000 m³
3. 14,700 cm³

PAGE 372 REVIEW EXERCISES **1.** 36 m
3. 105 cm **5.** 51.2 km **7.** 580.8 km

PAGES 375–377 WRITTEN EXERCISES
1. 5700 cm² **3.** 14.56 m² **5.** 1660 cm²;
2560 cm² **7.** 226 square units; 283 square
units **9.** 360 square units; 468 square units
11. 30 cubic units; 72 square units **13.** 5 cm
15. 6 **17.** 72 m²; 120 m² **19.** $n - 2$

PAGE 377 REVIEW EXERCISES **1.** 6
3. 105 **5.** 35 **7.** 38

PAGES 379–381 WRITTEN EXERCISES
1. 36π square units; 36π cubic units **3.** 144π
square units; 288π cubic units **5.** 400π square
units; $\frac{4000}{3}\pi$ cubic units **7.** $\frac{16}{3}\pi$ cubic units
9. 9.68π square units **11.** 51.84π square units;
62.208π cubic units **13.** 9 units; 324π square
units **15.** 8 units; $\frac{2048}{3}\pi$ cubic units **17.** 324π
cubic units **19.** The Earth's volume is about
49.3 times that of the moon. **21. a.** $2:3$
b. $2:3$ **c.** $2:3$

PAGE 381 REVIEW EXERCISES **1.** 2.1
3. 0.64 **5.** 3.5 **7.** 810

PAGE 381 CALCULATOR KEY-IN
1. About 126 times greater

PAGES 383–384 WRITTEN EXERCISES
1. 6300 **3.** 4300 **5.** 810 g **7.** 34 kg **9.** 460 t
11. 180 g **13.** 33.1 g **15.** 72.7 g **17.** 7460 kg

PAGES 384–385 PROBLEMS **1.** 13.3 kg
3. 81.1 g **5.** 3.91 t

PAGE 385 SELF-TEST B **1.** 41.8 **2.** 27,200
3. 9248; 9.248 **4.** 0.314 m³ **5.** 1200 m³
6. 10,800 cm³ **7. a.** 98 square units **b.** 122
square units **8. a.** 94.2 square units **b.** 251
square units **9. a.** 3024 square units **b.** 3672
square units **10. a.** 1296π cm² **b.** 7776π cm³
11. a. 144π m² **b.** 288π m³ **12.** 8240 g
13. 181.76 g

PAGE 387 ENRICHMENT **1.** New York

3. Rio de Janeiro **5.** Moscow **7.** Casablanca
9. 40°N, 105°W **11.** 55°N, 0° **13.** 15°N,
15°W **15.** 65°N, 165°W

PAGE 388 CHAPTER REVIEW **1.** b **3.** c
5. d **7.** 3864 cm³ **9.** 45.2 cubic units
11. 168; 266 **13.** 2300; 18400 **15.** 60.48 kg

PAGES 390–391 CUMULATIVE REVIEW
EXERCISES **1.** 5 **3.** 10 **5.** 12.5 **7.** −22.5
9. $\frac{37}{12}$, or $3\frac{1}{12}$ **11.** $\frac{2}{5}$ **13.** $\frac{52}{3}$, or $17\frac{1}{3}$ **15.** $-\frac{37}{4}$,
or $-9\frac{1}{4}$ **17.** All the numbers greater than 3
19. All the numbers less than or equal to 40
21. All the numbers greater than or equal to 9
23. 7 **25.** 21 **27.** 45°; 45° **29.** 8.1 **31.** 24%
33. 63,200 **35.** $y = 18 - 4x$ **37.** $y = x - 8\frac{1}{3}$
39. $y = \frac{20}{x}$ **41.** 196π cm² **43.** 15625π km²
45. $3,258,025\pi$ cm² **47.** 256π square units;
$\frac{2048}{3}\pi$ cubic units **49.** 5184π square units;
$62,208\pi$ cubic units

PAGE 391 CUMULATIVE REVIEW
PROBLEMS **1.** 1929 stories **3.** 25 m **5.** $\frac{1}{4}$
7. 5%

11 Applying Algebra to Right Triangles
PAGE 395 WRITTEN EXERCISES **1.** 6 and
7 **3.** −4 **5.** 1 **7.** −6 **9.** 7 and 8 **11.** 5
and 6 **13.** 3 and 4 **15.** 1 and 2 **17.** 3 **19.** 4
and 5 **21.** 9 **23.** > **25.** < **27.** = **29.** >
31. 81 **33.** 11

PAGE 395 REVIEW EXERCISES **1.** 6.57
3. 8.67 **5.** 11.95 **7.** 0.13

PAGE 398 WRITTEN EXERCISES **1.** 3.3
3. 5.7 **5.** 2.8 **7.** 5.1 **9.** 7.5 **11.** 9.5 **13.** 2.3
15. 3.0 **17.** 2.9 **19.** 1.9 **21.** 12.3 **23.** 26.5
25. 3.9 **27.** 8.4 **29.** 0.6 **31.** 0.2 **33.** 1.41
35. 2.23

PAGE 398 REVIEW EXERCISES **1.** 58
3. 6.72 **5.** 3.89 **7.** 93.57

PAGE 398 CALCULATOR KEY-IN **1. a.** 1
b. 10 **c.** 100 **3. a.** 8.3666002 **b.** 83.666002
c. 836.66002 **5. a.** 0.73484692 **b.** 7.3484692
c. 73.484692

PAGES 400–401 WRITTEN EXERCISES
1. 8.06 **3.** 7.48 **5.** 9.85 **7.** 64.03 **9.** 0.87
11. 22.25 **13.** 26.15 **15.** 59.40 **17.** 12.57
19. 0.37 **21.** 0.43 **23.** 2.43 **25.** 9.03

27. 2.95 **29.** 7.13 **31.** 27.15 **33.** 22.36
35. 19.49 **37.** 58.91

PAGE 401 PROBLEMS **1.** 9.22 m **3.** $21
5. 3.87 cm **7.** 5.92 m

PAGE 401 REVIEW EXERCISES **1.** 0.81
3. 0.0036 **5.** 13.69 **7.** 590.49

PAGE 404 WRITTEN EXERCISES **1.** 289
3. 400 **5.** Yes **7.** Yes **9.** Yes **11.** Yes
13. No **15.** $c = 10$ **17.** $a = 3.32$
19. $c = 11.40$ **21.** $b = 70$ **23.** $a = 27$, $b = 36$,
$c = 45$

PAGES 404–405 PROBLEMS **1.** 108.2 km
3. 55.7 m **5.** 7.1 cm **7.** 17.3

PAGE 405 SELF-TEST A **1.** 7 and 8
2. -9 **3.** 8 **4.** 7 **5.** 9.3 **6.** 4.2 **7.** 7.1
8. 3.1 **9.** 2.4 **10.** $c = 5$ **11.** $a = 28$
12. $b = 16$

PAGES 409–410 WRITTEN EXERCISES
1. RQ **3.** 9 **5.** 104° **7.** 25 **9.** 65°; 65°
11. $x = 5$, $y = 9$ **13.** $x = 27$, $y = 25$
15. $x = 46\frac{2}{7}$, $y = 14$ **17.** 180 cm **19. a.** 18
b. 18 **21.** $\angle CDA \cong \angle BCA$; $\angle A \cong \angle A$; so
$\angle B \cong \angle DCA$ **23.** Yes; angles congruent,
sides proportional **25.** Not necessarily; the
lengths of the sides may differ.

PAGE 410 REVIEW EXERCISES **1.** 519
3. 1562 **5.** 2.2454 **7.** 4.878 **9.** 3741.36

PAGES 413–414 WRITTEN EXERCISES
1. $\frac{3\sqrt{10}}{5}$ **3.** $\sqrt{3}$ **5.** $\frac{2\sqrt{x}}{x}$ **7.** $x = 3.2$, $y = 5.5$
9. $x = 7.4$, $y = 8.6$ **11.** $x = 3.2$, $y = 4.5$
13. $2\sqrt{2}$ **15.** $5\sqrt{3}$; $10\sqrt{3}$ **17.** $AB = 5.4$
19. $BC = 6.0$ **21.** $BC = 1.7y$ **23.** $x = 6$,
$y = 3$

PAGES 414–415 PROBLEMS **1.** 8.7 m
3. 20 m **5.** 56.6 cm **7.** 40; 28.3 **9. a.** 0.9 r
units **b.** 0.4 r² units² **11.** 5.2 m

PAGE 415 REVIEW EXERCISES **1.** 1.25
3. 0.$\overline{2}$ **5.** 1.1 **7.** 0.1$\overline{6}$

PAGES 418–419 WRITTEN EXERCISES
1. $\sin A = \frac{3}{5}$; $\cos A = \frac{4}{5}$; $\tan A = \frac{3}{4}$; $\sin B = \frac{4}{5}$;
$\cos B = \frac{3}{5}$; $\tan B = \frac{4}{3}$ **3.** $\sin A = \frac{80}{89}$;
$\cos A = \frac{39}{89}$; $\tan A = \frac{80}{39}$; $\sin B = \frac{39}{89}$; $\cos B = \frac{80}{89}$;
$\tan B = \frac{39}{80}$ **5.** $\sin A = \frac{a}{c}$; $\cos A = \frac{b}{c}$;

$\tan A = \frac{a}{b}$; $\sin B = \frac{b}{c}$; $\cos B = \frac{a}{c}$; $\tan B = \frac{b}{a}$
7. $x = 5$; $\tan A = \frac{5}{12}$ **9.** $x = \sqrt{21}$;
$\sin A = \frac{\sqrt{21}}{11}$ **11.** $x = 24$; $\cos A = \frac{12}{13}$
13. a. $\frac{\sqrt{3}}{2}$; 0.866 **b.** $\frac{1}{2}$; 0.500 **c.** $\sqrt{3}$; 1.732
15. a. 6.4 **b.** 2.7 **c.** 0.4 **17. a.** 3.8 **b.** 8.2
c. 0.5

PAGE 419 REVIEW EXERCISES **1.** b
3. a **5.** b **7.** b

PAGE 422 WRITTEN EXERCISES
1. 0.4226; 0.9063; 0.4663 **3.** 0.9994; 0.0349;
28.6363 **5.** 0.6293; 0.7771; 0.8098 **7.** 0.9613;
0.2756; 3.4874 **9.** 0.6428; 0.7660; 0.8391
11. 0.9063; 0.4226; 2.1445 **13.** 81° **15.** 1°
17. 76° **19.** 30° **21.** 60° **23.** 6 **25.** 58°
27. 25° **29.** 70° **31.** $c = 9.4$, $m\angle A = 32°$,
$m\angle B = 58°$ **33.** $a = 9.5$, $b = 3.1$,
$m\angle B = 18°$ **35.** $a = 8.1$, $m\angle A = 64°$,
$m\angle B = 26°$ **37.** $a = 41.3$, $c = 43.9$,
$m\angle A = 70°$ **39.** $a = 19.2$, $c = 22.6$,
$m\angle B = 32°$

PAGES 423–424 PROBLEMS **1.** 42.0 m
3. 11° **5. a.** 42.5 m **b.** 10.7 m **7.** 39° **9.** 67°

PAGE 424 SELF-TEST B **1.** ~ **2.** $\frac{TN}{TY}$
3. 7.5 **4.** = **5.** 6 cm **6.** $4\sqrt{3}$; $8\sqrt{3}$ **7.** $\frac{p}{q}$
8. $\frac{r}{q}$ **9.** $\frac{p}{r}$ **10.** $m\angle P = 60°$, $m\angle R = 30°$,
$p = 5.2$ **11.** $p = 23.5$, $q = 24.1$, $m\angle R = 12°$
12. $q = 8.7$, $r = 3.4$, $m\angle P = 67°$
13. $r = 20.1$, $p = 13.1$, $m\angle P = 33°$

PAGE 425 COMPUTER BYTE **1.** 3, 4, 5
3. 5, 12, 13 **5.** Output: THERE IS NO SUCH
TRIPLE.

PAGE 427 ENRICHMENT **1.** 3 **3.** 2 **5.** 4
7. There is no square root because a is
negative and n is even. **9.** -10 **11.** 5
13. $\sqrt{36} = 6$ **15.** $\sqrt[3]{64} = 4$ **17.** $\sqrt[4]{16} = 2$
19. $\sqrt[4]{81} = 3$ Calculator Activity
1. 2.1544347 **3.** 2.1867241 **5.** 1.4953488
7. About 9.4203395 π

PAGE 428 CHAPTER REVIEW **1.** 2
3. 5.35 **5.** 4.899 and 5 **7.** False **9.** False
11. F **13.** 45° **15.** $7\sqrt{2}$ **17.** A **19.** D **21.** F

PAGES 430–431 CUMULATIVE REVIEW
EXERCISES 1. $\frac{10}{27}$ 3. 3300 5. $-3\frac{1}{3}$
7. -100 9. 0 11. -200 13. 2.5 15. -1
17. $>$ 19. $<$ 21. 38 23. 2.5 25. $7\frac{1}{3}$ 27. 8
29. 12 31. $5\frac{3}{5}$ 33. 11.6 ft 35. 4 37. 10
39.

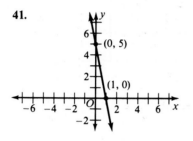

41.

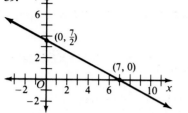

43. 55.5π 45. $\frac{5\sqrt{2}}{2}$ 47. $2\sqrt{n}$

PAGE 431 CUMULATIVE REVIEW
PROBLEMS 1. 40 dimes, 49 nickels, 52
quarters 3. $22.50 5. $2.17 7. 52 in. by
52 in.

12 Statistics and Probability

PAGES 436–437 WRITTEN EXERCISES
1. 100 million persons 3. approx. 400 million
5. 23%
7.

Highway Tunnels

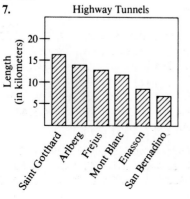

11.

Net Profit of XYZ Company

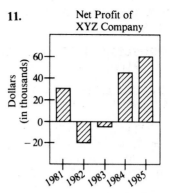

PAGE 437 REVIEW EXERCISES 1. 282
3. 354 5. 135 7. 131.4

PAGES 440–442 WRITTEN EXERCISES
1.

$\frac{1}{4}$		90°
$\frac{3}{10}$		108°
$\frac{1}{5}$		72°
$\frac{1}{4}$		90°
240	1	360°

Cards Sold

get well 72 | birthday 60
friendship 48 | thank you 60

3. Surface of Earth

Land 30%
Water 70%

5. Number of Cars Rented

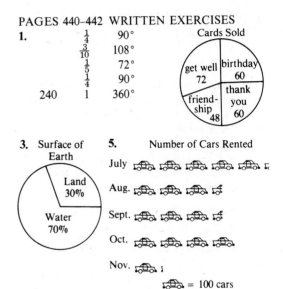

= 100 cars

9. People Living in U.S.

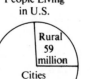

Rural 59 million
Cities 167 million

People Living in United States

Cities 👤👤👤👤👤👤👤
Rural 👤👤👤

👤 = 20 million people

15. a. Distribution of Library Grant

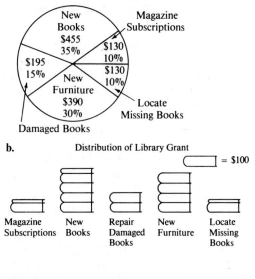

New Books $455 35%
Magazine Subscriptions $130 10%
$130 10%
$195 15%
New Furniture $390 30%
$130 10% Locate Missing Books
Damaged Books

b. Distribution of Library Grant

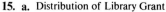

= $100

Magazine Subscriptions New Books Repair Damaged Books New Furniture Locate Missing Books

PAGE 442 REVIEW EXERCISES **1.** 0.84, 2.6, 3, 4, 7 **3.** -6, -5, $3\frac{1}{2}$, $4\frac{1}{4}$, 7 **5.** -12, -10, -9, -6, -2 **7.** 0.09, 0.9, 1.09, 1.1

PAGES 444–445 WRITTEN EXERCISES
1. 24; 23; 12 **3.** 16; 15; 19 **5.** 55.5; 55.5; 24 **7.** 3.2; 3.4; 0.9 **9.** -1; -2; 8 **11.** 0.3; 0.2; 2.1 **13.** $-2°$, $-1°$, 19° **15.** 16 **17.** 16 **19.** 94 **21.** It is increased by 5.

PAGE 445 REVIEW EXERCISES **1.** 6.1 **3.** 14.8 **5.** 14 **7.** 3

PAGES 447–448 WRITTEN EXERCISES
1. 4; 6.95; 7; 7 **3.** 20; 10; 10; 5 **5.** 6; 16.75; 17; 16 and 17

7.

x	f	
8	2	range = 8
6	1	mean = 3.9
5	4	median = 4
4	5	mode = 4
3	2	
1	3	
0	1	

9.

x	f	
20	6	range = 6
19	7	mean = 18.1
18	8	median = 18
17	5	mode = 18
16	2	
15	1	
14	1	

11.

x	f	
103	2	range = 6
102	2	mean = 100.4
101	6	median = 100
100	9	mode = 100
99	3	
97	1	

13. 72

PAGE 448 REVIEW EXERCISES **1.** The average of a set of data. **3.** The number from a set of data which occurs most often. **5.** An integer not evenly divisible by 2. **7.** A number greater than 1 whose only factors are 1 and itself.

PAGE 449 COMPUTER BYTE **1.** $18.\overline{3}$ **3.** $578.1\overline{6}$ **5.** approx. 4494.13042 **7.** 489,439.2

PAGES 451–452 WRITTEN EXERCISES
1. 15 **3.** 1 **5.** 9 **7.** 20 **9.** 34
11.

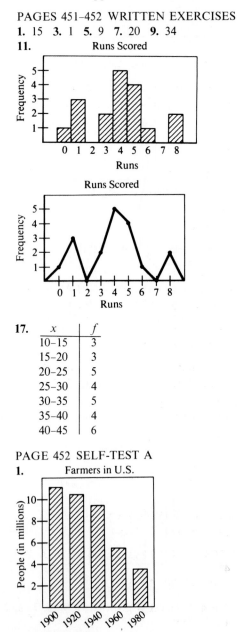

Runs Scored

Runs Scored

17.

x	f
10–15	3
15–20	3
20–25	5
25–30	4
30–35	5
35–40	4
40–45	6

PAGE 452 SELF-TEST A
1.

Farmers in U.S.

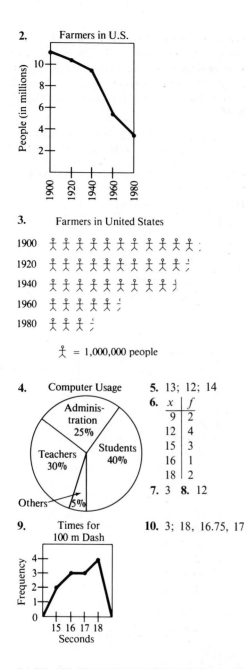

2. Farmers in U.S.

3. Farmers in United States

1900
1920
1940
1960
1980

☧ = 1,000,000 people

4. Computer Usage

Administration 25%
Teachers 30%
Students 40%
Others 5%

5. 13; 12; 14

6.

x	f
9	2
12	4
15	3
16	1
18	2

7. 3 **8.** 12

9. Times for 100 m Dash

10. 3; 18, 16.75, 17

PAGE 455 WRITTEN EXERCISES **1.** 120
3. 5040 **5.** 720 **7.** 40,320 **9.** 360 **11.** 74,046

PAGES 455–457 PROBLEMS **1.** 6 **3.** 24
5. 42 **7.** 24 **9.** 12 **11.** 5040 **13.** 720
15. 216 **17.** 20 **19.** 6

PAGE 457 REVIEW EXERCISES **1.** 7 **3.** 3
5. 12 **7.** 165

PAGES 459–460 PROBLEMS **1.** 15 **3.** 15
5. 210 **7.** 252 **9. a.** 4 **b.** 6 **c.** 4 **d.** 1
e. 15 **11.** 10,192

PAGE 460 REVIEW EXERCISES **1.** Any of two or more whole numbers that are multiplied to form a product. **3.** Any whole numbers that is divisible by 2. **5.** The product of a number by itself 3 times. **7.** One or less

PAGES 464–465 WRITTEN EXERCISES
1. $\frac{1}{6}$ **3.** $\frac{2}{3}$ **5.** 0 **7.** $\frac{1}{4}$ **9.** $\frac{1}{5}$ **11.** $\frac{1}{2}$ **13.** $\frac{3}{4}$
15. $\frac{2}{5}$ **17.** $\frac{3}{5}$ **19.** $\frac{1}{3}$ **21.** $\frac{1}{2}$ **23.** $\frac{1}{3}$ **25.** $\frac{2}{3}$ **27.** $\frac{1}{12}$
29. $\frac{1}{6}$ **31.** $\frac{1}{18}$ **33.** $\frac{2}{9}$ **35.** $\frac{5}{12}$ **37. a.** $\frac{1}{9}$ **b.** $\frac{5}{9}$
c. $\frac{4}{9}$ **d.** $\frac{8}{9}$ **e.** $\frac{4}{9}$ **39.** $\frac{1}{2}$

PAGE 465 REVIEW EXERCISES **1.** 0 **3.** $\frac{1}{3}$
5. $\frac{1}{2}$ **7.** $\frac{3}{4}$

PAGES 468–469 WRITTEN EXERCISES
1. 1 to 1 **3.** 1 to 2 **5.** 5 to 1 **7.** 2 to 3 **9.** 7 to 3 **11.** 1 to 1 **13.** 3 to 1 **15.** 4 to 1 **17.** 17 to 1 **19.** 17 to 1 **21.** 13 to 5 **23. a.** 2 to 1
b. 1 to 2 **25.** 11 to 25 **27.** 3 to 1 **29.** $\frac{1}{9}$

PAGE 469 REVIEW EXERCISES **1.** $\frac{23}{24}$
3. $\frac{11}{12}$ **5.** $\frac{25}{36}$ **7.** $\frac{71}{196}$

PAGE 469 COMPUTER BYTE **1.** Answers may vary; 1

PAGES 471–472 WRITTEN EXERCISES
1. $\frac{13}{15}$ **3.** 0.3 **5. a.** $\frac{1}{3}$ **b.** $\frac{1}{2}$ **c.** $\frac{5}{6}$ **7. a.** $\frac{1}{6}$ **b.** $\frac{5}{6}$
9. a. $\frac{1}{2}$ **b.** $\frac{1}{3}$ **c.** $\frac{5}{6}$ **11. a.** $\frac{1}{5}$ **b.** $\frac{2}{5}$ **c.** $\frac{3}{5}$
13. a. $\frac{1}{4}$ **b.** $\frac{3}{10}$ **c.** $\frac{11}{20}$ **15. a.** $\frac{1}{4}$ **b.** $\frac{3}{10}$ **c.** $\frac{2}{5}$
17. a. $\frac{1}{12}$ **b.** $\frac{11}{36}$ **c.** $\frac{11}{18}$ **19. a.** $\frac{1}{6}$ **b.** $\frac{1}{6}$ **c.** $\frac{1}{3}$
21. 9 to 11 **23.** 11 to 9

PAGE 473 SELF-TEST B **1.** 24 **2.** 120 **3.** 10
4. 210 **5.** $\frac{1}{8}$ **6.** $\frac{1}{2}$ **7.** $\frac{1}{4}$ **8.** 1 **9.** 1 to 3
10. 1 to 3 **11.** 3 to 1 **12.** $\frac{7}{12}$ **13.** 0.2

PAGE 475 ENRICHMENT **1. a.** 12 gal
b. −1, 1, −3, 3 **c.** 5 gal² **d.** 2.24 gal
3. a. 22.8 mi/gal **b.** −2.8, −3.8, −2.8, −0.8, 10.2 **c.** 26.96 mi/gal² **d.** 5.19 mi/gal

PAGE 476 CHAPTER REVIEW **1.** Sprint
3. broken line **5.** 8 **7.** 68.5 **9.** 2 **11.** 3
13. True **15.** True

PAGE 478 CUMULATIVE REVIEW
EXERCISES **1.** 49.5 **3.** 7.475 **5.** $m + 3n$
7. $1\frac{6}{35}$ **9.** $\frac{21}{32}$ **11.** $-3\frac{2}{3}$ **13.** 20 **15.** All the numbers greater than or equal to −2 **17.** 42
19. 13.3 **21.** 46.8 **23.** 20% **25.** 36

27. $C(-1, 4)$; $D(-7, 7)$; $m = -\frac{1}{2}$
29. $P = 468$ m; $A = 13308.75$ m^2
31. $P = 144$ m; $A = 756$ m^2 **33.** no

PAGE 479 CUMULATIVE REVIEW
PROBLEMS **1.** No **3.** 30% **5.** 9.9 cm
7. 180 m^2 **9.** $5\frac{1}{2}$ ft $\times 3\frac{1}{2}$ ft

Skill Review

PAGE 480 ADDITION **1.** 99 **3.** 43 **5.** 121
7. 741 **9.** 9.2 **11.** 367.43 **13.** 325.277
15. 46.119 **17.** 888 **19.** 522 **21.** 20.062
23. 8.156 **25.** 22.098 **27.** 18.50032 **29.** 95.83
31. 1396 **33.** 6.88 **35.** 155.072 **37.** 1497
39. 98.187 **41.** 1565 **43.** 1754 **45.** 1276.208
47. 54.7138

PAGE 481 SUBTRACTION **1.** 13 **3.** 26
5. 655 **7.** 613 **9.** 5.201 **11.** 11.744
13. 2.137 **15.** 1.892 **17.** 435.54 **19.** 0.074
21. 25 **23.** 62 **25.** 44 **27.** 48 **29.** 33
31. 40.13 **33.** 57.03 **35.** 0.063 **37.** 3162
39. 3549 **41.** 6925 **43.** 21.026 **45.** 2.6205
47. 0.8651 **49.** 73.403 **51.** 14,548

PAGE 482 MULTIPLICATION **1.** 26
3. 159 **5.** 141 **7.** 360 **9.** 1008 **11.** 4615
13. 942 **15.** 13,897.6 **17.** 44.53 **19.** 142.576
21. 600 **23.** 900 **25.** 72,000 **27.** 680,000
29. 141,000 **31.** 15,201 **33.** 5024 **35.** 55,380
37. 286.165 **39.** 18.8241 **41.** 75.295
43. 8840 **45.** 7914.7224 **47.** 0.1162779
49. 1.8574 **51.** 0.00869812

PAGE 483 DIVISION **1.** 17 **3.** 46 **5.** 16
7. 35.2 **9.** 0.76 **11.** 15.7 **13.** 10.8 **15.** 15.8
17. 13.3 **19.** 548.1 **21.** 49.6 **23.** 73.29
25. 81 **27.** 2.75 **29.** 2.63 **31.** 7.36 **33.** 1910
35. 0.25 **37.** 517.06 **39.** 129,413.33
41. 47.91 **43.** 534.27 **45.** 307.45 **47.** 610.67
49. 4900.53 **51.** 18.43 **53.** 3697.69 **55.** 0.01
57. 99.09

Extra Practice

PAGES 484–485 CHAPTER 1 **1.** 42.63
3. 0.16 **5.** 1 **7.** 24 **9.** 9 **11.** $\frac{1}{6}$ **13.** 40.8
15. 14 **17.** 2 **19.** 169 **21.** 1156 **23.** 16,807
25. 6561 **27.** 16,000 **29.** 3,456,000 **31.** 64
33. 1728 **35.** $(5 \times 10^2) + (1 \times 10^1) +$

$(6 \times 10^0) + \left(2 \times \frac{1}{10^1}\right) + \left(1 \times \frac{1}{10^2}\right)$

37. $(2 \times 10^1) + (5 \times 10^0) + \left(2 \times \frac{1}{10^1}\right)$

39. $(9 \times 10^1) + (1 \times 10^0) + \left(9 \times \frac{1}{10^1}\right)$

41. $(3 \times 10^2) + (0 + 10^1) + (7 \times 10^0) +$

$\left(0 \times \frac{1}{10^1}\right) + \left(0 \times \frac{1}{10^2}\right) + \left(9 \times \frac{1}{10^3}\right)$ **43.** 5.004

45. 9.0009 **47.** 0.0006 **49.** 113.9 **51.** 0.06
53. 45.55 **55.** 100 **57.** 1.84 **59.** 0 **61.** 8
63. 8 **65.** 112 **67.** 7 **69.** 11 **71.** 12 **73.** 31
75. 2448 **77.** 40 **79.** 52.1 s **81.** 1260 parts
83. 3 h

PAGES 486–487 CHAPTER 2 **1.** 3 **3.** 1
5. 6 **7.** 2 **9.** 9

11.

13.

15.

17. $^-8$, $^-2$, 0, 5, 6 **19.** $^-7$, $^-4$, $^-1$, 3, 5 **21.** $^-5$,
$^-4$, 0, 4, 5 **23.** $<$ **25.** 5, $^-5$ **27.** 0 **29.** 6, 5,
4, 3, 2, 1, 0, $^-1$, $^-2$, $^-3$, $^-4$, $^-5$, $^-6$
41. 9.9 **43.** 0 **45.** $^-404$ **47.** $^-2.9$ **49.** $^-2.3$
51. 20.9 **53.** 12.5 **55.** -0.6 **57.** 20.3
59. -13.5 **61.** -20.3 **63.** 5.2 **65.** 5.7
67. -3.2 **69.** -2.5 **71.** -8.9 **73.** 2.5
75. -4.1 **77.** -610 **79.** -0.91 **81.** 9100
83. -0.003 **85.** 0.5 **87.** -4.76 **89.** 50.02
91. 32.86 **93.** -25.434 **95.** -13.345
97. -15.66 **99.** 512 **101.** 128 **103.** 324
105. 144 **107.** $\frac{1}{16}$ **109.** $\frac{1}{1296}$ **111.** $\frac{1}{81}$
113. -1 **115.** $-\frac{1}{125}$ **117.** 10 **119.** $\frac{1}{16}$ **121.** $\frac{1}{9}$
123. 4

PAGES 488–489 CHAPTER 3 **1.** 1, 2, 3, 6
3. 1, 2, 5, 10 **5.** 1, 3, 5, 15 **7.** 1, 41 **9.** 1, 2,
4, 13, 26, 52 **11.** 1, 59 **13.** 5 **15.** 3, 9
17. 2, 4 **19.** 2, 3, 4, 5, 9, 10 **21.** 2, 3, 4, 5, 9,
10 **23.** none **25.** 2×5 **27.** 2×3^3
29. $2 \times 3 \times 5$ **31.** $\frac{1}{3}$ **33.** $1\frac{2}{5}$ **35.** $-1\frac{1}{2}$ **37.** $\frac{3}{5}$
39. $-1\frac{3}{4}$ **41.** $-\frac{7}{9}$ **43.** 1 **45.** $-\frac{1}{5}$ **47.** $-\frac{2}{7}$
49. 8 **51.** 5 **53.** 4 **55.** $\frac{17}{3}$ **57.** $-\frac{43}{10}$
59. $-\frac{57}{8}$ **61.** $\frac{25}{4}$ **63.** $\frac{20}{24}, \frac{9}{24}$ **65.** $\frac{12}{24}, \frac{10}{24}$
67. $-\frac{33}{84}, \frac{34}{84}$ **69.** $\frac{9}{13}$ **71.** $\frac{1}{3}$ **73.** $-\frac{179}{224}$
75. $-1\frac{17}{60}$ **77.** $3\frac{35}{48}$ **79.** $-5\frac{7}{12}$ **81.** $-\frac{3}{5}$
83. $-\frac{1}{2}$ **85.** $2\frac{4}{19}$ **87.** 2 **89.** $\frac{7}{30}$ **91.** $-\frac{5}{27}$
93. 0.375 **95.** $0.9\overline{54}$ **97.** $0.1\overline{6}$ **99.** $-0.5\overline{3}$
101. $0.7\overline{45}$ **103.** $-2.\overline{27}$ **105.** $\frac{3}{5}$ **107.** $1\frac{17}{50}$
109. $-3\frac{1}{40}$ **111.** $-2\frac{1}{11}$ **113.** $8\frac{7}{33}$

552 *Answers*

PAGES 490–491 CHAPTER 4 **1.** 50 **3.** 3
5. 62 **7.** 0.27 **9.** 4 **11.** 72 **13.** 4 **15.** 245
17. $\frac{1}{3}$ **19.** 4 **21.** $\frac{25}{108}$ **23.** 0.2 **25.** 90 **27.** 5
29. 4 **31.** 18 **33.** $18 - t$ **35.** $\frac{40}{m} - 16$
37. $3y + 11$ **39.** $6n = 54$ **41.** $n + 19 = 61$
43. $n = 152 - (-100)$ **45.** 395.77°C **47.** 5 h
49. 31 min to work; 24 min home

PAGES 492–493 CHAPTER 5
1. 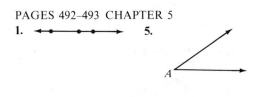 **5.**

7. 10,000 **9.** 900 **11.** 7,700 **13.** 1.5 **15.** 157.5
17. 200; 2000 **19.** right **21.** vertex **23.** obtuse
25. sides, angles **27.** right **29.** equilateral
31. True **33.** False **35.** False **37.** True
39. 352 mm **41.** 50.2 mm **43.** 4.11 m
45. $\overline{SR}$ **47.** $\overline{NM}$ **49.** $\angle N$ **51.** $\angle L$
53. $\triangle CAB \cong \triangle DAB$; SSS
55.

PAGES 494–495 CHAPTER 6 **1.** $\frac{1}{6}$ **3.** $\frac{1}{8}$
5. $\frac{1}{4}$ **7.** $\frac{3}{10}$ **9.** 6.25 km/h **11.** 24 eggs
13. 15¢ **15.** 9.5 **17.** 39 **19.** 72 **21.** 8
23. $52 **25.** $1.95 **27.** 44 km **29.** 63.2 km
31. 81.6 km **33.** 122 km **35.** $\frac{1}{10}$ **37.** $\frac{39}{100}$
39. $\frac{27}{100}$ **41.** 2 **43.** $2\frac{3}{20}$ **45.** 10% **47.** $12\frac{1}{2}\%$
49. $43\frac{3}{4}\%$ **51.** 144% **53.** 440% **55.** 0.71
57. 0.152 **59.** 0.024 **61.** 6.25 **63.** 2 **65.** 23%
67. 5% **69.** 0.25% **71.** 53% **73.** 12.5%
75. 0.25; 25% **77.** 0.625; 62.5% **79.** 1.375;
137.5% **81.** 8.75; 875% **83.** 5.2; 520%
85. 108.9 **87.** 500 **89.** 30% **91.** 240
93. 25 **95.** 3.0% **97.** 58 **99.** 48.96

PAGES 496–497 CHAPTER 7 **1.** 46.7%
3. 40% **5.** 400% **7.** 35% **9.** 80 **11.** 195
13. $1.92 **15.** 150% **17.** $38.16 **19.** 8.7%
21. $138,297.87 **23.** $81\frac{1}{4}\%$ **25.** $556.50
27. 13.8% **29.** $296.33 **31.** 51 boxes
33. $1.25 **35.** $510

PAGES 498–499 CHAPTER 8 **1.** 4 **3.** $\frac{1}{2}$
5. $\frac{3}{7}$ **7.** $\frac{1}{2}$ **9.** $1\frac{1}{3}$ **11.** $1\frac{1}{2}$ **13.** 1 **15.** 4 **17.** 4
19. $-\frac{1}{2}$ **21.** 3 **23.** $-1\frac{2}{3}$ **25.** sandwich: $2.60,
milk: $0.65 **27.** 15 ft, 45 ft **29.** $<$ **31.** $>$
33. $>$ **35.** $17 > 12$ **37.** $2n > 69$
39. $80 - 26 > 2(21)$ All the numbers: **41.** less
than or equal to -22 **43.** greater than $4\frac{5}{6}$
45. less than 7 **47.** greater than 7 **49.** less
than -4 **51.** less than -63 **53.** greater than
or equal to -55 **55.** less than 70 **57.** less
than or equal to $-4\frac{2}{7}$ **59.** less than or equal
to $11\frac{1}{5}$ **61.** greater than -5 **63.** greater than
or equal to -24 **65.** less than -9 **67.** less
than or equal to -3 **69.** 3 h

PAGES 500–501 CHAPTER 9 **1.** $(-6, 2)$
3. $(4, 4)$ **5.** $(-2, 4)$ **7.** G **9.** I **11.** J
13. c. rectangle **15.** c. triangle
17. c. right triangle
19. yes **21.** no **23.** yes **25.** yes **27.** yes
29. yes **31. a.** $y = 3x + 4$ **b.** $(-5, -11)$,
$(0, 4)$, $(5, 19)$ **33. a.** $y = \frac{3}{2}x + 3$ **b.** $(-2, 0)$,
$(0, 3)$, $(2, 6)$ **35. a.** $y = x - 3$ **b.** $(6, 3)$,
$(-1, -4)$, $(-3, -6)$
37.

39.

41.

43.

45.

47. 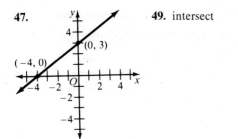 **49.** intersect

51. parallel **53.** intersect **55.** $y = 5x + 25$; slope is 5; 60¢

57. 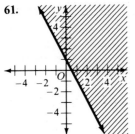 **59.**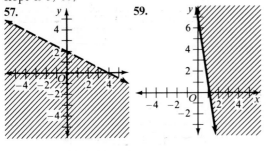

61.

PAGES 502–503 CHAPTER 10 **1.** 5000 m², 300 m **3.** 7625 cm², 372 cm **5.** 132 cm²
7. 119 km² **9.** 80.5 cm **11.** 135 m
13. 20 mm **15.** 380 m² **17.** 9850 m²
19.   **21.** 865 m³

23. 1260 mm³ **25.** 30 cm **27.** 3536 cm³
29. a. 1350 cm² **b.** 1890 cm² **31. a.** 900 cm²
b. 1350 cm² **33.** 1296π cm² **35.** 12 m
37. 2.64 kg **39.** 8530.2 g

PAGES 504–505 CHAPTER 11 **1.** 3 **3.** −6,
−5 **5.** 4, 5 **7.** 9 **9.** 7, 8 **11.** 5 **13.** 4
15. 9, 10 **17.** 4.9 **19.** 9.6 **21.** 7.1 **23.** 3.2
25. 6.1 **27.** 2.4 **29.** 2.83 **31.** 2.24 **33.** 4.90
35. 6.25 **37.** 5.57 **39.** 7.62 **41.** 3.97
43. 4.63 **45.** no **47.** no **49.** no **51.** yes

53. yes **55.** 6.40 **57.** 9 **59.** 9.90 **61.** 15
63. $x = 20$, $y = 40$ **65.** $x = 12$, $y = 12$
67. $x = 20$, $y = 10$ **69.** $\dfrac{2\sqrt{3}}{3}$ **71.** $\dfrac{x\sqrt{2a}}{2a}$

73. $\dfrac{x}{y}$ **75.** $\dfrac{y}{z}$ **77.** $\dfrac{x}{z}$ **79.** 0.4540, 0.8910,
0.5095 **81.** 0.9998, 0.0175, 57.2900 **83.** 26°
85. 53° **87.** 23°

PAGES 506–507 CHAPTER 12
1.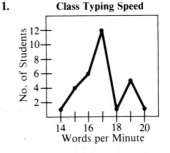

3. mean: 7; median: 8; range: 10 **5.** mean:
4.4; median: 3.5; range: 8 **7.** mean: 197;
median: 190; range: 95 **9.** mean: 5500;
median: 6500; range: 7000

11.

x	f
8	1
9	2
10	4
11	3
12	3
13	0
14	1
15	0
16	1

mean: 11; median: 11; range: 8; mode: 10

13.

x	f
1	3
2	5
3	3
4	3
5	4

mean: 3; median: 3; range: 4; mode: 2

15.

x	f
4.5–34.5	6
34.5–64.5	8
64.5–94.3	11

17. 720 **19.** 3,628,800 **21.** 120 **23.** 6 **25.** 20
27. 252 **29.** 1,326 **31.** $\frac{4}{7}$ **33.** 1 **35.** $\frac{5}{7}$
37. a. 7 to 1 **b.** 3 to 1 **c.** 3 to 1 **39. a.** $\frac{5}{18}$
b. $\frac{1}{36}$ **c.** $\frac{11}{36}$ **41.** $\frac{1}{2}$ **43. a.** $\frac{1}{6}$ **b.** $\frac{5}{36}$ **c.** $\frac{1}{36}$ **d.** $\frac{5}{18}$

Appendix A • Estimation

PAGES 512–513   EXERCISES   **1.** c
3. c **5.** b **7.** d **9.** c
PAGE 513   PROBLEMS   **1.** 1 hour
3. after the 8   **5.** $400

Appendix B • Stem-and-Leaf Plots

PAGE 515   WRITTEN EXERCISES

1. 1 | 4, 4, 8   **3.** 4 | 3, 4, 4, 4
  2 | 2, 5, 7, 9   5 | 0, 3
  3 | 1, 5   6 | 2, 5, 7
               7 | 2

5. 0 | 2, 5, 5, 7, 9 **7.** 5 | 3, 3, 6, 8
  1 | 0, 2, 3, 6   6 |
  2 | 3, 4, 7   7 | 7
  3 | 0   8 | 4, 7
               9 | 0, 1, 1, 2, 5

9. Car Wash Customers **11.** Basketball Point Totals
  3 | 0, 1, 2, 6   7 | 5, 7, 8
  4 | 2, 4, 5, 5, 6   8 | 0, 2, 2, 3, 3, 7, 7
  5 | 3, 4, 7   9 | 1, 4, 5
  6 | 10 | 1, 2
  7 | 2, 3

13. Since the data are all   4 | 6, 8, 9
multiples of ten, disregard 5 | 2, 3, 5, 7, 8
the last digit and use the   6 | 1, 4, 5
hundreds' digits as stems   7 | 2, 8
and the tens' digits as leaves.

Appendix C • Box-and-Whisker Plots

PAGE 517   WRITTEN EXERCISES

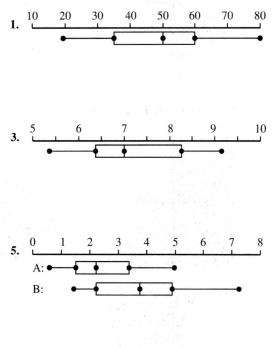

7. Example: 20, 40, 50, 55, 62, 65, 80